Bedside Clinics in
GYNECOLOGY

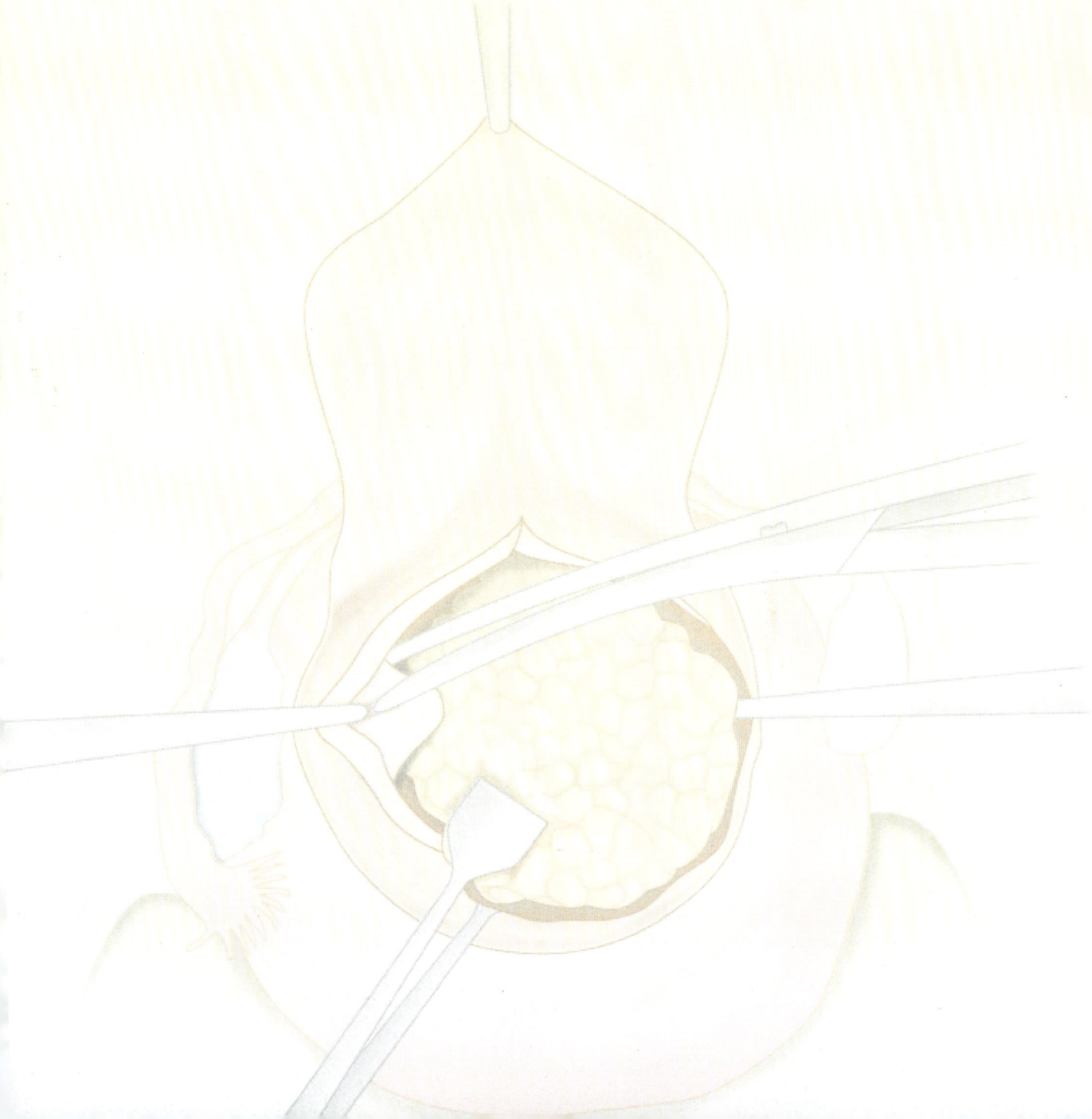

Bedside Clinics in GYNECOLOGY

Clinics to Care with Illustrations

Second Edition

Arup Kumar Majhi MD DNB FICOG

Professor, Department of Obstetrics and Gynecology
Santiniketan Medical College, Bolpur, Birbhum, West Bengal, India

Formerly, Head, Department of Obstetrics and Gynecology
RG Kar Medical College and Hospital, Kolkata
Professor and Head, Department of Obstetrics and Gynecology
Bankura Sammilani Medical College, Bankura
Associate Professor, Department of Obstetrics and Gynecology
Nil Ratan Sircar Medical College, Kolkata
Assistant Professor, Department of Obstetrics and Gynecology
Burdwan Medical College, Burdwan
West Bengal, India

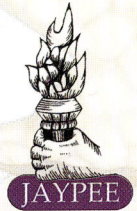

JAYPEE BROTHERS MEDICAL PUBLISHERS
The Health Sciences Publisher
New Delhi | London

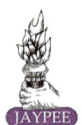
Jaypee Brothers Medical Publishers (P) Ltd.

Headquarters
Jaypee Brothers Medical Publishers (P) Ltd.
EMCA House
23/23-B, Ansari Road, Daryaganj
New Delhi - 110 002, India
Landline: +91-11-23272143, +91-11-23272703
+91-11-23282021, +91-11-23245672
Email: jaypee@jaypeebrothers.com

Corporate Office
Jaypee Brothers Medical Publishers (P) Ltd.
4838/24, Ansari Road, Daryaganj
New Delhi 110 002, India
Phone: +91-11-43574357
Fax: +91-11-43574314
Email: jaypee@jaypeebrothers.com

Overseas Office
J.P. Medical Ltd.
83 Victoria Street, London
SW1H 0HW (UK)
Phone: +44 20 3170 8910
Fax: +44 (0)20 3008 6180
Email: info@jpmedpub.com

Website: www.jaypeebrothers.com
Website: www.jaypeedigital.com

© 2023, Arup Kumar Majhi

The views and opinions expressed in this book are solely those of the original contributor(s)/author(s) and do not necessarily represent those of editor(s) and publisher of the book.

All rights reserved. No part of this publication may be reproduced, stored or transmitted in any form or by any means, electronic, mechanical, photocopying, recording or otherwise, without the prior permission in writing of the publishers.

All brand names and product names used in this book are trade names, service marks, trademarks or registered trademarks of their respective owners. The publisher is not associated with any product or vendor mentioned in this book.

Medical knowledge and practice change constantly. This book is designed to provide accurate, authoritative information about the subject matter in question. However, readers are advised to check the most current information available on procedures included and check information from the manufacturer of each product to be administered, to verify the recommended dose, formula, method and duration of administration, adverse effects and contraindications. It is the responsibility of the practitioner to take all appropriate safety precautions. Neither the publisher nor the author(s)/editor(s) assume any liability for any injury and/or damage to persons or property arising from or related to use of material in this book.

This book is sold on the understanding that the publisher is not engaged in providing professional medical services. If such advice or services are required, the services of a competent medical professional should be sought.

Every effort has been made where necessary to contact holders of copyright to obtain permission to reproduce copyright material. If any have been inadvertently overlooked, the publisher will be pleased to make the necessary arrangements at the first opportunity.

Inquiries for bulk sales may be solicited at: jaypee@jaypeebrothers.com

Bedside Clinics in Gynecology

First Edition: 2018
Revised Reprint: 2020
Second Edition: 2023

ISBN: 978-93-5696-120-3

Printed at: Samrat Offset Pvt. Ltd.

Dedicated
To
All the Students

FOREWORD

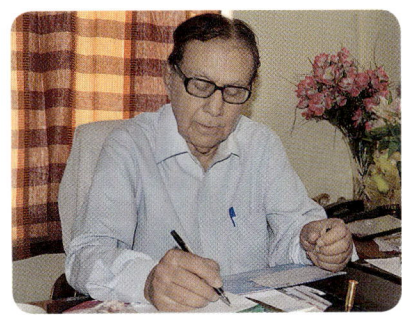

The art of presentation of updated knowledge, the science of application of rapidly developing modern gadgets in clinical practice and an interactive approach to patient care are the criteria for a good and successful teacher-cum-clinician. Prof Arup Kumar Majhi has shown wonderful and convincing evidences of these qualities in this book very efficiently and effectively.

The first chapter of this book covers the general scheme of clinical history taking and examination with detailed discussions of symptoms, signs, the perfect way of clinical methods of examination and to reach at probable diagnosis which are essential for every student to learn. A lot of illustrations on clinical methods, both live and diagrammatic has made this chapter very lucid and easy to learn. In fact, other than the treatment part almost all gynecological problems have been adequately covered in this chapter.

Every individual case in the respective chapter has been dealt with in a systematic protocol from clinical diagnosis to final diagnosis including all investigative procedures mentioning the latest technology. All varieties of management procedures have been discussed including surgical procedures, with newer developments, wherever necessary. The most attractive part of this book is a huge number of illustrations of various disease entities, operative findings and procedures, both original and diagrammatic. In some areas to simplify, Prof Majhi has made also question-answer format wherever necessary. The chapters of instruments, specimens and imaging will be very helpful for examinations purpose.

Research is invaluable in biomedical field for development of medical science. Development of clinical medicine always requires a sound platform of basic research and science. Through the chapter on basic research methodology, Prof Majhi has shown his foresightedness which will help not only the students but the upcoming research-minded teachers as well. The chapter on 'Examination of a Rape Victim: Procedures and Protocols' will enrich the knowledge how to tackle when a gynecologist encounters this issue.

A good teacher can impress the students by his presentation, but the success of medical teaching depends on how much a student can remember and will be able to apply this knowledge in clinical practice, communication and pass on for propagation to the next generation.

I am very excited and at the same time very proud as well to see that such a complete, informative, updated and illustrative book on clinical gynecology has been compiled by one of my students.

I am sure, like the author's Bedside Clinics in Obstetrics, this *Bedside Clinics in Gynecology* will also win the heart of both undergraduate and postgraduate students as well as practicing gynecologists.

BN Chakravarty
MO (Cal) FRCOG (Lond) DSc (Hon)
Director
Institute of Reproductive Medicine
Kolkata, West Bengal, India

PREFACE TO THE SECOND EDITION

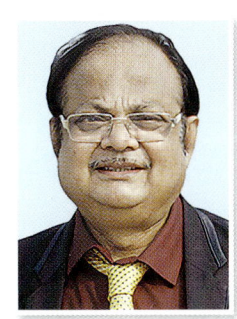

Since the release of first edition, many advancements in medical sciences have happened, along with release of newer guidelines, hence it was essential to update the book. Rise in popularity and demand on this style of book among the students have inspired me to release the updated edition.

In this second edition of *Bedside Clinics in Gynecology*, most of the chapters have been revised keeping the style same, especially change in staging of cancers, management, classifications of Müllerian anomaly and many more have been incorporated with recent ones. Some topics and areas which were essential to add have been included as well.

The steps of nondescent vaginal hysterectomy (NDVH) have been incorporated with the direct contribution by Prof Abhijit Rakshit, RG Kar Medical College, Kolkata. As imaging has come a long way in modern medicine both for diagnostic and therapeutic purposes, few newer sonographic images have also been incorporated for which I am grateful to Prof Kamal Oswal, Head, Department of Radiodiagnosis, VIMS, Kolkata.

Many original figures have been added so that the student and practitioners get a clear visual idea of every detail where description with text is not sufficient.

I am very indebted to my colleagues, juniors and the seniors for the constant encouragement and support that they have provided over the years. The book would not have been made possible, without the valuable inputs from many of my postgraduates.

It was not possible to edit the book without the active support of my wife Dr (Mrs) Swapna Majhi and son, Debanjan.

Lastly, I must thank Shri Jitendar P Vij (Group Chairman), Dr Madhu Choudhary (Director–Educational Publishing), Dr Aditya Tayal (Team Lead–UG Publishing), and Mr Sabyasachi Hazra (Head–Kolkata Branch), for their constant encouragement, appreciation and active support.

Hope this unique edition will be highly useful and acceptable to all categories of medical students as well as for practitioners.

Arup Kumar Majhi
Email: drarupkmajhi@yahoo.com

PREFACE TO THE FIRST EDITION

Since the publication of the book *Bedside Clinics in Obstetrics,* there was a tremendous and continuous demand from different corners to publish a similar book on gynecology. At present, in India, there is no dearth of gynecology books and many of them are of very standard quality. Every year lots of books on gynecology are coming in the field and in this perspective it was a great challenge to publish another book.

In spite of several other good books in obstetrics in market, my book on obstetrics became very popular among the students and practitioners. This made me an impression that a book of similar style is urgently needed especially for the students who have thirst for knowledge to fulfill their requirements. It was my dream from my early days in late eighties to compile a book for the students to make them competent in clinical acumen, with a clear idea of the disease processes, modern technology and their application besides they can do well in examination. After all, patient is a human being who deserves special attention from clinicians. Interaction, communication and sympathetic examination in most of the cases can explore not only the clue to diagnosis but also the patient becomes highly satisfied.

It cannot be denied that rapid developing modern technology and investigative procedures have enabled to diagnose the disease more easily. Development of newer surgical techniques and procedures like endoscopy, laser and many innovative methods has enriched the medical science tremendously. Today, approach to diagnose has become streamlined with the advent of evidence-based medicine. During the last few decades, there has been marked improvement in the areas of reproductive medicine including infertility management and management of cancer patients. Reconstructive and restorative operative techniques and procedures have enriched the medical science remarkably. New guidelines and protocols are coming in day-to-day practice.

In this rapid growing era, students are very often puzzled with the controversies and frequent change of protocol of management. What they will accept and how they will make good in examinations and also in clinical practice is a crucial issue for them.

Keeping all these aspects in mind and applying my experience of more than two and half decades as a teacher and a practitioner, I took the challenge of this herculean task of writing this clinical book on gynecology in very lucid manner with a lot of illustrations aided by updated information starting with clinical approach so that students can grasp very easily, retain for a long time, do good in examination and can apply in clinical practice.

During compilation, I have consulted various current and old books, publications and literature with latest guidelines. I have also consulted the experts of the respective fields and took extensive contribution from them wherever required.

My dream and hard work will be successful if this book fulfills the demands and requirements for both undergraduate and postgraduate students as well as for practicing gynecologists.

Arup Kumar Majhi
Email: drarupkmajhi@yahoo.com

ACKNOWLEDGMENTS

For writing this book, it is obvious that I have received enormous help, support, encouragement and blessings from many.

Firstly, I must mention the names of my teachers Prof BN Chakravarty and Prof BB Sarkar, who have always encouraged me from the start of writing books on both obstetrics and gynecology.

I am thankful to Prof Debashish Bhattacharya (Director of Medical Education, Government of West Bengal), Dr Ajay Chakraborty (Director of Health Service, Government of West Bengal), Prof Tamal Ghosh (Special Secretary, Department of Health and Family Welfare, Government of West Bengal), Prof Sudhhyodan Batabyal (Principal, RG Kar Medical College, Kolkata), and Prof Somnath Laha (Head, Department of Obstetrics and Gynecology, RG Kar Medical College, Kolkata, West Bengal, India), for their support for writing this book.

My special acknowledgment and thanks to Dr Abhijit Rakshit, Associate Professor, Department of Obstetrics and Gynecology, RG Kar Medical College, Kolkata, who has actively supported me to continue this work from the beginning.

Dr Rahul Karmakar, one of my students deserves special appreciation for his beautiful and complex drawings in many of the places in the book.

I am very much thankful to Prof RP Ganguly and Prof Debdutta Ghosh, RG Kar Medical College, Kolkata, for the huge input for the book.

I am deeply indebted to Prof Kamal Oswal (Department of Radiodiagnosis, Vivekananda Institute of Medical Sciences, Kolkata), Prof M Karmakar (Department of Radiodiagnosis, Institute of Postgraduate Medical Education and Research, Kolkata), and Dr Shuvro H Roychowdhury (Interventional Radiologist), for their contribution in imaging.

My sincere thanks to Dr Gopinath Barui (Associate Professor, Department of Pathology, RG Kar Medical College, Kolkata), Dr Anup Boler (Associate Professor, Department of Pathology), and Dr Tripti Das, for providing the microphotographs.

I am indebted to Dr Alok De (Associate Professor, Department of Obstetrics and Gynecology, RG Kar Medical College, Kolkata), Prof Kushagradhi Ghose (Director, Fetal Care Center), Dr Bani Mitra (Director, RG Center, Kolkata), Dr Subhas Halder (Consultant Gynecologist), and Dr Abhinibes Chatterji (Consultant Gynecologist), who have enriched the manual with endoscopic photographs.

I must acknowledge Prof Sukanta Misra (Head, Department of Obstetrics and Gynecology, Vivekananda Institute of Medical Sciences, Kolkata), Prof Subratalall Seal (RG Kar Medical College), Prof Subhas Chandra Biswas (Department of Obstetrics and Gynecology, Institute of Postgraduate Medical Education and Research, Kolkata), Prof Chandana Das (Head, Department of Obstetrics and Gynecology, Nil Ratan Sircar Medical College and Hospital, Kolkata), Dr Shyamal Dasgupta (Associate Professor, Department of Obstetrics and Gynecology), Dr Ramprasad Dey (Associate Professor, Department of Obstetrics and Gynecology, Chittaranjan Seva Sadan, Kolkata), Dr Subir Bhattacharyya (Associate Professor), Dr Prosenjit Banerji (Associate Professor, Department of Obstetrics and Gynecology, North Bengal Medical College, Kolkata), Dr Ranjan Basu (Associate Professor, KPC Medical College), Prof Asoke Biswas (Vivekananda Institute of Medical Sciences, Kolkata), Dr Rupali Modak (Assistant Professor), Dr Anindya Das (Assistant Professor), Dr Sanjoy Bhattacharyya (Assistant Professor), and Dr Monimmala Murmu (Assistant Professor), RG Kar Medical College, Kolkata, for enriching the illustrations.

Dr Jaydip Bhaumik (Senior Consultant, Gynecological Oncology, Tata Medical Center, Kolkata) and Dr Dipanwita Banerji (Assistant Professor, Chittaranjan National Cancer Institute, Kolkata), deserve special appreciation for their contributions of colposcopic pictures.

Dr Siddharta Chatterjee (Director, Fertility Mission), Dr Tulika Jha (Associate Professor, Department of Obstetrics and Gynecology), Dr Ajanta Samanta (RMO-cum-Clinical Tutor), Dr Sangita Dubey (RMO-cum-Clinical Tutor, RG Kar Medical College, Kolkata), Dr Chiranjit Ghose, Dr Sandos Saha, Dr Subrata Samanta (RMO-cum-Clinical Tutor), Dr Mallika Sengupta (Assistant Professor, RG Kar Medical College, Kolkata), Dr Debmalya Maiti (Assistant Professor, Nil Ratan Sircar Medical College and Hospital, Kolkata), Dr Pallab Mistri (Associate Professor, Medical College), Dr Anirban Mondal (Associate Professor, Bankura Sammilani Medical College), Dr Pradipto Sanyal (Senior Gynecologist), and Dr Manas Saha (Calcutta National Medical College, Kolkata), deserve special thanks for their input in various ways.

My acknowledgment to the legend of our speciality, Dr MN Parikh, who always tried to introduce research methodology in gynecology. My special thanks to Dr Tapabrata Guha Ray (Associate Professor, CM of RG Kar Medical College, Kolkata), for input in the chapter of "Research Questions" and Dr Navanil Biswas, for compiling this chapter and Dr Bijoy Kumar Bandopadhyaya (Associate Professor, Department of Anesthesiology) and Dr Abhishek Bhadra (Assistant Professor, Department of Obstetrics and Gynecology), for input in the chapter of "Postoperative Management".

Prof Sobhan K Das (Head, Department of Forensic Medicine and Toxicology), deserves special appreciation for the chapter on 'Rape'.

The junior brigades comprising Dr Sudipto Jana, Dr Arunasis Mullick, Dr Keka Monadal, Dr Amrita Rai and Dr Prajit Roy need special mention as they have done tremendous hard work and their day-to-day contribution has made this mammoth task successful.

My sincere thanks to Prof Tapan Lahiri (Principal, Medical College, Kolkata), Prof Arati Biswas (HOD, Calcutta National Medical College, Kolkata), Prof Partha Mukherji (HOD, Medical College, Kolkata), Prof Partha Chakraborty (HOD, Institute of Postgraduate Medical Education and Research, Kolkata), Prof Joydev Mukherji (HOD, North Bengal Medical College, Kolkata), Prof Tapan Naskar (Medical College, Kolkata), Prof Hiralal Konar (Calcutta National Medical College, Kolkata), Prof Amitava Das, Prof Rupkamal Das, Prof Nilanjana Chwodhury of RG Kar Medical College, Prof Ashis Mukhopadhyaya (MSVP, Chittaranjan Seva Sadan, Kolkata), Prof Narayan Jana (HOD, Chittaranjan Seva Sadan, Kolkata), Prof Subhendu Dasgupta (HOD, Bankura Sammilani Medical College), Prof Prabir Sengupta (HOD, Burdwan Medical College, Burdwan), Prof BN Sil (HOD, Murshidabad Medical College), Prof N Bhattacharyya (HOD, Malda Medical College), Prof Alauddin (HOD, Midnapore Medical College, Midnapore), Dr Hasibul Hassan (Assistant Professor, RG Kar Medical College), Prof GS Kamilya (Institute of Postgraduate Medical Education and Research, Kolkata), Prof Kakali Sinha Karmakar (HOD, Sagar Dutta Medical College), Prof Joydev Roychowdhury (Dean, ESI Hospital, Joka), Prof SM Bhattacharyya (KPC Medical College), Dr Somajita Chakraborty (Associate Professor, Medical College, Kolkata), Prof Sajal Dutta (Vivekananda Institute of Medical Sciences, Kolkata), Dr Monidip Pal (Associate Professor, Kalyani Medical College), Dr Sukumar Barik (Associate Professor, Haldia Medical College), Dr Biswajyoti Guha (Associate Professor, Haldia Medical College), Prof Amitava Pal (Burdwan Medical College), Prof Swapan Kundu (Kisangaunj Medical College), Prof Alka Kriplani (HOD, All India Institute of Medical Sciences), Prof Kallol Roy (All India Institute of Medical Sciences), Prof JB Sharma (All India Institute of Medical Sciences, New Delhi), Prof Sudha Prasad (Maulana Azad Medical College, New Delhi), Prof Pratima Mittal (HOD, Safdarjang Medical College, New Delhi), Prof Mala Srivastava (Sir Ganga Ram Hospital, New Delhi), Prof Santa Singh (Director, Regional Institute of Medical Sciences, Manipur), Prof Gokul Das, Prof Ashis Bhattacharyya (HOD, Gauhati Medical College and Hospital, Assam), Prof Pranay Nath, Prof Arun Pal Chowdhury (HOD, Silchar Medical College, Assam), Prof Robin Medhi (HOD), Prof Saswati Sanyal Chowdhury (Barpeta Medical College), Dr Pranay Phukon (Associate Professor, Dibrugarh Medical College, Assam), Prof Dilip Bhowmik (Jawaharlal Nehru Medical College, Wardha), and Prof Mamata Pradhan (HOD, Agartala Government Medical College, Tripura).

I like to express my thanks to Prof PC Mahapatra, Prof Shyama Kanungo, Prof Lucy Das, Prof Maya Padhi (Shri Ramachandra Bhanj Medical College, Cuttack, Odisha), Prof Tushar Kar (HOD), Dr Ojasini Patel (Associate Professor, Sambalpur Medical College, Odisha), Prof Gangadhar Sahoo (Dean, Institute of Medical Sciences and SUM Hospital, Odisha), for their constant encouragement and support for writing this book. I take this opportunity to thank Prof Anita Sinha, Prof Abharani Sinha and Prof Alka Pandey (Patna Medical College, Bihar), Prof Manju Gita Mishra of Patna, Prof LK Pandey, and Prof Sulekha Pandey (Banaras Hindu University), for their moral support for writing this book.

My sincere regards to Prof Ashok Mondal, Prof Gita Ganguly Mukherji, Prof AR Bhattacharyya, Prof Sudipto Bose, Prof Biman Chakraborty, Dr Sudip Chakraborty, Dr Kalidas Bakshi, Dr BD Mukherji and Dr Dilip Dutta, for their constant encouragement. I wish to thank Prof Sudhir Adhikary, Dr Sudarsan Ghose Dastidar, Dr Abinas Roy, Dr Suranjan Chakraborty, Dr Saktirupa Chakraborty, Prof Krishnendu Gupta, Dr Bhaskar Pal, Dr Basab Mukherji, Dr Mousumi De Banerji, Dr Jayita Chakraborty, Dr Chhabi Bose, and Dr Amit Chakraborty, RG Kar Medical College, Kolkata, for their support and encouragement.

I have received tremendous support from the team of Institute of Reproductive Medicine, Kolkata, for compiling many chapters in reproductive medicine in various ways namely Dr Souren Goswami, Dr Ratna Chatterji, Dr Sunita Sharma, Dr Sanghamitra Ghosh, and Dr Shovandeb Kalapahar.

Finally, I find myself extremely fortunate to have Shri Jitendar P Vij (Group Chairman), Mr Ankit Vij (Managing Director), Mr MS Mani (Group President), Dr Madhu Choudhary (Director–Educational Publishing), Ms Pooja Bhandari (Production Head), Ms Sunita Katla (Executive Assistant to Group Chairman and Publishing Manager), Ms Samina Khan (Executive Assistant to Director–Educational Publishing), Dr Aditya Tayal (Team Lead–UG Publishing), Mr Rajesh Sharma (Production Coordinator), Ms Seema Dogra (Cover Visualizer), Mr Kapil Dev Sharma (Typesetter), Ms Geeta Barik (Proofreader), Mr Manoj Pahuja (Senior Graphic Designer), and the team of M/s Jaypee Brothers Medical Publishers (P) Ltd, New Delhi, India, who have given tremendous efforts to release this book within stipulated time. I especially mention the staff of Kolkata branch, Mr Sabyasachi Hazra (Head), who has given relentless effort and constant encouragement for this project.

I express my gratitude and indebtedness to my enormous patients who have allowed me to learn the subjects and cooperated to collect the materials.

This would have never seen the light of the day without the support and sacrifice of my wife Dr Swapna Majhi, who has actively worked for this book including many complex drawings in addition to managing the all family burden and her professional liability. I am indebted to my son Debanjan (Sion), who has helped me in various ways, especially in crisis.

In spite of a long list of acknowledgment, I could not mention all the names individually who have helped and contributed in various ways.

I am grateful to the Department of Health and Family Welfare, Government of West Bengal, for giving me the permission to publish this book.

CONTENTS

SECTION 1: GYNECOLOGICAL HISTORY TAKING, EXAMINATION AND INVESTIGATIONS

1. Writing a Gynecology Case 3
- Structure of History Writing 3
- Detailed Parameters Under the Broad Headings 3
- Discussion of the Points Essential for Proper Case Taking and Writing 5
- Investigations Supplied or Required 33
- Summary of the Case 33
- Example of Writing a Summary (Sample Summary) 33
- Provisional Diagnosis 33
- Differential Diagnosis 33

2. Investigative Procedures in Gynecology and Imaging in Gynecology 34
- Investigations 34
- Imaging in Gynecology 37
- Role of Ultrasonography in Gynecology 37
- Role of USG According to Symptomatology 38
- Procedures Under Ultrasonography Guidance 38
- Computed Tomography Scan (CT Scan) 40
- Magnetic Resonance Imaging (MRI) in Gynecology 40
- Positron Emission Tomography (PET) 41
- X-ray—its Role in Gynecology 41
- Pipelle Biopsy 41

SECTION 2: CLINICAL CASES

3. A Case of Lump Abdomen (Ovarian Tumor) 45
- History Taking 45
- Physical Examination 46
- Gynecological Examination 46
- Summary of the Case (Sample Summary) 46
- Investigations Supplied or Required 46
- Provisional Diagnosis 47
- Differential Diagnosis 47
- Diagnosis of a Case of Benign Ovarian Tumor 48
- USG Features of Malignant Ovarian Tumor 50
- Tumor Markers in Ovarian Malignancy 51
- Classification of Ovarian Tumor 52
- Epithelial-Stromal Tumors 53
- Sex Cord—Stromal Tumors 53
- Germ Cell Tumors 53
- Secondary (Metastatic) Tumors 53
- Functional Cyst 53
- Follicular Cyst 54
- Corpus Luteum Cyst 54
- Theca Lutein Cyst 54
- Classification of Ovarian Tumor 54
- Benign Serous Cystadenoma 55
- Benign Mucinous Cystadenoma 55
- Brenner (Transitional) Tumor 56
- Dermoid Cyst of Ovary (Synonym: Benign Cystic Teratoma) 56
- Complications of Ovarian Tumor 58
- Pseudomyxoma Peritonei 59
- Management of a Case of Benign Ovarian Cyst and Tumor 59
- Steps of Laparotomy in a Case of Ovarian Tumor 60

Ovarian Cancer 62
- Screening of Ovarian Cancer 62
- Genetic Testing in Ovarian Cancer and its Utility 63
- Types and Pathology of Ovarian Cancer 63
- Diagnosis and Investigations of Ovarian Cancer 64
- Route of Spread of Epithelial Ovarian Cancers 66
- Stages of Ovarian Cancer 67
- Gradings of Ovarian Malignancy 68
- Management of Early-stage and Advanced Ovarian Cancer 68
- Steps of Surgical Staging 69
- Chemotherapeutic Agents Used in Ovarian Malignancy 71
- Recurrent Ovarian Cancer 71
- Borderline Ovarian Tumor (Synonym: Low Malignant Potential Tumor) 72

Fallopian Tube (FT) Cancer 73
- Germ Cell Tumors 74
- Sex Cord Stromal Tumors 77
- Management of a Case of Ovarian Tumor in Pregnancy 81

4. A Case of Uterine Leiomyoma (Uterine Fibroid) 82
- Patient's Particulars 82
- History 82
- Physical Examination 83
- Systemic Examination 83
- Gynecological Examination 83
- Summary of the Case (Sample) 83
- Investigations Supplied or Required 84

- Provisional Diagnosis 84
- Differential Diagnosis 84
- Diagnosis of Fibroid Uterus 84
- Wandering and Parasitic Fibroid 90
- Broad Ligament Fibroids 90
- Microscopical Features 92
- Degenerations of Uterine Fibroid 92
- Details of Management of Fibroid Uterus 94
- Surgery 97
- Hysteroscopic Myomectomy 97
- Laparoscopic Myomectomy 97
- Open Myomectomy 98
- Cervical Fibroid 102
- Broad Ligament Cysts and Tumors 105
- Uterine Polyp 107

5. **A Case of Abnormal Uterine Bleeding (Endometrial Hyperplasia)** 110
   - Patient's Particulars 110
   - History 110
   - Physical Examination 111
   - Gynecological Examination 111
   - Summary of the Case 111
   - Definition of AUB 112
   - Causes of Reproductive Tract Bleeding 113
   - Structural and Nonstructural Causes of AUB as Defined in PALM-COEIN Classifications by FIGO 2011 113
   - Dysfunctional Uterine Bleeding (DUB) 117
   - Postcoital Bleeding 117
   - Diagnosis of AUB 117
   - Case of AUB 118
   - Endometrial Biopsy—Different Methods 120
   - Management 121
   - Uterine Procedures 126
   - Heavy Menstrual Bleeding in Adolescents (Puberty Menorrhagia) 128
   - Metropathia Hemorrhagica 129
   - Isthmocele 130
   - Arteriovenous Malformation (AVM) 130
   - Myometrial Hypertrophy 130
   - Endometrial Hyperplasia 130
   - Classification 131

6. **A Case of Endometrial Carcinoma (Including Postmenopausal Bleeding) and Uterine Sarcoma** 133
   - Patient's Particulars 133
   - History 133
   - Physical Examination 134
   - Gynecological Examination 134
   - Investigations Supplied or Required 134
   - Summary of the Case (Sample) 134
   - Provisional Diagnosis 134
   - Differential Diagnosis 134
   - History 136
   - Management of Endometrial Carcinoma 140
   - Pyometra 144
   - Postmenopausal Bleeding (PMB) 144
   - Sarcoma of the Uterus 146

7. **A Case of Choriocarcinoma (Gestational Trophoblastic Neoplasia)** 149
   - Patient's Particulars 149
   - History 149
   - Physical Examination 150
   - Gynecological Examination 150
   - Summary of the Case (Sample) 150
   - Investigations Supplied or Required 150
   - Provisional Diagnosis 151
   - Differential Diagnosis 151

8. **A Case of Carcinoma Cervix and Premalignant Lesions of Cervix** 157
   - Patient's Particulars 157
   - History 157
   - Physical Examination 158
   - Stages of Cancer Cervix 161
   - Lymphatic Drainage of Cancer Cervix 165
   - Management of Cancer Cervix 166
   - Radical Hysterectomy 167
   - Premalignant Lesions of Cervix 170
   - Cervical Carcinogenesis 173
   - Colposcopy 177
   - Human Papilloma Virus Vaccine 183

9. **A Case of Carcinoma Vulva, Preinvasive Lesion of Vulva, and Vaginal Cancer** 185
   - Patient's Particulars 185
   - History 185
   - Physical Examination 186
   - Systemic Examination 186
   - Gynecological Examination 186
   - Summary of the Case (Sample) 186
   - Investigations Supplied or Required 187
   - Provisional Diagnosis 187
   - Differential Diagnosis (If H/P Not Available) 187
   - Diagnosis of Vulvar Carcinoma 187
   - Staging of Vulvar Cancer 190
   - Key Changes in FIGO Staging for Vulvar Cancer 2021 191
   - Management of Vulvar Cancer 191
   - Prognosis of Vulvar Cancer 195
   - Preinvasive Lesions of Vulva 196
   - Vulvar Intraepithelial Disease 198
   - Vaginal Cancer 199

10. Pelvic Organ Prolapse (Genital Prolapse) 202
- Genital Prolapse 202
- History Taking 202
- Physical Examination 203
- Gynecological Examination 204
- Summary of the Case (Sample Summary) 204
- Investigations Supplied or Required 205
- Provisional Diagnosis 205
- Differential Diagnosis 205
- Supports of Uterus and Vagina 207
- Etiologies of Pelvic Organ Prolapse 209
- Anatomical Classification of Pelvic Organ Prolapse 210
- Grading Systems of Pelvic Organ Prolapse 212
- Pelvic Organ Prolapse Quantification System (POP-Q) 214
- Surgicopathological Changes in Pelvic Organ Prolapse 216
- Diagnosis of Pelvic Organ Prolapse 217
- Demonstration of POP-Q Staging 220
- Demonstration of Enterocele 222
- Demonstration of Stress Incontinence 222
- Management of Pelvic Organ Prolapse 223
- Conservative Management 223
- Vaginal Pessary 223
- Surgery in Pelvic Organ Prolapse 225
- Surgeries Done in POP 225

Operative Details of Pelvic Organ Prolapse 226
- Anterior Colporrhaphy 226
- Posterior Colpoperineorrhaphy 231
- Fothergill's Operation (Manchester Operation) 233
- Ward Mayo's Operation (Vaginal Hysterectomy with Pelvic Floor Repair) 236
- Le Fort's Operation (Colpocleisis) 241
- Purandare's Abdominal Sling Operation (1956) 241
- Shirodkar's Abdominal Sling Operation (1960) 241
- Khanna's Abdominal Sling Operation 241
- Abdominal Sacrocolpopexy, Sacrocolpohysteropexy 241
- Sacrospinous Ligament Fixation 243
- McCall Culdoplasty 244
- Prevention of Pelvic Organ Prolapse 245
- Pregnancy with Pelvic Organ Prolapse 245

11. A Case of Infertility 247
- Patient's Particular 247
- History 247
- Physical Examination 248
- Gynecological Examination 248
- Investigations Supplied or Required 249
- Summary of the Case (Sample) 249
- Provisional Diagnosis 249
- Differential Diagnosis 249
- Contribution of Male and Female Partners 249
- Causes of Female Factor Infertility 249
- Etiologies of Male Factor Infertility 250
- Investigation (Evaluation) of a Case of Infertility 250
- History and Examination of Female Partner 250
- History and Examination of Male Partner 251
- Diagnosis or Detection of Ovulation 251
- Ovarian Reserve 257
- Tubal Patency Test 258
- Anovulation 261
- Cervical Factor Causing Infertility 261
- Causes of Tubal Block 262
- Causes of Infertility in Endometriosis 262
- History and Examination of Male Partner 262
- Semen Analysis 264
- Hormones Profile in Assessment of Male Infertility 266
- Reactive Oxygen Species 267
- Management of Female Infertility 268
- Management of Ovulatory Dysfunction 268
- Management of Diminished Ovarian Reserve 271
- Ovarian Hyperstimulation Syndrome 271
- Surgical Management in Anovulation/Oligoovulation 272
- Tubal Factor Infertility 272
- Assisted Reproductive Technology 275
- In Vitro Fertilization and Embryo Transfer 275
- Surrogacy (Gestational Carrier Surrogacy) 279
- Management of Male Factor Infertility 280
- Intrauterine Insemination (IUI) 280
- Intracytoplasmic Sperm Injection 283
- Treatment of Erectile and Ejaculatory Dysfunction 285
- Azoospermia 286
- Klinefelter Syndrome (47 XXY) 287
- Vaginismus 287
- Unexplained Infertility 287

12. A Case of Polycystic Ovarian Syndrome and Hirsutism 288

A Case of Polycystic Ovary Syndrome 288
- Patient's Particular 288
- History 288
- Physical Examination 289
- Gynecological Examination 289
- Investigations Supplied or Required 289
- Summary of the Case (Sample) 289
- Diagnosis of PCOS 290
- Clinical Presentations of PCOS 292
- Complications of PCOS 292
- Etiology of PCOS 292
- Endocrine Profile and Other Investigations in PCOS 293
- Diagnosis of Adolescent PCOS 293
- Management Outline in a Case of PCOS 294
- Outline the Management of Adolescent PCOS 294
- Management of PCOS in Elderly 295
- Discuss the Pathophysiology of PCOS 295

Hirsutism 297
- Exogenous Pharmacological Agents Causing Hirsutism 300
- Medications Causing Hirsutism and Hypertrichosis 300
- Idiopathic Hirsutism 300
- Androgen Synthesis in Female 300
- Different Androgens and their Sources 300
- Evaluation of Hirsutism 301
- Laboratory Investigations 302
- Further Investigations 302
- Imaging 302
- Summary of Recommendation for Evaluation of Hirsutism 303
- Outline the Management of Hirsutism 303
- Summary of Recommendation of Treatment 305
- Physiology of Hair 305
- Differential Diagnosis of PCOS 307

13. A Case of Primary Amenorrhea and Disorder of Sexual Development 308
- Writing a Case of Primary Amenorrhea 311
- Definition 312
- Etiologies of Primary Amenorrhea 313
- Common Causes of Primary Amenorrhea 313
- Diagnosis a Case of Primary Amenorrhea 314
- Discussion of Individual Cases 319
- Turner Syndrome 319
- Anatomical Defects Leading to Amenorrhea 321
- Creation of Neovagina 322
- Reifenstein Syndrome 325
- Swyer Syndrome 325
- Congenital Adrenal Hyperplasia (Adrenogenital Syndrome) 327

Disorder of Sexual Development (Intersex) 328
- Definition of DSD 328
- Gender Identity 328
- Sexual Differentiation: Mechanism 328
- Classification of Disorder of Sexual Differentiation 329
- Hermaphrodite 330
- Transgender 330
- New Nomenclature 330
- Gonads in Different DSDs 331
- Approach in a Case of Ambiguous Genitalia 331
- Diagnosis of a Case of Ambiguous Genitalia 331
- Management of a Case of DSD 332
- Gender Assignment 332
- Surgeries in DSDs 333
- Medical Management in DSDs 334

14. A Case of Secondary Amenorrhea 335
Case Taking in a Case of Secondary Amenorrhea 335
- Patient's Particular 335
- History 335
- Physical Examination 336
- Gynecological Examination 336
- Investigations Supplied or Required 336
- Summary of the Case (Sample Summary) 336
- Provisional Diagnosis 337
- Differential Diagnosis 337
- Definition of Secondary Amenorrhea 337
- Causes of Secondary Amenorrhea 337
- Diagnosis of Secondary Amenorrhea 338
- Approach to Diagnose a Case of Secondary Amenorrhea 339
- Hyperprolactinemia and Amenorrhea 339
- Thyroid Disorder and Amenorrhea 341
- Polycystic Ovarian Syndrome 342
- Obesity and Menstrual Abnormality 342
- Asherman Syndrome (Uterine Synechiae) 342
- Premature Ovarian Failure (Also Called Primary Ovarian Insufficiency) 342
- Late-onset Congenital Adrenal Hyperplasia 343
- Functional Hypothalamic Amenorrhea 343
- Amenorrhea in Androgen-producing Tumor 343

15. A Case of Precocious Puberty (Pediatrics and Adolescent Gynecological Problem) 345
A Case of Precocious Puberty 345
- Patient's Particulars 345
- History 345
- Detailed General Survey are Done and Noted 346
- Systemic Examination 346
- Gynecological Examination 346
- Investigations Supplied or Required 346
- Summary of the Case 346
- Provisional Diagnosis 346
- Differential Diagnosis (D/D) 346
- Evaluation of a Case of Precocious Puberty 348
- Onset of Puberty 350

Pediatric and Adolescent Gynecology (PAG) 351
- Common Gynecological Problems in Pediatric and Adolescent Group 351
- Labial Adhesion 352
- Vulvovaginitis 352
- Vaginal Bleeding in Prepubertal Girl 353
- Ovarian Neoplasms in Adolescents and Children 353
- Endometriosis in Adolescent 354
- Disorder of Sexual Differentiation (DSD) 354
- Adolescent Polycystic Ovary Syndrome 355
- Preventive Gynecology in Pediatrics and Adolescent 355

16. A Case of Endometriosis Adenomyosis 356
- Patient's Particulars 356
- History 356
- Physical Examination 357
- Gynecological Examination 357
- Investigations Supplied or Required 357
- Summary of the Case (Sample) 357

- Provisional Diagnosis 358
- Differential Diagnosis 358
- Adenomyosis 369
- Dysmenorrhea 373
- Chronic Pelvic Pain 375
- Ovarian Remnant Syndrome and Ovarian Retention Syndrome 376

17. A Case of Vesicovaginal Fistula and Urinary Incontinence 377
- History Taking 377
- Physical Examination 378
- Gynecological Examination 378
- Summary of the Case (Sample Summary) 378
- Investigations Supplied or Required 378
- Provisional Diagnosis 378
- Differential Diagnosis 378
- Summary of Diagnosis 380
- Ureterovaginal Fistula 385
- Urinary Incontinence 389

18. A Case of Old Complete Perineal Tear 400
- Patient's Particulars 400
- History 400
- Physical Examination 401
- Gynecological Examination 401
- Summary of the Case (Sample) 401
- Complete Perineal Tear 402
- Anatomy of Anal Canal and Anal Sphincter 402
- Anal Incontinence 403
- Diagnosis of Old Complete Perineal Tear 403
- Steps of Surgery for Repair of CPT 405

Rectovaginal Fistula (RVF) 408

SECTION 3: REPRODUCTIVE PHYSIOLOGY

19. Physiology of Ovulation, Menstruation, Spermatogenesis and Implantation 413
- Physiology of Ovulation 413
- Two-Cell, Two-Gonadotropin Theory 415
- Ovulation Phase 417
- Physiology of Menstruation 418
- Normal Composition of Semen 421
- Physiology of Spermatogenesis 422
- Implantation 426
- Premenstrual Syndrome (PMS) or Premenstrual Tension (PMT) 429

20. Menopause and its Management 431
Menopause 431
- Physiology of Menopause 432
- Management of Menopause 435

21. Development of Genital Organs and Müllerian Anomaly 438
- Development of Male Genital System 438
- Development of Female Genital System 438
- Müllerian Anomaly Classification 439
- ASRM Müllerian Anomaly Classification 2021 (MAC, 2021) 441
- Unicornuate Uterus 443
- Uterine Didelphys 445
- Bicornuate Uterus 446
- Septate Uterus 448
- Arcuate Uterus 449
- Transverse Vaginal Septum 449
- Longitudinal Vaginal Septum 450
- Cervical Agenesis 451
- Vaginal Agenesis 451
- Mayer-Rokitansky-Küster-Hauser Syndrome 451
- Surgical Methods in Müllerian Anomaly 453
- Uterine Transplantation 455

SECTION 4: BIRTH CONTROL AND POPULATION DEMOGRAPHY

22. Family Planning and Contraception 459
- Common Viva Questions on Contraceptives 459
- History of Birth Control 461
- Criteria of an Ideal Contraceptive 462
- Classification of Birth Control Methods 462
- WHO Tier Method (Groups) Classification 462
- Expression of Failure Rate 463
- Classification of Steroidal Contraceptives 464
- Combined Oral Contraceptives Pills 464
- Noncontraceptive Benefits of Combined Oral Pills 467
- Noncontraceptive Uses of COCs 467
- Medical Eligibility Criteria (MEC) Wheel for Contraceptive Use 468
- Missing Pill 468
- Progesterone-only Pill 471
- Centchroman 472
- Injectable Contraceptives 472
- Subdermal Implants 474
- Combined Hormonal Transdermal Patches 476
- Transvaginal Combined Hormonal Ring 476
- Progesterone Vaginal Ring 476
- Emergency Contraceptives (Synonyms: Morning After Pill, Postcoital Contraception) 476
- Intrauterine Contraceptive Devices (IUDs or IUCDs) 478
- Contraindications of Copper-containing IUDs 481

Postpartum IUCD 488
- Long-acting Reversible Contraceptive (LARC) 490
- Barrier Methods of Contraceptive 491

Permanent Contraception 495
- Pomeroy Technique 496
- Other Techniques of Tubal Sterilization 498
- Laparoscopic Sterilization 499
- Eligibility of Male Sterilization 506
- Other Male Contraceptives 507
- Antifertility Vaccine 508

23. **Demography and Family Planning Programs in India—Present Scenario** 509
    - Magnitude of the Problem 509
    - Fertility Indicators 509
    - Current Use of Family Planning Methods (Currently Married Women Age 15–49 Years) as Per NFHS-5 (2019-21) Data 510
    - Unmet Need in India 510
    - Milestones of Family Planning Program in India 510
    - Contraceptives Available at Present Through Government of India 511

SECTION 5: INSTRUMENTS AND OPERATION

24. **Identify the Instruments—Know Your Instruments** 515
    - Instruments at a Glance 515
    - Sponge Holding Forceps (Also Called Swab Holding or Ring Forceps) 528
    - Ovum Forceps 528
    - Female Metallic Catheter 528
    - Foley Catheter 529
    - Sims' Double-Bladed Posterior Vaginal Speculum 529
    - Single-Bladed (Universal) Posterior Vaginal Speculum 530
    - Cusco's Bivalve Self-retaining Speculum 530
    - Auvard's Self-retaining Speculum 531
    - Anterior Vaginal Wall Retractor 531
    - Allis Tissue Forceps 531
    - Multiple Teeth Vulsellum 531
    - Single Tooth Vulsellum 532
    - Uterine Sound 532
    - Cervical Dilators 533
    - Uterine Curette 534
    - Uterine Dressing Forceps 534
    - Lane's Tissue Forceps 534
    - Hysterectomy Clamp (Straight/Curve) 535
    - Babcock's Tissue Forceps 535
    - Myoma Screw 535
    - Bonney's Myomectomy Clamp 536
    - Landon's Bladder Retractor 536
    - Aneurysm Needle with Thread 536
    - Ring Pessary 536
    - Hodge–Smith Pessary 537
    - Hysterosalpingography Cannula 537
    - Ayre's Spatula 538
    - Cytobrush 538

25. **Operative Gynecology** 539
    - Hysterectomy 539
    - Classification of Hysterectomy in Relevance to Surgery of Cancer Cervix 540
    - Steps of Abdominal Approach of Total Hysterectomy 540
    - Indications of Hysterectomy 544
    - Justification of Salpingectomy During Hysterectomy 544
    - Nondescent Vaginal Hysterectomy (NDVH) 544
    - Wertheim's Operation (Abdominal Radical Hysterectomy) 545
    - Dilatation and Curettage 546
    - Surgery for Chronic Uterine Inversion 550
    - Surgery for Making Uterus Anteversion 551
    - Other Gynecological Surgeries are Described in the Respective Chapters as Below 551
    - Preoperative Assessment of a Patient Undergoing Gynecological Surgery 551

26. **Endoscopic Surgery: Laparoscopic/Hysteroscopic/Robotic Surgery** 553
    - Laparoscopic Surgery 553
    - Hysteroscope 559
    - Robotic Surgery 562

27. **Routine Postoperative Management in a Gynecological Surgery** 563
    - Postoperative Round in First Postoperative Day 563
    - Postoperative Round in Second Postoperative Day 564
    - Complications Anticipated in Postoperative Period 564
    - Alarming Signs in Postoperative Period 564
    - ERAS 566

SECTION 6: SPECIMENS

28. **Specimens** 569
    - Specimen 1: Submucous Fibroid 569
    - Specimen 2: Submucous Fibroid 570
    - Specimen 3: Multiple Fibroid 570
    - Specimen 4: Subserous Fibroid 570
    - Specimen 5: Large Cervical Fibroid 571
    - Specimen 6: Large Cervical Fibroid 571
    - Specimen 7: Pseudobroad Ligament Fibroid 571
    - Specimen 8: Simple Serous Cyst Ovary 572
    - Specimen 9: Benign Tumor 572
    - Specimen 10: Ovarian Cyst 572
    - Specimen 11: Dermoid Cyst of Ovary 572
    - Specimen 12: Benign Ovarian Tumor (TAH with BSO) 573
    - Specimen 13: Malignant Ovarian Tumor 573
    - Specimen 14A and 14B: Krukenberg Tumor 574
    - Specimen 15 and 15A: Cancer Cervix 574

- Specimen 16: Cancer Cervix 575
- Specimen 17: Endometrial Cancer 575
- Specimen 18: Cancer Vulva 576

SECTION 7: IMAGING

29. Hysterosalpingography Plates, X-ray Plates with IUCD and Other Imaging 579

Hysterosalpingography Plates 579
- Normal Scan 579
- Bilateral Tubal Block 580
- Left Side Tube Block 581
- Bicornuate Uterus 581
- Septate Uterus 582
- Unicornuate Uterus 582
- Arcuate Uterus 583
- Bicornuate Uterus 583

X-ray Plates 583
- Cu-T Intrauterine Contraceptive Device 583
- Inert IUCD 584

Sonography Plates 584
- IUCD in Uterine Cavity 584
- Displaced Cu-T 584
- 3D USG 585
- Chocolate Cyst Ovary 585

MRI Plates 585
- Fibroid Uterus 585

SECTION 8: MISCELLANEOUS

30. Research Questions for Students 589
- Types of Study 592
- Clinical Trials 592
- Randomized Control Trial (RCT) 592
- CONSORT 594
- Levels of Evidence 595
- Clinical Trials Registry—India 596

31. Examination of a Rape Victim: Procedures and Protocols 597
- Rape and Function of a Doctor 597
- Purpose of Medical Examination in Female Rape Victim 597
- Prerequisites for Examination of Victim 597
- Examination and Note of Findings 598
- Acknowledgments 599

32. Swellings of Vulva: Bartholin's Cyst and Abscess 600
- Classifications of Swellings 600
- Bartholin's Cyst and Abscess 601

33. Pelvic Inflammatory Disease, Sexually Transmitted Infections and Female Genital Tuberculosis 605
- Pelvic Inflammatory Disease (PID) 605
- Criteria Developed and Recommended (2015) by CDC for Initiation of Treatment of PID 607
- Sexually Transmitted Infections (STIs) 608
- Female Genital Tuberculosis (FGT) 612

Index 617

Section 1

Gynecological History Taking, Examination and Investigations

Section Outline

1. Writing a Gynecology Case
2. Investigative Procedures in Gynecology and Imaging in Gynecology

CHAPTER 1

Writing a Gynecology Case

Chapter Outline

- Structure of History Writing
- Detailed Parameters
- Discussion of the Points in Detail
  - History
- Physical Examination and Gynecological Examination
- Investigations
- Summary Writing and Diagnosis
  - Example of Writing a Summary (Sample Summary)

STRUCTURE OF HISTORY WRITING

A case should be written under the following broad headings:
I. Patient's particulars
II. History
III. Physical examination including systemic examinations
IV. Gynecological examinations
V. Investigations supplied or required
VI. Summary of the case
VII. Provisional diagnosis
VIII. Differential diagnosis

DETAILED PARAMETERS UNDER THE BROAD HEADINGS

Patient's Particulars

1. Name:
2. Age:
3. Address:
4. Occupation:
5. Married/unmarried:
6. History of infertility:
7. Husband's occupation:
8. Socioeconomic status:
9. Religion:
10. Parous/nulliparous:

Bed no.:
Date of admission:
Date of examination:

History

- *Chief complaint/complaints:*
- *History of present illness:*
- *Menstrual history:*
  - Last menstrual period (LMP)
  - Duration of menstruation
  - Interval in days
  - Age of menarche
  - Regularity of cycle
  - Pain during period/If pain relation with menstruation
  - Amount of bleeding
  - Clot
    - Intermenstrual bleeding (IMB)
    - Heavy menstrual bleeding [HMB (menorrhagia)]
    - Menopause or not—any postmenopausal bleeding
    - If amenorrhea—primary or secondary
- *Obstetric history* **(Table 1)**:
  - Parity
  - *Living issue (LI)*: Write "Nil" in nulliparous
  - Last child birth (LCB)
- *Past history:*
  - Medical
  - Gynecological
  - Surgical

SECTION 1: Gynecological History Taking, Examination and Investigations

Table 1: Obstetric history.

Serial no.	Year and month	Pregnancy events	Labor events	Mode of delivery	Puerperium or postabortal period	Baby
1.		• Duration of pregnancy • Antenatally cared or not • Complications if any • Treatment	• Spontaneous or induced • History of PROM • History of prolonged labor	• Vaginal delivery with/without episiotomy • Forceps/ventouse • LUCS—indications • Place of delivery • Who conducted delivery?	• Uncomplicated or complicated, e.g., PPH, sepsis, nonunion of episiotomy wound • History of blood transfusion • Hospital stay • History of intake of Rh anti-D immunoglobulin in Rh negative mother	• Living or dead • If dead—still birth—or neonatal death. If still birth fresh or macerated • Birth weight • Condition at birth • Sex • Breastfeeding • Immunization

Abbreviations: PROM, premature rupture of membranes; LUCS, lower uterine segment cesarean section; PPH, postpartum hemorrhage

- *Family history:*
- *Marital or sexual history:*
- *Functional history:*
  - Bowel
  - Bladder
  - Sleep
  - Appetite
- *Personal history:*
  - Personal hygiene
  - Smoking/alcohol
- *Contraceptive history:*
- *Drug history:*
  - History of any drug allergy
  - History of intake of corticosteroids, antiepileptic or other drugs (previous or present).

Physical Examination

Patient—alert, conscious and cooperative
- Build
- Nutrition
- Height
- Weight/body mass index (BMI)
- Edema
- Pallor
- Cyanosis
- Jaundice
- Clubbing
- Tongue, teeth, gum, and tonsil
- Secondary sexual character
- Facies and skin—presence of excessive pimple, hirsutism and acanthosis nigricans
- Neck veins
- Neck glands
- Leg veins
- Pulse
- Respiration
- Temperature
- Blood pressure.

Systemic Examination

- *Central nervous system*
- *Cardiovascular system:*
  - Auscultation of heart
- *Respiratory system:*
  - Auscultation of chest
- *Gastrointestinal system (during abdominal examination):*
  - Liver
  - Spleen
- *Examination of other systems:*
  - Examination of back and spines skeletal system
  - Neurological examination
  - Ophthalmoscopic examination
  - Urinary system
- *Examination of breasts and nipple*
- *Inspection*
- *Palpation.*

Gynecological Examination

- *Abdominal examination:*
  - Inspection
  - Palpation
  - Percussion
  - Auscultation
- *Vaginal examination*
- *Inspection and palpation of external genitalia*
- *Speculum examination*
- *Bimanual examination*
- *Rectovaginal examination and rectal examination.*

Summary of the Case

Investigations Supplied or Required

Provisional Diagnosis

Differential Diagnosis (D/D)

DISCUSSION OF THE POINTS ESSENTIAL FOR PROPER CASE TAKING AND WRITING

The following descriptions will be of immense help to write a clinical case in proper way.

Patient's Particulars

- **Age:** Dysfunctional uterine bleeding (DUB) is more common in menarcheal age and perimenopause whereas abnormal bleeding in reproductive age is mostly pregnancy-related bleeding. The average age of cancer cervix is 35–45 years and that of endometrial cancer is 55–70 years (mean 60 years). Age is no bar in ovarian malignancy but is more common in elderly or in younger age group.
- **Address:** If the patient is not in a position to tell her address properly one should write—rural, urban, urban slum or semiurban.
- **Parous/nulliparous:**
  - Parity means only previous pregnancy/pregnancies reaching beyond the age of viability.
  - *Nulliparous*: No history of any conception. Gravida means a pregnancy state *both* present and past *irrespective* of the period of gestation (not relevant in gynecological case).

  Cancer cervix and genital prolapse are more common in multiparous and endometrial cancer and endometriosis are mostly found in nulliparous or low parity women.
- It must be mentioned whether woman is a widow.

History

- *Chief complaints:* When the patient has definite chief complaints then write them in chronological order. If there is no definite complaint, it is to be enquired for which problem she was brought to hospital. The duration and character of symptoms with associated features if any and exaggerating or relieving factors should be recorded.
- *History of present illness:*
  - Elaborate the chief complaints with onset, duration, severity, etc.
  - Mention the important negative points
  - Mention any other relevant symptoms.

  Detailed queries related to the individual clinical cases are discussed in respective chapters. However, some important aspects of gynecological history should always be enquired like pelvic pain, vaginal discharge, menstrual abnormality and abnormal uterine bleeding, presence of urinary/fecal incontinence, something coming down per vagina, patient presenting with lump abdomen which are outlined below.

Pelvic pain
- If there is any pelvic pain, it should be enquired in detail and its relation with menstruation or association with bladder and bowel function should be searched for. The important causes of acute pelvic pain of gynecological origin are acute pelvic inflammatory disorder (PID), torsion of ovarian tumor, ectopic pregnancy, incomplete abortion and dysmenorrhea.
- Causes of chronic pelvic pain are endometriosis, adenomyosis, symptomatic leiomyoma, chronic pelvic infection, pelvic adhesions, etc. In pelvic pain, bowel and urologic cause must be considered.
- The characteristics of pelvic pain of different origin can be expressed by a mnemonic— SOCRATES—these are site, onset, character, radiation, associated feature, timing, exacerbating factor and severity to diagnose the cause as shown in **Table 2**.
- Pain is a subjective symptom and very difficult to quantify because it depends on individual's pain perception. To quantify discomfort pain scales have been developed which includes visual analog scale (VAS) and verbal descriptor scales (VDS).
- In visual rating scale 0—no pain, 1—mild pain, 2—moderate pain and 3—severe pain.

Table 2: Characteristics of pelvic pain of different origin (SOCRATES).

Origin	Site	Onset	Character	Radiation	Associated features	Timing	Exacerbating factors	Severity
Uterine	Midline	Prior period	Cramping	Thigh and lower back	Vaginal bleeding	Along with period	Nonspecific	Variable
Ovarian	Any iliac fossa	Acute, intermittent	Gripping	Groin, shoulder (if ascitis)	Pregnancy, ovarian cyst, irregular period	Cyclical	Positional	Severe
Pelvic infections/or adhesions	Lower abdomen, prominently one side	Gradual, acute or chronic	Shooting, gripping	Not specific	Fever, vaginal discharge, history of surgery	Acute, may be cyclical	Examination, coitus, movement	Severe intermittently
Endometriosis	Not definite	Gradual or sudden	Cramping, shooting	Not specific	Subfertility	During period	Cyclical, coitus	Variable

Vaginal discharge

- In case of discharge per vagina its amount, character, color, odor, presence of blood, associated with itching or not and relation with menstrual cycle are enquired. Association of itching with white discharge is mostly due to candidiasis/or trichomoniasis.
- **The causes may be physiological, infective, early cancer cervix or idiopathic,** etc. Before ovulation, there is physiological excessive cervical mucus discharge which is clear, transparent, copious and stretches like egg white and after ovulation the discharge becomes thick and less in amount. Infective causes are candidiasis, trichomoniasis and bacterial vaginosis.
- **The most common is candidiasis caused** by *Candida albicans*, a fungus. In candidiasis, it is creamy white, thick curdy discharge associated with marked vulvar itching and soreness. In trichomoniasis (caused by protozoa *Trichomonas vaginalis*), the discharge is fishy-odor, frothy, clean, sometimes yellowish green and associated with vulvar soreness and itching. In bacterial vaginosis (caused by *Gardnerella vaginalis*) the discharge is clear, homogeneous, whitish-gray and fishy smelling. In cancer cervix discharge may be mixed with blood.

Causes of dyspareunia: See below.

Causes of something coming down per vagina
Pelvic organ prolapse [uterine prolapse **(Fig. 1)**, cystocele, rectocele, and enterocele], Gartner's duct cyst, cervical polyp, chronic inversion of uterus, elongation of cervix and cervical growth (details in Page 205, Chapter 10).

Causes of incontinence of urine
Vesicovaginal fistula (VVF), ureterovaginal fistula (UVF), stress incontinence and urge incontinence (details in Page 389).

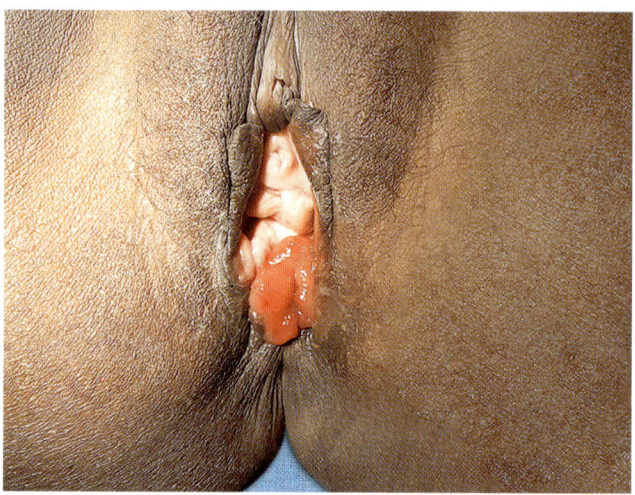

Fig. 2: Old complete perineal tear (CPT).
(24 years woman presented with incontinence of stool with history of home delivery 1 year back)

Causes of incontinence of stool
Old complete perineal tear (CPT) **(Fig. 2)**, rectovaginal fistula (details in Page 402).

Causes of lump lower abdomen
Full bladder, pregnancy, ovarian tumor **(Fig. 3)** uterine fibroid, large TO mass, Koch's peritonitis, etc. (details in Page 47)

Causes of amenorrhea
Primary amenorrhea, secondary amenorrhea and menopause (*see* below).

❖ *Menstrual history*
 Examples:
 - Last menstrual period (LMP): First day of last menstrual period.

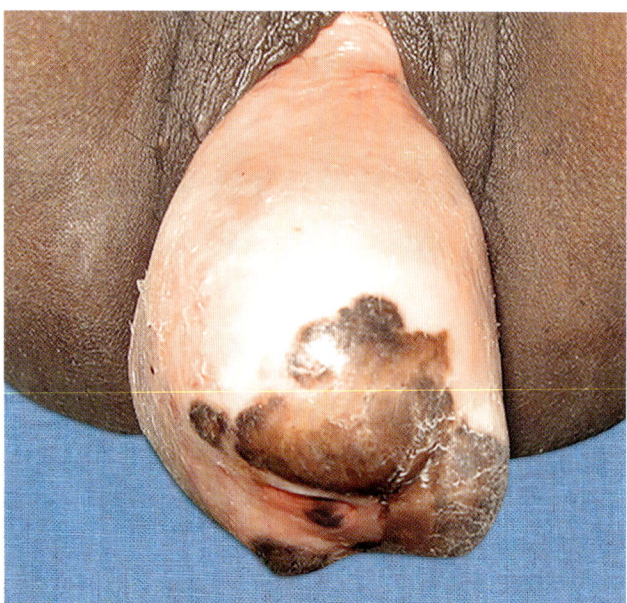

Fig. 1: Uterine prolapse.
(63 years parous postmenopausal woman presenting with something coming down P/V)

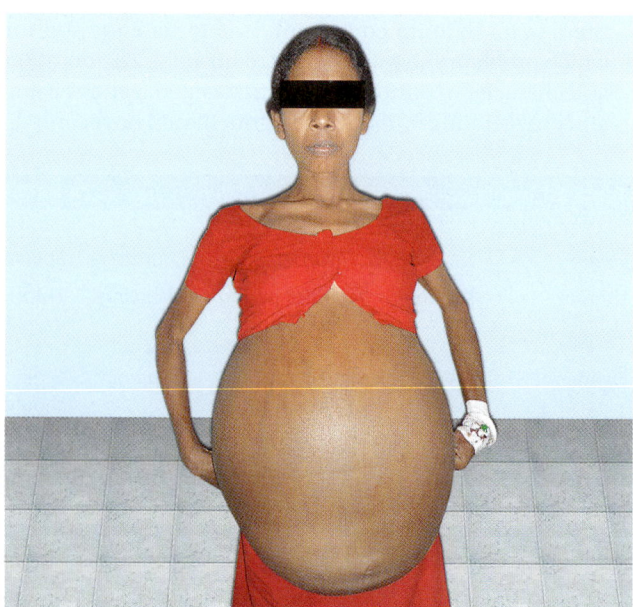

Fig. 3: Large ovarian tumor with ascites.
(32 years nulliparous woman married for 11 years presented with huge abdominal swelling. Subsequently, it was found to be a metastatic papillary serous cystadenocarcinoma of ovary)

- *Age of menarche*: 12 years.
- *Duration of menstruation*: 4–5 days.
- *Interval in days*: 28 ± 2 days.
- *Regularity of cycle*: Regular/irregular.
- *Pain during period*: Present, if present severity and relation with period.
- *Amount of bleeding*: Average, scanty or heavy.
- *Clot*: Present or not—occasionally.
- If there is IMB character of bleeding whether continuous, intermittent, spotting, etc.
- Any medication taken during period.

Menorrhagia
- Menorrhagia means excessive menstrual bleeding (>80 mL/cycle) in duration and/or amount where cycle length is normal. It is now named as "heavy menstrual bleeding" (HMB).
- **Important causes of HMB** are DUB, fibroid uterus, adenomyoma, endometriosis, PID and hereditary blood disorder (for details *see* Page 112).

Hypomenorrhea
Hypomenorrhea is defined as reduced flow either in amount or in duration or in both with cycle length normal (*see* Page 113).

Polymenorrhea or epimenorrhea (*see* Page 113)
- Polymenorrhea or epimenorrhea is characterized by short cycle (<24 days) resulting in frequent menstruation and, when associated with menorrhagia, it is called polymenorrhagia.
- When cycle length is long, more than 38 days, the condition is called oligomenorrhea.

Metrorrhagia
- Metrorrhagia refers to the IMB (Intermenstrual bleeding)—bleeding between periods suggesting hormonal, endometrial or cervical pathology.
- In recent International Federation of Gynecology and Obstetrics (FIGO) classification all above terminologies are abandoned except "HMB and IMB".

Postmenopausal bleeding (PMB) (*see* Page 144)
- Bleeding per vagina after 1 year of permanent cessation of menstruation is called "postmenopausal bleeding".
- **Common causes of PMB** are atrophic endometrium (the most common cause), endometrial cancer, cancer cervix, endometrial hyperplasia, endometrial polyp and decubitus ulcer.

Menopause
Menopause is declared at a point in time after 1 year of cessation of menstruation.

Primary amenorrhea
- Absence of menses by 13 years of age with no visible secondary sexual characteristic development or absence of menses by 15 years of age in the presence of normal secondary sexual characteristics.
- **Important causes** are constitutional delay (delayed puberty), Turner syndrome, Rokitansky-Küster-Hauser (RKH) syndrome, androgen insensitivity syndrome and adrenogenital syndrome (congenital adrenal hyperplasia).

Secondary amenorrhea
- The absence of menstruation for 6 months in a patient who had previously regular menses or absence for at least three previous cycles in a woman with previous irregular cycles.
- **Common causes** of secondary amenorrhea encountered are ovarian pregnancy, polycystic ovarian syndrome (PCOS), hypothalamic and hyperprolactinemia.

Dysmenorrhea
- Cyclical pain during period incapacitating to the woman from normal activity is called "dysmenorrhea".
- In **primary dysmenorrhea** no identifiable cause is detected and most intense just before and during period.
- **Secondary dysmenorrhea** is due to endometriosis, adenomyosis, PID, outlet obstruction, endometrial polyp and submucous fibroid.

Q. How will you assess the quantity of blood loss?

The different methods which are suggested are:
a. Measurement of Hb from sanitary napkins
b. Hb and hematocrit estimation
c. Number and type of pad or tampons and amount of passing clot and by using a scoring sheet
d. By maintaining menstrual calendar and putting the symbols against each day.

Clinically, it is said to be HMB or menorrhagia when there is:
1. Less than or equal to 3 hourly pad change
2. Change of pad at night time
3. More than 21 pads per cycle
4. Passage of clots greater than 1 inch
5. More than 80 mL blood loss in each menstrual period
6. Clinical anemia (for details *see* chapter of AUB).

- *Past obstetric history:* Write in the tabular forms.
  - Write "nil" if patient is nulliparous.
  - Endometriosis and endometrial cancer is common in nulliparous whereas in multiparous there is more chance of pelvic organ prolapse and cancer cervix.
  - Any history of infertility (mention if conception after treatment)
  - Write in chronological order the followings: Term delivery, preterm delivery
  - History of abortion (spontaneous or induced including MTP, place of termination), ectopic pregnancy and hydatidiform mole. PID may be sequel of unsafe abortion. Undiagnosed bleeding may be due to incomplete abortion or due to gestational trophoblastic neoplasia (GTN).
  - In vesicovaginal fistula (VVF), there may be history of obstructed labor. CPT is common in home delivery.

- ❖ *Past history*
  - ▪ Past medical history
    The following medical histories are important:
    - Diabetes—obese diabetic woman is high-risk subject for endometrial cancer
    - Hypertension
    - Bronchial asthma
    - Thyroid disorder—menstrual abnormality, amenorrhea, and infertility are common
      - Hyperprolactinemia with/without galactorrhea may cause amenorrhea and infertility
    - *Tuberculosis:* In genital tuberculosis, there may be history of pulmonary tuberculosis.
    - Renal disease
    - Cardiac disease
    - Epilepsy/seizure disorder
    - Rheumatic fever
    - Sexually transmitted diseases (STD)/PID/puerperal sepsis
    - History of blood transfusion
    - History of chemotherapy and radiation
    - History of coagulation disorder in young girl may present with abnormal uterine bleeding (von Willebrand disease)
  - ▪ Past gynecological history
    - *Gynecological disease:* History of PID, STDs, pelvic pain, endometriosis, and genital prolapse.
    - *Gynecological surgery:*
      - *Abdominal:* Hysterectomy, myomectomy, and oophorectomy
      - *Vaginal:* Vaginal hysterectomy (VH) with/without PFR, VVF repair, Fothergill's operation, amputation of cervix, and CPT repair.
  - ▪ Past surgical history
    The following are to be enquired for:
    - Cholecystectomy
    - Appendicectomy
    - Any laparotomy
    History of anesthetic difficulties in previous surgery.
- ❖ *Family history*
  The following family histories are relevant:
  - ▪ Medical disorder
    - Diabetes
    - Hypertension/dyslipidemia/ischemic heart disease
    - History of birth of baby with congenital anomalies or chromosomal disorder
    - Tuberculosis
    - Blood dyscrasia.
  - ▪ Genetic disorder: Androgen insensitivity syndrome, Turner syndrome, premature menopause may run in family.
  - ▪ Cancer predisposition in family: Breast, endometrial and ovarian cancer. Risk of endometrial cancer occurs in *hereditary nonpolyposis colorectal cancer (HNPCC)* group. *BRCA* mutation carrier may suffer from breast cancer syndrome.

- ❖ *Marital and sexual history*
  Sexual history is very important so far as infertility is concerned.
  - ▪ **Dyspareunia** means pain during intercourse.
  - ▪ **Causes of deep dyspareunia** are pelvic endometriosis, prolapsed ovary and pelvic infection.
  - ▪ **Superficial dyspareunia** is usually due to introital infection or trauma. Vaginal dryness is common cause of dyspareunia in menopause.
    - **Vaginismus** is pain on penetration due to involuntary contraction of pelvic floor mostly of psychological origin.
- ❖ *Functional history*
  It should be taken in details, e.g.
  - ▪ Bowel: Constipation is common in enterocele and cervical fibroid. Tenesmus is found in deep endometriosis. Pelvic abscess may cause diarrhea. History of bleeding piles, etc.
  - ▪ Bladder: History of stress incontinence, frequency and retention of urine.
    Retention of urine may be due to pelvic organ prolapse, cervical fibroid and in cryptomenorrhea due to imperforate hymen.
  - ▪ Sleep
  - ▪ Appetite: Sudden loss of weight and anorexia is common in ovarian malignancy. In young girl, loss of weight with anorexia and amenorrhea may occur in anorexia nervosa.
- ❖ *Social history*
  This is taken in very sensible way. Her occupation, her living standard, whether she is in a relationship, any pertinent family or social problem, wherefrom she will get support if surgery is advised, especially in case of elderly woman. Any addiction for drug, smoking and alcohol is enquired. Screening of intimate partner violence (IPV) or depression is done in relevant situation.
- ❖ *Contraceptive history*
  Duration and types are to be enquired. Past history of sterilization, use of oral contraceptive (OC) pills and intrauterine contraceptive device (IUCD) or any other methods used are to be enquired. IUCD may cause menorrhagia, OC pills break through bleeding and LNG-IUS is associated with amenorrhea.
- ❖ *Drug history*
  History of intake of steroids, antihypertensive, antidiabetic, anticoagulants, thyroxine and any other hormone like estrogen. Estrogen and aspirin should be stopped before surgery. Estrogen therapy may be a cause of abnormal uterine bleeding. History of drug allergy should always be asked for.

Physical Examination

- ❖ Build
  It can be expressed as average/short stature/tall stature. Build is actually a "skeletal framework" of a person.

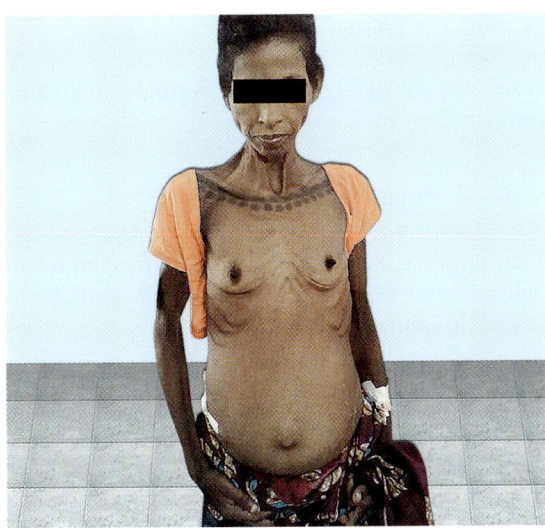

Fig. 4: Ovarian cachexia.

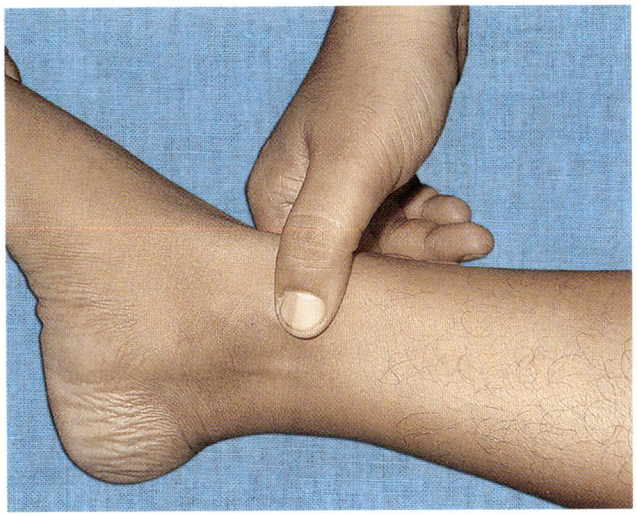

Fig. 5: Edema demonstration.

❖ **Nutrition:** It can be expressed as average/good/poor or malnourished/looks obese.
Nutrition is clinically assessed by (a) measuring the skinfold thickness between index or middle finger or by calipers, (b) by seeing the mid upper arm circumference (<22 cm—malnourished, >30 cm—likely obese), (c) mid-thigh circumference and (d) examining the features of vitamin deficiency.
Typical cachectic look is a feature of ovarian malignancy **(Fig. 4)**.

❖ **Height:** Measured either in *centimeter* or *foot and inches*. When large measuring scale is not available in the examination hall ask the patient to stand by the side of any wall, mark the highest point and measure from floor to this point with your measuring tape.
Short stature may be due to Turner syndrome. Other physical stigmas are looked for.

❖ **Weight:** Write in *kg*. Assess overweight or thin/underweight.
Body mass index (BMI) = Weight in kg/Height in meter^2
BMI <18.5—Underweight, 25–29.9—Overweight, >30—Obesity
Obesity with menstrual abnormality in young girl may be due to PCOS. Middle-aged women with obesity, hypertension and diabetes are subjects for corpus cancer syndrome (endometrial cancer).

❖ **Edema:** Write as "*present*" or "*absent*". Pitting edema or nonpitting edema like myxedema.
  ▪ Primary sites to examine:
    • Just above the medial malleolus elicited by pressing with the tip of right thumb at least for 15 seconds **(Fig. 5)**
    • Anterior surface of the lower third of shin bones
    • The dorsum of foot.
    • Other sites:
    • Facial edema
    • Over the sacrum
    • Parieties (abdomen)
    • Over the vulva **(Fig. 6)**.

❖ **Anemia:**
Present or absent—mild moderate or severe
  ▪ Primary site to see:
    • Lower palpebral conjunctiva—retract both the lower eyelids at a time and tell the patient to look upward **(Fig. 7)**.
  ▪ Other sites:
    • Dorsum and tip of the tongue
    • Soft palate
    • Nail beds
    • Palm and soles
    • Skin.

Anemia and pallor are not synonymous. Anemia is one cause of pallor. Pallor may be due to anemia or shock of any origin.

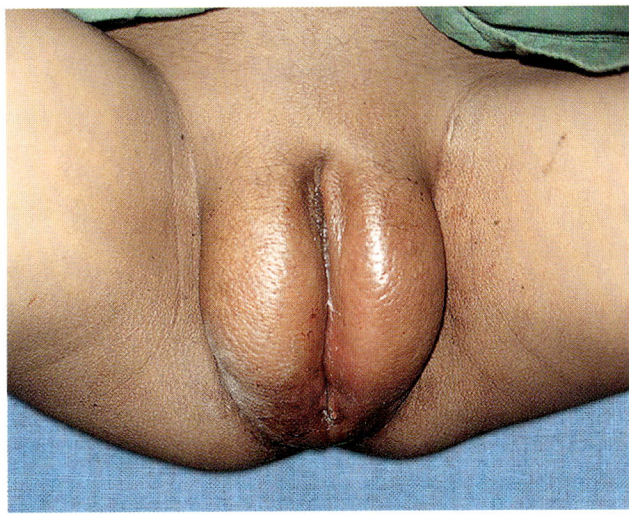

Fig. 6: Edema vulva.

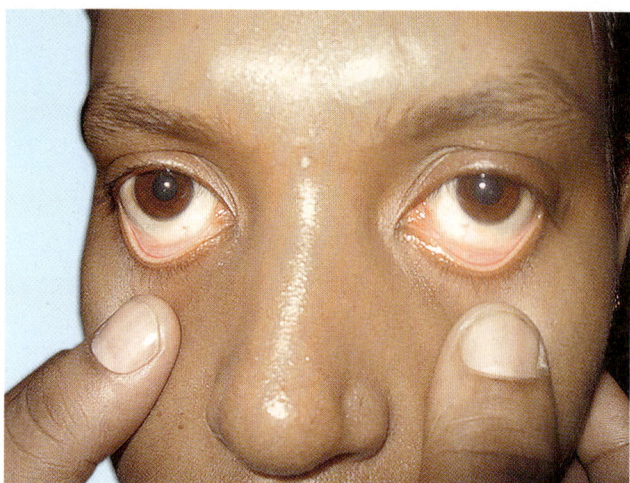

Fig. 7: Anemia demonstration.

You can write pallor instead of anemia on physical examination.

Clinically, anemia is categorized as *mild, moderate* and *severe* and may not be associated with laboratory findings always. The arbitrary gradings are:
- Mild: 10–10.9 g%
- Moderate: 7–<9.9 g%
- Severe: <7 g%
- Very severe: 4 g%.

In case of abnormal uterine bleeding (AUB) status of pallor reflects the severity of bleeding.

The **common causes of anemia** are iron deficiency, AUB, repeated pregnancy, bleeding piles, thalassemia and hook worm infestation.

❖ Cyanosis

Absent or present
Types: Peripheral and central.
- Sites to detect cyanosis:
  - *Peripheral*:
    - Tip of nose
    - Ear lobule
    - Outer surface of lips, cheek and chin
    - Tips of fingers and toes
    - Nail beds
  - *Central*:
    - Tongue
    - Inner surface of lips
    - Gum, soft palate, cheeks
    - All sites of peripheral cyanosis.

❖ Jaundice

Expressed as *present or absent*
- Sites to detect:
  - *Upper bulbar conjunctiva:* The patient is asked to look downward and upper eyelids are retracted to *see* the bulbar conjunctiva well.
  - Under surface of tongue
  - Soft palate
  - Sole and palm
  - Skin.

Jaundice is always checked in sunlight near an open window.

❖ Clubbing

❖ Tongue, teeth, gum and tonsils

Write *healthy* or any specific lesion present.
- The mouth is examined for features of malnutrition like glossitis, stomatitis, presence of any septic focus like tonsillitis and caries teeth.

❖ Examination of secondary sexual characters

Breasts, axillary hair and pubic hair—This is important in primary amenorrhea and intersex.

❖ Examination of facies and skin

Excessive pimples over face, excessive growth of hair over face and other body areas (hirsutism) **(Fig. 8)**, *acanthosis nigricans* (pigmentation of skin) **(Fig. 9)** are features of androgen excess commonly PCOS.

❖ Neck veins

Generally examined to *see* whether these are engorged or not.

❖ Neck glands

The neck is examined for presence of any enlarged gland. Supraclavicular glands are palpated for enlargement. Virchow's gland (enlarged left supraclavicular, also known as Troisier's sign) may be palpable in advanced ovarian malignancy.

Thyroid gland is also inspected and palpated for any enlargement or any other pathology.

❖ Examination of inguinal lymph nodes which may be involved in pelvic cancers or in infections.

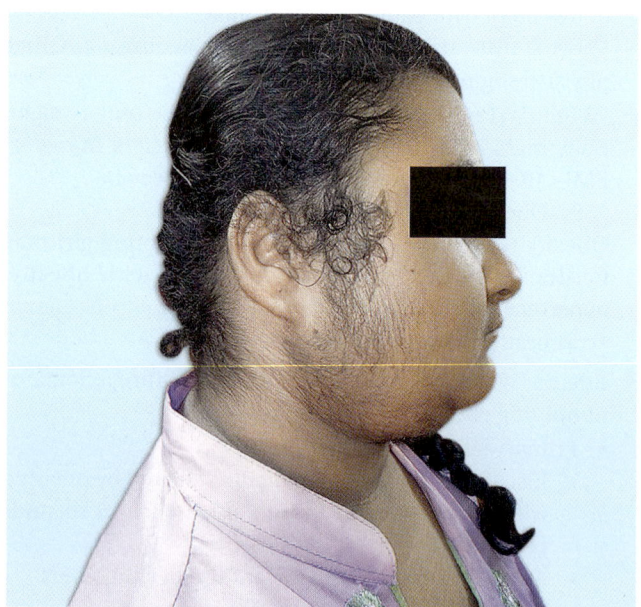

Fig. 8: Hirsutism.
(21 years unmarried girl presented with long cycle interval menstrual period, obesity and hirsutism)

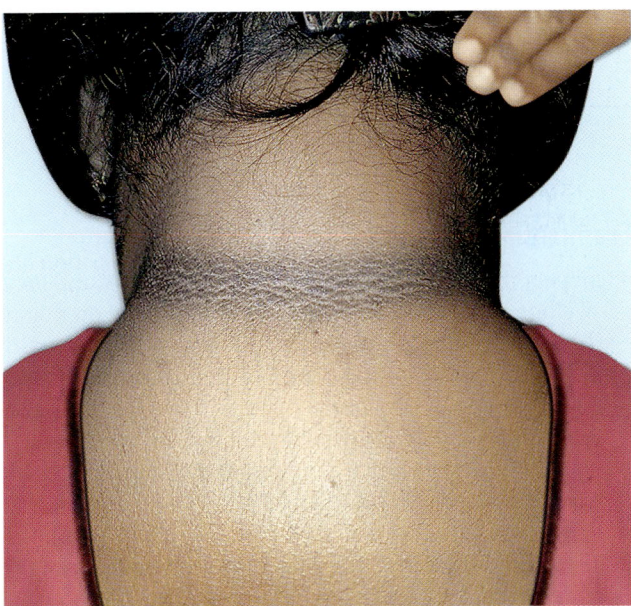

Fig. 9: Acanthosis nigricans.

❖ **Leg veins**
Note the presence of tortuosity of veins, varicose veins or presence of any pigmentation or ulcer. Prominent leg veins are features of ovarian malignancy.

❖ **Pulse**
Radial pulse is palpated at the wrist, lateral to the flexor carpi radialis tendon by the pulp of three fingers with the patient's forearm semipronated and wrist slightly flexed.
Write:
- *Rate:* Normal rate is 60–90 beats per minute (bpm). Less than 60 bpm is called bradycardia and tachycardia is rate of more than 100 bpm.
- *Volume:* It reflects pulse pressure. Volume can be expressed as normal, low volume or large (increased) volume. Feeble indicates very low volume pulse. Increased volume is seen in advanced age, arteriosclerosis, hypertension, anemia and thyrotoxicosis. Low pulse volume occurs in LFV, hypovolemia and peripheral arterial disease.
- *Rhythm:* Regular or irregular.
- *Any special character:* Character refers to the waveform or shape of the arterial pulse.
- *Other pulses:* Other than radial pulse brachial, carotid, femoral, popliteal, posterior tibial and arteria dorsalis pedis can be palpated in special situations.
- *Any difference of upper and lower limb pulses:*
In **Turner syndrome**, pulses of both upper and lower limbs should be examined. In Turner syndrome, there may be congenital coarctation of aorta which is narrowing of aorta distal to the left subclavian artery and pulses of upper limb are usually normal with reduced lower limb pulses which are delayed in relation to pulses of upper limb, i.e. radiofemoral delay. **Radiofemoral delay** can be checked by palpation of radial and femoral artery simultaneously. **Radio-radial delay** is found in presubclavian coarctation of aorta.

❖ **Respiration**
- Rate: —/min
- Rhythm:—
- Type: Abdominal or thoracic
- Any special variety: —

❖ **Temperature:**
Temperature is best recorded by thermometer.

❖ **Blood pressure**
- Expressed as systolic/diastolic mm of Hg.
- Normal BP is defined as less than 130/85 mm of Hg (British Hypertension Society). Optimal BP is less than 120/80 mm of Hg.

Importances of blood pressure measurement in gynecological practice:
(1) BP measurement is a routine procedure to assess the general health of a woman, (2) may be associated with some gynecological diseases like AUB and endometrial cancer and (3) also as a part of preoperative evaluation for surgery.

Procedure of Measurement of Blood Pressure

Patient should take rest at least for 5 minutes before measurement.

Position of the patient
BP can be measured either in *sitting or lying down* posture in relaxed attitude supporting the patient's arm comfortably at the *level of heart*. The sphygmomanometer cuff is applied over the upper arm, with the center of the bladder on brachial artery. There should not be no tight clothing constricting the upper arm; loose thin clothing usually makes no difference.

Systolic pressure
Systolic pressure is first assessed roughly by palpation of radial pulse or brachial pulse after inflating the cuff till it becomes impalpable. In auscultation technique, diaphragm is placed gently over the brachial pulse which is situated medial to the biceps Brachii tendon, over the elbow joint. The cuff is initially inflated to a pressure 20–30 mm of Hg higher than the estimated systolic pressure determined by palpation. Then the cuff is deflated 2 mm/sec until a regular tapping sound **(Korotkoff phase I: K1)** is heard. Blood pressure is read to the nearest 2 mm of Hg.

Diastolic pressure
The cuff is deflated slowly until the sounds disappear. The pressure is recorded as diastolic pressure at which the sound completely disappears **(Korotkoff phase V: K5)**. Sometimes muffled sounds persist **(Korotkoff phase IV: K4)** and do not disappear, then the point of muffling (K4) is taken as diastolic pressure.

It is better to measure BP in both arms. If different the higher one is considered and noted.

Size of BP cuff

The bladder should be at least 80% of the length and 40% of the width of upper arm circumference. A standard adult cuff has a bladder 13 cm × 30 cm and suits an arm circumference of 22–26 cm. In obese patients with an arm circumference of more than 32 cm may give false high readings in normal sized cuff, therefore larger cuff (bladder 16 cm × 38 cm) or thigh cuff (20 cm × 42 cm) is needed for those patients.

Systemic Examination

- *Cardiovascular system:* Palpation of precordium and auscultation of heart are done in different areas.
  Write:
  - Palpation of precordium: No abnormality detected.
  - Auscultation: Normal heart sounds.

  If any lesion is detected or suspected detailed examination of different areas is done and noted. In Turner syndrome, there may be coarctation of aorta.

- *Respiratory system:*
  - Position of trachea
  - Palpation, percussion and auscultation done on both sides. Pleural effusion may be present due to abdominal ascites.
    Write: No abnormality detected
         Breath sounds are normal
         No adventitious sound.
    If any abnormality is detected—then write in detail.

- *Gastrointestinal system:* Liver and spleen are palpated routinely for any enlargement and tenderness (*see* below).
  Write: *Not enlarged* or *just palpable* or *enlarged* (fingers as the measurement is).

- *Other systems:*
  - Neurological systems:
    - Higher function
    - Cranial nerves
    - Sensory function
    - Motor function
  - Ophthalmoscopic examination—not done.

- Urinary system:
  - Kidney
  - **Renal angle tenderness:** Renal angle tenderness is elicited at the junction of lower border of 12th rib and lateral (outer) border of erector spinae (*see* **Figs 22 and 23**, Page 16).

Examination of Breasts

- Inspect the skin, areola, nipple, sizes of breasts and local swelling in different positions: (a) arms resting on thighs, (b) arms pressing on hips, (c) arms over the head and (d) leaning forward to make breasts pendulous. Compare both sides for any asymmetry **(Figs. 10A to D)**.
- Breasts are palpated in lying down position. With head on one pillow and patient's hand under the head on the side to be examined **(Figs. 11A and B)**.
- Palpate each breast systematically **(Figs. 12A to C)** over all the quadrants from periphery toward nipple. Presence of any lump and tenderness is noted. If there is any mass its characteristics are noted (size, position, consistency, fixity, surface, margins, inflammation and tenderness). Palpate the nipple for any abnormality or discharge—watery, bloody or milky (galactorrhea). Palpate also the axillae for any extension of breast (axillary tail) between thumb and finger and presence of nodes. Palpate also the supraclavicular group of lymph nodes.
- In case of primary amenorrhea, development of breast is staged according to Tanner's staging (*see* **Fig. 19A**, Chapter 13, Page 318).
- Clinical breasts examination (CBE) is performed by healthcare professionals and self breast examination (SBE) is done by the patient herself.

Per Abdominal Examination

Before gynecological examination (abdominal and vaginal) the following preparatory procedures are done:
- Ask the patient to evacuate her bladder
- Always keep one female attendant/chaperone
- Stand on right side of the patient **(Figs. 13 to 15)**

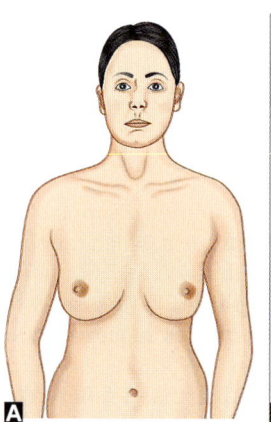 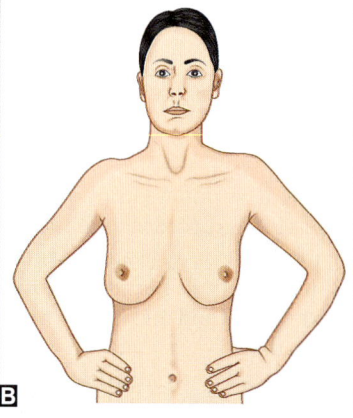 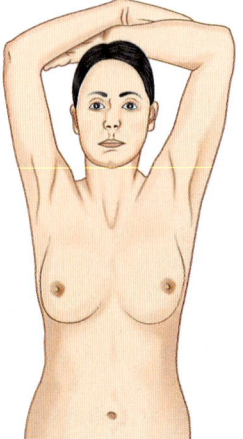 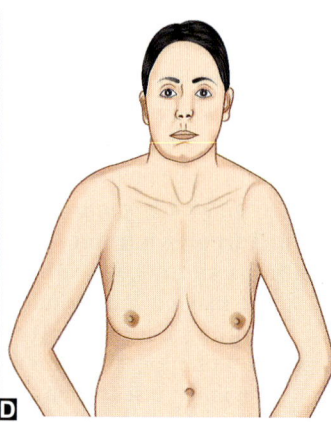

Figs. 10A to D: Examination of breasts. (A) Arms resting on thighs; (B) Arms pressing on hips; (C) Arms over the head; (D) Leaning forward to make breasts pendulous.

CHAPTER 1: Writing a Gynecology Case

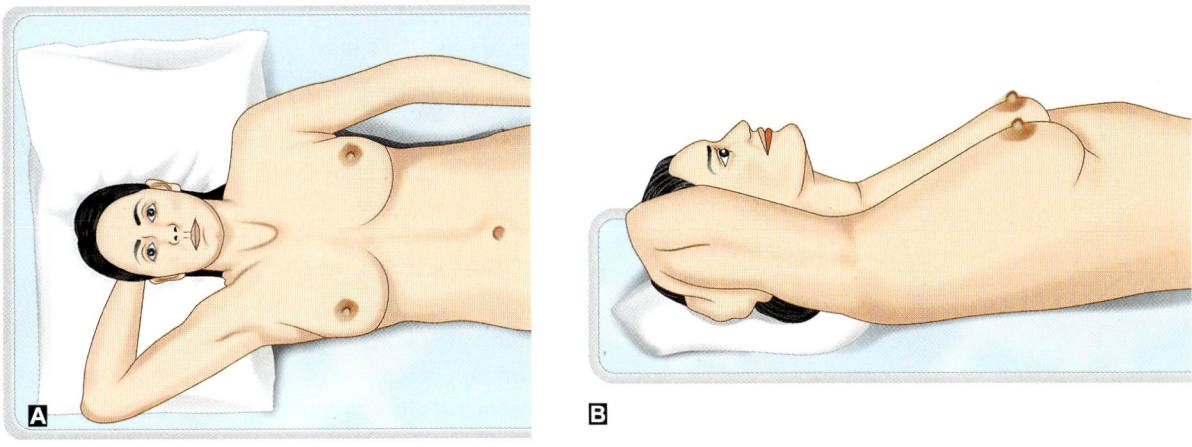

Figs. 11A and B: Palpation of breasts in lying down position. (A) With head on one pillow; (B) Patient's hand under the head on the side.

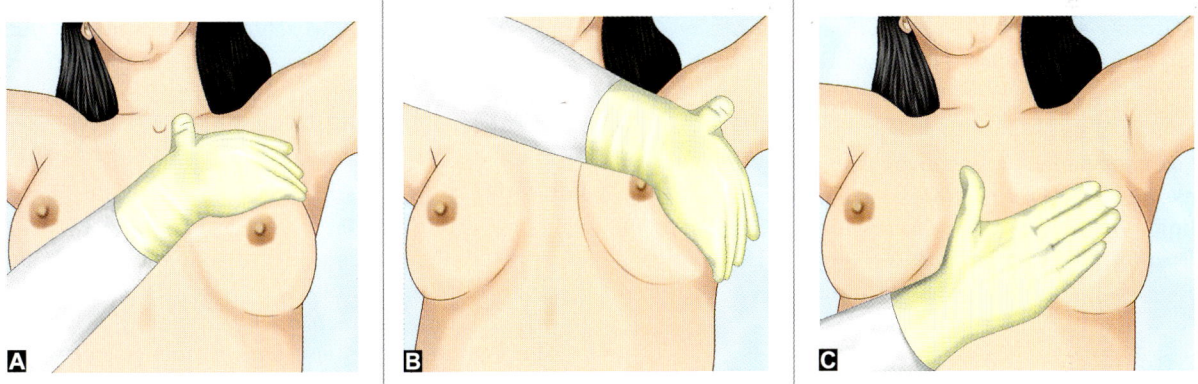

Figs. 12A to C: Palpation of each breast systematically.

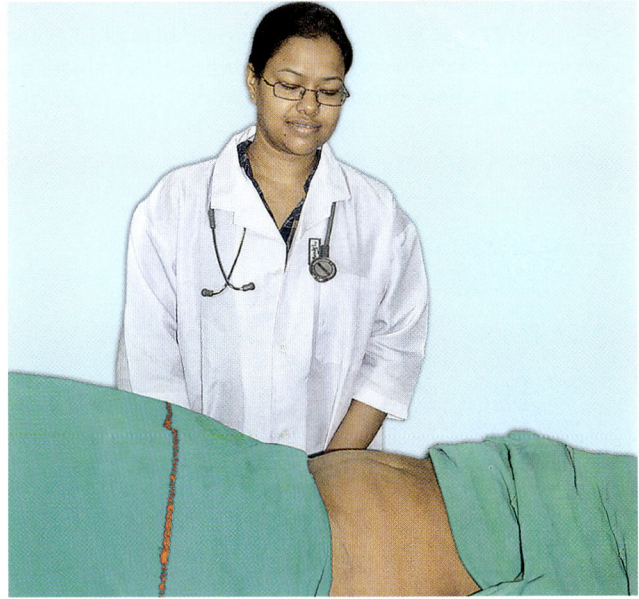

Fig. 13: Inspection of the abdomen: Position of the patient—dorsal supine position with partial flexion of knees and thighs.

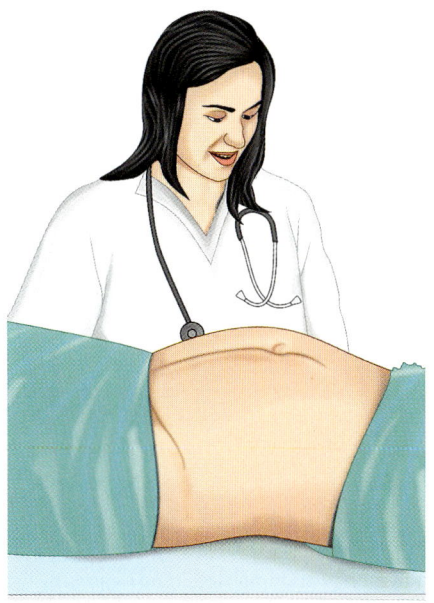

Fig. 14: Inspection of the abdomen.

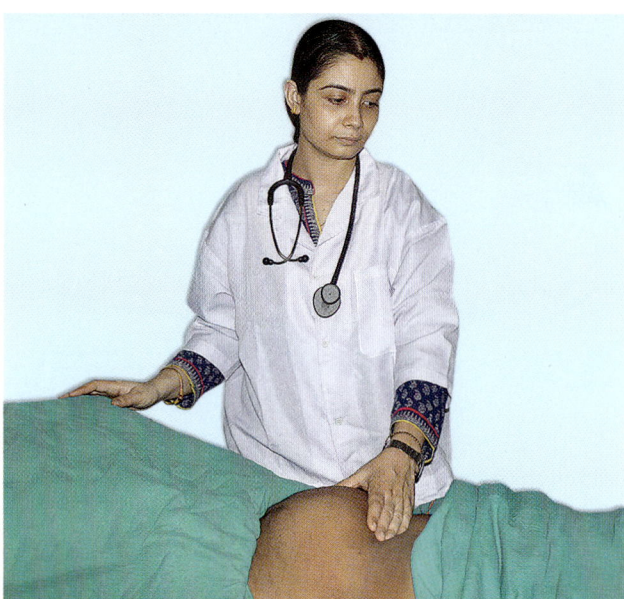

Fig. 15: Position of the patient—dorsal supine position with partial flexion of knees and thighs.

- Explain the patient what you are going to do
- Make **dorsal supine position,** head is supported by a small pillow—***partial flexion of knees and thighs facilitate relaxation of abdominal muscles*** (Figs. 13 to 15).
- Abdomen is exposed fully and other parts are covered well.

Gynecological Examination

- *Abdominal examination*
  Regions of abdomen (**Fig. 16**)

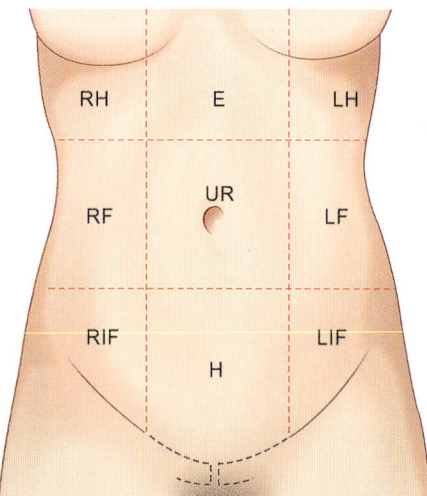

Fig. 16: Subdivision of abdomen into nine regions by two horizontal and two vertical lines or planes.

Abbreviations: RH, right hypochondrium; E, epigastrium; LH, left hypochondrium; LF, left flank or lumbar region; LIF, left iliac fossa; H, hypogastrium or suprapubic region; RIF, right iliac fossa; RF, right flank or lumbar region; UR, umbilical region

Abdomen is subdivided into *nine regions* by two horizontal and two vertical lines or planes (**Fig. 16**). The upper horizontal line joins the tips of the 9th costal cartilages on either side and the lower horizontal line is drawn from highest points of the iliac crests (transtubercular). The vertical lines on either side are drawn vertically upward from midclavicular points.

Inspection (*see* Figs. 13 and 14)

- Contour of abdomen
- Condition of skin
- Condition of umbilicus—everted/flushed/inverted
- Presence of any scar and its description
- Presence of any lump or fullness of the abdomen. Both in ovarian tumor and ascites abdomen is enlarged. In case of ascites flanks are also full and in ovarian tumor center is only full (*see* below). In ascites enlargement of abdomen is equal in both sides laterally, but in ovarian cyst enlargement on two lateral sides are usually unequal.
- Presence of sites of hernia—coughing impulse if any
- Enlarged inguinal lymph nodes, testes in inguinal region (androgen insensitivity syndrome).

Palpation

Palpation is done by flat of the hand and finger movements must be gentle and from metacarpophalangeal joints and not interphalangeal joints (**Figs. 15 to 18**).

- *Superficial palpation:* By superficial palpation temperature, tenderness, parietal edema, localized lump, divarication of recti and fluid thrill are elicited.
- *Deep palpation:* Abdomen is palpated deeply with flat of the dominant hand as well as the fingers while patient is asked to breathe quietly. All the surgical areas (**Fig. 16**) of the abdomen are palpated symmetrically either clockwise or anticlockwise starting from the right hypochondrium for any mass or enlarged organ. It is better to palpate the region at the end which is tender. Sometimes in difficult

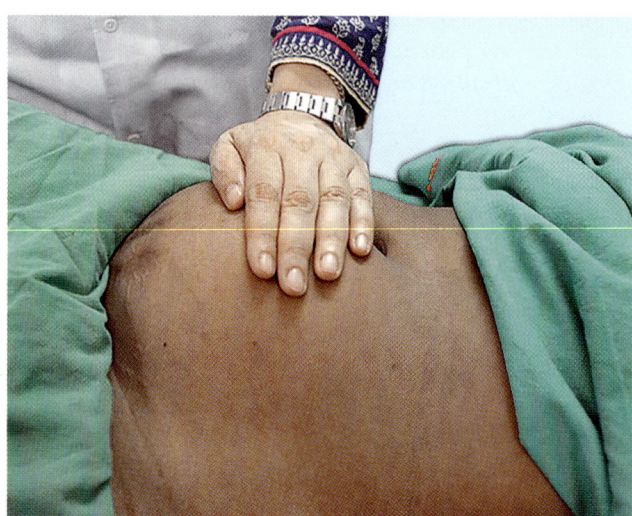

Fig. 17: Palpation of abdominal lump.

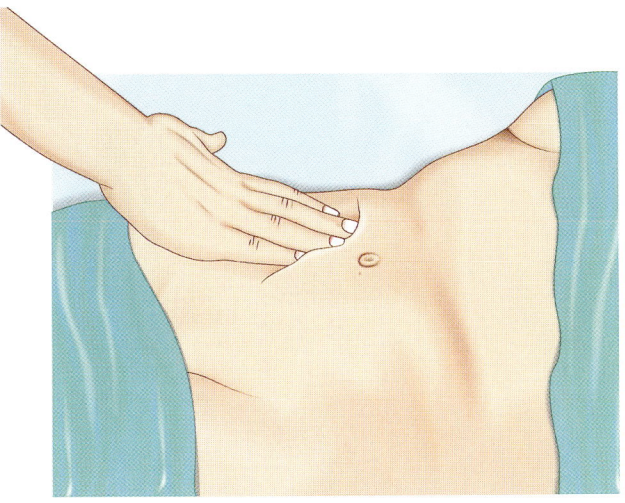

Fig. 18: Palpation of abdomen (diagrammatic).

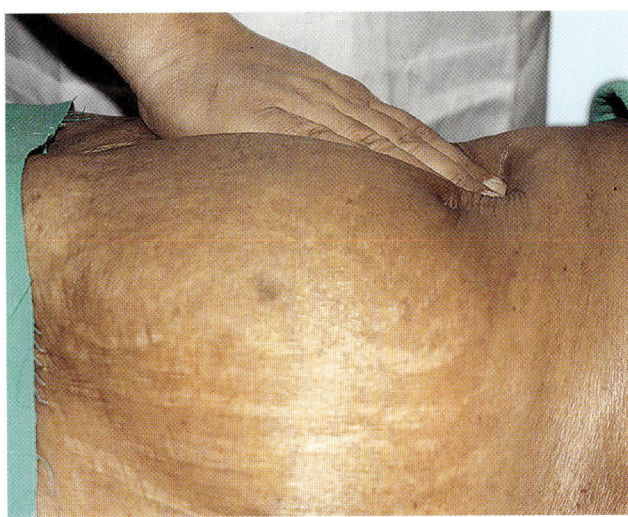

Fig. 19: Palpation of liver.

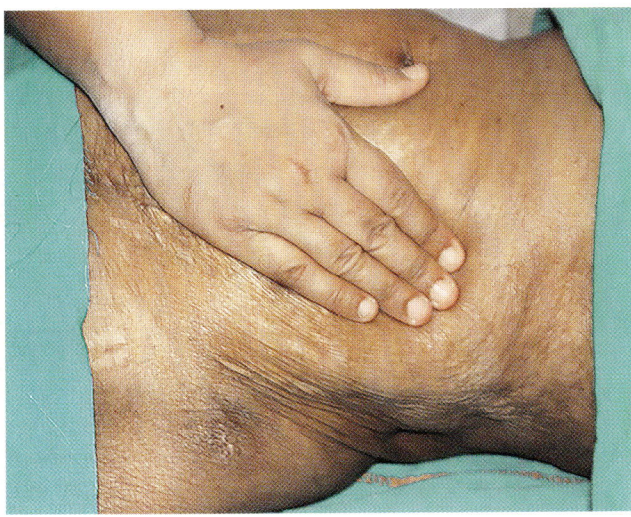

Fig. 20: Palpation of spleen.

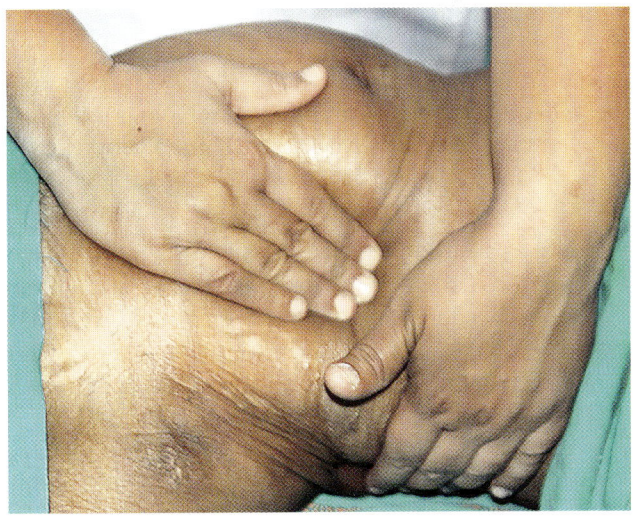

Fig. 21: Palpation of spleen.

palpation like in obesity and ascites, etc., the left hand is placed over right hand to feel deeply.
- *Liver and spleen are palpated (Figs. 19 to 21):* Patient is asked to take deep breath during palpation.
- *Palpation of kidney:* The site of kidney is palpated and renal angle is elicited keeping hand behind near the junction of lateral border of erector spinae and lower border of 12th rib **(Figs. 22 and 23)**.
- All surgical areas are palpated—presence of any lump, tenderness, rigidity and muscle guarding are looked for.
- *Rebound tenderness* is elicited by complain of severe pain abdomen after giving pressure over the abdomen and then taking off the hands suddenly.
- In presence of any lump note its:
  a. Site
  b. Shape
  c. Size
  d. Surface
  e. Margins
  f. Consistency
  g. Tenderness
  h. Mobility.
- In pelviabdominal mass note whether lower margin can be reached or not. If it is not reached you can write *"cannot get below the lump".* In pelvic mass, it can be moved from side to side, but difficult to move vertically.
- Inguinal area is palpated to look for enlarged lymph nodes and if any its character is noted.

Q. How would you test a lump is parietal or intra-abdominal?

Leg raising test: Any mass whether it is intra-abdominal or parietal is determined. Patient is asked to lift up both extended legs together on lying down position. In case of intra-abdominal mass, it will disappear and in case of intraparietal it will be prominent.

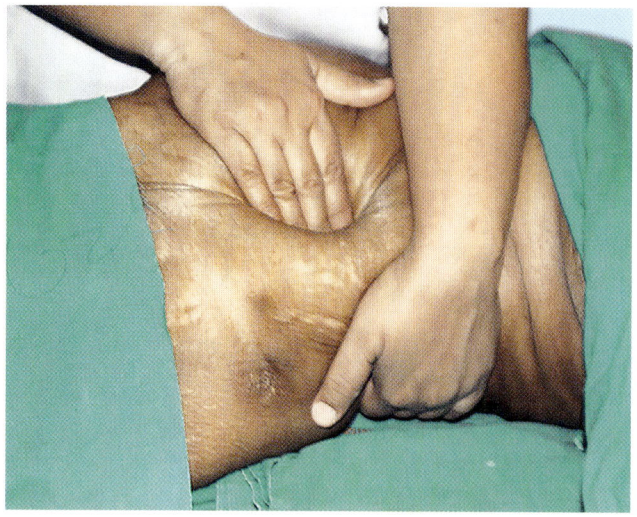

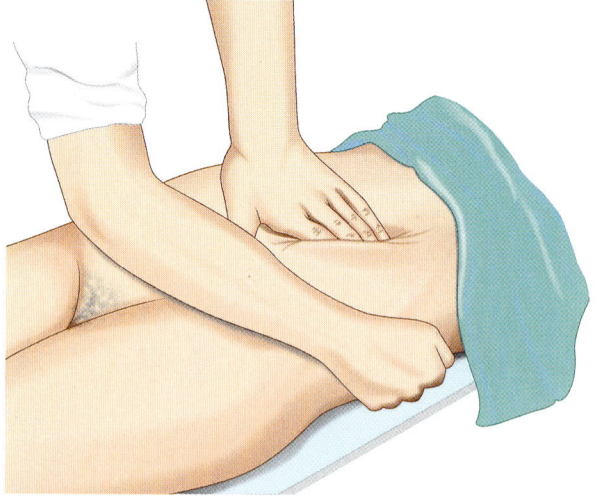

Fig. 22: Palpation of kidney.

Fig. 23: Palpation of kidney (diagrammatic).

Q. How would you determine a lump is retroperitoneal or intra-abdominal?

Knee elbow position to rule out retroperitoneal lump—in intra-adominal lump, it will be prominent and in case of retroperitoneal mass, it will become not prominent.

Percussion

- Percussion can differentiate abdominal mass and ascites.
- In ascites midline (A) is resonant, flanks are dull on percussion, and "shifting dullness" is positive **(Fig. 24A)**.
- Whereas in mass like ovarian tumor without ascites midline (A) is dull on percussion and flanks are resonant **(Fig. 24B)**.
- If ovarian cyst is associated with gross ascites the midline will be resonant, flank is dull **(Fig. 24C)** and "shifting dullness" becomes positive.
- Fluid thrill is present in huge ascites and is also present in large ovarian cyst and in encysted fluid.

Demonstration of shifting dullness (Figs. 25 to 27)

In supine position, percuss from the midline out to the flanks. Any change from resonant to dull is noted along with the areas of dullness and resonance. Finger on the site of dullness is kept and patient is asked to turn on to her side and a pause of 10–30 seconds is given. Then again percussion is done. If the dull and tympanic areas are reversed "shifting dullness" is said to be positive.

Demonstration of fluid thrill (Figs. 28 and 29)

It is done when abdomen is tensely distended. The palm of the left hand flat is placed against the left side of the patient's abdomen. The patient or an assistant is asked to place of the edge of hand on the midline of abdomen. The right side of the abdomen is flicked by a finger of right hand, if a ripple is felt against left hand "fluid thrill", is said to be present.

Auscultation

Intestinal peristaltic sound is usually heard. Fetal heart sound is excluded in any lump abdomen. Absent peristalsis indicates peritonitis and increase peristalsis is heard in intestinal obstruction.

Vaginal Examination

- *Preparatory procedures*
  - Ask the patient to evacuate her bladder before examination except in case where there is history of stress incontinence.
  - Woman will lie in *dorsal supine position*, thigh flexed and knee flexed keeping the feet on extended foot rests so that buttock comes to the margin of table which facilitates the introduction of speculum **(Figs. 30 and 31)**. Some schools prefer to do it in *dorsal lithotomy* position **(Fig. 32)** which is not comfortable for the patient and not practiced in all setup.
  - Keep one female attendant/chaperone
  - Stand on right side of the patient near the leg ends
  - Ask the patient what you are going to do and take consent for that. In case of minor, consent from legal guardian is taken.
  - Examination is done in good light.
- *Other positions in different situations*
  - *Sims' semi-prone position:* Left lateral position with left leg extended and right thigh and knee partially flexed **(Figs. 33A and B)**. This position is very useful for inspection of lesions of anterior vaginal wall lesion like VVF using Sims' speculum to retract posterior vaginal wall **(Figs. 33 and 34)** and rectal examination.
  - *Squatting position:* This position is sometimes necessary for proper visualization of genital prolapse if not demonstrated in dorsal position. Even genital prolapse sometimes needs *standing position* to visualize well (*see* **Figs. 40 and 41**, Chapter 10, Page 218).

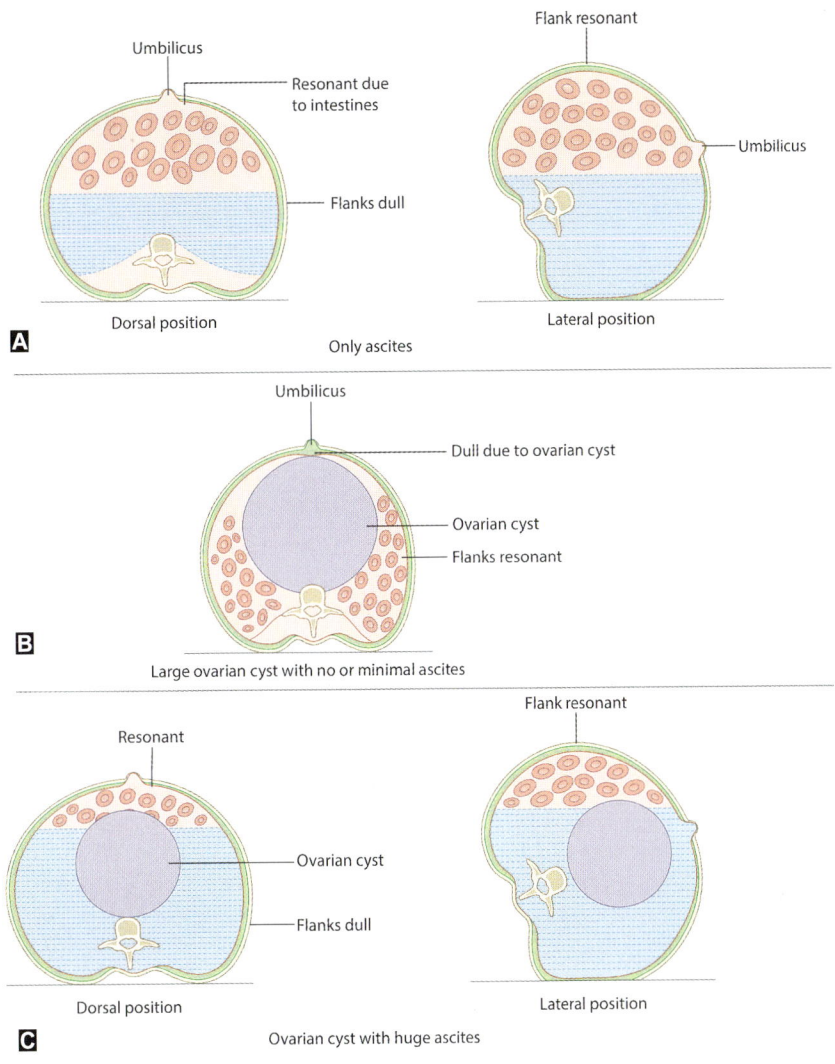

Figs. 24A to C: (A) Only ascites; (B) Large ovarian cyst; (C) Ovarian cyst with huge ascites.

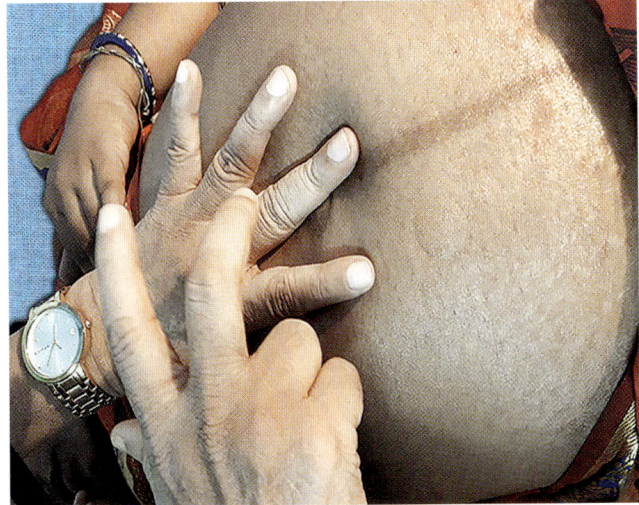

Fig. 25: Percussion on midline in dorsal position.

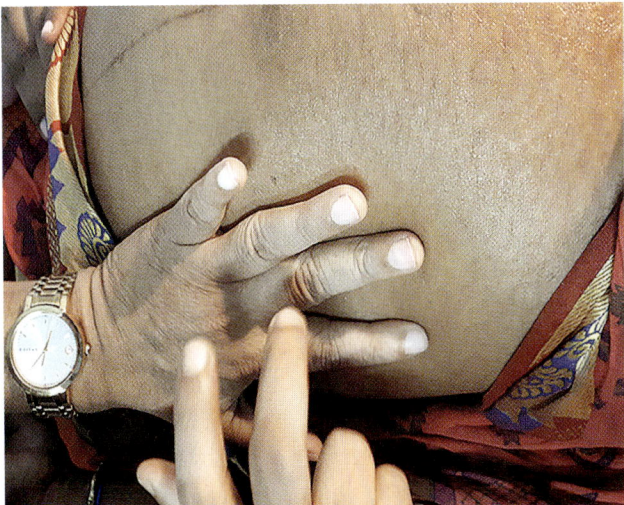

Fig. 26: Percussion from midline towards the flank in dorsal position.

SECTION 1: Gynecological History Taking, Examination and Investigations

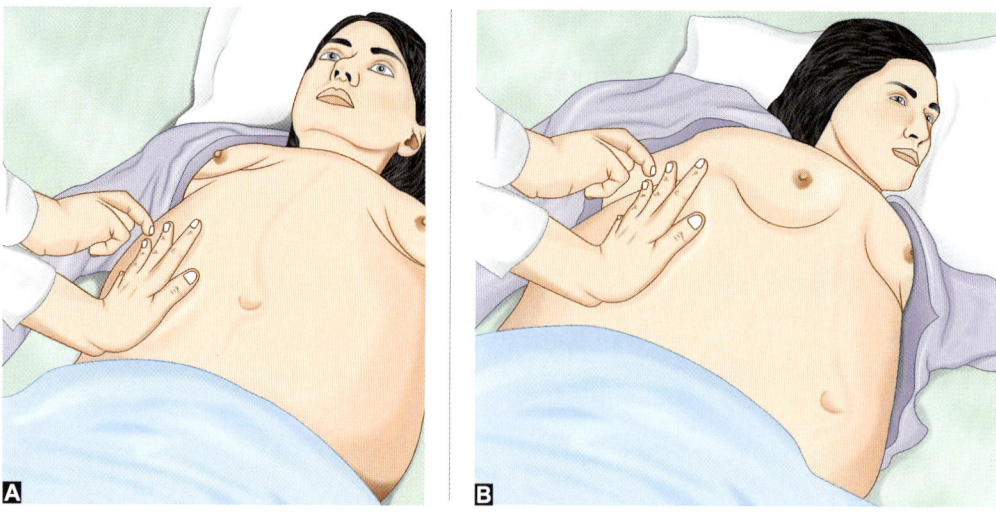

Figs. 27A and B: Demonstration of shifting dullness: (A) Dorsal position; (B) Lateral position.

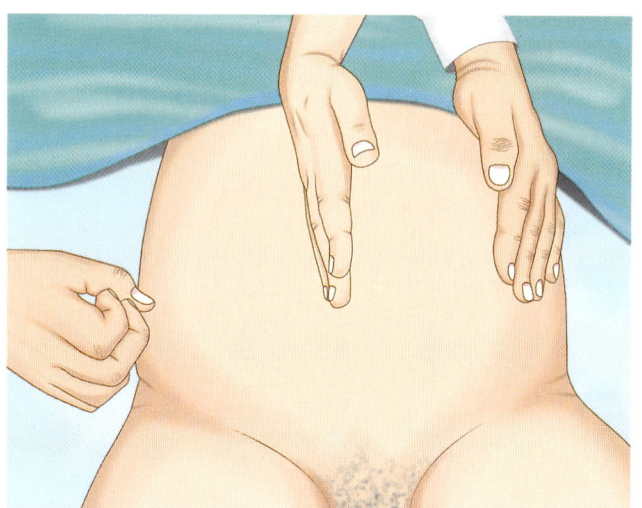

Fig. 28: Demonstration of fluid thrill (diagrammatic).

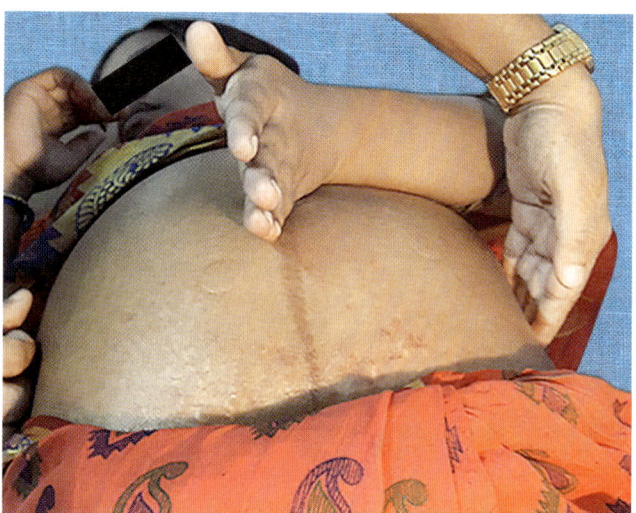

Fig. 29: Demonstration of fluid thrill.

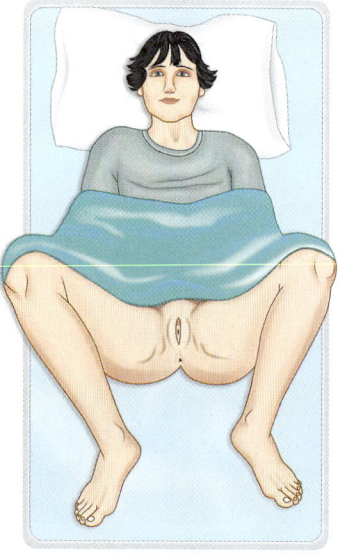

Fig. 30: Dorsal supine position (diagrammatic).

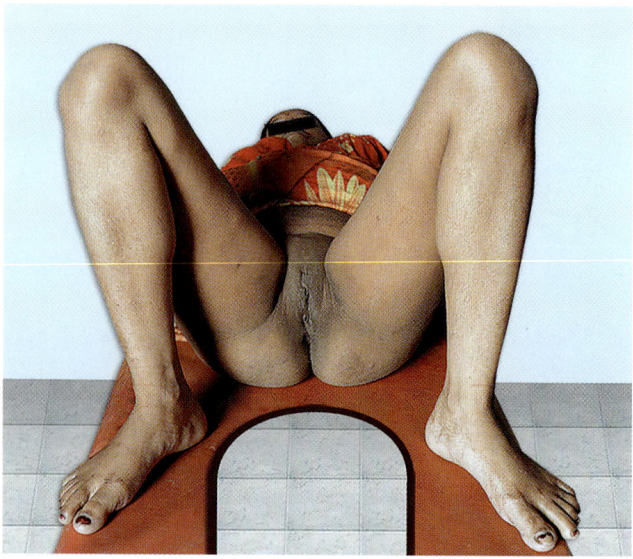

Fig. 31: Dorsal supine position.

CHAPTER 1: Writing a Gynecology Case

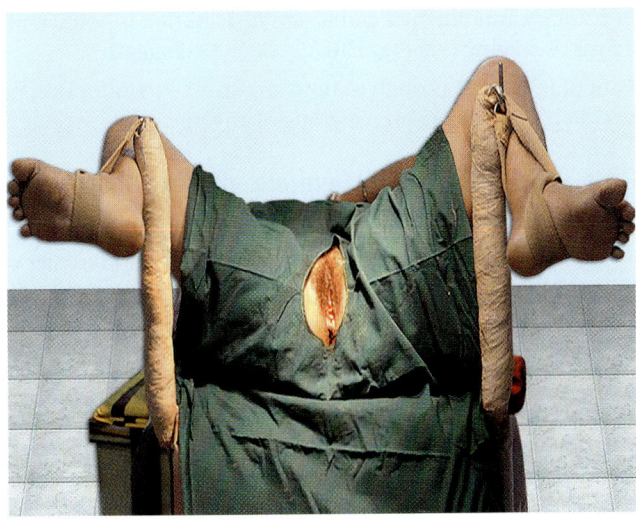

Fig. 32: Dorsal lithotomy position.

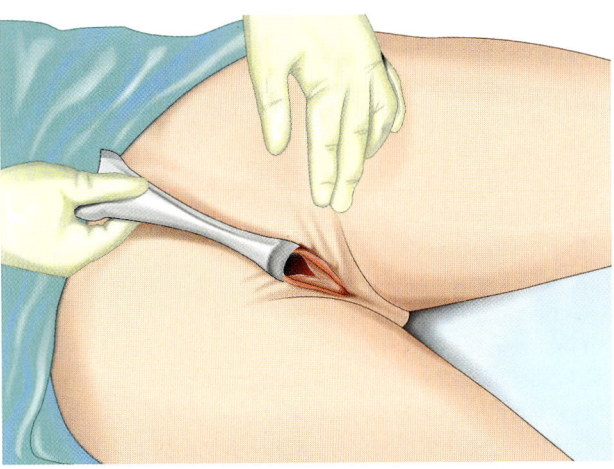

Fig. 34: Sims' speculum to retract posterior vaginal wall to visualize the anterior wall.

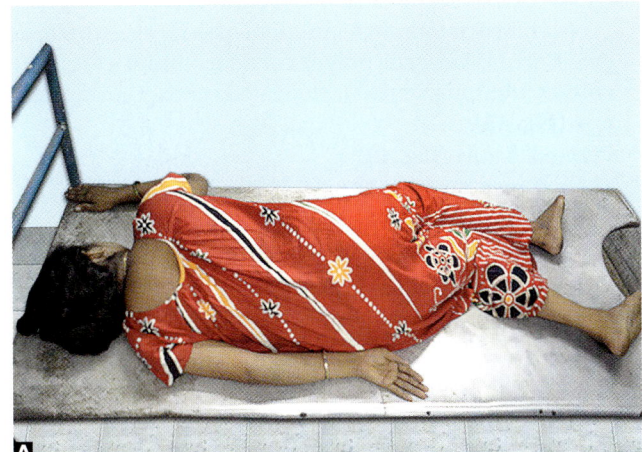

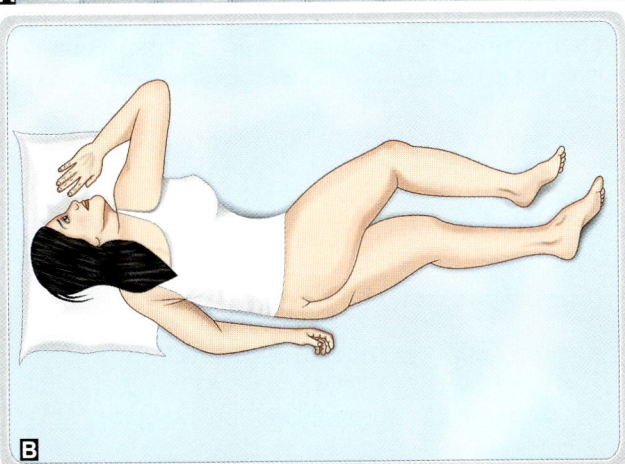

Figs. 33A and B: Sims' semi-prone position (left lateral position with left leg extended and right thigh and knee partially flexed).

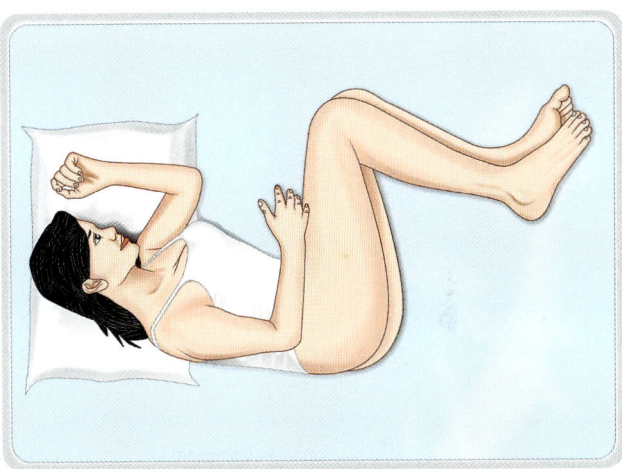

Fig. 35: Left lateral position.

Hence, the different positions for gynecological examinations are:
1. Dorsal position (*see* Figs. 30 and 31)
2. Dorsal lithotomy position (*see* Fig. 32)
3. Sims' semi-prone position (*see* Figs. 33A and B)
4. Left lateral position (Fig. 35).

Sequence of Vaginal Examination
- Inspection of external genitalia
- Palpation of external genitalia and vagina
- Speculum examination
- Bimanual examination.

Inspection of External Genitalia

Inspect the vulva visually **(Fig. 36)** one by one the following structures **(Fig. 37)**:
- Labia majora and labia minora
- Clitoris
- Urethra
- Fourchette
- Vaginal introitus
- Bartholin's gland
- Anus
- Gynecological perineum.

Observe for any discharge, lesions, ulcers, scratch mark, discoloration, redness, any growth, swelling of vulva like sebaceous cyst, enlargement of clitoris, ambiguous genitalia, old perineal tear, and protruding masses like genital prolapse.

In primary amenorrhea, pubic hair distribution is noted with Tanner's staging (see **Fig. 19B**, Chapter 13, Page 318).

Patient is asked to cough to note any stress incontinence, or to watch for impulse on coughing of any mass.

Observations of External Genitalia and Probable Causes

- Red lesion—contact dermatitis, tinea cruris
- White lesion—leukoplakia **(Fig. 38)**, lichen sclerosus et atrophicus, squamous cell hyperplasia, squamous cell carcinoma
- Papules—molluscum contagiosum, condyloma acuminata (vulvar warts) **(Figs. 39 and 40)**
- Cyst/swelling—lipoma **(Fig. 41)**, sebaceous cyst **(Fig. 42)**, indirect inguinal hernia, Bartholin cyst **(Fig. 43)**/abscess **(Fig. 43)**, vulvar fibroma **(Fig. 44)**
- Ulcers/erosion—herpes, chancre
- Discharge—trichomonas, candidiasis **(Fig. 45)**, bacterial vaginosis
- Large growth—vulvar cancer **(Fig. 46)**
- Deficient perineum—complete perineal tear (see **Fig. 2**)
- Protruding mass through introitus—pelvic organ prolapse (see **Fig. 1**), cervical polyp, cervical fibroid **(Fig. 47)**, chronic uterine inversion, elongated cervix, Gartner duct cyst **(Fig. 48)**
- Perineal fistula **(Fig. 49)**
- Vaginal agenesis **(Fig. 50)**
- Imperforate hymen **(Fig. 51)**
- Vaginal septum **(Fig. 52)**
- Enlarged clitoris with fused labia **(Fig. 53)** (congenital adrenal hyperplasia).

Swellings of vulva including Bartholin cyst are described in Chapter 32.

Palpation of External Genitalia and Vagina

Digital examination is done to palpate the vulva and vagina for accurate diagnosis of the lesion and presence

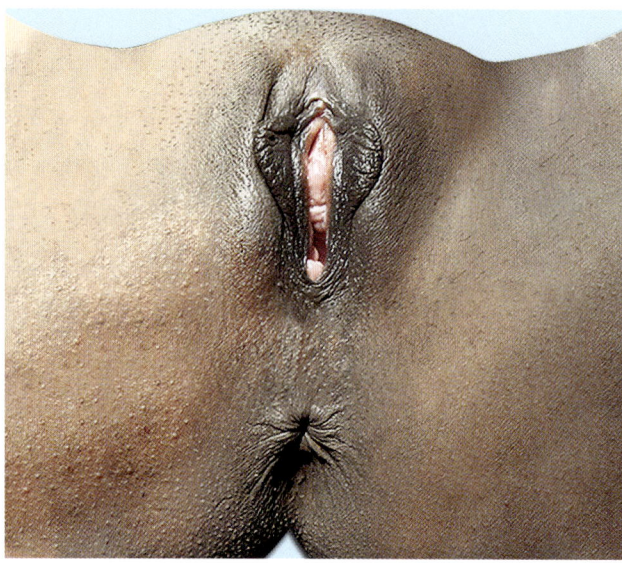

Fig. 36: Female external genitalia.

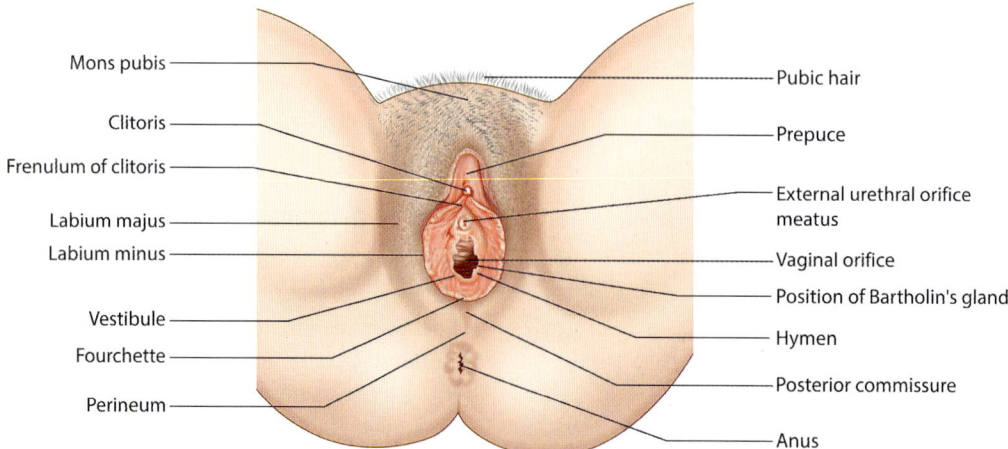

Fig. 37: Inspection of the female external genitalia.

CHAPTER 1: Writing a Gynecology Case

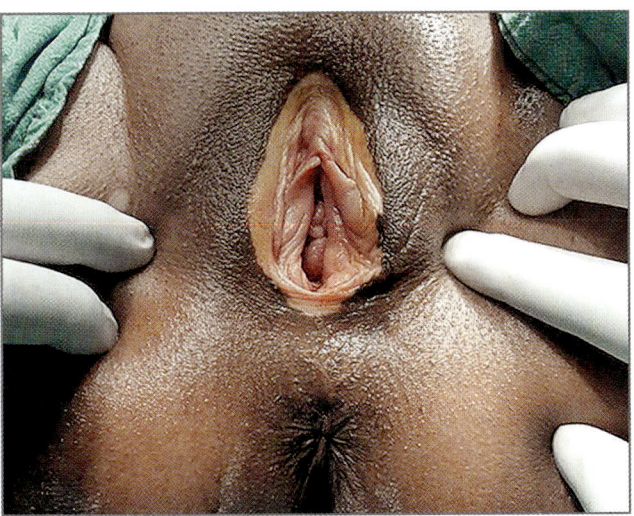

Fig. 38: Leukoplakia vulva.

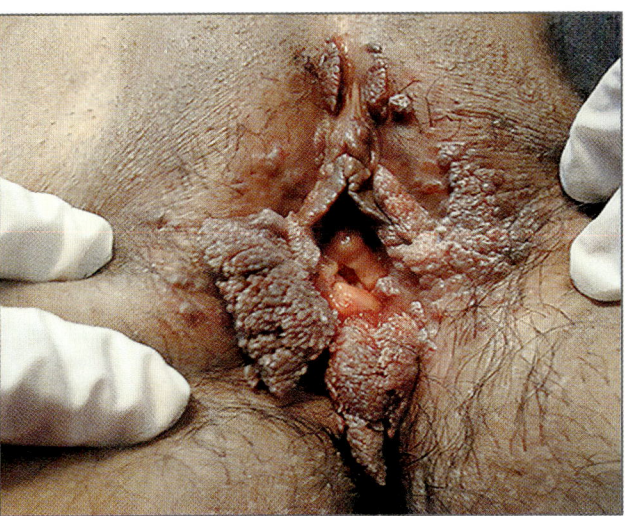

Fig. 39: Vulvar warts (condyloma acuminata).

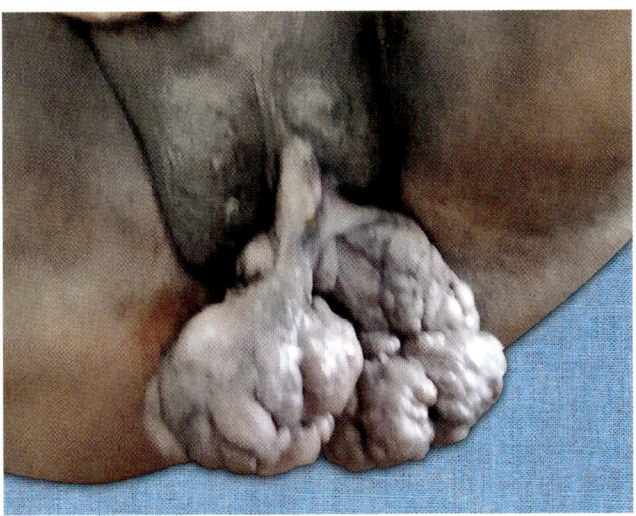

Fig. 40: Vulvar warts.

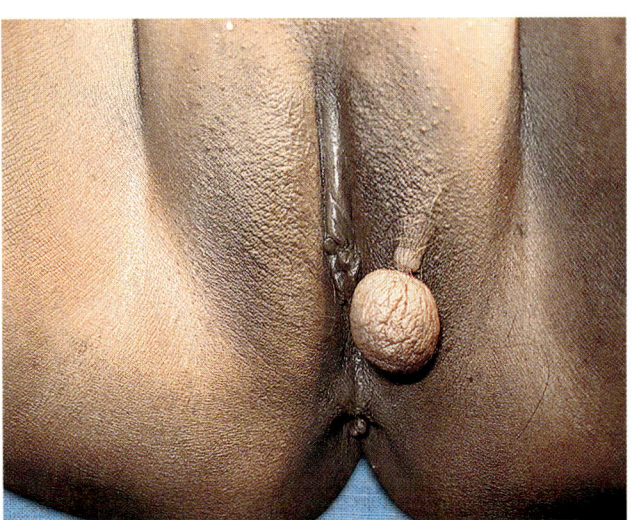

Fig. 41: Vulvar lipoma.

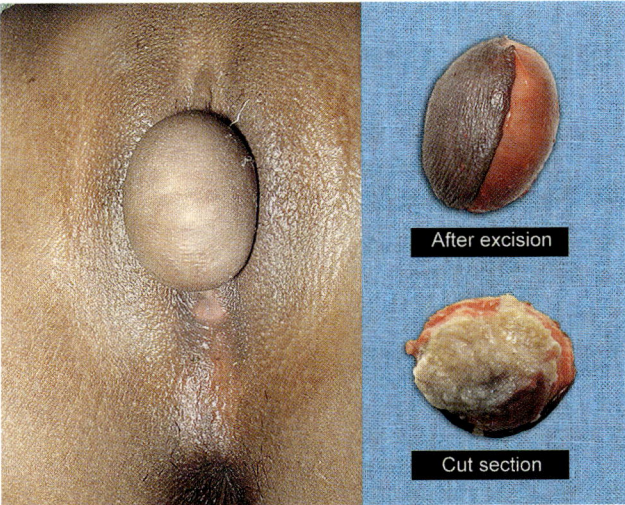

Fig. 42: Sebaceous cyst of vulva.

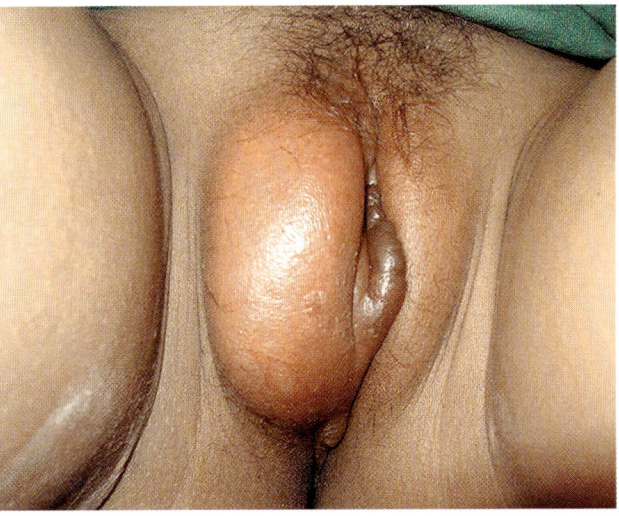

Fig. 43: Bartholin abscess.

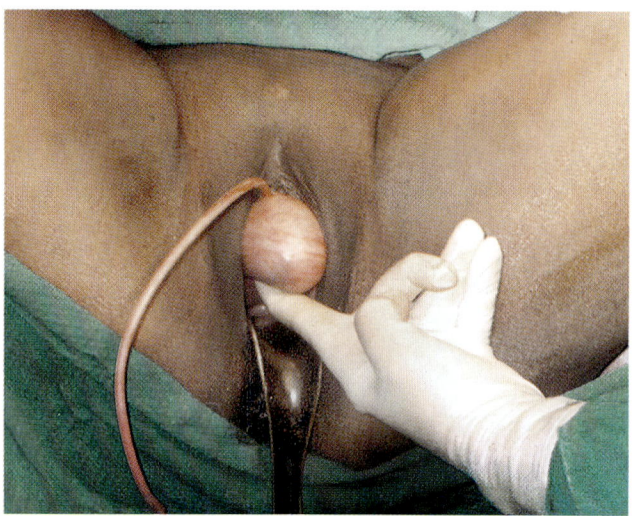

Fig. 44: Vaginal fibroma.

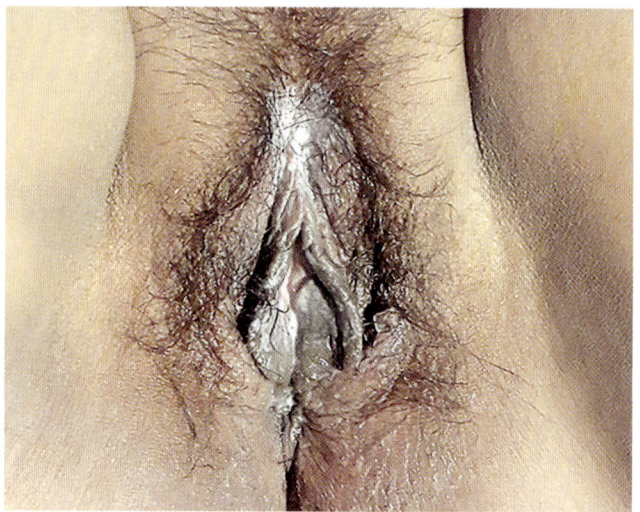

Fig. 45: Vulvar candidiasis.

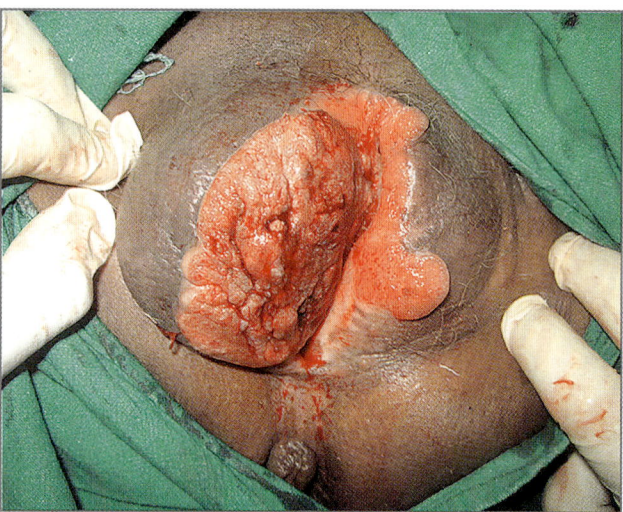

Fig. 46: Vulvar cancer.

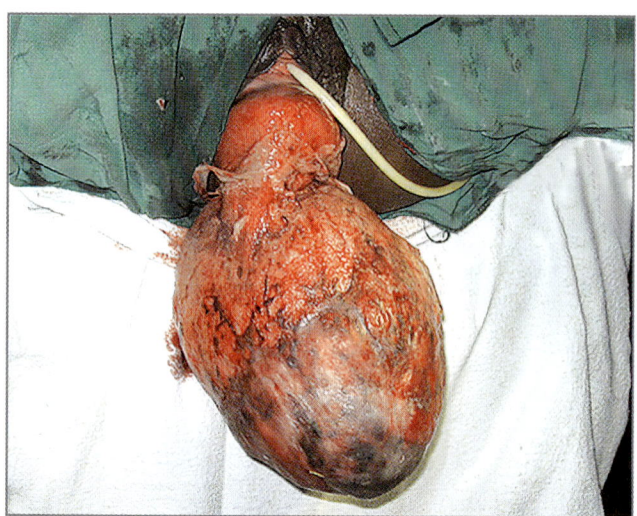

Fig. 47: Large cervical fibroid from portio vaginalis.

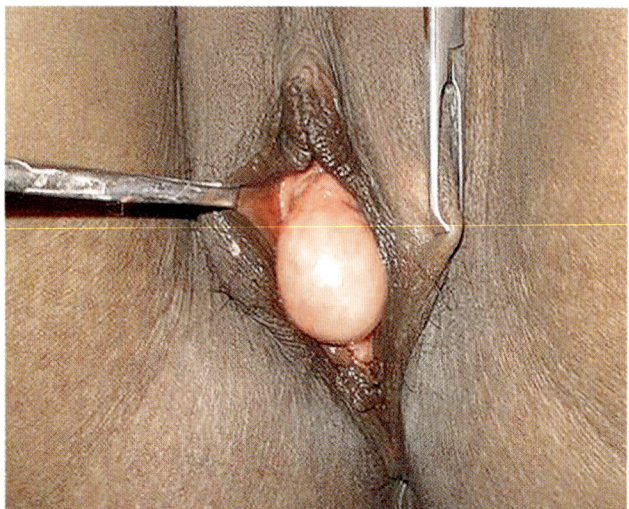

Fig. 48: Gartner duct cyst.

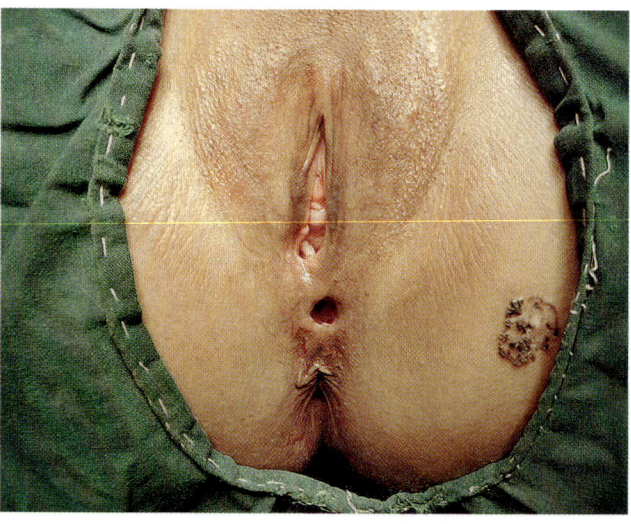

Fig. 49: Vagino-perineal fistula (tubercular).

CHAPTER 1: Writing a Gynecology Case

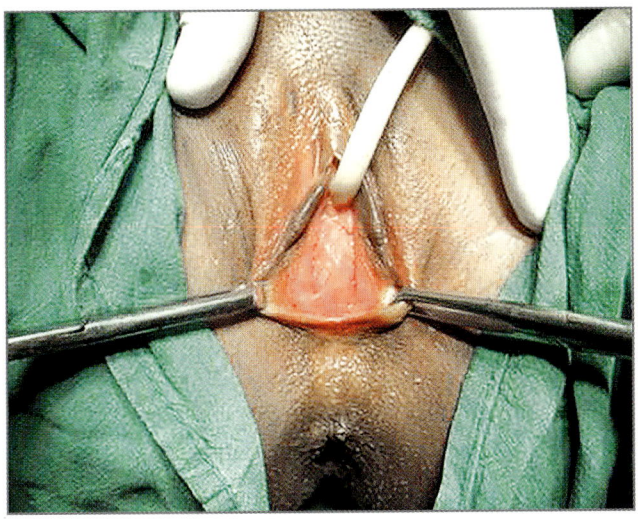

Fig. 50: Imperforate hymen.

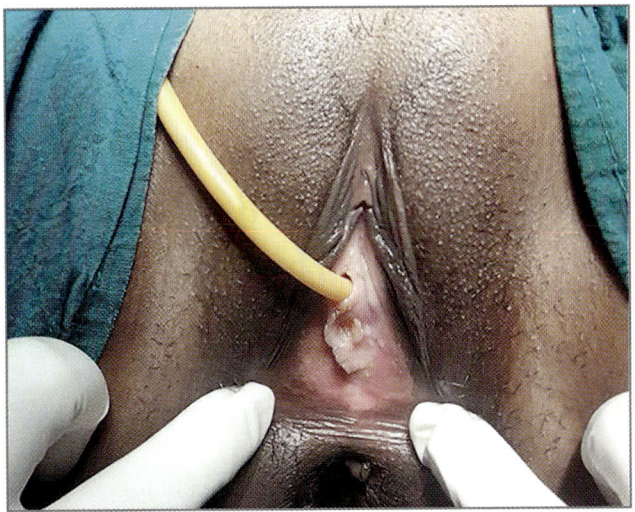

Fig. 51: Vaginal agenesis.

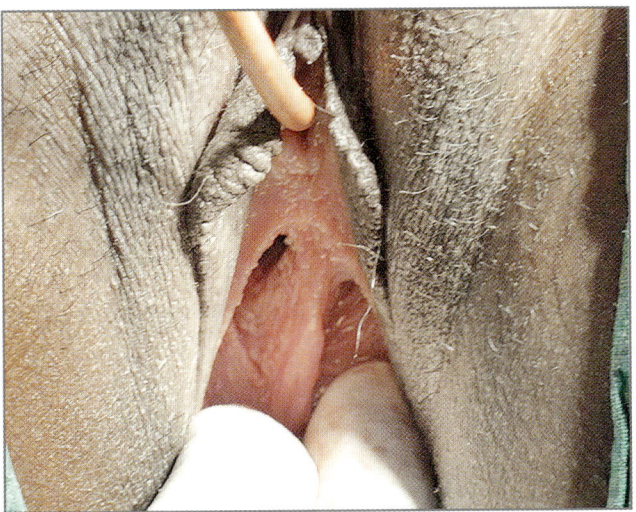

Fig. 52: Vaginal septum.

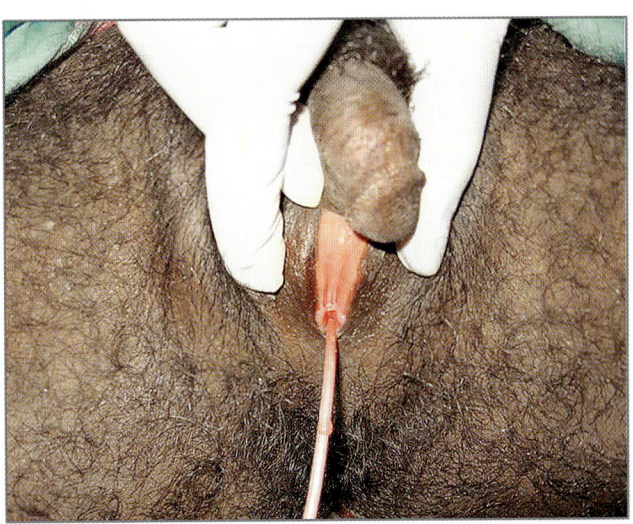

Fig. 53: External genitalia in congenital adrenal hyperplasia (CAH)—enlarged clitoris with fused labia.

of tenderness. Urethra and Bartholin gland are squeezed to express any discharge. Bartholin gland is situated in posterior third of introitus deep to bulbospongiosus on two lateral sides (**Figs. 54A and B**).

In genital prolapse cervix is dragged. Uterus is palpated to determine the degree of prolapse. Perineal body and levator ani are palpated to assess the tone (details in Chapter 10).

Speculum Examination

Speculum examination is usually done in dorsal position (lithotomy by some school) with a bivalve Cusco's speculum (**Fig. 55**) or single or double bladed Sims' speculum (**Fig. 56**) before bimanual examination.

How to Introduce Cusco's Speculum?

❖ After separating the labia with left thumb and index finger (**Figs. 57 to 61**) transverse blades of Cusco's speculum (lubricated by jelly) is introduced in anteroposterior direction (as vaginal introitus is anteroposterior slit depressed from side to side) and is then rotated 90° to bring the transverse blades transversely (upper part of vagina transversely enlarged).

❖ During introduction one should be cautious that speculum does not touch roughly the urethral meatus which is very sensitive.

❖ After opening the blades cervix is well visible (**Figs. 60 and 61**). If cervix is not visible speculum is angled 30° to

SECTION 1: Gynecological History Taking, Examination and Investigations

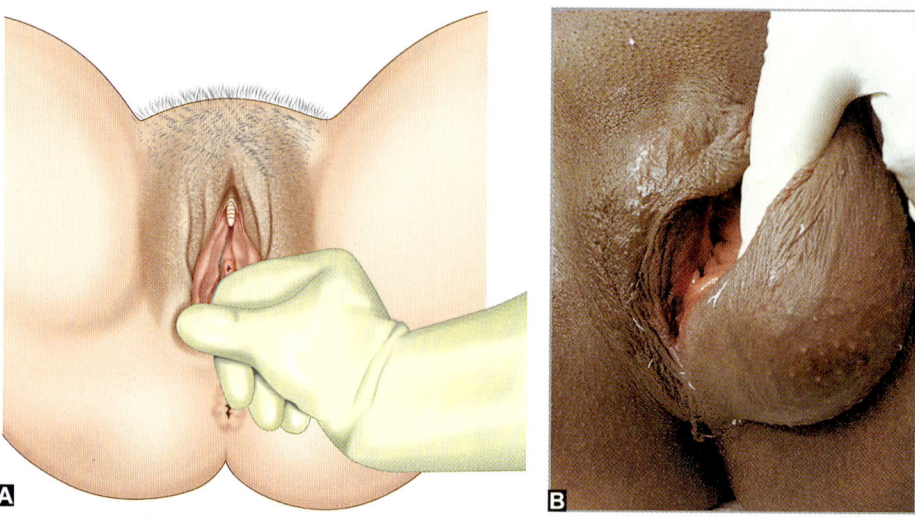

Figs. 54A and B: (A) Palpation of vulva; (B) Palpation of Bartholin cyst (left side).

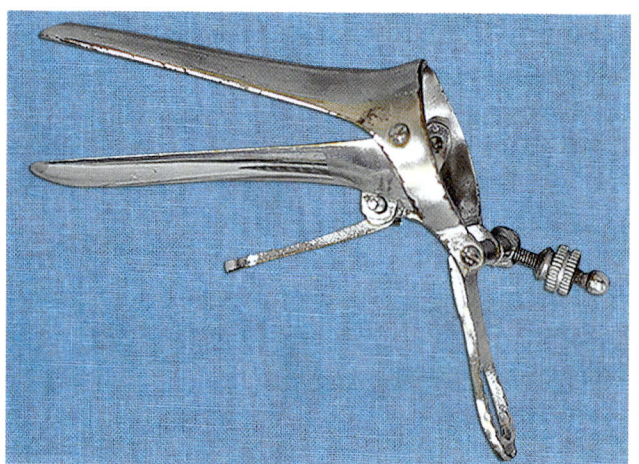

Fig. 55: Cusco's speculum.

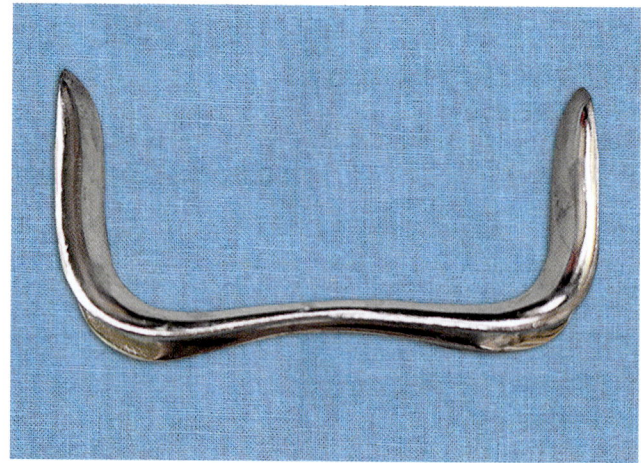

Fig. 56: Double-bladed Sims' speculum.

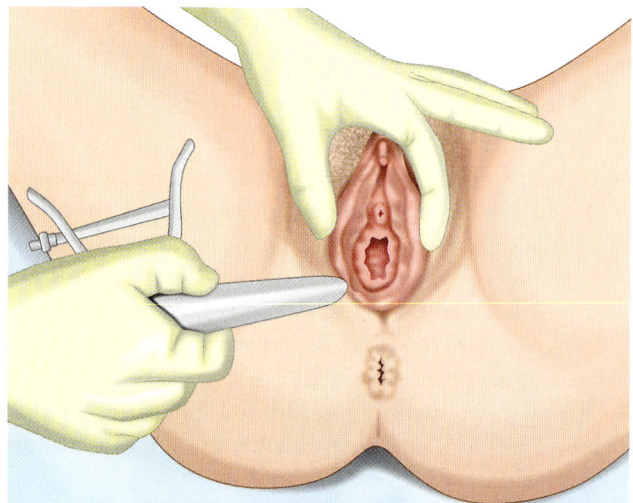

Fig. 57: Diagrammatic representation of introduction of Cusco's speculum.

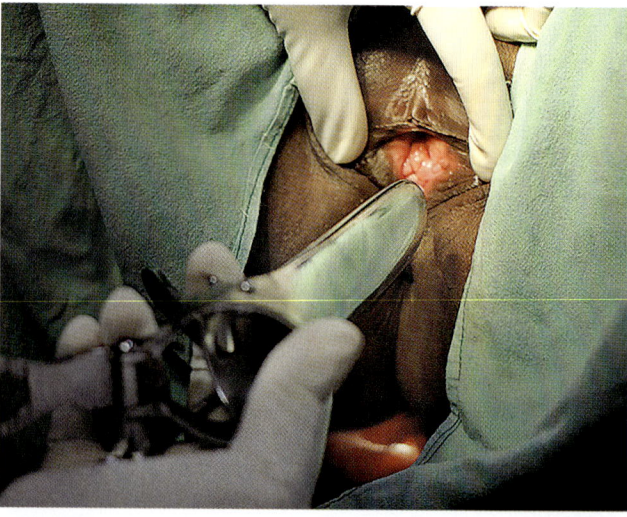

Fig. 58: Showing separation of labia with left thumb and index finger for introduction of Cusco's speculum—transverse blades of Cusco's speculum is introduced in anteroposterior direction and is then rotated 90° to bring the transverse blades transversely.

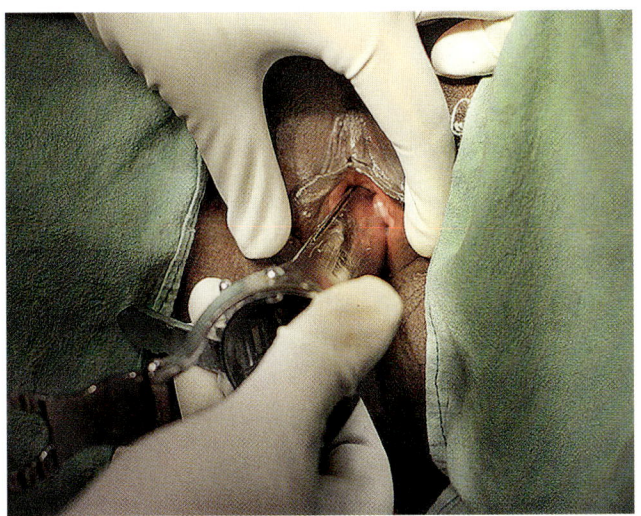

Fig. 59: Introduction of Cusco's speculum.

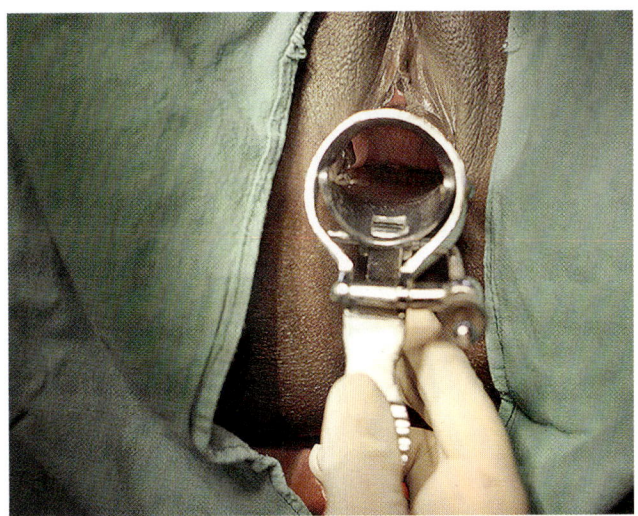

Fig. 60: Introduction of Cusco's speculum (handling posteriorly—commonly used).

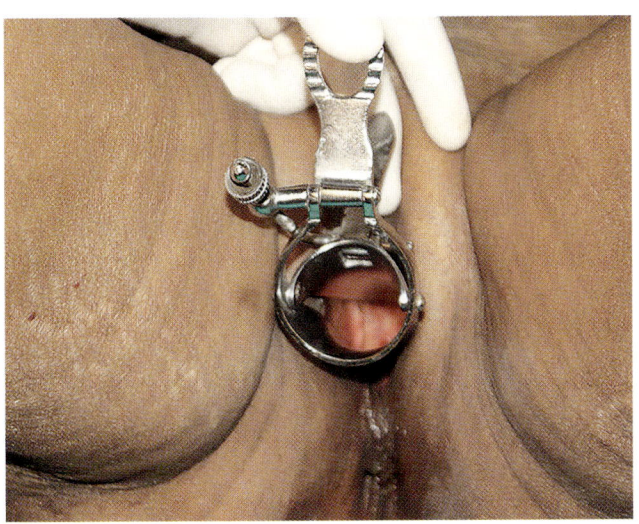

Fig. 61: Cusco's handling anteriorly (occasionally needed).

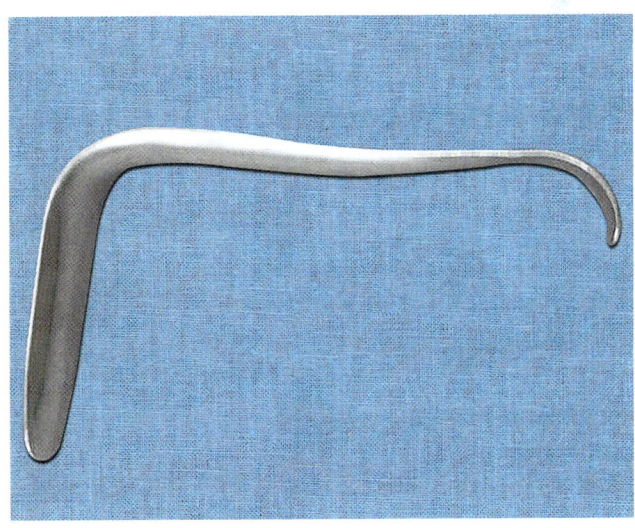

Fig. 62: Single bladed posterior vaginal speculum.

visualize cervix as in anteverted uterus (most common) cervix lies posteriorly.
- Lateral vaginal walls and cervix are visible well with Cusco's speculum. Both anterior and posterior vaginal walls are not visible as obscured by two blades.
- The handle of the Cusco's speculum can be kept anterior (Fig. 61) or posterior (Fig. 60) which will be convenient for proper visualization for cervix. The retaining screw can be tightened to allow the speculum self-retained without any support.

Insertion of Sims' Speculum

- To visualize the anterior vaginal wall Sims' speculum either double bladed (see Fig. 56) or single bladed (Fig. 62), is used, best in Sims' semiprone left lateral position (Fig. 63A) but can be done also in dorsal supine position (Fig. 63B) provided back of the patient is brought to the edge of table.
- Like Cusco's speculum Sims' speculum may also be needed to insert laterally first and then to rotate 90° posteriorly to retract the posterior vaginal wall.
- With this instrument anterior vaginal wall, lateral vaginal wall and cervix are visualized.
- If there is cystocele, it is retracted with anterior vaginal wall retractor (Fig. 64), to visualize the cervix and vault of the vagina (Figs. 64 and 65).
- In Sims' position, the lesion of anterior vaginal wall like VVF (Fig. 66) or cystocele is well visualized. After introduction of speculum the structures are seen and findings are noted.

SECTION 1: Gynecological History Taking, Examination and Investigations

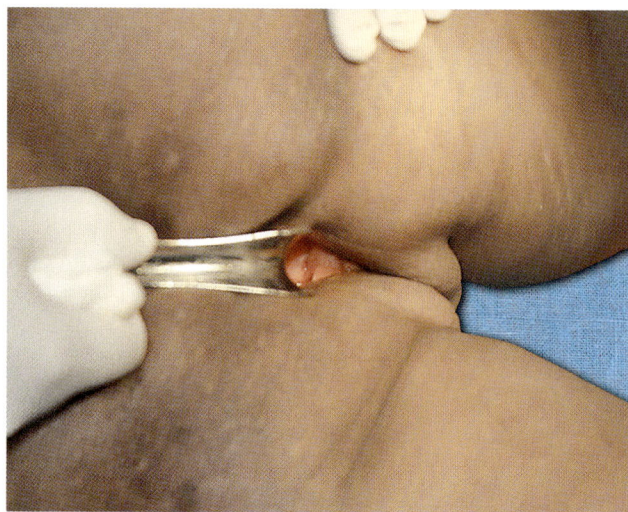

Fig. 63A: Introduction of Sims' speculum—Sims' position.

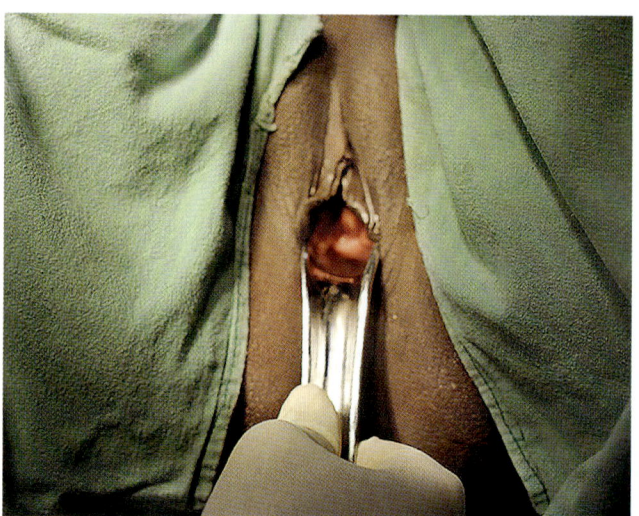

Fig. 63B: Introduction of Sims' speculum—dorsal supine position.

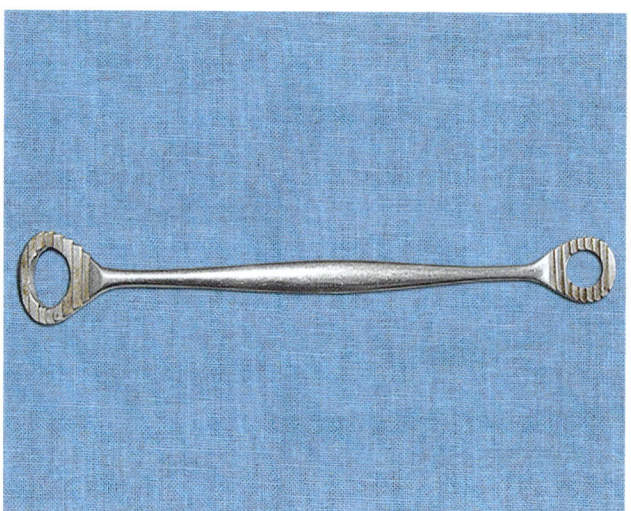

Fig. 64: Anterior vaginal wall retractor.

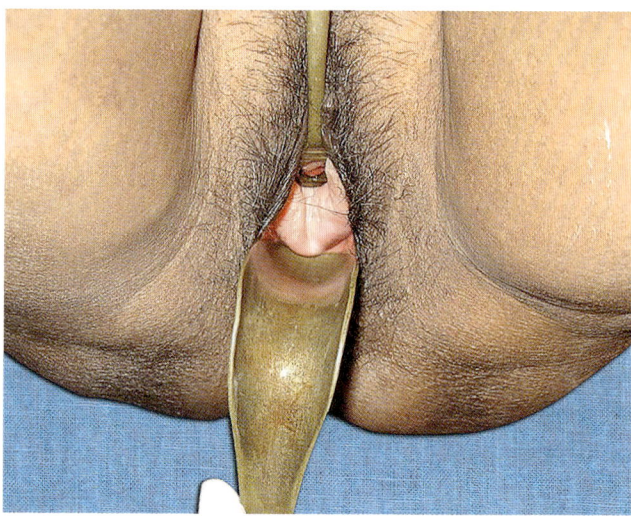

Fig. 65: To *see* the enterocele by retracting the posterior vaginal wall by Sims' speculum and retracting the anterior vaginal wall by anterior vaginal wall retractor.

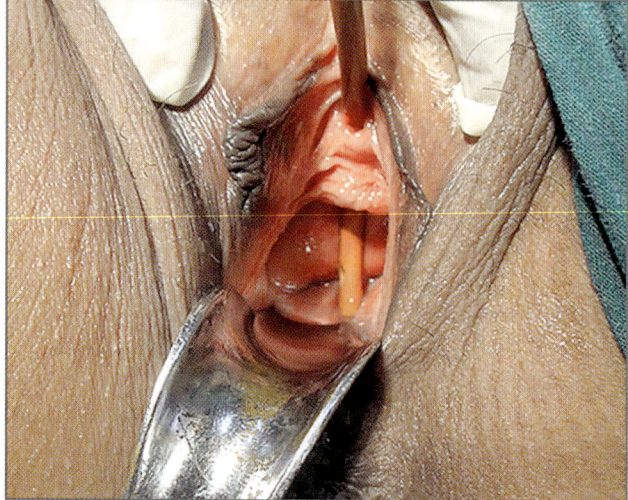

Fig. 66: Vesicovaginal fistula (VVF). Catheter is seen through the fistula opening.

Findings of Vagina on Inspection and Speculum Examination

What to see?	Findings of vagina
Vagina is noted for character of mucosa, its moistness, any abnormal discharge, any infection, any lesion or growth	❖ *Normal finding*—the mucosal color is pink, there is small mucous discharge. In reproductive age, vagina is rugosed ❖ In *postmenopausal period*, vaginal mucosa becomes atrophied, dry and there may be features of senile vaginitis ❖ In *candidiasis*, there is creamy white, thick curdy discharge. In *trichomoniasis* the discharge is fishy-odor, frothy, clear and sometimes yellowish green, whereas in *bacterial vaginosis* the discharge is clear, homogeneous whitish-gray and fishy smelling. ❖ Vaginal wall becomes keratinized, pigmented and even ulcerated in pelvic organ prolapse ❖ There may be nodules and/or papules in condyloma acuminata, chancre and in vaginal carcinoma. Reddish polypoid nodule is seen in vaginal adenosis and adenocarcinoma. Large growth in vaginal carcinoma may occasionally be visible (**Fig. 67**) ❖ Gartner's duct cyst is usually situated on anterolateral wall of vagina. Cystocele is situated on anterior vaginal wall and rectocele on posterior vaginal wall. Any congenital anomaly of vagina is also noted (*see* **Fig. 52**)

Cervical Findings on Speculum Examination

What to look for?	Findings of cervix
❖ Cervix is inspected for its color, any discharges, character of external os, tear, hypertrophy, cervicitis, erosion, ectropion, entropion, cervical polyp—mucus or fibroid, cyst, Nabothian cyst and growth	❖ *Normal findings:* Normal cervix is deep pink in color. External os is pinhole or round in nulliparous and it is transverse slit like in multiparous (**Fig. 68A**). The squamocolumnar junction is situated in between the pink squamous epithelium of ectocervix and bright—red columnar epithelium of the endocervix and situated near the external os at reproductive age. Preovulatory cervical mucus is clear, transparent, abundant and stretchable ❖ *Old tear of cervix* is usually sequel of vaginal delivery. Polyp may be mucous, fibroid or placental (rarely). Fibroid polyp (**Fig. 68B**) may originate from cervix or may arise from uterus and protrudes through external os. Hypertrophy is common in uterine prolapse. Cervix becomes wide and barrel shaped in endocervical cancer ❖ *Discharge*—like that of vagina (candida, trichomonas and bacteria vaginosis). There may be mucopurulent cervical discharge in STDs like gonorrhea and chlamydia. Strawberry appearance of cervix can be seen in trichomoniasis due to punctate hemorrhagic spots
❖ Cervix	❖ *Malignant growth:* The cervical carcinoma may be ulcerative, cauliflower or hypertrophic (**Fig. 69**) ❖ Tuberculous growth (rare) of cervix may mimic cancer cervix (*see* **Fig. 7**, Chapter 33).

Cervical smear is taken for PAP smear from the surface of cervix by Ayer's spatula and from the cervical canal by cytobrush. If there is any discharge that should be collected for microscopical examination. PAP smear should be taken before vaginal examination.

Bimanual Examination (Pelvic Examination or Bimanual Examination)—Procedure

❖ Index and middle fingers of gloved right hand is introduced gently through the vagina after retracting the labia minora

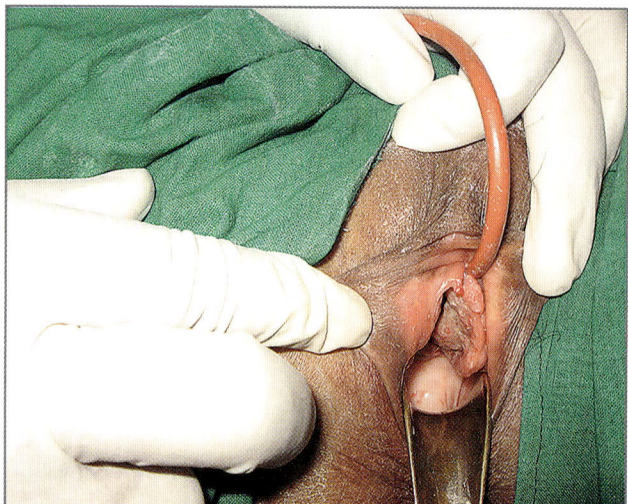

Fig. 67: Vaginal cancer.

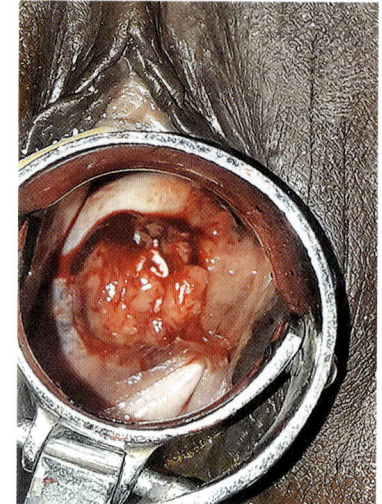

Fig. 69: Cancer cervix—endocervical adenocarcinoma.

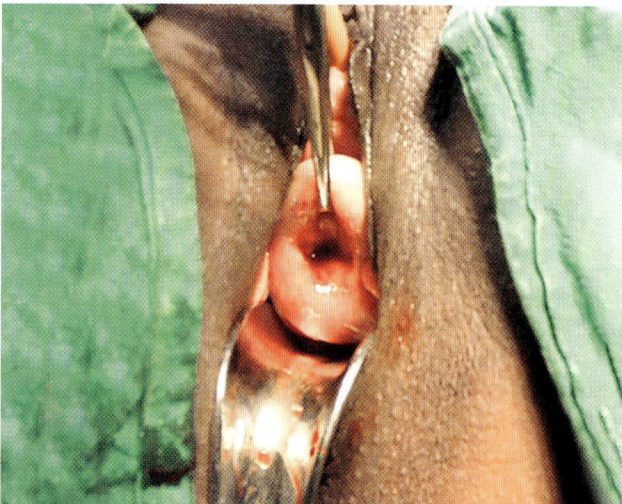

Fig. 68A: Normal looking cervix.

with left thumb and index finger after using any lubricating jelly until the cervix is palpable **(Figs. 70 to 75)**.

❖ In *anteverted uterus* (which occurs in most of the cases) cervix is directed posteriorly and so anterior lip is touched first **(Fig. 76)**.

❖ When the uterus in *midposition* touching of both lips of cervix together are likely **(Fig. 77)**.

❖ In *retroverted uterus* (15%) cervix is directed anteriorly, so posterior lip is palpated first **(Fig. 78)**.

❖ Cervix is palpated first. Then the other hand is placed over the patient's abdomen over the suprapubic region to do the bimanual examination to palpate the uterus and the fornices (two lateral, anterior and posterior) to note the findings.

❖ The different positions of uterus are anteverted (most common), midposition and retroverted (15%) and is shown in **Figure 79**.

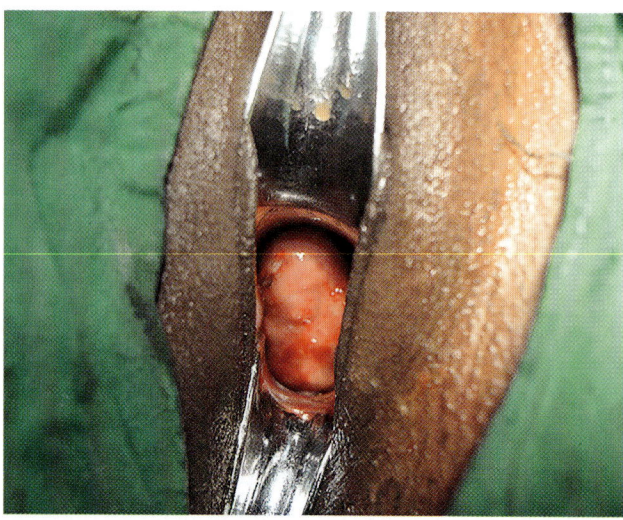

Fig. 68B: Fibroid polyp.

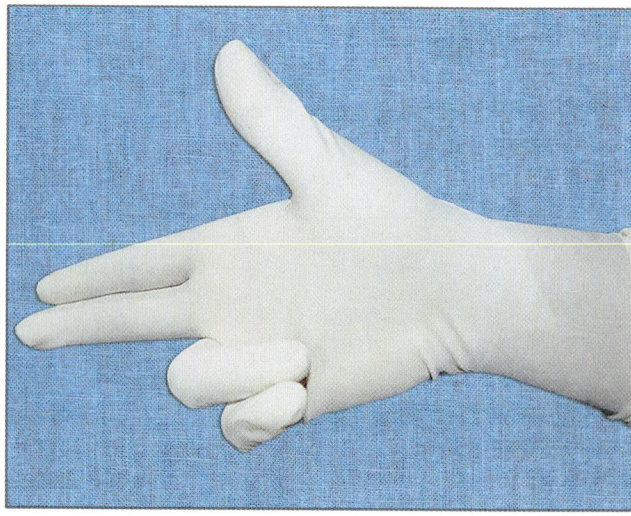

Fig. 70: Examining fingers.

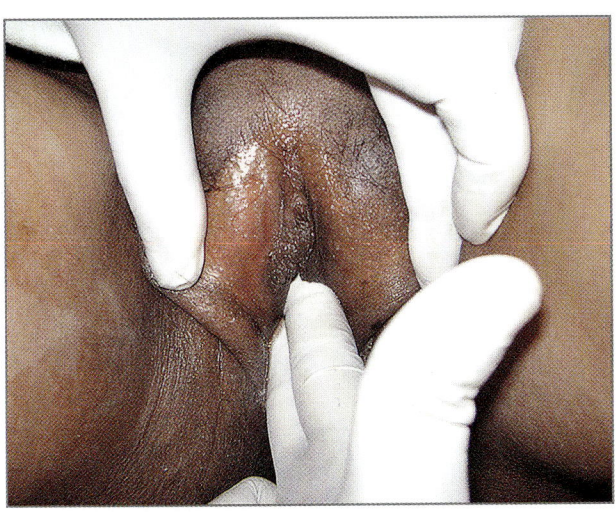

Fig. 71: Per vaginal examination—index and middle fingers are introduced by retracting the labia.

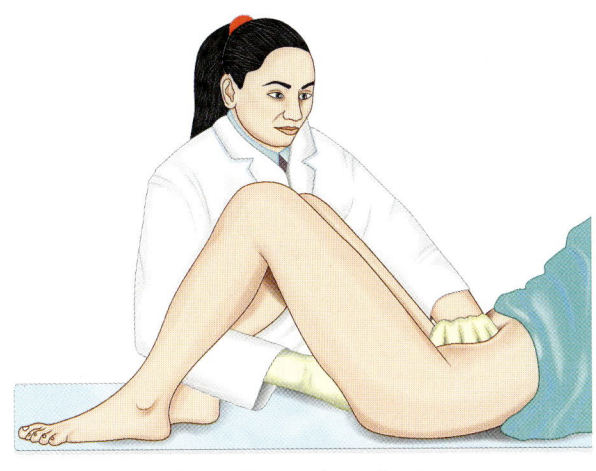

Fig. 74: Bimanual examination.

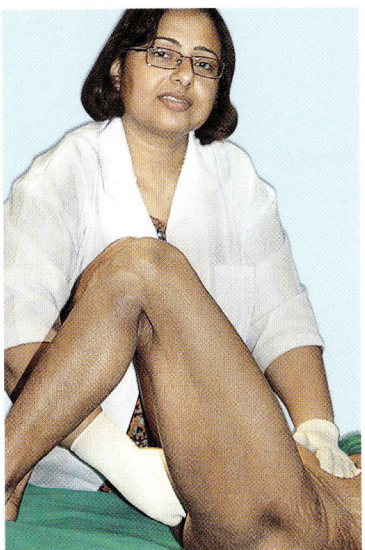

Fig. 72: Bimanual examination—left hand over the suprapubic region.

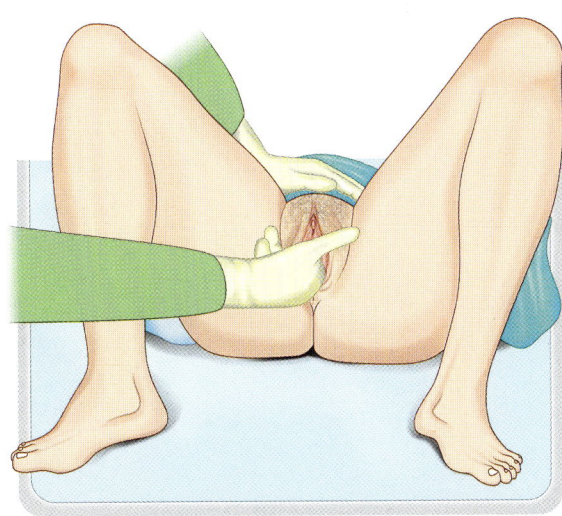

Fig. 75: Bimanual examination. Left hand over suprapubic region (diagrammatic).

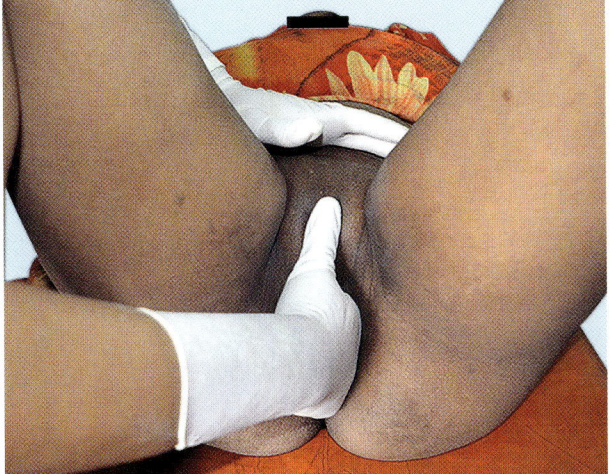

Fig. 73: Bimanual examination—left hand over the suprapubic region.

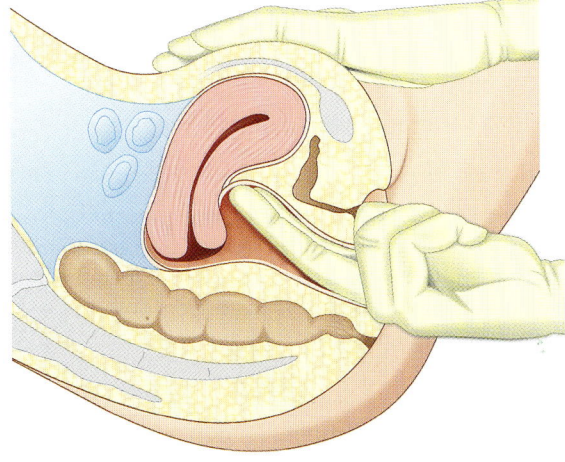

Fig. 76: Bimanual examination in anteverted uterus (anterior lip of cervix is felt first).

SECTION 1: Gynecological History Taking, Examination and Investigations

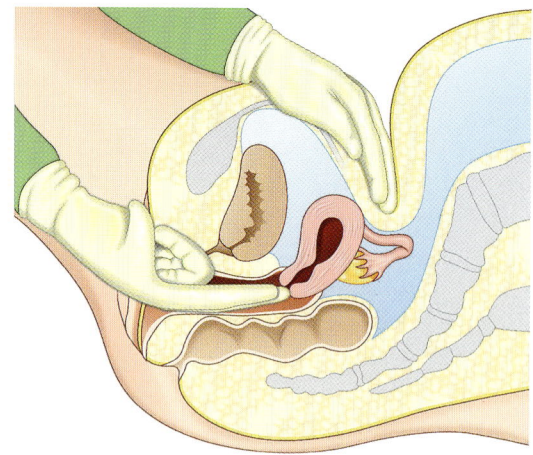

Fig. 77: Bimanual examination—uterus in mid-position (both lips of cervix is felt together).

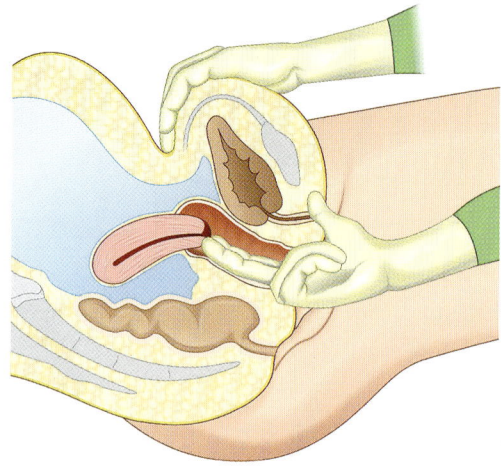

Fig. 78: Bimanual examination—in retroverted uterus (posterior lip of cervix felt first).

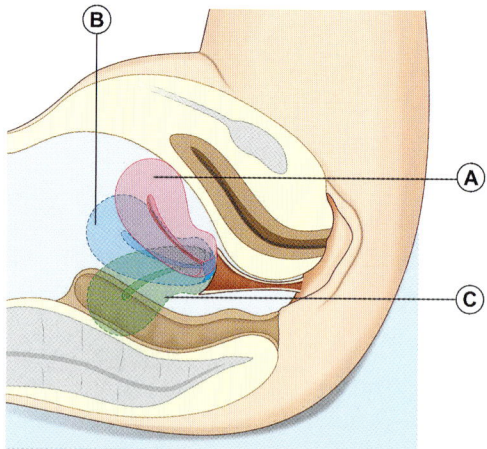

Fig. 79: Different positions of uterus (A— anteverted, B—mid-position, and C—retroverted).

Bimanual Examination and What to See

Palpation of cervix	Findings
Cervix is palpated to note size, consistency, mobility, and to diagnose any pathology, whether there is any bleeding on touch and cervix is moved to note any tenderness	Bleeding on touch may signify malignancy. Tenderness on movement is found in: ❖ Ectopic pregnancy and ❖ Acute pelvic inflammatory disease

Bimanual Examination and What to See

Palpation of uterus	Findings
The other hand is placed over the patient's abdomen over the suprapubic region and tried to reach behind the uterus and uterus is palpated in between the two hands keeping fingers both in anterior fornix and posterior fornix to note: ❖ Position ❖ Consistency ❖ Size ❖ Mobility ❖ Shape ❖ Any tenderness	Normal uterus is firm in consistency and size is 7.5 cm × 5 cm × 2.5 cm, anteverted, and anteflexed with good mobility. Uterus is uniformly enlarged in: ❖ Pregnancy ❖ Fibroid ❖ Hematometra ❖ Adenomyosis ❖ Pyometra ❖ Endometrial polyp ❖ Endometrial carcinoma. Uterus is irregularly enlarged in fibroid uterus. Mobility of uterus is restricted in: ❖ PID ❖ Endometriosis ❖ Malignancy

Bimanual Examination and What to See

Mass in pelvis	Findings
Palpated bimanually—internal fingers are directed to the fornices toward the abdominal fingers to palpate any mass in between If there is a mass it is uterine origin or adnexal origin—How will you understand?	Uterine mass usually lies in midline whereas adnexal mass on any lateral fornix. If any mass is palpated, first it is assessed whether it is separated from the uterus or not. ❖ If there is a cleft in between the uterus and the mass it is most likely adnexal mass (commonly ovarian tumor) **(Figs. 80A and B)**. And in uterine fibroid there is no such cleft **(Figs. 81A and B)**.

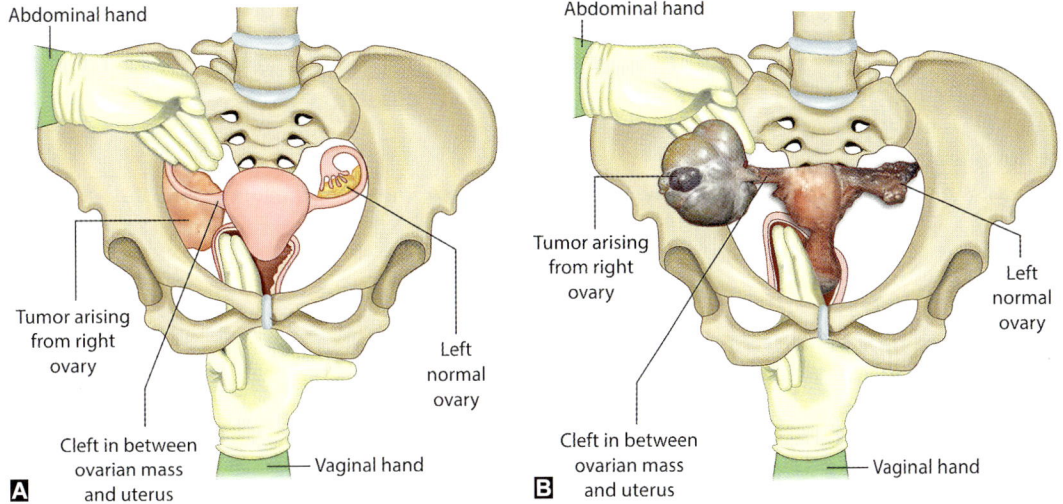

Figs. 80A and B: Cleft (groove) in between the uterus and the mass indicate mass is adnexal origin commonly ovarian tumor.

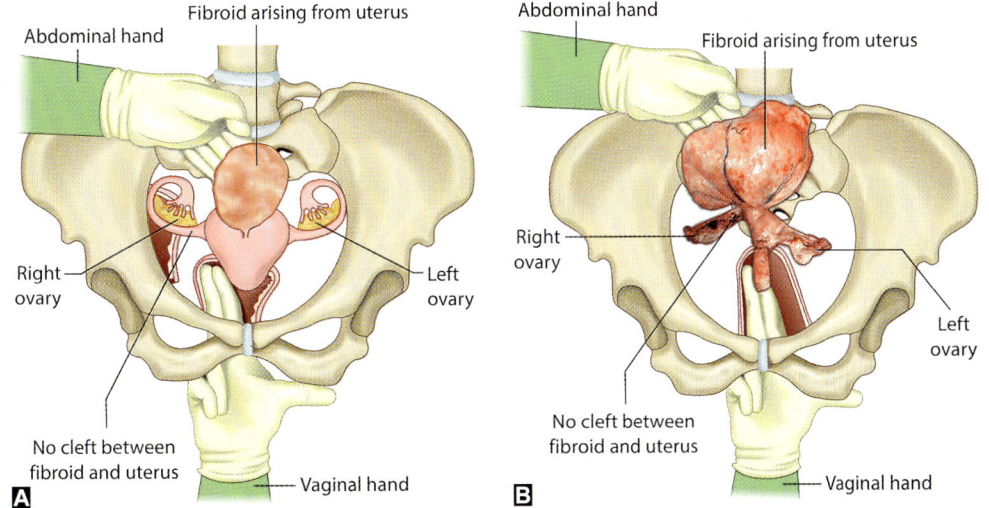

Figs. 81A and B: There is no cleft (groove) between the mass and the uterus which is not separately palpable indicating mass originating from uterus, likely to be fibroid.

Bimanual Examination and What to See

	Findings
Relation of movement of cervix with the uterus and vice-versa	❖ On movement of the cervix upward if the mass also moves, the origin of mass is uterus and in that case if uterus is pushed down cervix also moves down.

SECTION 1: Gynecological History Taking, Examination and Investigations

Lateral fornix: Palpation Normally fallopian tubes and ovaries are not easily palpable. Normal ovaries can be palpable in very slim patient and if palpable a characteristic painful sensation of ovary occurs	Adnexal swelling in lateral fornix may be: ❖ Ovarian tumor ❖ Tubo-ovarian mass ❖ Chocolate cyst of ovary ❖ Broad ligament tumor ❖ Paraovarian or fimbrial cyst ❖ Ectopic pregnancy
Posterior fornix is palpated for any, nodule, mass, tenderness or any collection. Causes of mass or nodule in posterior fornix (in pouch of Douglas)—may be due to: ❖ Retroverted uterus ❖ Prolapsed ovary ❖ Posterior lower uterine fibroid ❖ Tubo-ovarian (TO) mass ❖ Mass of rectovaginal wall.	The typical nodular structure in POD may be: ❖ Metastatic nodule of ovarian cancer ❖ Endometriosis ❖ Tuberculosis ❖ Scybella (hard stool) Fluctuating mass in posterior fornix—may be due to collection of blood or pus
Anterior fornix: What are the masses you may get on anterior fornix?	The masses in anterior fornix are due to: ❖ Ovarian cyst (commonly dermoid) ❖ Fibroid uterus ❖ Chronic ectopic ❖ Broad ligament fibroid ❖ Mass related to urinary bladder

Rectal Examination and Rectovaginal Examination

Procedures	Findings
Rectovaginal area (gynecological perineum)—inspection and palpation It is a wedge-shaped area extending from fourchette to anus. Average normal length is 4 cm (*see* **Figs. 36 and 37**).	Length is reduced in perineal tear and to some extent in posterior vaginal wall prolapse. In complete perineal tear gynecological perineum is almost absent and replaced by a horizontal bridge of rectovaginal septum and incontinence of stool (*see* **Fig. 2**).

Rectal Examination (Rectoabdominal)

Procedures	Findings
Done by gloved index finger lubricated with jelly (**Fig. 82**). Gynecological indications of rectal examination are: ❖ Cancer cervix ❖ Posterior vaginal wall prolapse ❖ Endometriosis ❖ Ovarian malignancy ❖ Adolescent girl ❖ Primary amenorrhea (vaginal agenesis) ❖ Stenosed vagina	Findings Carcinoma cervix In carcinoma cervix: (a) involvement of parametrium and lateral pelvic wall is felt better, (b) shape of cervix can be assessed, and (c) involvement of rectal mucosa can be diagnosed Genital prolapse: To differentiate between rectocele and enterocele Pelvic endometriosis: Involvement of uterosacral ligament and POD (nodular) Ovarian malignancy: Metastatic nodule in POD In young virgins: In absence of ultrasonography.
Rectal examination has become less important nowadays due to the availability of ultrasound	In *vaginal agenesis* rectal examination helps to identify the presence of uterus In *stenosed vagina* pelvic examination is done by rectoabdominal method.

Rectovaginal Examination

It is done by keeping index finger in vagina and middle finger in rectum (**Fig. 83**) Rectovaginal examination is done to palpate rectovaginal septum, POD, posterior surface of uterus, fornices and uterosacral ligaments	It can differentiate the enterocele and rectocele (*see* Chapter 10, Page 222) and any lesion in rectovaginal septum like endometriosis or growth can also be diagnosed. Piles, rectal polyp and cancer can be detected. Tone of perineal body can be assessed.

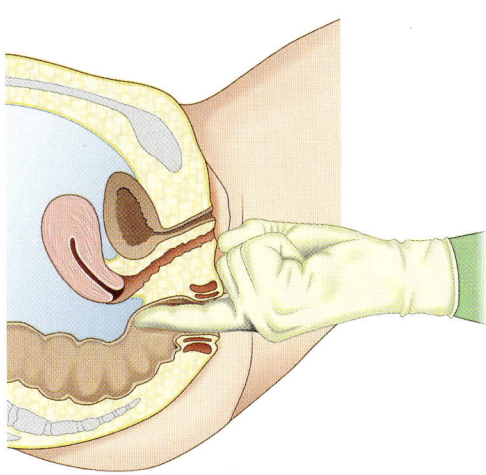

Fig. 82: Rectal examination.

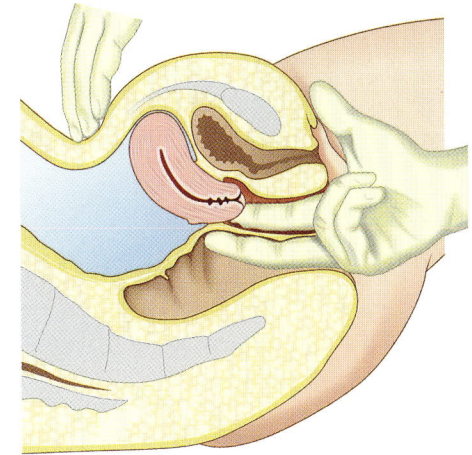

Fig. 83: Rectovaginal examination.

INVESTIGATIONS SUPPLIED OR REQUIRED

Investigations are done for two purposes:
1. Firstly for confirmation of diagnosis and to assess the extent of disease and
2. Others for preoperative investigations for patient's surgical fitness.
3. Routine screening

These are:
- *Routine preoperative investigations:* Routine blood examination—Hb%, TC, DC, and ESR, blood sugar (fasting and postprandial), renal function test (urea and creatinine), urine—routine examination and culture, liver function test, serology (hepatitis B and C, HIV) X-ray chest, ECG.
- *Investigations in gynecology which are done for the confirmation of diagnosis* and/or to assess the extent of disease as suggested by clinical diagnosis are given in Chapter 2 (*see* Page 34).
- *Papanicolaou test (PAP test)* is done routinely in gynecological cases. *STD (sexually transmitted disease) screening* is one essential part in gynaecology (described in Page 36, Chapter 2 and Page 608, Chapter 33).

SUMMARY OF THE CASE

Summary will contain the following points:
- Patient's profile and complaints
- Significant or relevant history—positive and negative
- Important physical examination findings including vital signs (always write vital signs even if they may be normal)
- Gynecological examination findings
- Investigations supplied or required.

EXAMPLE OF WRITING A SUMMARY (SAMPLE SUMMARY)

Mrs XY aged 35 years parity three, living issue 3, tubectomy done 4 years back was admitted on—with complain of lump abdomen progressively increasing for last 3 months duration. Her LMP was—period is regular, almost monthly interval and duration of 4–6 days. She has no pain abdomen or any other significant symptom. There is no significant past and family history.

On general examination, her height is 5 feet, weight 54 kg, GC—average, Pallor—mild, edema— nil, neck glands not enlarged, Pulse/min, BP mm of Hg (or may write normotensive) and any other positive findings. Breasts examination revealed no abnormality.

On abdominal examination, there is a lump lower abdomen almost globular, corresponding to 24 weeks pregnancy size, surface smooth, well-defined margin, nontender and mobile. Shifting dullness is negative and there is no fluid thrill, no Braxton Hicks contraction, no fetal parts palpable and fetal heart sound not audible.

On pelvic examination revealed a large pelviabdominal mass separated from the uterus which is of normal size and retroverted.

In investigating report her hemoglobin level is 11 g%, blood group—A positive, CA 125-21 U/mL, USG is suggestive of ovarian cyst of 20 cm × 15 cm size with uterus of normal size without any ascites.

PROVISIONAL DIAGNOSIS

A case of ovarian tumor probably benign in nature in a 35-year multiparous woman.

DIFFERENTIAL DIAGNOSIS

Write the differential diagnosis like in case of lower abdominal lump—it will be uterine fibromyoma, mesenteric cyst, full bladder and pregnancy, etc. (*see* Chapter 3, Page 45).

CHAPTER 2

Investigative Procedures in Gynecology and Imaging in Gynecology

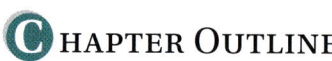

Chapter Outline

Investigations done in gynecology for diagnosis of the disease and for assessment of their extent

- Pap Test
- Vaginal Discharge Evaluation
- Pipelle Biopsy—Procedure, Advantages and Disadvantages

Imaging in Gynecology:
- Role of Ultrasonography
- Saline Infusion Sonography, Transvaginal Sonography and Three-Dimensional Sonography
- Role of CT Scan
- Role of Magnetic Resonance Imaging, Positron Emission Tomography
- Role of X-ray

INVESTIGATIONS

Q. What are the investigations done in gynecology for diagnosis of the disease and for assessment of their extent?

- The list of the investigative procedures is enumerated below.
- The relevant investigations are discussed in the respective chapters.
- This chapter deals here some of the common subjects and some procedures are highlighted.

Investigations in gynecology which are done for the confirmation of diagnosis and/or to assess the extent of disease as suggested by clinical diagnosis.

These are:
- Ultrasonography, CT scan, MRI, PET scan for assessment of pelvic organs and mass
- Hormones (TSH, prolactin, gonadotropins, sex steroids) in amenorrhea, hirsutism and infertility cases
- Tumor markers
- High vaginal swab in pelvic and vaginal infection
- Vaginal discharge examination—hanging drop preparation for *Trichomonas vaginalis* shows motile protozoal organism with typical flagella (cone-shaped flagellated organism in the center, with a terminal spike and four flagella), *Candida albicans* can be diagnosed by wet film examination or Gram stain showing speckled gram-positive spores. Clue cell detection for bacterial vaginosis and gram-negative diplococci (gonorrhea) in Gram staining.
- Biopsy in vulva, vagina and cervix in obvious or suspected growth
- Pipelle biopsy for endometrial lesion:
  - Hysterosalpingography (HSG)/sonohysterosalpingography for tubal patency
  - Hysteroscopy in intrauterine pathology
  - Laparoscopy—diagnosis of pelvic pathology and intervention
  - Colposcopy—assessment of premalignant changes in cervix.

Of these investigations, the procedures which are done during the gynecological examinations are:

1. Pap smear

2. Collection and study of vaginal discharge and
3. Endometrial sampling.

Papanicolaou Testing (Pap Test) (Figs. 1 to 3)

Afrer George Nicholas Papanicolaou (1883–1962)

Pap smear is now a routine gynecological procedure done with the gynecological examination. Three types of device are used for cervical cytology *cytobrush* (**Fig. 1**), *spatula* (**Fig. 2**), and *broom* (**Fig. 3**).

The details including colposcopy are described in the Chapter 8 (Carcinoma Cervix, Page 175).

Vaginal Discharge Evaluation—Approach to a Case of Vaginal Discharge

On gynecological examination, discharges are commonly found from the vagina and also from cervix and may be associated with vulvovaginitis.

Q. What do you mean by leukorrhea?

The term *leukorrhea* is a symptom of pouring out of white discharge per vagina.

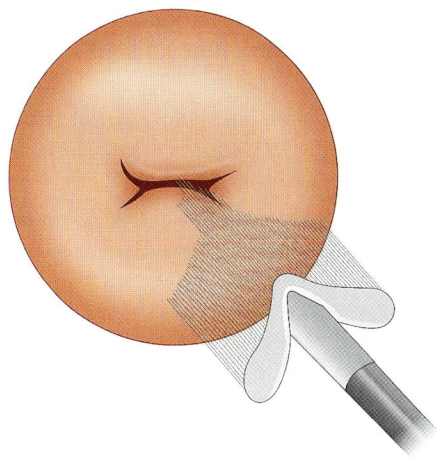

Fig. 3: Cervical cytology by plastic broom.

Causes of Leukorrhea

Physiological

There may be normal vaginal discharge, physiological increase of discharge from the cervix immediately before ovulation and early pregnancy due to effect of estrogen.

Pathological

- It varies according the phase of woman's life.
- White discharge frequently may be of infective in origin.
- *In children,* vulvovaginitis, foreign body, and worm infestation are common etiological factors, poor general health is a causative factor in young girl.
- *In married woman,* infective and sexually transmitted diseases (STDs) are important. In parous woman, chronic cervicitis and cervical erosion are the important causative factors. Combined oral pill and intrauterine contraceptive device (IUCD) may increase white discharge per vagina.
- *In perimenopausal woman,* uterine polyp, endometrial cancer, and early cancer cervix may present with white discharge.
- *In postmenopausal woman,* with white discharge senile vaginitis, genital cancer, decubitus ulcer, and retained pessary are to be enquired.

Infective cause is common in reproductive age group

- The most common is *candidiasis* caused by *Candida albicans*, a fungus. In candidiasis, it is creamy white, thick curdy discharge associated with marked vulvar itching and soreness.
- *In trichomoniasis* (caused by protozoa *Trichomonas vaginalis*), the discharge is fishy-odor, frothy, clean, sometimes yellowish-green and associated with vulvar soreness and itching. The vagina looks strawberry appearance due to hemorrhagic punctum.
- *In bacterial vaginosis* (caused by *Gardnerella vaginalis*), the discharge is clear, homogenous, whitish-gray and fishy smelling. There may be mucopurulent cervical discharge in gonorrhea and chlamydia, both are STD and may have history of contact bleeding.

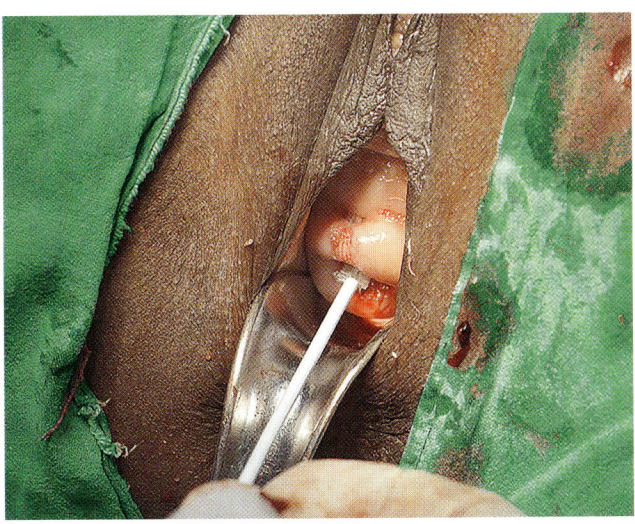

Fig. 1: Pap smear from endocervical canal by cytobrush.

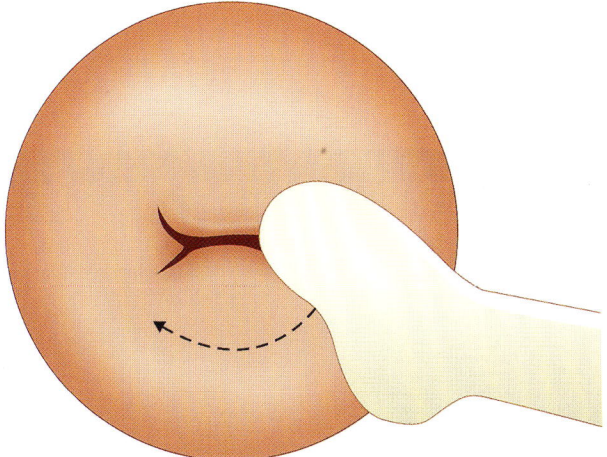

Fig. 2: Cervical cytology by Ayre's spatula.

- Normal vaginal discharge contains exfoliated vaginal epithelial cells and Doderlein's bacilli, large rod-like lactobacilli.

For final diagnosis, *wet film preparation, mixing with potassium hydroxide (KOH) solution, Gram stain*, and *culture* in respective culture media are needed.

Diagnosis of trichomoniasis—*hanging drop preparation*:

For hanging drop preparation, the discharge is collected from the posterior fornix by speculum and one drop is taken on glass slide and mixed with a drop of saline and covered with cover glass and examined under microscope.

In *trichomoniasis*, motile protozoal organism with *typical flagella* (cone-shaped flagellated organism in the center, with a terminal spike) and four flagella is detected **(Fig. 4)**.

Feinberg-Whittington or Diamond's media is used for culture of *Trichomonas vaginalis*.

Diagnosis of candidiasis—*adding with 10% KOH*:

In another small container, vaginal discharge is collected and equal amount of 10% KOH solution is added. One drop of mixture is taken and examined under microscope under cover slip. *Typical hyphae* and *budding spores* (yeast-like organism) are seen in *candidiasis*. Candida is also diagnosed by Gram staining showing speckled Gram-positive spores.

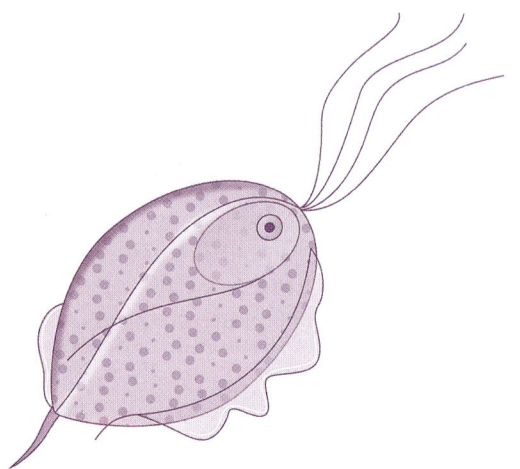

Fig. 4: Trichomona with four flagella.

For culture of *Candida albicans* culture Nickerson-Sabouraud media is used.

Diagnosis of bacterial vaginosis—*wet film preparation*:

Clue cells are detected in wet film of vaginal discharge under microscope in case of bacterial vaginosis. Clue cells are epithelial cells covered with bacteria showing characteristic stippled appearance. A fishy smell after mixing the discharge with KOH indicates bacterial vaginosis.

Amsel criteria for diagnosing bacterial vaginosis—any three of four:

1. Presence of clue cells on microscopy
2. Creamy grayish white discharge
3. Vaginal pH more than 4.5
4. Characteristic fishy odor on addition of alkali.

Diagnosis of gonorrhea—*Gram staining of discharge*:

Gonorrhea, caused by Gram-negative diplococcus, *Neisseria gonorrhoeae* may be asymptomatic or may present with increase vaginal discharge, pelvic pain, dysuria, and endocervical and urethral mucopurulent discharge.

Gonococcal infection is diagnosed with Gram staining of discharge collected from cervix, Bartholin's gland, and urethra by detecting *Gram-negative intracellular diplococci*. It is cultured in agar medium containing antibiotic to reduce growth of other organism, which is commonly associated with gonorrhea. It is also diagnosed by nucleic acid amplification test (NAAT).

Diagnosis of gonorrhea—*nucleic acid amplification technique from a vulvar swab or a first void urine*:

Chlamydial infections, one of most common STDs, caused by *Chlamydia trachomatis*, an obligate intracellular bacterium may be asymptomatic or there may be contact bleeding, intermenstrual bleeding, and mucopurulent discharge from cervix or urethra with dysuria.

It is *diagnosed by NAAT* from a vulvar swab or a first void urine sample. The intracellular organism is seen under microscope. Diagnosis is confirmed by staining by an immunofluorescence technique. It contains both deoxyribonucleic acid (DNA) and ribonucleic acid (RNA). It multiplies like bacteria, but only inside cell as viruses. Culture is very expensive.

*Diagnosis of causative organisms of vaginal discharge is summarized in **Table 1**.*

Table 1: Summary of diagnosis of causative organisms of vaginal discharge.					
	Candidiasis	Trichomoniasis	Bacterial vaginosis	Gonorrhea	Chlamydia
Causative organism	Candida albicans, a fungus	Trichomonas vaginalis, which is protozoa	Bacteria Gardnerella vaginalis	Gram negative intracellular diplococcus Neisseria gonorrhoeae	Chlamydia trachomatis, an obligate intracellular bacterium
Wet prep		Motile protozoal organism with typical flagella	Clue cells	—	—

Contd...

Contd...

	Candidiasis	Trichomoniasis	Bacterial vaginosis	Gonorrhea	Chlamydia
Mixing with KOH solution	Typical hyphae and budding spores (yeast like organism)	—	Characteristic fishy smell	—	—
Gram stain	Speckled Gram-positive spores			Gram-negative intracellular diplococci	
Culture	Nickerson–Sabouraud medium	Feinberg–Whittington or Diamond's media		Agar medium containing antibiotic to reduce growth of other organism and also diagnosed by nucleic acid amplification test (NAAT)	Culture is very expensive. It is diagnosed by nucleic acid amplification technique or Aptima Combo 2 and BD Probetec. The intracellular organism is seen under microscope. Diagnosis is confirmed by staining by an immunofluorescence technique.

Abbreviation: KOH, potassium hydroxide

Sexually Transmitted Infections and their Causative Organisms

Pelvic inflammatory (PID), sexually transmitted infections (STIs) and female genital tuberculosis (FGT) are discussed with their management in Chapter 33, Page 608.

IMAGING IN GYNECOLOGY

Use of imaging technology has become inevitable in day-to-day gynecological practice. The rapid progress of technological improvement has done miracle in the clinical practice.

- Ultrasound is very effective for diagnosis of gynecological disease.
- Computed tomography (CT) scan, positron emission tomography (PET), and magnetic resonance imaging (MRI) have some specific roles especially for extend of the disease.
- The use of X-ray has now limited role in gynecology and its use is restricted to hysterosalpingography (HSG), X-ray chest, intravenous pyelogram (IVP) and straight X-ray abdomen and some special clinical situations.

Approach of Ultrasonography

- Transabdominal sonography (TAS)—always full bladder is necessary
- Transvaginal sonography (TVS)—commonly preferred
- Transperineal
- Transrectal—in case of virgin or where vaginal approach is not possible.

Other than conventional sonography, color Doppler/3D ultrasound has come with tremendous advantages.

ROLE OF ULTRASONOGRAPHY IN GYNECOLOGY

(Details are described with illustration in the respective Chapters. Here general indications are highlighted)

For detection of pathology of specific organ **(Fig. 5)**:

- *Uterine abnormality*: Pregnancy, fibroid, adenomyosis, Mullerian anomaly, hematometra/pyometra, cervical fibroid, cervical pregnancy, cornual pregnancy, and gestational trophoblastic disease.

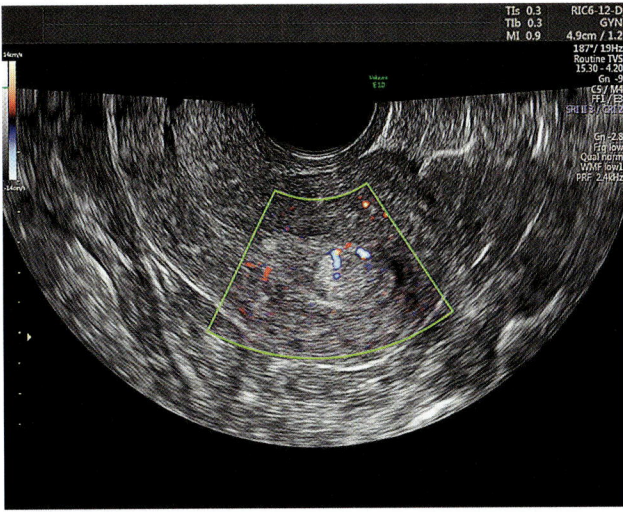

Fig. 5: Transvaginal ultrasonography (TVS) with color Doppler—endometrial polyp.

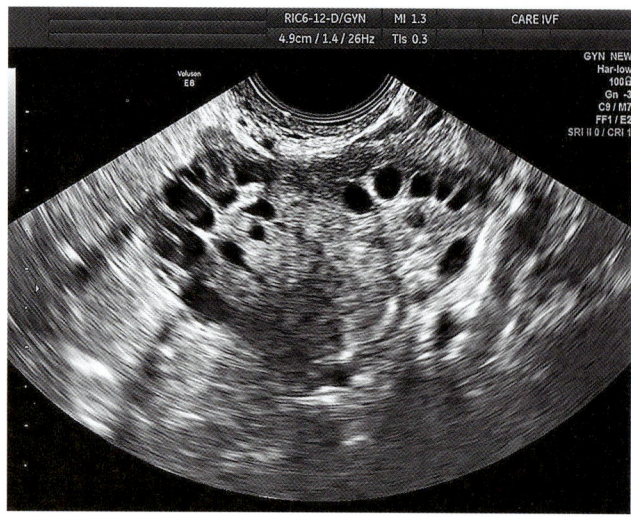

Fig. 6A: Transvaginal ultrasonography (TVS) showing polycystic ovarian morphology with multiple small hypoechoic cysts.

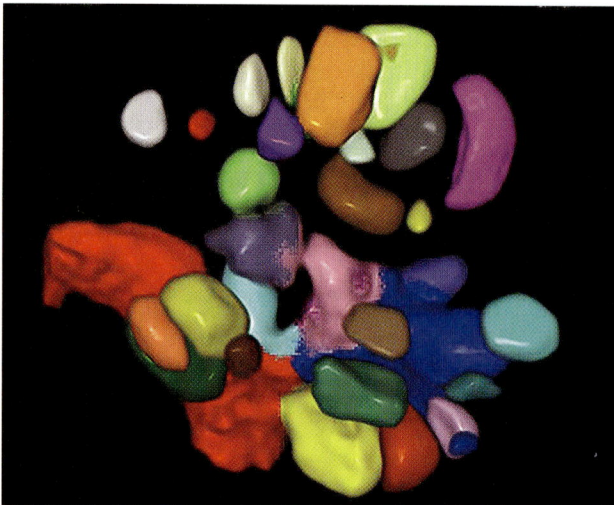

Fig. 6B: Sonography-based automated volume count follicle (SonoAVC) 3D picture of polycystic ovary showing multiple follicles.
Courtesy: Professor Kamal Oswal, VIMS, Kolkata

- *Endometrial pathology*: Polyp **(Fig. 5)**, submucosal leiomyoma, hyperplasia, endometrial cancer, synechia, missing IUCD, and infertility evaluation.
- *Ovarian pathology*: Functional cyst, neoplastic cyst, torsion of ovarian cyst, ovarian malignancy, endometriotic cyst, polycystic ovarian disease **(Figs. 6A and B)**, in infertility–ovarian volume and presence of follicles, presence of ovulation folliculometry.
- *Tubal disease*: Diagnosis of hydrosalpinx, ectopic pregnancy, and Fallopian tube carcinoma.
- *Pelvic inflammatory disease/pelvic abscess.*

ROLE OF USG ACCORDING TO SYMPTOMATOLOGY

- Abnormal uterine bleeding (AUB)
- Acute and chronic pelvic pain
- Suspected ectopic pregnancy and ovarian torsion
- Amenorrhea
- Primary amenorrhea, precocious puberty, intersex, and hirsutism.
- *Infertility*: Tubal patency (hysterosonosalpingography), ovarian reserve, and ovulation monitoring.
- *ART*: in ART, it is inevitable—oocyte retrieval, monitoring, and detection of ovarian hyperstimulation syndrome (OHSS).
- To exclude pregnancy.
- Recurrent abortion and preterm labor.
- Pelvic and abdominopelvic mass—suspected or obvious—to know the nature of mass.

PROCEDURES UNDER ULTRASONOGRAPHY GUIDANCE

- Ultrasound-guided biopsy and fine-needle aspiration cytology (FNAC)
- USG-guided cyst aspiration/drainage of ascites
- Oocyte retrieval in in vitro fertilization (IVF) program, even transfer of embryo.

Role of 3D Ultrasonography (Figs. 7 and 8A)

- Endometrial cancer
- Ovarian malignancy **(Fig. 7)**
- Ovarian torsion
- Ectopic pregnancy
- Leiomyoma
- Endometrial polyp **(Fig. 8A)**
- Mullerian anomaly **(Fig. 8B)**
- Arteriovenous malformation.

Role of Transvaginal Ultrasonography in Abnormal Uterine Bleeding

- For assessment of AUB, TVS is chosen as first-line investigative tool.

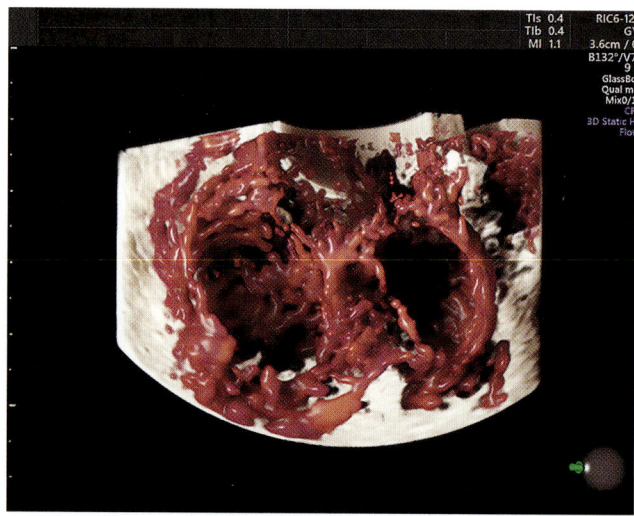

Fig. 7: 3D image of vascularity inside ovarian malignancy.
Courtesy: Professor Kamal Oswal, VIMS, Kolkata

CHAPTER 2: Investigative Procedures in Gynecology and Imaging in Gynecology

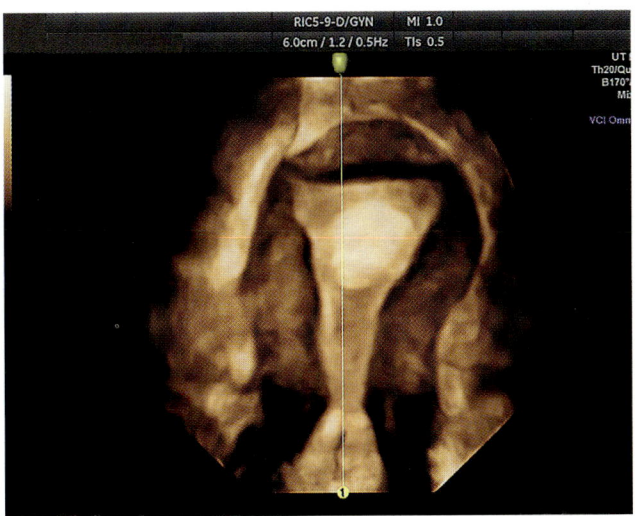

Fig. 8A: Endometrial polyp in 3D 33-year woman presented with abnormal uterine bleeding (AUB).
Courtesy: Professor Kamal Oswal, VIMS, Kolkata

The interpretation of characteristic findings of endometrium by TVS is as follows:
- Cystic endometrial changes → suggestive of polyps
- Homogeneous thickened endometrium → indicates hyperplasia
- Heterogeneous structural pattern → suspicious of malignancy.

The most common disadvantage of TVS is high false-negative rate for focal intrauterine pathology detection.

Saline Infusion Sonography (Figs. 9 and 10)

Saline infusion sonography (SIS), also called sonohysterography or hysterosonography, is helpful to diagnose the pathology of endometrial cavity like submucous fibroid, endometrial polyp, blood clot associated with uterine bleeding. It is done when in general TVS endometrial thickening or mass is detected. It is also useful in infertility workup for tubal patency test.

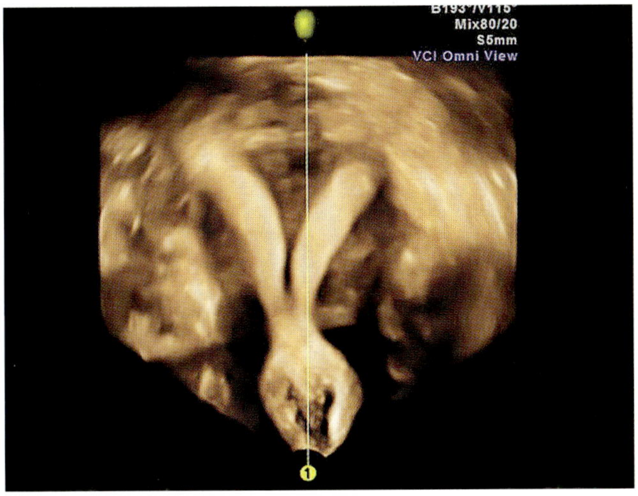

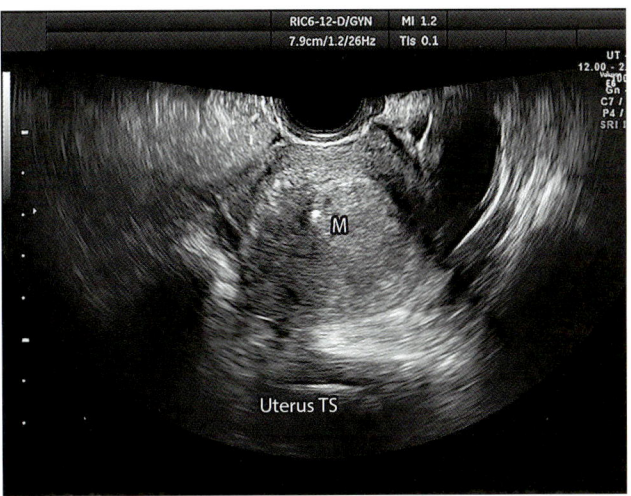

Fig. 8B: 3D ultrasonography (USG) suggestive of complete septate uterus.
Courtesy: Professor Kamal Oswal, VIMS, Kolkata

Fig. 9: Saline infusion sonography (SIS)— transverse section (TS).

- Myometrium and endometrium can be assessed by TVS, not by hysteroscopy or endometrial biopsy.
- Patient feels less discomfort in comparison to other.
- Postmenopausal endometrial hyperplasia and cancer detection by TVS is comparable to other tool. If the thickness is more than 4 mm hysteroscopy and biopsy is warranted in postmenopausal women. If the thickness is less than or equal to 4 mm cancer is less likely and is usually associated with atrophic endometrium and immediate evaluation of endometrium is not needed. In premenopausal women, cut off value is yet to determine, however, above 10-mm ET further evaluation is needed. There is no consensus on ET threshold in this age group and other risk factors for hyperplasia are evaluated.

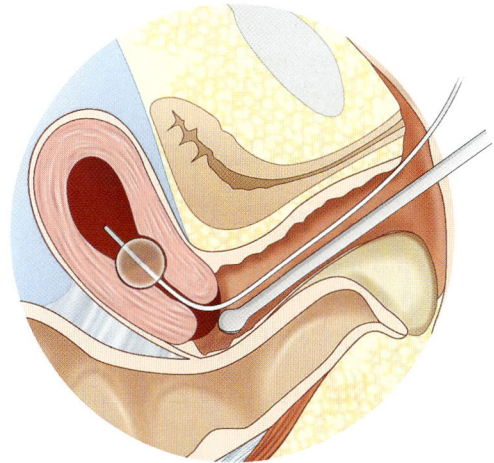

Fig. 10: Saline infusion sonography (SIS) (schematic diagram).

SECTION 1: Gynecological History Taking, Examination and Investigations

Procedure

- After evacuation of bladder, a TVS is done. Posterior vaginal speculum is inserted and a small catheter (usually 7 or 8 size Foley) is introduced through the cervical os. Prior holding the anterior lip with tenaculum facilitates the procedure.
- Then 20–40 mL of normal saline is injected into the uterine cavity through the catheter during which cavity is seen through TVS and detailed sonography scan is done in longitudinal and transverse plane.
- During withdrawal after deflation of balloon, cervical canal and upper vagina (sonovaginography) are also visualized.
- It is done within 10 days preferably 4–6 days of period to overcome the missing of endometrial pathology by thickened endometrium.
- Complications like pelvic infection are very less. Prophylactic antibiotic is preferred by many.

Contraindications

These are hematometra, active pelvic infection, and pregnancy.

Advantages and Disadvantages

Saline infusion sonography is superior to only TVS to differentiate the endometrial, submucous, or intramural. However, it is not superior in diagnosis of cancer where hysteroscopy is the gold standard. It is also cycle dependent to avoid false positive and false negative in diagnosis of uterine cavity pathology.

COMPUTED TOMOGRAPHY SCAN (CT SCAN)

Computed tomography scan is two-dimensional high-resolution imaging technology with or without contrast. Multiple slices picture can be obtained with very close interval (few mm). It has severe radiation hazard.

Role of CT in gynecology are:

- Pituitary (micro or macro) adenoma in case of hyperprolactinemia.
- Extent of malignant ovarian tumor and other malignancy—lymph node involvement, liver metastasis, and presence of ascites **(Fig. 11)**.
- Parametrial infiltration in Ca cervix
- Cerebral metastasis in choriocarcinoma
- Detection of intraperitoneal collection
- Diagnosis of dermoid cyst.

MAGNETIC RESONANCE IMAGING (MRI) IN GYNECOLOGY

- No radiation hazard.
- It is used in many gynecological conditions where diagnosis is inconclusive in sonography.
- It has special role in following conditions:
  - Mullerian anomaly to diagnose bicornuate, septate, and unicornuate uterus.
  - To differentiate between fibroid uterus and adenomyosis **(Fig. 12)**.
  - Endometrial carcinoma—better than CT (*see* Chapter 6) **(Fig. 13)**.

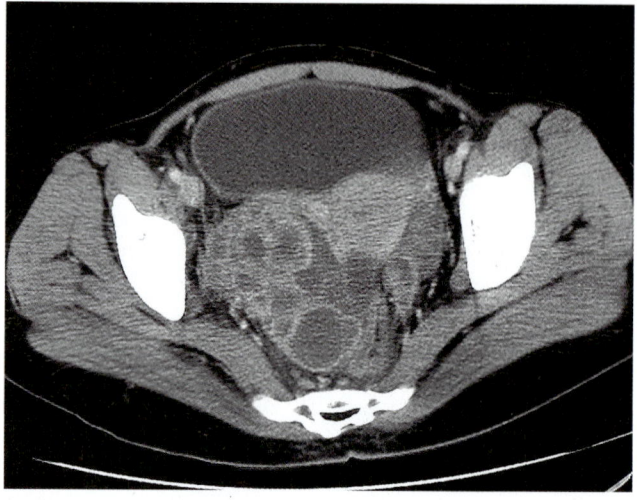

Fig. 11: Computed tomography scan of pelvis showing malignant ovarian tumor with septation.

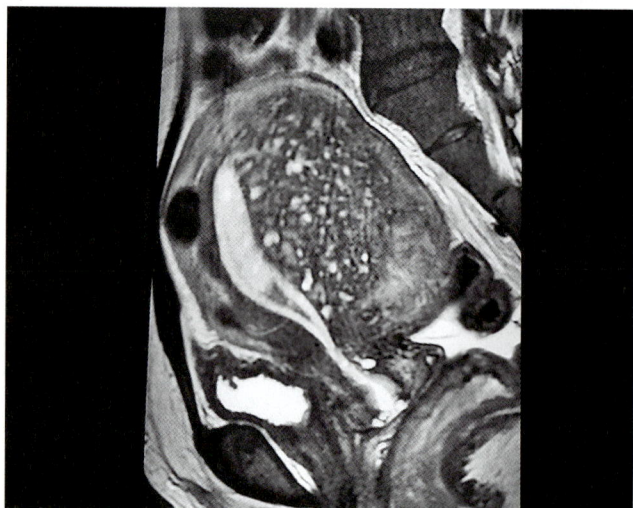

Fig. 12: Magnetic resonance imaging—adenomyosis.
Courtesy: Professor M Karmakar

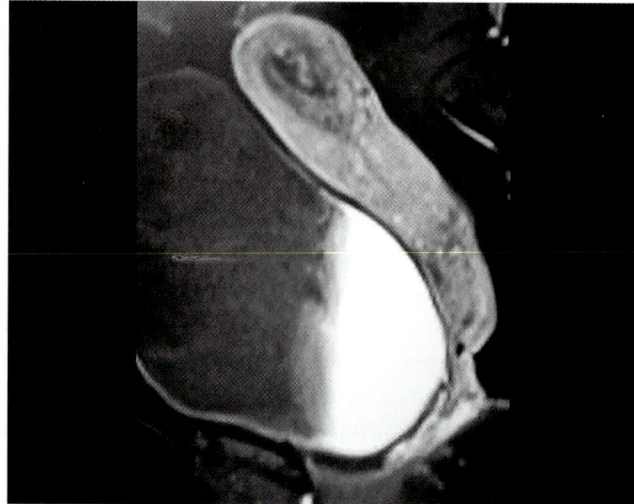

Fig. 13: Magnetic resonance imaging—endometrial cancer invading the adjacent inner myometrium at the fundoposterior region (Stage 1B).

- For uterine artery embolization (UAE) in leiomyoma uterus (*see* Chapter 4).

POSITRON EMISSION TOMOGRAPHY (PET)

Useful in early detection of recurrence of cancer. Use in primary cancer is debatable.

X-RAY—ITS ROLE IN GYNECOLOGY

- ❖ Hysterosalpingography **(Fig. 14)** is the usual procedure in infertility workup for tubal patency test. It is discussed in detail in infertility chapter (*see* Chapter 11) and in instrument chapter (*see* Chapter 24) and chapter of Imaging (*see* Chapter 29)
- ❖ Plain chest X-ray is done as a routine preoperative evaluation of patient
- ❖ Detection of lung metastasis
- ❖ Straight X-ray abdomen is done to detect IUCD in missing thread, it can detect also dermoid cyst by visualization of calcified elements like teeth and mandible.

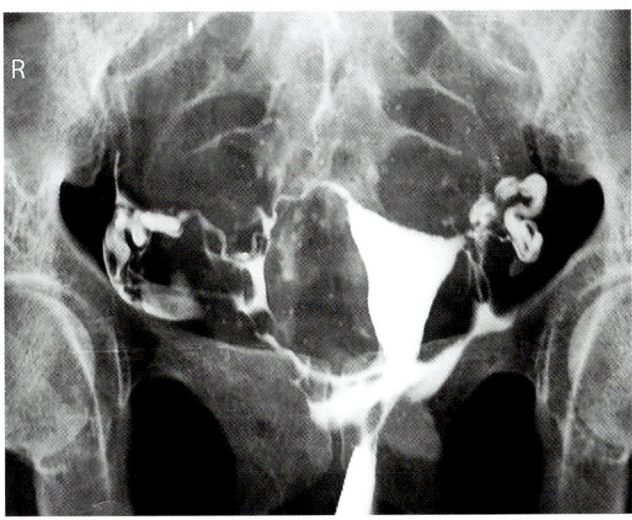

Fig. 14: Hysterosalpingography—bilateral patent tubes.

PIPELLE BIOPSY

Q. How will you do endometrial sampling by aspiration with pipelle (Fig. 15)? Describe of advantages and disadvantages.

Procedure

- ❖ It is an office procedure, less painful and little discomfort with minimal risk. Usually nonsteroidal anti-inflammatory drug (NSAID) is sufficient before procedure.

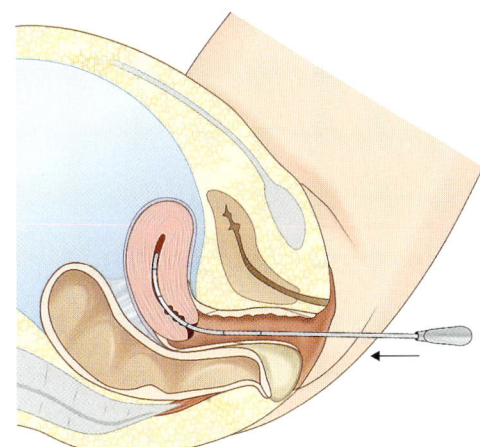

Fig. 15: Pipelle biopsy.

- ❖ After antiseptic swabbing of cervix, pipelle is introduced through the cervix. Usually, a tenaculum is needed to stabilize the anterior lip.
- ❖ Pipelle is introduced till resistance is felt. Pipelle stilette inside is retracted to create suction and it is withdrawn (up to internal os) and introduced many times gently for thorough sampling.

Advantages of Pipelle

- ❖ In D and C, anesthesia is needed, there are surgical risk, risk of perforation, discomfort and pain during and after surgery, and in metal curette—there is discomfort, risk of injury, and infection.
- ❖ Hence, plastic sampler is used with equal efficacy for histological diagnosis. Diagnostic accuracy is 90–98% when compared with findings of D and C or hysterectomy.

Disadvantages of Pipelle

- ❖ In atrophic endometrium, sample is inadequate to test. Negative histological report is not always cancer free, as there is negative failure rate of 1%.
- ❖ In endometrial polyp, negative sampling may occur.
- ❖ In cervical stenosis, device cannot be introduced then dilatation and curettage and hysteroscopic biopsy is needed.

Section 2

Clinical Cases

Section Outline

3. A Case of Lump Abdomen (Ovarian Tumor)
4. A Case of Uterine Leiomyoma (Uterine Fibroid)
5. A Case of Abnormal Uterine Bleeding (Endometrial Hyperplasia)
6. A Case of Endometrial Carcinoma (Including Postmenopausal Bleeding) and Uterine Sarcoma
7. A Case of Choriocarcinoma (Gestational Trophoblastic Neoplasia)
8. A Case of Carcinoma Cervix and Premalignant Lesions of Cervix
9. A Case of Carcinoma Vulva, Preinvasive Lesion of Vulva and Vaginal Cancer
10. Pelvic Organ Prolapse (Genital Prolapse)
11. A Case of Infertility
12. A Case of Polycystic Ovarian Syndrome and Hirsutism
13. A Case of Primary Amenorrhea and Disorder of Sexual Development
14. A Case of Secondary Amenorrhea
15. A Case of Precocious Puberty (Pediatrics and Adolescent Gynecological Problem)
16. A Case of Endometriosis Adenomyosis
17. A Case of Vesicovaginal Fistula and Urinary Incontinence
18. A Case of Old Complete Perineal Tear

CHAPTER 3

A Case of Lump Abdomen (Ovarian Tumor)

Chapter Outline

Writing a case of lump abdomen and how to present the case?

- Differential Diagnosis of Ovarian Tumor
- How to Differentiate Ovarian Tumor and Fibroid Uterus
- Diagnosis of Benign and Malignant Ovarian Tumor
- Complications of Ovarian Tumor
- Classification of Ovarian Neoplasm
- Benign and Malignant Epithelial Tumor
- Staging of Ovarian Tumor
- Description of Individual Ovarian Tumor
- Management of Benign and Malignant Ovarian Tumor
- Borderline Ovarian Tumor
- Fallopian Tube Cancer
- Germ Cell Tumor
- Sex Cord Stromal Tumor

HISTORY TAKING

Patient's Particulars
As usual.

History

- *Chief complaint or complaints*: Patient usually presents with lump abdomen. Patient may complain of gastrointestinal (GI) symptoms.
- *History of present illness*: Elaborate the chief complaints including the duration. Whether the mass has been noticed suddenly. You must enquire about any bowel and bladder symptom.
- *Menstrual history*: Routine history is taken. In ovarian tumor, there is usually no history of menstrual abnormality except in case of hormone producing tumor and malignant neoplasm. If menopausal-duration of menopause, whether there is any postmenopausal bleeding to be enquired.
  Early menarche and late menopause are risk factors of ovarian cancer.
- *Obstetric history*:
  - Parity—ovarian tumor is more common in nullipara
  - Living issue—write "Nil" if patient is primi.
  - Last child birth:
    - Breastfeeding for more than 1 and half years reduces ovarian cancer
    - It is taken in tabular form in usual manner.
- *Past history*:
  - Medical
  - Surgical
  - Gynecological: Endometriosis is a risk factor for ovarian cancer.
- *Family history*: History of ovarian and breast cancer in family is very relevant in ovarian cancer. *BRCA1* and *BRCA2* carriers are risk factors.
- *Functional history*: Bowel, bladder, sleep and appetite.
- *Personal history*: Ovarian cancer is found in women who take fatty diet more. Cigarette smoking increases the chance of mucinous cystadenoma.
- *Contraceptive history*: Oral contraceptive pill reduces ovarian carcinoma and functional cysts.
- *Drug history*.

PHYSICAL EXAMINATION

- Detailed general survey is recorded.
- Anemia and signs of malnutrition are looked for; ovarian cachexia is the typical feature of ovarian malignancy.
- Neck veins, neck glands (especially supraclavicular glands—Virchow's gland) and leg veins are looked for.

Systemic Examination

- Routinely cardiovascular system, respiratory system, GI systems and urinary system (kidney and renal angle tenderness) are examined.
- There may be metastasis in lung in advanced malignancy.
- On the other hand primary of secondary ovarian tumor may be in stomach or other GI sites.

Examination of Breasts

It is very vital in case of ovarian malignancy as in secondary metastatic ovarian tumor breast may be the primary site.

GYNECOLOGICAL EXAMINATION

Before examination preparatory procedures are undertaken as written in Section 1 Chapter 1.

Abdominal Examination

- *Inspection*:
  - Contour of abdomen, condition of skin, condition of umbilicus, presence of any scar are noted.
  - There is fullness of abdomen and if there is fullness on flanks it indicates presence of ascites.
  - There may be unequal enlargement of flanks due to only ovarian tumor; in ascites flanks look equally full.
- *Palpation*:
  - There is usually a lower abdominal mass, tensely cystic or solid or partly solid and partly cystic, surface smooth or nodular.
  - Size and shape are noted. Mobility is tested from side to side and above below.
  - Lower margin may be reached.
  - Fetal parts are not palpable. Braxton Hicks contraction is not palpable.
- *Percussion* (*see* **Figs. 24A to C**; Chapter 1, Page 17)
  - In ovarian tumor without ascites midline (top) is dull on percussion and flanks are resonant.
  - In ascites flanks are dull on percussion, midline (top) is resonant and shifting dullness is positive in case of ascites.
- If ovarian cyst is associated with gross ascites the midline will be resonant, flank is dull and "shifting dullness" becomes positive.
- Fluid thrill is present in huge ascites and is also present in large ovarian cyst and in encysted fluid.
- *Auscultation*: Fetal heart sound is excluded.

Vaginal Examination

- Inspection and palpation of vulva and perineum is done to note any abnormality.
- Per speculum examination is done to visualize the cervix and to see any discharge.
- Bimanual examination is done as usual manner.
- The mass is felt pelvic or pelviabdominal and lower pole of the mass is felt through any fornix.
- Uterus is felt separately from the mass and of normal size.
- A cleft is felt in between the mass and the uterus.
- On movement of the cervix upward the mass does not move and on movement of the mass per abdominally cervix does not move which are elicited in uterine fibroids.
- Posterior fornix is palpated for presence of any nodule.
- Rectal examination is done to confirm the vaginal findings and to note the nodules in pouch of Douglas (POD).
- Rectovaginal examination is done to note any mass, nodule and metastatic deposit.

SUMMARY OF THE CASE (SAMPLE SUMMARY)

Mrs XY 56-year-old parous woman menopause for 8 years, housewife, coming from low socioeconomic status presented with lump abdomen for 6 months and flatulence, dyspepsia, anorexia and loss of weight for last 3 months. She has no significant past and family history, she is mother of three children, all vaginal delivery last child birth 26 years back and husband is well. She had tubectomy immediately after third issue.

On physical examination her weight is____, height_____, looks cachectic, nutrition poor, pallor present, no cervical gland enlargement, pulse rate 84 beats/min, normotensive, leg veins prominent, chest clear and heart sounds normal.

On examination of breasts no abnormality was detected. On per abdominal examination:

- On inspection, abdomen is uniformly enlarged including the fullness of flanks, veins are prominent, umbilicus everted, small lower abdominal scar mark of ligation.
- On palpation, liver and spleen are not palpable. There is a lower abdominal mass almost spherical shape of ....X.... cm size, surface nodular, mobility restricted, consistency firm no tenderness, lower margin could be reached with difficulty and ascitic fluid present.

On vaginal inspection, no significant finding detected.

- Bimanual examination revealed a large pelviabdominal mass which is not freely mobile but separated from small uterus. Adnexae are not separately palpable. Few nodules may be palpable in POD.
- Per rectal examination finding is consistent with the presence of lower abdominal lump and presence of nodules in POD.

INVESTIGATIONS SUPPLIED OR REQUIRED

- Investigations include Hb%, routine blood count (TC, DC, ESR), urine analysis, ABO, Rh factor, urine examination, blood sugar, urea, creatinine, X-ray of chest and ECG.

- Ultrasonography (USG) report and/or any CT scan.
- Tumor marker level like CA 125 (cancer antigen 125), etc.

PROVISIONAL DIAGNOSIS

A 56-year-old parous postmenopausal woman with a lump lower abdomen probably ovarian tumor with a possibility of malignant nature.

DIFFERENTIAL DIAGNOSIS

For differential diagnosis of lump abdomen, *see* below.

Q. What is your case?
Tell the summary of the case.

Q. What is your diagnosis?
Tell the provisional diagnosis.

Q. What are the causes of lump lower abdomen?
The causes are:
- Full bladder
- Pregnancy
- Ovarian tumor
- Fibroid uterus or broad ligament fibroid
- Large tubo-ovarian mass
- Large chocolate cyst in endometriosis
- Mesenteric cyst
- Koch's peritonitis
- Ascites

Other causes are:
- Renal lump
- Splenic enlargement
- Retroperitoneal lymphoma
- Gastrointestinal lump
- Huge splenic enlargement and
- Any retroperitoneal mass like lymphoma, lipoma, etc.

They are differentiated as follows:
- **Full bladder (Fig. 1):**
  - Patient usually complains of retention of urine and pain lower abdomen.
  - Soft midline swelling lower abdominal and tenderness on pressure.
  - She is asked to pass urine. If the lump persists catheterization is done and bladder is deflated and lump disappears.
- **Pregnancy:**
  - There will be presence of amenorrhea and other symptoms and signs (breasts) of pregnancy.
  - On palpation fetal parts and fetal movements are palpable and there will be presence of Braxton Hicks sign. Fetal heart sound is audible.
  - Serum or urinary β human chorionic gonadotropin (hCG) will be high. Pregnancy is confirmed by sonography.
- **Ovarian tumors (Fig. 2):**
  Ovarian tumors are mostly asymptomatic in early stage and symptoms appear in late when it becomes bigger. Symptoms are enlargement of abdomen, lower abdominal heaviness, discomfort or sometimes dull aching pain and respiratory discomfort in huge tumor. Usually no menstrual disturbance is found in benign ovarian tumor except in hormone producing tumor. No characteristic sign is seen in early period. Ovarian cachexia is a typical feature of ovarian malignancy.
  Abdominal examination shows lower abdominal mass, usually spherical and may extend to upper abdomen depending on size. In benign tumor surface is smooth, may be irregular in multiloculated cyst, margins well defined except lower end, consistency—tense cystic, very rarely solid.
  On vaginal bimanual examination lower part of the tumor is palpable through one of the vaginal fornices and uterus may be palpable separately. There is a cleft between the mass and the uterus (*see* Chapter 1, **Figs. 80A and B**, Page 31). On movement of mass per abdominally cervix does not move and vice versa. USG confirms the diagnosis.
- **Fibroid uterus or broad ligament fibroid (Fig. 3):**
  - Menstrual abnormality in the form of menorrhagia is usual in uterine fibroid and there may be presence of pallor if the bleeding is excessive. History may be of long duration.

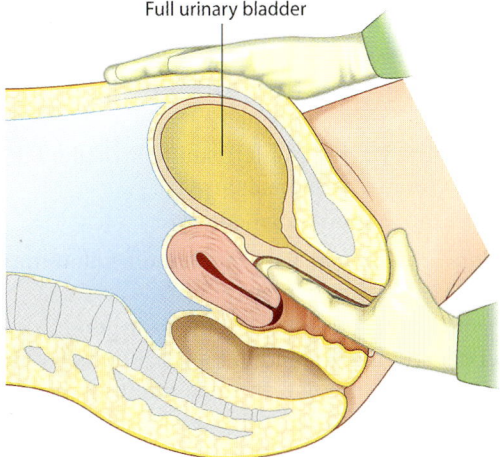

Fig. 1: Full urinary bladder.

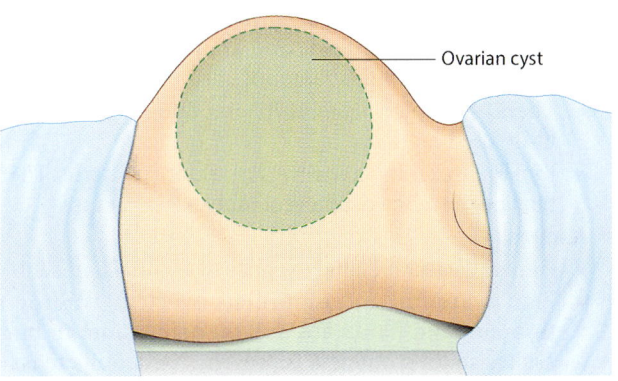

Fig. 2: Ovarian cyst.

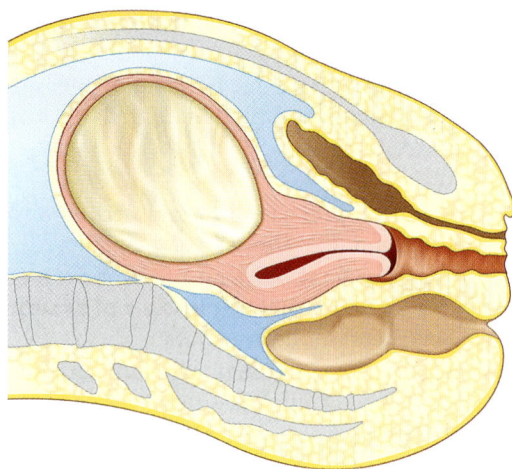

Fig. 3: Uterine fibroid.

- On per abdominal examination lump is felt firm in consistency and mobile from side to side and lower border could not be reached.
- On per vaginal examination mass seems to be arisen from the uterus and there is no cleft or groove in between the mass and the uterus (*see* Chapter 1, **Figs. 81A and B**, Page 31). On movement of the cervix lump moves and vice versa.

❖ **Large Tubo-ovarian Mass**
Pain in lower abdomen, menorrhagia and dysmenorrhea may be present.
Lump is not so large and may not be sufficiently large enough to be palpable abdominally and margins are not well defined. It arises from one or both adnexa and separated from the uterus, tender and fixed on bimanual examination.

❖ **Large chocolate cyst in endometriosis:**
- There may be severe dysmenorrhea and also menorrhagia.
- Mass is not so large and may have infertility.
- On bimanual examination mass is not so large, may be bilateral and mobility restricted and separated from the uterus.

❖ **Mesenteric cyst:** Mass is cystic in consistency and wall is smooth. It is mobile perpendicular to mesenteric line and not along the line.

❖ **Koch's peritonitis:**
- History of long-standing fever, cough, history of pulmonary tuberculosis and anorexia. There may be loss of weight and patient looks ill.
- There is a large vague lump with doughy feeling with ill-defined margins.
- Bimanual examination reveals normal size uterus. There may be presence of bilateral tubo-ovarian mass.

❖ **Ascites:**
- General feature related to cause of ascites is present.
- Flanks are full and umbilicus everted. Midline is resonant and flanks are dull on percussion. In huge ascites shifting dullness is present. No definite mass is palpable even on deep palpation.
- Bimanual examination can exclude presence of any ovarian mass associated with ascites.

Q. How will you confirm your diagnosis of ovarian tumor?
By USG and/or by CT scan and MRI and finally by surgery.

DIAGNOSIS OF A CASE OF BENIGN OVARIAN TUMOR

Q. How will you diagnose a case of benign ovarian tumor?

Symptoms: Many neoplastic ovarian tumor are asymptomatic and symptoms appear in late when it becomes bigger. Sometimes it is diagnosed on routine health check up and is found incidentally or due to any complications arising out of the tumor like torsion or rupture.

❖ *Age*: Usually in reproductive age group or postmenopausal. In children and in adolescent mostly germ cell tumor. Parity has no definite relation. The usual symptoms in absence of emergency are as follows:
- Gradually increasing enlargement of abdomen, lower abdominal heaviness, discomfort or sometimes dull aching pain, respiratory discomfort in huge tumor.
- Pain is unusual in uncomplicated tumor. Torsion, rupture, intracystic hemorrhage and adhesions may rise to pain.
- Dyspepsia and loss of appetite are commonly the features of malignant tumor but may be presenting symptoms in large benign tumor.

❖ *Menstrual history*: Usually no menstrual disturbance is found in benign ovarian tumor. Menstrual irregularity is common in estrogen producing tumor like granulosa cell tumor and amenorrhea is a feature of arrhenoblastoma.

❖ *Symptoms due to pressure effects:*
- Urinary retention due to impacted tumor in POD, urinary frequency and overflow incontinence may also occur due to pressure over bladder.
- Constipation due to pressure on rectum, edema legs, varicosities and venous prominence over abdomen due to pressure over veins and lymphatics are not unusual.

Signs:
❖ No characteristic sign in early period.
❖ Ovarian cachexia is a typical feature of ovarian malignancy, but may be present in large benign ovarian tumor.
❖ There may be pallor and edema.
❖ Neck gland (Virchow's—left supraclavicular) is always searched for in ovarian malignancy.
❖ Breasts examination is mandatory.

Abdominal examination: For examination, follow the general principles as given in Chapter 1.
❖ *Inspection*: Lower abdominal enlargement, usually spherical and may extend to upper abdomen depending on size. Flanks are flat. In huge swelling there may be prominent veins and umbilicus everted **(Fig. 4)**.
❖ *Palpation*: Both superficial and deep palpation are done (*see* Chapter 1).

CHAPTER 3: A Case of Lump Abdomen (Ovarian Tumor)

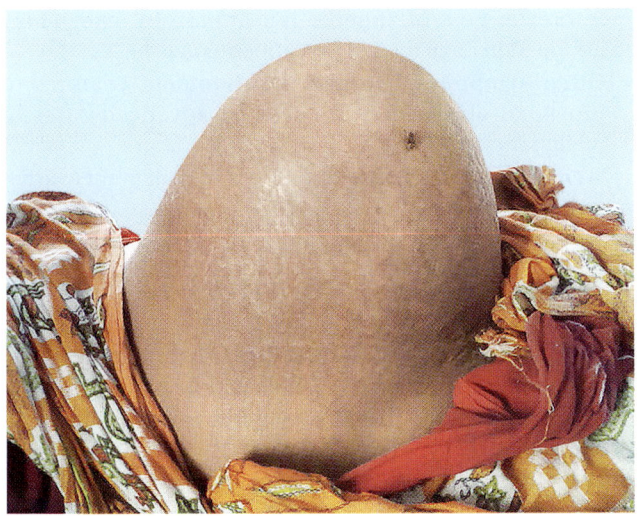

Fig. 4: A 32-year-old parous woman (living issue 1) presenting with huge abdominal enlargement which showed benign serous cystadenoma following surgery.

Site, shape and size and surfaces are described. In benign tumor surface is smooth, may be irregular in multiloculated cyst, margins well defined except lower end which may be palpable when the tumor comes out of the pelvis due to long pedicle, consistency—tense cystic, very rarely solid like in benign tumor like Brenner tumor, mobility present except huge size and it is nontender.

Tenderness may appear in torsion and in infection.

❖ *Percussion*: Shifting dullness and fluid thrill are done as needed to differentiate ascites, ovarian cyst with no or minimal ascites and ovarian tumor with significant ascites as written above in case discussion and also demonstrated in Chapter 1, **Figs. 24 to 29** (*see* Pages 16 to 17).

❖ *Per vaginal examination*: On bimanual examination lower part of the tumor is palpable through one of the vaginal fornices and uterus may be palpable separately if the tumor is small. Benign tumors are usually unilateral. There is a cleft between the mass and the uterus (*see* Chapter 1, **Figs. 80A and B**, Page 31). On movement of mass per abdominally cervix does not move and vice versa.

❖ *Investigations:*
  ▪ USG, CT scan and MRI.
  ▪ Simple X-ray can detect teeth and bones in dermoid cyst.
  ▪ Tumor markers are estimated to exclude malignant varieties and *hormones* in suspected hormone producing tumors.

Q. Where does the ovarian tumor lie in pelvi-abdominal cavity?

❖ A small size tumor lies to the side of uterus in pelvis (**Figs. 5A to D**).
❖ A moderate size lies usually behind the uterus in POD.

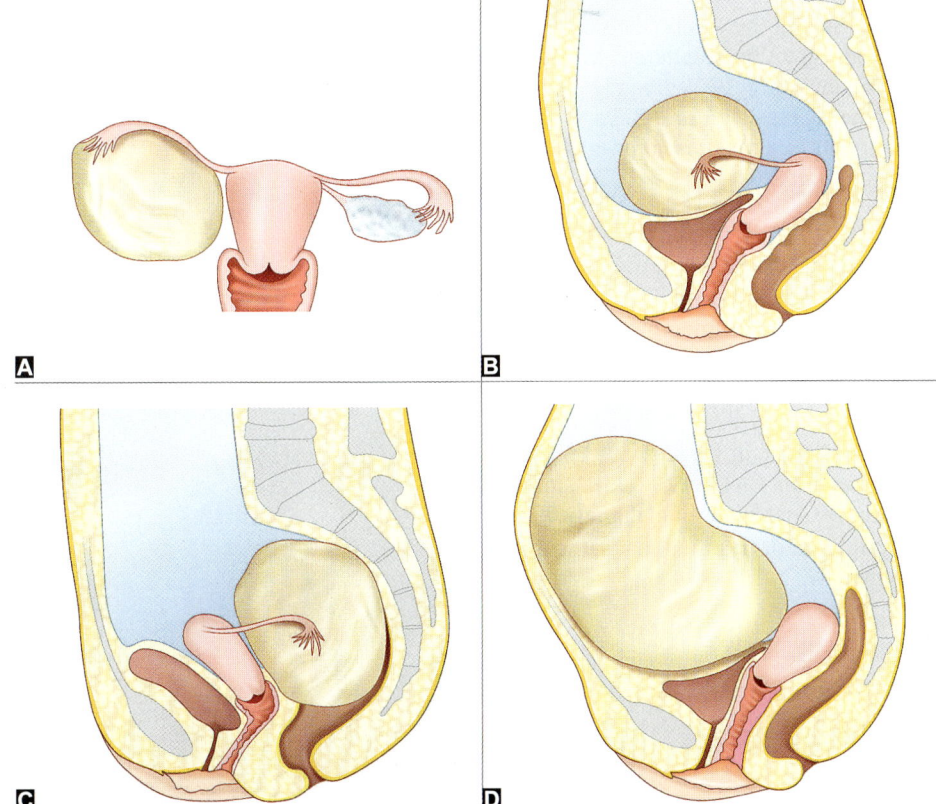

Figs. 5A to D: (A) A small size tumor lies to the side of uterus in pelvis; (B) A small or moderate size tumor may lie in front of uterus and chance of torsion is more; (C) A moderate size lies usually behind the uterus in pouch of Douglas; (D) A large tumor occupies upper abdomen above the uterus.

- A small or moderate size tumor may lie in front of uterus and chance of torsion is more as the pedicle is large.
- A large tumor occupies the upper abdomen and lies above the uterus.

Q. Clinically, how can you say it is an ovarian tumor, not uterine fibroid?

- Fibroids are mostly in reproductive age group. Ovarian tumor may occur in any age group, tumor in postmenopausal age is likely of ovarian origin.
- Uterine fibroid is a slow growing tumor; ovarian tumor is rapid growing. Fibroid grows in years whereas ovarian tumor grows in months.
- Fibroids are more symptomatic than ovarian tumor. Menstrual irregularity in the form of menorrhagia is common in fibroid and presence of menstrual abnormality almost excludes ovarian tumor.
- In fibroid there may be presence of pallor if the bleeding is excessive; cachectic look is a feature of ovarian malignancy and may be in huge ovarian tumor.
- On abdominal examination, fibroid lump is felt firm in consistency and mobile from side-to-side and lower border could not be reached. In ovarian tumor, it varies from tense cystic to hard irregular depending on the type of tumor. Ascitis is common association with malignant ovarian tumor, sometimes with large benign ovarian tumor but never in fibroid uterus.
- On per vaginal examination in fibroid mass seems to be arisen from the uterus and there is no cleft or groove in between the mass and the uterus whereas in ovarian tumor a cleft is felt and mass may be separately palpable from uterus (*see* Chapter 1, **Figs. 80A and B**, Page 31). In fibroid, on movement of the cervix lump moves and vice versa but not in ovarian tumor.

Q. How can you say it is a benign or malignant in nature?

- From the history and clinical examination
- Investigations: By USG with color Doppler, X-ray of chest, CT scan, MRI, positron emission tomography (PET), CT scan. Presence of ascites and metastasis needs prompt oncologist referral.
- Measurement of tumor marker: Premenopausal increase of CA 125 >200IU/mL or OVA1 score ≥5.0 and postmenopausal increase of CA125 CA >35IU/mL or OVA1 score ≥5.0 should be suspicious of malignancy.
- RMI >200 in premenopausal or postmenopausal woman is suspicious of malignancy.
- From surgical findings
- To be confirmed by histopathology.

Q. What history and clinical findings suggest it to be malignant in nature not benign?

History

- Duration: Rapid increase of tumor is suggestive of malignancy.
- Age of patient: Though no age is bar malignancy commonly occurs in aged women or in young adolescents.
- Anorexia: Loss of appetite is common in malignancy although in large benign cyst appetite may be less.
- Other symptoms like pain in abdomen: Features of intestinal obstruction are seen in advanced cases of malignancy.
- Weight: Rapid loss of weight occurs in malignant ovarian tumor.

Physical examination

- Typical ovarian cachexia (**Fig. 31**), emaciated body, and anemia are characteristic of malignancy.
- Virchow's gland (left supraclavicular lymph nodes) may be palpable in malignancy. There may be lump in breasts.
- Pleural effusion: Its presence indicates malignancy (except Meigs' syndrome, *see* below).
- Leg edema is more common in malignancy.

Abdominal examination

- Swelling is solid or variegated, may be bilateral, irregular surface, ill-defined margin, and mobility restricted in malignancy.
- Ascites: Presence of ascites is in more favor of malignancy.
- Liver may be enlarged.

Bimanual examination: There may be nodules in POD and mobility of tumor is restricted.

Rectal examination and rectovaginal examination: It is done to confirm the vaginal findings and to note the nodules in POD and metastatic deposit in malignancy.

USG FEATURES OF MALIGNANT OVARIAN TUMOR

Q. What are the findings in USG from which malignant ovarian tumor is differentiated from a benign one?

In transvaginal sonography (TVS), the following findings are suggestive of malignancy (**Fig. 6**).

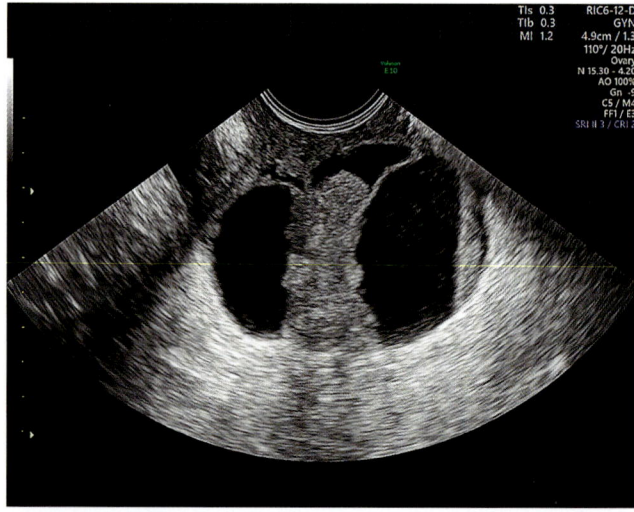

Fig. 6: Sonographic features of malignancy showing multilocularity, solid areas, and papillary projections.
Courtesy: Professor Kamal Oswal, Department of Radiodiagnosis, VIMS, Kolkata

Adnexal mass of:
- Bigger size (>5 cm)
- Multiple echogenic pattern (solid)
- Mutilocular
- Presence of multiple irregular thick septae
- Nodularity
- Neovascularization in color Doppler and papillary projections is likely to be malignant.

RMI Score

Q. What is RMI score?

The meaning of RMI is risk of malignancy index.

This score is determined by the multiplication *of ultrasound score (U) × menopausal score (M) × CA 125 level in U/mL*.

There are two types of RMI score—RMI 1 and RMI 2.

In RMI 1 type, RMI score above 200 indicates high malignancy risk and in RMI 2 type (NICE) 250 is regarded as cut off value. RMI 1 scoring system is widely accepted.

The score is determined according to **Table 1**.

Table 1: Risk of malignancy index.

Ultrasound features and score	
Multilocular cyst	No abnormality = 0
Presence of solid areas	One abnormality = 1
Bilaterality of lesions	Two or more
Presence of ascites	abnormality = 3
Presence of intra-abdominal metastasis	
Menopausal score	
Premenopause	1
Postmenopause	3
CA 125 score	
CA 125 level	U/mL

Postmenopause means 1 year after cessation of menstruation or age above 50 years after hysterectomy. RMI = *Ultrasound score (U) × Menopausal score (M) × CA 125 level in U/mL*.

Q. What is ROMA and what is ROCA?

- The term *ROMA* means risk of ovarian malignancy algorithm.
- Risk of ovarian malignancy algorithm is a numerical score in assessing the risk of ovarian cancer in women with a pelvic mass based on the patient's *human epididymis protein 4 (HE4) and CA 125 levels* and their menopausal status.
- Risk of ovarian malignancy algorithm should always be interpreted in conjunction with an independent clinical and radiological assessment.
- The term *ROCA* means risk of ovarian cancer algorithm. It is prepared on the slope of serial CA 125 measurements drawn at regular interval.

Q. What is OVA1 panel?

It is a serum test for prediction of ovarian cancer in woman with pelvic mass. OVA1 panel involves measurement of 5 biomarkers: *transthyretin, apolipoprotein A-1, β_2-microglobulin, transferrin, and CA 125*.

Using software a score is generated by multivariate index assay algorithm. A score of 5 or higher in premenopausal woman and a score of 4.4 or higher in postmenopausal woman are considered high probability for malignancy. US Food and Drug Administration (FDA) has recently approved this test.

Q. What is IOTA rule of ovarian tumor?

It is purely based on USG criteria (2008). IOTA means International Ovarian Tumor Analysis Group **(Table 2)**.

Table 2: Benign and malignant features of ovarian tumor.

Benign features	Malignant features
Unilocular	Irregular solid tumor
Presence of solid components with largest diameter <7 mm	Presence of ascites
Presence of acoustic shadows	At least four papillary structures
Smooth multilocular tumor with largest diameter <100 mm	Irregular multilocular solid tumor with largest diameter ≥100 mm
No blood flow on color Doppler	Very strong blood flow on color Doppler

Q. What is the role of CECT and MRI?

- The CECT of whole abdomen has role to determine extent of the disease like in liver, omentum, and retroperitoneal spread or other intraabdominal areas (*see* **Figs. 35 and 36**). This is helpful for planning of surgical cytoreduction.
- However, CT has little value in detecting lesion less than 1 to 2 cm in diameter.
- Accuracy of CT is poor in differentiating benign from malignant tumor limited to pelvis and TVS is better.
- Both MRI and PET have limited information and not routinely recommended except in advance cases.

TUMOR MARKERS IN OVARIAN MALIGNANCY

Q. What is tumor marker? What are the different tumor markers and what are their significances? What is sensitivity and specificity?

- Tumor markers are proteins which are liberated by the tumor cells or produced in the body by the effect of tumor cells.
- Different tumor markers are CA 125, serum alpha-fetoprotein (AFP), β-hCG, lactate dehydrogenase (LDH), placental alkaline phosphatase (PLAP), carcinoembryonic antigen (CEA), and cancer antigen 19-9 (CA19-9) and Inhibin A and B.

Q. What are the different tumor markers specific for individual type of ovarian tumors?

Epithelial ovarian cancer (EOC)	:	CA 125
Mucinous epithelial ovarian carcinoma	:	CEA and CA19-9

Dysgerminoma	:	LDH and PLAP, β-hCG ±
Yolk sac tumor (endodermal sinus tumor)	:	AFP
Embryonal carcinoma	:	AFP, β-hCG
Choriocarcinoma	:	β-hCG
Immature teratoma	:	AFP ±
Polyembryoma	:	β-hCG ±, AFP ±
Mixed germ cell tumor	:	β-hCG ±, AFP ±
Granulosa cell tumor	:	Inhibin A and B, estradiol
Sertoli-Leydig cell tumor	:	Inhibin A and B, AFP (sometimes)
Sex cord tumor with annular tubules	:	Inhibin A and B

Q. What is the importance of determination of serum CA 125 in ovarian tumor?

Cancer antigen 125 is elevated in 90% cases of malignant nonmucinous epithelial tumors and a useful marker to differentiate malignant and nonmalignant tumor, especially in postmenopausal age.

There is 96% positive predictive value for malignancy in a postmenopausal adnexal mass with a very high serum CA 125 level (>200 U/mL).

In premenopausal age, the specificity of serum value of CA 125 is low because elevated value (false-positive) is found in many benign conditions like endometriosis, PID, leiomyoma, pregnancy, and also during menstrual period.

On the other hand, in general, 50% cases of stage I ovarian cancers have a normal (false-negative) CA 125 value.

Value of CA 125 should not be considered alone for evaluation of pelvic mass. RMI is based on the level of CA 125, patient is premenopausal or postmenopausal and ultrasound findings (described above).

Serial determination of CA 125 is important in follow up in malignant tumor under chemotherapy. When CEA is high the ratio of CA 125: CEA is considered to determine the primary site of ovarian tumor. If the CEA is elevated a gastric or colonic primary with metastatic to ovary is considered. If CA125: CEA is more than 25:1 ovarian primary is likely, though it does not rule out the primary at GI tract.

Q. What are the surgical findings from which you can suspect the malignant nature of the tumor (Figs. 7 and 8)?

- On opening the abdomen ascites is present and may be mixed with blood; however, clear ascitic fluid may be present sometimes in benign ovarian tumor.
- Involvement of both sides likely to be malignant.
- Surface nodular and irregular, there may be breakage of capsule and prominent vessels over the surface.
- Consistency—solid to mixed variety.
- Adhered with the adjacent structures.
- Metastatic deposits may be seen over the parieties, intestines, undersurface of diaphragm, and superior surface of liver.
- Aortic, paraaortic, and pelvic lymph nodes may be palpable.

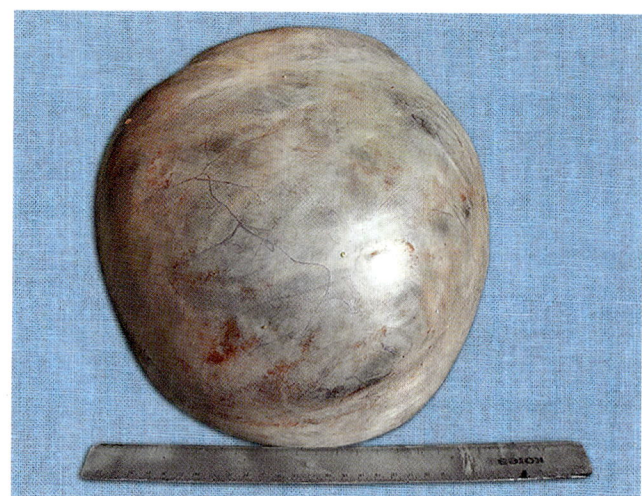

Fig. 7: Benign ovarian tumor—smooth surface, no adhesion, no breakage of capsule, and purely cystic (serous cystadenoma).

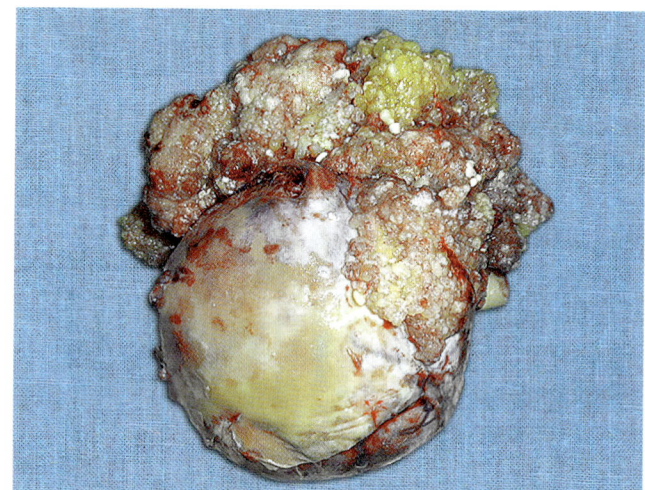

Fig. 8: Malignant ovarian tumor—irregular surface, breakage of capsule protruding fungating growth with solid areas and hemorrhages.

Q. What are the causes of ovarian masses?

The causes are:
- Non-neoplastic or neoplastic
- Most of the masses are cystic
- Cystic masses are either neoplasm, functional cyst or endometrioma
- Neoplasms are commonly benign. In reproductive age, benign comprises 90% of ovarian neoplasm. In aged women and young girls, malignancy is more common.

CLASSIFICATION OF OVARIAN TUMOR

Q. How will you classify the ovarian neoplasms (based on WHO histological classification)?

The classification of ovarian tumor is based on the types of tissue from where they arise **(Fig. 9)** namely, *epithelial*, *connective tissue* of ovary (sex cord stromal) or *germ cells*. In addition, there are some metastatic tumors of ovary and

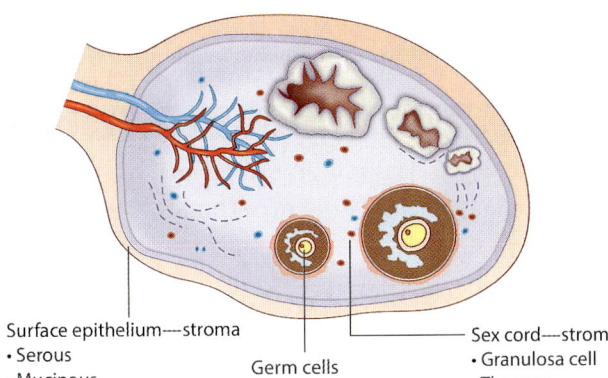

Fig. 9: Tumors of ovary arising from three cell lines, e.g. surface epithelial, germ cells, and sex cord—stromal cells.

- Surface epithelium—stroma
  - Serous
  - Mucinous
  - Endometroid
  - Clear cell
  - Transitional cell
- Germ cells
  - Dysgerminoma
  - Yolk sac
  - Embryonal carcinoma
  - Choriocarcinoma
  - Teratoma
- Sex cord—stroma
  - Granulosa cell
  - Thecoma
  - Fibroma
  - Sertoli cell
  - Sertoli-Leydig cell
  - Steroid

there are some very rare varieties of tumor which originate from the ovary.
- Epithelial-stromal tumors (80%)
- Sex cord-stromal tumors (10%)
- Germ cell tumors (10%)
- Metastatic and others.

EPITHELIAL-STROMAL TUMORS

Different varieties are:
- *Serous tumors:*
  - Benign—serous cystadenoma, papillary cystadenoma, and serous cystadenomafibroma
  - Borderline
  - Serous cyst adenocarcinoma, papillary adenocarcinoma, cystadenocarcinofibroma, etc.
- *Mucinous tumors*, endocervical like, intestinal type:
  - Benign—mucinous cystadenoma and mucinous cystadenofibroma
  - Borderline
  - Malignant—mucinous cystadenocarcinoma.
- *Endometrioid tumors:*
  - Benign
  - Borderline
  - Malignant epithelial.
- *Clear cell tumors:*
  - Benign
  - Of low malignant potential (LMP)
  - Malignant.
- *Transitional cell epithelial tumors:*
  - Benign-Brenner tumor
  - Borderline Brenner tumor
  - Malignant—malignant Brenner tumor and transitional cell carcinoma (non-Brenner variety).
- *Squamous cell tumors*
- *Mixed epithelial tumors*—benign, borderline, and malignant
- *Undifferentiated carcinoma.*

Types of ovarian cancer is detailed in Page 63.

SEX CORD—STROMAL TUMORS

Different varieties are:
- *Granulosa-stromal cell tumors: Granulosa cell tumors and thecoma-fibroma.*
- *Sertoli-stromal cell tumors*, androblastoma: Well differentiated, Sertoli–Leydig cell tumor of intermediate differentiation, Sertoli–Leydig cell tumor of poorly differentiated, retiform.
- *Sex cord tumor with annular tubules*
- Gynandroblastoma
- Unclassified
- *Steroid (lipid) cell tumors:* Stromal luteoma, Leydig cell tumor, unclassified.

GERM CELL TUMORS

- *Dysgerminoma*
- *Yolk sac tumors (endodermal sinus tumor)*
- *Embryonal carcinoma*
- *Polyembryoma*
- *Choriocarcinoma*
- *Teratomas:* Immature, mature, monodermal, mixed germ cell.

Others:
- Gonadoblastoma
- Germ cell sex cord-stromal tumor of nongonadoblastoma type
- Tumors of the rete ovarii
- Mesothelial tumors
- Tumors of uncertain origin, miscellaneous tumors
- Gestational trophoblastic diseases
- Soft tissue tumors not specific to ovary
- Malignant lymphomas, leukemias and plasmacytomas
- Unclassified tumors.

SECONDARY (METASTATIC) TUMORS

Krukenberg tumor.

FUNCTIONAL CYST

Q. What are the different varieties of functional cyst?
- Follicular cyst
- Corpus luteum cyst
- Theca lutein cyst.

Q. What are the characteristics of functional cyst?
- Usually bilateral

- Size is usually not more than 8 cm and does not increase with time
- Regresses spontaneously: Role of combined oral contraceptives (COC) in regression is challenged
- Histology gives the specific diagnosis.

FOLLICULAR CYST

Follicular cyst is the most common type of functional cyst and formed due to accumulation of fluid within follicular antrum which remains unruptured. There is a hormonal imbalance. The cyst is lined by granulosa cells and is not associated with cellular proliferation. It may be single or multiple in one or both ovaries. Prolong estrogen production is often found resulting amenorrhea followed by excessive bleeding, mimicking metropathia hemorrhagica. Follicular cyst has been found with progesterone—only pill use and also where dominant follicle is formed in response to gonadotropin but without ovulation.

Ultrasonographic finding shows completely rounded anechoic lesions with regular, thin walls.

If asymptomatic, treatment is expectant with regular follow up. Combined oral contraceptive is often used to prevent and to treat follicular cyst, but its role is challenged recently. If persistent or size increases surgical evaluation by laparoscopy is needed.

CORPUS LUTEUM CYST

Corpus luteum cyst is formed following ovulation due to hemorrhage in the corpus luteum which usually regresses spontaneously. There may be pain due to excessive bleeding inside the cyst. Rarely, rupture occurs resulting profuse intraperitoneal hemorrhage which needs immediate surgical intervention *(ovarian apoplexy)* which usually occurs within 21–25 days of the cycle.

Picture is like ectopic pregnancy. Corpus luteum cyst may be associated with pregnancy. Sonographic appearance of corpus luteum cyst is variable depending on the time of imaging. Immediately after intracystic hemorrhage it appears echogenic. After retraction of clot a linear ring is formed between clot and serum. Due to peripheral vascularity Doppler shows a bright red colored ring *(ring of fire)* around the cyst.

No treatment is needed in majority of the cases and spontaneous regression occurs.

THECA LUTEIN CYST

These are special variety of follicular cysts commonly found in the conditions where there is excess β-hCG stimulation. The conditions are *gestational trophoblastic disease, multifetal pregnancy*, etc. Theca lutein cysts may be of larger size. These are rarest among functional cysts.

On USG, they look multiloculated. Usually asymptomatic and spontaneous regression occurs following withdrawal of β-hCG. Sometimes torsion may occur.

This type of cysts may also occur in ovarian hyperstimulation syndrome following ovulation induction.

CLASSIFICATION OF OVARIAN TUMOR

Q. How would you classify ovarian teratoma?

Ovarian teratomas belong to germ cell tumor. *"Teras"* means monster.

Classification:
- *Mature*: (A) Mature cystic teratoma also called benign cystic teratoma and dermoid cyst; (B) mature solid teratoma, and (C) homunculus forms or fetiform teratoma.
- *Immature teratoma*: Malignant neoplasm.
- *Monodermal and highly specialized*: Struma ovarii (thyroid tumor), neuroectodermal tumor, squamous cell or adenocarcinoma, melanocyte type, sebaceous, and carcinoid.

Struma ovarii: It is a monodermal teratoma, benign in nature, solely composed predominantly of thyroid tissue.

Q. What are the different varieties of benign ovarian cyst not necessarily neoplastic?

- *Functional cyst*: Follicular, corpus luteal, and theca lutein cyst.
- *Inflammatory*: Tubo-ovarian abscess. Endometrioma (not strictly inflammatory).
- *Germ cell tumor*: Benign cystic teratoma (dermoid cyst).
- *Epithelial cell*: Serous and mucinous.

Of these functional and inflammatory are not neoplastic.

Name the benign ovarian tumors:
- Epithelial: Serous, mucinous, and Brenner
- Germ cell: Dermoid, mature solid teratoma
- Sex cord stromal: Fibroma, theca cell tumor.

Q. What are the different varieties of pure solid ovarian tumor?

- Brenner tumor, sex cord-stromal tumors, Krukenberg tumor, ovarian fibroids and leiomyosarcoma, primary lymphoma, and carcinoid tumor may present as solid masses.
- If the tumor is completely solid, it is likely to be benign nature. However, they should be removed as chance of malignancy cannot be ruled out.
- Malignant tumors are usually mixed variety containing both cystic and solid component.
- Benign tumors are commonly cystic.

Q. Which one is the most common variety of ovarian tumor?

Epithelial tumor—of them most common is serous cystadenoma.

Q. Which may be the largest one?

Largest sizes are serous cystadenoma and pseudomucinous cystadenoma and the latter becomes more larger.

Q. Which tumor is the most common variety in pregnancy and why?

- Dermoid cyst, serous cystadenoma, and papillary cystadenoma in order as all are more prevalent in reproductive age group.
- Dysgerminoma is the most common ovarian malignancy during pregnancy also due to age-related prevalence.

BENIGN SEROUS CYSTADENOMA (FIGS. 10 TO 12)

- The most common benign tumor
- Bilateral in *20%* cases
- Moderate size and spherical shaped with a pedicle
- Surface smooth, in papillary variety papillary growth
- Unilocular, may be multilocular
- Consistency—cystic or solid papillomatous in papillary type. Thin wall cyst contains serous fluid. Epithelium secretes serous fluid.
- On H/P, cysts are lined by single layer low columnar epithelial cells mimicking those of fallopian tube. *"Psammoma bodies"* are areas of calcified granulation present within the tumor and may be radiopaque.
- *Chance of malignancy is 25%*. 5-10% borderline malignant potential.

BENIGN MUCINOUS CYSTADENOMA (FIGS. 13 TO 15)

- Second common benign tumor
- Bilateral in *10–15%* cases
- Small to huge size, spherical shaped with a pedicle

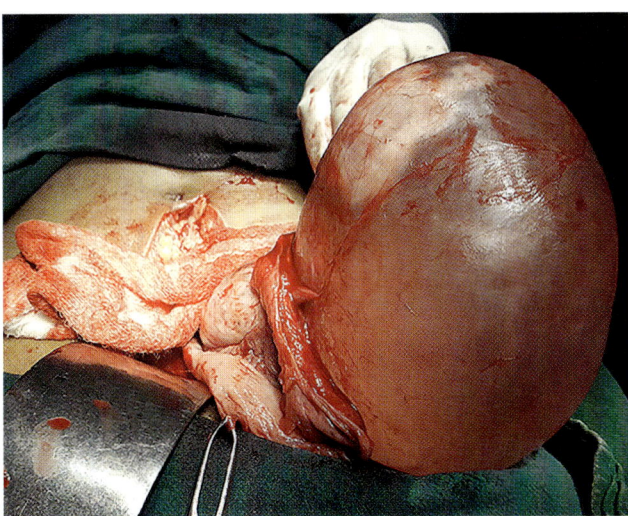

Fig. 10: Simple clear serous cystadenoma of left ovary in a 22-year-old nulliparous woman— cystectomy done.

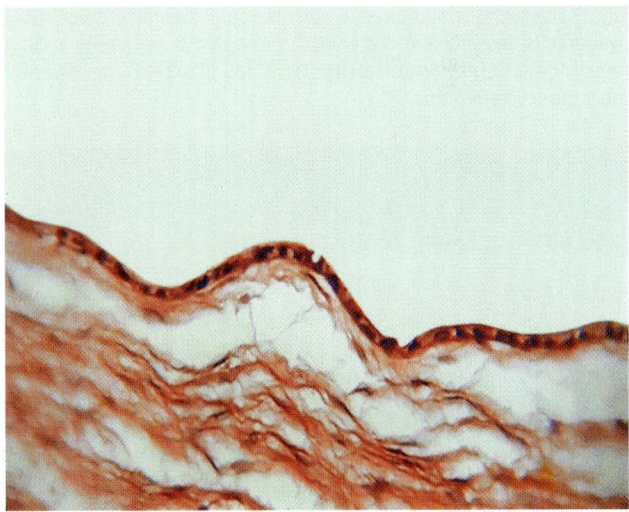

Fig. 11: Microphotography of serous cystadenoma ovary showing single layer low columnar epithelium (H&E, X400).
Courtesy: Professor Gopinath Barui, Department of Pathology

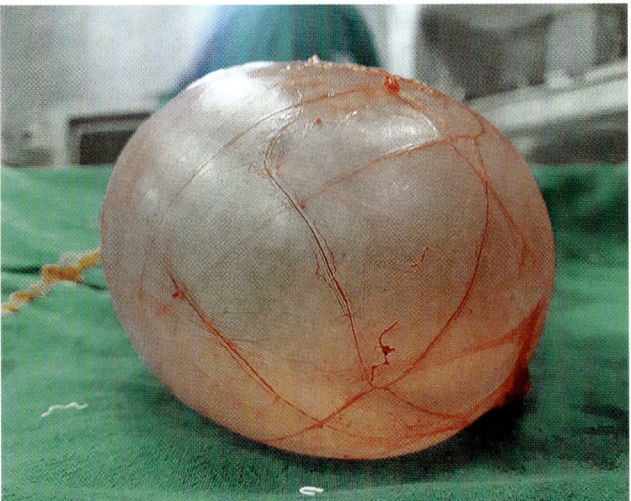

Fig. 10A: Simple cyst following cystectomy.

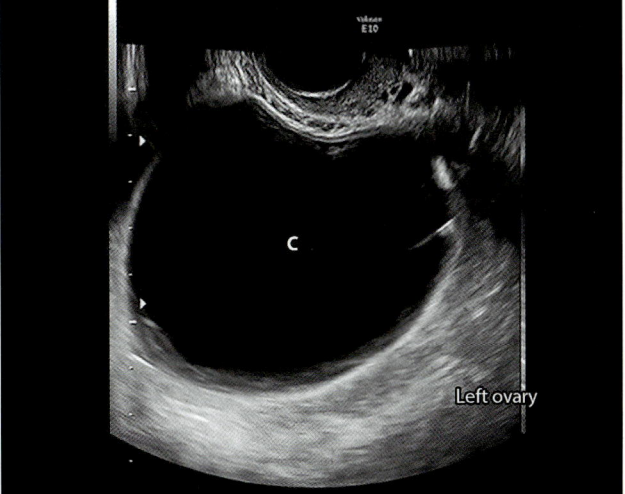

Fig. 12: Sonography showing unilocular ovarian mass with anechoic fluid—likely benign serous cystadenoma.
Courtesy: Professor Kamal Oswal, Department of Radiodiagnosis, VIMS, Kolkata

SECTION 2: Clinical Cases

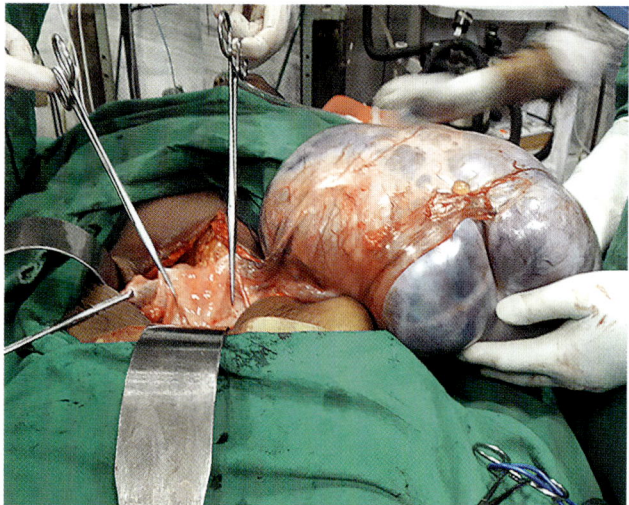

Fig. 13: Laparotomy finding in a case of large unilateral multiloculated ovarian cyst in a 40-year-old woman. Note peritoneal cavity is clear, free of any adhesion, and no ascites. It was found to be a case of benign mucinous cystadenoma.

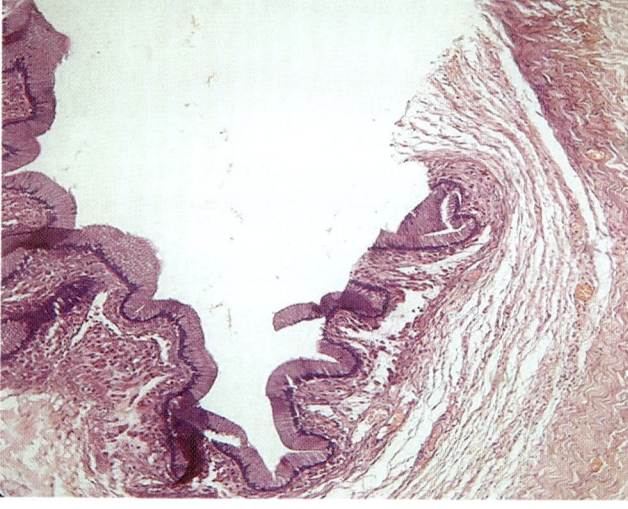

Fig. 15: Microphotography of mucinous cystadenoma ovary showing single columnar layer containing cells with abundant mucin (H&E, X400).
Courtesy: Professor Gopinath Barui, Department of Pathology

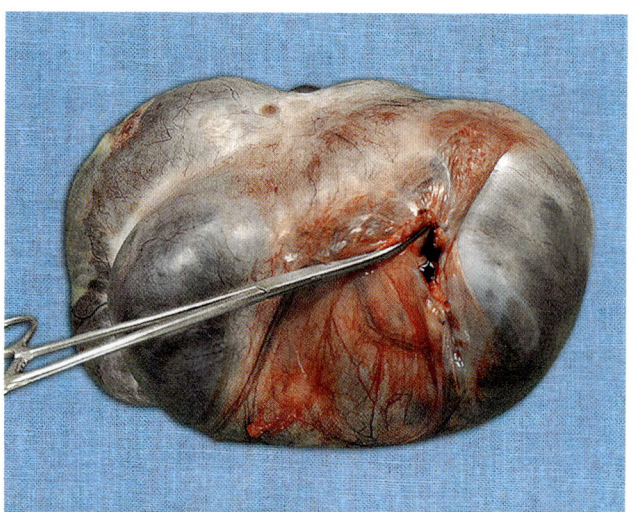

Fig. 14: Multiloculated mucinous cystadenoma.

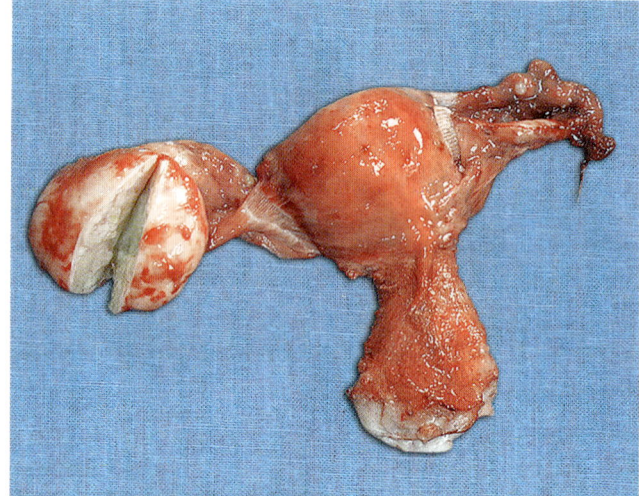

Fig. 16: Left-sided Brenner tumor (solid epithelial tumor)—total abdominal hysterectomy with bilateral salpingo-oophorectomy done, almost always unilateral, patient was 49 years postmenopausal.

- Surface smooth to lobulated and multilocular
- Consistency—partly cystic and partly solid. Wall is thick containing mucoid viscid fluid.
- Histopathology—wall is lined by single columnar layer containing cells with abundant mucin
- *Chance of malignancy is 5–10%.* Malignant mucinous tumors are very difficult to differentiate from metastatic GI malignancies.

BRENNER (TRANSITIONAL) TUMOR (FIG. 16)

- Epithelial benign solid ovarian tumor
- Well circumscribed rubbery mass with tan to yellow color
- Histopathology—consists of islands of clear epithelial cell nests of transitional type epithelial cells in fibrous stroma resembling *"Walthard bodies"*

- Almost always *unilateral* with small size
- Cut surface—slightly yellowish, smooth bosselated
- Frequent in postmenopausal age
- Oophorectomy is done in younger age and TAH-BSO (total abdominal hysterectomy with bilateral salpingo-oophorectomy) done in postmenopausal age.

DERMOID CYST OF OVARY (SYNONYM: BENIGN CYSTIC TERATOMA) (FIGS. 17 TO 20)

- It is mature cystic teratoma also called benign cystic teratoma. It is called "dermoid" due to the prevalence of dermal elements.
- Dermoid cyst which is the *most common variety of germ cell tumor* comprising 95% of all germ cell tumors.

CHAPTER 3: A Case of Lump Abdomen (Ovarian Tumor)

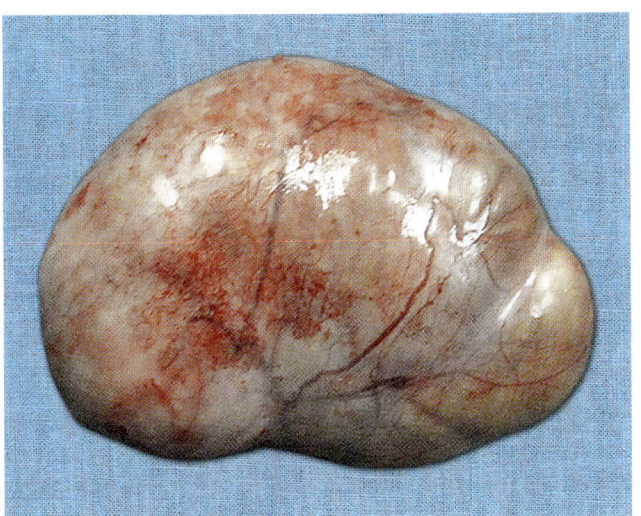

Fig. 17: Dermoid cyst of ovary (benign cystic teratoma) after cystectomy in a 27-year-old woman.

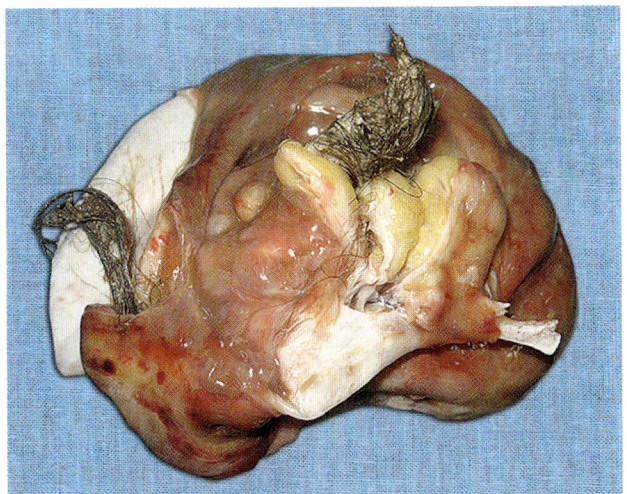

Fig. 18: Dermoid cyst—cut section of the same specimen as shown in Figure 17 shows sebaceous materials, hair, bones, etc.

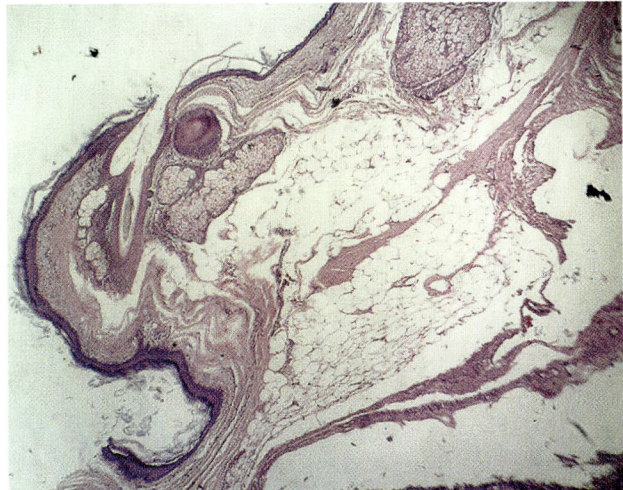

Fig. 19: Microphotography of dermoid cyst ovary showing all elements, predominantly ectodermal.

Courtesy: Dr Tripti Das, Department of Pathology

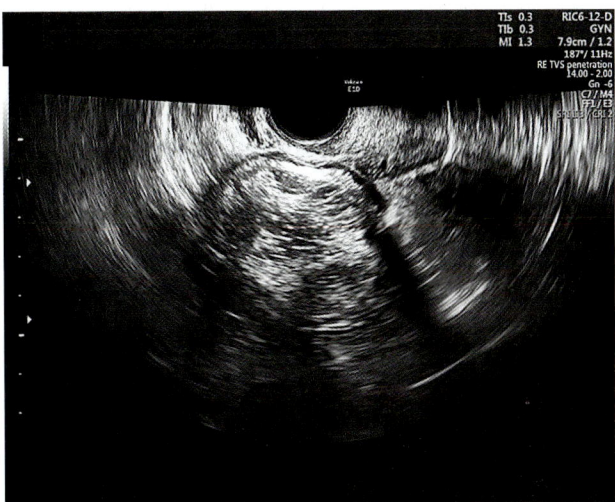

Fig. 20: Sonography showing features of dermoid cyst of ovary, predominantly hyperechoic (see text).

Courtesy: Professor Kamal Oswal, Department of Radiodiagnosis, VIMS, Kolkata

- Common in reproductive age though no age is immune. The most *common in pregnancy.*
- 10–20% of all ovarian neoplasms and 60% of benign ovarian tumors.
- Size small to moderate with a pedicle—5–10 cm.
- Bilateral 10% smooth surface, tense cystic.
- Unilocular cut section shows *Rokitansky protuberance* which is a localized growth which protrudes into the cystic cavity. This protuberance is also called dermoid plug, dermoid process, dermoid mamilla or embryonal rudiment. The cavity contains hair, fat, cartilage, bone, teeth and sebaceous material.
- Histopathology—all elements ectodermal, endodermal or mesodermal components found but predominantly ectodermal. Rokitansky protuberance is covered with keratinized squamous epithelium with sweat and sebaceous glands.
- Karyotype—46XX.
- Complication: Chance of *torsion* is more as it is of moderate size, heavy tumor with long pedicle and torsion occurs in *15%* cases and rupture is uncommon for its thick wall.
- *Malignant transformation: 1–3%* and mostly (80%) squamous cell carcinoma.
- Diagnosis—clinical: No specific symptoms and sign and features are like other benign ovarian cyst.
- X-ray may show bone and teeth.
- Sonography—"*tip of iceberg*" sign is formed by amorphous echogenic interfaces of fat, hair, and tissues. Fat-fluid or hair-fluid levels are found as linear demarcation. Rokitansky protuberance of 2–4 cm is seen as a hyperechoic area.
- Treatment:
  - Ovarian cystectomy or ovariotomy by laparotomy or through laparoscopy.
  - Ovarian cystectomy is almost always possible. Even preserving a small amount of ovarian cortex is beneficial in young woman.

Q. What will you do if an ovarian tumor is diagnosed?

Surgical removal.

Q. Why ovarian tumor is to be removed as early as possible it is diagnosed?

Due to its complications.

COMPLICATIONS OF OVARIAN TUMOR

Q. What are the complications of ovarian tumor?

- Torsion—the most common
- Rupture
- Intracystic hemorrhage
- Infection
- Adhesions
- Malignant transformation (5–10%)
- Pseudomyxoma peritonei
- Adhesions with adjacent structures.

Torsion of ovarian cyst (Figs. 21 and 22):

It is the *most common complication* of ovarian tumor—10 to 15%.

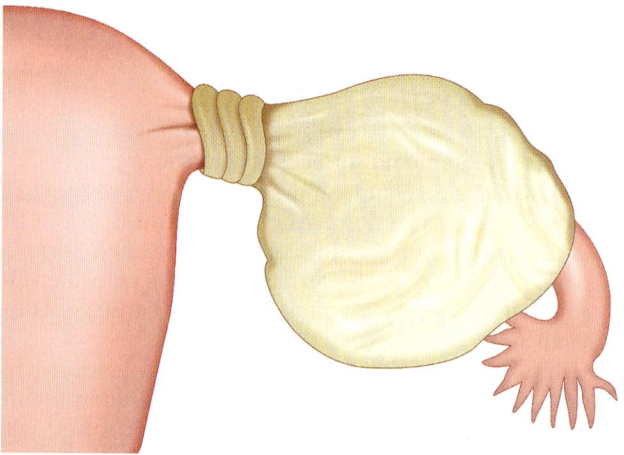

Fig. 21: Torsion of ovarian cyst.

Heavy tumor, moderate size, long pedicle, and lax abdomen favor torsion. Maximum torsion occurs in a mass of 6–10 cm and more commonly on right side.

In order of frequency the *most common variety* undergoing torsion is *dermoid cyst*, then pseudomucinous cystadenoma, simple serous cystadenoma, and papillary cystadenoma.

More common in pregnancy and puerperium as in pregnancy it becomes abdominal organ and gets more space for torsion. Of all torsions 25% occurs in pregnancy. In puerperium after sudden empty of abdominal cavity ovarian mass gets a large space for movement.

Pathology and morbid changes—commonly single turn occurs and in initial phase torsion and detorsion occur. There may be two and more turn. Initially venous obstruction results in congestion and edematous. Intracystic hemorrhage and lymph exudate result adhesion with surrounding structures. Finally ovarian arterial occlusion which occurs rarely may lead to gangrenous necrosis of the cyst. Infection may supervene.

Q. How would you diagnose torsion?

- *Clinical presentation* may be subacute or acute.
  In acute variety, there may be acute abdomen with features of sudden severe pain, vomiting with/without fever, tachycardia, and even there may be features of shock; abdominal tenderness with muscle guard and lump abdomen.
  In subacute variety recurrent attacks of pain occur with intermittent relieve due to untwisting of pedicle.
- *Sonography*: Specific findings of torsion are: (1) multiple follicle rimming an enlarged ovary (indicating congestion and edema), (2) *Bull's eye target, whirlpool, or snail shell* which is rounded hyperechoic structure with (3) multiple, inner, concentric hypoechoic rings (feature of twisted pedicle) and disruption of vascular flow of adnexa in color Doppler **(Fig. 23)**. CT and MRI may be helpful.

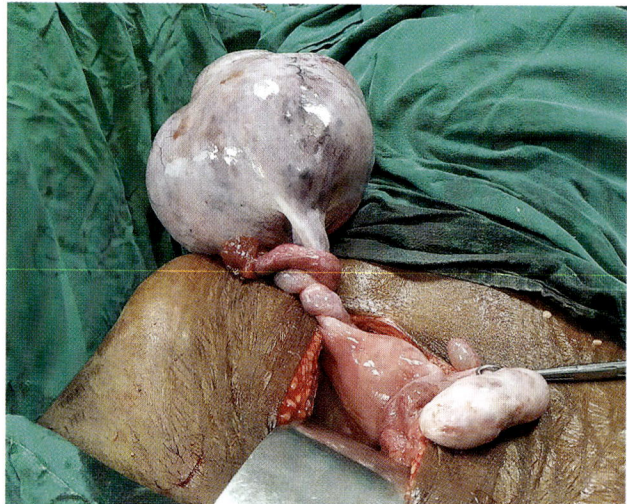

Fig. 22: Torsion of ovarian cyst.

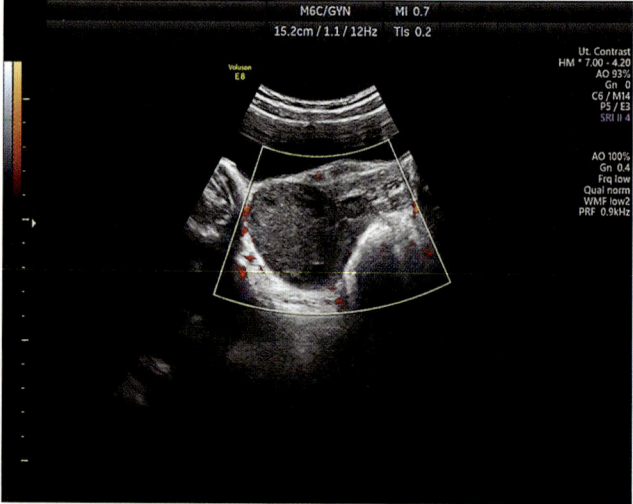

Fig. 23: Power Doppler showing ovarian mass with reduced vascularity—feature of ovarian torsion.
Courtesy: Professor Kamal Oswal, Department of Radiodiagnosis, VIMS, Kolkata

Q. How would you manage if torsion is suspected or diagnosed?

- Immediate laparotomy with simultaneous resuscitation with IV fluid and antibiotic followed by ovariotomy is treatment in case of necrosis or rupture.
- Laparoscopy is a good option for evaluation of torsion and treatment.
- Ovarian cystectomy following detorsion with preservation of ovary can be done with good outcome in early torsion in absence of necrosis.
- Oophoropexy (shortening of ovarian ligament or fixing the ovarian ligament or ovary with uterus, broad ligament or lateral pelvic wall) can be done to prevent recurrence of torsion.

Q. What is parasitic cyst?

When pedicle atrophies following torsion and the tumor gets its circulation from adjacent structure it is called parasitic cyst—a very rare event.

Rupture of ovarian cyst (Fig. 24)

Rupture of ovarian cyst may occur spontaneously or traumatic by blow, kick, and fall. Spontaneous rupture may occur in papillary and pseudomucinous cystadenoma. Sometimes, rupture may occur during surgical removal. In few cases, there may be hemorrhage.

Patient may present with acute abdomen or sometimes with regression.

Management is the treatment of shock and laparotomy followed by removal of ruptured cyst. Ovarian tumor should be removed in intact and in accidental rupture thorough peritoneal toileting is done.

PSEUDOMYXOMA PERITONEI

Q. What is pseudomyxoma peritonei?

- A rare complication due to rupture of benign or malignant pseudomucinous cystadenoma.
- This results from implantation of epithelium with subsequent huge production of jelly like mucoid substance inside the peritoneal cavity.
- Removal of rupture ovary with removal of mucoid material as far as possible from the peritoneal cavity is the treatment.
- But this is notorious for recurrence and repeat laparotomy for drainage may be needed.
- Even external radiation and chemotherapy have been attempted with less success.
- The prognosis is poor.
- Mucocele appendix and intestinal carcinoma may result also similar condition.

Q. What is the chance of malignant transformation of benign ovarian cyst?

- May occur in 5-10% cases in benign cystic neoplasm.
- Highest chance of malignant change occurs in papillary cystadenoma (>25%), least in simple serous cystadenoma, and in case of dermoid, it is 2%.

Infection of ovarian cyst: Transmitted from bowel or infected appendix, salpingitis, more common in puerperium and also following torsion.

Pain in abdomen, rise of temperature, abdominal tenderness and rigidity, and high leukocytosis are the features.

Antibiotics, analgesics, and laparotomy after localization of sepsis are the treatment.

Adhesion of ovarian cyst:

- Adhesion with the bowel, omentum, and broad ligament is a common problem especially in a twisted cyst. It can be encountered during laparotomy.
- *Management*: In majority of the cases, adhesions can be separated by gentle dissection and ovariotomy becomes possible. In rare instances where adhesiolysis may injure the important structure due to dense adhesion removal of cyst content with removal of capsules as far as possible or marsupialization of the cyst is done. Hemorrhage is secured in every case. Help of general surgeon is always sought for.

MANAGEMENT OF A CASE OF BENIGN OVARIAN CYST AND TUMOR

Q. How will you manage a case of benign ovarian cyst and tumor?

Once ovarian neoplasm is diagnosed, treatment is surgical removal.

Depending upon the type and bilaterality of the tumor and the patient's profile (age, parity, future fertility desire), it may be:

- Cystectomy
- Oophorectomy or salpingo-oophorectomy
- Total hysterectomy and bilateral salpingo-oophorectomy.
  Commonly, it is done by laparotomy.

Now, laparoscopic removal of benign ovarian tumor has been accepted as a standard acceptable procedure.

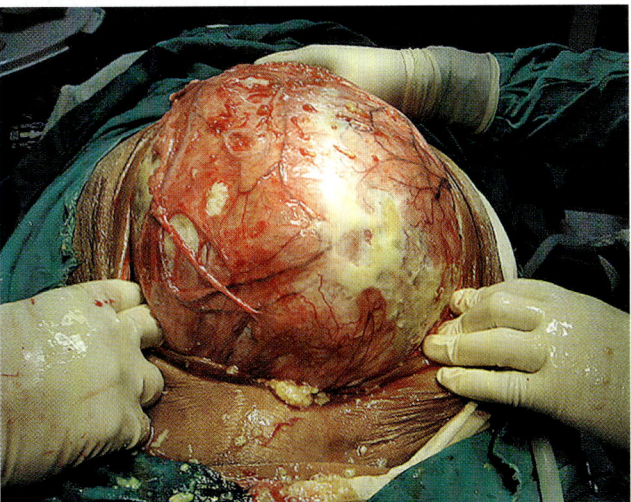

Fig. 24: Ruptured ovarian cyst showing mucinous materials coming out (laparotomy finding—old partial rupture).

Ovarian cystectomy (Figs. 25 to 27):

- Enucleation of cyst retaining the healthy ovarian tissue **(Fig. 26)**.
- *Indication*: Young woman desiring fertility having unilateral benign cyst—serous cystadenoma, mucinous cystadenoma, and dermoid cyst.
- *Procedure*: With light and gentle incision, enucleation of cyst **(Fig. 25)** is done and bed is repaired with complete hemostasis.

Oophorectomy or salpingo-oophorectomy (see Figs. 14, 29 and 30):

- Removal of ovarian tumor with the affected ovary.
- *Indication*: Large benign ovarian tumor or benign ovarian cyst where cystectomy is difficult to do like in torsion of ovarian cyst.
- Steps—*see* below.
- Removal of healthy or unhealthy ovary is called "oophorectomy". Previously, removal of diseased

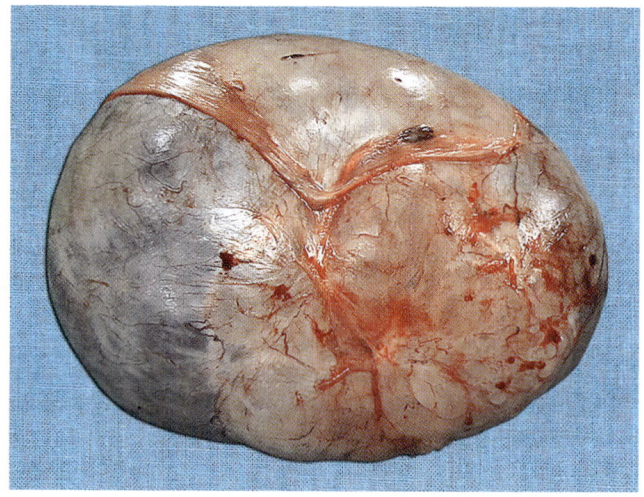

Fig. 27: Ovarian cyst following cystectomy.

ovary was meant to say "ovariotomy", but now the term "ovariotomy" is rarely used. When fallopian tube is also removed it is called salpingo-oophorectomy.

Total hysterectomy and bilateral salpingo-oophorectomy (Figs. 28A and B):

- Removal of uterus, bilateral tubes, and ovaries including the tumor on one or of both sides.
- *Indication*: Peri- or postmenopausal women, bilateral tumor or in case of suspected malignancy.

STEPS OF LAPAROTOMY IN A CASE OF OVARIAN TUMOR

Q. Tell the steps of laparotomy in a case of ovarian tumor.

- Preoperative check-up done by anesthesiologist clinically and from investigation reports.
- Patient in supine position.
- Catheterization done.
- Antiseptic dressing and draping done.

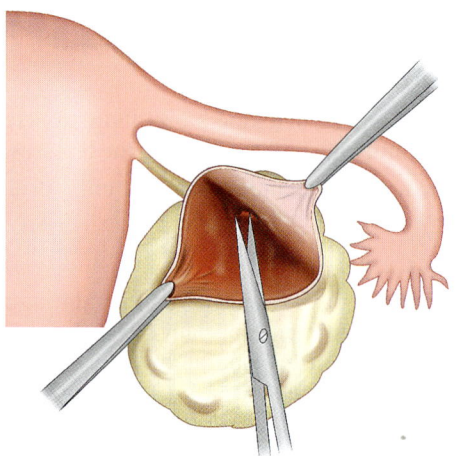

Fig. 25: Ovarian cystectomy.

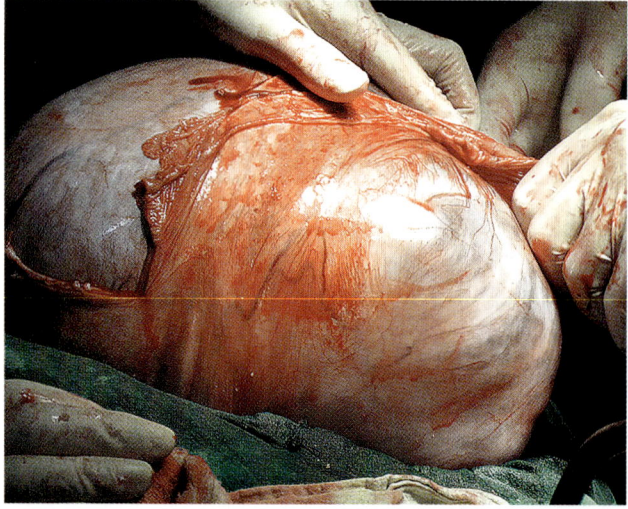

Fig. 26: Large serous cystadenoma on the process of enucleation (cystectomy) in a 31-year-old nulliparous woman clinically seems to be benign in nature.

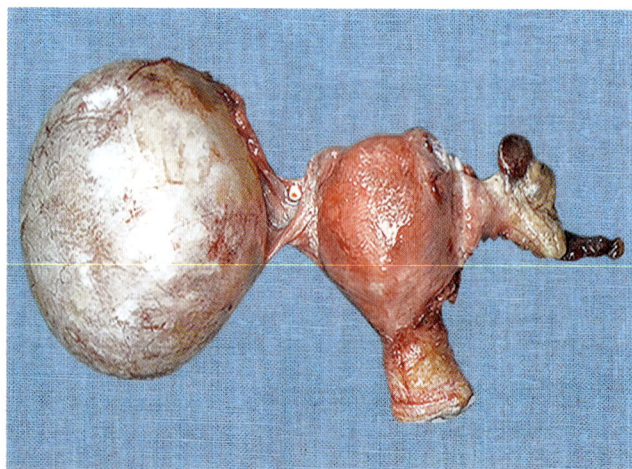

Fig. 28A: Specimen of total hysterectomy with bilateral salpingo-oophorectomy (TAH with BSO) in a left-sided ovarian cyst in postmenopausal woman (even in benign tumor TAH with BSO is the treatment of choice in postmenopausal age).

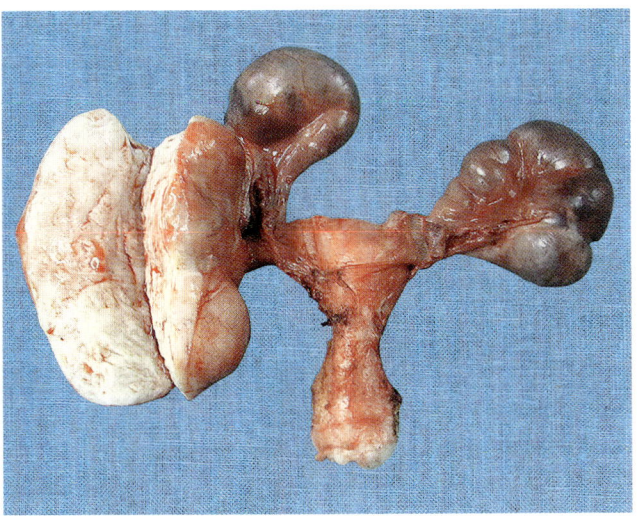

Fig. 28B: Specimen of total hysterectomy with bilateral salpingo-oophorectomy (TAH with BSO) in a right-sided ovarian tumor (fibroma) with bilateral hydrosalpinx in a 45-year-old woman.

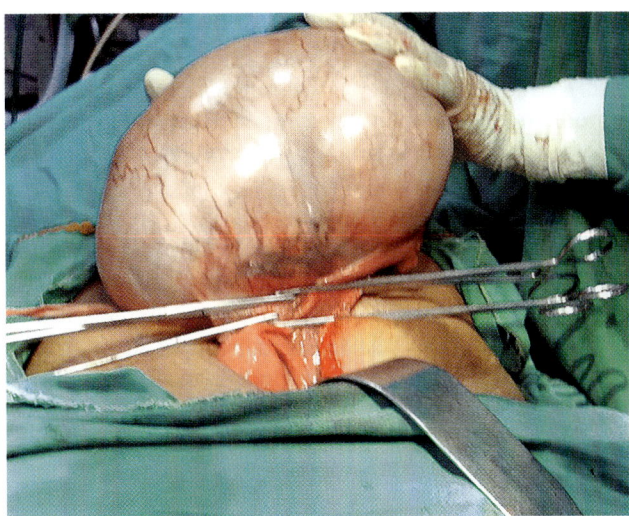

Fig. 30: Clamping of ovarian pedicle (ovarian ligament, mesovarium, and infundibulopelvic ligament from medial to lateral) for salpingo-oophorectomy in left-sided ovarian tumor.

- Midline or paramedian longitudinal incision is done from umbilicus to symphysis pubis and may be extended above the umbilicus depending upon the size of the tumor, *principle is that ovarian cyst is not ruptured during removal*. Skin, subcutaneous tissue, and the rectus sheath are cut; rectus muscle separated, extraperitoneal tissue and parietal peritoneum are cut to open the abdomen. There is no posterior layer of rectus sheath below the umbilicus.
- If ascitic fluid is present fluid is collected for cytological and biochemical examination. If not present peritoneal washing with 100 cc of normal saline is done and collected.
- The tumor mass is thoroughly assessed and opposite adnexa is examined. Under surface of diaphragm, superior surface of liver, parieties, paracolic gutter, intestines, and whole abdomen were explored for presence of any deposits and metastasis which are unlikely in benign disease. Lymph nodes are palpated for any enlargement.
- Decision of extent of surgery is taken. If there is torsion of tumor, it is untwisted slowly and if there is adhesion with the adjacent structures, it is gently separated. If densely adhered, assistance of general surgeon is sought for.
- Following definitive surgery, complete hemostasis is done and abdomen is closed in layers. (For more of detailed surgical staging of ovarian cancer *see* later in Page 69).

Q. How would you clamp the pedicle in oophorectomy or salpingo-oophorectomy?

- The pedicle of ovarian tumor contains ovarian ligament, mesovarium and infundibulopelvic ligament containing ovarian vessels **(Figs. 29 and 30)**.
- The pedicle is clamped in two halves—medially ovarian ligament, fallopian tube, laterally the infundibulopelvic ligament and in the middle part mesovarium by pair of two clamps **(Figs. 29 and 30)**.
- On the side of the tumor another two pairs of clamps are put and pedicle is incised in between the clamps and tumor with whole ovaries and fallopian tube are removed **(Fig. 30)**. The clamps are separated after transfixation suture with absorbable sutures commonly with 1-0 Vicryl.

Q. During oophorectomy fallopian tube should be removed or not?

Present opinion is that fallopian tube should be removed with neoplastic ovary provided the other tube is healthy where fertility is a concern. *Many high-grade serous cyst adenocarcinomas which were thought to be arisen from ovary or peritoneum are now believed to take origin from fallopian tube fimbriae* (*see* later).

Bilateral salpingectomy performed along with other procedure to reduce high-grade serous cystadenoma is called *opportunistic salpingectomy*.

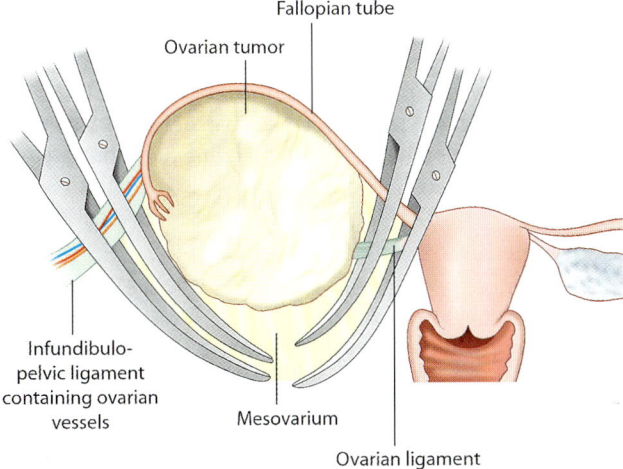

Fig. 29: Pedicle of ovarian tumor—ovarian ligament, fallopian tube, mesovarium, and infundibulopelvic ligament from medial to lateral.

Q. Is there any role of conservative (expectant) management in ovarian cyst?

In all cases of functional cysts which occur in prepubertal and reproductive age women expectant management is the rule.

In **postmenopausal women**, expectant management can be done in following circumstances:
* Cyst diameter is less than 5 cm
* Cyst is unilocular, and thin walled by USG
* CA 125 level—normal
* Close follow-up
* No increase of cyst size during follow-up.

American College of Obstetricians and Gynecologists (ACOG) (2013) states that simple thin-walled cyst up to 10 cm size can safely be followed up by sonographic surveillance even in postmenopausal women.

OVARIAN CANCER

Q. What is true about epithelial ovarian cancer (EOC)?

* Deaths from ovarian cancer are more than the combined deaths of all other gynecological malignancies. Ovarian cancer is the fifth leading cause of death from all cancers
* Ovarian malignancy (all varieties) is the second most common gynecological malignancy next to cancer cervix (in India) and fifth cause of malignancy in female.
* Epithelial ovarian cancer comprises 90–95% of all ovarian malignancies. Malignant germ cell tumors and sex cord—stromal tumors contribute less than 5% cases.
* Of ovarian malignancy cases only 1% occurs in childhood and adolescent and the most common variety of malignant ovarian tumor in this age group is germ cell tumor.
* More than 50% of epithelial cancers are serous type, endometrioid 15–20%, mucinous 5–10%, clear cell 5–10%, transitional (Brenner) below 1%, and undifferentiated below 1%.
* Only 25% EOC are diagnosed in Stage 1 disease with excellent survival.
* Two-thirds of EOC are diagnosed in advanced stage with poor prognosis. Reasons are asymptomatic in early stages and there is no effective screening strategy till date.
* In Stage 1A, or Stage 1B, grade 1 and 2 EOC only surgery is adequate. Other cases surgery plus chemotherapy for 3–6 courses are needed (*see* below). Aggressive debulking with chemotherapy results clinical remission in advanced stages. Chemotherapy of choice is combination of carboplatin and paclitaxel in epithelial carcinoma (whereas in germ cell tumor BEP regime—bleomycin, etoposide, and cisplatin are preferred).
* Relapse occurs in 90% cases in advanced EOC.
* Overall 5-year survival of all stages of EOC is 45% whereas those of uterine cancer is 85%, and cervical cancer is 75%.

In macroscopic appearance, there is no such gross difference among the different varieties of epithelial cancers. Each has solid and cystic components.

Q. Why death from ovarian cancer is so high in comparison to other genital malignancies?

* Asymptomatic in nature in early stage.
* When it is diagnosed, it is almost in advanced stage.
* Only 25% of all ovarian cancers are diagnosed in early stage and 75% in advanced stage.
* There is no standard method of screening like cancer cervix.
* Rapid spread of the diseases.
* High recurrence (90%) in advance disease.

SCREENING OF OVARIAN CANCER

Q. How will you screen ovarian cancer?

There is no routine standard method of screening strategy of ovarian cancer. Screening procedure involves the following components.

Detection of high-risk women: Most important risk factors are: (1) *BRCA1* or *BRCA2* carriers and (2) strong family history of breast and ovarian cancer. Others are given below:
* Serum markers CA 125
* Transvaginal sonography
* Pelvic examinations
* CA125 and ROCA. CA125 singly is a poor marker for ovarian cancer detection. ROCA which is based on the slope of CA125 with serial screening, if exceeds 1% there is risk of ovarian cancer.

Risk factors for ovarian cancer:
* White women
* History of breast cancer(own)
* Family history—breast cancer and ovarian cancer
* Nulliparity—H/O Infertility
* Early menarche
* Increasing age up to mid-70s.
* *Genetic*: (a) Mutation of *BRCA1* (80%) and *BRCA2* (15%) genes—10–15% of epithelial cancer has genetic link. (b) Inherited deleterious mutation in *BRCA1* and *BRCA2* major genetic risk factor. (c) Lynch syndrome is **hereditary nonpolyposis colorectal cancer (HNPCC)** and is associated with endometrial cancer and 10% risk of ovarian cancer and (d) low to moderate penetrance genes.
* Late menopause
* PID
* Endometriosis
* Postmenopausal hormone therapy (Schorge, 2010)
* High fat diet.
* Regular use of perineal talc.

Ovarian cancer is reduced in:
* Late menarche
* Early menopause
* Multiparity
* Hysterectomy and tubal ligation

- Low fat and high-fibre diet.
- Oral contraceptive—decreases ovarian cancer by 50%.
- Breastfeeding more than 1 and half year.
- IUCD reduces reduce risk of ovarian cancer.

GENETIC TESTING IN OVARIAN CANCER AND ITS UTILITY

BRCA mutation testing or multi-gene panel testing are the two genetic testing for hereditary breast and ovarian cancer syndrome. Multi-gene panel includes *BRCA and other genetic mutations.* Genetic testing helps to identify women with deleterious mutations and guides for prophylactic surgery to prevent ovarian cancer.

Q. What is *BRCA1* and *BRCA2* genes?

These are tumor-supressor genes that produce two proteins *BRCA1* and *BRCA2*. These two proteins do DNA repair by homologous recombination (HR) to maintain intact chromosomal structure. Mutation of these *BRCA1* and *BRCA2* genes lead to dysfunction of *BRCA1* and *BRCA2* proteins which cause genetic instability resulting more risk of malignant transformation.

Role of Prophylactic Surgery

- Routine oophorectomy is not recommended to prevent ovarian Clinical trial is going on to determine prophylactic salpingectomy- delayed oophorectomy
- However, in *BRCA1* or *BRCA2* carriers prophylactic bilateral salpingo-oophorectomy (BSO) is effective in preventing ovarian cancer in 90% cases. In HNPCC, it is 100%. Prophylactic BSO should be offered to women with BRCA1 carriers in age group 35-40 years and for BRCA2 carriers BSO is recommended between 40-45 years and for other HR deficiency (BRIP1, RAD51C) carriers BSO is recommended in age group 45-50 years women (ACOG 2017).
- *Many high-grade serous cyst adenocarcinomas which were thought to be arisen from ovary or peritoneum are now believed to take origin from fallopian tube fimbriae. For which, during oophorectomy, fallopian tubes are also removed.*
- It is also postulated that prophylactic BSO reduces the breast CA in 50% cases and TAH-BSO reduces the chance of endometrial CA in women with HNPCC.
- *Opportunistic bilateral salpingectomy* is considered along with other gynaecologic procedure or in place of tubal ligation to reduce high-grade serous cystadenoma (ACOG 2019).

Q. Suppose you found one woman who has family history of ovarian cancer. What will be your approach?

- Refer the woman to genetic clinic for assessment of family tree.
- Hereditary cancer genetic testing for *BRCA1* and *BRCA2* genes.
- Screening the women over the age of 35 years by TVS and CA 125.
- Prophylactic salpingo-oophorectomy has role in women who have completed family and genetic history.

TYPES AND PATHOLOGY OF OVARIAN CANCER

Histologically, tumors are categorised as benign, borderline, or malignant. According to WHO ovarian carcinoma is classified histologically as:
- Serous adenocarcinoma (>50%)
- Endometrioid adenocarcinoma (15–20%)
- Mucinous adenocarcinoma (5–10%)
- Clear cell adenocarcinoma (5–10%)
- Transitional cell carcinoma (<5%)
- Malignant Brenner tumor
- Squamous cell carcinoma—rare
- Mixed epithelial and mesenchymal [adenocarcinoma and carcinosarcoma (<1%)]—highly aggressive
- Small cell carcinoma—rare
- Undifferentiated carcinoma—rare

Pathogenesis

The postulated theory for development of epithelial cancer is that the ovarian carcinogenesis occurs by two ways:

1. Type I: The first postulation is that tumor develops from either benign extraovarian lesions that incorporate into ovary and transformed into malignant change or from the surface epithelium of ovary which is entrapped in the cortex of the ovary. Subsequently, metaplastic changes occur in those entrapped tissue in the cortex resulting formation of endometrioid, mucinous or low grade serous carcinoma and malignant Brenner tumor. They tumors usually present as unilateral, large cystic tumor without ascites and less virulent.

2. Type II: High grade serous carcinomas arise from the fallopian tube fimbria contradicting the previous theory that they arise from the ovarian or peritoneal surfaces. This group is more common. Serous tubal intraepithelial carcinoma (STIC) occurs first which is followed by development of ovarian carcinoma after several years, but with rapid metastasis. In 50% of these cancers mutation of the genes is involved in the HR pathway of DNA repair particularly BRCA1 and BRCA2. High grade serous tumours are very aggressive and responsible for 90% of deaths from ovarian cancer.

Pathology of Individual Ovarian Cancers

Serous adenocarcinoma: These are most common varieties (>50%) of all ovarian cancers. Low grade serous carcinoma is characterized by well differentiated pattern resembling epithelium of fallopian tube. High grade neoplasms are characterized by solid sheets of cells, nuclear pleomorphism and mitotic activity. **Psammoma bodies** are present in 80% cases of serous carcinoma and pathognomonic. These tumors need grading.

Endometrioid adenocarcinoma (Fig. 31): It is the second most common variety. Endometrial tumor demonstrates all

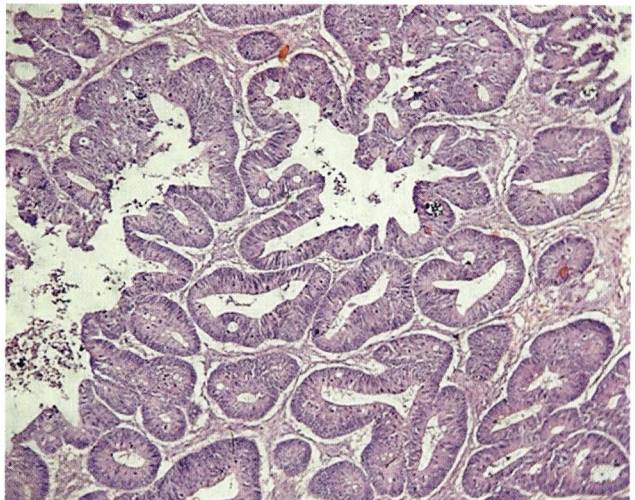

Fig. 31: Microphotography of endometrioid adenocarcinoma ovary (H&E, X400).
Courtesy: Professor Gopinath Barui, Department of Pathology

the features of endometriosis. The malignant potentiality of endometriosis is low though transition may occur from ovarian endometriosis. It is characterized by markedly glandular pattern resembling variations of epithelia found in the uterus. It is associated with endometrial adenocarcinoma in 15–20% case for which it is called 'synchronous' tumor. They may be associated with pelvic endometriosis.

Mucinous adenocarcinoma: Confined to the ovary in more than 90% cases and bilateral in 8–10% cases. Histology resembles mucin secreting adenocarcinoma of intestine or endocervix in well differentiated cases. As most of the ovarian metastatic mucinous carcinomas contain enteric-type cells it is difficult to differentiate from the metastasis from GI tract on the basis of histology only and clinical corelation is needed. Primary ovarian neoplasms rarely metastasize to the mucosa of bowel, but involve the serosa. On the other hand the metastasis occurs more commonly from the bowel to ovary. **Pseudomyxoma peritonei** (*see* Page 58) are almost metastatic than primary as ovarian mucinous carcinoma with ascites rarely develops this. Hence in presence of pseudomyxoma peritonei appendix or other intestinal source is to be excluded. Appendicectomy and histological evaluation is indicated in presence of pseudomyxoma peritonei. *Disseminated peritoneal adenomucinosis* is said when when peritoneal epithelial cells look benign or borderline.

Clear cell adenocarcinoma: This is most frequently associated with pelvic endometriosis. These tumors are typically limited to ovary and surgery alone is sufficient. But in advance disease prognosis is poor. Clear and hobnail cells are present which project their nuclei into atypical cytoplasm. As high-grade nuclei are invariably present it cannot be graded.

Transitional cell carcinoma: Transitiona cell carcinoma is referred to primary ovarian carcinoma resembling primary bladder carcinoma. This is considered as high grade serous carcinoma but has better prognosis.

Malignant Brenner tumor: Very rare tumors containing benign Brenner or borderline Brenner tumor coexisting with transitional cell carcinoma. They carry a better prognosis than pure transitional cells carcinoma.

Primary squamous cell carcinoma of ovary is extremely uncommon and has poor prognosis. Squamous cell carcinoma may arise from dermoid cyst and is under malignant germ cell tumor. Metastasis from cervical carcinoma may also occur. Small cell carcinomas are highly malignant, but very rare.

Undifferentiated carcinomas are poorly differentiated and cannot to be categorized into a group. They are very rare and carry poor prognosis.

Primary Peritoneal Cancer

Peritoneal cancers are indistinguishable from ovarian and fallopian cancers histologically. Of the typically described epithelial cancers at least 15% are primary peritoneal carcinomas which arise from the peritoneal lining of pelvis or abdomen. The ovaries must be normal or less involved, instead uterosacral ligament, pelvic peritoneum and omentum are found involved. The extraovarian size involvement will be larger than the involvement of the surface of the ovary. Primary peritoneal carcinoma may arise many years after bilateral salpingo-opherectomy. Histologically, peritoneal carcinoma is mostly papillary serous carcinoma, moderately to poorly differentiated. Clinical behavior, staging, treatment and prognosis are like those of epithelial ovarian carcinoma.

DIAGNOSIS AND INVESTIGATIONS OF OVARIAN CANCER

Q. Diagnosis and investigations of ovarian cancer (*see* also benign vs malignant as written above (Page 51).

- From the history and clinical examination.
- **Investigations**: By USG with color Doppler, X-ray of chest, CT scan, MRI, and PET scan.
- Measurement of tumor marker.
- Cytology and biopsy
- From surgical findings.
- To be confirmed by histopathology.

History of malignant ovarian tumor:

Age of patient— though no age is bar, malignancy commonly occurs in aged women or in young adolescent. Average age is 55-60 years.

Medical history: Possible risk factors, h/o other cancers and h/o cancer in the family.

Symptoms

Ovarian cancer lacks specific symptoms and signs in early stage for which it is diagnosed late. Though symptoms develop for several months these are like mostly common problems occurring normally like gastrointestinal symptoms indigestion, bloating, etc. The symptoms which occur in ovarian malignancy are as follows:

- Abdominal distension, feeling of lump, pain and discomfort of abdomen, anorexia, indigestion, nausea, vomiting, bloating, sometime features of subacute intestinal obstruction, constipation, back pain, and urinary urgency.
- Duration—rapid increase of tumor.
- Weight—rapid loss of weight occurs in malignant ovarian tumor.

Physical examination:
- Typical ovarian cachexia, emaciated body **(Fig. 32A)**, and anemia are characteristic of malignancy.
- Virchow's gland (left supraclavicular lymph nodes) may be palpable in malignancy. There may be lump in breasts.
- Examination of chest for pleural effusion. Its presence indicates malignancy.
- Leg edema and varicosity.

Abdominal examination (Fig. 32B):
- Swelling is solid or variegated, may be bilateral, irregular surface, ill-defined margin and mobility restricted in malignancy. Upper abdominal mass may be due to omental cake of advanced malignancy.
- Ascites is almost invariably present in ovarian malignancy.
- Liver may be enlarged.
- An umbilical nodule may be rarely palpable in umbilicus indicating spread from infraumbilical malignancy

Bimanual examination:
- A pelvi-abdominal mass is palpable separately from the uterus.
- There may be nodules in POD and mobility of tumor is restricted.

Rectal and rectovaginal examination: This is to detect nodules in POD, and involvement of uterosacral ligament and rectovaginal septum.

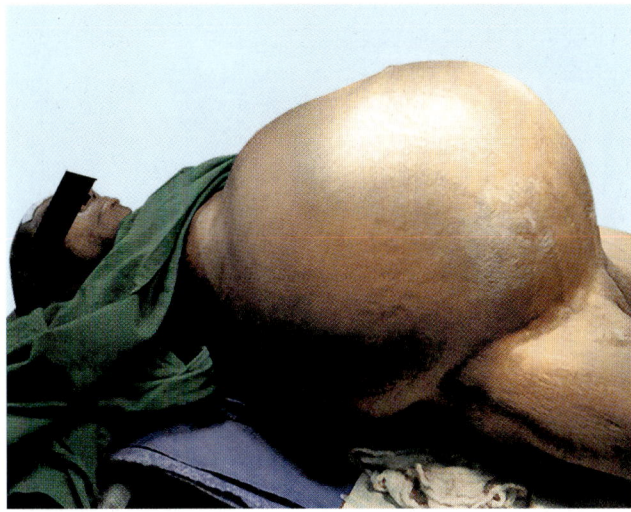

Fig. 32B: Hugely distended abdomen with lump and ascites—laparotomy showed malignant ovarian tumor.
Courtesy: Dr Shyamal Dasgupta, Associate Professor, Obstetrics and Gynecology

Investigations:
- Laboratory: Complete blood count, electrolytes, LFT, Kidney function test. There may be thrombocytosis and low serum sodium.
- Tumor markers CA 125, CA19-9, HE4CEA, (*see* details in Pages 51 and 52).
- Imaging **(Figs. 33 to 36)**: (a) X-ray of chest for pleural effusion and for metastasis, (b) USG, (c) CT scan, MRI, and PET. Barium enema may be helpful to detect colon cancer, diverticular disease and rectosigmoid involvement in cancer ovary. For TVS finding *see* Page 50 and role of CT, MRI *see* Page 51.
- RMI scoring, OVA1 panel, ROMA, and ROCA.
- Paracentesis of ascitic fluid.
- Fine needle aspiration cytology (FNAC) (doubtful value).

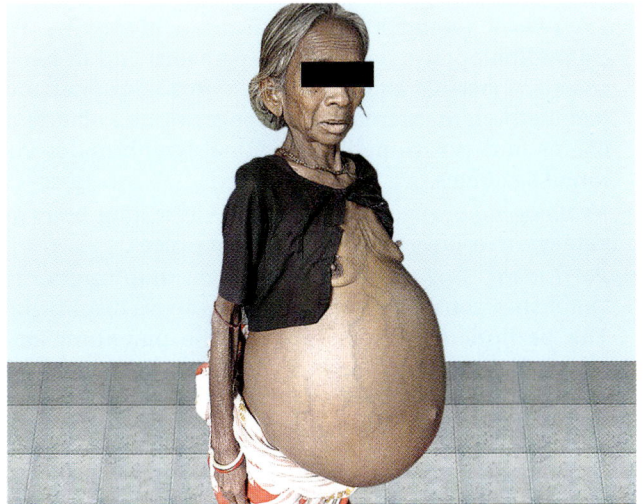

Fig. 32A: Ovarian cachexia with hugely enlarged abdomen with prominent veins over abdomen in a 63-year-old woman— features suspicious of malignancy.

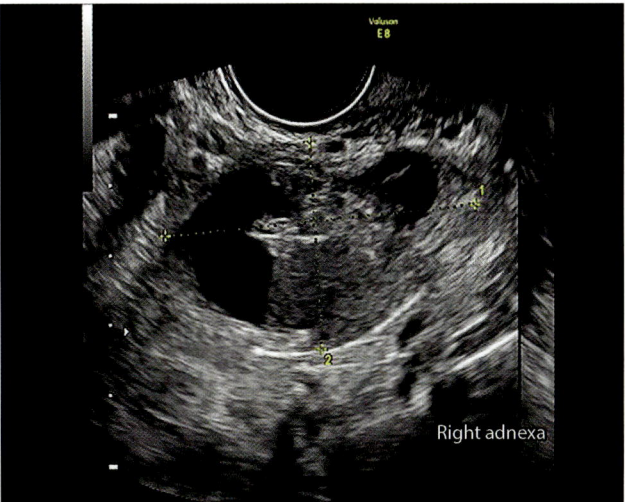

Fig. 33: Sonography showing ovarian tumor with solid and cystic areas suggestive of malignancy.
Courtesy: Professor Kamal Oswal, Department of Radiodiagnosis, VIMS, Kolkata

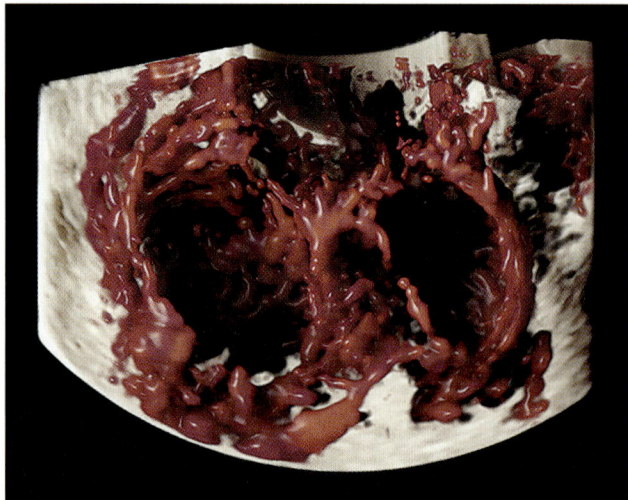

Fig. 34: 3D image of ovarian tumor showing vascularity indicating malignancy.
Courtesy: Professor Kamal Oswal, Department of Radiodiagnosis, VIMS, Kolkata

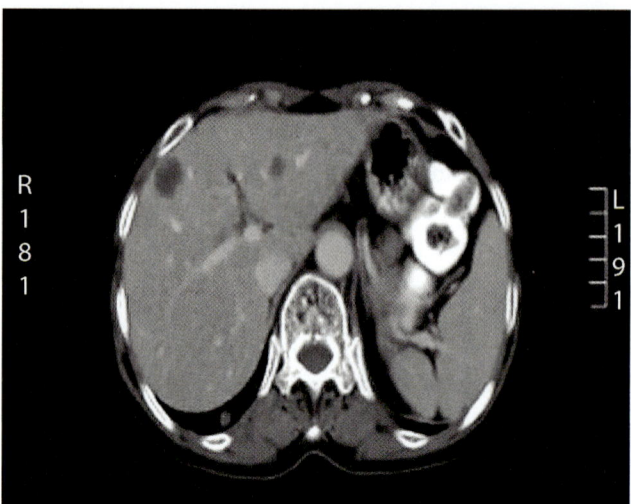

Fig. 36: CT scan of abdomen showing hepatic metastasis in malignant ovarian tumor.
Courtesy: Professor Kamal Oswal, Department of Radiodiagnosis, VIMS, Kolkata

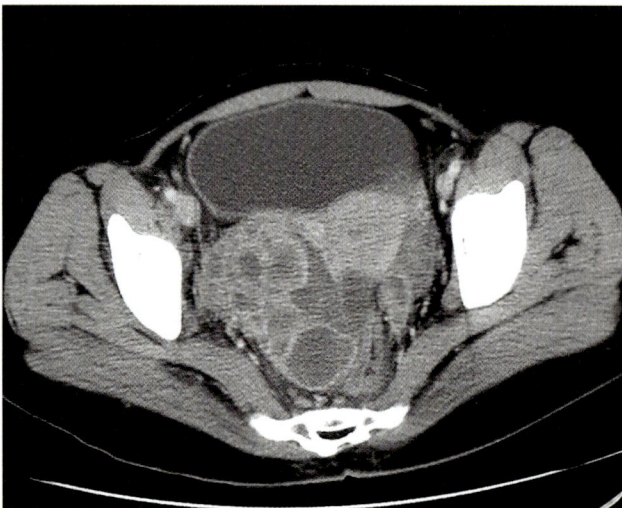

Fig. 35: CT scan of pelvis showing ovarian tumor with septation suggestive of malignancy.
Courtesy: Professor Kamal Oswal, Department of Radiodiagnosis, VIMS, Kolkata

- Upper GI and lower GI endoscopy and stool for occult blood test.
- Mammography.

Cytology and Biopsy
- *FNAC*: FNAC is still not universally accepted due to its diagnostic inaccuracy, dissemination of malignant cells with the rupture of cyst. However, due to its low risk of complication and detection of malignant cell without major surgery it is advised in many settings.
- *TRU-Cut biopsy or core biopsy*: Core biopsy from the metastatic or primary growth is indicated before starting neoadjuvant therapy where primary surgery is not possible either in medically compromised patient or inoperable growth in preoperative assessment and FNAC inconclusive.
- *Paracentesis and cytological diagnosis*: Often nonspecific and there is chance of metastasis in abdominal wall at needle entry site. Suggested in presence of ascites and absence of a pelvic mass. However, biochemical test of ascitic fluid may gives clue to diagnosis of abdominal tuberculosis. It has added advantage of volume reduction and relieve of symptoms.
- *Histopathological diagnosis including frozen section biopsy.*

ROUTE OF SPREAD OF EPITHELIAL OVARIAN CANCERS

- *Direct spread* to pelvic peritoneum, adjacent structures like uterus, fallopian tubes, rectum, and sigmoid colon.
- *Exfoliation* from the surface of capsule of tumor and implants metastasize in peritoneal cavity, omentum, diaphragm, and intestines. Epithelial ovarian cancers mostly, especially serous tumors metastasise by exfoliation.
- *Lymphatic spread* along the ovarian blood vessels (infundibulopelvic ligament) to paraaortic up to renal vessels. Others go laterally through broad ligament and parametrium to external iliac, hypogastric and obturator chains and occasionally to inguinal lymph nodes via round ligaments.
- *Hematogenous* spread to distal organs liver, lung, brain or kidneys in recurrent and most advance cases.
- *Peritoneal surfaces* drain through diaphragmatic lymphatics, thus major venous vessels above diaphragm. The peritoneum which includes the omentum and abdominal viscera is the most common site for spread of ovarian and fallopian tube cancers. This includes the diaphragmatic and liver surfaces.

Q. What is the reason of ascites and pleural effusion in ovarian malignancy?

Ascites is due to excessive production of fluid from cancer cells and also obstruction of lymph channels resulting less clearance. Malignant pleural effusion is due to passage of fluid through diaphragm.

STAGES OF OVARIAN CANCER

Q. What are the different stages of ovarian cancer?

International Federation of Gynecology and Obstetrics (FIGO) ovarian cancer staging, 2014 (Fig. 37) which has revised the staging of ovarian cancer **incorporating ovarian, fallopian tube, and peritoneal cancer** into the same system.

Staging of cancer ovary is surgical, done according to findings during surgery before removal.

Broad FIGO (2014) staging of the ovary, fallopian tube and primary peritoneal carcinoma

Stage I: Tumor confined to ovaries.

Stage II: Tumor involves one or both ovaries or fallopian tubes with pelvic extension (below the pelvic brim) or primary peritoneal cancer.

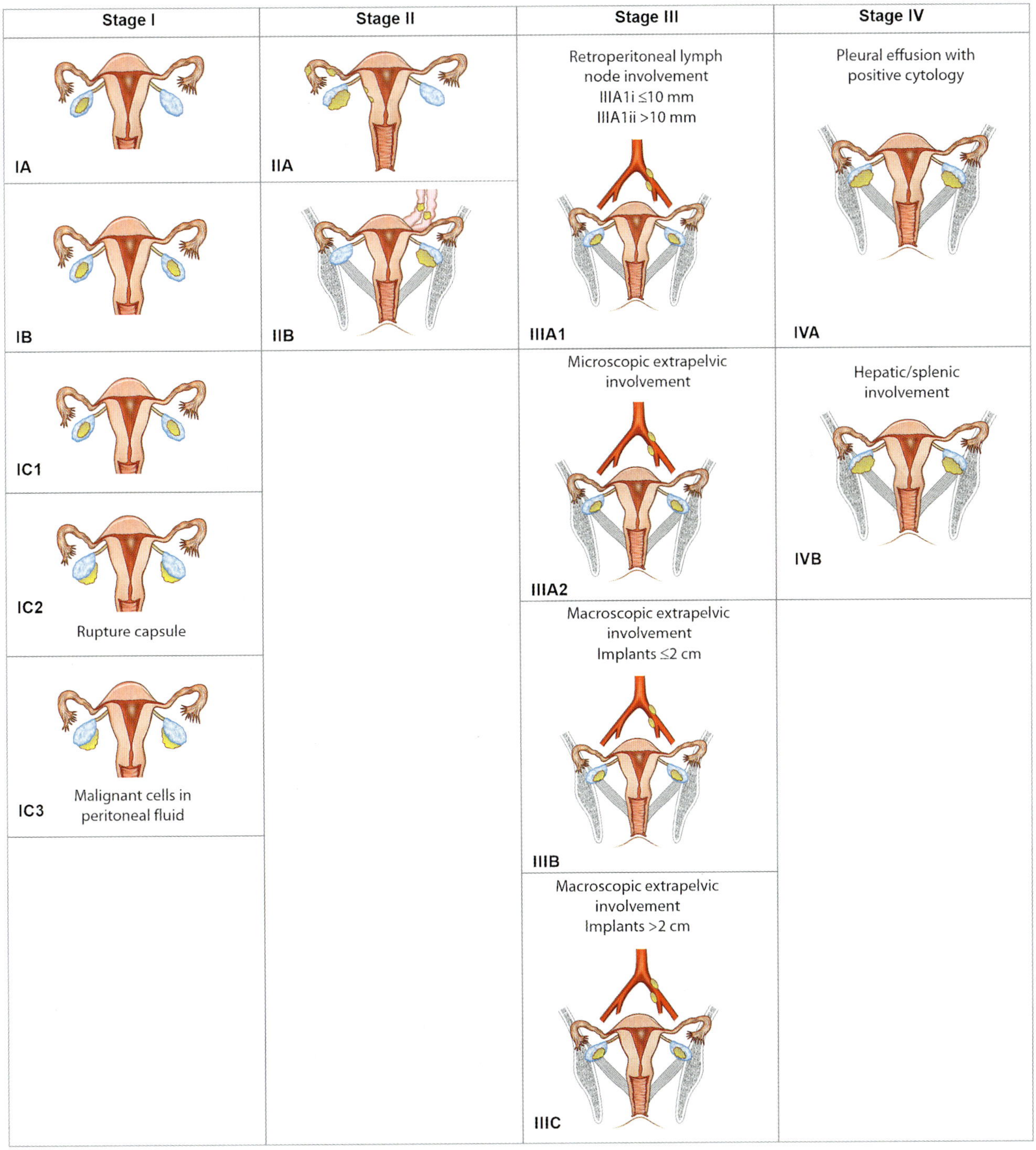

Fig. 37: Ovarian cancer staging (FIGO 2014).

Stage III: Tumor involves one or both ovaries or fallopian tubes or peritoneal cancer with cytologically or histologically confirmed spread to the peritoneum outside the pelvis and/or metastasis to the retroperitoneal lymph nodes.

Stage IV: Distant metastasis excluding peritoneal metastasis.

FIGO (2014) staging of the ovary, fallopian tube and primary peritoneal carcinoma **(Fig. 37)** are given in **Table 3** in detail.

Other major recommendations (FIGO 2014) are as follows:
- Histologic type including grading should be designated at staging.
- Primary site (ovary, fallopian tube or peritoneum) should be designated where possible.
- Tumors that may otherwise qualify for Stage I but involved with dense adhesions justify upgrading to Stage II if tumor cells are histologically proven to be present in the adhesions.

GRADINGS OF OVARIAN MALIGNANCY

Malignant tumors are graded as well differentiated (grade 1), moderately differentiated (grade 2) and poorly differentiated (grade 3). Only in early-stage disease of ovarian cancer grade has important prognostic factor.

Accordingly, it is also called low grade serous cancer (LGSC) and high grade serous ovarian cancer (HGSOC). The grading system is not applied for nonepithelial tumor.

According to FIGO staging two-third of patients are detected in advanced stage disease (stage III and stage IV) and one third in early stage (stage I and stage II) disease. In one study of 4,825 cases stage I was found to be in 28% cases, stage II in 8%, stage III in 50% and stage IV in 13% cases (FIGO annual report, 2006).

Q. Which stages are called early ovarian cancer and which are advanced ovarian cancer?
- *Early ovarian cancer*: Stage I and stage II—comprises one-third of cases.
- *Advanced ovarian cancer*: Stage III and stage IV—two-thirds of cases.

MANAGEMENT OF EARLY-STAGE AND ADVANCED OVARIAN CANCER

Q. Outline the management of early-stage ovarian cancer and advanced ovarian cancer.

Principle:
- All established cases of malignant or suspected malignancy of ovarian mass primary aim is to do surgery.
- *During surgery*:
  - Accurate surgical staging is done and
  - Primary surgery is performed.

Table 3: Staging of the ovary, fallopian tube and primary peritoneal carcinoma (FIGO 2014).

Stage I: Tumor confined to ovaries	
IA	Tumor limited to one ovary, capsule intact, no tumor on surface, and negative washings
IB	Tumor involves both ovaries (or both tubes) otherwise like IA
IC	Tumor limited to one or both ovaries (or tubes) with any of the followings:
IC1	Surgical spill
IC2	Capsule rupture before surgery or tumor on ovarian or fallopian tube surface
IC3	Malignant cells in the ascites or peritoneal washings
Stage II: Tumor involves one or both ovaries or fallopian tubes with pelvic extension (below the pelvic brim) or primary peritoneal cancer	
IIA	Extension and/or implant on uterus and/or fallopian tubes and/or ovaries
IIB	Extension to other pelvic intraperitoneal tissues
Stage III: Tumor involves one or both ovaries or fallopian tubes or peritoneal cancer with cytologically or histologically confirmed spread to the peritoneum outside the pelvis and/or metastasis to the retroperitoneal lymph nodes	
IIIA	Positive retroperitoneal lymph nodes and/or microscopic metastasis beyond the pelvis
IIIA1	Positive retroperitoneal lymph nodes only IIIA1 (i) Metastasis ≤10 mm IIIA1 (ii) Metastasis >10 mm
IIIA2	Microscopic, extrapelvic (above the brim) peritoneal involvement ± positive retroperitoneal lymph nodes
IIIB	Macroscopic, extrapelvic, peritoneal metastasis ≤2 cm ± positive retroperitoneal lymph nodes. Includes extension to capsule of liver or spleen
IIIC	Macroscopic, extrapelvic, peritoneal metastasis >2 cm ± positive retroperitoneal lymph nodes. Includes extension to capsule of liver or spleen
Stage IV: Distant metastasis excluding peritoneal metastasis	
IVA	Pleural effusion with positive cytology
IVB	Hepatic and/or splenic parenchymal metastasis, metastasis to extra-abdominal organs (including inguinal lymph nodes and lymph nodes outside of the abdominal cavity)

Removal of lymph nodes is important in staging and its effect on survival benefit is controversial.

- Following surgery need of *chemotherapy (adjuvant)* and duration of chemotherapy is determined by the stage of the disease.
- Chemotherapy of choice is combination of carboplatin and paclitaxel and of 3–6 months duration.
- *Neoadjuvant chemotherapy* (preoperative) is given either in (1) medically compromised patient or (2) inoperable growth or anticipated incomplete removal in preoperative assessment after cytological diagnosis.

STEPS OF SURGICAL STAGING (FIGS. 38 TO 42)

Q. What are the steps of surgical staging (Figs. 38 to 41)?

- Large longitudinal incision is given.
- Ascitic fluid or in its absence peritoneal washing (100 cc) is collected.
- All peritoneal surfaces, parities and intestines, colon, paracolic gutter, under surface of diaphragm and capsules of liver including superior surface, omentum, and retroperitoneal areas are thoroughly inspected and palpated in systematic manner.
- In addition to suspicious sites peritoneal scraping and biopsies are taken randomly from peritoneal surface of bladder, POD, paracolic gutter, both pelvic walls and subdiaphragmatic surfaces.
- If ovary is primary tumor surface is examined for capsule rupture.
- Total hysterectomy with bilateral salpingo-oophorectomy is usually done.
- Infracolic omentectomy (if not possible biopsy is taken).
- Pelvic and para-aortic lymphadenectomy **(Fig. 39B)** done.
- Appendicectomy for mucinous cystadenoma.
  Fertility sparing surgery—unilateral adnexectomy is done in young and Stage 1A disease (*see* later).

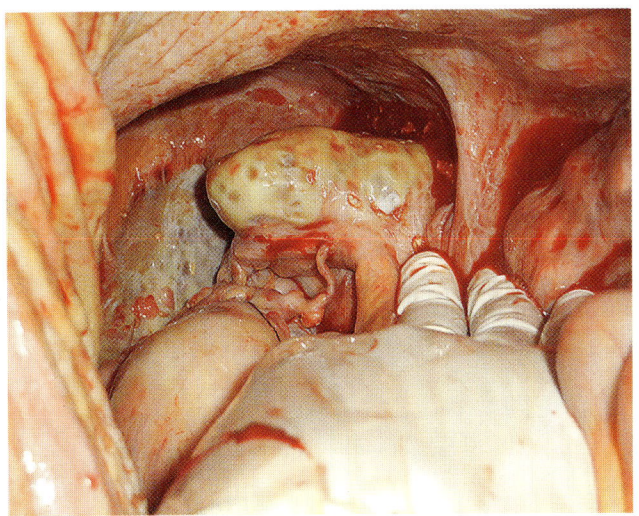

Fig. 39A: Metastasis over peritoneum, liver, and over inferior surface of diaphragm in advanced epithelial carcinoma.

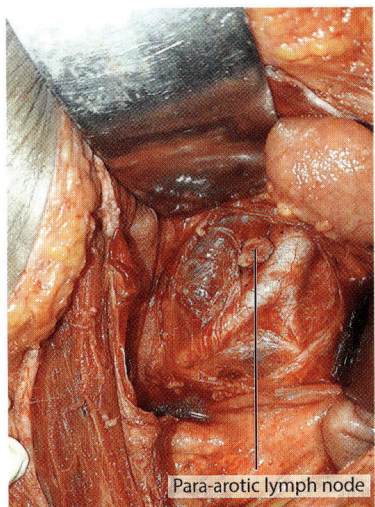

Fig. 39B: Para-aortic lymph node dissection—showing a large lymph node in between aorta and inferior vena cava.

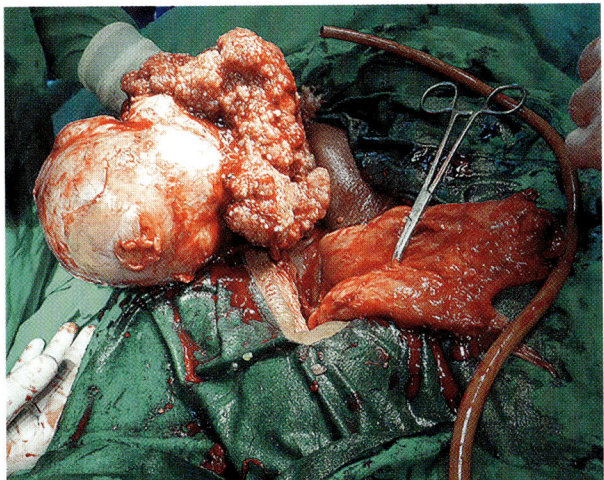

Fig. 38: Advanced epithelial ovarian carcinoma during laparotomy—on the process of removal.

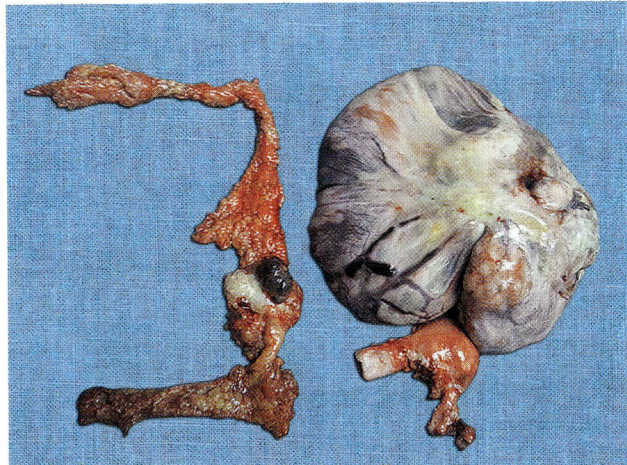

Fig. 40: Total abdominal hysterectomy with bilateral salpingo-oophorectomy with infracolic omentectomy done in ovarian malignancy. Note the formation of omental cake due to metastasis.

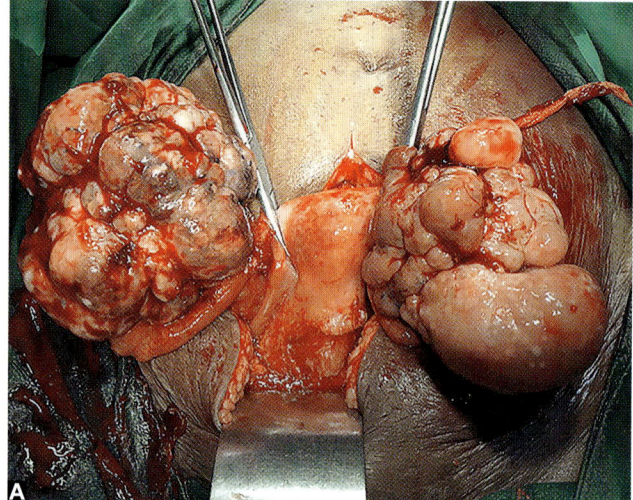

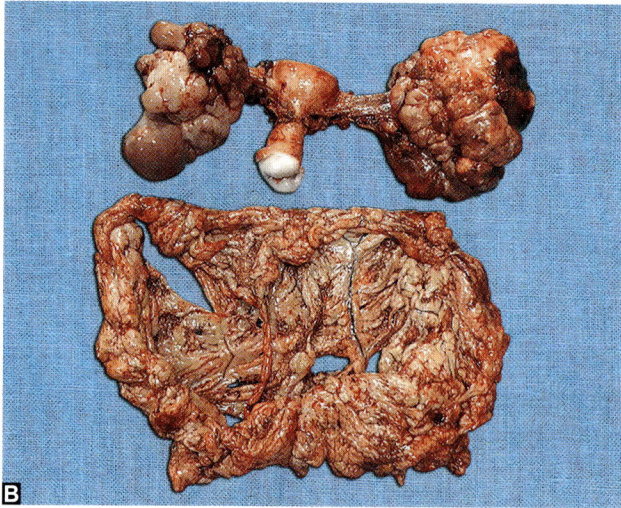

Figs. 41A and B: Bilateral malignant ovarian tumor. Note that on opening of uterovesical fold of peritoneum bladder was found not involved; (B) Specimen of the same patient as (A) who was a parous 37-year-old woman. TAH BSO with omentectomy done. Biopsy report shows serous cystadenocarcinoma. Following three courses of chemotherapy patient responded well.

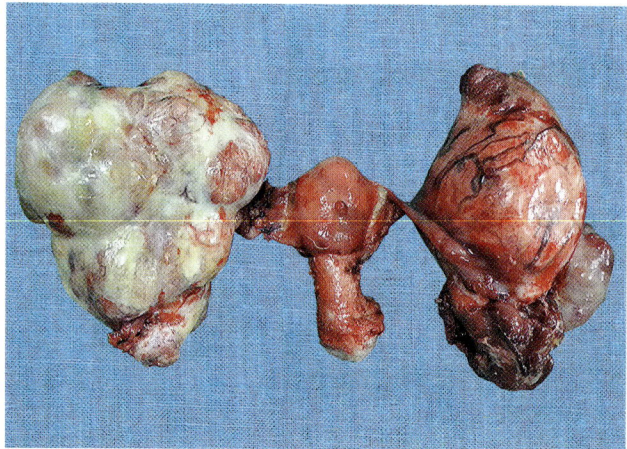

Fig. 42: Bilateral malignant ovarian tumor—a 55-year-old nulliparous with h/o infertility. There was huge ascites, omental and paraaortic lymph node metastasis. Serous adenocarcinoma of ovary.

Frozen section biopsy from any suspicion lesion is performed based on which definite surgery is planned. Excised specimen (usually TAH and BSO), omentum, tissues from all areas and lymph nodes are sent for histopathological examination **(Fig. 31)**.

Management of Early Epithelial Ovarian Cancer

Stage 1A, or Stage 1B, grade 1 and 2: Surgery only by TAH-BSO and infracolic omentectomy—no adjuvant chemotherapy.

For fertility preservation in Stage 1A unilateral salpingo-oophorectomy (USO) with long term survival.

Stage 1A or 1B grade 3, Stage 1C and Stage II: Surgery followed by 3–6 cycles of chemotherapy (carboplatin and paclitaxel).

20% of women with early stage disease recurs within 5 years even after chemotherapy.

Role of MIS (minimal invasive surgery)

In an apparent Stage I early stage ovarian cancer laparoscopic staging (MIS) is valuable as a primary treatment.

Follow up

Following complete treatment patient with early-stage disease is followed up 3 months for two years, then six monthly for another three years and then annually. In each follow up complete physical and pelvic examination is done. Serum CA125 is monitored if it was high initially. If recurrence is suspected by clinical examination and serum CA125 level imaging is advised for confirmation.

Management of Advanced Ovarian Cancer (Approximately Two-Thirds)

Primary debulking

- *Primary surgery* if possible—TAH-BSO, omentectomy, and debulking by surgical cytoreduction.
- *Additional surgery* like large or small bowel resection, appendicectomy, splenectomy, diaphragm stripping or resection may also be needed.
- *Chemotherapy* for 6 cycles (*see* Page 71 for details)

Interval debulking surgery (IDS)

- *Neoadjuvant chemotherapy* (NACT) for 3–4 courses followed by interval debulking, which is followed by three courses of chemotherapy. Indications are patients of poor performance status, significant comorbidities, gross ascites and/large pleural effusion and visceral metastasis.
- If in primary surgery complete debulking is not possible, following a course of chemotherapy a second debulking procedure is performed.

Q. What should be the aim of cytoreduction?

In cytoreduction, the aim is to make debulking so that none of individual area of tumor left measures more than 2 cm.

Survival rate is increased related to the size of residual disease left, it becomes less than 1.5 cm, 1 cm or less than

0.5 cm and there is longest survival if no residual disease remains.

Optimal debulking means individual residual tumor size is less than 1 cm. Currently, there is growing consensus that the optimal debulking means presence of no gross residual disease.

Systemic lymphadenectomy is beneficial if complete debulking and clearance is possible. Usual route of chemotherapy is intravenous. Result of intraperitoneal route is also encouraging (*see* HIPEC and PIPAC therapy).

CHEMOTHERAPEUTIC AGENTS USED IN OVARIAN MALIGNANCY

Epithelial Ovarian Cancer

Intravenous Chemotherapy

Standard adjuvant chemotherapy is 6 cycles of intravenous platinum-based combination chemotherapy with carboplatin or cisplatin and paclitaxel or docetaxel.

Dose of Intravenous Chemotherapy

- Carboplatin [starting dose AUC (area under curve) 5-6], and paclitaxel (175 mg/m^2) every 3 weeks.
  Or
- Carboplatin AUC 6 every 3 weeks for 6 cycles and weekly paclitaxel 80 mg/m^2 (18 weeks).

The dose of carboplatin is calculated by Calvert formula depending on the age, body weight, and creatinine clearance (AUC = area under curve). In an average 60 kg weight woman of 50 years with normal creatinine clearance each dose of carboplatin is about 500 mg.

Intraperitoneal Chemotherapy

Intraperitoneal (IP) chemotherapy is used in selected patients at stage III following optimal debulking. The concept of intraperitoneal chemotherapy is that epithelial tumor spreads mostly along peritoneal surfaces ang likely to highly effective. With IP chemotherapy toxicity is higher and problems due to catheter is common. Instead of traditional IP therapy Hyperthermic intraperitoneal chemotherapy has been introduced with better result.

Dose of Intraperitoneal Chemotherapy

Paclitaxel 135 mg/m^2 intravenously on day 1, followed by cisplatin 100 mg/m^2 intraperitoneally on day 2, followed by paclitaxel 60 mg/m^2 intraperitoneally on day 8, every 3 weeks for 6 cycles. In patients who may not tolerate combination chemotherapy because of medical comorbidities or advanced age, use single-agent, intravenously administered carboplatin (AUC 5-6). In patients who have a significant hypersensitivity reaction to paclitaxel, an alternative active drug can be used (e.g. docetaxel or nanoparticle paclitaxel).

Q. What is HIPEC therapy?

Hyperthermic intraperitoneal chemotherapy—concentrated, heated chemotherapy is delivered directly to the abdomen during surgery. Cisplatin is commonly used. Overall survival rate is extended for significant period.

Q. What is PIPAC?

Pressurized intraperitoneal aerosol therapy (PIPAC) is a potential tool for peritoneal carcinomatosis and for the palliative treatment in peritoneal metastasis where systemic chemotherapy is not effective.

Q. What is chemotherapy response score (CRS)?

CRS is a histopathological score to measure the response to neoadjuvant chemotherapy based on three-tier system. A CRS 3 which means complete or near complete pathological response is associated with better prognosis.

Q. What is targeted therapy?

The purpose of treatment is to identify and to attack the cancer cells with minimal damage to normal cells. Angiogenesis inhibitors and PARP (poly ADP- ribose polymerase) inhibitors are used for this purpose.

Bevacizumab is one angiogenesis inhibitor and given intravenously. It is the first drug used as targeted therapy to show significant single-agent activity in ovarian cancer. Bevacizumab 7.5 to15 mg/kg can be added to other conventional IV or IP chemotherapeutic agents in selected patients with advanced ovarian cancer. However, the cost is very high. Olaparib and rucaparib are examples of PARP inhibitor given orally. Pazopanib, an oral multikinase inhibitor of vascular endothelial growth factor receptor is emerging as an effective maintenance therapy. PARP inhibitors have great role in recurrent ovarian cancer and in patients with BRCA mutations and in tumor with homologous recombination deficiency (HRD).

Treatment assessment of epithelial ovarian cancer

Following optimal cytoreductive surgery and subsequent chemotherapy for epithelial ovarian cancer most women have no evidence of disease. The parameters of treatment assessment are periodical clinical examination, tumor markers, radiological assessment and second look surgery. Tumor markers and radiology are not so sensitive to exclude the presence of subclinical disease .The second look surgery which is important historically is abandoned due to lack of meaningful benefit

RECURRENT OVARIAN CANCER

Recurrent ovarian cancer is diagnosed by gradual elevation of CA 125 on follow up or appearance of symptoms.

Patients are categorized as three types—(1) platinum refractory, (2) platinum resistant, and (3) platinum sensitive.

"Platinum refractory" means where tumor progresses during chemotherapy.

"Platinum resistant" signifies where relapse occurs within 6 months.

"Platinum sensitive" means where relapse occurs 6–12 months after primary therapy.

In the first two groups, prognosis is worse and nonplatinum chemotherapy is the only option but response is poor and response is only 5–10%.

Secondary Cytoreductive Surgery

The term Secondary cytoreductive surgery is applied to the attempt of cytoreductive surgery in recurrent ovarian cancers where debulking is done as much as possible. It works best in platinum sensitive cases, solitary site recurrence, absence of ascites and prolonged disease free interval.

Salvage Chemotherapy

Salvage chemotherapy means retreatment with platinum-based drug irrespective of secondary cytoreductive surgery and is the preferable treatment for recurrent platinum sensitive cases. *Carboplatin along with paclitaxel* or other drug like *pegylated liposomal doxorubicin* is attempted with reasonable success. Now few newer single chemotherapeutic drugs have been attempted with equal success. In neurotoxicity instead of paclitaxel gemectabine or liposomal doxorubin is given.

Second Look Surgery

Second look surgery is done principally for surveillance of ovarian cancer and it was once said to be "gold standard" for detection of residual disease. But it is considered now to have little value.

Purpose
- To assess completeness of treatment response
- Resection of residual tumor if any.

Components
- Ascitic fluid or cytological washings should be collected if not biopsy proved
- Visual inspection of all peritoneal surfaces including diaphragm
- Resection of any suspicion nodules, tumors or adhesions
- Biopsy from the residual omentum, and peritoneal surfaces if no gross disease is found
- Lymph node sampling (pelvic and paraaortic) unless initially not done

Procedure—either laparoscopically or laparotomy

Benefits of second look surgery—several studies show that there is no survival benefit on second look surgery. Only benefit is to assess the effectiveness of treatment within an experimental protocol. If no recurrent disease is revealed it can be said it has improved survival rate.

Summary—second look surgery was performed previously to evaluate treatment assessment, but almost abandoned now as there is no meaningful benefit to the patients as evidenced by various studies. The other assessment procedures like imaging and tumor markers are available now.

BORDERLINE OVARIAN TUMOR (SYNONYM: LOW MALIGNANT POTENTIAL TUMOR)

Low malignant potential (LMP) tumors or borderline tumors are intermediate in between benign cyst and frank invasive carcinoma.

It constitutes *10–15% of epithelial ovarian carcinoma*. There is lot of dilemma of diagnosis and management of LMP tumors. 75% are at the stage I at the time of diagnosis.

Histological diagnostic criteria: Presence of at least two of the followings:
- Nuclear atypia
- Stratification of the epithelium
- Cellular pleomorphism
- Microscopic papillary projections or
- Mitotic activity.

And there is no stromal invasion like invasive cancer. However, 10% of LMP may have microinvasion less than 3 mm.

Clinical Features

These are like other pelvic masses, e.g. abdominal distension, pain lower abdomen or asymptomatic diagnosed incidentally. Tumor size may be small to very large of 30 cm in mucinous variety. Sonography and CT scan are to diagnose and to exclude frank malignancy and invasion. CA 125 is nonspecific.

Management

It depends on age and future desire of fertility.

In young premenstrual aged women fertility sparing surgery like USO is performed.

In postmenopausal women TAH-BSO is done.

As preoperatively, it is not possible to diagnose preparation for surgical staging and counseling for advance surgical procedure is done and proceeded like other epithelial carcinoma. If it is really LMP, it is not possible to differentiate from benign mass and invasive cancer.

Staging biopsy should be performed and staged as FIGO staging of EOC. Frozen section should always be done but not confirmatory until and unless histology from the excised mass is done. However in doubtful cases minimum surgery should be performed primarily. Laparoscopic approach is useful in many cases.

In borderline ovarian tumor, it is always advisable to take opinion of gynecologic oncologist for further therapy including chemotherapy.

Prognosis

Prognosis is excellent in LMP tumor. 10 year survival rate is 95%. Overall survival is above 80% in cases of Stage I disease. Recurrence is 15% on opposite side when fertility sparing surgery is done. Prognosis of epithelial ovarian, fallopian and peritoneal malignancies depends on (a) stage of the cancer at diagnosis, (b) histological type and grading, and (c) maximum diameter of the residual disease after cytoreduction.

Prognosis of Epithelial Ovarian Cancer
- Stage I disease (one quarter) has excellent long-term survival.

- In advanced stages (two-thirds cases) relapse occurs in 80% patients after treatment.
- Overall 5-year survival of all stages of EOC is 45%, that of uterine cancer is 85% and cancer cervix is 75%.
- Prognosis is excellent in LMP tumor.

5-year survival rate of EOC according to stage:
- Stage I: 70–90%
- Stage II: 80%
- Stage III: 30%
- Stage IV: 10–20%.

Q. What are the important favorable prognostic factors for ovarian cancer?
- Young age
- Good health
- Lower the FIGO staging better is the prognosis
- *BRCA* carriers have better prognosis due to good platinum sensitivity
- No ascites
- Cell type other than mucinous and clear cell
- Well-differentiated tumor
- Smaller tumor size prior surgery
- Least residual size after primary cytoreduction.

FALLOPIAN TUBE (FT) CANCER (FIGS. 43A AND B)

Overview
- Fallopian tube cancer contributes 0.3% of all gynecological malignancies. Historically, primary fallopian tube cancer was considered to be much less. As many high-grade serous carcinoma is said to originate from fimbrial end of fallopian tube, real incidence of FT cancer probably is high.
- FT cancer may be primary which is more common and secondary from ovary, endometrium, GI tract and breast. To diagnose primary fallopian tube cancer the tumor must be visible macroscopically within the tube and fimbria, uterus and ovary will be free of any tumor or if present they should be clearly distinguishable.
- Mostly epithelial frequently serous variety.
- Risk factors, spread, histology, character, staging and treatment are like ovarian cancer, hence diagnosis and management are similar to ovarian cancer.
- In FIGO staging (2014) fallopian tube cancer has been incorporated in common Staging of the Ovary, Fallopian tube and Primary peritoneal carcinoma (FIGO 2014) given in **Table 3**, Page 68.

Diagnosis
- **Mean age 60 years.**
- Women with germ line mutations in *BRCA1* and *BRCA2* are higher risk, hence prophylactic removal is justified.
- Vaginal discharge or bleeding is most common symptom (>50%). The classic triad of fallopian tube carcinoma

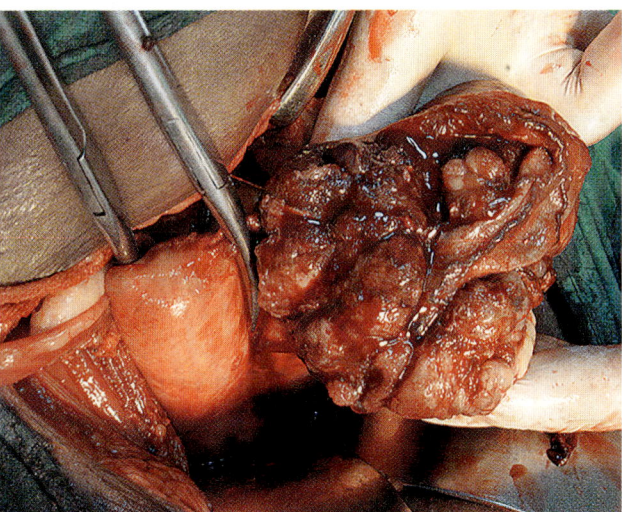

Fig. 43A: Fallopian tube cancer.

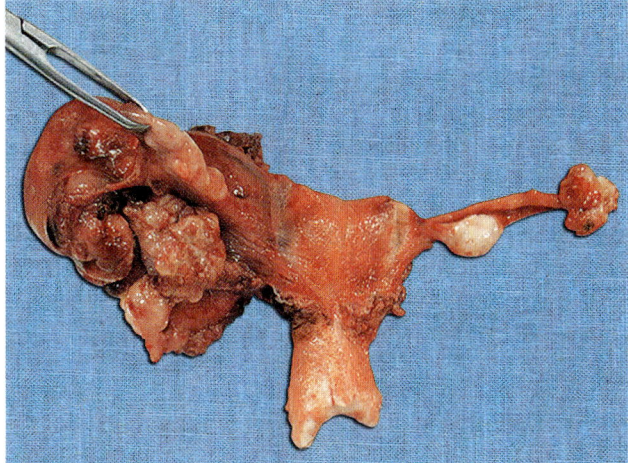

Fig. 43B: Specimen of TAH with BSO in fallopian tube cancer.

(Fig. 56) is (a) watery vaginal discharge (hydrops tubae profluens), (b) pelvic pain, and (c) pelvic lump is found in 15% cases.
- Pelvic mass is definitely palpable in bimanual examination and may be palpable abdominally if mass is large. There may be presence of ascites.
- **Spread** is like ovarian cancer spread.
- All investigations are done in the line of epithelial ovarian cancer (tumor markers, imaging).
- **The staging** is surgical staging and included in common staging of the ovary, fallopian tube and primary peritoneal carcinoma (FIGO 2014).

Management
- **Like ovarian cancer.**
Surgery is the primary treatment. Staging laparotomy (**Fig. 43A**) is done. TAH and BSO with removal of primary tumor with omentectomy (**Fig. 43B**) followed by platinum-based chemotherapy and cytoreductive surgery and evaluation of retroperitoneal lymph nodes in advanced disease.

Survival Rate

Overall 5 year survival rate of fallopian tube cancer is 40%.

GERM CELL TUMORS

Varieties of germ cell tumors are (classify germ cell tumor):
- Dysgerminoma
- Yolk sac tumors (endodermal sinus tumor)
- Embryonal carcinoma
- Polyembryoma
- Choriocarcinoma
- *Teratomas*: Immature, mature, monodermal, and mixed germ cell.

Varieties of teratoma are described before (*see* Page 53). Dermoid cyst which is a benign cystic teratoma is described in detail before (*see* Page 56).

Facts about Germ Cell Tumor

- Germ cell tumors originate from the primordial germ cell of ovary and comprising *one-third of all ovarian neoplasms*.
- *Dermoid cyst* which is benign mature cystic teratoma is the *most common variety* of germ cell tumor comprising 95% of all germ cell tumors.
- *Immature teratomas* are now the *most common malignant germ cell tumor* comprising half of malignant germ cell tumors.
- *Dysgerminoma* is the most common variety to be *bilateral* of all malignant germ cell tumor (15–20%).
- Of all *malignant* ovarian tumors malignant *germ cell tumors contribute only 3% cases*. Most common is EOC—90 to 95%, others are sex cord-stromal tumors (nearly 2%).
- In *childhood and young adolescents, the most common* ovarian malignancy is germ cell malignant tumors.
- Surprisingly, during last few decades the *incidence of dysgerminoma has decreased* and that of immature teratoma is increased by two folds.
- From clinical points of view malignant germ cell tumors are *different* from the epithelial tumors in three respects.
  1. They are mostly diagnosed at *early stage* so fertility preservation surgery is possible.
  2. Mostly present in very *young age* groups (adolescent or early 20s).
  3. *Prognosis* is excellent. In advanced stage, prognosis is also good due to *highly chemosensitivity*. Staging laparotomy or laparotomy is done to determine the extent of disease and need for adjuvant chemotherapy. Staging is not required in fibroma, thecoma, gynandroblastoma, well-differentiated Sertoli–Leydig cell tumor, and sclerosing stromal tumor.

Diagnosis of Germ Cell Tumors

Clinical

Symptoms and signs: Subacute abdominal pain may present as acute abdomen in 10% cases. There may be menstrual abnormalities. Asymptomatic and incidental diagnosis in one-fourth cases. Young woman with amenorrhea developing pelvic mass may have dysgenetic gonads which develop gonadoblastoma or dysgerminoma.

There may be pelviabdominal mass or pelvic mass. As the patients mostly are adolescents vaginal examination is not often possible and *examination under anesthesia* is needed. Ascites, pleural effusion, and other organomegaly may be detected in advanced malignancy.

Sonography is essential though transvaginal route is difficult to do in young adolescents. Typical features of dermoid cyst become evident in USG, CT, and MRI. Color Doppler is useful for detection of malignant masses. Chest X-ray is indicated in suspected metastasis and pleural effusion.

Specific tumors like serum hCG and AFP are indicated in suspected germ cell tumors. AFP is definitely raised in Yolk cell tumor and embryonal carcinoma and may be raised in immature teratoma, mixed germ cell tumor, and polyembryoma. hCG is obviously raised in choriocarcinoma and embryonal carcinoma and may be in dysgerminoma, mixed germ cell tumor and in polyembryoma but not in all cases.

Ultrasonography-guided or CT-guided percutaneous biopsy has little role as excision is required for confirmatory diagnosis for *Histopathology*.

Immunohistochemistry may be required in many cases.

Treatment of Germ Cell Tumor

In prepubertal girl, any mass of more than 2 cm and in postmenopausal woman more than 8 cm surgical exploration is needed.

Surgery is the treatment. In suspected malignancy staging is done on laparotomy. In most cases, cystectomy or oophorectomy is the treatment which is required. More radical surgery is needed in advanced cases and in bilateral involvement. Opposite ovary must be examined meticulously. Laparoscopy is safe and alternative method in small mass in stage I disease.

Chemotherapy

Stage IA dysgerminoma and Stage IA grade 1 immature teratoma—no chemotherapy. Other advanced and histological varieties:

Chemotherapy: Combination of bleomycin, etoposide, and cisplatin *(BEP)*—5 days course every 3 weeks for 3–4 cycles—3 for fully resected and 4 for incompletely resected germ cell tumors.

Chemotherapeutic Agents used in Germ Cell Tumor

The recommended chemotherapy regimen (BEP) is as follows:
- Bleomycin 30,000 IU IV/IM on days 1/8/15 for 12 weeks.
- Etoposide 100 mg/m^2 IV per day for 5 days every 3 weeks for 3 cycles.

- Cisplatin 20 mg/m² IV per day for 5 days every 3 weeks for 3 cycles. If bleomycin is omitted, then 4 cycles of EP are commonly used.

Drugs	Mechanism of action	Side effects
Bleomycin	Prevent DNA synthesis	Fever, weight loss, rash, and pulmonary fibrosis
Etoposide	Topoisomerase inhibitor act by damaging DNA	Low blood count, vomiting, loss of appetite, diarrhea, and hair loss
Cisplatin	Inhibit DNA replication	Marrow suppression, kidney problem, vomiting, and hearing problem
Paclitaxel	Interfere with normal function of microtubules during cell division	Hair loss, bone marrow suppression, allergic reaction, diarrhea, and numbness

Dysgerminoma (Figs. 44 and 45)

- Dysgerminoma which was the most common malignant germ cell tumor few decades back is now next to immature teratoma (*see* above) in incidence. It comprises of more than one-third of all malignant germ cell tumor. Recently, its incidence has declined. It is the most common malignant ovarian tumor encountered in pregnancy.
- "Dys" means two—occurs in both sexes.
- *Bilateral in 15–20%*, bilaterality is uncommon in other germ cell tumor.
- *Gross appearance*: Size—5 to 15 cm, appearance variable, solid with rubbery consistency, grayish to pink to cream color and lobulated (Fig. 44).
- *Microscopic*: Large polyhedral clear cells resembling primordial germ cells (Fig. 45) and identical to seminoma testis histologically. Choriocarcinoma, yolk cell tumor may be mixed with dysgerminoma.

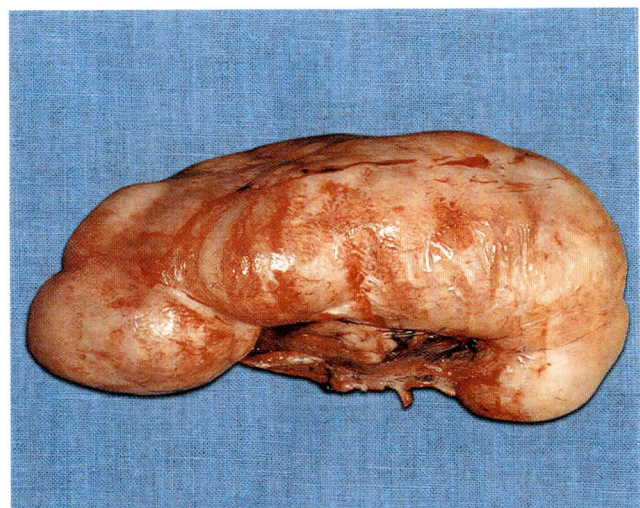

Fig. 44: Dysgerminoma of ovary—a 16-year-old girl presented with lump abdomen. Unilateral salpingo-oophorectomy done as it was diagnosed in Stage IA. On 5 years follow-up, she was well.

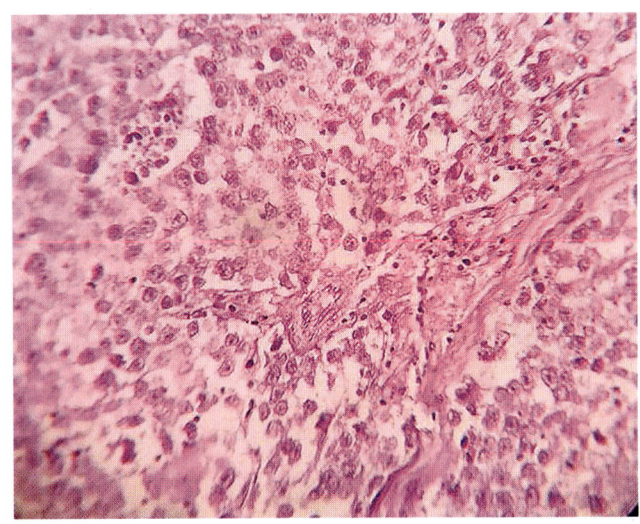

Fig. 45: Microphotography of dysgerminoma of ovary (H&E, X400) showing large polyhedral cells resembling primordial germ cells.
Courtesy: Professor Gopinath Barui, Department of Pathology

- Dysgerminoma may also arise (5%) from the gonad with abnormal karyotype particularly in presence of Y chromosome like mosaic Turner syndrome and Swyer syndrome.

  Dysgerminoma may arise in *gonadoblastoma*, a benign tumor in dysgenetic gonad. 50% of gonadoblastoma may turn into dysgerminoma if untreated.

- *Diagnosis*: Commonly occurs in younger age group, less than 30 years. History, clinical evaluation, imaging, laparoscopy, laparotomy, and finally histopathology reach the diagnosis. *LDH is useful for monitoring of the disease.* Beta-hCG may be elevated in some cases. PLAP and LDH are secreted by dysgerminoma up to 95% cases.
- *Treatment*: Common treatment is USO as dysgerminomas are mostly diagnosed in Stage I in two-thirds of cases and patients are young.

  In rare cases, ovarian cystectomy is performed.

  In elderly and advance cases, TAH with BSO is done. Lymphadenectomy is especially considered as metastasis is highest (30%) in dysgerminoma among all malignant germ cell tumors. Though tumors are highly radiosensitive, radiotherapy is rarely used nowadays due to good response to chemotherapy *(BEP)* and fertility problem in young patient.
- *Prognosis*: *Best prognosis* among all malignant germ cell tumors. 5-year survival is 99% in Stage I and more than 98% in stage II-IV disease with platinum-based chemotherapy, commonly BEP.

Immature Teratoma (Figs. 46 and 47)

Immature teratomas are now the *most common malignant germ cell tumor* comprising half of malignant germ cell tumors.

Bilaterality is less.

Macroscopically spherical, soft to firm, lobulated often breakage of capsule and chance of adhesion to adjacent structures, so less chance of torsion (Fig. 46).

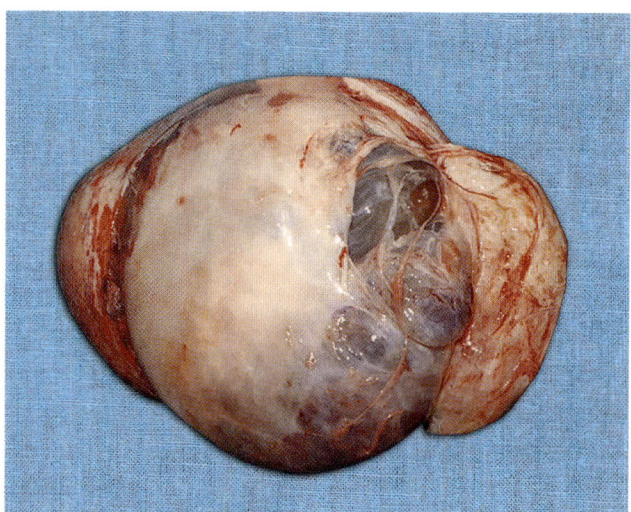

Fig. 46: Immature teratoma—a 29-year-old nulliparous woman presented with lump abdomen. On laparotomy one ovary was involved, there was few breakage of capsule, other ovary was healthy, no malignant cell on peritoneal washing (Stage IC2). Unilateral salpingo-oophorectomy done followed by adjuvant therapy.

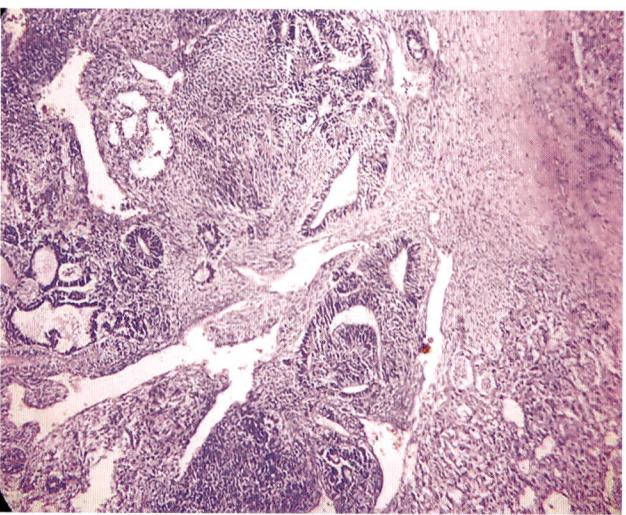

Fig. 47: Microphotography of immature teratoma of ovary showing all elements of all germ cell layers.
Courtesy: Dr Anup Boler, Associate Professor, Department of Pathology

Cut section shows solid to cystic containing cartilage, bone and sebaceous material.

Composed of tissues derived from all germ layers—ectoderm, endoderm, and mesoderm. Microscopically (**Fig. 47**) round malignant cells, immature neuroectodermal tissues with variable nature. Grades are done 1 and 2 (low) and 3 (high).

Treatment

Unilateral salpingo-oophorectomy is treatment of choice in younger women. Adjuvant therapy is not needed in early stage.

Growing teratoma syndrome is an entity where immature teratoma contains mature tissue implants over peritoneum benign in nature which do not increase the stage or no impact on survival but do not respond to chemotherapy and may increase in their way. Second-look surgery is needed to resect for excluding diagnosis of recurrence.

Prognosis depends on grade of tumor. Prognosis is excellent in Stage 1A grade I tumor. In Stage II–IV, disease with complete therapy 5-year survival rate is above 70%.

Yolk Sac Tumor (Old Name: Endodermal Sinus Tumor)

It is called yolk sac carcinoma as derived from primitive yolk sac and the third most frequent germ cell tumor.

Yolk sac tumor is the *deadliest malignant tumor* of ovary, always (100%) unilateral, solid, yellow and friable, and tendency to rupture.

Microscopically cystic degeneration with focal necrosis, reticular pattern with irregular spaces lined by epithelial cells. *Schiller–Duval bodies* are characteristic.

Alpha fetoprotein is frequently raised and serves as reliable tumor marker.

This is the ovarian tumor where *chemotherapy is essential in all stages* even Stage I due to its rapid spread in all routes and recurrence.

More than 50% are diagnosed in Stage I and 5-year survival rate is above 90%. 5-year survival rate ranges from 60 to 90% in stage II–IV disease. Recurrence may occur within 1 year and almost unresponsive to treatment.

Choriocarcinoma

Nongestational choriocarcinoma (NGC) arises from germ cell of ovary.

It can be differentiated from metastatic gestational choriocarcinoma by history of pregnancy and presence of other germ cell component on histology. This differentiation is important as prognosis of NGC has poorer prognosis though clinical features are same.

Sexual precocity in prepubertal girl and abnormal vaginal bleeding in reproductive age group may be the presenting features.

Diagnosed by very high serum hCG.

Embryonal Cell Carcinoma

Rare germ cell tumor containing epithelial cells looking like embryonic disk with sheets of anaplastic gland-like spaces and papillary structures.

Both hCG and AFP become high.

Mostly found in younger and peripubertal age.

Mixed Germ Cell Tumor

Incidence is half to one-third in all ovarian germ cell tumors.

Dysgerminoma is the most common component and others are yolk sac tumor and immature teratoma.

Chance of bilaterality is high due to preponderance of dysgerminoma.

When hCG and AFP level are raised in any apparently dysgerminoma review of histopathology is done to search for other germ cell component as prognosis depends on the presence of other elements.

SEX CORD STROMAL TUMORS

Common varieties are:
- Granulosa-stromal cell tumors: Granulosa cell tumors and thecoma-fibroma
- Sertoli-stromal cell tumors, androblastoma: Well differentiated, Sertoli–Leydig cell tumor of intermediate differentiation, Sertoli–Leydig cell tumor of poorly differentiated, retiform
- Sex cord tumor with annular tubules
- Gynandroblastoma.

Facts about the Sex Cord Stromal Tumors

- Sex cord stromal tumors arise from ovarian matrix and *mostly hormone producing* either estrogen, androgen or both.
- *Most rare* form of ovarian malignancy, incidence is half of gem cell malignancy (<5%). May occur in all ages.
- Major varieties are granulosa-stromal cell tumors or Sertoli-stromal cell tumors, androblastoma. *70% are granulosa cell tumor*.
- Clinical features are mainly abdominal mass with occasional pain abdomen with symptoms and signs of hormone excess either isosexual precocious puberty in prepubertal age, menstrual abnormality and amenorrhea, virilization in reproductive age group and postmenopausal bleeding with androgen excess in menopausal women.
- *Imaging:* USG, CT or MRI is helpful to diagnose. *Serum androgen* may be higher in virilizing tumor. *Inhibin* is excess in granulosa cell tumor.
- Final diagnosis is done by histopathology of excised specimen.
- Immunostaining may be needed sometimes to confirm nature of tumor.
- Most of these tumors are *LMP, indolent growth pattern, unilateral, and localized.*
- Recurrence is less and if occurs relapse is in late.
- Primary treatment is surgical removal: Total abdominal hysterectomy with bilateral salpingo-oophorectomy is performed who have completed family and USO is done in localized and young patients.
  Adjuvant chemotherapy is needed in Stage I disease if the tumor size is large, rupture, surface break, incomplete staging, high mitotic index, and equivocal pathology. In stage II–IV diseases adjuvant therapy is given usually *with BEP regime* for 3–4 course as first-line chemotherapy. Currently radiotherapy has limited role.
- Prognosis is excellent as mostly diagnosed early and confined to one ovary.

Granulosa Cell Tumor (Figs. 48 and 49)

This is the most common variety (70%) of sex cord stromal tumors (SCSTs).

This type of tumor arises from sex cords and mostly estrogen producing. There are two types—adult type and juvenile type.

Mostly occurs after the age of 30 years.

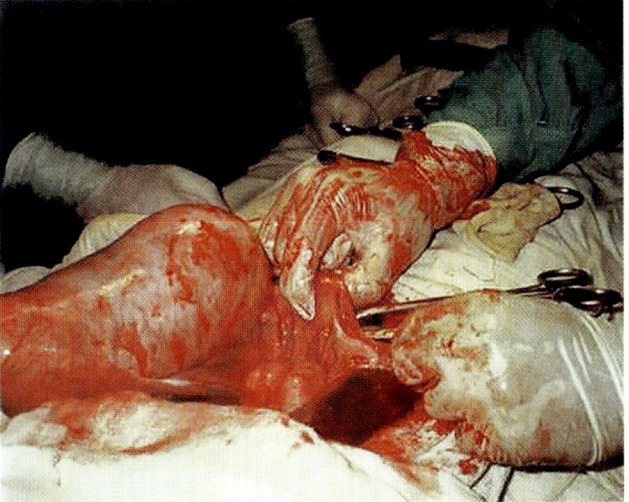

Fig. 48: Granulosa cell tumor in a 7 years and 6 months old girl who presented with precocious puberty and unilateral Stage IA tumor. Unilateral salpingo-oophorectomy done. Her breast regressed and menstruation ceased after surgery (*see* Chapter 15 of Precocious Puberty).

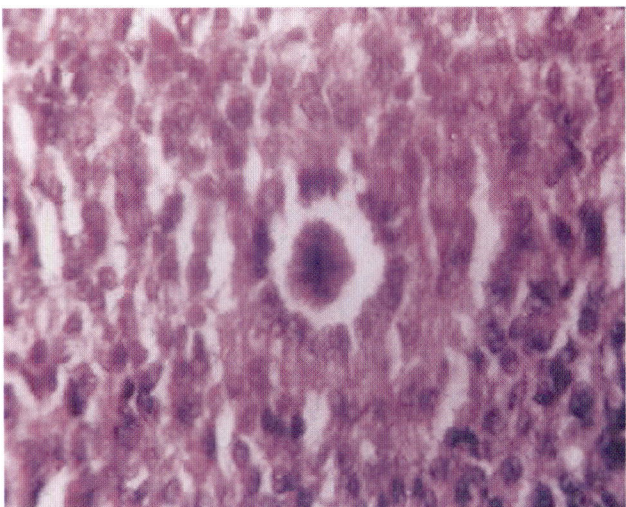

Fig. 49: Microphotography of granulosa cell tumor showing rosette arrangement of cells.

Diagnosis

- Juvenile type 90% diagnosed before puberty.
- It is diagnosed by presenting symptoms, e.g., lump abdomen sometimes with pain abdomen, sometimes acute variety (torsion, rupture), menometrorrhagia, postmenopausal bleeding associated with breast enlargement and tenderness.
- In children, there may be *precocious puberty* with development of breasts, other secondary sexual characters, primary or secondary amenorrhea, or early menarche and vaginal discharge. Tumor marker *inhibin B* is raised.
- These tumors are low-grade malignancies, 95% unilateral and up to *90% Stage I* during diagnosis.

Macroscopic appearance (see Fig. 48)—large, average diameter is 12 cm. Surface edematous, adhered with adjacent structures, high possibility of rupture during removal.

On cut section variable—solid to cystic with hemorrhage and gelatinous material.

Histology (see Fig. 49) shows mostly granulosa cells with grooved pale "coffee bean" nuclei. A *rosette arrangement* of cells around a central cavity resembling primordial follicles called *"Call-Exner bodies"* is a characteristic *Sertoli-stromal cell tumors* which may not be present in adult type.

Unilateral oophorectomy is possible many a times. Following surgery features of precocious puberty may regress in young girl.

More radical surgery is needed in advanced stage and elderly women with *use of chemotherapy*.

Prognosis is excellent, 5-year survival in Stage I is 90–95% in both adult and juvenile group. Advance stage prognosis is poor—30 to 50%. In juvenile variety, in advanced stages, tumor is more aggressive.

Sertoli-stromal cell tumors may be isolated Sertoli cell tumors or Sertoli–Leydig cell tumor, latter is more common.

Sertoli–Leydig Cell Tumor (Figs. 50 to 53)

Sertoli–Leydig tumor which was previously called *arrhenoblastoma or androblastoma* a male hormone producing tumor is the *second most common* type among all *SCST* next to granulose cell tumor with an incidence of less than 0.2% of ovarian cancer.

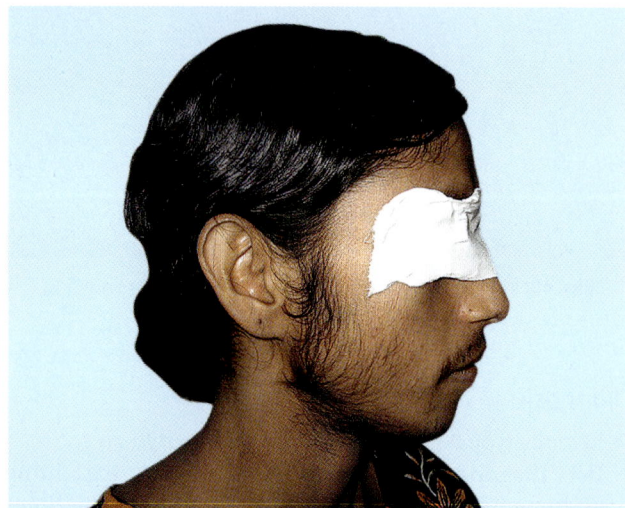

Fig. 50: Hirsutism due to Sertoli–Leydig cell tumor—a 19-year-old married woman presented with lump abdomen, amenorrhea, hirsutism, hoarseness of voice, and enlarged clitoris (Figs. 51 to 53). On laparotomy, tumor was multiloculated, 18 cm × 15 cm but in Stage IA. Unilateral salpingo-oophorectomy done. Patient was lost in follow-up without taking any chemotherapy and surprisingly she came back after 1 year with pregnancy of 10 weeks with regressed features of hyperandrogenism. She delivered by cesarean section a healthy female baby of 2.7 kg (*see* Fig. 17 of Chapter 12, Page 300).
Courtesy: Professor Anita Roy and Dr Subir Bhattacharyya, Associate Professor, Obstetrics and Gynecology

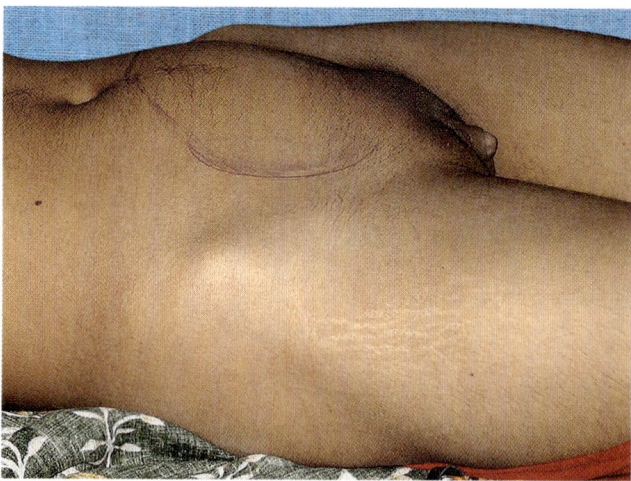

Fig. 51: Lump abdomen and enlarged clitoris in Sertoli–Leydig cell tumor in the same woman (*see* Fig. 50).

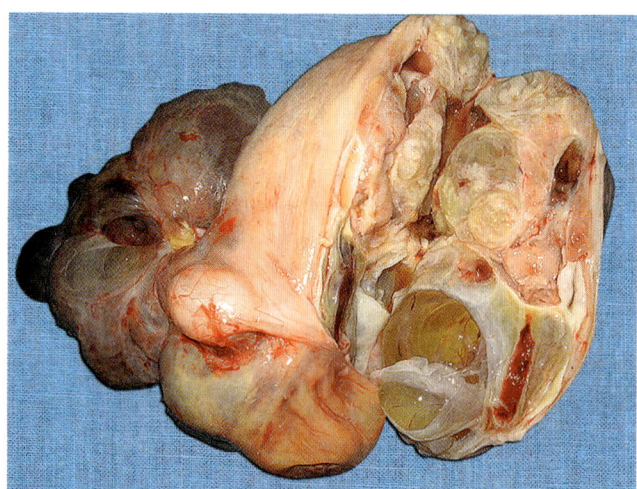

Fig. 52: Cut section of the Sertoli–Leydig cell tumor (partly solid and partly cystic) of the same patient (*see* Fig. 50).

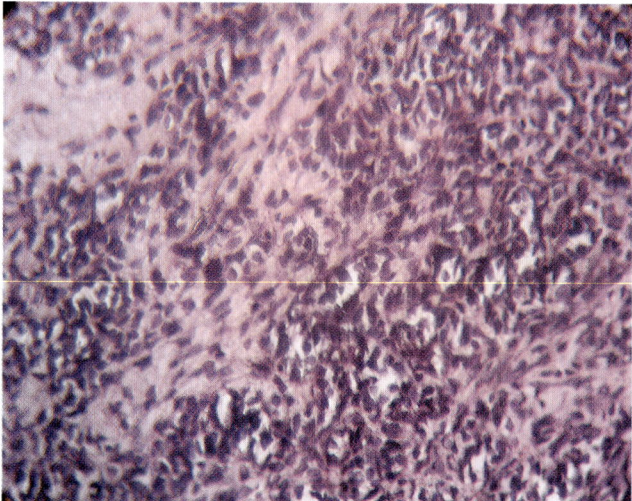

Fig. 53: Microphotography of Sertoli–Leydig cell tumor with intermediate differentiation.
Courtesy: Professor Tamal Ghosh, Department of Pathology

Sertoli–Leydig cell tumors are *rarely bilateral* (<1%).

90% cases are diagnosed in Stage I. 15–20% are clinically malignant.

Clinical Presentation

These tumors occur most frequently in the third and fourth decade of life, 75% of the patients are less than 40 years of age.

About 70–85% women may present with abdominal mass with *features of virilization* like oligomenorrhea followed by amenorrhea, breast atrophy, acne, hirsutism (**Fig. 50**), clitoromegaly (**Fig. 51**), deepening of voice and a receding hairline.

Serum testosterone becomes high and serum testosterone–androstenedione ratio is elevated.

Gross appearance: Sizes vary from an impalpable small nodule to a larger tumor of average 14 cm, solid, yellow surface and are often lobulated (**Fig. 52**).

Histologically (**Fig. 53**), there may be five subtypes of differentiation—well, intermediate, poor, retiform, and heterologous. Well differentiated are clinically benign. Well-differentiated tumors consist of hollow tubules separated by Leydig cells. In intermediate variety more primitive Sertoli cells are found to be arranged in cord whilst in poorly differentiated varieties cells resembling spindle cell sarcoma are found.

Sertoli–Leydig cell tumors are *mostly low-grade malignancies* and have tendency to late recurrence and occasionally a poorly differentiated variety may behave more aggressively.

Treatment

Premenarchal girls or women of reproductive age group usually present in Stage I disease. An unilateral salpingo-oophorectomy (USO) (*see* **Fig. 30**) is the appropriate therapy for these patients.

For perimenopausal and postmenopausal women, total hysterectomy with bilateral salpingo-oophorectomy is the treatment of choice.

Efficacy of *chemotherapy* is not well documented due to rarity of tumor.

Prognosis depends on stage and degree of tumor differentiation. In *Stage I tumors*, 5-year survival rates of *about 90%* have been reported and recurrences are not common.

In advanced disease, Sertoli–Leydig cell tumors are associated with bad prognosis.

Krukenberg Tumor (Figs. 54 and 55)

Krukenberg tumor is *secondary metastatic tumor* of ovary. It comprises of one-third of all metastatic tumors of ovary.

The *primary* of Krukenberg tumor is the intestine, *characteristically stomach*. Other less common primary sites are breasts, colon, and gallbladder.

The tumor is almost *bilateral*.

The *route of spread* is not clearly known, may be by transperitoneal spill, retroperitoneal lymphatic permeation or through blood stream.

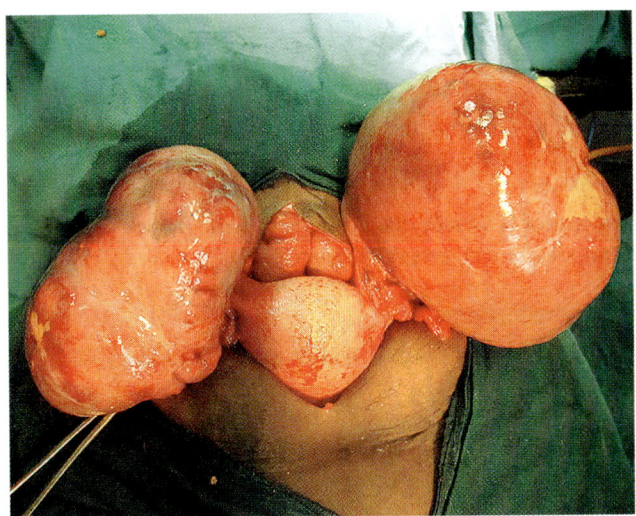

Fig. 54: Krukenberg tumor—a 51-year-old postmenopausal woman presented with lump abdomen. Primary site was found to be at stomach.
Courtesy: Dr Prosenjit Banerjee, Associate Professor; Dr Pradipto Sanyal, Senior Consultant, Obstetrics and Gynecology

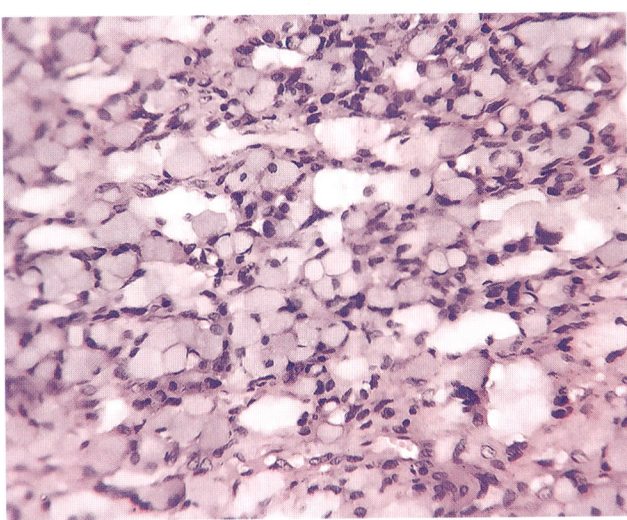

Fig. 55: Microphotography of Krukenberg tumor showing signet ring appearance (H&E, X400).
Courtesy: Professor Gopinath Barui, Department of Pathology

Tumor is almost always *bilateral* moderate size, like the shape of enlarged ovary or kidney, surface smooth, white, capsule not infiltrated, solid and lobulated (**Fig. 54**).

Cut surface shows solid and cystic spaces with area of degeneration.

Histology

It is mucinous or signet ring cell adenocarcinoma (**Fig. 55**). Signet ring cells are ovoid-shaped cells with granular cytoplasm and the nucleus is displaced by intracytoplasmic mucin globule resembling *signet-ring appearance*.

Investigations are like other epithelial carcinoma, but *primary site is always searched* for preoperatively.

Management

Management includes surgery and chemotherapy. During surgery, primary site is also explored and managed accordingly. In few cases, primary tumor is never found.

Prognosis

The tumor is usually discovered when the primary disease is advanced and so *prognosis is poor*.

Gynandroblastoma

It is the rarest variety of sex cord stromal tumor with low malignant potential.

It is a *mix variety* SCSTs mainly of granulosa cells and Sertoli cells along with theca or Leydig cells. Patients are usually in early 30s and present with features of sex hormone excess and menstrual irregularity.

Thecoma-Fibroma of Ovary

Thecoma

Solid tumors composed of cells resembling theca cells, with androgen secretion capability. They are not uncommon variety and clinically benign.

They occur mostly in postmenopausal age group and presenting symptoms are pelvic mass and or with

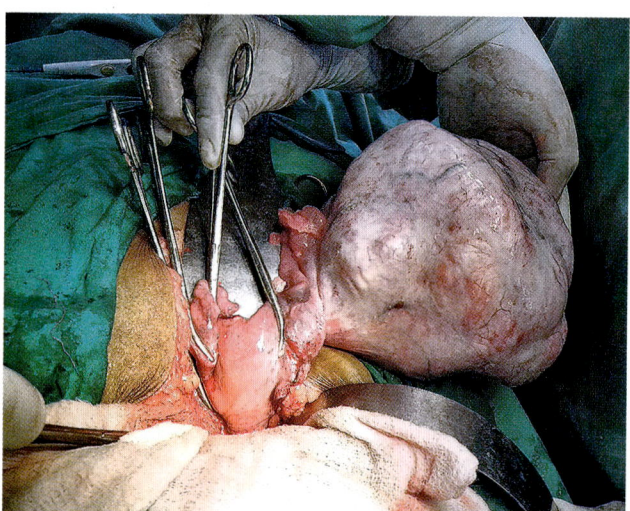

Fig. 56: Laparotomy findings in a 58-year-old woman P4+0 Living issue 4, last child birth 24 years back menopause for 14 years who attended with h/o gradual pain and swelling lower abdomen for 2 years. Right sided solid ovarian tumor.
Courtesy: Dr Pranati Kasyapi and Prof Debdutta Ghose, RG Kar MCH, Kolkata

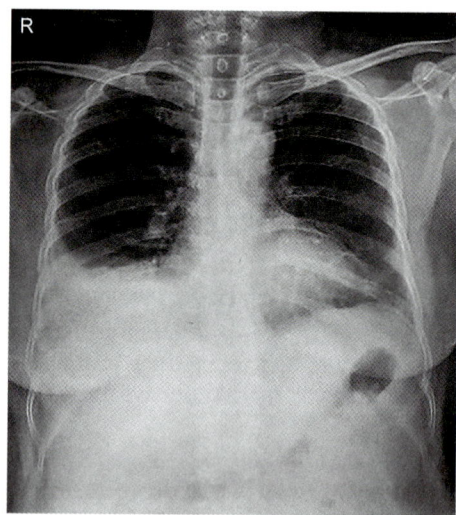

Fig. 58: X-ray chest showing right sided pleural effusion in the patient undergoing laparotomy as shown in Figure 56.

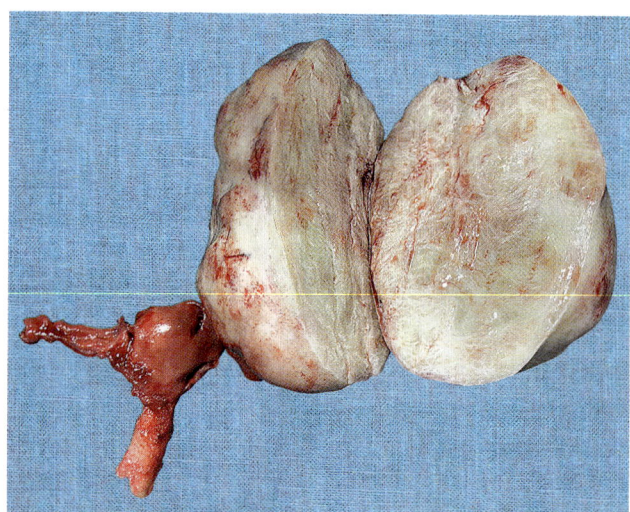

Fig. 57: Hysterectomy specimen following total hysterectomy with bilateral salpingectomy as in the patient shown in Figure 56. Cut open to show the right sided solid ovarian tumor (fibroma).

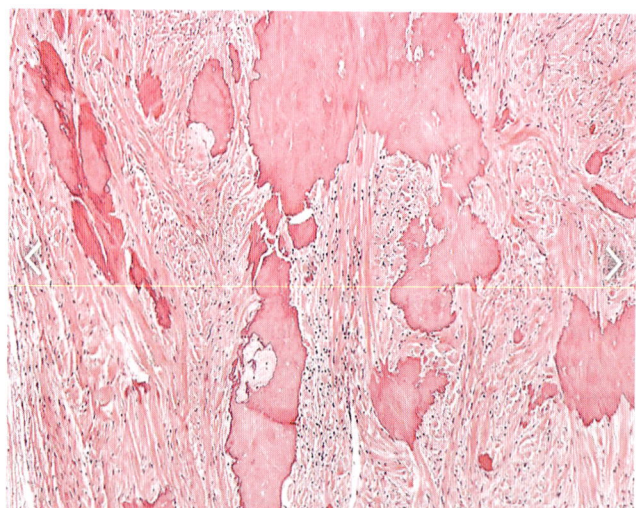

Fig. 59: HP consistent with ovarian fibroma of the specimen in Figure 57.

postmenopausal or irregular vaginal bleeding and because of solid nature mimic subserous fibroid of uterus.

They may be associated with endometrial hyperplasia and CA.

Fibroma

They are hormonally inactive, occurs in same age group like thecoma.

They are solid and benign; very few cases may be low malignant and 1% chance of fibrosarcoma. A special variety of fibroma is Meigs' syndrome described above.

As thecoma-fibroma are mostly benign, treatment is simple excision.

Q. What do you mean by Meigs' syndrome (J V Meigs 1937)?

Ovarian fibroma associated with ascites and right-sided pleural effusion is called Meigs' syndrome *(triad of solid ovarian mass, pleural effusion, and ascites)*. Origin of pleural fluid is likely to be from ascitic fluid which is transudate. Removal of ovarian tumor results disappearance of both ascitic and pleural fluid (*see* **Figs. 56 to 59**).

MANAGEMENT OF A CASE OF OVARIAN TUMOR IN PREGNANCY

See author's Bedside Clinics in Obstetrics, Fifth edition, Academic Publishers.

CHAPTER 4

A Case of Uterine Leiomyoma (Uterine Fibroid)

CHAPTER OUTLINE

Writing a case of fibroid uterus and how to present the case?

- Differential Diagnosis
- How to Differentiate from Ovarian Tumor?
- Diagnosis of Fibroid Uterus
- Complications of Uterine Fibroid
- Types of Uterine Fibroid—Recent Classifications
- Management of Fibroid Uterus
- Description of Uterine Artery Embolization
- Steps of Myomectomy
- Cervical Fibroid
- Broad Ligament Fibroid
- Uterine Polyp

PATIENT'S PARTICULARS

1. Name:
2. Age: Commonly in reproductive age group mostly in between 30 years and 40 years
3. Address:
4. Occupation:
5. Married/unmarried:
6. History of infertility: Association is common
7. Husband's occupation:
8. Socioeconomic status:
9. Religion:
10. Parous/nulliparous: Nulliparous or low parity

Bed No.:
Date of Admission:
Date of Examination:

HISTORY

1. *Chief complaint/complaints*: Heavy menstrual bleeding (HMB), menorrhagia, lump abdomen, pain in abdomen, dysmenorrhea, and infertility.

2. *History of present illness*: Elaborate the chief complaints. Menorrhagia is more common, whether there is any intermenstrual bleeding, whether there is any pain in lower abdomen is searched for. Any pressure symptoms, frequency, urgency of urine present or not is enquired. Is there any palpitation or weakness?

3. *Menstrual history*: Details to be noted as in fibroid uterus this is the main complaint.
   - Last menstrual period (LMP):
   - Duration of menstruation:
   - Interval in days:
   - Age of menarche: Early menarche favors uterine fibroid
   - Regularity of cycle:
   - Pain during period/if pain relation with menstruation—there may be dysmenorrhea
   - Amount of bleeding—to be enquired as written in Chapter 1 (*see* Page 7)
   - Clot: HMB (menorrhagia) is common in uterine fibroid
   - Intermenstrual bleeding—common in submucous fibroid or other pathology

4. *Obstetric history*:
   - Parity—nulliparous or low parity/may be history of infertility

- Living issue (LI)—Write "Nil" if patient is primi
- Last child birth (LCB):
  Write down in tabular form as in Chapter 1.
5. *Past history*:
   - Medical
   - Surgical: Any previous history of surgery for fibroid or anything else
6. *Family history*: Seen in families, but specific gene is not identified
7. *Sexual history*:
8. *Functional history*:
   - Bowel—constipation may be present due to posterior low corporeal or cervical fibroid
   - Bladder—any pressure symptom—retention of urine
   - Sleep
   - Appetite
9. *Personal history*:
   - Personal hygiene
   - Smoking or alcohol
10. *Contraceptive history*:
11. *Drug history*:
    - History of any drug allergy
    - History of intake of iron, corticosteroids, antiepileptic or other drugs (previous or present)
    - History of blood transfusion if any.

PHYSICAL EXAMINATION

Patient—alert, conscious, and cooperative
- Build
- Nutrition
- Height
- Weight/body mass index (BMI)
- Edema
- Anemia—present
- Cyanosis
- Jaundice
- Clubbing
- Tongue, teeth, gum, tonsil
- Neck veins
- Neck glands
- Leg veins
- Pulse
- Respiration
- Temperature
- Blood pressure: High BP may be associated with fibroid.

SYSTEMIC EXAMINATION

- *Central nervous system*
- *Cardiovascular system*:
  - Auscultation of heart
- *Respiratory system*:
  - Auscultation of chest
- *Gastrointestinal system:*
  - Liver
  - Spleen
- *Examination of other systems:*
  - Examination of back and spines skeletal system
  - Neurological
  - Ophthalmoscopic examination
  - Urinary system
- *Examination of breasts and nipple:*
  - Inspection
  - Palpation.

GYNECOLOGICAL EXAMINATION

Abdominal Examination

- *Inspection*: There may be lump lower abdomen or suprapubic fullness. Flanks are flattened.
- *Palpation:*
  - Site, size, shape, surface—smooth, margins—well-defined all sides except lower margin, consistency—firm to hard, tenderness, mobility—present from side to side, lower pole— could not be reached
  - No fetal parts, no Braxton Hicks sign—felt
  - Rising test—intra-abdominal swelling
  - Sometimes fibroid may not be palpable abdominally or there may be only suprapubic fullness. Size of 14 weeks or above palpable abdominally.
- *Percussion*: Dull over the lump. No free fluid in abdomen.
- *Auscultation*: Silent.

Vaginal Examination

- Inspection and palpation of external genitalia, vulva, vagina—normal
- Speculum examination—look for any pathology over cervix and any polyp
- Bimanual examination.
  Mass seems to be arisen from the uterus, mass moves with the movement of cervix and vice versa. Mass may be nodular in multiple fibroids. Fornices may be clear or tubo-ovarian swellings may be palpable. There is no cleft or groove in between uterus and mass (*see* Page 27, Chapter 1).
- Examination of rectovaginal area and rectal examination.

SUMMARY OF THE CASE (SAMPLE)

Mrs XY aged 39 years P1+ 0 housewife coming from low socioeconomic status was admitted with history of heavy menstrual period and lump lower abdomen for last 8 months. Her LMP was—, period is regular but persisting for 8–10 days, occurring 28–30 days interval. Patient felt lower abdominal swelling for last 6 months.

On examination she is normotensive, pulse 80 beats/min, and moderate pallor.

On abdominal examination there was a lower abdominal swelling, situated midline, almost globular, firm in consistency extending up to umbilicus, margins are well defined except lower margins which could not be reached, surface smooth, dull on percussion.

Vaginal examination revealed vulva, vagina normal, cervix looks healthy on speculum examination. Bimanual examination shows a pelviabdominal large mass seems to be arisen from the uterus extending up to the umbilicus. Both fornices are clear.

INVESTIGATIONS SUPPLIED OR REQUIRED

The investigations required are hemoglobin (Hb)% and ultrasonography (USG). The other investigations required if any are noted.

PROVISIONAL DIAGNOSIS

Fibroid uterus in a 39-year-old woman.

DIFFERENTIAL DIAGNOSIS

Differential diagnosis (D/D) of lump lower abdomen (written in Chapter 3, Section 2 of Ovarian Tumor, Page 47) includes:
- Full bladder
- Pregnancy
- Ovarian tumor
- Fibroid uterus/broad ligament fibroid
- Large tubo-ovarian mass
- Large chocolate cyst in endometriosis
- Mesenteric cyst
- Adenomyosis
- Koch's peritonitis
- Ascites.

Other causes are:
- Renal lump
- Splenic enlargement
- Retroperitoneal lymphoma
- Gastrointestinal lump
- Huge splenic enlargement and
- Any retroperitoneal mass like lymphoma, lipoma, etc.

In small fibroid D/D of abnormal uterine bleeding (AUB) with enlarged uterus, e.g., dysfunctional uterine bleeding (DUB), endometrial carcinoma (CA).

Q. How to differentiate adenomyosis from fibroid uterus? (Features of adenomyosis)

- In adenomyosis the size of the uterus is usually not more than 12–14 weeks size
- In adenomyosis uterus is uniformly enlarged in contrast to uterine fibroid except in case of single fibroid
- Dysmenorrhea and dyspareunia are present in adenomyosis in contrast to fibroid
- On bimanual examination uterus is uniformly enlarged, soft and tender in adenomyosis
- Sonography can differentiate and MRI is more useful to diagnose. By MRI in adenomyosis junctional zone (JZ) is at least 12 mm and/or ill-defined low signal intensity myometrial area whereas there is a well-circumscribed mass related to leiomyoma (*see* Page 372, Chapter 16).
- In between the leiomyoma and myometrium there is a pseudocapsule and myoma can be easily shelled out during myomectomy (**Fig. 37–40**, *see* Page101) but there is no such plane in adenomyosis and difficult to enucleate. In diffuse adenomyosis glands and stroma are scattered in myometrium and in focal adenomyosis a focal nodular collection is seen.

Q. Why are you saying this is a case of fibroid uterus?

- Menstrual abnormality in the form of heavy menstrual bleeding (menorrhagia)
- Presence of pallor
- On abdominal examination a lump is felt which is firm in consistency and mobile from side to side and lower border could not be reached.
- On per vaginal examination mass seems to be arisen from the uterus and there is no cleft or groove in between the mass and the uterus. On movement of the cervix lump moves and vice versa.

Q. What are the other nomenclatures of uterine fibroid?

Most appropriate is leiomyoma, often called myoma, fibromyoma, and colloquially known as fibroids.

The term fibroid is misnomer because the tumor contains smooth muscle cells within elastin, collagen, and extracellular matrix proteins.

Q. How will you confirm the diagnosis?

Diagnosis will be confirmed by USG and other imaging technique.

DIAGNOSIS OF FIBROID UTERUS

Q. How would you diagnose fibroid uterus?
- Symptoms
- Signs
- Investigations.

Symptoms

- Majority of women with fibroid is asymptomatic. But more than 25% are symptomatic.
- Age: Mostly reproductive age group 30–40 years
- Abnormal uterine bleeding (most common symptom)
  - Menorrhagia (HMB) is the most common type of abnormal bleeding and may be as high as 30–50%
  - Other types are metrorrhagia (intermenstrual bleeding) and polymenorrhea
- Lump abdomen

- Pelvic pressure, low back pain, pain in abdomen, dysmenorrhea and dyspareunia
- Pressure symptoms—urinary frequency, incontinence and constipation
- Palpitation and weakness due to anemia
- White discharge due to submucous fibroid
- Infertility: Fibroid is responsible for 2–3% cases of infertility only.

Signs
On physical examination—pallor—present.

Per Abdominal Examination
- *Inspection:* There may be lump lower abdomen or suprapubic fullness. Flanks are flattened.
- *Palpation:*
  - Site, size, shape, surface—smooth, margins—well-defined all sides except lower margin, consistency—firm to hard, tenderness, mobility—present from side to side, lower pole— could not be reached
  - No fetal parts, no Braxton Hicks sign felt
  - Rising test—intra-abdominal swelling
  - Sometimes fibroid may not be palpable abdominally or there may be only suprapubic fullness. Size of 14 weeks or above palpable abdominally.
- *Percussion: No free fluid inside abdomen*
- *Auscultation: Nothing special.*

Vaginal Examination
- Per speculum examination—sometimes, a fibroid polyp can be seen from the cervical canal, presence of any bleeding looked for
- Bimanual examination shows a pelviabdominal large mass seems to be arisen from the uterus. Both fornices are clear. No cleft or groove between the uterus and mass.

Investigations for Diagnosis
- Examination under anesthesia (EUA)
- Ultrasonography (USG), sonohysterography
- Magnetic resonance imaging (MRI)
- Laparoscopy
- Hysteroscopy.

Routine Investigations
It includes Hb%, total count (TC), differential count (DC), erythrocyte sedimentation rate (ESR), blood grouping, typing, kidney function, postprandial sugar, and others include thyroid stimulating hormone (TSH), triiodothyronine (T3), and thyroxine (T4).

Management Options of Uterine Leiomyoma
- Expectant (observation)
- Medical
- Radiological intervention: Uterine artery embolization (UAE) and magnetic resonance-guided focused ultrasound
- Surgery: Myomectomy, hysterectomy, myolysis, and laparoscopic uterine artery occlusion.

Indication of Observation
See later, for indication of observation (Page 94).

Indication of Surgical Intervention
See later, for indication of surgical intervention (Page 97).

Medical Management Options
- Hematinic
- *Nonhormonal*: Tranexamic acid, nonsteroidal anti-inflammatory drugs (NSAIDs), and aromatase inhibitors
- *Hormones*: Combined oral contraceptives (COCs), progestins—DMPA (depot medroxyprogesterone acetate), LNG-IUS (levonorgestrel-intrauterine system), GnRH (gonadotropin-releasing hormone), androgens, danazol, gestrinone, SPRMs (selective progesterone receptor modulator)—mifepristone and ulipristal acetate. For details of management, *see* further Page 94.

Q. What are the causes of menorrhagia (HMB) in fibroid uterus?

- Increase of endometrial surface—normal surface area of endometrial cavity is 15 cm^2
- Endometrial hyperplasia
- Increase vascularity of uterus
- Abnormal uterine contractility
- Increase congestion due to impaired venous drainage by compression with fibroid
- Dysregulation of growth factor causing disordered angiogenesis and vasodilatation.
  Heavy menstrual bleeding may occur in intramural, submucous, and even also subserous variety.

Q. What is the cause of intermenstrual bleeding (metrorrhagia) in fibroid uterus?

- Due to submucous fibroid with ulceration and necrosis of underlying endometrium
- Rarely, due to associated endometrial CA.

Cause of Pain in Uterine Fibroid
Pain is not a common symptom in fibroid uterus but may occur.

The causes are due to degenerative changes especially red degeneration, torsion of pedicle, prolapsing leiomyoma or associated infection.

Prolapse of tumor (submucous variety) from the endometrial cavity will cause cramping or acute pain as the tumor stretches the endocervical canal during passing through.

Dysmenorrhea: It is due to submucous fibroid or associated pelvic and adnexal inflammation.

Cause of Excessive Discharge

White discharge is due to excessive surface area, bloody discharge for submucous variety, and offensive discharge due to ulceration and necrosis of submucous fibroid.

Cause of Infertility in Fibroid Uterus

Uterine fibroid contributes *only 1–3%* cases of infertility. The causes are:
- Occlusion of tubal ostia due to pressure effect
- Alteration of uterine contraction that propels sperm and ova
- Distortion of uterine cavity which diminishes implantation and sperm transport
- Disruption of implantation due to endometrial inflammation and vascular changes
- Ovum pick up may be hampered due to corporeal fibroid distorting the tube. Subfertility is more associated with submucous variety than other type. Spontaneous abortion and pregnancy wastage is increased in uterine fibroid. Other factors are evaluated first for diagnosing fibroid as a cause of infertility.

Q. What is *myomatous erythrocytosis syndrome*?

In patient of leiomyoma, erythropoietin production is increased by the kidney or by the leiomyoma themselves in 5% cases. Following hysterectomy red cell mass returns to normal.

Q. What is *leiomyomatosis*?

Leiomyomatosis is extrauterine smooth-muscle tumors, which are benign, yet infiltrative developed in women concurrently or with history of prior uterine leiomyoma.

Q. What is pseudo-Meigs syndrome?

Uterine fibroid with ascites and pleural effusion is called pseudo-Meigs syndrome. Discordancy between the arterial supply and the venous and lymphatic drainage from the leiomyoma is the probable etiology. Removal of tumor or hysterectomy cures the condition.

Q. What are the findings of leiomyoma in sonography (Figs. 1 to 5)?

Ultrasonography should always be done to confirm the diagnosis.

Larger one can be done transabdominally but smaller can be done by transvaginal route (**Figs. 1A and B**).
- It looks enlarged uterus with patchy echogenicity.
- It varies from hypo- to hyperechoic depending on ratio of smooth muscle to connective tissue.
- USG color Doppler shows the vascularity mainly in the periphery in fibroid (**Fig. 2**). Calcification shows hyperechoic ranging from a rim to diffuse hyperechogenicity whereas cystic degeneration shows hypoechoic or anechoic areas.

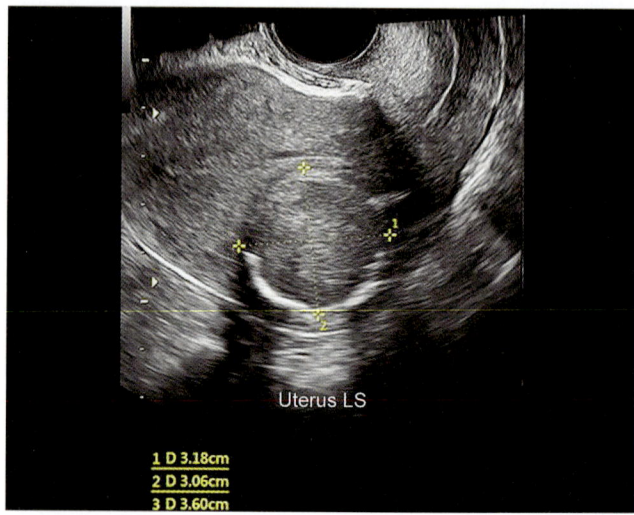

Fig. 1A: Transvaginal sonography showing a solitary fibroid in posterior wall of uterus compressing the endometrial cavity.
Courtesy: Professor Kamal Oswal, VIMS, Kolkata

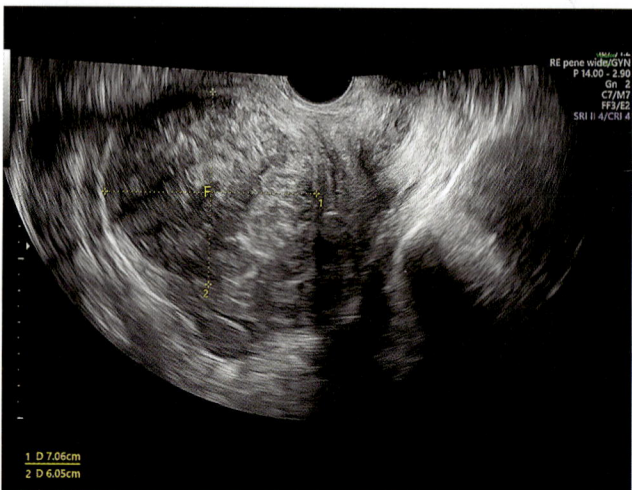

Fig. 1B: Sonograpphy showing intramural fibroid (7.06 cm × 6.05 cm).
Courtesy: Professor Kamal Oswal, VIMS, Kolkata

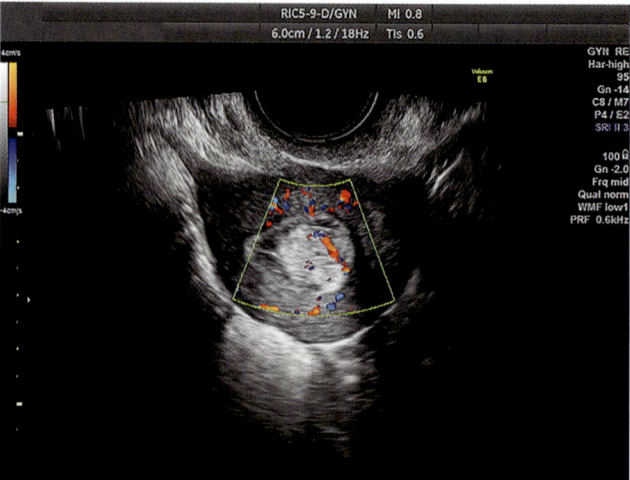

Fig. 2: Endometrial polyp with Doppler.
Courtesy: Professor Kamal Oswal, VIMS, Kolkata

- Serial USG is necessary when expectant or medical management is continued. Volume of fibroid is measured by the formula $4/3\pi r^3$ where r is the radius.
- In submucous leiomyoma endometrium looks thick or irregular by transvaginal sonography (TVS) **(Fig. 3)**.
- Saline infusion sonography (SIS) **(Fig. 4)** and hysteroscopy **(Fig. 6)** can diagnose better.
- Three-dimensional (3D) TVS **(Fig. 5)**, 3D SIS, and color Doppler are very informative.

Role of Hysteroscopy in Diagnosis of Uterine Fibroid (Fig. 6)

Hysteroscope is valuable to diagnose submucous myoma **(Fig. 6)** and surgery can be done simultaneously for Grade 0 and Grade 1, leiomyoma as FIGO (International Federation of Gynecology and Obstetrics) classification with optimal diameter <3 cm and >50% in cavity.

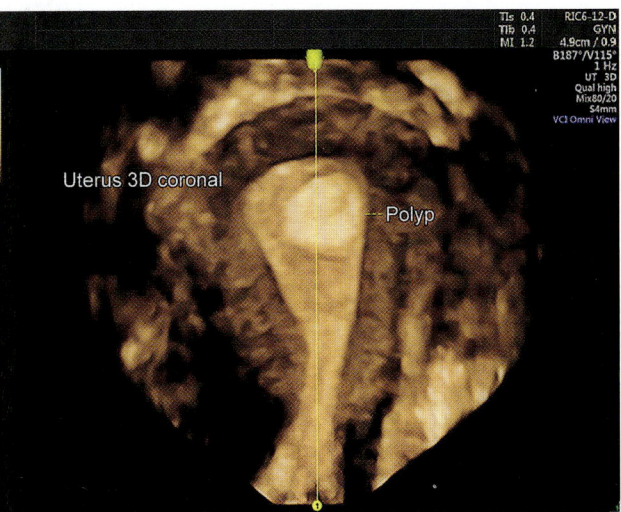

Fig. 5: 3D ultrasonography showing endometrial polyp inside endometrial cavity.
Courtesy: Professor Kamal Oswal, VIMS, Kolkata

Role of MRI in Diagnosis of Uterine Fibroid (Fig. 7)

- An MRI is useful tool to assess accurately the number, size, and location of fibroids.
- MRI is a useful tool to plan the therapy especially before UAE **(Fig. 7)**.
- To *differentiate between myoma and adenomyosis MRI is most suitable diagnostic tool as in later enucleation during surgery is not possible due to lack of proper cleavage plane.*
- Malignancy can be predicted from MRI by age > 45 years, menopausal status, endometrial thickening, intramoral hemorrhage, signal heterogenicity and nonmyometrial origin.

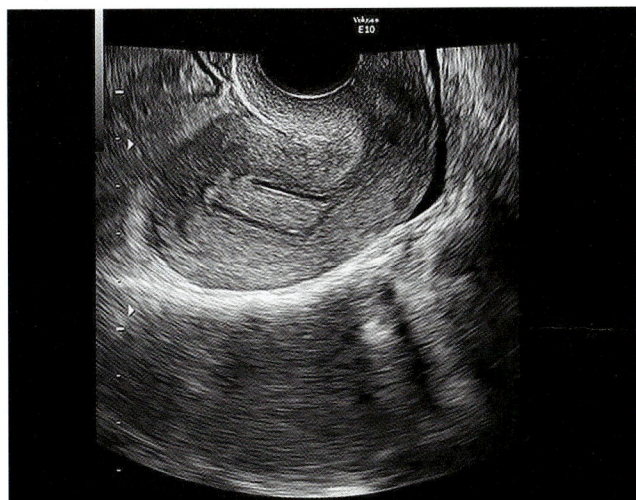

Fig. 3: Transvaginal sonography showing endometrial polyp inside endometrial cavity.
Courtesy: Professor Kamal Oswal, VIMS, Kolkata

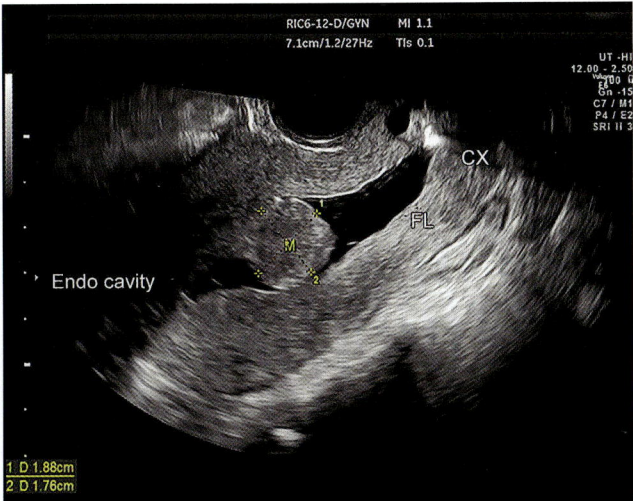

Fig. 4: Saline infusion sonography showing endometrial polyp inside endometrial cavity.
Courtesy: Professor Kamal Oswal, VIMS, Kolkata

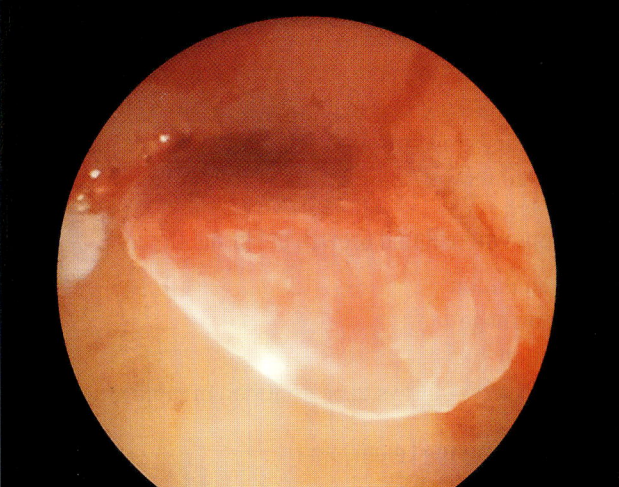

Fig. 6: Hysteroscopic view of endometrial cavity with submucous fibroid.
Courtesy: Dr Bani Mitra, Kolkata

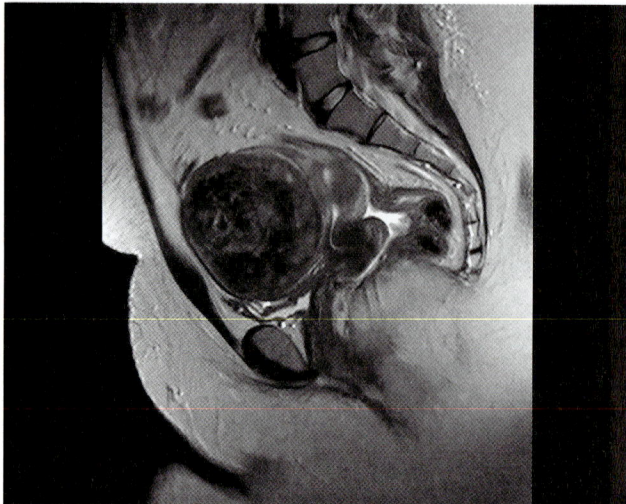

Fig. 7: Sagittal T2-weighted MRI of pelvis of a 42-year-old lady with symptomatic large intramural and subserosal fibroids with a distorted endometrium. This compresses the urinary bladder anteriorly and causes frequency and urgency during periods.
Courtesy: Dr Shuvro H Roy-Choudhury, Consultant Interventional Radiologist

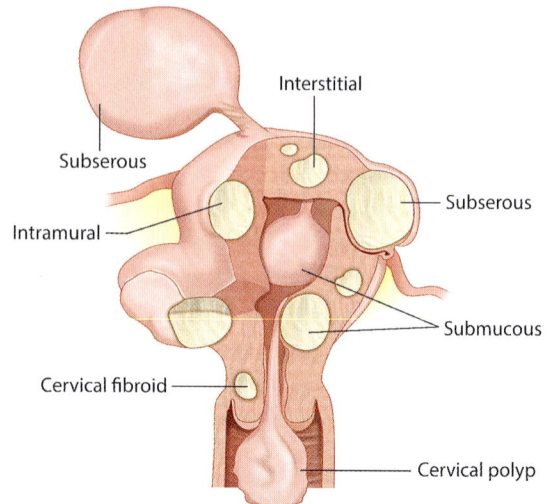

Fig. 8: Varieties of fibroid.

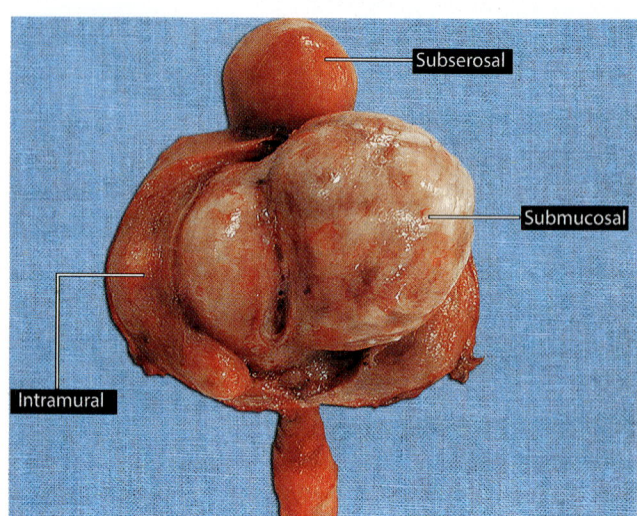

Fig. 9A: Subserosal, intramural, and submucous fibroid together.

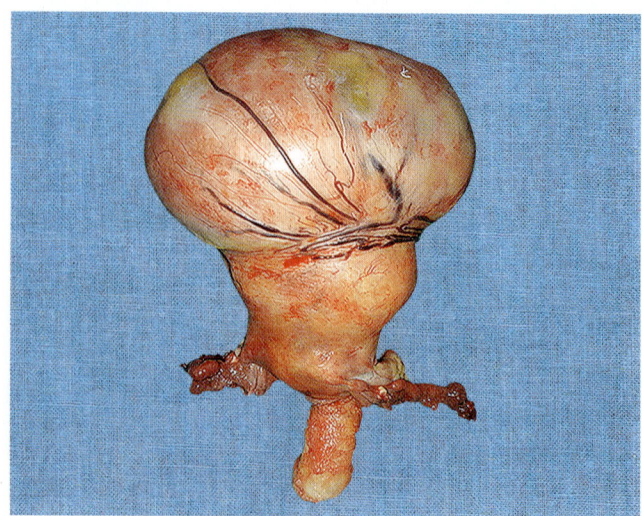

Fig. 9B: Sessile subserosal fundal fibroid.

Role of Laparoscopy

Laparoscopy is of clinical value in a pelvic lump less than 12 weeks size especially in infertility and pelvic pain where clinical and USG findings fail to diagnose clearly.

It can differentiate a pedunculated fibroid from ovarian tumor.

Additionally presence of endometriosis, pelvic inflammatory disease (PID), and tubal pathology can be revealed.

Rate of Growth of Abdominopelvic Lump

- Leiomyoma grows in years—average growth is 0.5 cm/year in diameter, in some patient up to 3 cm/year has been observed. It takes 3 years to reach the size of an orange. To be palpable abdominally, it takes 5 years.
- Ovarian tumor grows in months
- Pregnancy grows in weeks
- Full bladder (retention of urine) grows in days

Situations where Rapid Growth of Fibroid Occurs

- Degeneration
- Hemorrhage
- Infection
- Malignancy—always to be excluded in rapid growth.

Location of Uterine Leiomyoma

- Corporeal **(Figs. 8 and 9)**
- Cervical (1–2%) **(Fig. 8)**.

Types of Uterine Leiomyoma (Fig. 8)

- Subserosal: 20% (subgroup—sessile, pedunculated, parasitic or wandering)
- Intramural or interstitial—most common 60%
- Submucosal: 20%.

Fibroids may be multiple **(Figs. 8 and 9)** or may be single **(Fig. 10)**.

Submucosal

Less common, more than 50% projects inside the uterine cavity and covered by endometrium, usually single **(Figs. 10 and 11)**. It may be sessile or pedunculated. Intermenstrual bleeding is special feature **(Figs. 12A and B)**.

A submucosal fibroid may prone to be infected and sloughing, may form a polyp and a pedunculated type with large stalk, may prolapse through cervical canal **(Fig. 8)**, and may rarely cause inversion **(Fig. 13)** of uterus during expulsion. According to detailed FIGO classification system 0, 1, and 2 are submucosal (*see* Page 91, Table 1).

Intramural (Figs. 14A and B)

More than 50% fibroid mass lie within the myometrium. It is said that all leiomyoma starts growing as intramural, then remains as intramural or becomes subserosal or submucosal. According to detailed FIGO classification system 3 and 4 are intramural.

Subserosal (Fig. 15)

It projects outward from the uterine surface more than 50% and covered by peritoneum. They may be sessile or pedunculated. Subserosal fibroid may grow inside broad

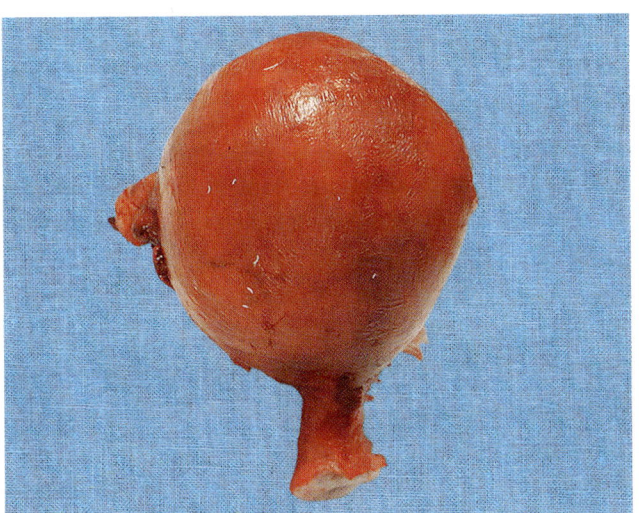

Fig. 10: Intramural single fibroid.

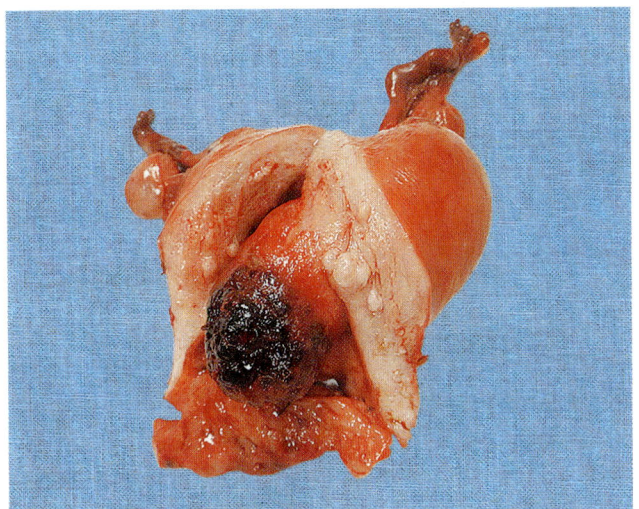

Fig. 12A: Submucous fibroid—source of bleeding (intermenstrual bleeding).

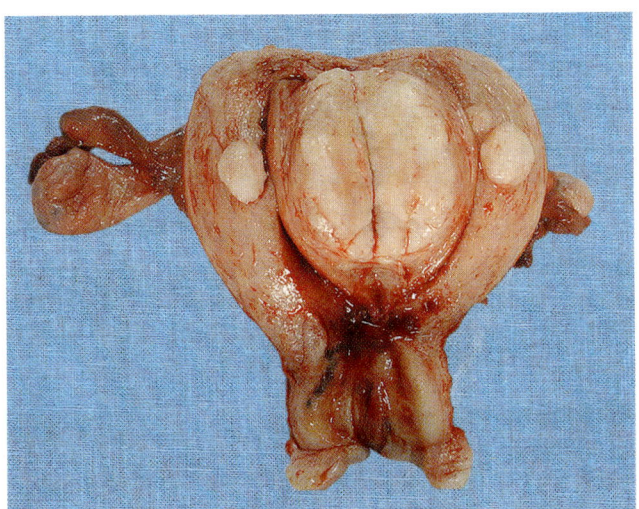

Fig. 11: Submucous fibroid showing in the cavity.

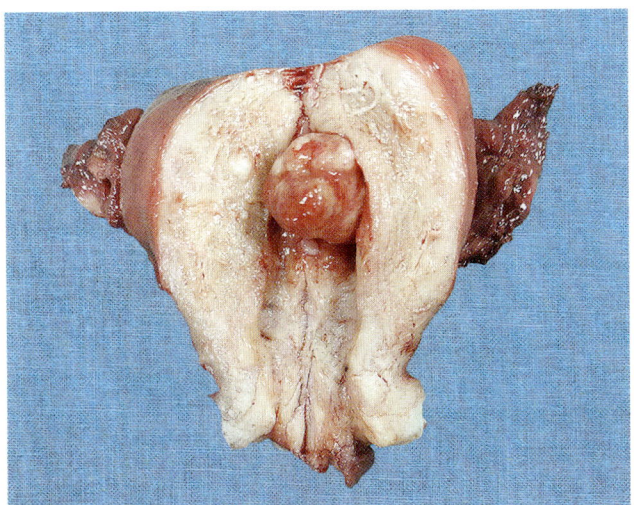

Fig. 12B: 38 years P2+0, LI-2 attended with history of Heavy menstrual bleeding, submucus polyp Type 1 ideal for hysteroscopic resection less than 3 cm diameter 50% intracavitary if patient is younger woman and would be desirous of child.

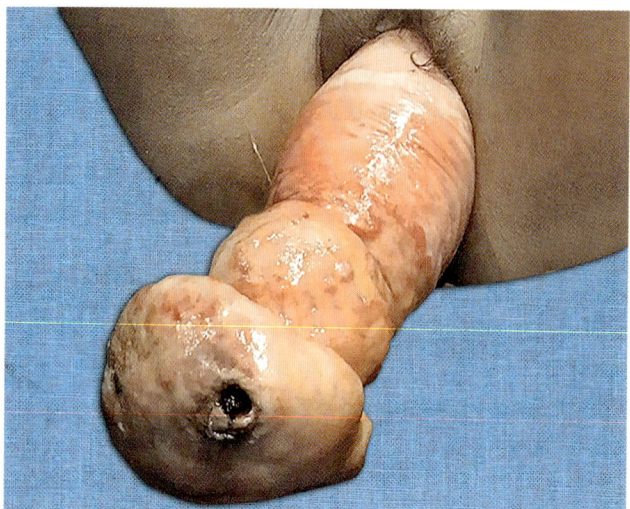

Fig. 13: Fundal submucous large fibroid causing uterine inversion (there was maggots over the tumor).
Courtesy: Dr Shyamal Dasgupta, Associate Professor and Dr Kasmira Majumdar, Department of Obstetrics and Gynecology, RG Kar Medical College

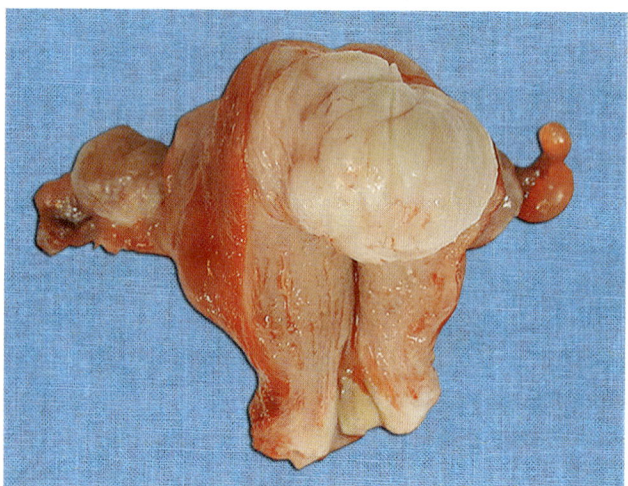

Fig. 14A: Intramural fundal fibroid.

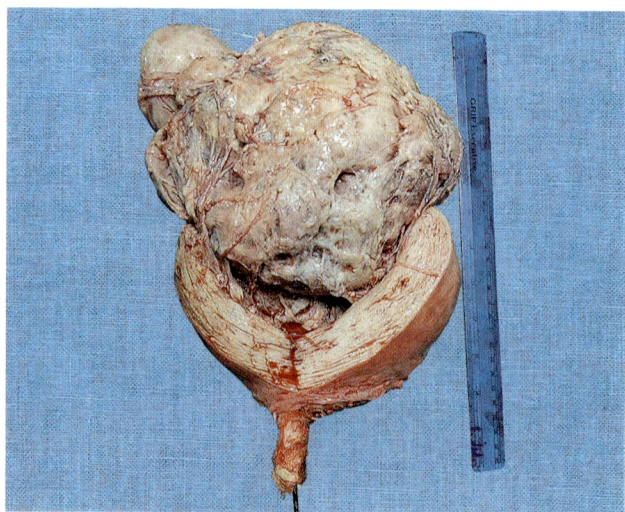

Fig.14B: Cut section of uterus showing degeneration in intramural fibroid.

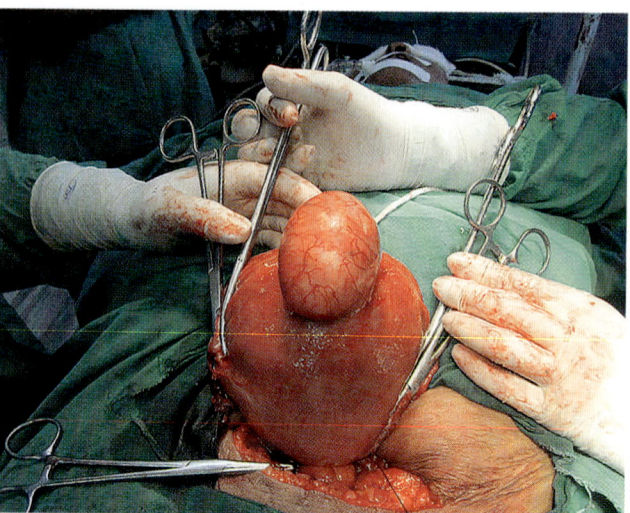

Fig. 15: Subserous fibroid.

ligaments called pseudo broad ligament fibroid (*see* further) or rarely may be detached from the original site called *parasitic or wandering fibroid* (*see* further). Subserosal fibroid with long pedicle may undergo torsion arising emergency. Rupture of vessels from surface of subserosal fibroid may result intraperitoneal hemorrhage. According to detailed FIGO classification system 5, 6, and 7 are subserosal.

Q. What is the FIGO new classification of uterine fibroids?

In new leiomyoma subclassification system, total nine types are described **(Table 1)** from 0 to 8 **(Fig. 16)**.

Fibroids may also be extrauterine, may arise from anywhere where there is any Müllerian tissue:
- Round ligament fibroid
- Ovarian ligament
- Uterosacral ligament
- Vagina
- Vulva
- Broad ligament fibroid— (1) True and (2) Pseudo
- Parasitic or wandering

WANDERING AND PARASITIC FIBROID

Q. What is wandering or parasitic fibroid?

They are subserosal pedunculated type of fibroid which become attached with the adjacent structures, e.g., intestine, omentum deriving blood supply from them with or without detachment from the uterus by axial rotation.

BROAD LIGAMENT FIBROIDS (FIG. 17)

There are two types: (1) true and (2) pseudo broad ligament fibroid (*see* Page 105).

True broad ligament fibroid arises from smooth muscle fibers of round ligament, ovarian ligament or perivascular connective tissue. Pseudo broad ligament fibroid arises from the lateral wall of the uterus, grows inside the two layers

Table 1: Nine types of uterine fibroids (FIGO classification).

	Submucosal (SM)	0	Pedunculated intracavitary
		1	<50% intramural
		2	≥50% intramural
		3	Contacts endometrium; 100% intramural
		4	Intramural
		5	Subserosal ≥50% intramural
		6	Subserosal <50% intramural
		7	Subserosal pedunculated
		8	Other (specify, like, cervical and parasitic)
	Hybrid leiomyomas (impact both endometrium and serosa)		Two numbers are listed separated by a hyphen. The first refers to the relation with endometrium and second refers to the relation with serosa by convention, e.g., 2–5 submucosal and subserosal, each with less than half the diameter in the endometrial and peritoneal cavities, respectively

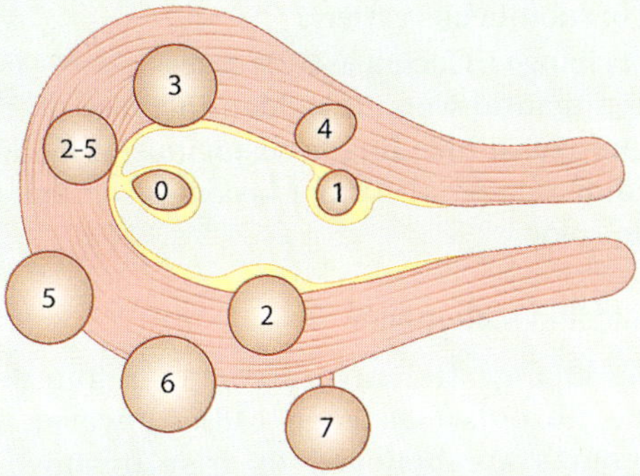

Fig. 16: FIGO subclassification of leiomyoma.

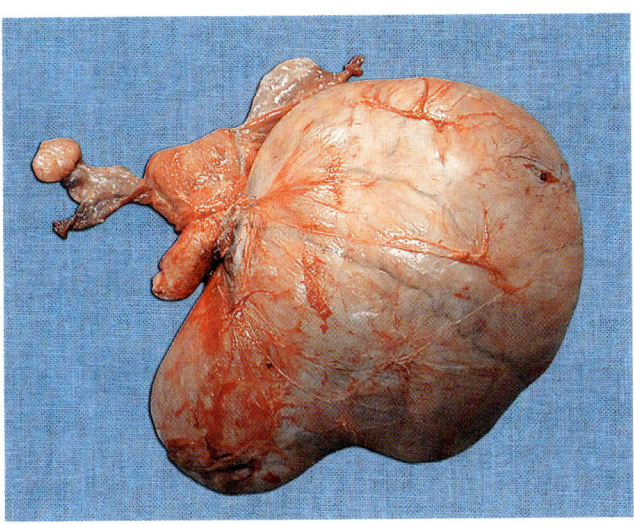

Fig. 17: Large broad ligament fibroid.

of broad ligament and connected with the uterus by thick structure and the former lacks any attachment with uterus.

During removal ureter is vulnerable to be injured in broad ligament fibroid (*see* later with **Fig. 55**—relation between ureter and broad ligament fibroid).

Macroscopic Features of Uterine Leiomyoma (Fig. 18)

They are:
- Spherical
- Rubbery tumors, normally firm, felt firmer than normal myometrium, may be soft due to degeneration, hard due to calcification
- Usually multiple in number, may be single
- Size varies from seedling to large occupying whole abdomen
- Cut section shows typical whorl appearance, the center is paler than the periphery **(Fig. 19)**
- Blood supply comes from periphery to center which makes the center less vascular. Vascularity of myoma is less in comparison to surrounding myometrium sometimes leading to hypoperfusion and ischemia causing acute pain which usually happens in degeneration.

Q. What is pseudocapsule or false capsule?

The leiomyoma is distinct from the surrounding compressed myometrium by a thin connective tissue layer. This is called

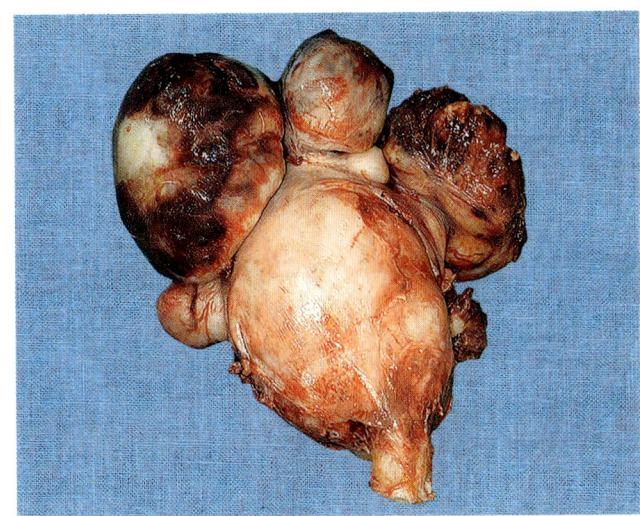

Fig. 18: Multiple fibroids.

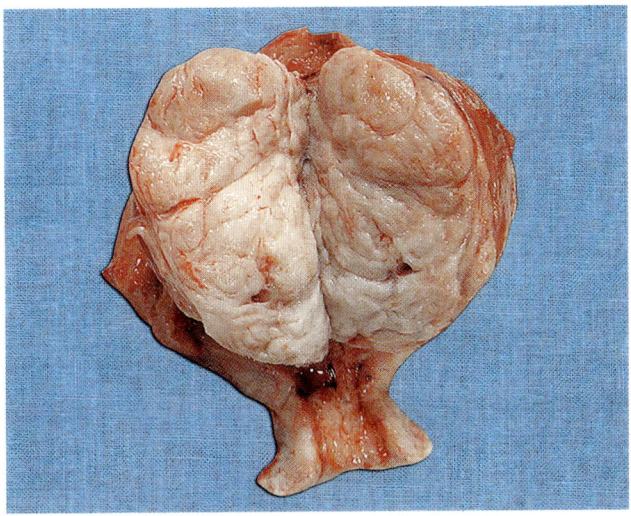

Fig. 19: Cut section shows whorl appearance.

"pseudocapsule" or "false capsule" deep to which there is a plane of cleavage which allows fibroid to be easily shelled from the uterus during myomectomy.

In adenomyoma there is no such capsule making difficulty in its enucleation.

An MRI can differentiate best (*see* **Fig. 7**).

MICROSCOPICAL FEATURES (FIG. 20)

Leiomyomas are benign smooth muscle neoplasm containing spindle-shaped smooth-muscle cells arranged in dense bundles with intervening bundles of fibrous connective tissue. Absence of mitotic activity differentiates benign nature from leiomyosarcoma. At periphery there is connective tissue with blood vessels. Degenerative changes alter the typical appearance of leiomyoma.

Q. What are the changes in uterus and adjacent organs due to uterine fibroid?

Uterus: Size of the uterus increased, endometrial cavity becomes distorted and increased in submucous and interstitial variety.

There is myometrial hypertrophy, endometrium become edematous, and congested except over submucous myoma where it becomes thin, and even necrosed. There may be associated endometrial hyperplasia. All vasculature becomes dilated.

There is increase incidence of endometrial CA found with uterine fibroid.

Ureter: It may be compressed by broad ligament fibroid resulting hydronephrosis.

Common Associations of Uterine Fibroid

Endometriosis and adenomyosis are common association.

Q. What are the secondary changes in uterine fibroid?

- Degenerations: Different varieties
- Vascular changes

- Infection: Infection may occur in submucous variety or subserous variety due to adhered bowel, sometimes areas of red degeneration may be infected.
- Necrosis: It occurs due to vascular obstruction. More common in submucous variety.
- Malignant changes: Occurs in 0.2% cases.

In postmenopausal woman sudden increase of fibroid and postmenopausal bleeding is suspicious of malignant changes (leiomyosarcoma). Tumor becomes soft and looks yellow gray in color.

Uterine Fibroid and Malignancy

Sarcomatous change (leiomyosarcoma) is found only 0.2% uterine fibroids (*see* Page 146). However, most leiomyosarcomas are believed to arise de novo, not related to existing benign tumor. Until proven otherwise sarcomatous transformation in a fibroid is a 'myth'. Removal of asymptomatic fibroid on ground of malignant transformation cannot be justified.

DEGENERATIONS OF UTERINE FIBROID

Q. What are the different degenerations on uterine fibroid?

In process of degeneration smooth muscle is replaced by varieties of degenerative substances after necrosis.

These are: (A) Hyaline, (B) Fatty, (C) Red degeneration, (D) Calcification, (E) Cystic, (F) Myxoid, and (G) Atrophic.

It may be asymptomatic or there may be pain of varying degree.

Hyaline degeneration: Most common degeneration, common after menopause, due to impairment of blood supply. Feels like soft elastic. Cut section shows homogenous appearance.

Fatty degeneration: Fat globules appear in the cells (**Fig. 21**).

Red degeneration: Also called "carneous" degeneration *mostly found in pregnancy;* coagulative necrosis results hemorrhagic, meaty, pigmented cut surface and areas of cystic degeneration and mucinous change (**Figs. 22A to C**).

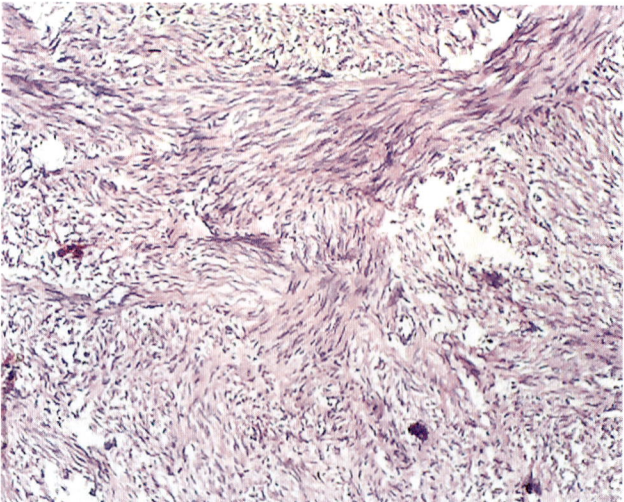

Fig. 20: Microphotograph of leiomyoma.

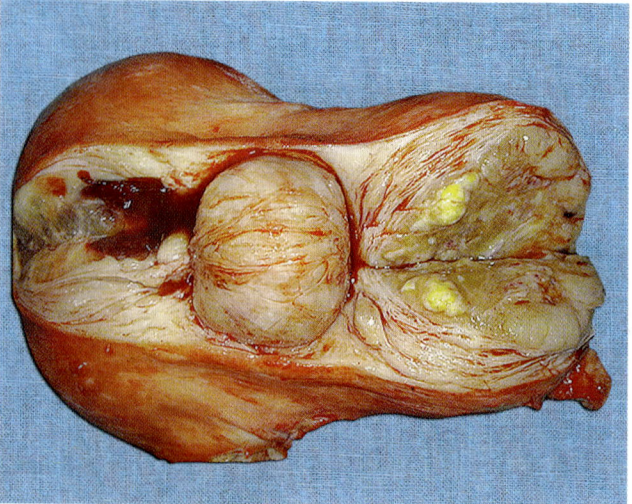

Fig. 21: Fatty degeneration of fibroid.

CHAPTER 4: A Case of Uterine Leiomyoma (Uterine Fibroid)

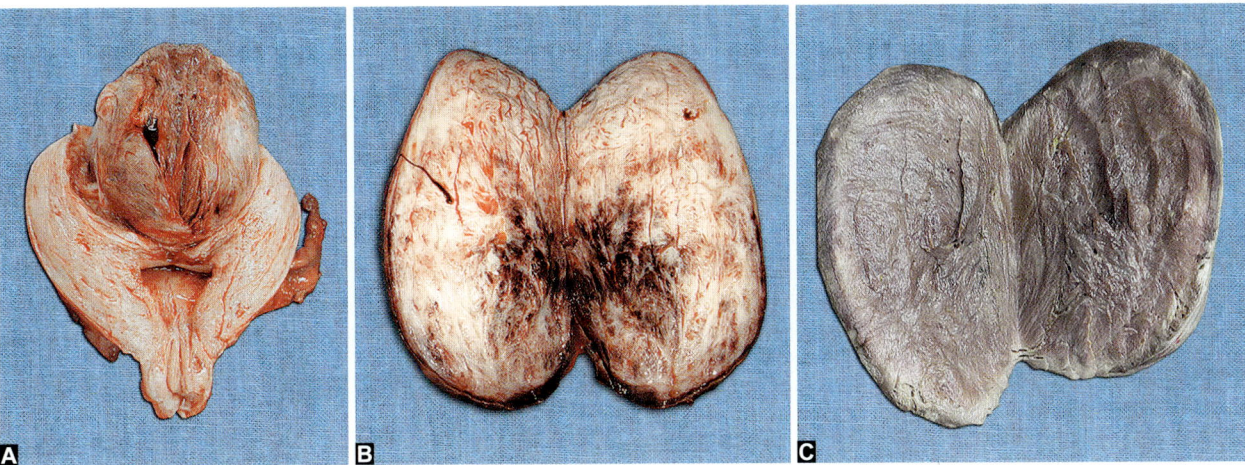

Figs. 22A to C: (A and B) Red degeneration in intramural fibroid; (C) Old red degeneration of fibroid.

The cause is not known exactly, probably due to obstruction of vascular supply, necrosis with hemolysis of RBCs result of "vascular accident".

Patient may present with severe pain in abdomen and mild fever, leukocytosis, high ESR and treated with NSAIDs. Sometimes patient needs admission due to acute abdomen like presentation.

Calcification: Fatty changes and calcification occurs especially in postmenopausal women and in subserous type.

Cystic degeneration: Due to liquefaction of hyalinized or necrosed areas, the tumor becomes soft **(Fig. 23)**.

Myxoid Degeneration

Atrophic degeneration: It may occur after menopause. But probably never regress completely.

Q. What are the complications of uterine fibroids?

The complications are:
- Hemorrhage and anemia
- Degeneration particularly red degeneration causing severe pain

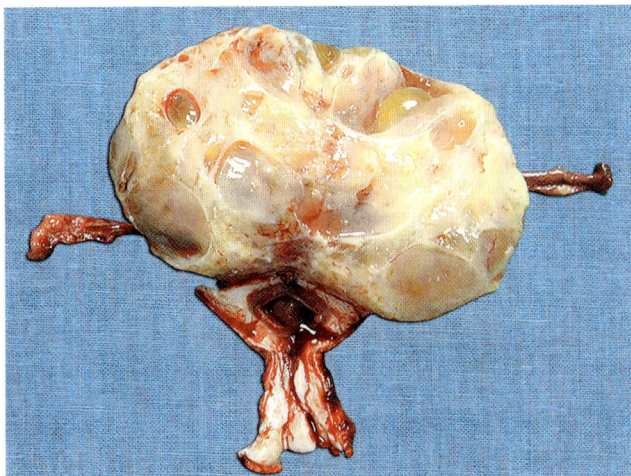

Fig. 23: Cystic degeneration of fibroid.
Courtesy: Dr Alok De, Associate Professor, Obstetrics and Gynecology

- Torsion of subserosal fibroid presenting acute abdomen
- Rupture of vessels from subserosal fibroid resulting intraperitoneal hemorrhage
- Malignancy—0.2% cases
- Infection: Submucosal variety, in puerperium more chance of infection
- Uterine inversion by submucosal large fibroid polyp
- Impaction of lower uterine or cervical fibroid causing retention of urine, constipation, and obstructed labor.

Gynecological emergencies those may arise due to uterine fibroid:
- Torsion
- Impaction causing retention of urine
- Red degeneration causing severe pain
- Severe vaginal hemorrhage and subperitoneal hemorrhage
- Inversion.

Incidence of Uterine Leiomyoma

Fibroids are the most common benign tumor of the uterus and the most common pelvic tumor in women.

Generally 20–25%, may be as high as 70–80% if USG and histopathology (H/P) are considered.

Risk Factors and Etiology of Uterine Fibroid
- *Age*: Latter half of reproductive age 30–40 years
- *Race*: 3–5 times more common in black women than white, Asian or Hispanic women
- *Early menarche*
- *Parity*: More common in nulliparous, low parity, pregnancy has protective effect
- *Familial hereditary factors* are considered in fibroid though specific gene is not identified
- *Genetic factors* (*see* further)
- *Caffeine and alcohol increases while smoking decreases* the risk due to reduction of estrogen level
- *Obesity, diabetes mellitus, polycystic ovarian syndrome, and high blood pressure* increase risk of fibroids

❖ *Estrogen*: Fibroid growth is both estrogen and progesterone dependent disease. Local concentration of estrogen is more than that of normal myometrial tissue. Both estrogen and progesterone receptors are found to be increased in fibroid tissue. In contrary to earlier study COC has no association of fibroid growth.

Recent Genetic View

Fibroid is developed from a progenitor myocyte and each tumor of same uterus has independent cytogenetic origin. Defects in some chromosomes and specific gene mutations are related with tumor growth. Of these mutations fumarate hydratase gene mutations, though rare may lead to the hereditary leiomyomatosis and renal cell cancer which also includes cutaneous cancer (2015).

DETAILS OF MANAGEMENT OF FIBROID UTERUS

Parameters Considered for Management

- Age
- Size and location
- Symptoms
- Desirous of fertility
- Availability of facility
- Experience of provider

Management Options of Uterine Leiomyoma

- Expectant (observation)
- Medical
- Radiological intervention: Uterine artery embolization (UAE) and magnetic resonance-guided focused ultrasound
- Surgery: Myomectomy, hysterectomy, myolysis, and laparoscopic uterine artery occlusion

Expectant Management

Indication

- Asymptomatic fibroids (as 50% of fibroid are)
- 12 weeks or less size. However removal of more than 12 weeks size otherwise asymptomatic has been challenged now as spontaneous regression occurs in menopause.
  As already discussed, sarcomatous changes in untreated fibroid is a myth.
  Recent view is an observation in asymptomatic fibroid irrespective of size but surveillance with annual pelvic examination. In case of difficult and inconclusive pelvic examination annual sonographic monitoring is suggested.

Medical Management

Objectives

- To relieve the symptoms
- Complete regression of fibroids
- Fertility achievement if desired

Limitation of medical management: Complete regression does not occur and recurrence is common after withdrawal of treatment.

Medical Agents

- *Hematinic*: Iron with vitamin C is prescribed to improve anemia as there is HMB (Hb% estimation is must)
- *Nonhormonal*:
  - Tranexamic acid (TXA) is an antifibrinolytic agent. Oral TXA is Food and Drug Administration (FDA) approved for the treatment of ovulatory AUB and there is some evidence to use it in fibroid related bleeding. Dose is 650 mg two tablet thrice daily orally for first 5 days of menstrual period.
  - Nonsteroidal anti-inflammatory drugs (NSAID) like ibuprofen and naproxen: Their use as sole agent in myoma related bleeding is less clear but helpful for myoma-related dysmenorrhea. They reduce blood loss but less effective than TXA.
  - Aromatase inhibitor like letrozol and aristozol have been studied in myoma-related bleeding with success as aromatase levels are higher in myoma but not fully established. It is effective in fibroid in postmenopausal women.
- *Hormonal*:
  - *Combined oral contraceptives (COC)*: Current thought is that *lower estrogen containing pill* is a reasonable treatment option to treat myoma-related symptoms as higher dose of estrogen was alleged to increase fibroid size. COC reduces blood loss. However, close monitoring of fibroid and uterine size is recommended by American College of Obstetricians and Gynecologists (ACOG) (2012) due to unpredictable effect of progesterone on myoma.
  - *Progesterone*:
    - *Injection DMPA* has been tried to reduce uterine bleeding in fibroid
    - LNG-IUS is most effective medical treatment of myoma-related menorrhagia, however, less efficacious than used in DUB. There is higher expulsion rate in comparison to use in AUB in normal uterus. LNG-IUS should not be used in patients with fibroids which distort the uterine cavity.
  - *Gonadotropin releasing hormone (GnRH) agonist*:
    - Creates profound hypoestrogenic by hypogonadotropic state by downregulation of GnRH receptors
    - Reduces the size of uterine fibroid significantly and relieves menorrhagia
    - Induces endometrial atrophy and amenorrhea and helps to improve anemia
    - Uterine volume is reduced by 30–60%, and volume is reduced by 35% after 3 months and 60% by 6 months with little change thereafter anemia is improved in women with HMB and fibroids. Leuprolide

acetate is FDA approved for short-term use in the preoperative treatment of uterine leiomyomata.
- Their use as primary treatment is hampered by rapid recurrence after withdrawal and menopausal symptoms and loss of bone density on long-term treatment.
- Subcutaneous goserelin induces atrophy and amenorrhea usually among premenopausal women within 3-4 weeks of the drugs administration. Leuprolide acetate 3.75 mg IM monthly or 11.25 mg IM every 3 month is given. It should be commenced on midluteal phase for quick pituitary downregulation.
- Duration is limited to 6 months only due to side effects of menopausal symptoms including vasomotor symptoms, vaginal atrophy, dryness, depression, and bone loss.
- Add back therapy (E+P) is indicated if used more than 6 months.

■ *Gonadotropin releasing hormone (GnRH) antagonists*:
- Elagolix and relugolix are nonpeptides and available for oral use. They reduce moth bleeding and myoma size. Advantage is absence of initial flare of gonadotropin. These are not yet approved by FDA for use in fibroid.

■ *Antiprogestins*: Various antiprogestogen agents and SPRMs are used to treat myoma on the basis that progesterone is essential for myoma growth.
- *Mifepristone (RU-486)*: An antiprogestin reduces the volume of fibroid by half. Dose is 2.5–10 mg given orally for 3–6 months.
  Side effects: Vasomotor symptoms and antiprogestational effects on endometrium which ranges from simple hyperplasia to newly described "progesterone-receptor modulator-associated endometrial change".
- *Ulipristal acetate*: A SPRM has similar effect like mifepristone. It induces apoptosis in fibroid cells. Amenorrhea occurs in 75% cases within 10 days and uterine volume is reduced to 40% after 3 months. Dose is 5–10 mg daily. Treatment is limited to 3 months for continuous use. Hepatotoxicity is recent concern and contraindicated in liver disease. Liver function test is done before a treatment, monthly during treatment and then 2–4 weeks after treatment finally. *"Progesterone-receptor modulator-associated endometrial change"* is found in two-thirds women during treatment but resolves within 6 months after discontinuation. Endometrial concern prevents its use for long-term and limits its use as adjunct before surgery.

■ Selective estrogen receptor modulators (SERM) has no role in fibroid management.

■ Other androgenic hormones, danazol and gestrinone, reduce the size of fibroid and treats menorrhagia, but their side effects restrict their long-term routine use.

Uterine Artery Embolization (Figs. 24 to 26)

In this procedure, polyvinyl alcohol particles (500–700 mm) or other particulate emboli are injected into the both uterine arteries to occlude by interventional radiologist. Under regional anesthesia an angiographic catheter is introduced into uterine arteries through femoral artery under fluoroscope guidance **(Figs. 24 and 25)**. Catheter is removed after occlusion which is confirmed by angiography. The particles are placed toward to the tumor sparing the normal myometrium. The procedure takes approximately 1 hour and only 20 rads are exposed. Pregnancy must be excluded. Fibroids supplied by end arteries undergo necrosis whereas the normal myometrium is escaped due to colateral circulation.

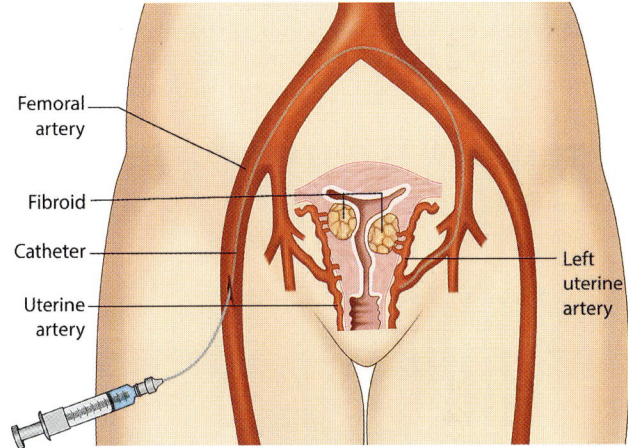

Fig. 24: Uterine artery embolization—introduction of catheter (schematic diagram).

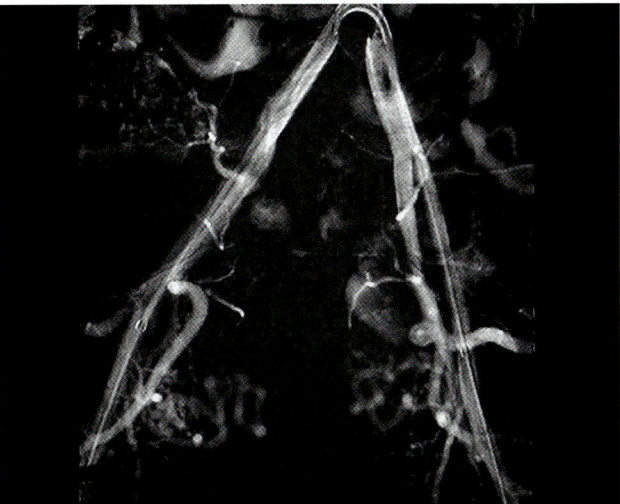

Fig. 25: Standard bilateral common iliac artery roadmap image done prior to selective cannulation of the uterine arteries. The tortuous uterine arteries are seen. The origin of the right uterine artery is well seen but a further oblique image was required to demonstrate the left uterine artery origin.

Courtesy: Dr Shuvro H Roy-Choudhury, Consultant Interventional Radiologist

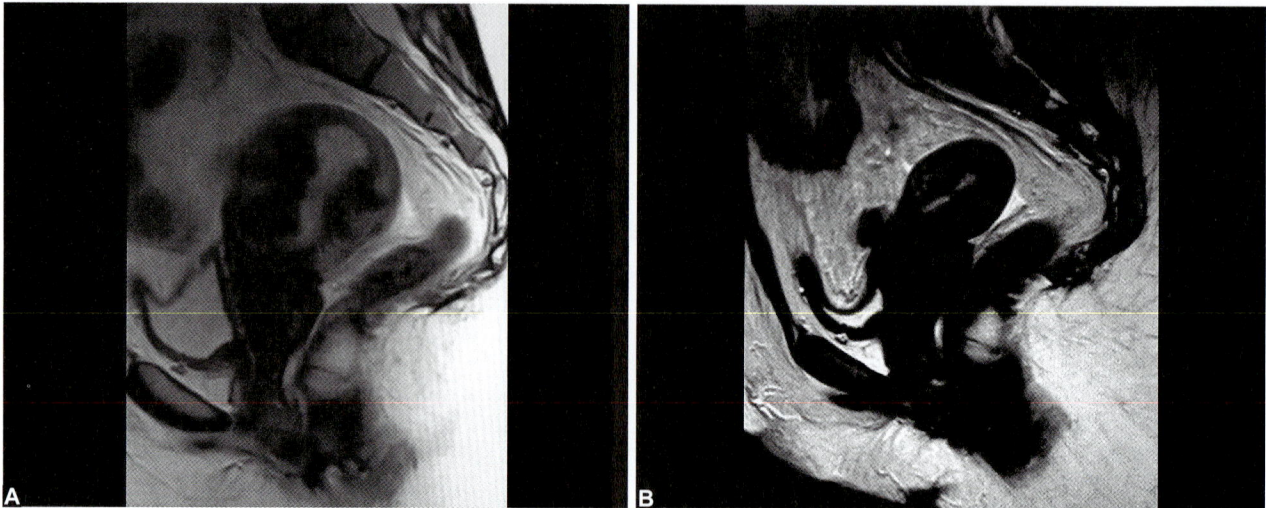

Figs. 26A and B: Reconstitution of distorted endometrium, reduction in uterine size and disappearance of multiple uterine fibroids 9 months after embolization in a 36-year-old school teacher with symptomatic fibroids (A) before embolization and (B) after 9 months of embolization.
Courtesy: Dr Shuvro H Roy-Choudhury, Consultant Interventional Radiologist

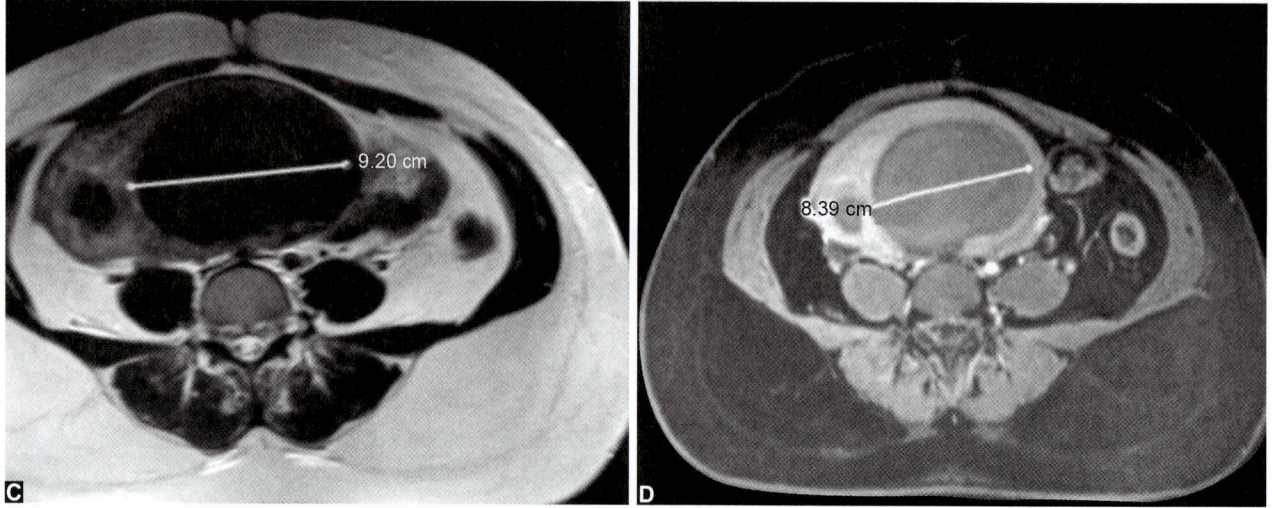

Figs. 26C and D: (C) Pre-embolization T2W axial MRI of a 36-year-old nulliparous lady who was advised embolization after full counseling by the gynecology team. This shows a dominant fibroid with a length of 9.3 cm and smaller other fibroids; (D) Postembolization T1W axial post-gadolinium MRI of the same lady. This shows the dominant fibroid with no enhancement indicating complete necroses with a length of 8.4 cm. This lady subsequently went on to deliver a full-term baby.
Courtesy: Dr Shuvro H Roy-Choudhury, Consultant Interventional Radiologist

Indication of UAE

Women with leiomyoma, treatment failure with medical method who otherwise may be considered for hysterectomy or myomectomy. *Patient desires of child should be treated with myomectomy rather than UAE.*

Contraindications

Absolutes are active infection, pregnancy and suspected malignancy. Relative contraindications are pretreatment with GnRH, family not completed, coagulopathy, renal failure, uterine size more than 24 weeks, salpingectomy, hydrosalpinx, and dye allergy.

Advantages

Shorter (1 day) hospital stay, higher patient satisfaction and faster (1 week) return to job. Low major complication and high symptom relief score. Efficacy—85% reduction of HMB, 50% reduction of fibroid size, and 80% patient satisfaction for 5 years.

Complications

Groin hematoma, failure in cannulation, severe pain following procedure, excessive uterine discharge, expulsion of necrosed myoma especially in submucosal variety (sometimes need dilatation and removal), uterine sepsis, amenorrhea, premature ovarian failure may occur due to ovarian artery embolization.

In few cases postembolization syndrome comprising of lower abdominal pain, fever, nausea and leukocytosis may occur and persists for not more than one week. Analgesics and supportive care cure the condition.

In post UAE cases the pregnancy complications are high, e.g. miscarriage, preterm labor, fetal growth restriction, malpresentation, increase cesarean section (CS) rate and postpartum hemorrhage and treatment failure in 25% cases.

Magnetic Resonance Imaging (MRI)-guided Focused Ultrasound (MRgFUS)

In this method high intensity ultrasound is directed to a precise area of tissue via MRI. It helps in (1) locating fibroid and (2) thermal mapping.

It causes temperature rise and incites coagulation necrosis of the selected myoma. This causes controlled thermal ablation of fibroid leaving the normal myometrium undamaged.

Advantages: It is noninvasive, the procedure takes 3 hours, only conscious sedation done in lying down in prawn position, discharged after 1 hour and can return to work after 48 hours. Quality of life score is good and well-tolerated.

Complications are skin burn, adjacent healthy tissue damage, pain from sciatic nerve irritations and thromboembolism.

The procedure needs prolong evaluation and not recommended for women who wish to preserve fertility.

SURGERY

Indications of Surgery

- Persistent symptom in spite of conservative treatment
- Large size. Solely size is not an indication of myomectomy in contrast to previous belief. Conservation with regular surveillance is recent opinion.

Types of Surgery

Q. What are the surgeries which may be done in uterine fibroids?

- Hysterectomy
- Myomectomy
- Endometrial ablation
- Myolysis—by heat, laser and by focused energy delivery sytem

Hysterectomy

Indications: Family completed, late reproductive age, myomectomy contraindicated, associated pathology like PID, endometriosis, suspected sarcoma, and endometrial CA.

Types: (A) Abdominal (laparotomy); (B) Vaginal; (C) Laparoscopy (total laparoscopic hysterectomy, LAVH)

Vaginal hysterectomy is the preferred method when possible.

Prophylactic salpingectomy is considered to prevent ovarian cancer.

Myomectomy

Indication: Symptomatic fibroids: (A) Where fertility preservation is needed; (B) Does not want hysterectomy.

Routes of myomectomy

- Abdominal open method (laparotomy)
- Vaginal myomectomy
- Laparoscopic myomectomy
- Hysteroscopic resection of submucosal myoma
- Robotic myomectomy

HYSTEROSCOPIC MYOMECTOMY

Q. When will you do hysteroscopic myomectomy?

For submucosal (intracavitary fibroids) hysteroscopic myomectomy is the gold standard procedure.

Indications are HMB, recurrent miscarriage, and infertility.

By hysteroscopy Grade 0 and Grade 1 fibroids (optimal size <3 cm and >50% tumor intracavitary) can be removed easily but *in Grade 2 fibroids* it is difficult to resect by hysteroscopy as most of the fibroid lies inside the myometrium and the safety depends on the thickness of myometrium between fibroid and serosa in Grade 2 fibroid.

Hysteroscopic resection adjunct with endometrial ablation is a good choice to reduce menstrual blood loss when fertility is not concern.

LAPAROSCOPIC MYOMECTOMY (FIG. 27)

During last decade laparoscopic myomectomy has gained huge popularity and has become an acceptable alternative approach for myomectomy.

Q. Laparotomy/laparoscopic myomectomy—which one is preferred?

The choice depends on the availabilities of facility, expertise of surgeons, and tumor number, size, and location. For subserosal and intramural leiomyoma laparoscopic approach is a good option. Submucous fibroids are best treated by hysteroscopic resection.

In comparison to conventional open myomectomy laparoscopic approach is associated with *longer operative time*, *less blood loss*, *less postoperative pain*, and *fewer complications*.

In symptomatic fibroids where future childbearing is concern laparoscopic myomectomy is considered as best option.

In presence of huge size and multiple fibroids conventional open myomectomy has advantages over laparoscopy.

Tissue extraction following laparoscopic myomectomy by power morcellation is a matter of great concern now due to possibility of peritoneal leiomyomatosis, parasitic myoma, de novo endometriosis and worsening of patient's

SECTION 2: Clinical Cases

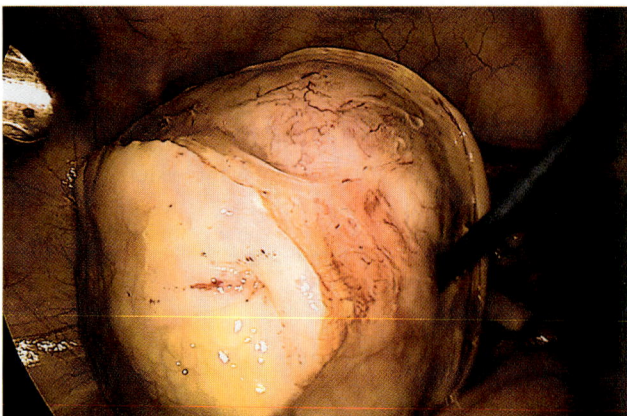

Fig. 27: Laparoscopic myomectomy.
Courtesy: Dr Abhinibes Chatterjee, Advanced Laparoscopic Surgeon, Kolkata

prognosis in occult uterine sarcoma. Alternative methods of tissue extraction are minilaparotomy or colpotomy. Closed bag morcellation is attempted to avert the complications for which bag is specially designed.

Robotic myomectomy is also gaining popularity in recent days.

Vaginal myomectomy is needed sometimes in cases of cervical fibroid.

Q. What preoperative consent, counseling and precautions to be taken before myomectomy?

To be explained that there are some risks of myomectomy particularly *severe hemorrhage* and sometimes due to uncontrolled hemorrhage and extensive myometrial injury it may end into *hysterectomy* (now 0-2%). Consent of hysterectomy is taken preoperatively.

- Few units of blood should be kept ready
- There may be persistence of symptoms (20-25% cases) following myomectomy
- There is chance of adhesion formation
- There may be recurrence of leiomyoma (10-30% cases)
- In case of infertility pregnancy is not guaranteed following myomectomy. When myomectomy is done solely for infertility other factors should be evaluated
- Incidence of CS is more and scar rupture is little more following pregnancy
- In abnormal uterine bleeding preoperative D&C or hysteroscopy is suggested by many.
- May need hysterectomy later (10% go for hysterectomy within 5-10%)

Q. How would you prepare the patient for surgery?

As the patient is usually anemic and there is chance of intraoperative blood loss hemoglobin status is improved before surgery by iron therapy. GnRH and progesterone antagonist have some benefits.

OPEN MYOMECTOMY

Steps of abdominal myomectomy by open myomectomy (Figs. 28 to 41):

- Supine position
- Anesthesia—regional or general anesthesia
- Foley catheterization
- Antiseptic dressing and draping
- Skin incision: Pfannenstiel incision. If the size is more than 14 weeks, midline vertical incision is given.
- Uterus with fibroid is exteriorized after careful inspection of any other pelvic pathology.
- Leiomyomas are identified by inspection of uterine serosal surface. By squeezing palpation intramural and submucosal myomas are identified.

Hemostasis

Tourniquets of Foley catheter or simple rubber catheter is passed through the avascular area of broad ligaments on both sides at the level of isthmus and tied in front to occlude

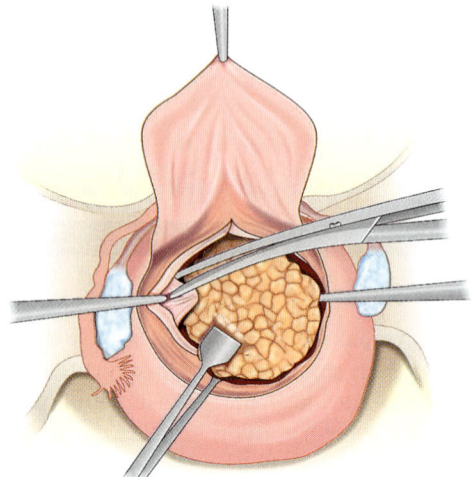

Fig. 28: Myomectomy.

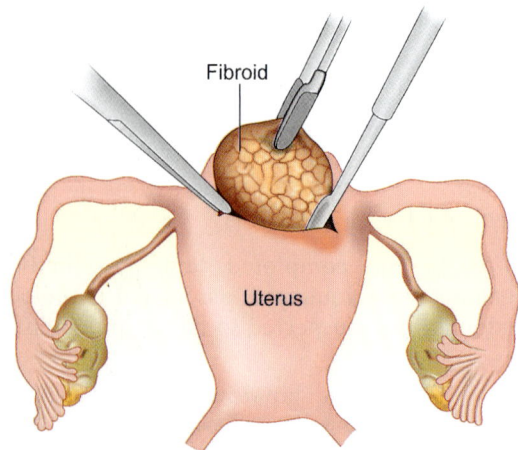

Fig. 29: Removal of solitary myoma.

CHAPTER 4: A Case of Uterine Leiomyoma (Uterine Fibroid)

both uterine arteries. Tourniquet is released half hourly. Many suggest to occlude also ovarian and infundibulopelvic (IP) ligaments to occlude ovarian arteries.

Previously *Bonney's myomectomy clamp* **(Fig. 36A)** was used to occlude uterine arteries. Currently, *local vasopressin (pitressin) injection* is used to prevent blood loss 20 units (one vial of 1mL) is diluted in 30–100 cc of normal saline and injected along the planned line of incision.

Half-life is 10–20 minutes. However, one should be very cautious about inadvertent intravascular injection. It is contraindicated in cardiovascular and pulmonary disease. Prior to infiltration anesthetist is informed and consulted.

Incision over Uterus

Incision is made over serosa either with cold knife or cutting diathermy.

Principle is to place *vertical incision* on the anterior wall as midline as possible and to enucleate as many number of myomas as possible through a single incision. More the number of incisions and incision over posterior wall are associated with more postoperative adhesion. The length of the incision is such that through it largest tumor can be evacuated. For lateral tumors lateral myometrial incision can be given through original central incision. Sometimes multiple incisions are needed to remove all the tumors.

In case of large posterior myoma *Bonney's hood operation* is performed **(Figs. 33 and 34)**.

In this technique, a transverse incision is given posterior to fundus and just above the level of tubal attachment, enucleation of myoma done followed by suturing the redundant flap (hood) on the lower part of anterior wall. This will avoid adhesion formation.

Primary posterior incision may also be needed for myoma situated posterior lower part. By transcavitary approach with deliberate opening of cavity to remove the fibroid from posterior wall has risk of postoperative uterine adhesion.

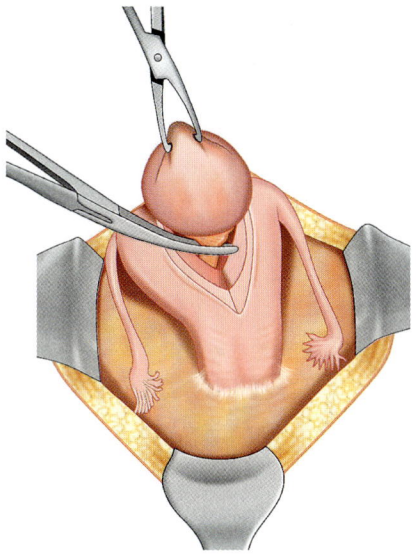

Fig. 30: Stalk of the myoma is grasped with the artery forceps before cutting.

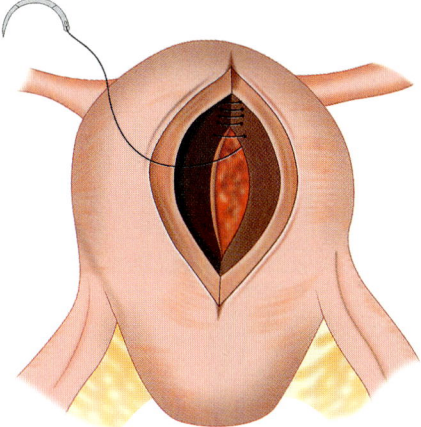

Fig. 31: Closure of myoma bed.

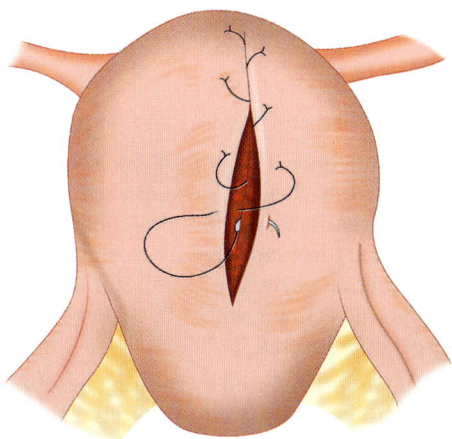

Fig. 32: Suturing of serosal coat of uterus (final closure).

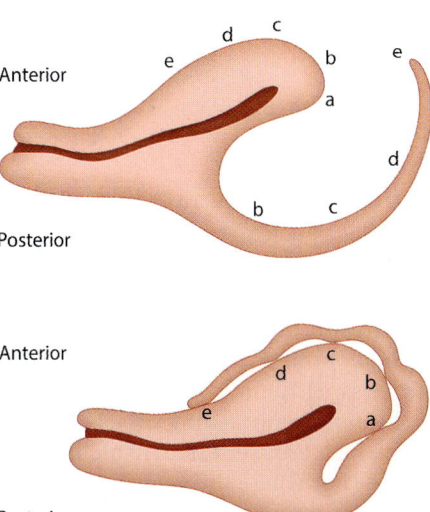

Fig. 33: Bonney's hood operation.

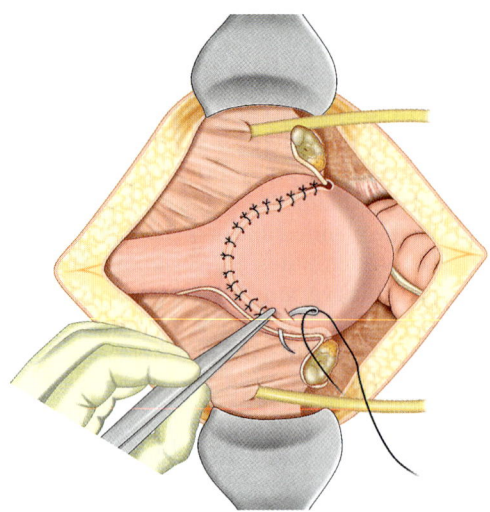

Fig. 34: Repair of flap over the anterior surface of uterus (Bonney's hood operation).

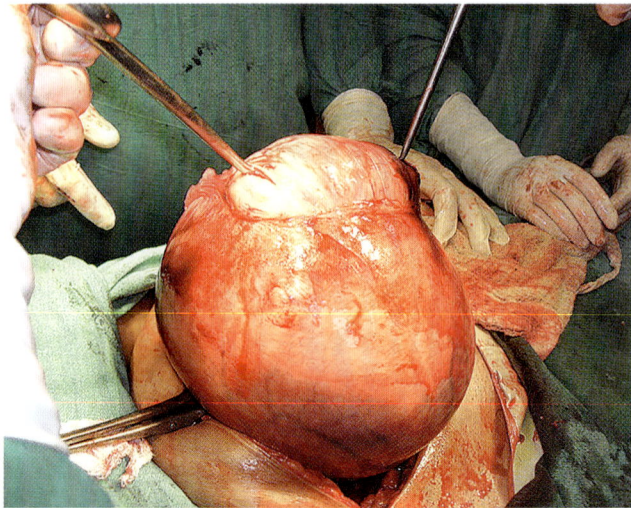

Fig. 35: Myomectomy—after incision holding the myoma with myoma screw and tenaculum.
Courtesy: Dr Abhijit Rakhshit, Associate Professor, Department of Obstetrics and Gynecology

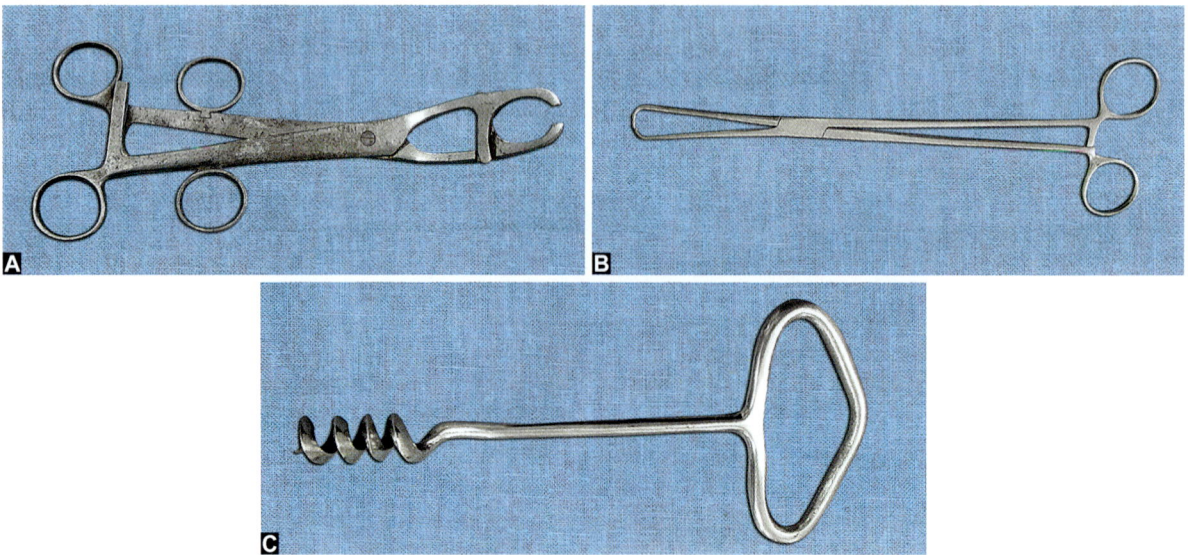

Figs. 36A to C: (A) Bonney's myomectomy clamp; (B) Single tooth tenaculum (vulsellum); (C) Myoma screw.

Enucleation (Figs. 28 to 30 and 36 to 39)

Depth of the incision is up to the myoma wall which is identified by whitish color. Traction is given by myoma screw **(Figs. 36C, 38 and 39)** or single tooth tenaculum **(Fig. 36B)** outward and a plane between myometrium and tumor is identified. By sharp and blunt dissection (finger and scissor) tumor is enucleated from the bed. During enucleation some feeding vessels (usually 2–4) are encountered which are identified, ligated, and cut. There are no definite sites where the vessels are situated. Every effort is made to remove all palpable myomas cutting through myometrium.

Closing of Myoma Bed and Serosal Layer (Figs. 31, 32 and 40)

After enucleation bleeding points are secured and the myometrium (myoma bed) is closed in several layers with 1-0 delayed absorbable suture for perfect hemostasis and to prevent hematoma formation. Before closing search is made whether endometrial cavity is opened. If it is opened repair of endometrial wall is made with 3-0/4-0 even finer running delayed absorbable sutures.

Finally serosal wound is closed by running baseball stitch or subserosal or subcuticular running stitches using delayed absorbable suture (*see* **Fig. 32**).

CHAPTER 4: A Case of Uterine Leiomyoma (Uterine Fibroid)

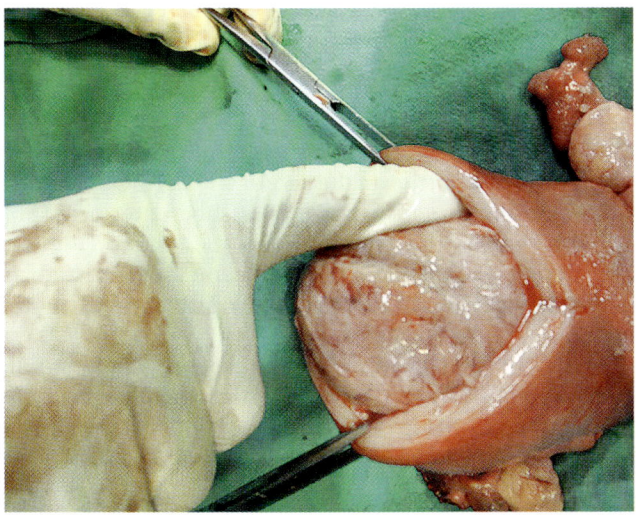

Fig. 37: Demonstration of enucleation of myoma in a hysterectomy specimen.

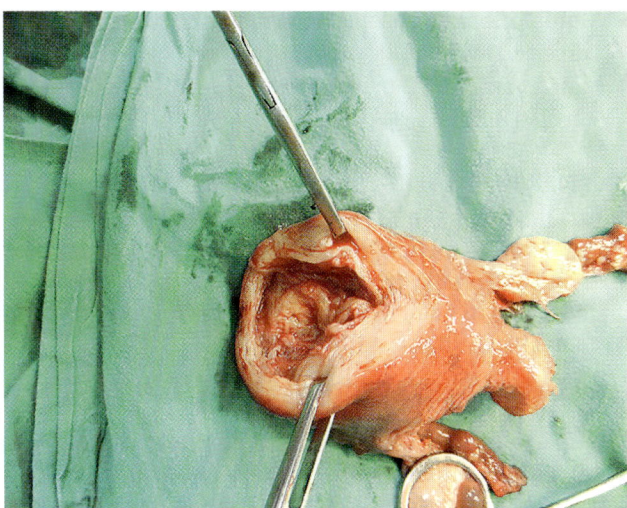

Fig. 40: Myoma bed after enucleation.

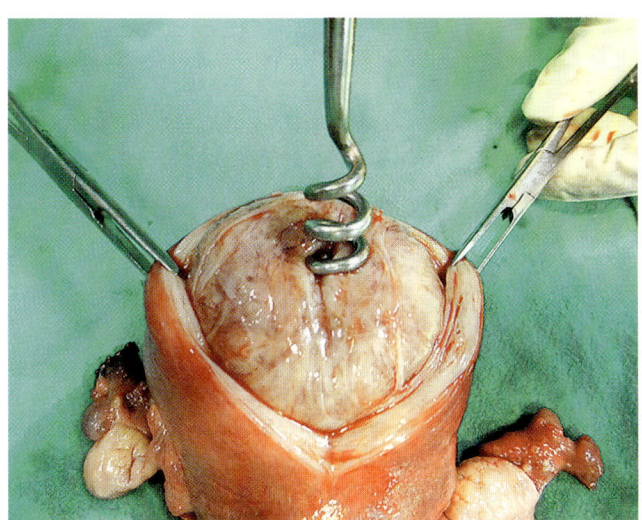

Fig. 38: Traction of myoma with myoma screw.
Courtesy: Dr Chiranjit Ghosh

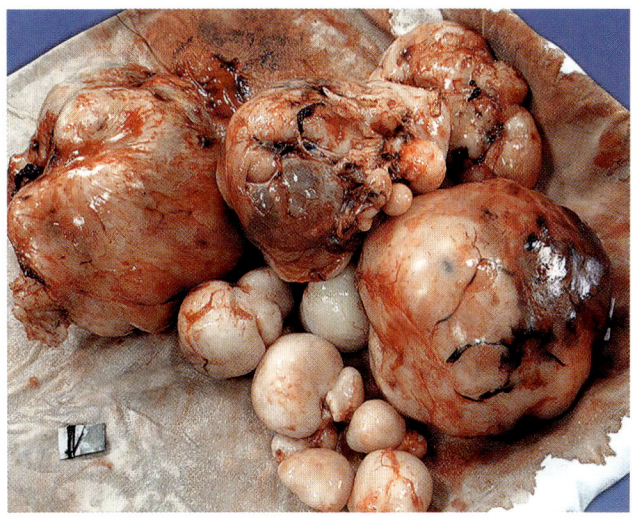

Fig. 41: Multiple fibroids after myomectomy.

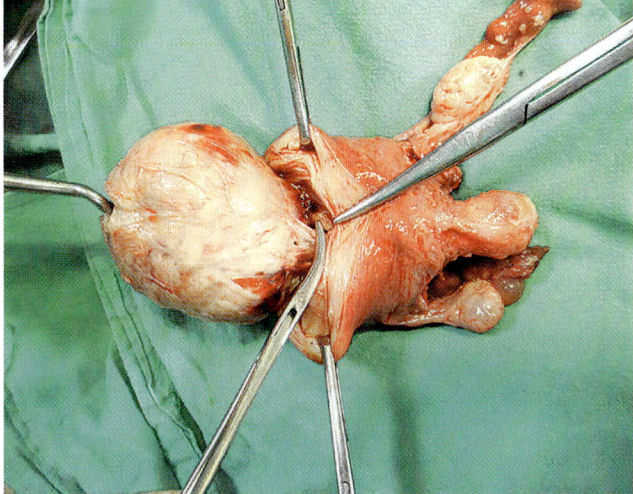

Fig. 39: Clamping the stalk at the end of myomectomy.

Abdomen is closed in layers after counting and final look of the abdominal cavity and operative area.

Disadvantages of Myomectomy

- Hemorrhage (both preoperative and postoperative)
- Persistence and recurrence of menorrhagia (20–25% cases)
- Recurrence of myoma(10–30% cases)
- Adhesion formation
- Scar rupture following pregnancy (rare, chance of pregnancy is 40% following myomectomy).
- Need for hysterectomy in 10% cases within 10 years

Situations where hysterectomy may be needed on attempt of myomectomy:

- Excessive uncontrolled hemorrhage
- Other pathology like bilateral large tubo-ovarian mass, severe endometriosis

- Multiple fibroids making the repair impossible
- Large cervical fibroid
- Malignancy
- Infected fibroid.

Endometrial Ablation

This is the treatment of choice in AUB due to endometrial dysfunction. In myoma-related bleeding, its failure rate is high (40%). It is efficacious when submucous myoma is less than or equal to 3 cm. As an adjunct following hysteroscopic resection it may improve HMB better.

Myolysis

This newer approach involves *myoma puncture* with tools to incite myoma necrosis and subsequent shrinkage by cautery, cryotherapy or laser vaporization. It can be done laparoscopically.

Laparoscopic Uterine Artery Occlusion

This is the method by which occluding uterine arteries laparoscopically achieve avascularity and necrosis of the fibroids. Treatment failure rate is high. This method is still not popular.

CERVICAL FIBROID

Q. What is the incidence of cervical fibroid?

About 1–2% of uterine fibroids may be located in the cervix usually to its supravaginal portion.

Q. What are the different varieties of cervical fibroid?

Cervical fibroid belongs to type 8 category in the new FIGO fibroid classification system (*see* Page 91, **Fig. 16**).
- Supravaginal—most common **(Fig. 42)**
- Vaginal **(Figs. 43 to 45)**.

Cervical fibroids may be:
1. Anterior
2. Posterior
3. Lateral
4. Central in location involving either the vaginal or supravaginal portion of the cervix.

In anterior variety, bladder is pushed anteriorly **(Fig. 46)** and in posterior type it pushes the rectum **(Fig. 47)** and pouch of Douglas (POD) becomes obliterated, in lateral cervical fibroid uterus expands laterally close to the ureter.

In central cervical fibroid, cervix expands all around the circumference **(Fig. 48)** occupying the whole pelvic cavity and the uterus lies top over the cervical fibroid mass looking like "*Lantern on dome of St. Paul's*" **(Figs. 42 and 49)**.

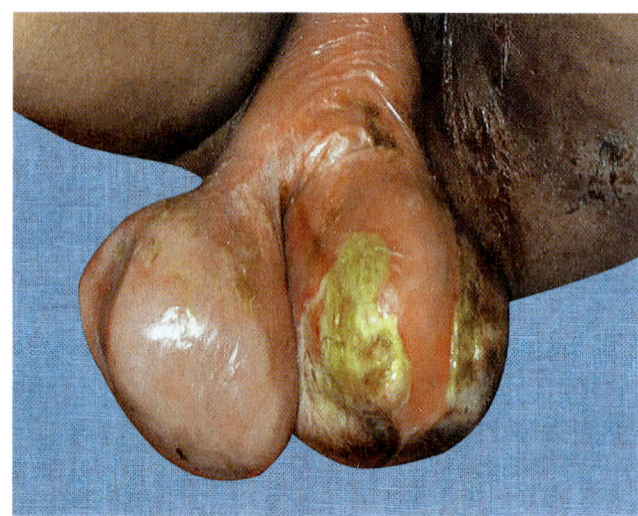

Fig. 43: Cervical fibroid arising from vaginal part of cervix—a 41-year-old parous woman came with something coming down per vagina, Ward Mayo's operation (vaginal hysterectomy with pelvic floor repair done).

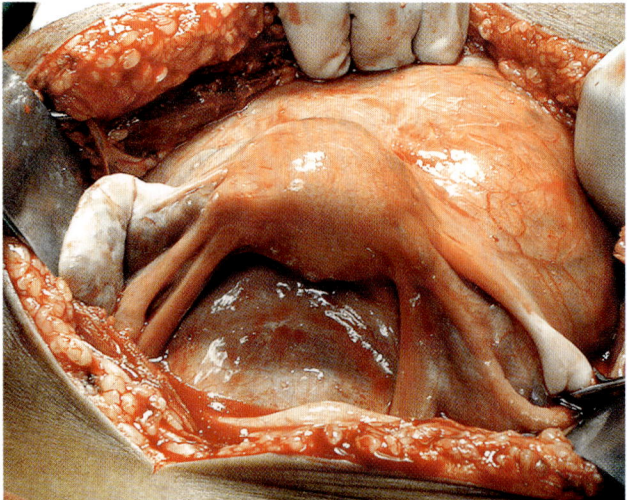

Fig. 42: Cervical fibroid central—"Lantern on Dome of St. Paul's".
Courtesy: Professor Shukanta Mishra, HOD, VIMS, Kolkata

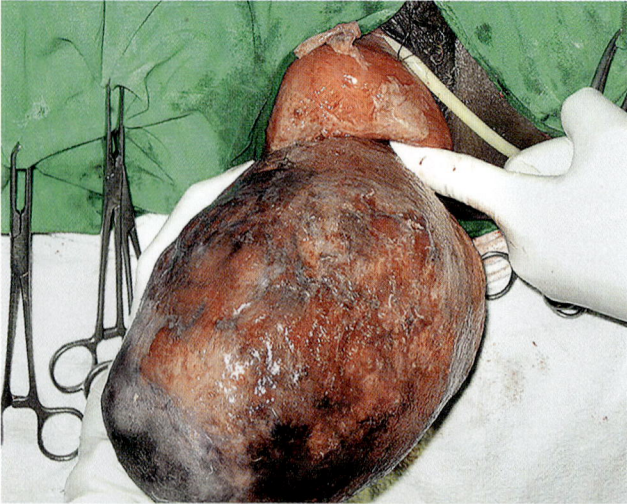

Fig. 44: Cervical fibroid from right lateral part of anterior lip of cervix in a 34-year-old nulliparous woman—myomectomy done vaginally.

CHAPTER 4: A Case of Uterine Leiomyoma (Uterine Fibroid)

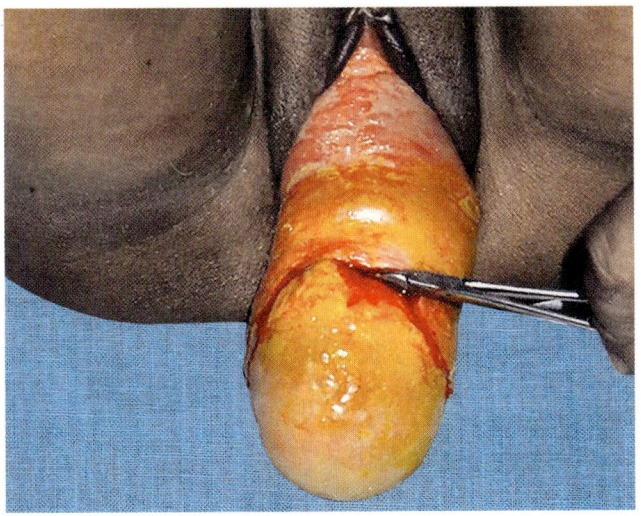

Fig. 45: Cervical fibroid arising from posterior lip of cervix in a 43-year-old parous woman. Vaginal hysterectomy with pelvic floor repair done.

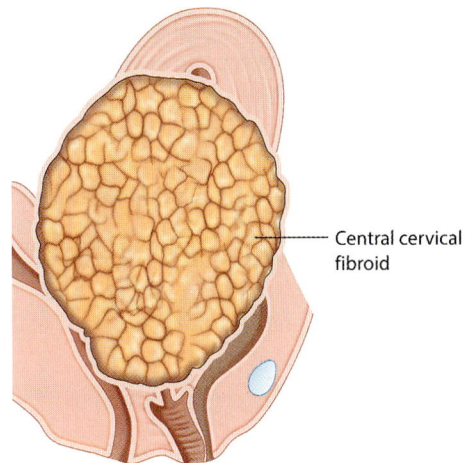

Fig. 48: Central cervical fibroid.

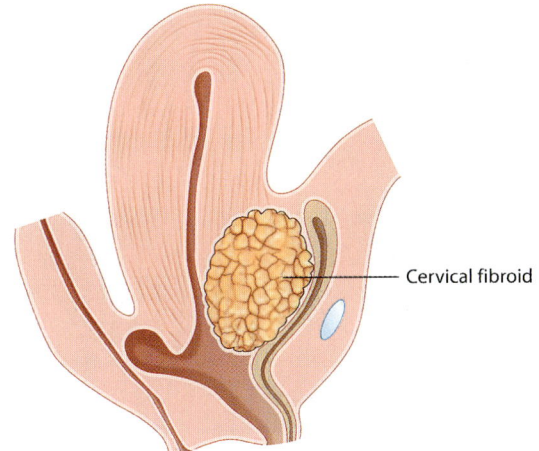

Fig. 46: Anterior cervical fibroid.

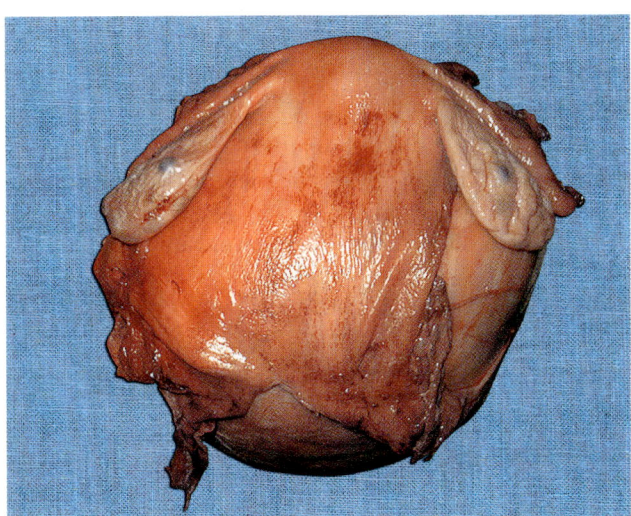

Fig. 49: Central cervical fibroid—looks like "Lantern on dome of St. Paul's". Fibroid is removed along with uterus. This is very risky procedure as during clamping of uterine artery there is chance of ureteric injury for which myomectomy followed by hysterectomy is considered safe (*see* Figs. 50 and 51).

Sometimes, rarely submucous uterine fibroid may burrow downwards to lie in the position of the cervix which is expanded and is called pseudocervical fibroid.

Large fibroid arising from the vaginal part of the cervix may protrude through the vagina forming a *cervical polyp*. Sometimes, it is confused with chronic inversion of uterus.

Q. How would you diagnose cervical fibroid?

Cervical fibroid would be diagnosed from symptoms, signs, and investigations.

Symptoms

Heaviness of pelvis (pelvic discomfort) and usually bladder and bowel pressure symptoms—frequency and retention of urine, constipation, and difficulty in defecation.

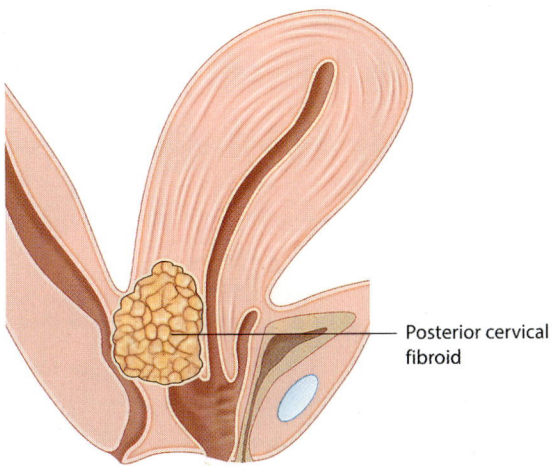

Fig. 47: Posterior cervical fibroid.

In pure cervical fibroid, there is no menstrual abnormality except in cervical polyp.

Chance of infertility is less except resulting from difficulty in coitus due to cervical polyp, however obstructed labor may occur.

Signs

- Per abdominally larger one is palpable but may not be palpable if it is small
- Per speculum examination: Cervix is broad.
- Bimanual examination—enlarged firm mass in pelvis, attached with cervix and immobile and body of the uterus above the mass.

Diagnostic clinical criteria of cervical fibroid is:

- Cervical attachment
- Firm
- Fixity
- Pelvic position.
  Rectal examination shows the expanded cervix.

Investigations

- Ultrasonography confirms the diagnosis. There may be hydronephrosis and hydroureter.
- Intravenous pyelography is helpful to *see* the location of ureter.
- Urine analysis and kidney function are always done.

Management of Cervical Fibroid

Small asymptomatic fibroid in supravaginal part needs no treatment. Symptomatic fibroid is treated mostly by surgery.

Surgery

Large cervical fibroids may be managed by surgery:

- Myomectomy alone or
- Hysterectomy—with or without prior enucleation (myomectomy) **(Figs. 50 and 51)** depending upon the need for fertility desire of the patient and/or its location and size. Injury of ureter during hysterectomy with the tumor is of concern and prior myomectomy before hysterectomy is a safe option.
  Surgery can be done by laparotomy or by laparoscopy. Opening of cervical canal during myomectomy is a concern. Hemisection of uterus followed by myomectomy is practiced by many **(Fig. 52)**.
- Route may be abdominal, vaginal or abdominovaginal
- Cervical fibroid from vaginal part is removed vaginally
- Fibroid polyp protruded through vagina is tackled vaginally
- Very rarely abdominovaginal approach is needed.

Other Treatments

The newer modalities of treatment such as *medical therapy* with GnRH or SPRM, UAE, MRI-guided focused ultrasound tend to decrease the mortality and morbidity of the patient and preserve the fertility.

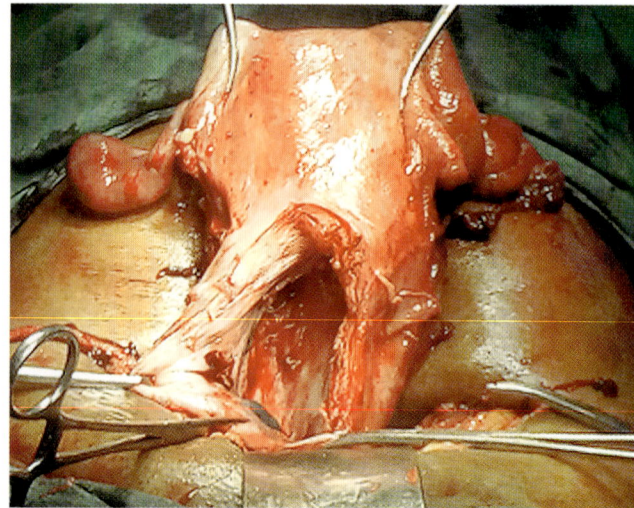

Fig. 50: Cervical fibroid is removed first followed by hysterectomy.

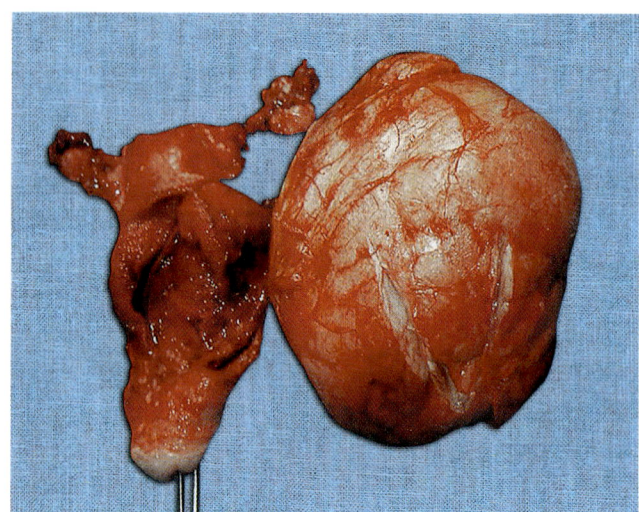

Fig. 51: Central cervical fibroid. Hysterectomy done after enucleation.

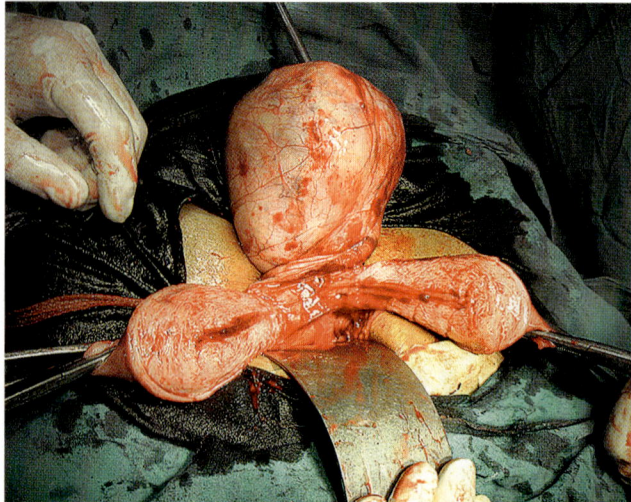

Fig. 52: Cervical fibroid central—enucleation done after hemisection of uterus.

Myomectomy for Cervical Fibroid

The principle of surgery is to excise the tumor intracapsular to avoid injury of ureter.

In anterior fibroid, bladder is pushed down after cutting uterovesical fold of peritoneum. By vertical or transverse incision myomectomy is performed, myoma bed closed, and uterovesical fold of peritoneum is repaired.

In case of posterior fibroid, myomectomy is done through transverse or vertical incision over posterior wall. In every case one should be vigilant about the opening of cervical canal, if it occurs it should be repaired maintaining the patency of canal.

In central cervical fibroid one option is to do hemisection of uterus **(Fig. 52)**, enucleation followed by repair of bisected uterus.

Hysterectomy

Direct hysterectomy is avoided as there is chance of injury of ureter. Instead, hysterectomy is performed following enucleation of myoma (myomectomy) which makes the procedure easier and safe.

BROAD LIGAMENT CYSTS AND TUMORS

Q. What are the broad ligament cysts and tumors?

Broad ligament cysts **(Fig. 53A)** are the cysts arising from the structures of broad ligament.

Pseudo broad ligament cyst is ovarian cyst burrowing inside the broad ligament **(Fig. 53B)**.

Parovarian cyst arises from the vestigial structure, parovarium namely epoophoron, paroophoron, and Wolffian duct. This mass is tensely cystic structure growing in between the layers of broad ligament. The cyst contains clear fluid and lined by cubical epithelium. *Fimbrial cysts* are commonly unilateral, may be bilateral **(Fig. 54)**, translucent cystic mass lined by cubical epithelium initially pedunculated, then burrowing into the layers of broad ligament. The tube is stretched over

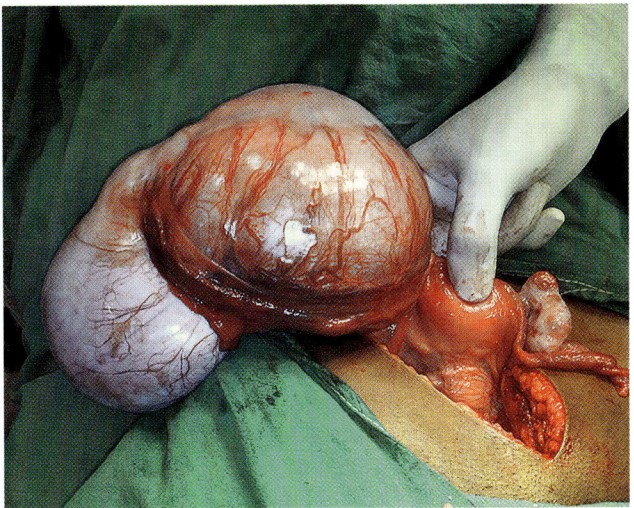

Fig. 53B: Pseudo broad ligament cyst—look that cyst has arisen from the ovary and buried into broad ligament.

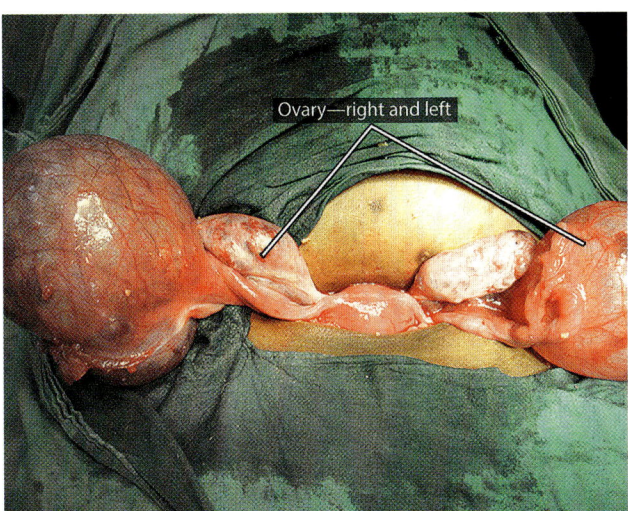

Fig. 54: Bilateral fimbrial cysts—note that both the ovaries are normal and cysts have origin from fimbrial ends.

the cyst and ovary looks normal. There may be torsion of the cyst.

- Broad ligament cysts do not become malignant
- Symptoms may be pelvic pain or pressure symptom if cyst is large. Per abdominally it may be palpable above inguinal ligament. On per vaginal examination, parovarian cyst is palpable on lateral fornix and fimbrial cyst like ovarian cyst.
- Treatment is shelling out after giving gentle incision over avascular area usually in front and parallel to fallopian tube. Cyst bed is closed by stitches. Caution is to be taken to avoid injury to ureter.

Broad ligament tumors may be fibromyoma (fibroid), fibroma, and lipoma, but they are rare.

Broad ligament fibroids are of two types:

1. True broad ligament fibroid
2. Pseudo broad ligament fibroid

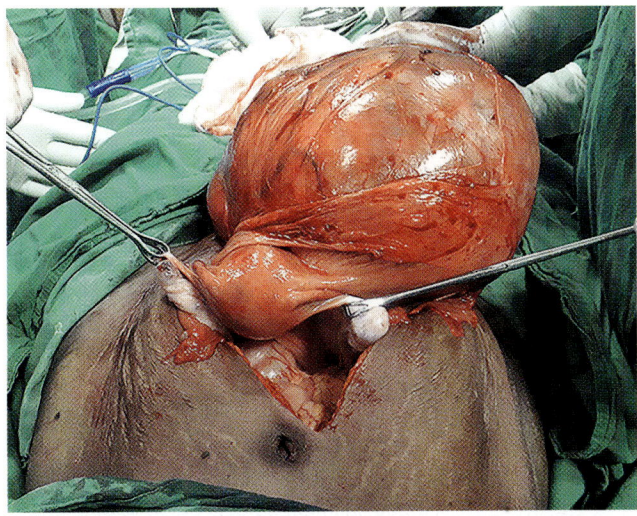

Fig. 53A: True broad ligament cyst (both ovaries normal).

SECTION 2: Clinical Cases

True broad ligament fibroid

True broad ligament fibroid arises from smooth muscle fibers of round ligament, ovarian ligament or perivascular connective tissue.

Pseudo broad ligament fibroid

Pseudo broad ligament fibroid arises **(Figs. 55 and 56)** from the lateral wall of the uterus, grows inside the two layers of broad ligament and connected with the uterus by thick structure and the former lacks any attachment with uterus.

During removal ureter is vulnerable to be injured in broad ligament fibroid.

In case of true broad ligament fibroid ureter lies medially and below to it but in case of pseudo broad ligament ureter may lie laterally, or below the tumor at the base of broad ligament or rarely above the tumor depending upon the site of uterus from where it arises **(Fig. 55)**.

Diagnosis of broad ligament fibroid is based on clinical features like palpable swelling in very large size and feeling of firm to solid mass in lateral fornix.

Treatment of broad ligament fibroid is enucleation by avoiding the injury of ureter.

A *"postbox"* incision is given on an avascular area in between the round ligament and fallopian tube **(Fig. 57A)** and enucleation is done in between the layers of broad ligament. Hemostatic suture is given on the bed if there is bleeding taking care of avoiding ureteric inclusion in suture. In case of hysterectomy, enucleation of broad ligament is done first, then hysterectomy is performed **(Figs. 57B and C)**. This will make the hysterectomy easier and will avoid injury to ureter.

Rarely, broad ligament fibroid is removed during vaginal hysterectomy **(Fig. 58)** with taking care of ureter.

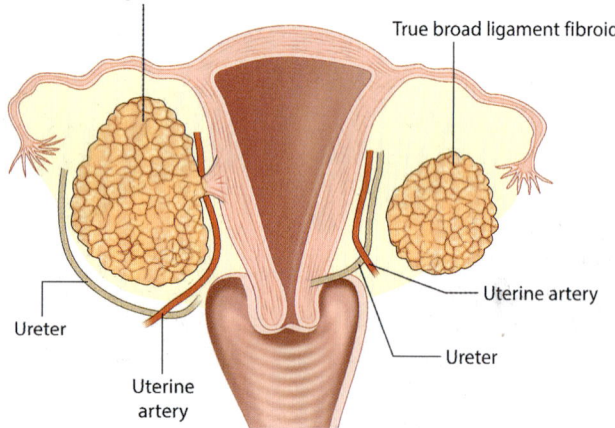

Fig. 55: Broad ligament fibroid—pseudo on left side and true on right side. Note the relation with the ureter in both types.

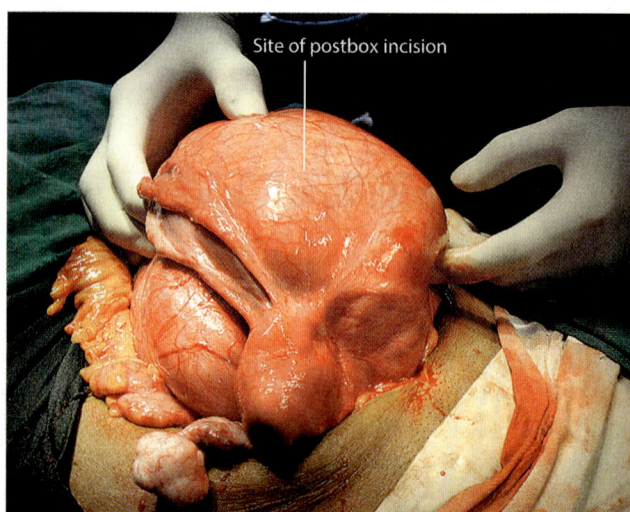

Fig. 57A: Broad ligament fibroid (left side)—postbox incision is given in between fallopian tube and round ligament for enucleation for safe removal. The line of incision is shown by right thumb.

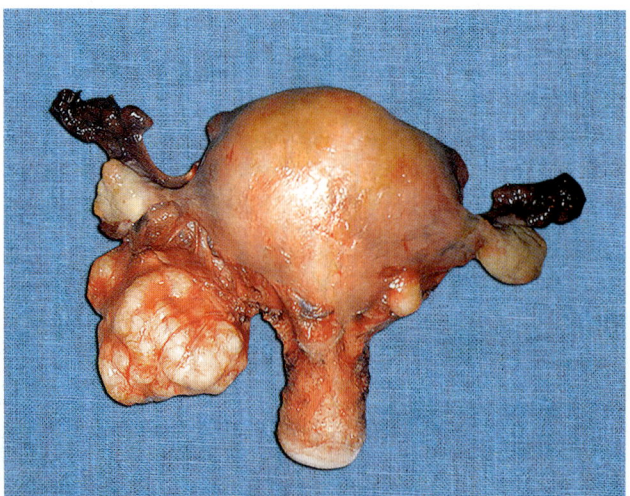

Fig. 56: Small pseudo broad ligament fibroid—note that it is actually fibroid originating from body of uterus and buried into layers of broad ligament.

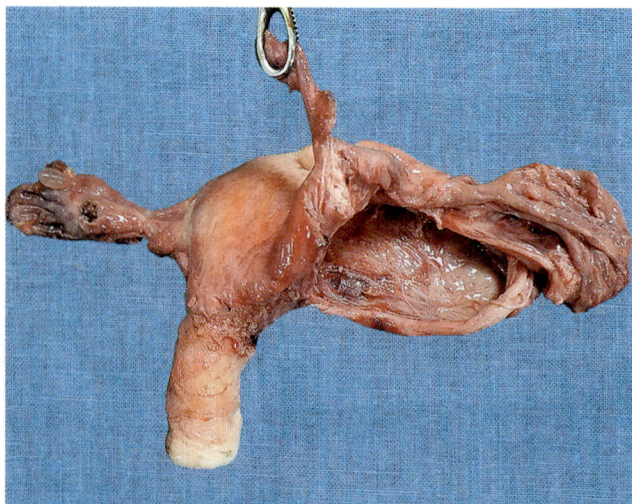

Fig. 57B: Hysterectomy done after enucleation of broad ligament fibroid.

CHAPTER 4: A Case of Uterine Leiomyoma (Uterine Fibroid)

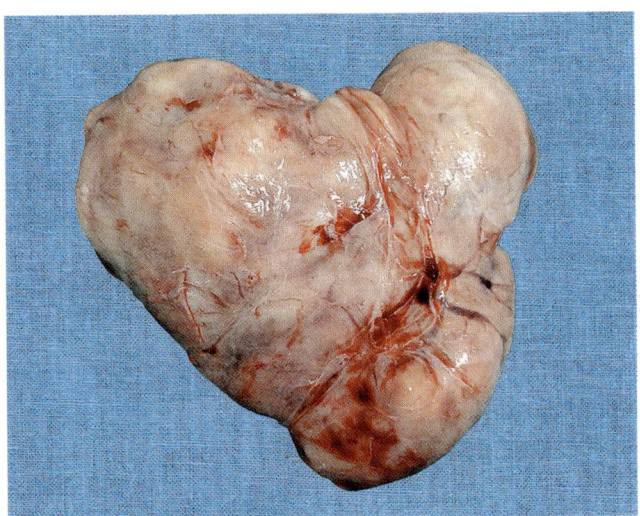

Fig. 57C: Broad ligament fibroid removed first before hysterectomy.

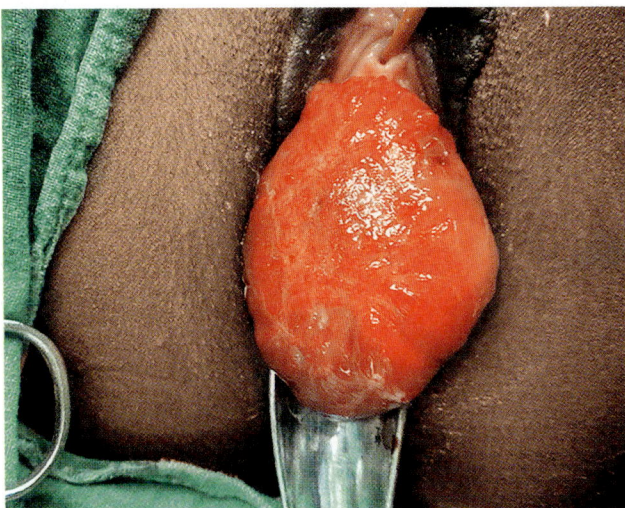

Fig. 59: Cervical polyp—a 27-year-old nulliparous woman presented with abnormal uterine bleeding and something coming down per vagina. The stalk was inside uterine cavity indicating pedunculated submucous fibroid arising from cavity.

Fibroid Polyp (Fig. 59)

It develops by extrusion from submucous fibroid, either from body or from cervix of uterus. Size may be moderate to huge sometimes obliterating whole vagina. Usually single, pedunculated or sessile, firm in consistency, surface becomes congested red with patchy white areas.

Microscopically, capsule of fibroid breaks and is covered by mucous membrane of endometrium and cervix and leiomyoma lies centrally. In pedunculated type the stalk is covered by mucosa with remnant of leiomyomatous tissue with central vasculature. There may be ulceration and infection on large polyp.

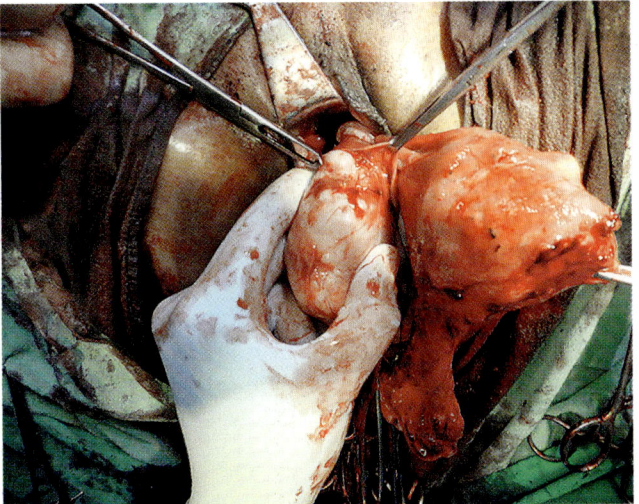

Fig. 58: Broad ligament fibroid removed through vagina during vaginal hysterectomy—a rare event.
Courtesy: Professor Debdutta Ghosh, Department of Obstetrics and Gynecology, RG Kar Medical College, Kolkata

Placental Polyp (Fig. 60)

It develops from nonseparated retained bits of placental tissue following an abortion or child birth. Always sessile, not pedunculated, usually single, small to moderate size, dark red in color, spongy to firm and friable.

Microscopically, degenerated chorionic tissue, degenerated decidua with old hemorrhage without a capsule.

UTERINE POLYP

Q. What do you mean by polyp?

Polyp is a pedunculated growth. In uterine polyp, it arises either from uterine cavity or cervix.

Q. What are the different types of polyp?

Polyp may be benign (mucous polyp, fibroid polyp, and placental polyp) and malignant.

Mucous Polyp

It arises from endometrium or endocervix. Size is small usually of pea size, usually multiple, soft, bright-red look, and pedunculated. Structure is like mucosa of uterus and component of adenofibroma may be present. Malignancy is rare.

Malignant Polyp

Malignant polyps are primary or secondary to fibroid or mucous polyp. Sarcomatous is more than carcinoma in case of malignant polyp. Size varies from small to large occupying whole vagina, soft, friable, and bleeds on touch. It is confirmed by biopsy.

Q. What are clinical presentations of uterine polyp?

Polyps are diagnosed mostly in reproductive age, few in postmenopausal women.

SECTION 2: Clinical Cases

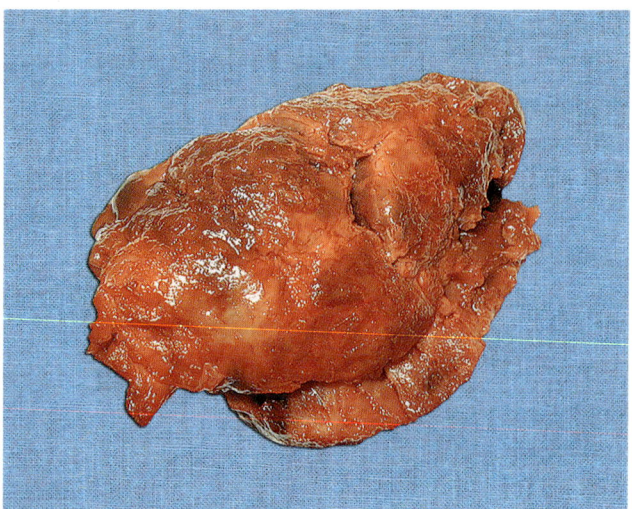

Fig. 60: Placental polyp—a 27-year-old woman P1+1 presented with irregular bleeding per vagina for 2 months following midtrimester abortion 5 months back. USG was suggestive of uterine fibroid. Myomectomy attempted and this submucous mass removed which showed placental tissue on histopathology.

Symptoms:
- Bleeding per vagina, intermenstrual bleeding (metrorrhagia) is the typical bleeding pattern, there may be HMB (metrorrhagia);
- White discharge, in infection and necrosis there may be offensive discharge;
- Postmenopausal bleeding;
- Dysmenorrhea, pain lower abdomen, and
- Something coming down per vagina.

Signs:
There may be anemia, per abdomen there may be associated large uterine fibroid.

Vaginal examination:
Large polyp is seen outside the vagina and presents with something coming per vagina.

Speculum examination (Fig. 61):
A polypoid growth may be seen to come out through external os, red in color, cervical wall becomes thin and stretched due to polyp inside cervical canal. There may be bleeding per vagina.

Bimanual examination:
Uterus may be bulky in intrauterine polyp and placental polyp.
Sonography is helpful to diagnose. EUA may be needed.

Management of Uterine Polyp

Management depends on the type and the size.

Q. How would you remove a fibroid polyp (Fig. 61) protruding through the external os (steps of polypectomy)?
- Patient in lithotomy position

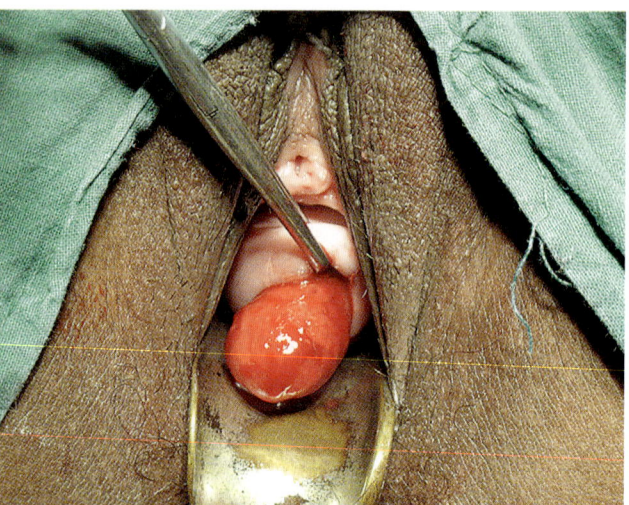

Fig. 61: Cervical polyp—a 38-year-old woman P2+0, presented with irregular and heavy menstrual bleeding for last 1 year.

- General or regional anesthesia or paracervical with deep sedation
- Antiseptic dressing, draping, and catheterization done
- Bimanual examination is done to note the size, position, mobility of uterus and status of both adnexae
- Sims' speculum is introduced to retract posterior vaginal wall
- Anterior lip is held by Allis tissue forceps or vulsellum
- Polyp **(Fig. 61)** is grasped either by Allis tissue forceps **(Fig. 62)** or sponge holding forceps **(Fig. 63)** or multiple teeth vulsellum **(Fig. 64)** and twisted followed by removal. In case of large stalk, incision may be necessary with a stitch at route to occlude feeding vessel.

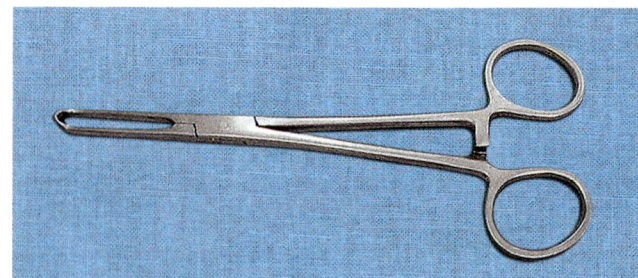

Fig. 62: Allis tissue forceps.

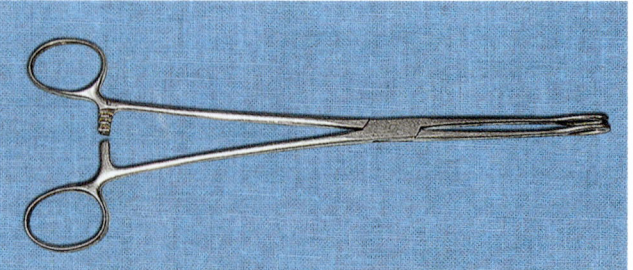

Fig. 63: Sponge holding forceps.

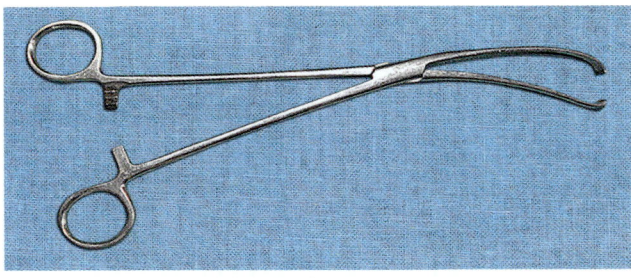

Fig. 64: Multiple teeth vulsellum.

- Dilatation and curettage is always done to remove any endometrial polyp. A small ovum forceps may be needed to remove endometrial polyp.
- Excised polyp and curetted materials are sent for histopathology.

Pregnancy with Uterine Fibroid

Read from the author's *Bedside Clinics in Obstetrics,* Fifth edition, Academic Publishers.

CHAPTER 5

A Case of Abnormal Uterine Bleeding (Endometrial Hyperplasia)

Chapter Outline

Writing a case of abnormal uterine bleeding (dysfunctional uterine bleeding) and how to present the case?

- Types of Abnormal Menstruation Including HMB and IMB
- Causes of Abnormal Uterine Bleeding
- PALM-COEIN Classification with Significance
- Diagnosis of AUB
- Place of Dysfunctional Uterine Bleeding in New System
- Investigations of AUB
- How to Approach a Case of AUB?
- Management of AUB—Management Based on New Classification
- Details of Hormonal Management
- Uterine Procedures in Management of AUB
- Puberty Menorrhagia
- Isthmocele
- Arteriovenous Malformation
- Endometrial Hyperplasia—Types, Significance and Management

PATIENT'S PARTICULARS

1. Name:
2. Age: 39 years
3. Address:
4. Occupation: Housewife
5. Married/unmarried: Married
6. History of infertility: Nil
7. Husband's occupation:
8. Socioeconomic status: Middle
9. Religion:
10. Parous/nulliparous: Parous

Bed No.:
Date of admission:
Date of examination:

HISTORY

- *Chief complaint/complaints*: Complaint of irregular vaginal bleeding for last 1 year.
- *History of present illness*: Written in detail—duration of abnormality, any clot, amount, number of pad used during the bleeding phase, the bleeding pattern, any intermenstrual bleeding, heavy menstrual bleeding (HMB), associated with pain, and associated with coitus or not.
- *Menstrual history*:
  - Last menstrual period: Last normal menstrual period
  - Duration of menstruation:
  - Interval in days:
  - Age of menarche:
  - Regularity of cycle:
  - Pain during period/if pain relation with menstruation:
  - Amount of bleeding:
  - Clot:
    - Intermenstrual bleeding:
    - Any amenorrhea
- *Obstetric history:*
  - Parity
  - Living issue:
  - Last child birth (LCB):

CHAPTER 5: A Case of Abnormal Uterine Bleeding (Endometrial Hyperplasia)

Serial no.	Year and Month	Pregnancy events	Labor events	Mode of delivery	Puerperium or postabortal period	Baby

- ❖ *Past history*:
  - Medical: No such
  - Surgical: Nil.
- ❖ *Family history*:
- ❖ *Sexual history*:
- ❖ *Functional history*:
- ❖ *Personal history*:
  - Personal hygiene
  - Smoking/alcohol
- ❖ *Contraceptive history*: Tubectomy long back at the age of 29 years. In other abnormal uterine bleeding (AUB) patients, history of intrauterine contraceptive device (IUCD) or hormonal contraceptive should be taken.
- ❖ *Drug history or treatment history*:
  - History of any drug allergy
  - History of intake of corticosteroids, antiepileptic or other drugs (previous or present)
  - History of nonsteroidal anti-inflammatory drugs (NSAIDs) or hormone intake should be taken.

PHYSICAL EXAMINATION

Patient—alert, conscious, and cooperative.
- ❖ Build:
- ❖ Nutrition:
- ❖ Height:
- ❖ Weight/body mass index (BMI): Obesity causes anovular bleeding, endometrial hyperplasia, and endometrial carcinoma
- ❖ Edema: May be present
- ❖ Anemia: Present
- ❖ Cyanosis
- ❖ Jaundice
- ❖ Clubbing
- ❖ Tongue, teeth, gum, tonsil: Increase gingival bleeding
- ❖ Bruising over skin in coagulopathy
- ❖ Neck veins
- ❖ Neck glands: Enlarged thyroid (goiter and exophthalmos)
- ❖ Leg veins
- ❖ Pulse
- ❖ Respiration
- ❖ Temperature
- ❖ Blood pressure.

Systemic Examination

Examination of breasts and nipple:
- ❖ Inspection
- ❖ Palpation: Presence of galactorrhea.

GYNECOLOGICAL EXAMINATION

- ❖ *Abdominal examination*:
  - *Inspection*:
  - *Palpation*:
  - *Percussion*:
  - *Auscultation*:
- ❖ *Vaginal examination*:
  - Inspection and palpation of external genitalia
  - Speculum examination
  - Bimanual examination
  - Examination of rectovaginal area and rectal examination.

SUMMARY OF THE CASE

A 39-year-old woman coming from middle class family having 2 children, one of 16 years, the other 13 years has been admitted with chief complain of irregular bleeding per vagina for last 1 year. Patient complains that this problem was started 2 years back when she noticed that bleeding during period was excessive and often persisted for 8–10 days for which she has to take medicine. During last 1 year bleeding is irregular and she feels weakness. She had occasional pain lower abdominal pain during period. She is nondiabetic.

On general examination, she has pallor, BMI—overweight; on per abdominal examination, no significant finding is noted.

On per vaginal examination, cervix looks healthy, uterus slight bulky uniformly enlarged on bimanual examination and fornices are free without any tenderness.

Her Hb is 10 g%, urinary pregnancy test is negative, and transvaginal sonography of pelvis (TVS) shows bulky uterus, homogeneous myometrial pattern with a rounded hyperechoic mass within the cavity.

Investigations Supplied or Required

Investigations supplied include complete hemogram, sonography, for any other like coagulation disorder.

Provisional Diagnosis

A 39-year-old parous woman with Abnormal uterine bleeding probably endometrial polyp (AUB-P).

Differential Diagnosis

Q. What is your diagnosis?

Tell the provisional diagnosis.

Q. What is your case?

Tell the summary.

Q. Why are you saying this is a case of AUB-P?

She has AUB and a rounded hyperechoic mass within the cavity by TVS.

Q. Why not it is a case of submucous leiomyoma?

It is difficult to differentiate from submucous leiomyoma with the available findings. Here there is no such other pathology in myometrium and endometrium shown in TVS. However, TVS with colour Doppler or power Doppler can differentiate. Submucous leiomyoma gets blood flow from several blood vessels from the inner myometrium, whereas endometrial polyp receives supply from single feeding vessel.

Q What are the different varieties of uterine polyp?

See the Chapter 4 of uterine fibroid

DEFINITION OF AUB

Q. How will you define AUB?

Any deviation of frequency, regularity, amount or duration of flow from the normal menstrual flow is called abnormal uterine bleeding.

Bleeding in prepubertal age, in menopause, and following coitus are also regarded as AUB. (For definition of acute AUB and chronic AUB see later).

Q. What is the prevalence of AUB?

Abnormal uterine bleeding occurs in 10–30% of reproductive age women and 50% in perimenopausal women.

Q. When do you call normal menstruation?

- *Interval:* Varies from 21 days to 35 days. Average 28 days
- *Duration:* 2 days to 6 days, average 5 day, more than 7 days is abnormal
- *Blood loss:* 20–60 mL, average 40 mL. It is called heavy menstrual bleeding when total amount of bleeding per day exceeds 80 mL.

Menstrual Parameters -Recommended Terminologies

Table 1 depicts about the menstrual parameters defined by FIGO (2011).

Q. How will you assess menstrual blood loss?

Two ways of blood loss are subjective self-reporting or objective estimation of blood loss

Table 1: FIGO (2011) menstrual parameters.

Menstruation	Terms used	Limits
Frequency	• Frequent • Normal • Infrequent	• <24 days • 24–38 days • >38 days
Regularity of mens (cycle to cycle variation in 12 months)	• Absent • Regular • Irregular	• No bleeding • <7–9 days variation in 12 months • >10 days variation in 12 months
Duration of flows	• Prolonged • Normal • Shortened	• >8 days • 4.5–8 days • <4.5 days
Monthly blood loss (volume)	• Heavy • Normal • Light	• >80 mL • 5–80 mL • <5 mL

It is very difficult to assess quantitative blood loss. The different methods which are suggested are as follows:

- *Measurement of Hb from sanitary napkins*: Adding sodium chloride it is converted to hematin and measured spectrophotometrically. However, it is practically not possible in clinical set up.
- *Hb and hematocrit estimation*: Hb value below 12 g/mL is called menorrhagia. However normal value does not mean patient has no menorrhagia.
  Number and type of pad or tampons and amount of passing clot and by using a scoring sheet. Lightly stained pad = 1 point, moderately stained = 5 points, completely soaked = 20 points. Small clots = 1-point, large clots = 5. More than 100 points in each menstruation is above 80 mL.
- *Menstrual calendar*: By maintaining menstrual calendar and putting the symbols against each day, e.g., X = normal, / = light, ▪ = Heavy, S = Spotting, P = Provera.

Q. When do you call HMB or menorrhagia in clinically practice?

Clinically, it is said to be HMB or menorrhagia when there is:
- Less than or equal to 3 hourly pad change
- Change of pad at night time
- More than 21 pads per cycle
- Passage of clots more than 1 inch
- Above 80 mL blood loss in each menstrual period
- Clinical anemia.

Q. What are the different types of abnormal menstrual pattern?

- *Menorrhagia*: Now the term is replaced by HMB (see below)
- *Metrorrhagia*: Intermenstrual bleeding (IMB)
- *Menometrorrhagia*: Both menorrhagia and metrorrhagia in combination
- *Irregular bleeding:* When the length of cycle varies ≥10 days from cycle to cycle
- *Breakthrough bleeding*: Type of metrorrhagia that typically occurs during hormone administration
- *Hypomenorrhea*: Diminished flow or of short duration (normal interval is 28 ± 7 days)
- *Infrequent bleeding (Oligomenorrhea)*: Interval more than 38 days
- *Frequent bleeding (Polymenorrhea)* : Regular cyclical cycle length less than 21 days
- *Withdrawal bleeding*: Expected bleeding after abrupt decrease of progesterone
- *Spotting:* Bleeding not requiring any sanitary pad.

Heavy Menstrual Bleeding or Menorrhagia

- Menorrhagia is defined as when bleeding occurs cyclically in regular intervals but excessive in amount and/or duration which affects the physical, mental, and social aspects of life of a woman. Bleeding persists for more than 7 days or more than 80 mL of blood loss per cycle in regular interval. Term is recently called heavy menstrual bleeding.

- Causes of menorrhagia are:
  - *DUB*: 50% cases
  - *Pelvic causes*: Fibroid uterus, endometrial polyp, adenomyoma, endometriosis, pelvic inflammatory disease (PID), endometrial hyperplasia, and arteriovenous malformation.
  - *Systemic causes*: Hypothyroidism, coagulation disorder—von Willebrand disease, thrombocytopenia, systemic lupus disease (SLE), liver, and chronic renal disease.
  - *Iatrogenic*: IUCD, anticoagulant, other drugs—antipsychotic and antiepileptic. (For oral—DUB, fibroid uterus, adenomyoma, endometriosis, and PID)

Intermenstrual Bleeding or Metrorrhagia

Type of AUB which is acyclical and irregular.

Causes are fibroid polyp, endometrial cancer, cervical cancer, cervical polyp, cervical vascular erosion, decubitus ulcer, and irregular hormone intake.

Menometrorrhagia

Irregular heavy bleeding. Submucous fibroid is important cause.

Infrequent Bleeding or Oligomenorrhea

- Cycle interval is more than 38 days, may be irregular.
- Its causes are polycystic ovary syndrome (PCOS), hypothyroidism, hyperprolactinemia, menopausal transition, and menarche (like secondary amenorrhea). It is usually anovular.

Hypomenorrhea

- Scanty period lasting for less than 2 days with regular, cyclical bleeding.
- Its causes are endometrial Kochs, partial synechia following vigorous dilatation and curettage (D&C) and dilation and evacuation (D&E).

Frequent Bleeding (Polymenorrhea, Epimenorrhea)

- *Frequent bleeding (Polymenorrhea):* Regular cyclical cycle length less than 21 days
- Cycle is shorter than 21 days
- Its causes are menopausal transition and PID.

Q. What are the recent nomenclatures of type of bleeding pattern by FIGO?

All the nomenclatures are replaced by only two terms: (1) HMB (previously menorrhagia) and (2) Intermenstrual bleeding (previously metrorrhagia)

CAUSES OF REPRODUCTIVE TRACT BLEEDING

Q. What are the causes of reproductive tract bleeding?

- Pregnancy related bleeding is responsible for 15–20% of AUB. It is not included in PALM-COEIN classification
- Structural and nonstructural causes according to PALM-COEIN classification for AUB
- Other causes of bleeding from lower genital tract
- Bleeding due to systemic disorder

Pregnancy-related Bleeding

- Implantation bleeding
- Abortion
- Hydatidiform mole
- Ectopic pregnancy
- Postabortal or postpartum causes.

Pregnancy related bleeding should always be excluded from history and by determination of urine or serum βhCG. Spontaneous miscarriage is associated with excessive or prolonged bleeding. Unintented pregnancies are common and in women more than 40 years and adolescents.

Structural and nonstructural causes as defined in **PALM-COEIN** classifications described later

Other Causes of Bleeding from Lower Genital Tract

- Trauma—over vulva, vagina and forgotten foreign body
- Malignancy—vulva, vagina, fallopian tube, hormone producing tumour of ovary
- Outlet obstruction of genital tract—longitudinal or partial transverse septum
- Others—vaginal adenosis, granulation tissue following surgery.

Bleeding due to Systemic Disorder

- *Endocrinal disorder*: Hypothyroidism or hyperthyroidism, adrenal disorder, PCOS, diabetes mellitus, and obesity.
- Hormone intake: Sex steroids and corticosteroids
- Coagulopathy
- Hepatic failure and chronic renal failure.

STRUCTURAL AND NONSTRUCTURAL CAUSES OF AUB AS DEFINED IN PALM-COEIN CLASSIFICATIONS BY FIGO 2011

PALM-COEIN Classification

PALM-COEIN classification for causes of AUB by FIGO 2011 has been described in **Flowchart 1**.

Q. What is PALM-COEIN classification?

Due to the general inconsistency in the nomenclature used to describe AUB and lack of proper classification system *FIGO (2011)* has developed a classification system, which can be used by clinicians, investigators, and even patients to facilitate communication, clinical care by fostering a common language for research, known as *PALM-COEIN classification system* for AUB in *nongravid women of reproductive age*.

The causes of AUB are divided into two groups: (1) PALM and (2) COEIN consisting of total *9 main categories*, which are arranged according to the acronym PALM-COEIN. *PALM*

Flowchart 1: PALM-COEIN classification for causes of AUB.

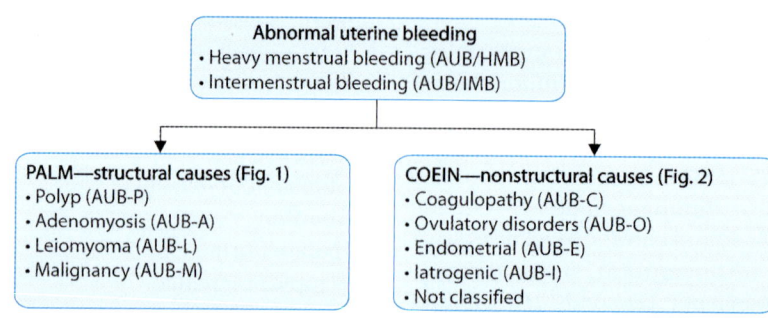

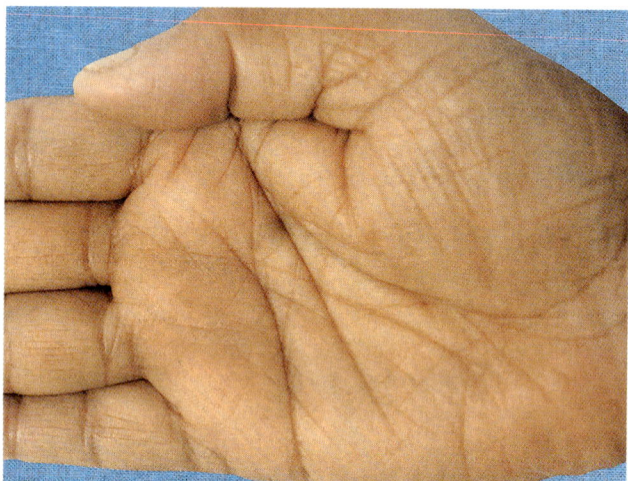

Fig. 1: PALM.

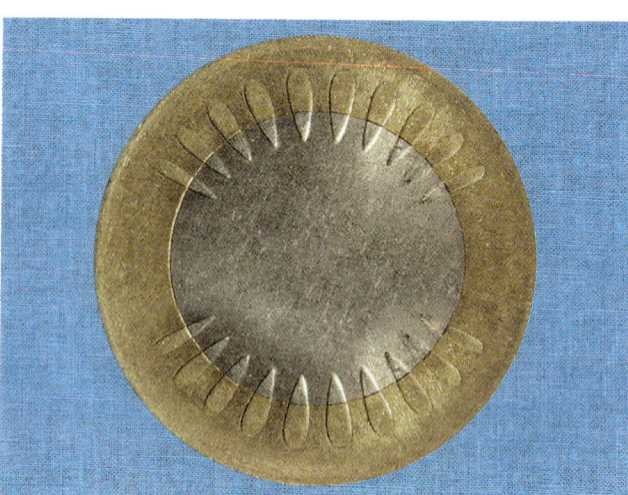

Fig. 2: COEIN.

group are discrete (structural) entities that can be identified visually with imaging techniques and/or histopathology. *COEIN group* is related to entities that are not diagnosed by imaging or histopathology (nonstructural).

PALM

Polyp (Fig. 3): Endometrial, endocervical

Adenomyosis (Fig. 4)

Leiomyomas (Figs. 5 and 6)

Malignancy (Fig. 7): CIN, EIN (premalignant hyperplasia) and cervical cancer, endometrial cancer and sarcoma

COEIN

Coagulopathy

Ovulatory (ovulatory dysfunction)

Endometrial

Iatrogenic

Not yet classified

- Each parameter is designed to facilitate the development of subclassification systems, as necessary. The subclassifications would be most relevant at specialist and research levels, e.g., the primary classification system (AUB-L) reflects only the presence or absence of 1 or more leiomyomas, regardless of the location, number, and size. In the secondary system, it is essential to distinguish [submucosal (SM)] from others (O) because submucosal lesions are the most likely to cause AUB. In the tertiary classification system of the PALM-COEIN, it includes submucosal, intramural, and subserosal leiomyomas

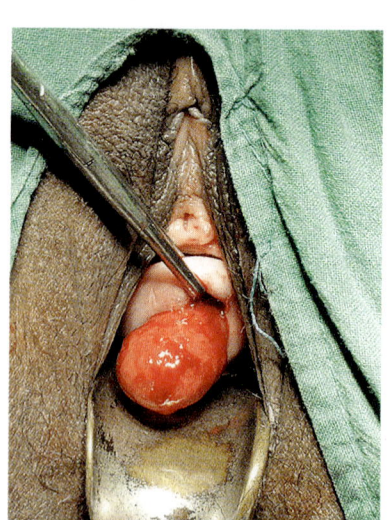

Fig. 3: Polyp (P) (cervical)—detected on clinical examination.

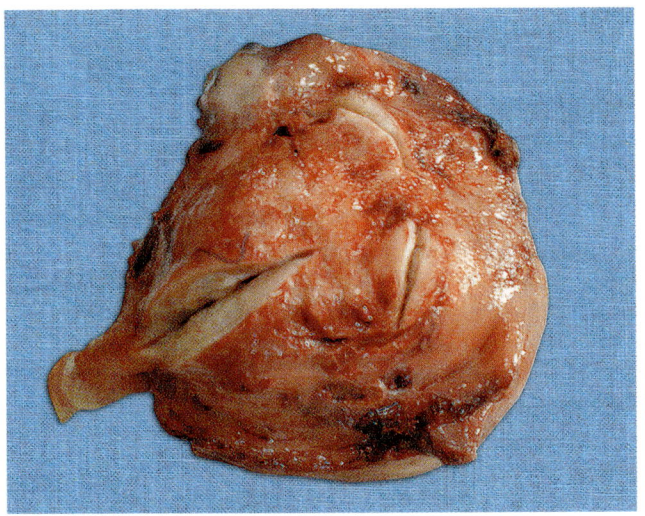

Fig. 4: Adenomyosis (A).

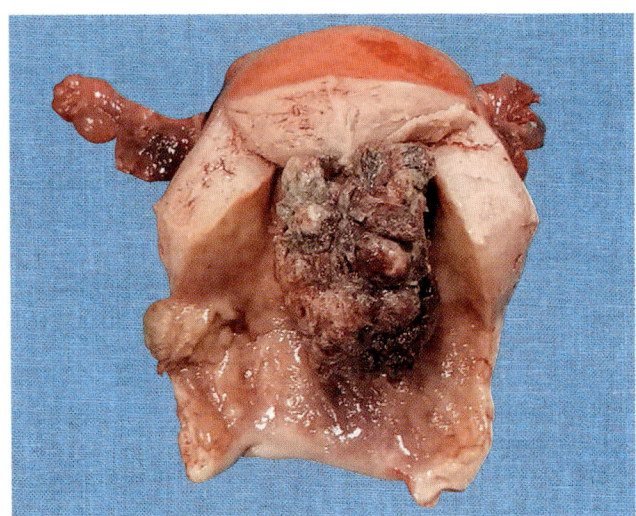

Fig. 7: Malignancy (M)—endometrial carcinoma.

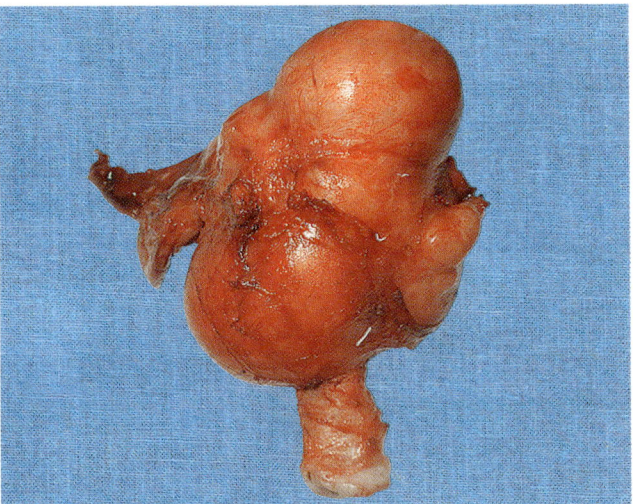

Fig. 5: Leiomyoma (L).

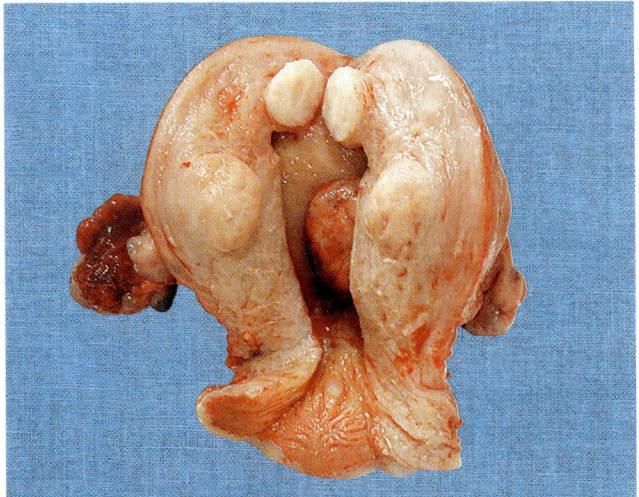

Fig. 6: Leiomyoma (L)—hysteroscope can diagnose only the submucous fibroid but transvaginal sonography can diagnose all types of fibroid.

from 0 to 8 (9 categories) and more detail is given in the Chapter 4: A Case of Fibroid Uterus; **Table 1**, **Fig. 16**.

- In the new system most of the older terminologies are abandoned including DUB. Only two terminologies *heavy menstrual bleeding (HMB)* in place of menorrhagia and *intermenstrual bleeding (IMB)* in lieu of metrorrhagia are recommended in new system.
- The system was developed recognizing that any patient could have one or several entities that could result or contribute to AUB.
- Each component is addressed for all patients. In all cases, the presence or absence of each criterion is noted using "0" if absent, "1" if present, and "?" if not yet assessed.
  Example: A woman with AUB having one submucous fibroid and with ovular dysfunction can be expressed as AUB $P_0 A_0 L_{1(SM)} M_0 - C_0 O_1 E_0 I_0 N_0$. As it is cumbersome to write, it is easier to write as AUB-LSM; O.
- PALM-COEIN classification is an ongoing process with potentiality of expansion.

AUB-P (see Fig. 3): It includes both endometrial and endocervical polyp which causes abnormal bleeding. It is difficult to differentiate from submucous leiomyoma. TVS with color Doppler or power Doppler can differentiate. Submucous leiomyoma gets blood flow from several blood vessels from the inner myometrium, whereas endometrial polyp receives supply from single feeding vessel. Endometrial polyps result heavy menstrual bleeding, intermenstrual bleeding, irregular bleeding and postmenopausal bleeding and dysmenorrhea. Majority of endometrial polyps are asymptomatic. Use of tamoxifen is associated with endometrial polyp.

AUB-A (see Fig. 4): AUB caused by adenomyosis though relation between adenomyosis and abnormal bleeding is less clear. As MRI is not accessible to all, sonographic criteria for adenomyosis are accepted in PALM-COEIN system.

AUB-L (see Figs. 5 and 6): Leiomyoma is an important cause of AUB. As submucous variety most likely causes AUB, it is grouped in secondary subclassification system of this

PALM-COEIN and in tertiary system all leiomyoma are classified into nine groups (see Chapter 4: A Case of Fibroid Uterus)

AUB-M (see Fig. 7): It not only includes malignancy but also the *premalignant conditions* CIN, EIN (premalignant hyperplasia) and cervical cancer, endometrial cancer and sarcoma. Diagnosis is confirmed by biopsy.

AUB-C: It encompasses spectrum of systemic disorder of hemostasis contributing about 13% of all AUB. Causes are congenital, acquired-hepatic failure and immunological. Most important is von Willebrand disease. It is confirmed by hematological test if screen is positive.

AUB-O: Ovulatory disorder or anovulation are important cause of AUB. Causes of anovulation are puberty, perimenopause, PCOS (5–10%), obesity, hypothyroidism, hyperthyroidism, hyperprolactinemia, premature ovarian failure, pituitary and hypothalamic disorder, CAH, Cushing syndrome, stress, anorexia, excessive exercise and some drugs. It is common at puberty and at menopause transition. Ovulatory status and physical features are the cornerstones of diagnosis.

AUB-E: AUB is due to primary disorder in endometrium in typical ovulatory cycle. Causes are intrinsic defect, endometrial hyperplasia, endometrial atrophy, chronic endometritis. It is diagnosed when no other cause is identified (diagnosis by exclusion).

AUB-I: Many medical or surgical interventions may cause AUB. These are exogenous hormones, IUCD, anticoagulant and sodium valproate, etc.

AUB-N: Many unclassified causes are pelvic inflammatory disease, cervicitis, genital tuberculosis, arteriovenous malformation, isthmocele, myometrial hypertrophy and partial uterine synechia. AUB-N is the conditions which are still not cause of AUB conclusively.

Etiology of AUB According to Age

- *Childhood*: Vulvovaginitis, foreign body, trauma, and malignancy.
- *Adolescent*: Anovulation, coagulation disorder (von Willebrand disease) NASIDs, and aspirin should not be taken frequently for dysmenorrhea as they cause platelet dysfunction.
- *Reproductive age:* Pregnancy, fibroid, and endometrial polyp.
- *Perimenopause:* Anovulatory bleeding, benign or malignant growth.
- *Menopause:* The most common cause is atrophic endometrium, endometrium cancer must be considered as it is common in this age group. Vulval, vaginal, and cervical lesion may be considered.

Common Causes of AUB

Common causes of AUB in premenarchal age is foreign body, in reproductive age is pregnancy related and in postmenopausal age is atrophy. The common cause in menarche and perimenopause is anovular. However, in menarche coagulation defects (like von Willebrand disease) and in menopause malignancy should always be excluded.

Mechanism of Normal Menstrual Bleeding (*see* also Chapter 19)

Shedding of functional layers of endometrium due to ischemic necrosis, physiology of ovulation, menstruation as a result of withdrawal of estrogen and progesterone is termed as *menstruation*. In absence of implantation sex steroids are withdrawn, spiral arterioles are highly coiled and vascular spasm of spiral artery results endometrial ischemia. Prostaglandins are produced maximum throughout men. PGF2α causes vasoconstriction which is also responsible for vasospasm. Myometrial contraction due to the effect of PGF2α removes sloughed out endometrial tissue. Breakdown of lysosomes and release of proteolytic enzymes promote local tissue destruction.

Mechanisms of Abnormal Bleeding in Related to Ovulatory Status

Anovular abnormal bleeding: No ovulation → no progesterone production → excessive proliferation of endometrium → endometrium hyperplasia → instability.

It is associated with stromal breakdown, decreased spiral arteriole density, and dilated and unstable venous capillaries and bleeding.

Ovular abnormal bleeding: Bleeding is mainly due to vasodilatation alone. Endometrial vessels become markedly dilated due to *autocrine and paracrine defects*. Imbalance of prostaglandins F2 alpha (PGF2α) (vasoconstrictor): PGE2 (vasodilator) and thromboxane A2 (constrictors): PGI2 (vasodilators) decreased resulting severe bleeding. Angiogenic factors like vascular endothelial growth factor (VEGF) and fibroblast growth factors are major angiogenic factors which are related to DUB.

Pattern of Bleeding in Anovular AUB

Pattern of bleeding in anovular AUB is described in **Table 2**.

Difference between Anovulatory and Ovulatory Abnormal Bleeding

Table 3 shows the difference between anovulatory and ovulatory bleeding.

Table 2: Pattern of bleeding in anovular AUB.	
Insufficient follicular development	*Menstrual pattern*
- Low estrogen - Short cycle - Inadequate proliferative or atrophic endometrium	- Polymenorrhea - Metrorrhagia
Persistent follicle like in polycystic ovary syndrome	
- Unopposed estrogen - Deficient progesterone - Proliferative or hyperplastic endometrium	- Oligomenorrhea - Metropathia hemorrhagica

CHAPTER 5: A Case of Abnormal Uterine Bleeding (Endometrial Hyperplasia)

Table 3: Difference between anovulatory and ovulatory bleeding.

Anovulatory (AUB-O)	Ovulatory (AUB-E)
90%	10%
Common at puberty, menopause transition, and other anovulatory condition	At reproductive age group
Bleeding pattern—irregular	Regular. HMB with premenstrual dysmenorrhea
Dysfunction of HPO axis leading to anovulation	Local endometrial defect—autocrine paracrine defects leading to imbalance of prostaglandins
Causes: Puberty, perimenopause, PCOS (5–10%), hypothyroidism, hypothyroidism, hyperprolactinemia, and some drugs	No specific entity known—any woman at reproductive age group
Hormonal treatment is the first choice. Nonhormonal drugs are not recommended	Can be managed both by hormonal and nonhormonal treatments

Abbreviations: AUB, abnormal uterine bleeding; HMB, heavy menstrual bleeding; HPO, hypothalamic–pituitary–ovarian; PCOS, polycystic ovary syndrome

DYSFUNCTIONAL UTERINE BLEEDING (DUB)

Q. Status of Dysfunctional Uterine Bleeding in New FIGO PALM-COEIN Classification System

Following new FIGO Classification System of PALM-COEIN the term DUB has now been abandoned and should no longer be used. Women who fit the description of DUB, in the new system generally have one or a combination of coagulopathy (AUB-C), disorder of ovulation (AUB-O), or primary endometrial disorder (AUB-E)—the last of which is most often a primary or secondary disturbance in local endometrial hemostasis.

Q. How DUB was defined previously?

Dysfunctional uterine bleeding is regarded as excessive bleeding of uterine origin, not related to any systemic disease or complications of pregnancy (European Society of Human Reproduction and Embryology). About 50% of AUB is contributed by DUB. Anovular bleeding comprises 90% and ovular bleeding 10%.

POSTCOITAL BLEEDING

Bleeding following intercourse:
- *Causes*: The most common is typically benign. In two-thirds cases, no pathology detected.
- *Others are*:
  - Cervical erosion—one-fourth cases
  - Endocervical polyp
  - Cervicitis
  - Endometrial polyp
  - Cervical or other genital tract cancer.

Women with cancer cervix may present with postcoital bleeding but common cause of postcoital bleeding is not cervical cancer.

Q. How would you evaluate a case of patient with AUB?

The initial step is to determine whether bleeding is acute or chronic.

Q. What do you mean by chronic AUB and acute AUB?

- *Chronic AUB* can be defined as bleeding from the uterine corpus that is abnormal in volume, regularity, and/or timing, and has been present for the majority at least for past 6 months. Chronic AUB would not, require immediate intervention.
- *Acute AUB* may present in the context of existing chronic AUB or might occur without such a history. Acute AUB requires immediate intervention.

DIAGNOSIS OF AUB

Q. How will you reach at diagnosis in a case of AUB?

The diagnosis is done by:
- *Clinical*: History, general physical examination, abdominal examination, and vaginal examination.
- *Investigations*: Laboratory, imaging, endometrial biopsy, and hysteroscope.

The purpose is to:
- Exclude pregnancy
- To exclude or to detect any local pathology
- To detect or to exclude any systemic disorder.
- If no cause is detected DUB is diagnosed.

History

- *Age:* Puberty, premenarcheal, reproductive age, perimenopausal, and menopausal: In every age group, the etiology of AUB is different as described above. In menarche, adolescent, and in perimenopausal age bleeding is due mostly of anovular. In reproductive age pregnancy-related bleeding or other uterine and nonuterine pathology may be the cause.
- *Type of abnormal bleeding and relation with menstruation*: Bleeding pattern, frequency, irregularity, HMB, intermenstrual bleeding, association with dysmenorrhea, premenstrual symptoms, relation with coitus. Assessment of amount of bleeding by number of pads used, change of pad at night, and passage of clots.
- *Any bleeding preceded by amenorrhea* may be due to pregnancy-related bleeding or anovular bleeding like PCOS. Severe dysmenorrhea is suggestive of endometriosis or PID. Intermenstrual bleeding may be due to submucous uterine or cervical polyp.

- *Pelvic pain*: Infection and endometriosis.
- *Dyspareunia*: Endometriosis, PID, and postcoital bleeding indicate local pathology.
- Symptoms of anemia, e.g., palpitation, breathlessness, and weakness.
- *Obstetric history*: History of infertility is associated with PCOS, endometriosis. History of recent pregnancy loss, medical termination of pregnancy.
- *Past history*: Diabetes, hypertension, thyroid disorder, history of bleeding manifestation (coagulation disorder).
- *Family history*: Coagulation disorder, endometrial cancer. Other risk factors of endometrial cancer must be enquired—obesity, PCOS, diabetes, nulliparity, and perimenopausal age.
- *Contraceptive history*: IUCD, combined oral contraceptive (COC) and its irregular intake.
- *History of hormone intake and other drugs* like antipsychotic, corticosteroids, and anticoagulants like warfarin and heparin. NSAID using for dysmenorrhea further increases bleeding by platelet dysfunction.
- *Treatment history*: History of blood transfusion.
- *Personal history*: Quality of life, social life.

General Physical Examination

- Anemia
- Edema
- Weight—obesity—BMI high. In thyrotoxicosis, there may be weight loss
- Features of PCOS: Hirsutism, acne, and acanthosis nigricans
- Skin: Bruising, petechial hemorrhage in coagulation defects
- Eye-exophthalmos in thyrotoxicosis
- Enlarged thyroid (goiter)
- Gum (gingival) bleeding in coagulation defects
- Breasts: Galactorrhea.

Per Abdominal Examination

- *Upper abdomen:* Enlarged liver and spleen.
- *Lower abdomen:* Any mass—uterine fibroid, pregnancy, ovarian tumor (hormone producing tumor may cause AUB).

Gynecological Examination

- Vulva, vagina, urethra, anal canal to look for any source of bleeding.
- Per speculum examination: Cervix—cervicitis, erosion, endocervical polyp, fibroid polyp, any growth (cancer).
- Bimanual examination—enlarged uterus due to pregnancy, fibroid, adenomyosis, endometrial cancer, and uterine sarcoma.
- Tenderness with fixed uterus with enlarged adnexae—endometriosis and PID.
- Presence of thread of Cu-T through external os.

Investigations

Laboratory Testing

- Serum or urinary β-human chorionic gonadotropin (β-hCG) testing is done first to exclude pregnancy
- Complete hemogram to see the degree and type of anemia
- Screening for coagulation disorder especially in adolescents with menorrhagia—CBC, platelet, PTT, PT, and screening for von Willebrand disease.
- *"Wet prep"* examination of cervical secretions: Microscopic examination of cervical secretion in saline shows neutrophils and red blood cells in chronic cervicitis and infection.
- *Pap smear screening*: Commonly abnormal squamous cells from cervix and less frequently to see abnormal endocervical gland and endometrial cells.
- *Others:* Hormone assays as clinically indicated—TSH, free testosterone, prolactin, and progesterone.

Ultrasonography

- Transabdominal or transvaginal sonography (TVS) **(Fig. 8)**
- SIS (saline infusion sonography) **(Fig. 9)**
- Transvaginal color Doppler sonography (TV-CDS) **(Fig. 10)**.

Endometrial Biopsy (EMB)—Endometrial Sampling

(If Clinically Indicated) can be done by
- D&C
- Metal curettes
- Flexible plastic samplers (Pipelle) by aspiration.

Hysteroscopy and Hysteroscopic-guided Biopsy

(if clinically indicated)

CASE OF AUB

Q. How to approach a case of AUB?

Exclude pregnancy first by history and urinary or serum β-hCG.

Be sure bleeding is of uterine origin and chronic in nature by history and clinical examination. The structural causes

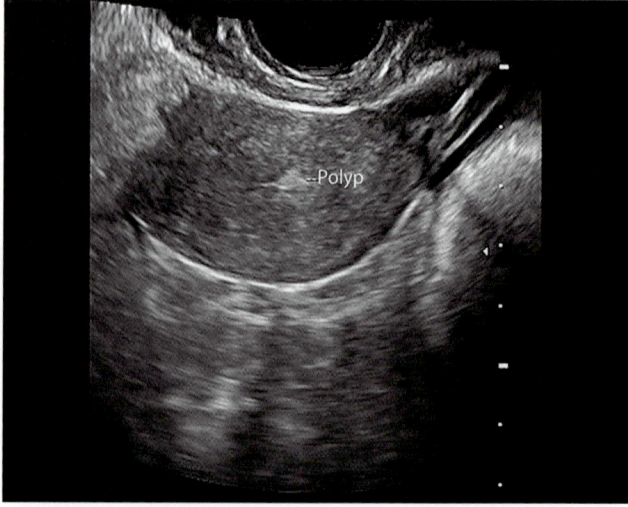

Fig. 8: Small endometrial polyp 0.49 cm.

CHAPTER 5: A Case of Abnormal Uterine Bleeding (Endometrial Hyperplasia)

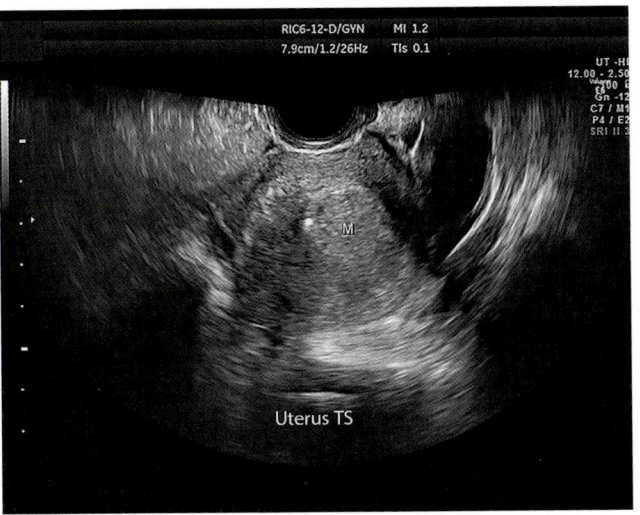

Fig. 9: Saline infusion sonography transverse section.

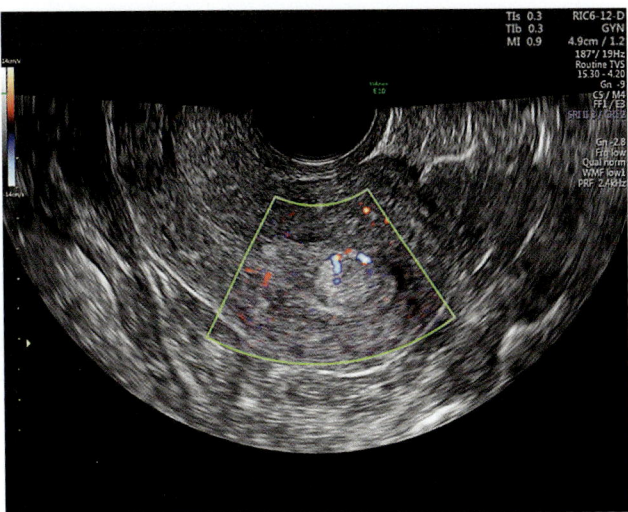

Fig. 10: Transvaginal sonography of endometrial polyp with color Doppler.
Courtesy: Professor Kamal Oswal, VIMS, Kolkata

(PALM—polyp, adenomyosis, leiomyoma and malignancy including premalignant hyperplasia) are diagnosed by clinical examination and the procedures such as TVS, SIS, hysteroscopy which one is needed. Biopsy is done if required.

Nonstructural causes (COEIN—coagulopathy, ovulatory dysfunction, endometrial, iatrogenic and not yet classified cause) are searched for if structural cause excluded or presence of nonstructural cause is suspected (there may be multiple cause of AUB). For diagnosis of AUB-C screening of coagulation disorder is done first followed by confirmatory test in screen positive cases. AUB-O is diagnosed by determination of ovulatory dysfunction by history particularly menstrual pattern and clinical examination considering the etiological conditions of anovulation such as peripubertal, perimenopausal age group woman, PCOS, hyperprolactinemia, hypothyroidism, obesity, extreme weight loss, etc. AUB-I is determined by iatrogenic causes of bleeding like any drug interfering dopamine metabolism, sex steroid hormones, IUCD or surgery. AUB-N is the condition which is still not cause of AUB conclusively. AUB-E, ovulatory bleeding with primary disorder of endometrium, is diagnosed by exclusion of other causes.

Approach to Diagnose AUB

For approach to diagnose AUB, *see* **Flowchart 2**.

Flowchart 2: Approach to diagnose AUB.

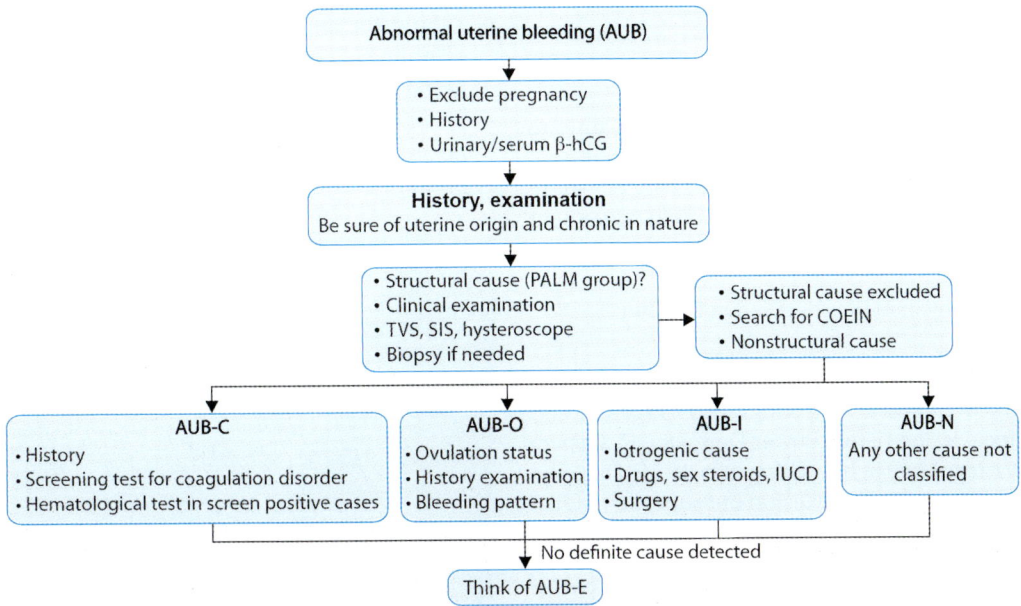

Abbreviations: AUB, abnormal uterine bleeding; hCG, human chorionic gonadotropin; TVS, transvaginal sonography; SIS, saline infusion sonography; IUCD, intrauterine contraceptive device

Role of TVS in Diagnosis of AUB (see Fig. 8)

For assessment of AUB, TVS is chosen as first-line investigative tool.

Myometrium and endometrium can be assessed by TVS, and by hysteroscope or endometrial biopsy.

Patient feels less discomfort in comparison to other.

Postmenopausal endometrial hyperplasia and cancer detection by TVS is comparable to other tool. If the thickness is more than 4 mm, hysteroscopy and biopsy are warranted in postmenopausal women. If the thickness is less than or equal to 4 mm cancer is less likely and is usually associated with atrophic endometrium and immediate evaluation of endometrium is not needed. In premenopausal women, cut off value is yet to determine; however above 10 mm ET, further evaluation is needed. There is no consensus on ET threshold in this age group and other risk factors for hyperplasia are evaluated.

The interpretation of characteristic findings of endometrium by TVS is as follows:

- Cystic endometrial changes → suggestive of polyps
- Homogeneous thickened endometrium → indicates hyperplasia
- Heterogeneous structural pattern → suspicious of malignancy.

The most disadvantage of TVS is high false negative rate for focal intrauterine pathology detection.

Role of Saline Infusion Sonography (SIS), also Called Sonohysterography or Hysterosonography (see Fig. 9)

Saline infusion sonography (SIS) is helpful to diagnose the pathology of endometrial cavity like submucous fibroid, endometrial polyp, and blood clot associated with uterine bleeding. It is done when in general TVS endometrial thickening or mass is detected. It is also useful in infertility workup.

The detailed procedure of SIS is described in Chapter 2: Investigative Procedures in Gynecology and Imaging in Gynecology.

Saline infusion sonography is superior to TVS only to differentiate the endometrial, submucous or intramural. However, it is not superior in diagnosis of cancer where hysteroscope is the gold standard. It is also cycle dependent to avoid false positive and false negative diagnosis cavity pathology.

Role of sonography in AUB is detailed in Chapter 2.

Other Imaging in AUB

Color and pulsed Doppler/3D sonography **(Fig. 11)** can delineate the focal lesion better. Power Doppler can suspect malignancy by irregularity in branching vessels. MRI is rarely needed in detecting endometrial lesion but superior to CT.

Q. Why endometrial biopsy is important in AUB?

Endometrial cancer presents with AUB near 90% cases. Some risk factors warrant for endometrial biopsy. These are women older than 45 years with AUB, younger women

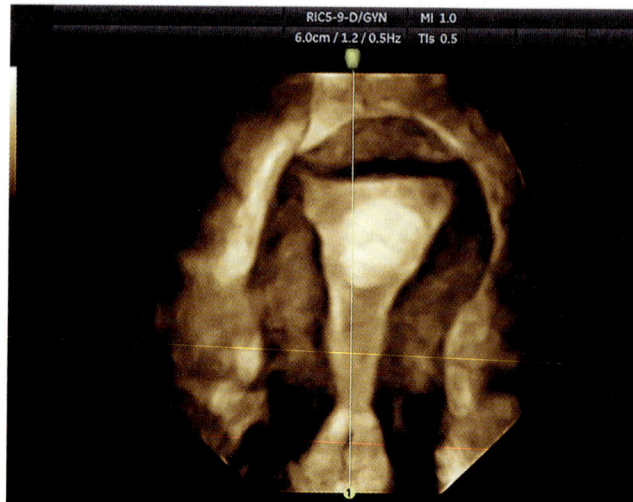

Fig. 11: Endometrial polyp in 3D; a 33-year-old woman presented with abnormal uterine bleeding.

not responding to medical management, PCOS, diabetes, tamoxifen users, and genetic predisposition to uterine cancer (Lynch syndrome).

Q. In which cases of AUB you will do endometrial biopsy (ACOG 2012)?

Any woman more than 45 years of age with AUB.

Before 45 years where there is unopposed estrogen exposure, such as PCOS, obesity, and the cases not responding to medical management and persistent AUB and genetic predisposition to uterine cancer (Lynch syndrome).

ENDOMETRIAL BIOPSY—DIFFERENT METHODS

Q. What are the different methods of endometrial biopsy and which one is preferred?

- Dilatation and curettage—D&C is used for years for sampling of endometrium.
- Metal curette (Sharman's curette) **(Fig. 12)**
- Flexible plastic curette (Pipelle device). Pipelle device is a flexible plastic curette provided with *suction system* and is preferred for various reasons.

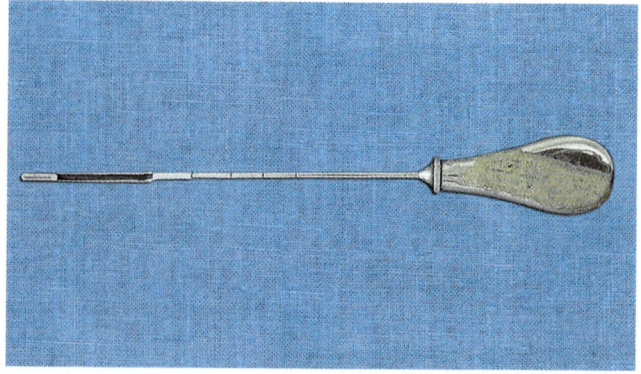

Fig. 12: Sharman's metallic curette for endometrial biopsy (not popular now).

Q. How will you do endometrial sampling by aspiration with pipelle? Advantage and disadvantage (Fig. 13) (*see* also Chapter 2).

Procedure

It is an office procedure, less painful and little discomfort with minimal risk. Usually, NSAID is sufficient before procedure.

After antiseptic swabbing of cervix, pipelle is introduced through the cervix. Usually, a tenaculum is needed to stabilize the anterior lip. Pipelle is introduced till resistance is felt. Pipelle stilette inside is retracted to create suction and it is withdrawn (up to internal os) and introduced many times gently for thorough sampling.

Procedure of D&C is discussed in Chapter 25: Operative Gynyecology.

In D&C anesthesia is needed, there are surgical risk, risk of perforation, discomfort and pain during and after surgery, and in metal curette—there is discomfort, risk of injury, and infection.

Hence plastic sampler is used with equal efficacy for histological diagnosis. Diagnostic accuracy is 90-98% when compared with findings of D&C or hysterectomy.

Disadvantages of Pipelle device are:

- In atrophic endometrium, sample is inadequate to test.
- Negative histological report is not always cancer free as there is negative failure rate of 1%.
- In endometrial polyp, negative sampling may occur.
- In cervical stenosis, device cannot be introduced then D&C and hysteroscopic biopsy is needed.

Hysteroscopy for Assessment of AUB

Q. Hysteroscopy in assessing AUB, a gold standard—why (Fig. 14)?

Uterine cavity is distended by 3–5 mm diameter hysteroscope to visualize the endometrial cavity with an added advantage of taking biopsy from suspicious lesion and also in the same sitting many lesions can be removed.

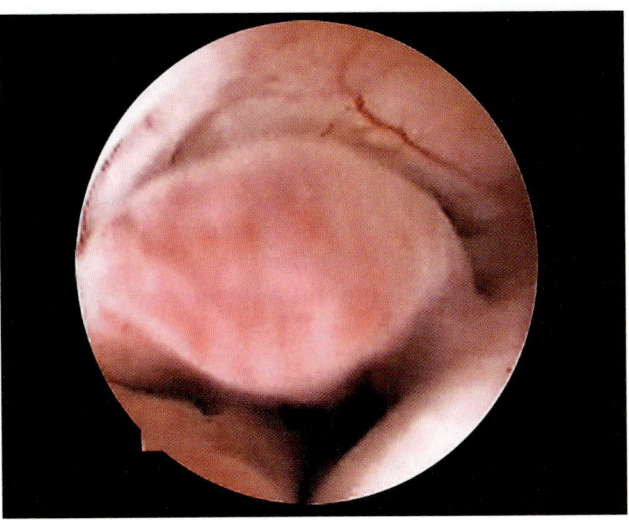

Fig. 14: Hysteroscopic view of endometrial polyp.
Courtesy: Dr Alok De, Associate Professor

TVS versus SIS

Advantage to TVS and SIS is that many small lesions like polyp or leiomyoma is not missed which may happen in the latter.

The disadvantage is invasiveness, cost, less value in diagnosis of hyperplasia, and peritoneal contamination of endometrial cancer cells through fallopian tube.

Q. Which procedure to be done first to evaluate endometrial pathology?

There is no clear cut sequence amongst endometrial biopsy, TVS, SIS, and hysteroscopy. Transvaginal sonography is accepted as first to do as low cost, better tolerated, and strip thickness can be determined well.

For focal lesion SIS or hysteroscope is better usually guided from the finding of TVS.

In suspected cancer or hyperplasia hysteroscopic biopsy has obvious advantages over the others.

MANAGEMENT

Management of Abnormal Uterine Bleeding

It includes: (1) the treatment of specific diseases depending upon causes and (2) treatment of DUB.

Q. What are the different modalities of management of AUB?

- General health management including blood transfusion and iron therapy
- Medical management
- Uterine artery embolization/Foley catheter tamponade
- Surgical management:
  - D&C
  - Endometrial resection or ablation
  - Hysterectomy
- Other specific management according to etiology.

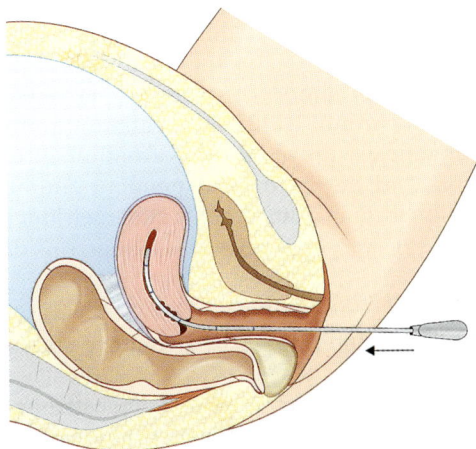

Fig. 13: Pipelle biopsy.

Medical Management

- NSAIDs
- Tranexamic acid (TXA)
- Iron therapy
- Hormone: Progesterone, COCs, only estrogen, oral progestins, injectable estrogen, Danazol, gonadotropin-releasing hormone (GnRH) agonists, and selective progesterone receptor modulator
- Hormone containing intrauterine system (IUS) (levonorgestrel-IUS).

Surgical Management

- D&C
- Endometrial ablation or resection
- Myomectomy—hysteroscopy
- Hysterectomy.

Nonsteroidal Anti-inflammatory Drugs

Nonsteroidal anti-inflammatory drugs acts by altering the types of prostaglandins in endometrium and commonly used to treat AUB-E. Mefenamic acid and naproxen are the two most widely studied NSAIDs in the treatment of HMB and equally effective. NSAIDs could be beneficial in combination with other medical therapies. They improve dysmenorrhea which is a common association with HMB. They have lower side effects.

Tranexamic Acid

It acts by competitively blocking plasminogen binding sites, preventing plasma formation, fibrin degradation, and clot degradation. Oral TXA is FDA approved for the treatment of ovulatory AUB (AUB-E). In the treatment of HMB, it is superior to placebo, mefenamic acid, and luteal-phase progestins.

The dose is 1–1.3 g orally every 6–8 hours during menstruation.

Desmopressin

Desmopressin is used in bleeding disorders like von Willebrand disease, during episodes of acute AUB in consultation with hematologist. It is synthetic analog of vasopressin. It is used only when all other hormonal and nonhormonal therapies fail.

Use of Estrogen-Progesterone Contraceptives in AUB

Combined estrogen-progesterone (E-P) are very effective in reducing menstrual blood loss and affords cycle control.

- *Various routes*: Oral pill (COC), vaginal ring, and transdermal patch.
- *Mechanism of actions*: Estrogen in oral contraceptives (OCs) prevents follicle-stimulating hormone (FSH) secretion and formation of a dominant follicle. It also gives endometrial stability and growth and enhances the progestational action. The progesterone prevents the LH surge and inhibits ovulation and makes endometrial lining atrophy, thereby decreases overall blood loss at the time of menstruation (withdrawal bleeding).
- *Effectivity:* Monophasic pills are very effective in both acute and chronic AUB. Short-term multidose regime is very effective. A triphasic combination successfully treats HMB and IMB in women with ovulatory dysfunction.
- Extended (12 week cycle) or continuous (365 days) regime, prevents the monthly blood loss and improves anemia. Dysmenorrhea and pelvic pain are also improved.

High Dose Estrogen in AUB

- Heavy bleeding results thin, denude endometrium, and progesterone or E-P is unlikely to work, high dose estrogen is best initial treatment.
- Mechanism is less clear. May not be specific to endometrium. Effective also in GI bleeding and otolaryngeal bleeding.
- High-dose causes rapid growth of the endometrial epithelium and stroma; stimulating vasospasm of uterine arteries; promoting platelet aggregation and capillary clotting; increasing fibrinogen, factor V and factor XI; and increasing the production of both estrogen and progesterone receptors.
- Highly effective—71%.
- Antiemetic is recommended as in up to 40% cases, there is nausea and vomiting in this high dose.
- In high dose of estrogen risk of thromboembolism increases and better to be avoided with a past history or family history of thromboembolism.
- *Dose of estrogen*: In acute AUB 25 mg IV equine estrogen every 4–6 hourly for 24 hours followed by high-dose oral estrogen therapy 2.5 mg conjugated estrogen or more commonly COCs (containing 30 µg EE) every 6 hourly till bleeding is stopped or markedly diminished (*see* later for detail, Page 127).

Progesterone-only Preparation

- *Indication:* In contraindication to estrogen, it is an ideal alternative.
- *Mechanism of action:* It inhibits the growth of the endometrium by triggering apoptosis; prevents angiogenesis; promotes conversion of estradiol to the less active estrone. It inhibits ovulation and ovarian steroidogenesis, prevents the formation of estrogen receptors and the estrogen-dependent endometrium stimulation leading to an atrophic endometrium.
- *Route:* May be oral, injectable or as intrauterine device.

Regimen of Oral Progesterone

Oral regimen is determined by ovulatory status of the women.

In women with ovulatory AUB, oral progesterone is taken *cyclically* (starting on day 5 of menstruation for 21 days) or continuously provides cycle control and reduction of menstrual blood loss. Only *luteal-phase progesterone* is not effective in the treatment of ovulatory HMB.

In women with anovulatory bleeding, a *cyclic progesterone for 12–14 days* each month, leads to regulation of the menstrual cycle in 50% of women. In acute AUB, a multidose progesterone [i.e., medroxyprogesterone acetate (MPA) 20 mg 3 times daily for 1 week, followed by single or double (5–10 mg) daily dose for 3 weeks] can significantly reduce menstrual blood loss.

Injectable Progesterone: Depot Medroxyprogesterone Acetate (DMPA)

- Depot medroxyprogesterone acetate (DMPA) is one useful option for maintenance therapy in women who have difficulty with or cannot take E-P contraceptives.
- Depot medroxyprogesterone acetate has no place in acute management of abnormal bleeding.
- Once given cannot be withdrawn and if unsuccessful its effects can be difficult to overcome.
- *Side effects*: Weight gain and breakthrough bleeding. Breakthrough bleeding can be managed by estrogen. Dose is 150 mg IM 3 monthly.
- There is a lack of clinical data on the utility of DMPA for the treatment of acute or chronic AUB.
- Because of its prolonged action and difficulty in predicting the time of withdrawal bleeding DMPA is not recommended in secondary amenorrhea or DUB. In these conditions, oral therapy is recommended.

Intrauterine Progestogen-releasing Systems: The Levonorgestrel-releasing Intrauterine System (LNG-IUS; Mirena) (Fig. 15)

- Primarily used as long-acting reversible contraception (LARC).
- *Mechanism of action*: Releases the progestogen levonorgestrel (initial release rate of 20 μg/day), reduces ET and the mean uterine vascular density. Makes endometrium atrophy. In some women, ovulation is also inhibited.
- It remains effective as a contraceptive and treatment for HMB for 5 years. Menstrual blood loss is reduced near more than 90% after 3 months in HMB. Dysmenorrhea is also improved.
- The LNG-IUS is superior to luteal phase oral progesterone, DMPA, COCs, and mefenamic acid in treatment of HMB. LNG-IUS is superior to or comparable with endometrial ablation when menstrual loss and quality of life are considered. LNG-IUS when compared with hysterectomy for the treatment of HMB, quality of life seems similar after years later but cost of the LNG-IUS is low. However, above 40% patents using LNG-IUS eventually underwent hysterectomy by 10 years.
- It is particularly useful for reproductive aged women with AUB-O and AUB-E who wish to retain fertility.
- *AUB-A*: Insertion of LNG-IUS after endometrial resection is effective treatment for menorrhagia caused by adenomyosis.
- *AUB-M*: LNG-IUS is a reliable preference for younger patients with *endometrial hyperplasia without atypia* and wish to preserve their uterus. If fertility is not desired, women should be encouraged to retain the LNG-IUS for up to 5 years.
- *AUB-L*: LNG-IUS significantly reduces mean uterine volume in women with menorrhagia, and reduces menstrual blood loss (MBL) in women with uterine leiomyomas. Uterine cavity distortion is a contraindication.
- It can be used as first line of treatment in all span of reproductive age especially AUB-O.

Danazol

- Danazol has a weak androgenic influence and causing thinning or atrophy of endometrial tissue. It is a synthetic steroid ethisterone that inhibits pituitary secretion of FSH and LH.
- In the treatment of HMB, danazol is superior to luteal-phase oral progesterone and mefenamic acid. Danazol reduces menstrual blood loss by as much as 80%.
- More adverse effects, including weight gain, acne, and androgenic effects, than other medical therapies restrict its routine use.
- Dose is 100–400 mg daily orally.
- Vaginal use of danazol in low dose is being considered as a way to preserve the benefits of the drug while reducing systemic side effects.

GnRH Agonist

- Creates profound hypoestrogenic by hypogonadotropic state by downregulation of GnRH receptors.
- Induces endometrial atrophy and amenorrhea and helps to improve anemia. Randomized controlled trials have explored the efficacy of GnRH agonists in the treatment of AUB.
- It is highly effective when associated with leiomyoma and adenomyosis.
- Leuprolide acetate is FDA approved for short-term use in the preoperative treatment of uterine leiomyomata.

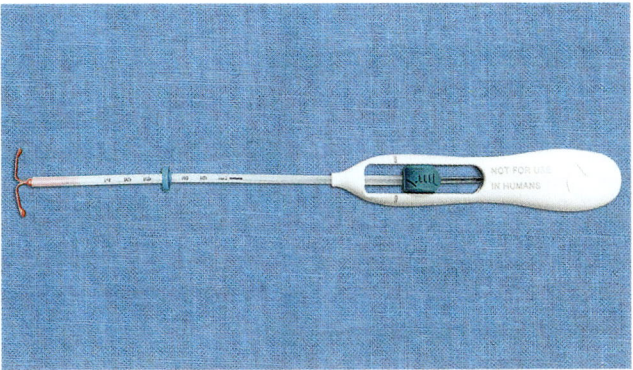

Fig. 15: Mirena with applicator.

Uterine volume is reduced by 30–60%, and anemia is improved in women with HMB and fibroids.
- Subcutaneous goserelin acetate also has FDA approval for the induction of endometrial atrophy prior to ablation for AUB. Atrophy and amenorrhea usually occur among premenopausal women within 3–4 weeks of the drug's administration.
- Leuprolide acetate 3.75 mg IM monthly or 11.25 mg IM every 3 month is given.
- Duration is limited to 6 months only due to side effects of menopausal symptoms including vasomotor symptoms, vaginal atrophy, dryness, depression, and bone loss.
- Add back therapy (E + P) is indicated if used more than 6 months.

Hormonal Agents used in AUB with Doses, Contraindications, Adverse Effects, and Efficacy

These hormonal agents are listed in **Table 4**.

Table 4: Hormonal agents used in AUB.

Agents	Dose	Contraindications	Adverse effects	Efficacy
CEE	Acute: 25 mg IV every 4–6 hourly for 24 hours	Pregnancy, history of thromboembolic disorder, breast cancer	Nausea, headache, mastalgia, breakthrough bleeding, TE, CVA, IHD	High
COC	Acute: Monophasic pill containing 35 μg estrogen 3 times daily for 1 week, then once daily for 3 weeks HMB: Cyclic monophasic or triphasic pills, extended or continuous, transdermal patch Vaginal ring can also be used	Pregnancy, smoking history of multiple risk factors for cardiovascular disease (i.e., elderly, smoking, diabetes, and hypertension), diabetic retinopathy, nephropathy, breast cancer, liver disorder, history of thromboembolic disease, IHD, stroke, valvular heart disease, SLE with vascular disease, nephritis, or antiphospholipid syndrome	Nausea, headache, mastalgia, breakthrough bleeding, TE, CVA, IHD	High
Oral progesterone	Acute: MPA 20 mg 3 times a day for 7 days HMB: Oral MPA (2.5–10 mg), norethindrone (2.5–5 mg), or micronized progesterone (200–400 mg) Without ovulatory dysfunction, take 1 tablet daily from 5th for 21 day In ovulatory dysfunction, 1 tablet daily for 2 weeks in every 4 weeks	Pregnancy, liver disease or tumor, breast cancer, history of IHD	Irregular bleeding	High
LNG-IUS	Used in HMB not in acute bleeding. Can be kept intrauterine for 5 years, releases progesterone 20 μg daily	Pregnancy, unexplained vaginal bleeding, liver disease, cancer cervix or uterus/uteri (untreated), breast cancer large or distorted uterine cavity, uterine abnormality, history of PID, STI within 3 months	Nausea, mood disturbance, acne spotting, irregular bleeding and spotting, mastalgia, pelvic cramping	High

Contd...

Contd...

Agents	Dose	Contraindications	Adverse effects	Efficacy
DMPA (depot medroxy-progesterone acetate)	HMB: Injection 150 mg IM every 3 months	Pregnancy, smoking history of multiple risk factors for cardiovascular disease (i.e., elderly, smoking, diabetes, and hypertension), breast cancer, liver disorder, IHD, disease, stroke	Irregular bleeding, amenorrhea, bone loss, weight gain, bloating, fluid retention, mastalgia	Low
GnRH (leuprolide acetate)	HMB: 3.75 mg IM monthly or 11.25 mg IM every 3 month	Pregnancy	Menopausal syndrome-like symptoms, e.g., hot flashes, sweating, and vaginal dryness, bone loss when used for more than 6 months	High
Danazol	HMB: 100–400 mg orally daily (in divided doses)	Pregnancy, unexplained uterine bleeding, impaired cardiac, liver, renal function	Weight gain, androgenic effect, acne, blackening of skin	Low

Abbreviations: CEE, conjugated equine estrogen; TE, thromboembolism; CVA, cerebrovascular accident; IHD, ischemic heart disease; COC, combined oral contraceptive; HMB, heavy menstrual bleeding; SLE, systemic lupus erythematosus; MPA, medroxyprogesterone acetate; LNG-IUS, levonorgestrel-releasing intrauterine system; PID, pelvic inflammatory disease; STI, sexually transmitted infection; GnRH, gonadotropin-releasing hormone

Nonhormonal Agents used in AUB with Doses, Contraindications, Adverse Effects, and Efficacy

These nonhormonal agents are listed in **Table 5**.

Table 5: Nonhormonal agents used in AUB.

Agents	Dose	Contraindications	Adverse effects	Efficacy
Tranexamic acid	*Acute:* 1.3 g orally every 8 hourly for 5 days. It is given in ovulatory women AUB	History of thromboembolic disease, impaired color vision (cannot be used with COC)	Nausea, vomiting, diarrhea, headache, myalgia	High
NSAIDs	Meclofenamate sodium: 100 mg 3 times daily Ibuprofen: 600–800 mg every 6–8 hourly	Pregnancy, GI hemorrhage, bowel disease, renal disease, bronchial asthma, cardiovascular disease	Bleeding, ulceration, and perforation of GI tract, alters platelet function and increases asthma	Moderate

Abbreviations: AUB, abnormal uterine bleeding; COC, combined oral contraceptive; NSAIDs, nonsteroidal anti-inflammatory drugs; HMB, heavy menstrual bleeding; GI, gastrointestinal

Q. What are the different medical management options in different clinical situations of AUB?

Different medical management options in different AUB are discussed in **Table 6**.

Table 6: Different medical management options in different clinical situations of AUB.

Clinical situation	Options of medical management
Acute AUB (no structural cause of uterus and no systemic disorder)	(1) Intravenous conjugated equine estrogen; (2) Oral tranexamic acid; (3) Multidose combined monophasic OC; (4) Multidose oral progesterone; (5) GnRH agonist with aromatase inhibitor or antagonist (to prevent initial estrogen flare). Intrauterine Foley catheter for tamponade can be used during acute period

Contd...

Contd...

Clinical situation	Options of medical management
HMB (no structural cause of uterus and no systemic disorder)	Ovulatory AUB: (1) LNG-IUS; (2) Tranexamic acid; (3) Combined OC (cyclic, extended, or continuous); (4) Cyclic or continuous oral progesterone (e.g., norethisterone), starting on day 5 for 21 days; (5) Injectable progesterone (DMPA); (6) NSAIDs; (7) GnRH agonist; (8) Danazol AUB with ovulatory dysfunction: (1) Combined OC; (2) MPA (for 2 weeks in every 4 weeks) An NSAID is considered in combination with any of the above agent
Leiomyomas with AUB	(1) LNG-IUS (approved by the FDA in women with an undistorted uterine cavity size); (2) Combined OCs; (3) NSAIDs; (4) Danazol; (5) Tranexamic acid Other medications are mifepristone, asoprisnil, ulipristal acetate, and epigallocatechin gallate Others: When medical therapy fails, surgical intervention, uterine artery embolization, MRI-focused ultrasound may be suggested
Inherited bleeding disorder	(1) Tranexamic acid; (2) Combined OC; (3) LNG-IUS; (4) DMPA; (5) Danazol; (6) GnRH agonist; (7) Desmopressin (in von Willebrand disease)
AUB due to anticoagulation therapy	(1) LNG-IUS; (2) Oral progesterone; (3) Depo-Lupron

Abbreviations: AUB, abnormal uterine bleeding; OC, oral contraceptive; GnRH, gonadotropin-releasing hormone; HMB, heavy menstrual bleeding; LNG-IUS, levonorgestrel-releasing intrauterine system; DMPA, depot medroxyprogesterone acetate; MPA, medroxyprogesterone acetate; NSAIDs, nonsteroidal anti-inflammatory drugs

UTERINE PROCEDURES

Q. What are the uterine procedures for management of AUB when medical management fails or withdrawn for adverse effects?

The procedures are:

* *Dilatation and curettage*: Done to remove thickened endometrium and arrest severe HMB not responding to high dose estrogen. Preoperative TVS is mandatory to exclude thin endometrium.
* *Endometrial resection or ablation*: To remove and destroy the endometrial lining permanently by using thermal, electrical, radiofrequency, and laser energy.
* *Uterine artery embolization (UAE)*: Mostly done when associated with leiomyoma, less done in emergency acute excessive HMB not responding to conservative method.
* *Uterine tamponade*: A Foley catheter is introduced with inflation of 30 mL fluid and kept for 24 hours to arrest acute episode of bleeding.
* *Myomectomy*: Indication is large fibroid with pressure symptoms in woman willing to conceive.
* *Hysterectomy*: Not advised as first-line therapy and discouraged due to availability of alternate methods. It is reserved in failure of medical and other procedures in women of more than 40 years of age. It is done in half of the cases within 5 years of seeking treatment for AUB. Overall patient satisfaction and complete cure are the advantages. Intraoperative and postoperative complications compared to other methods and hospitalization, cost, and recovery times are the disadvantages.

Ablative Surgery in AUB

Principle: To destroy the endometrium to a depth so that endometrium cannot regenerate.

Indication:

* Resistant to medical treatment and the patient does not want child as following ablation there is chance of preterm delivery and morbid adhesion of placenta.
* Uterus is not more than 10 weeks size and fibroids if present should be less than 3 cm.

Methods of Ablative Procedures

First generation: Transcervical resection of the endometrium (TCRE)—hysteroscopic ablation by resectoscope, roller ball coagulation, loop, and laser.

Second generation: (A) Thermal balloon therapy; (B) Radiofrequency-induced thermal ablation (RITEA); (C) Microwave ablation; (D) Impedance controlled endometrial ablation (Novasure). Second generation is preferred nowadays as they are safe, simple, effective even more than TCRE, takes less time and can be performed as OPD procedure.

Transcervical Resection of the Endometrium (TCRE)

Hysteroscopic resection can destroy the endometrium 4–5 mm and is done by general anesthesia and can also be done in paracervical block and best done immediately after menstruation (pretreatment endometrium thinning). Now instead of monopolar electrode bipolar electrode Versapoint is used.

Thermal Balloon Therapy

This procedure is now done as a first-line therapy. A thermal balloon containing hot normal saline (85–90°C) is used to destroy endometrium for 8–10 minutes duration. No dilatation is needed, no general anesthesia is needed and can be done as outpatient procedure and the result is comparable to other methods.

Radiofrequency-induced Thermal Ablation

A metallic probe of .6 mm is inserted through the external os under general anesthesia and endometrium is destroyed by radiofrequency electromagnetic thermal energy by rotating 360° for 15–20 minutes. No hysteroscope is needed, less risky, and needs less expertization.

Microwave Ablation

Endometrium is ablated with the applicator using the magnetic energy at a temperature of 80° for 2–3 minutes under local anesthesia. Hysteroscopy is not needed and the result is like TCRE. *Novasure* is impedance controlled endometrial ablation.

It is used recently and takes only 90 seconds to perform using bipolar radiofrequency to vaporize endometrium.

Result of Ablative Therapy

40% become amenorrheic, 40% significant improvement, and 20% not responding.

Complications: Uterine perforation and infection.

Management of AUB-C, AUB-O, and AUB-E

- Once malignancy and significant pelvic pathology excluded in AUB-C, AUB-O, or AUB-E, first-line therapy is medical treatment in order to decrease blood loss.
- Medical therapy includes hormonal therapy and nonhormone therapies.
- Endometrial ablation and hysterectomy are the two surgical options for AUB.
- Hormone therapies are COC, progestin given during luteal phase or in an extended regimen, LNG-IUS, and GnRH agonist and nonhormone therapies are NSAIDs and TXA.

Management of AUB-C

- AUB-C is best managed in a multidisciplinary approach including gynecologist and hematologist.
- Medical agents used are same used in women with normal coagulation except NSAIDs. This may include oral contraceptive pill (OCP) and LNG-IUS.
- If the first-line treatment fails specific treatment with desmopressin or factor replacement can be given.
- Surgical treatments (endometrium ablation/hysterectomy) may be needed and should be planned along with a hematologist, normalizing coagulation factors pre-, intra-, and postoperatively.

Management of AUB-O

- Ideally, AUB-O is reversed by correcting ovulation (weight loss and insulin sensitizers for PCOS, treating thyroid or prolactin disorders).
- Hormonal treatment is the first choice. *Nonhormonal drugs are not recommended.*
- *For chronic management* women who require contraception COCs, progestin-only pills, LNG-IUS, DMPA, and etonogestrel subdermal implant are options. Individual not requiring contraception cyclical progesterone [oral 10 days in cycle MPA—5 to 10 mg, norethindrone acetate (NETA) 5–10 mg or micronized progesterone 200–400 mg daily] is prescribed.
- GnRH is also used but less frequently which has advantages to permit severely anemic women to rebuild red cell mass.
- In 13–18-year-old girl, cyclical COCs is recommended.

Severe Acute HMB Requiring Acute Intervention in AUB-O

- Fluid resuscitation with simultaneous medical treatment to slow the bleeding.
- Conjugated equine estrogen (CEE) is given intravenous in 25 mg doses every 4 hours for up to three doses, may need even up to 24 hours.
- Once bleeding has slowed high-dose oral estrogen therapy 2.5 mg conjugated estrogen or more commonly COCs (containing 30 μg EE) are given every 6 hours is given till bleeding is stopped or markedly diminished, then one tablet 8 hourly for next 2–7 days then, one tablet 12 hourly for 2–7 days, then continued once daily for several weeks.
- Alternative to high dose estrogen high dose MPA, norethisterone or injection DMPA can be used.
- Intrauterine Foley balloon can be used with the medication in brisk hemorrhage to act as tamponade.
- Surgery is rarely indicated in AUB-O, indications are if medical therapy fails or contraindicated, intolerated or concomitant significant uterine structural lesion is present.
- Endometrial ablation is not recommended in AUB-O as first-line therapy as chronic anovulation is associated with increased risk of endometrial cancer compared with women who are treated with medical therapy.

Medical Management of AUB-O Based on Age Groups

Table 7 depicts the medical management of AUB-O based on age groups.

Management of AUB-E (Primary Endometrial Dysfunction)

- This ovulatory AUB is due to primary endometrial dysfunction and predominantly from endometrial vasodilatation. There is no clear diagnostic feature and AUB-E is a diagnosis of exclusion.
- Acute medical treatment is like that of acute heavy bleeding in AUB-O.
- Chronic treatment options are LNG-IUS, COCs, sustained progestins, TXA, NSAIDs, androgens (Gestrinone and Danazol), and GnRH agonists. Both hormonal and non-hormonal are effective. Best is LNG-IUS.
- Abnormal uterine bleeding-E can be managed both by hormonal and nonhormonal treatments. LNG-IUS seems to be the most effective choice in regard to reduction

Table 7: Medical management of AUB-O based on age groups.

Age group	Cause	Therapy
13–18 years	Poorly developed HPO axis, bleeding disorder, and obesity	Acute: Parenteral equine estrogen HMB: Low-dose COC and weight reduction
19–39 years	Obesity, PCOS, premalignant or malignant endometrial condition	Acute: Parenteral equine estrogen/oral progesterone HMB: Low-dose COC, progesterone including LNG-IUS, and weight reduction
40 years to menopause	Infrequent ovulation, premalignant or malignant endometrial condition	Acute: Multidose progesterone HMB: Cyclic progesterone, LNG-IUS, COC, and weight reduction

Abbreviations: AUB, abnormal uterine bleeding; HPO, hypothalamic–pituitary–ovarian; COC, combined oral contraceptive; PCOS, polycystic ovary syndrome; LNG-IUS, levonorgestrel-releasing intrauterine system

of menstrual bleeding, LNG-IUS (71–95% reduction), COCs (35–69% reduction), extended cycle oral progestins (87% reduction), TXA (26–54% reduction), and NSAIDs (10–52% reduction) were all effective therapy. The LNG-IUS, COCs, and antifibrinolytics are all superior to luteal-phase progestins. LNG-IUS is the best treatment, and it has been shown that it is superior to combined OCPs and NSAIDs. TXA (antifibrinolytics) is superior to NSAIDs.

* Surgery (hysterectomy and endometrial ablation) is performed when medical management fails, noncompliance of medical therapy, significant anemia not improving by medical management and also for quality of life, and concomitant uterine structural cause.

Management of AUB-L

* A patient with leiomyoma with AUB, it is not always clear whether fibroid is the cause of AUB except in some obvious cases like submucous fibroid. "Fibroids are passenger or problem"?
* The different modalities of treatment are: (1) Medical management; (2) Uterine artery embolization; (3) Focused ultrasound surgery, (4) Radiofrequency ablation, and (5) surgical—myomectomy or hysterectomy.

Medical management of AUB associated with fibroids includes:
* GnRH agonists: Approved by the FDA to reduce the size and volume (30–50%) of leiomyomas before surgical intervention and to reduce perioperative bleeding.
* LNG-IUS (FDA approved for the treatment of HMB in women with an undistorted uterine cavity.
* Combined OCs
* NSAIDs
* Danazol
* Tranexamic acid: Reduces menstrual blood loss significantly and causes fibroid necrosis and infarction.
* Other medications, such as mifepristone, asoprisnil, ulipristal acetate, and epigallocatechin gallate. Ulipristal is a selective progesterone receptor modulator that causes apoptosis and prevents cell growth and vascularization.

Medical management is mostly successful in absence of submucous myoma:

* Other procedures are done when medical methods fail.
* If patients want fertility, choice is myomectomy.
* If no desire of child but want to preserve uterus, the options are myomectomy, uterine artery embolization, MRI-guided focused ultrasound surgery or radiofrequency ablation.
* Hysterectomy is the last option.

HEAVY MENSTRUAL BLEEDING IN ADOLESCENTS (PUBERTY MENORRHAGIA)

Q. How to define heavy menstrual bleeding (HMB)?

Heavy menstrual bleeding (HMB) or menorrhagia is defined as when bleeding occurs cyclically in regular intervals but excessive in amount and/or duration which affects the physical, mental, social or material quality of life (*see before*).

Q. Prevalence of bleeding disorders in adolescent.

In general population the frequency of bleeding disorders is about 1–2%, but that incidence is 20% among adolescent girls who come with HMB and bleeding disorder is found in 33% of adolescent girls hospitalized for HMB.

Q. What are the causes of HMB in adolescents?

Adolescent heavy menstrual bleeding is also classified according to the PALM-COEIN system like in adult, i.e., polyp, adenomyosis, leiomyoma, malignancy and hyperplasia, coagulopathy, ovulatory dysfunction, endometrial, iatrogenic, and not classified.

Anovulation and immaturity of the hypothalamic–pituitary–ovary axis, cycles is the most common cause of HMB at menarche and in adolescent. Bleeding disorder is the second common cause. Structural causes of HMB are less common in adolescent age group.

Common bleeding disorders in adolescent

The most common bleeding disorders in adolescent with HMB are von Willebrand disease, platelet function defects, thrombocytopenia (congenital or acquired) and clotting factor deficiencies. Others are immune thrombocytopenic purpura or thrombotic thrombocytopenic purpura.

CHAPTER 5: A Case of Abnormal Uterine Bleeding (Endometrial Hyperplasia)

Q. How would you evaluate and diagnose HMB in adolescents?

Symptoms and signs
Regular heavy menses are commonly associated with bleeding disorders, but adolescents may have prolonged period or irregular bleedings due to superimposed anovulation. Girl suffers from fatigueness and headache doue to anaemia. Bleeding disorders sometimes may cause corpus luteum rupture with hemoperitoneum.

Medical history
History of pad count, assessment of bleeding. Pictorial blood assessment chart is useful to assess blood loss and to record treatment response.

The screening for bleeding disorder is considered positive if any one of following four criteria is met (Philipp CS et al AJOG 2011).

(i) Menstruation persists for 7 days or more or there is bleeding through the tampon or napkin within 2 hours in most cycle or 'flooding', (ii) F/H of bleeding disorder, (iii) H/O treatment of anaemia and (iv) Any H/O excessive bleeding during delivery, miscarriage and any surgery, tooth extraction.

Physical examinations
Vitals (pulse, BP, pallor, blood loss), presence of bruises and petechial hemorrhage over skin sexual maturity (Tanner staging)- breasts and pubic hair.

P/A, hepatosplenomegaly, any mass or distention.

Bleeding per vagina. Any trauma to be excluded. In adolescent P/S examination is avoided.

Laboratory investigations and imaging
Urinary HCG, Hb%, blood grouping and typing, complete blood count, serum ferritin, presence of any endocrine disorder responsible for anovulation, e.g., TSH, in suspeted PCOS testosterone level, DHES, prolactin, laboratory tests for bleeding disorder, e.g., PT, PTT, INR, Fibrinogen, von Willebrand antigen, von Willebrand activity, factor VIII level.

Gonorrhoea, chlamydia screening in sexually active individual. Routine sonography is not recommended until initial management fails as structural cause is rare in this group. Transabdominal is preferred to TVS in this age group.

Management of acute bleeding
First line: Medical management and surgery only when unresponsive

Hospitalization: If hemodynamically unstable or heavily active bleeding Hematologists consulted. IV infusion with crystalloid started. Blood transfusion is considered in hamodynamically unstable adolescenst. USG is considered.

In acute bleeding conjugated estrogen 25 mg IV 4–6 hourly for 24 hours is given. After bleeding becomes less or stops then tapering with COC or, monophasic combined oral contraceptive pills (OCPs) (in 30 of estrogen oral medroxy progesterone high dose 10–20 mg every 6–12 hours or norethindrone acetate 5–10 mg every 6 hour still bleeding stops then tapering. DMPA is not first line therapy.

Antifibrinolytics like tranexamic acid or aminocaproic acid (oral and IV) can be used to stop bleeding. 1.3 g orally or 10 mg/kg iv (maximum maximum 600 mg/dose) three times daily for 5 days.

After management of acute bleeding COC, progestins injection, or levonorgestrel-releasing intrauterine system (LNG-IUS) can be used as maintainance therapy.

Simultaneously iron therapy is given. During discharge oral iron is given but intravenous therapy is considered in noncompliance.

Nonmedical procedures
If bleeding is not controlled nonmedical procedures like examination under anesthesia may be needed. USG can guide the procedural management. Invasive procedures like endometrial ablation, uterine artery embolization, and hysterectomy should not be done.

In thickened endometrium suction evacuation or suction curettage (machine or mannual) may be considered. Sharp curettage is avoided. The purpose of curettage is to remove fragile bleeding endometrium, fecilitate regeneration of the endometrium. Concomitant hysteroscopy may be helpful in suspected intrauterine pathology. a levonorgestrel-releasing intrauterine device (LNG-IUD) can also be placed for long-term management.

Intrauterine balloon tamponade is one effective, low cost and readily available option.

Counseling
All adolescent patients with a bleeding disorder is counseled about safe medication use and future problems during surgery. Drugs like aspirin or nonsteroidal anti-inflammatory drugs which prevent platelet aggregation should be used with cautions, and before any surgery of adolescent with bleeding disorder all precautions should be taken for haemostasis and by keeping sufficient blood products in hand.

METROPATHIA HEMORRHAGICA

This is an old terminology, previously known as **Schroeder's disease** after a German Gynecologist, Schroeder.

It is an abnormal excessive uterine bleeding due to persistence of follicular phase as a result of anovulation. There is amenorrhea for short duration followed by excessive uterine bleeding due to proliferation and thickening of endometrium.

This happens as a result of continuous production of estradiol and the endometrium becomes cystic glandular hyperplastic type typically called **"swiss cheese"** which comes under simple endometrial hyperplasia. The endometrium becomes so much of thickened that a cast-like structure may be shed off very rarely **(Fig. 16)**.

Ovaries may be cystic with absence of corpus luteum and uterus may be enlarged due to myohyperplasia **(Fig. 17)**.

This type of bleeding pattern is more common in adolescent and perimenopausal age group when anovulation is common.

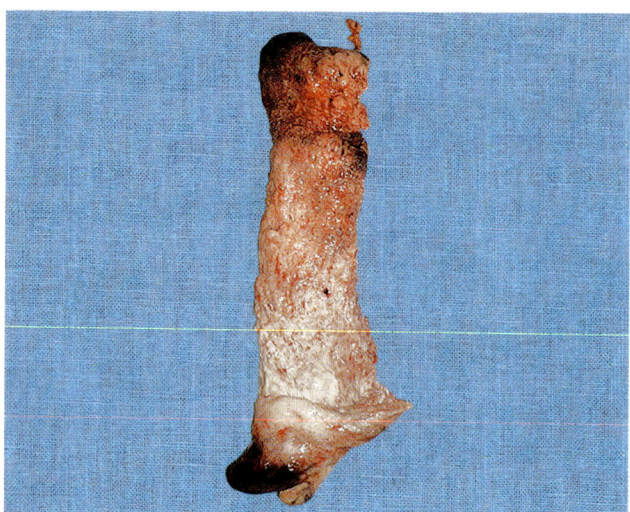

Fig. 16: Thickened endometrium is expelled spontaneously as cast in a woman suffering from dysfunctional uterine bleeding.
Courtesy: Dr Pradipto Sanyal, Senior Gynecologist

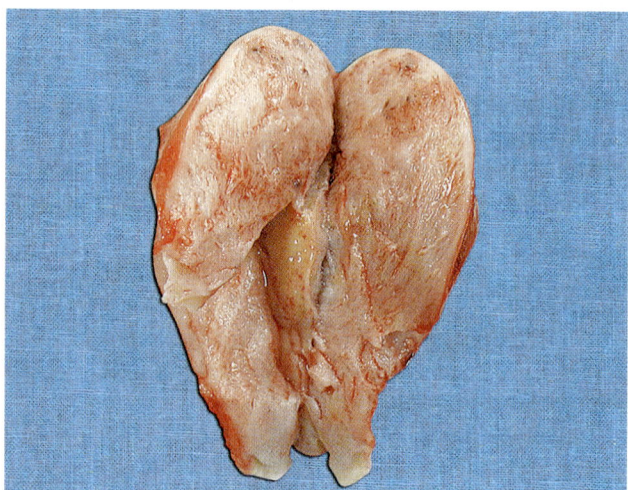

Fig. 17: Myohyperplasia with endometrial hyperplasia (associated with adenomyosis).

Diagnosis is done by history of painless bleeding pattern and sonography. In perimenopausal age, endometrial biopsy is needed.

Treatment is to address anemia and **progesterone therapy**. **Ablative surgery** may be needed and rarely hysterectomy in elderly group is performed.

ISTHMOCELE

Isthmocele is acquired sacculation (diverticulum) in the endometrial cavity due to the defect following caesarean delivery. This is also called caesarean scar defect.

Patient may complain of bleeding following menstruation or intermenstrual bleeding. Blood is reposited in these niches and after the menstruation is over blood comes out in postmenstrual days. Scar ectopic pregnancy may also occur on that site and in later months of pregnancy morbid adhesion of placenta (PAS) complicates the pregnancy.

These defects are diagnosed by TVS, saline infusion sonography (SIS) or by hysteroscopy. MRI is also useful to diagnose.

Management options are medical and surgical. Combined OC, progestogens and LNG-IUS are tried but not so useful. Surgical options are hysteroscopic resection, ablation after shaving the scar edges, excision of thin myometrium and approximation by stitches by laparoscopic approach and hysterectomy if other method fail. Perforation is one possibility with hysteroscopic ablation when the myometrium is thin.

The other cause of uterine diverticula is congenital, due to mullerian defect which is very rare.

ARTERIOVENOUS MALFORMATION (AVM)

This rare entity is one cause of AUB. There are structural abnormalities of fistulous communication of arterial, venous and small capillary channels. It occurs more commonly in uterine body than cervix.

Etiology is congenital or acquired. It may be consequence of surgery of endometrial cavity or myometrium. It may be found in patients of cancer cervix, cancer endometrium, GTD and IUCD users.

Symptoms are heavy menstrual bleeding or intermenstrual bleeding, either mild variety or sometimes patients may present with life threatening sudden torrential bleeding. Spontaneous or induced abortion, D&C and endometrial surgery may ignite the bleeding.

It is diagnosed by TVS which shows anechoic tubular structures in myometrium. It is not uncommon that it is diagnosed as an incidental finding in TVS without any symptom. SIS, color Doppler, power Doppler and angiogyaphy, CT scan and MRI are other diagnostic modalities. Angiography not only confirms, in the same sitting embolization of AVM can be done. Definitive treatment of arteriovenous malformation is hysterectomy.

MYOMETRIAL HYPERTROPHY (FIGS. 18 AND 19)

Myometrial hypertrophy is the generalized enlargement of uterus without any obvious pathology. Nulliparous uterine weight >130 g and multiparous uterine weight >210 g are regarded as hypertrophy. It commonly occurs in multigravia and due to pregnancy. Common complaint is heavy menstrual bleeding.

ENDOMETRIAL HYPERPLASIA

Q. What do you mean by endometrial hyperplasia? What is its importance?

Endometrial hyperplasia is defined as thickening of endometrium due to proliferation of irregularly sized and shaped glands with increases glands to stromal ratio. It is the only known direct precursor of endometrial carcinoma.

CHAPTER 5: A Case of Abnormal Uterine Bleeding (Endometrial Hyperplasia)

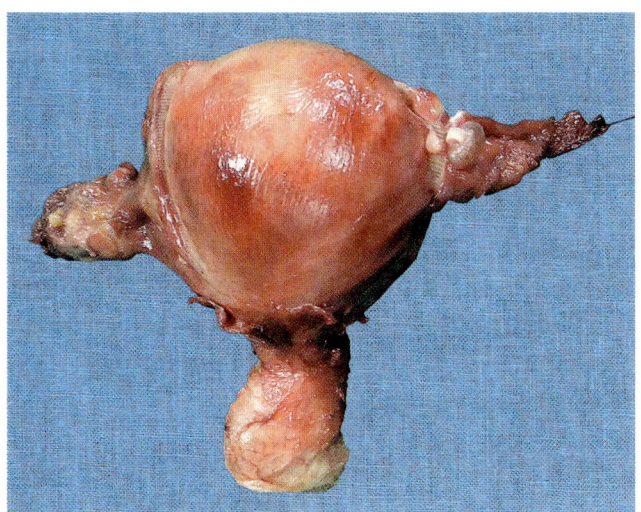

Fig. 18: Enlarged uterus due to myohypertrophy. 45 years multigravida P3+0 with persistent menorrhagia for last 2 years with diabetes. TAH with BSO done.

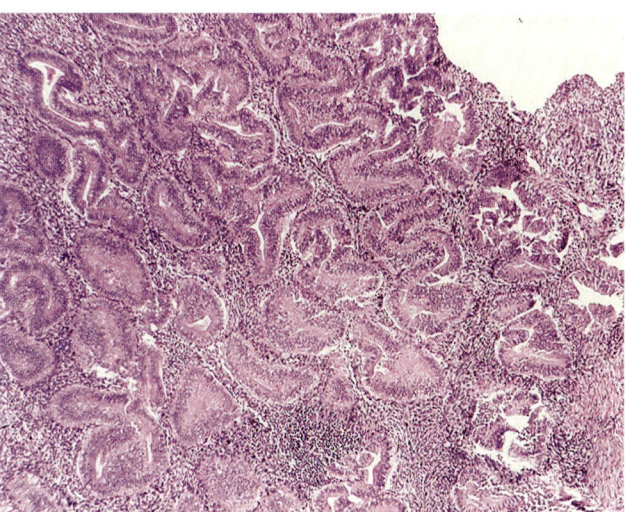

Fig. 20: Endometrial hyperplasia: Photomicrograph showing crowding of glands, increased gland to stroma ratio with prominent variability in size of glands, glandular budding with no cytologic atypia— (Photomicrograph: H&E, 400X).
Courtesy: Dr Tripti Das, Pathology

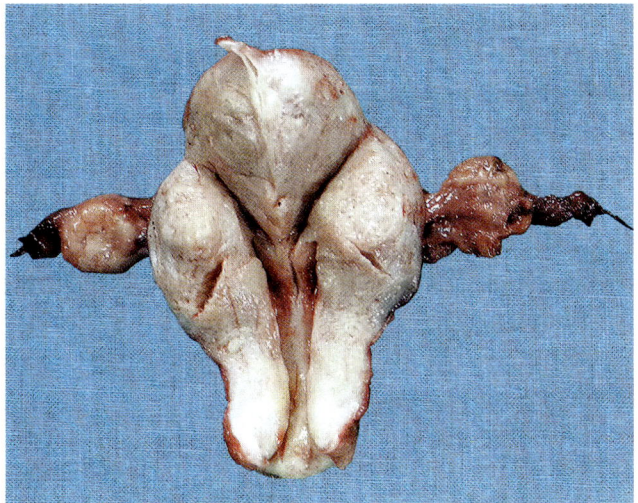

Fig.19: Cut section of the uterus to show myohypertrophy in the same specimen as in Figure 18.

Endometrial hyperplasia with atypia progresses to endometrial carcinoma in 30% cases. Without atypia the chance is very low—1 to 3%.

CLASSIFICATION

Q. What are the different varieties of endometrial hyperplasia? Describe each of them.

Based on architectural and cytological features and the presence or absence of nuclear atypia endometrial hyperplasia is of four varieties. Architectural abnormalities are gland crowding and complexity.

- *Simple hyperplasia:* Endometrium is thickened with normal tubular shape or mild abnormalities of gland shape and modestly crowded glands, increased gland to stroma ratio with prominent variability in size of glands, glandular budding with no cytologic atypia (**Fig. 20**). Simple hyperplasia progresses to cancer 1%.
- *Complex hyperplasia:* Glands are severely crowded and architectural abnormalities like papillary infoldings, but the gland profiles are fairly regular. Complex hyperplasia progresses to cancer 3%.
- *Simple hyperplasia with atypia:* Glands show occasional nuclear atypia characterized by nuclear rounding and visible nucleoli and glands are mildly crowded. *Simple hyperplasia with atypia* progresses to cancer 8%.
- *Complex hyperplasia with atypia:* Glands are severely crowded with presence of papillary folding in some glands and the nuclei show variable atypia. *Complex hyperplasia with atypia* progresses to cancer near 30%.

The revised WHO 2014 classification is categorized into two groups based upon the presence of cytological atypia, i.e., (1) hyperplasia without atypia and (2) atypical hyperplasia, the complexity of architecture is no longer part of the classification.

Q. What do you mean by endometrial intraepithelial neoplasia (EIN)?

The term endometrial intraepithelial neoplasia (EIN) is introduced in another system to emphasize premalignant nature like cervical intraepithelial neoplasia, vulvar intraepithelial neoplasia, and vaginal intraepithelial neoplasia.

The EIN diagnostic scheme comprises three categories— benign (endometrial hyperplasia), premalignant (a diagnosis of EIN based upon five subjective histological criteria), and malignant (endometrial cancer).

In this system, endometrial hyperplasia means anovulatory or prolonged estrogen exposed endometrium without atypia and EIN is considered as premalignant lesion with distinct morphological features. The diagnosis of EIN in the new WHO classification is considered interchangeable with atypical hyperplasia.

Q. How will you diagnose endometrial hyperplasia?

Endometrial hyperplasia is a **histological diagnosis (Fig. 20)**. Patients usually present with postmenopausal bleeding or premenopausal patient with AUB. She may have history of unopposed estrogen exposure.

Endometrial sampling is done by pipelle endometrial biopsy or outpatient D&C. **Transvaginal sonography** is a feasible method to detect endometrial hyperplasia by measuring ET in women with AUB. In postmenopausal women with vaginal bleeding ET less than or equal to 4 mm is usually associated with atrophic endometrium, more than 4 mm warrants biopsy.

Cystic endometrial changes are suggestive of polyps; *homogeneous thickened endometrium* indicates hyperplasia and malignancy is suspected in *heterogenous structural pattern*.

In premenopausal women cut off value is yet to determine; however above 10 mm ET, further evaluation is needed. There is no consensus on ET threshold in this age group and other risk factors for hyperplasia are evaluated.

Other diagnostic tool hysteroscope is more sensitive to focal lesions and poor sensitive for diagnosis of endometrial hyperplasia.

Rarely estrogen producing ovarian tumor can be a cause which can be clinically diagnosed.

Q. How will you manage endometrial hyperplasia?

Traditional treatment is surgery. Other option is oral, injectable progesterone or the LNG-IUS. The management protocol is as described next:

- In premenopausal women in absence of atypia **progesterone** is the treatment and regression occurs. Cyclic MPA orally for 12–14 days with daily oral dose of 10–20 mg daily for 3–6 months is the standard treatment. Continuous daily dose of 10 mg can be given and may be more effective. Cyclical COC is another option. LNG-IUS is effective and first line of medial management (RCOG, 2016). Cyclical progesterone is not used. On follow up after 6 months surveillance regression treatment may need to continue till menopause to protect endometrium.
- In postmenopausal women without atypia, **progesterone** is the treatment but should be used with very caution so that atypia is not missed in sampling. In follow-up endometrial biopsy is recommended in every 3–6 months.
- In both the groups regression with progesterone is 70–80%. In persistent hyperplasia higher dose of progesterone (MPA 40–100 mg daily or megestrol 160 mg daily) may be needed. In patients not responding to medical management hysterectomy is done.
- In atypical hyperplasia **hysterectomy** is the treatment of choice as it progresses to cancer in 30% cases and even there may be co-existent cancer. Total abdominal hysterectomy with bilateral salpingo-oophorectomy is done in postmenopausal group and in premenopausal age hysterectomy is performed. Salpingectomy is considered to reduce cancer risk.
- In premenopausal women with atypia in deserving fertility conservative management with high dose progesterone can be considered but with intense follow up is needed by serial biopsy and switched over to hysterectomy in persistent cases. Review with biopsy in 3 monthly interval until 2 consecutive negative biopsy obtained, then 6–12 monthly biopsy is done until hysterectomy is performed.

CHAPTER 6

A Case of Endometrial Carcinoma (Including Postmenopausal Bleeding) and Uterine Sarcoma

CHAPTER OUTLINE

Writing a case of endometrial cancer and postmenopausal bleeding and how to present the case?

- How to Diagnose Endometrial Carcinoma?
- Sonography, Biposy and Hysteroscopy—Role of Each Tool
- Role of MRI/CT
- Risk Factors of Endometrial Cancer
- Spread and Stages of Endometrial Carcinoma— How to Stage Endometrial Carcinoma

- Management Modalities—Role of Adjuvant Therapy
- Pyometra
- Postmenopausal Bleeding—Causes, Diagnosis and Management
- Sarcoma of Uterus

PATIENT'S PARTICULARS

1. Name: Bed No.:
2. Age: 53 years   Date of admission:
3. Address: Date of examination:
4. Occupation: Housewife
5. Married/unmarried: Married/no children
6. History of infertility: Present
7. Husband's occupation:
8. Socioeconomic status: Middle
9. Religion:
10. Parous/nulliparous: Nulliparous

HISTORY

- *Chief complaint/complaints*: Bleeding per vagina for last 10 days following menopause two years back.
- *History of present illness*: She states that she had menopause for two years. She suddenly felt that she had vaginal bleeding 10 days back and continued for 7 days which was painless and it has no relation with coitus. She had similar episodes of bleeding twice during last three months.
- *Menstrual history*: It was regular before menopause.
  - *Last menstrual period*: 2 years back
  - History of delayed menopause at 51 years.
- *Obstetric history*: History of infertility:
  - Parity—nulliparous
    - If parous, write in chronological order in tabular form.
- *Past history*:
  - Medical—diabetes and history of intake of oral antidiabetic medication present, history of hypertension taken, history of breast cancer or any other cancer and tamoxifen therapy. Any history of cancer previously and therapy.
  - Surgical—nothing significant.
- *Family history*: Nothing significant.
- *Sexual history*: Infrequent coitus.
- *Functional history*: All normal:
  - Bowel
  - Bladder
  - Sleep
  - Appetite

- ❖ *Personal history*:
  - Personal hygiene
  - Smoking/alcohol.
- ❖ *Contraceptive history*: History of hormone (estrogen) therapy if any.
- ❖ *Drug history*:
  - History of any drug allergy
  - History of intake of hormone replacement therapy, corticosteroids, antiepileptic or other drugs (previous or present)—she has no such.

PHYSICAL EXAMINATION

Patient—alert, conscious, and cooperative.

- ❖ Build
- ❖ Nutrition
- ❖ Height
- ❖ Weight/body mass index (BMI)—obese or not, write down exact BMI
- ❖ Edema
- ❖ Anemia—present
- ❖ Cyanosis
- ❖ Jaundice
- ❖ Clubbing
- ❖ Tongue, teeth, gum, and tonsil
- ❖ Neck veins
- ❖ Neck glands
- ❖ Leg veins
- ❖ Pulse
- ❖ Respiration
- ❖ Temperature
- ❖ BP = 120/84 mm Hg.

Systemic Examination

- ❖ *Central nervous system*
- ❖ *Cardiovascular system:*
  - Auscultation of heart
- ❖ *Respiratory system:*
  - Auscultation of chest
- ❖ *Gastrointestinal system:*
  - Liver
  - Spleen
- ❖ *Examination of other systems:*
  - Examination of back and spines skeletal system
  - Neurological examination
  - Ophthalmoscopic examination
  - Urinary system.
- ❖ *Examination of breasts and nipple*: Enquire whether any breast CA and tamoxifen therapy
  - Inspection
  - Palpation—for any breast lump.

GYNECOLOGICAL EXAMINATION

- ❖ *Abdominal examination*: Look for any lump abdomen.
  - Inspection
  - Palpation
  - Percussion
  - Auscultation
- ❖ *Vaginal examination*:
  - Inspection and palpation of external genitalia—any lesion over vulva or vagina.
  - Speculum examination—any cervical polyp, any growth over cervix or vagina. Usually cervix small and no growth. Blood may be visible at external os.
  - Bimanual examination—size of the uterus is enlarged, usually no adnexal lump.
  - Examination of rectovaginal area and rectal examination.

INVESTIGATIONS SUPPLIED OR REQUIRED

Investigations include Hb 10 g%, postprandial blood sugar 134 mg%, transvaginal sonography (TVS) reveals endometrial thickness 7 mm, uterus 10 cm × 7 cm × 4 cm and adnexae normal.

SUMMARY OF THE CASE (SAMPLE)

A 53-year-old nulliparous married woman coming from middle class family has been admitted on .... with history of bleeding per vagina which is of moderate amount for last 10 days duration for evaluation. She had similar episode of bleeding twice before in last 3 months. She had menopause 2 years back. She is diabetic controlled by antidiabetic drug, past history and family history nothing significant.

On examination, she is obese with BMI..., mild pallor, pulse rate 76 beats/minute, normotensive, systemic examination revealed no abnormality, breasts examination shows no abnormality. On per abdominal examination, abdomen is soft and no mass palpable and nontender.

On vaginal examination in vagina and vulva no lesion found, on per speculum examination cervix looks healthy and blood tickles through external os. Bimanual examination shows bulky uterus which is retroverted and mobile.

Transvaginal sonography report shows thickened (7 mm) endometrium.

PROVISIONAL DIAGNOSIS

A 53-year-old married nulliparous woman with postmenopausal bleeding (PMB) possibly due to endometrial cancer.

DIFFERENTIAL DIAGNOSIS

- ❖ Atrophic vaginitis—most common cause of PMB
- ❖ Endometrial cancer—10% case of PMB
- ❖ Cancer cervix
- ❖ Endometrial hyperplasia
- ❖ Endometrial polyp.

CHAPTER 6: A Case of Endometrial Carcinoma (Including Postmenopausal Bleeding) and Uterine Sarcoma

Q. How can you say this is a case of endometrial carcinoma?

It can only be confirmed by biopsy, but the points in favor of endometrial cancer are:
- Patient has presented with PMB
- Predisposing factors like obesity, diabetes, and nulliparity present
- Transvaginal sonography shows thickened endometrium.

Q. How will you confirm the diagnosis?

By biopsy—Pipelle office biopsy, dilatation and curettage (D&C) or hysteroscopic biopsy.

Q. What are common causes of PMB? Which is most common?

- Atrophic vaginitis—most common cause of PMB
- Endometrial cancer—10% case of PMB
- Cancer cervix
- Endometrial hyperplasia
- Endometrial polyp.

Q. How much of PMB is contributed by endometrial carcinoma?

About 10% is contributed by endometrial carcinoma.

Incidence of Endometrial Cancer

- 95/100,000 women (age-related)
- It contributes 25–30% of all gynecological malignancies in developed country. In developing countries including India, the incidence is 5–8% of all gynecological malignancies due to high incidence of cervical cancer, the incidence of which is low in developed country due to prevention by screening.

Age and Endometrial Cancer

- Average age of diagnosis is early 60s, peak is 55–70 years. After the age of 80 years incidence declines sharply.
- Chance increases after 45 years. Mostly (80%) postmenopausal, only 5–8% before 45 years, rest perimenopausal.

Q. Which is the most common gynecological malignancy?

In the world, endometrial cancer is the most common gynecological malignancy. In female, it ranks fourth next to breast, colon, and lung. In India, cancer cervix is the commonest (80%) gynecological malignancy.

Etiology, Risk Factors and Predisposing Factors

The exact cause is not known, however there is strong relation of unopposed estrogen to increase chance of endometrial cancer.

Etiology and Risk Factors

- Early menarche and late menopause above 52 years
- Nulliparous or low parity
- Obesity
- Polycystic ovary syndrome (PCOS)
- Unopposed estrogen therapy, hormone replacement therapy
- Tamoxifen therapy
- Feminizing ovarian tumor
- Hereditary—history of ovarian cancer and colorectal cancer [hereditary nonpolyposis colorectal cancer syndrome (HNPCC)]
- Age—older age (see above)
- Associated medical disorder, e.g., hypertension, diabetes, and gallbladder disease (obesity, hypertension, and diabetes are present in 30% cases of endometrial cancer)
- Western and higher societies—more.

Most of the above factors can be explained by estrogenic factors.

In *obesity*, there is more conversion of androgen to estrogen in adipose tissue and reduction of sex hormone-binding globulin in obesity increases free estrogen in circulation. Oligoovulation—anovulation also results unopposed estrogen exposure in obesity.

In *PCOS*, there is anovulation with high estrogen resulting endometrial hyperplasia and increase chance of endometrial cancer. In diabetes, there is interaction of insulin-like growth factor and insulin.

Tamoxifen which is used to prevent recurrent breast cancer increases chance of endometrial hyperplasia and cancer by 2.5 fold. It is a selective estrogen receptor modulator (SERM) and acts by blocking estrogen receptor in the breast. Raloxifene, a new generation SERM, has low or no effect on the endometrium.

In unopposed *hormone replacement therapy (HRT)*, there is increase in endometrial hyperplasia and cancer. The dose and duration of exposure of estrogen is related to the incidence of cancer and the risk may persist even after 10 years.

Genetic and hereditary factors are explored more recently. In Lynch syndrome, endometrial cancer is the most common extracolonic manifestation. *HNPCC*, autosomal dominant inheritance, is linked with colorectal, ovarian, endometrial, and urothelial tumors. Gene mutation promotes carcinogenesis. Lynch syndrome contributes to 2–5% of endometrial cancer and mostly premenopausal.

Q. Name the agents which protect endometrial cancer.

- Combined oral contraceptive or progesterone-only pill reduces the risk by 30–50%; and protective effect extends up to 10–20 years. Adding progesterone for 10–12 days in month to estrogen therapy decreases risk to 2%.
- Smoking—due to antiestrogenic effect of tobacco.

Q. How would you diagnose endometrial cancer?

- History
- Examination
- Investigations.

HISTORY

Age—mostly (80%) postmenopausal (see above)

Parity—low or nil

Chief complaints—postmenopausal bleeding or irregular vaginal bleeding. Pattern may be intermenstrual bleeding, heavy menstrual bleeding, blood-stained vaginal discharge, rarely dyspareunia, and pain in lower abdomen in advanced stage. Offensive discharge is a late symptom due to pyometra. About 10% of PMB is due to endometrial cancer. Initially, there may be excessive white discharge (hydrorrhea). Pain in the hypogastrium and iliac fossa called Simpson pain (15%) tends to appear at a particular time every day lasting for 1–2 hours.

Asymptomatic in 5–10% cases.

There may be history of risk factors—PCOS, HRT, hypertension, diabetic, history of breast cancer and tamoxifen therapy.

General Examination

- Pallor depending upon severity of bleeding
- Obesity, hypertension, and diabetics.

Corpus cancer syndrome—obesity, hypertension, and endometrial cancer.

Examination of Breasts

Search for any lump.

Per Abdomen Examination

Usually nothing evident, lump may be due to large fibroid or pyometra only in advanced cases. Enlargement of liver and ascites may be found in metastatic disease. There may be inguinal lymph nodes enlargement.

Per Vaginal Examination

Per speculum—cervix healthy, blood may come through os, in advance case cervix may be involved and growth may be seen on cervix which may be enlarged.

Vagina and vulva are also examined to detect any lesion. There may be metastatic nodule over anterior vaginal wall on suburethral region.

Bimanual examination—uterus usually enlarged and soft, may be of small size (postmenopausal) or normal size. Enlargement may be due to growth, fibroid or pyometra. In endometrial growth and pyometra, the enlargement is uniform and soft. In early cases, mobility is not restricted. Adnexal mass and nodules in pouch of Douglas (POD) are looked for.

Rectal Examination

In early case no abnormality, and in late case involvement of rectum or parametrium.

Investigations

- Endometrial biopsy
- Ultrasonography
- Hysteroscopy.

Endometrial Biopsy

Endometrial cancer can only be definitely diagnosed by histological examination of biopsy material.

Biopsy can be done by: (A) Office aspiration biopsy; (B) Traditional fractional curettage or (C) Hysteroscopy.

A. Office aspiration biopsy of endometrium is accepted as *first step* in case of abnormal uterine bleeding or suspected endometrial pathology. It is done usually by Pipelle curette, or by Vabra aspirator. As an OPD procedure and no dilatation is needed. Diagnostic accuracy is 90–98% when compared with findings of D&C or hysterectomy.

Fractional curette (D&C) and hysteroscopic biopsy are done when aspiration cytology cannot be performed due to cervical stenosis or patient's noncooperation or bleeding recurs even after negative report.

B. Traditional fractional curette (D&C) **(Figs. 1A and B)** starts with scraping of endocervical canal, dilatation of cervix followed by curettage from isthmus, and body of the uterus and fundus separately **(Figs. 1A and B)**. Missing of endometrial pathology occurs in 10% cases in this method.

Curettage of endometrial carcinoma has following characteristics:

- Profuse cheesy material
- Dark color
- Failure to grate during curettage.
  If pus comes during curettage, pus is allowed to drain by dilatation of cervix and curettage is kept abeyance and done in later date.

C. Hysteroscopy and biopsy enables to visualize the entire endometrium and to take biopsy from the selected area and chance of missing is less except in early lesion. Spillage into the peritoneal cavity is a concern of this technique.

Hysteroscopy is more sensitive for focal endometrial lesions and less helpful in diagnosing early endometrial carcinoma.

The histopathology report should mention the cancer type (I or II) and the grade of tumor. This will help to determine the treatment planning and extent of surgery.

Ultrasonography (Figs. 2 and 3)

Transvaginal sonography: It is done to assess the endometrial thickness (ET) and ovarian status. Other endometrial pathology like polyp, collection of fluid in endometrial cavity that may be due to pyometra and also extension to cervix can be detected.

If the thickness is more than 4 mm hysteroscopy biopsy is warranted in *postmenopausal women*. If the thickness is less than or equal to 4 mm cancer is less likely and

CHAPTER 6: A Case of Endometrial Carcinoma (Including Postmenopausal Bleeding) and Uterine Sarcoma

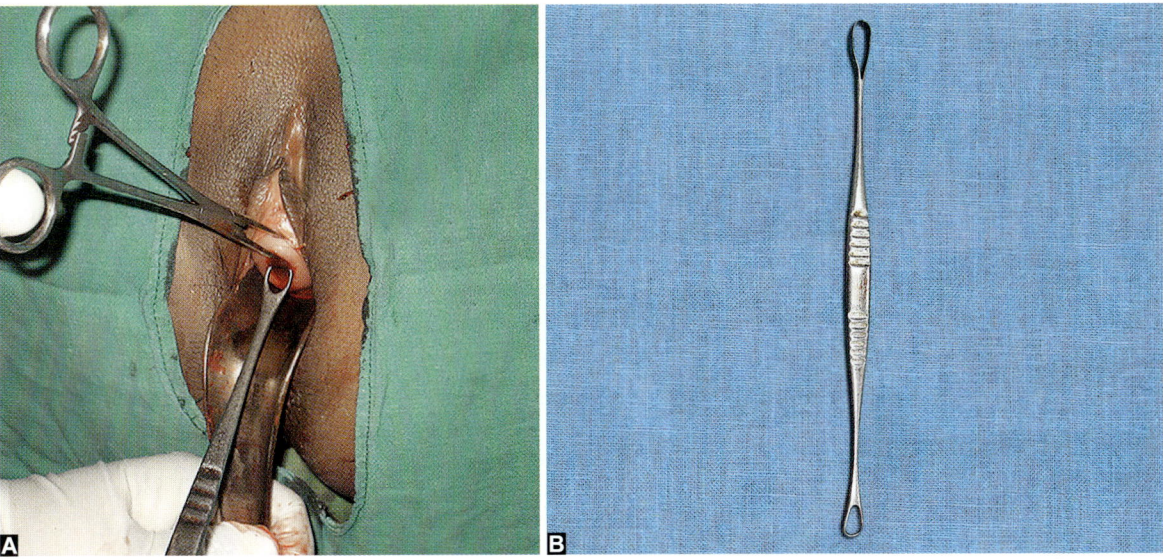

Figs. 1A and B: (A) Curettage of endometrium; (B) Uterine curette.

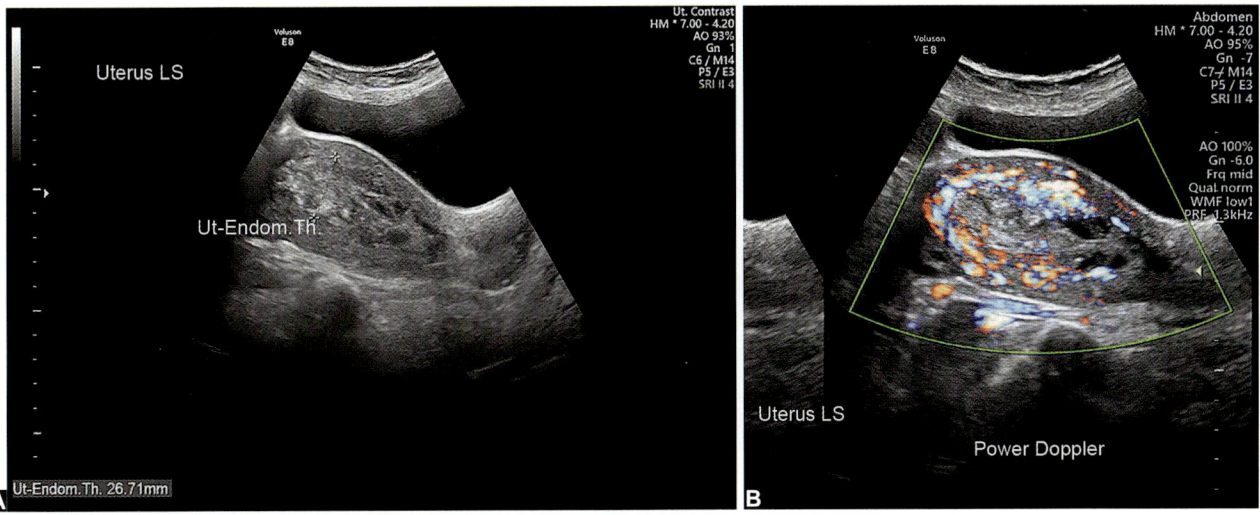

Figs. 2A and B: (A) Thickened heterogeneous (26.71 mm) endometrium; (B) Power Doppler of same patient as in Figure 2A.
Courtesy: Professor Kamal Oswal, VIMS, Kolkata

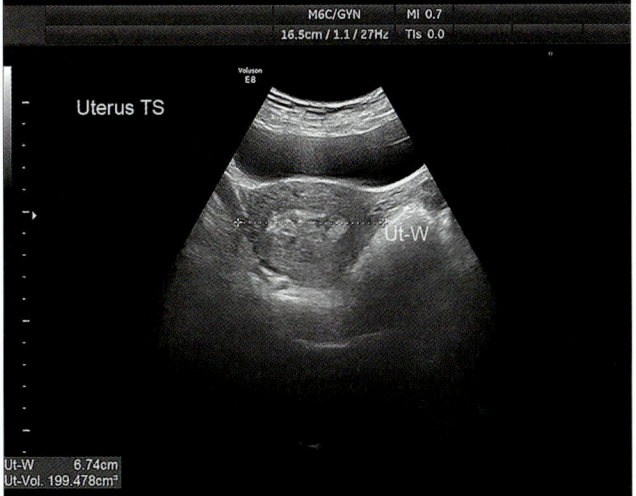

Fig. 3: Thick endometrium—transverse section view of uterus (same patient of Figures 2A and B).

immediate evaluation of endometrium is not needed. If the bleeding is recurrent biopsy is essential in spite of ET 4 mm or less.

In *premenopausal women*, cut off value is not determined, however in 10 mm and above further evaluation is needed. There is no consensus on ET threshold in this age group and other risk factors are considered.

The interpretation of characteristic findings of TVS is as follows:
- Cystic endometrial changes → suggestive of polyps
- Homogeneous thickened endometrium → indicates hyperplasia and
- Heterogeneous structural pattern → suspicious of malignancy **(Figs. 2A and 3)**.

Sonohysterography is an adjunct to TVS only to detect endometrial pathology like polyp. TVS cannot differentiate always thickened endometrium and endometrial polyp.

Color Doppler: In endometrial cancer, low resistance index of 0.37–0.7 or below is found **(Fig. 2A)**.

Role of Pap Stain

A Pap testing is not indicated for diagnosis of endometrial carcinoma as 50% cases of endometrial carcinoma has normal finding. However, atypical glandular cells found in Pap needs further evaluation to exclude cervical and endometrial malignancy.

Other Investigations for Preoperative Evaluation to Plan the Extent of Surgery

Imaging: CT/MRI/PET-CT/Chest X-ray

Imaging is useful to detect the spread of the disease, e.g., depth of myometrium, extension to cervix, lymph node involvement, and extrapelvic spread.

A CT or MRI are not routinely recommended and indicated for detection of extraendometrial involvement.

A CT is helpful in higher grade disease preoperatively to assess lymph node involvement or metastatic disease. It is superior to MRI to detect ascites, bowel, and omental metastasis.

An MRI is best to detect cervical extension and can distinguish between the endometrial cancer with cervical extension from primary endocervical adenocarcinoma. MRI is superior to CT in detection of myometrial involvement **(Fig. 4)** and nodal enlargement and no radiation hazard. A low density zone is detected in between endometrium and myometrium junction normally and its intactness indicates no myometrial involvement (Stage I).

Positron emission tomography (PET)-CT: It is gold standard for staging.

Chest X-ray: Chest radiography is done to detect lung metastasis in advanced disease.

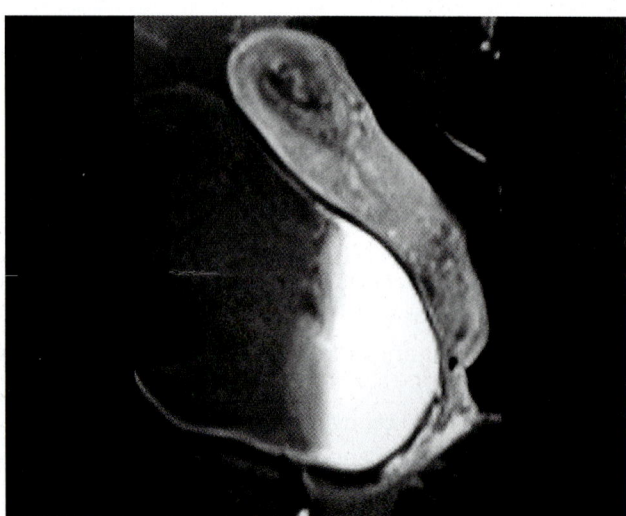

Fig. 4: MRI—endometrial cancer invading the adjacent inner myometrium at the fundoposterior region (Stage 1B).
Courtesy: Professor M Karmakar, IPGMER

Laboratory Testing

CA-125: Its role is limited. Elevated level (>35 IU/mL) indicates advanced disease. It is useful for monitoring in advanced disease and serous subtype.

Routine Preoperative (Preanesthetic) Investigations

These investigations include complete blood count, renal function, blood sugar, etc.

Q. Discuss the pathology.

Macroscopical Features

Endometrial cancer may look as localized lesion in the form of localized growth, polyp, nodule or diffuse lesion covering the whole endometrial cavity (*see* **Figs. 7 to 14**).

Microscopical Features

Q. What are the different histopathological types of endometrial cancer and how they differ?

There are two pathogenic types of endometrial cancer.

Type I (endometrioid adenocarcinoma) with good prognosis and *Type II* with poor prognosis.

Subtypes are given next.

Type I

Endometrioid adenocarcinoma—80%

Variants of endometrioid adenocarcinoma
- Squamous differentiation*
- Villoglandular
- Secretory
- Ciliated cell variant

*Previously endometrioid carcinomas with benign squamous areas were called adenoacanthoma and those with malignant squamous elements were called adenosquamous carcinomas. Now the two terms are replaced by single term "endometrioid adenocarcinoma with squamous differentiation" as tumor behavior depends on the glandular component.

Type II
- Papillary serous adenocarcinoma (5–10%)
- Clear cell adenocarcinoma (<5%)
- Mucinous adenocarcinoma (2%)
- Squamous cell carcinoma (rare)
- Carcinosarcoma
- Undifferentiated carcinoma (1–2%)
- Mixed carcinoma (Type I and Type II together—10%).

Characteristics of Type I cancers:
- Account for near 80% of endometrial adenocarcinoma
- Estrogen dependent
- Starts from atypical hyperplastic endometrium
- Found in younger age
- Well differentiated
- Low grade

- Histologically endometrioid adenocarcinoma
- Good prognosis.

Type I carcinoma develops from unopposed endometrium though a path of proliferative endometrium, then hyperplasia, atypical hyperplasia and finally endometrial carcinoma.

Characteristics of Type II cancers:

- Accounts for 10% of endometrial cancers only (mixed variety—10%)
- Nonestrogen dependent
- Not associated with hyperplasia, arises from atrophic endometrium
- Occurs in elderly, postmenopausal, and thin women
- Less differentiated
- Histologically papillary serous and clear cell carcinoma
- Aggressive clinical course
- Much poorer prognosis.

Type II carcinomas have no precursor lesion.

Q. How would you grade endometrial carcinoma on histological criteria?

It is according to FIGO (International Federation of Gynecology and Obstetrics) depending on differentiation, glandular architecture, and anaplasia.

- *Grade 1:* Less than 5% nonsquamous or nonmorular growth pattern
- *Grade 2:* 6–50% nonsquamous or nonmorular growth pattern
- *Grade 3:* More than 50% nonsquamous or nonmorular growth pattern.

Grade 1 type has little potentiality to spread outside the uterus, Grade 2 with intermediate progression and Grade 3 has increased potentiality to invade myometrium and metastasis.

The FIGO grading related only to Type I carcinoma (all endometrioids) as Type II (serous and clear cells carcinoma) is always considered as high grade.

Histology

Endometrioid adenocarcinoma **(Fig. 5):** This type I tumor comprises >80% cases of endometrial carcinoma and composed of neoplastic glands looking like those of normal endometrium. Cells are tall columnar with atypia of mild to moderate variety. There is no myometrial invasion. With decrease of glandular components it may be transformed into higher grade with potentiality to invasion. It may show different variants, e.g., squamous differentiation, villoglandular, secretory and ciliated cell variant.

Serous carcinoma: This type II carcinoma is known as uterine papillary serous carcinoma (UPSC) comprising 5–10% and very aggressive in nature. Cells have marked atypia in a complex pattern of papillary growth. It looks like ovarian epithelial tumor and also secretes CA125 for which difficult to differentiate from epithelial ovarian CA.

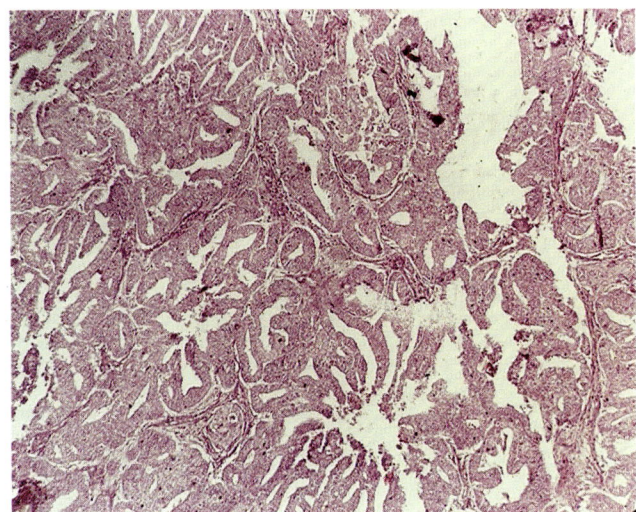

Fig. 5: Endometrial adenocarcinoma—photomicrograph (H&E, 400X) showing irregular complex glandular structures lined by pleomorphic stratified columnar cells with pleomorphic nuclei.
Courtesy: Professor Gopinath Barui, Pathology

Carcinosarcoma: This mixed tumor contains both epithelial and stromal components and also called malignant mixed Mullerian tumor. In contrast to previous belief, it is now established that this tumor is epithelial component driven and sarcomatous elements are derived from metaplasia of the epithelial element. Macroscopically, it is either sessile or polypoid and may occupy the whole endometrial cavity, sometimes through cervical os. They are high grade and spreads are like UPSC.

Clear cell carcinoma: There is no characteristic gross appearance, microscopical appearance features show papillary, solid, cystic or tubular appearance. These tumors are high grade, invasive, aggressive and have poor prognosis in advanced stage.

Spread of Endometrial Cancer (Fig. 6)

Type I spreads commonly in order like:

- *Direct spread*: Invasion to stroma, myometrium, and lastly perforation of serous coat. Tumor on body spreads to tubes and ovary and tumor of lower body involves cervix. In advanced stage, growth may directly invade to adjacent bladder, bowel, and vaginal vault.
- *Lymphatic spread*: Metastasis to pelvic and para-aortic nodal chains haphazardly in contrast to spread of cancer cervix. Metastasis to suburethral region occurs through lymphatic spread or vascular spread.
  Para-aortic lymph nodes are involved via ovarian lymphatics, internal, external, and common iliac via uterine lymphatics, occasionally through round ligaments to superficial inguinal lymph nodes **(Fig. 6)**.
- *Hematogenous spread*: Commonly to lung, less commonly liver, bone, brain, liver, and other sites like in the pelvis and low in the anterior vaginal wall.
- *Intraperitoneal exfoliation*: Transtubal transport of cancer cells.

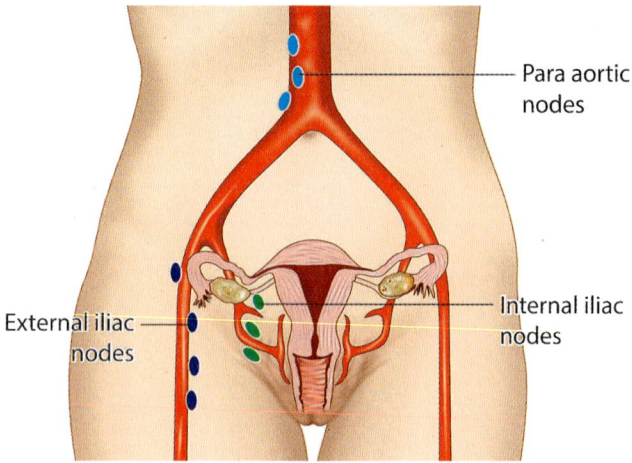

Fig. 6: Lymphatic spread of endometrial cancer.

Table 1: FIGO (International Federation of Gynecology and Obstetrics) staging of carcinoma of endometrium (2009).

Stage*	Characteristics
Stage I:	Tumor confined to the corpus uteri
• IA	No or <50% invasion
• IB	>50% invasion
Stage II	Tumor invades the cervical stroma, but does not extend beyond the uterus**
Stage III:	Local or regional spread of the tumor
• IIIA	Invades serosa of uterus and/or adnexae***
• IIIB	Vaginal and/or parametrial involvement***
• IIIC:	Metastasis to pelvic and/or para-aortic lymph nodes***
– IIIC1	Positive pelvic nodes
– IIIC2	Positive para-aortic lymph nodes with/without positive pelvic lymph nodes
Stage IV:	Tumor invades bladder and/or bowel mucosa, and/or distant metastases
• IVA	Tumor invasion of bladder and/or bowel mucosa
• IVB	Distance metastases, including intra-abdominal metastases and/or inguinal lymph nodes

*Either G1, G2, G3.
**Endocervical glandular involvement should only be considered as Stage 1.
***Positive cytology is to be reported separately without changing the stage

- Port site metastasis and following morcellation metastasis is less but reported.

Type II endometrial cancer spreads like ovarian cancer with extrauterine propensity.

Higher the grade and much is the depth of invasion of myometrium and risk of lymph node metastasis (pelvic and para-aortic) is more.

Even when, there is no myometrial invasion but tumor grade is 3 pelvic lymph node involvement is 16% and para-aortic involvement is 5%.

In grade 1 without myometrial invasion pelvic and para-aortic involvement is 1% in both cases.

State the FIGO Staging of Endometrial Carcinoma

The current FIGO staging is surgical. Clinical staging should be performed only in patients where surgery is not possible due to medical condition; the number of such cases is less now. The FIGO staging of carcinoma of endometrium (2009) have been listed in **Table 1**.

Q. What is distribution of different stages of endometrial carcinoma at diagnosis based on FIGO staging (2009)?

Almost 75% cases of endometrial carcinoma is diagnosed in stage I, 10% in stage II, 12% in stage III, and 3% in stage IV.

This is the reason for good prognosis of endometrial carcinoma.

MANAGEMENT OF ENDOMETRIAL CARCINOMA

Treatment Modalities
- Surgery
- Surgery with adjuvant therapy (radiotherapy/chemotherapy)
- Palliative

Q. How a case of carcinoma endometrium is managed?

Surgery is the mainstay of treatment as majority (75%) diagnosed in stage I disease.

Extent of surgery depends on the grade of disease, preoperative imaging, and surgicopathological staging.

Adjuvant therapy is given depending on the merit of the case.

Procedure of Surgical Staging

- On opening, the abdomen peritoneal washing is done with 50–100 mL of sterile saline and collected for cytological examination. If ascitic fluid is present, there is no need of peritoneal washing.
- Then thorough pelvic and intra-abdominal exploration is done and biopsy or excision of any suspicious lesion is done.
- Total abdominal hysterectomy (TAH) and bilateral salpingo-oophorectomy (BSO) are done **(Fig. 12)**.
- Hysterectomy specimen is taken away and uterus is opened to see the myometrial invasion by gross examination or by microscopic frozen section biopsy.
- Depending on the findings along with the preoperative tumor grading decision of pelvic and para-aortic dissection was taken.
- Surgical specimens following surgery of some of the cases of endometrial carcinoma are shown in **Figures 7 to 14**.

Indication of Pelvic Lymphadenectomy and Para-aortic Lymphadenectomy

- Performing routine systemic lymphadenectomy is controversial because therapeutic benefit of lymphadenectomy is not well proved. Lymphadenectomy

CHAPTER 6: A Case of Endometrial Carcinoma (Including Postmenopausal Bleeding) and Uterine Sarcoma

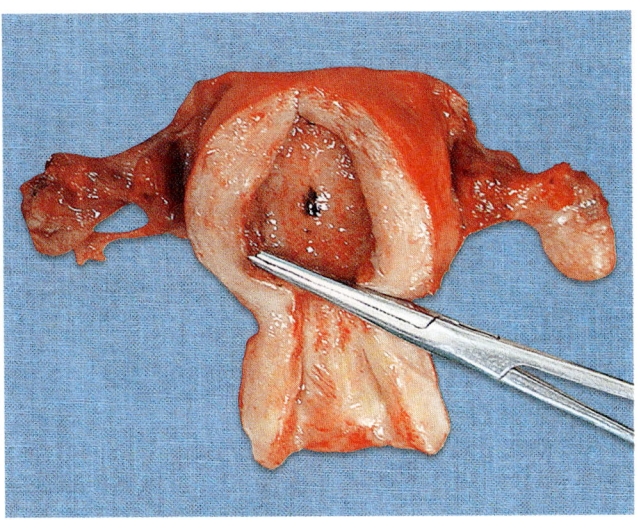

Fig. 7: Endometrial cancer—small localized growth less than 50% invasion (stage I).

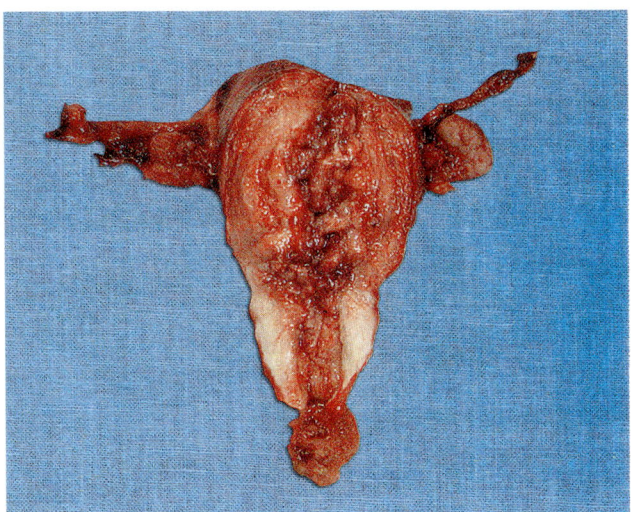

Fig. 10: Endometrial cancer more than 50% invasion of myometrium and involving cervix (stage II).

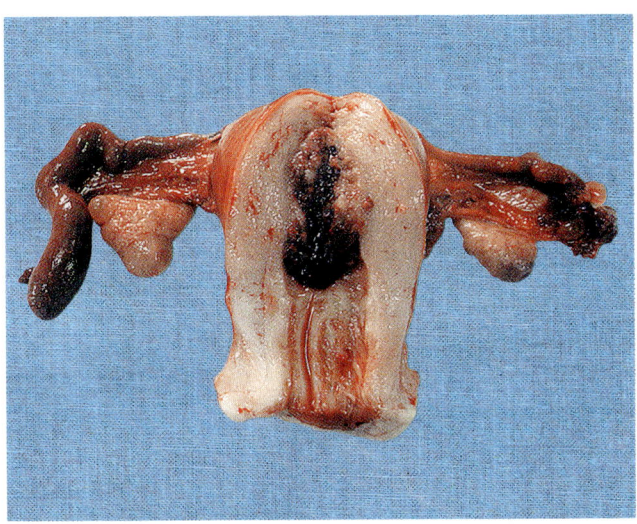

Fig. 8: Endometrial cancer confined to corpus uteri.

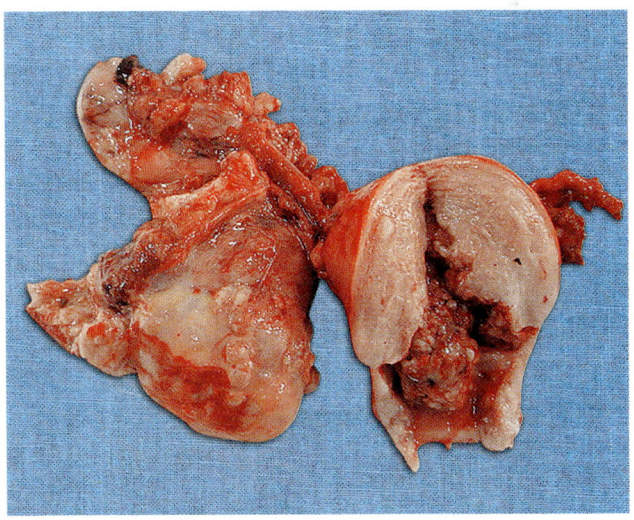

Fig. 11: Endometrial cancer with cancer ovary (stage III).

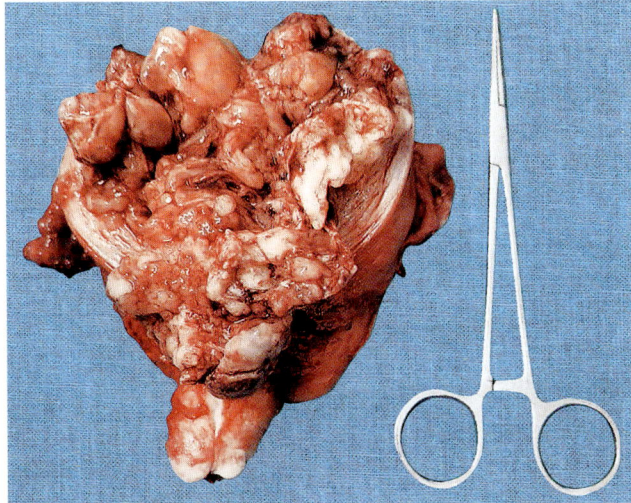

Fig. 9: Endometrial cancer—Cavity studded with growth invading more than 50% myometrium.
Courtesy: Dr Anirban Mondal, Associate Professor, Bankura Sammilani Medical College, West Bengal

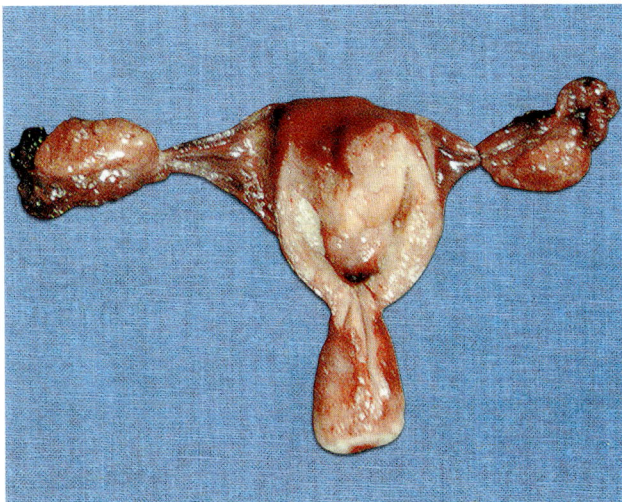

Fig. 12: Endometrial cancer—in a 51-year-old postmenopausal woman. Tubes are tied with silk suture to prevent spillage during surgery.

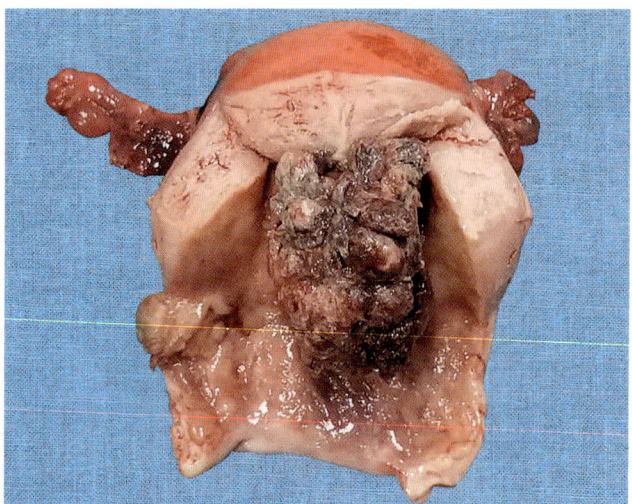

Fig.13: Hysterectomy specimen with a polypoidal growth of 7 cm in a 63-year-old P4+0 woman having complain of postmenopausal bleeding with pain lower abdomen. TAH+BSO with pelvic lymphadenectomy (radical hysterectomy) done. Histology: Carcinomatous growth admixed with sarcomatous element. Carcinomatous element shows high grade endometrial carcinoma. Tumor invades endocervical stroma and one ovary. Right external iliac and left internal iliac lymph nodes show metastasis. No parametral metastasis. Depth of myometrial invasion was 0.6 cm out of 2.4 cm total myometrial thickness.
Courtesy: Professor Abhijit Rakhsit, Dr Amrita, RG Kar Medical College, Kolkata

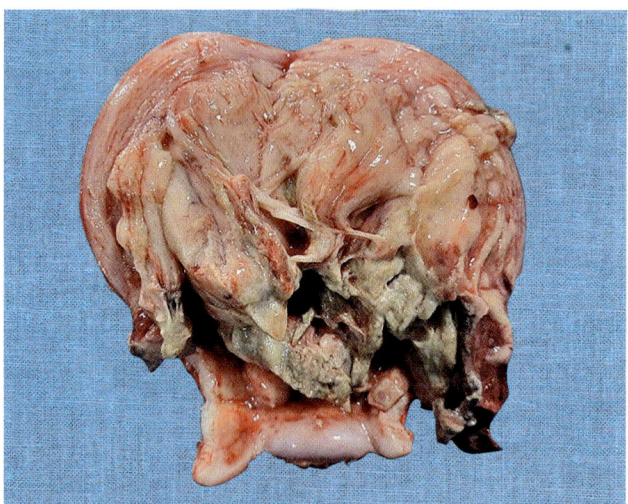

Fig. 14: Hysterectomy specimen of 60 years women who presented with postmenopausal bleeding. MRI shows gross thickening of endometrium, heterogenous lesion with loss of junctional zone. Macroscopically, a polypoid growth occupying the whole endometrial cavity. Histology: Carcinosarcoma, Stage Ia. Less than half myometrial involvement. Cervix, fallopian tube and parametrium are not involved. Lymphovascular involvement present.
Courtesy: Dr Monimala Murmu (Assistant Professor), Dr Madhurima Kar, RG Kar Medical College, Kolkata

  is done to determine staging and to determine whether subsequent need of adjuvant therapy is needed or not.
- Recently, selective and tailored lymph node assessment including sentinel lymph node biopsy has been suggested instead of comprehensive pelvic and para-aortic lymphadenectomy (NCCN, 2019).
- In general, pelvic lymphadenectomy is recommended in stage II and stage III disease and also in selected cases of stage I (IA G3, IB G1, G2, and G3).
- Para-aortic lymphadenectomy is done in case of positive pelvic nodes, enlarged para-aortic nodes which are palpable, extension to cervix or adnexal involvement.
- According to type: Type I—high-risk grade I endometrioid cancer and all cases G2, G3, and all type II endometrial cancers.

Management According to Stage

Stage I

Stage I low-risk [no or less than 50% myometrial invasion (stage IA) Grade 1, 2 endometrioid carcinoma, and tumor size <2 cm in diameter]: *Total extrafascial hysterectomy with bilateral salpingo-oophorectomy. No lymphadenectomy is needed. No further treatment is needed.*

Stage I all other cases [Grade 3 endometrioid carcinoma and/or ≥50% myometrial invasion (stage IB), and/or >2 cm in diameter or lymph nodes are palpably enlarged or Type II (serous papillary or clear cell) carcinoma]: *Total extrafascial hysterectomy with bilateral salpingo-oophorectomy and lymphadenectomy followed by postoperative radiotherapy.*

Of the second group Stage IA G3 and Stage IB G1, 2 are called Stage I intermediate risk—*only vaginal brachytherapy is given following total extrafascial hysterectomy with bilateral salpingo-oophorectomy and lymphadenectomy.* The others of this second group are regarded as *Stage I high risk and need both brachytherapy and teletherapy.* In this high-risk group, adjuvant chemotherapy may be considered in selected patients.

Stage II

In this stage, involvement of cervix is detected clinically or by MRI/USG. The options are:
- Modified radical hysterectomy (TAH with BSO with removal of parametrium, paracolpos and 1–2 cm upper vagina with lymphadenectomy)
- Radiation followed by surgery: External pelvic radiation and brachytherapy and TAH with BSO done after 6 weeks.

Stage III

Surgical resection of all metastatic disease followed by external beam radiotherapy and/or chemotherapy.

Stage IV

Only in intra-abdominal spread stage IV disease is treated by cytoreduction so that there remains no residual tumor. This is followed by platinum-based chemotherapy. In cases of extra-abdominal metastasis platinum-based chemotherapy or hormonal therapy (progesterone/LNG-IUS) is given. Only few patients are candidates for radiotherapy with curative intent.

General Principle of Adjuvant Therapy in Endometrial Carcinoma

- In low-risk early stage disease, surgery is adequate treatment.
- Radiotherapy after surgery reduces the local recurrence but does not improve survival.
- Intermediate risk group needs only vault brachytherapy following surgery.
- In high-risk group postoperatively high dose radiotherapy is given to the vaginal vault over a short period of time followed by external beam radiotherapy.
- Primary radiotherapy is selected rarely for exceptionally poor surgical candidates.
- Chemotherapy is given to metastatic disease to prevent the distant spread and reasonable option for in advanced endometrial cancer. The agents are platinum-based cisplatin, doxorubicin, and praclitaxel or carboplatin and paclitaxel combination.

Q. What are the indications of hormone therapy?

Endometrial cancer is hormone responsive tumor.

Indications are:

- Cases who are not the surgical candidates
- Young premenopausal women who desire fertility
- Recurrent diseases are also treated by progestogens.

Progesterone orally (medroxyprogesterone), intramuscularly (17α-hydroxyprogesterone or norethisterone) or in the form intrauterine system (levonorgestrel-releasing IUD) can be given. Combination with tamoxifen improves efficacy of progesterone.

Route of Surgery

Laparotomy is standard procedure. Laparoscopic and robotic surgical staging are now acceptable for surgical staging and proceed. Vaginal hysterectomy with/without bilateral salpingo-oophorectomy without surgical staging in comorbid patient is another option.

Q. How to follow-up a case of endometrial cancer after treatment?

Follow-up schedule: Lifelong follow up is needed every 3 months for 2 years, 6 monthly for 3 years and yearly for rest of life.

Components of follow-up are:

- Appearance of symptoms like vaginal bleeding, pain, abdominal swelling, and weight loss
- Examination including pelvic and vaginal examination in every check-up
- Vaginal cytology initially for 6 months then annually.

Prognosis of Endometrial Cancer

Overall survival rate is 80%.

In young women, endometrial cancer is well differentiated and prognosis is excellent whereas in postmenopausal women, it is poorly differentiated and prognosis is also poor.

Stage-wise Average 5 Year Survival Rate

Stage	Stage I	Stage II	Stage III	Stage IV
Five year survival (%)	88	75	55	15

Adverse prognostic factors:

- Age above 70 years
- High BMI
- Advanced surgical stage
- Grade 3
- Papillary serous or clear cell cancer (Type II)
- Increased tumor size
- Peritoneal cytology positive for cancer cells
- Lymphovascular space involvement
- Lymph node metastasis and distant metastasis
- Low tumor expression levels of estrogen receptors and progesterone receptors.

Prevention of Endometrial Cancer

- Education to alter the risk factors for endometrial cancer is important. Obesity and PCOS can be managed by diet and exercise.
- Prolonged anovulatory cycles should be treated either by ovulation inducing agent or cyclical progesterone.
- In intact uterus, estrogen therapy should be combined with 10–12 days of progesterone in a cycle.
- At the time of menopause, women are counseled about the risks and symptoms of endometrial cancer.
- Oral contraceptives give protection against endometrial cancer.
- Routine PAP smear is inadequate for endometrial cancer screening. Routine screening for hyperplasia is not advocated.
- Identification of women with Lynch syndrome is essential. Lynch syndrome cancers include colon, endometrium, kidney, ureter, and small bowel. Women with Lynch syndrome endometrial biopsy are recommended every 1–2 years and are candidates for genetic testing. Recent suggestion of prophylactic hysterectomy in women with Lynch syndrome is justified but not widely accepted.

Recurrent Endometrial Carcinoma

Recurrence occurs in 25% of patients treated for early endometrial cancer. More than 50% recurrence occurs within 2 years and 75% within 3 years.

Recurrence may be in the vaginal vault, lymph nodes, lateral pelvic wall, and distal sites like lung, liver, bone, and brain. The most common site is vaginal vault.

Distal metastasis is more common in case of initial combination therapy of surgery and radiotherapy. Best curable condition is vault recurrence in unradiated patient and it responds well to external beam therapy.

Local pelvic recurrence or nodal recurrence is treated by teletherapy if not previously irradiated. Cytoreductive surgery may be an option.

In disseminated relapse chemotherapy with praclitaxel and carboplatin is the choice. Progestogens with/without tamoxifen can be given in selected cases and this has less adverse effect. High dose MPA 100 mg thrice daily or megestrol acetate 80 mg thrice daily is continued at least for 3 months to get the response and continued according to the need.

Fertility Sparing Conservative Management in Endometrial Carcinoma

In young women with well differentiated type I endometrial carcinoma **hormonal treatment without hysterectomy** to preserve fertility is an option in exceptional cases.

Interestingly PCOS and chronic anovulation which cause infertility may lead to endometrial carcinoma. Selection of case is vital by diagnostic hysteroscope, D&C, and imaging to exclude deep myometrial invasion and extrauterine disease. It should be well differentiated, grade 1, type I, no myometrial invasion and have no extrauterine spread.

The aim of progesterone treatment is to reverse the lesion. Counseling regarding risk and follow-up is essential. Megestrol acetate160 mg daily orally, oral or intramuscular MPA, and LNG-IUS are the different progestogens used to treat.

Monitoring with repeated biopsy/D&C even 3 monthly interval may be needed to observe the regression and dosage adjustment or to switch over to hysterectomy if needed.

Conception and live birth is possible in patients who respond to treatment. In postpartum period again surveillance is needed and hysterectomy should be undergone.

PYOMETRA (FIGS. 15 AND 16)

Q. What are the causes of pyometra?

The most common cause (50%) is malignancy—endometrial or endocervical carcinoma. Others are atrophic endometritis, tubercular endometritis, and following radiotherapy. Cervical stenosis results pyometra.

Diagnosis

Symptoms of foul smelling discharge preceded by vaginal bleeding. On bimanual examination, uterus is enlarged. TVS is done to diagnose the collection of fluid in uterus.

Management

Management can be done by dilatation, drainage, curette, and biopsy **(Fig. 14)**. Chance of perforation is high during curettage and sometimes the procedure is kept abeyance to do in later date. Repeat dilatation is needed. Antibiotic or antitubercular drug is given accordingly.

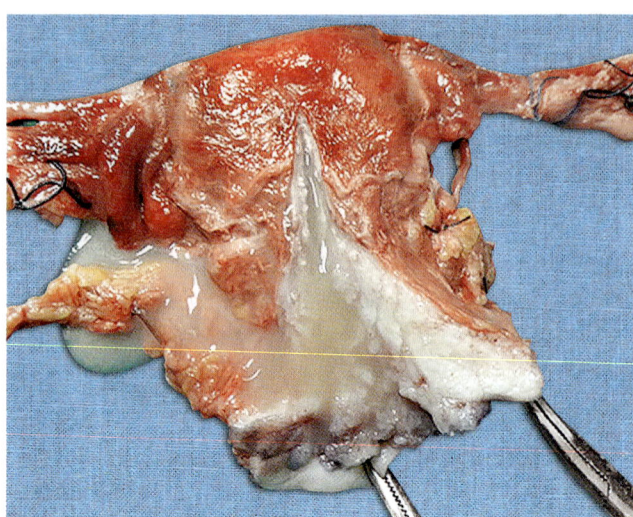

Fig. 15: Pyometra in a case of cancer cervix with cancer endometrium in a postmenopausal women—radical hysterectomy done.
Courtesy: Dr Arunasis Mullick

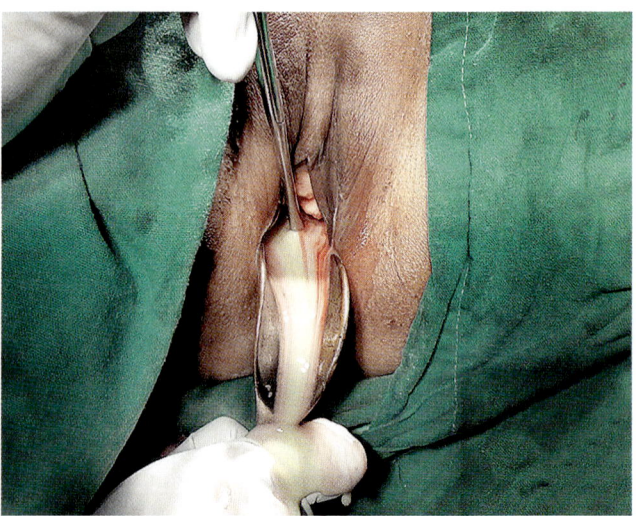

Fig. 16: Drainage of pyometra.
Courtesy: Professor Sukanta Misra, HOD, VIMS, Kolkata

POSTMENOPAUSAL BLEEDING (PMB)

Q. What do you mean by postmenopausal bleeding?

Bleeding per vagina after one year of permanent cessation of menstruation is called postmenopausal bleeding (PMB).

Q. What are the causes of postmenopausal bleeding?

Common Causes of PMB

- Atrophic endometrium—commonest cause of PMB
- Endometrial cancer—10% case of PMB
- Cancer cervix (20%) in India
- Endometrial hyperplasia
- Endometrial polyp
- Estrogen intake

CHAPTER 6: A Case of Endometrial Carcinoma (Including Postmenopausal Bleeding) and Uterine Sarcoma

Causes of PMB in Detail

- Uterine cause—atrophic endometrium, endometrial hyperplasia, dysfunctional uterine bleeding (DUB), endometrial cancer, estrogen therapy, endometrial polyp, uterine fibroid, endometritis, pyometra, sarcoma
- Cervical cause—cancer cervix, chronic cervicitis, cervical polyp, prolapse with decubitus ulcer
- Vaginal cause—atrophic (senile) vaginitis, vaginal cancer, forgotten pessary ulcer, radiation ulcer, trauma
- Estrogen intake
- Vulval cause—vulvovaginitis, vulval cancer, trauma
- Ovarian cause—ovarian malignancy, estrogen secreting tumor (granulosa cell tumor)
- Fallopian tube—carcinoma
- Blood dyscrasia
- Rectal bleeding or bleeding from urinary bladder may be confused with vaginal bleeding. Urinary tract—urethral caruncle, bladder papilloma and carcinoma.

Q. Do you want to investigate a case of postmenopausal bleeding immediately ? Why?

Yes. There is chance of endometrial carcinoma (in PMB 10% cases are due to endometrial cancer) and cervical carcinoma which need to be excluded though majority of postmenopauasal bleeding cause is benign. In 2/3rd cases single episode of bleeding is found and is mostly benign in nature.

Q. How would you investigate a case of postmenopausal bleeding?

(A) History, (B) Clinical examination, (C) Special investigations

History

- Pattern of bleeding, duration of bleeding and amount of bleeding. History of persistent PMB which is defined as presence of bleeding for more than one month.
- Early menarche, late menopause, nulliparous, obesity, diabetes, hypertension—are risk factors of Ca endometrium.
- Family history: Genetic and hereditary—in Lynch syndrome endometrial cancer is the most common extracolonic manifestation. *HNPCC (hereditary nonpolyposis colorectal cancer syndrome),* autosomal dominant inheritance is linked with colorectal, ovarian, endometrial, and urothelial tumors.
- Something coming down per vagina (prolapse), associated pain, postcoital bleeding,
- History of hormone intake, tamoxifen therapy, history of bleeding disorder. Tamoxifen, a selective estrogen receptor modulator which is used for adjuvant therapy in breast cancer has mild estrogenic effect on endometrium and associated with 2-6 fold increased risk of endometrial cancer.

Q. What do you mean by recurrent postmenopausal bleeding?

It is defined as two attendances to PMB clinic with two negative pipelle biopsy report for malignancy more than 6 months apart in the last 2 years.

Examination

- *General*: Pallor
  - High BMI/ hypertension
  - Breast examination to exclude Ca
- *Abdominal:* Any abdominal mass like ovarian mass, uterine enlargement (fibroid, pyometra), inguinal lymph node enlargement
- *Examination of vulva and vagina:* Any growth, ulcer, vulvovaginitis, any pelvic organ prolapse, decubitus ulcer
- *Per speculum examination:* Cervical polyp or growth, atrophic vaginitis, a Pap smear taken, bleeding through external os, vaginal metastasis
- *Bimanual examination:* Size of uterus, any other pelvic mass, adnexal lump, nodules in POD
- *Per rectal examination:* Parametrial involvement in cancer cervix, rectal involvement

Investigations

Q. What are the primary investigations? What are the other investigations?

(1) Pap smear of cervix, (2) TVS of pelvis, (3) Endometrial biopsy

Pap smear of cervix is advised as initial screening.

Pap smear is very informative for detection of abnormal cervical cytology (Page 176). Pap testing is not indicated for diagnosis of endometrial carcinoma as 50% cases of endometrial carcinoma has normal finding. However, atypical glandular cells found in Pap needs further evaluation to exclude cervical and endometrial malignancy (Page 138). *Ultrasound scan*, best is TVS.

Q. What would you see in TVS in PMB?

- Endometrial thickness (ET)
- Suspected polyps
- Presence of fibroids
- Uterine size
- Cervix
- Adnexal (ovary and fallopian tube) morphology
- Presence of ascites

If TVS is not possible a transabdominal scan (TAS) can be done in order to assess adnexal masses. As measurement of endometrial thickness (ET) is less accurate by TAS it should not be used for endometrial assessment.

Endometrial thickness (ET) is measured as anteroposterior (AP) 2-layer thickness in the sagittal plane near the fundus.

Endometrial thickness 4 mm or less in postmenopausal woman is unlikely to be endometrial CA, in ET > 4 mm further endometrial evaluation (biopsy) is needed. A cut off of 4 mm ET in woman with PMB produces a sensitivity of 95% and specificity of 55% for detection of endometrial cancer.

In women with ET <4 mm the incidence of endometrial cancer is 0.6% hence, do not require a biopsy.

Cystic endometrial changes are suggestive of polyps, homogeneous thickened endometrium indicates hyperplasia and malignancy is suspected in heterogeneous structural pattern.

Endometrium becomes thickened, cystic and irregular on tamoxifen therapy and warrants endometrial biopsy. PMB in woman with tamoxifen therapy needs endometrial biopsy under vision of hysteroscopy (ACOG).

If the endometrium is thickened endometrial biopsy is taken.

If histology shows no atypia or cancer conservative management is done. By TVS presence of adnexal mass is also evaluated.

Endometrial Biopsy

A Pipelle biopsy (endometrial sampling) is done. Pipelle provides a sensitivity of 99% and 88% for detection of endometrial cancer and atypical endometrial hyperplasia in postmenopausal women respectively.

Indications of endometrial biopsy

Endometrial biopsy is done when:
- ET ≥4 mm
- ET is not visualized due to any reason, e.g., fibroids*
- Persistent PMB irrespective of endometrial thickness
- Suspicion of polyp or mass on TVS irrespective of endometrial thickness
- ET ≥3 mm with fluid in the endometrial cavity (fluid is excluded in the measurement)

*Sometimes endometrium is obscured by fibroids, a Pipelle biopsy is attempted and hysteroscopy is suggested if definitive diagnosis cannot be made from the biopsy.

Q. Which should be done first? TVS or biopsy?

TVS should be done first for the following reasons:
- Endometrial biopsy may affect the appearance of the endometrium and if biopsy is done beforehand, ultrasound should not be done within 2 weeks.
- Other than endometrial thickness TVS can provide other information in PMB as mentioned above.

Pipelle biopsy (endometrial sampling) is recommended by some school as *first line of investigation.*

Q. When to do hysteroscopy in PMB?

- When Pipelle device could not be negotiated
- Biopsy material inadequate
- Suspected polyp
- Insufficient visualization of endometrium
- Recurrent PMB
- PMB with previous history of endometrial ablation

In pre/perimenopausal woman if endometrial biopsy is normal, ET >11 mm alone is not an indication for hysteroscopy due to the huge fluctuation of ET in this age group. Outpatient hysteroscopy or office hysteroscopy is preferred to GA.

Q. In asymptomatic women, if thickened endometrium is found as a coincidental finding on ultrasound scan what would you do?

- No endometrial biopsy is needed unless the ET is more than 11 mm. However, risk factors like obesity and diabetes are taken into account in managing such cases.
- The presence of intrauterine fluid per se, in otherwise asymptomatic women is also not an indication for a biopsy.

Incidental findings of ET ≥11 mm in asymptomatic women on tamoxifen therapy with negative hysteroscopy in the last 12 months do not need any further investigation.

Colposcope—in suspected cervical pathology
Cervical biopsy—in cervical lesion
CT and MRI—in obvious cervical and endometrial malignancy as may be needed
Cystoscopy and proctoscopy—may be needed when no cause detected and suspicious of bladder or rectal pathology.

Management Outline of Postmenopausal Bleeding According to Cause

- *Atrophic vaginitis:* Estrogen cream, estrogen pessaries or ring
- *Endometrial cancer:* Surgical staging. TAH-BSO with or without adjuvant therapy
- *Endometrial hyperplasia:* (*see* also Page 130)
  - Simple: Oral progestogen or LNG-IUS
  - Complex: Oral progestogen or LNG-IUS
  - Atypical: TAH
- *Endometrial polyp:* Hysteroscopic removal
- *Cervical polyp:* Polypectomy
- *Cervical cancer:* Radical hysterectomy in early stage, radiotherapy as per stage (*see* Page 166).

SARCOMA OF THE UTERUS (FIGS. 17 TO 19)

Incidence

It is 4–5% of all uterine cancer and contributes not more than 1% of all gynecological malignancies.

Varieties

According to the site of origin sarcomas are of four types:
1. Intramural, arises from myometrium
2. From endometrial stroma
3. From the benign leiomyoma
4. From cervix—grape-like sarcoma of cervix.

Histological Types

1. Pure mesenchymal tumors
   a. Leiomyosarcoma
   b. Endometrial stromal sarcoma
2. Mixed epithelial and mesenchymal tumors: Carcinosarcoma

Homologous means tissues normally found in the uterus and heterologous sarcoma means to tissue foreign to the uterus. Pure sarcomas are almost homologous.

Heterologous sarcomas are rare and contain the sarcomatous tissues like bone, cartilage, and striated muscle which are not found in the uterus. Common type is highly malignant rhabdomyosarcoma found in children presenting with grape-like mass from cervix and watery discharge. Distal metastasis is common with high recurrence.

Smooth muscle tumor of uncertain malignant potential (STUMP): There is some worrisome histological features, but cannot be diagnosed reliably whether benign or benign.

Gross Pathology

Uterus becomes enlarged, hard to firm and there may involvement of adjacent structures. Cut section shows heterogenous, solid areas with degenerative changes and hemorrhage **(Figs. 17 to 19)**.

Diagnosis

- **Leiomyosarcoma** may be primary or rarely secondary from benign tumor (<1%) (*see* Page 92). Preoperative diagnosis is difficult.
  Rapid growing pelvic mass with pain, enlarged uterus with softness on bimanual examination, and necrosis on MRI are the suspicious features. Vascular metastasis to distal site is common.
- **Endometrial stromal sarcoma** occurs mostly in perimenopausal age presenting with abnormal uterine bleeding with soft enlarged uterus and mostly of low grade.
- **Carcinosarcoma** (epithelial sarcomas), also called malignant mixed Müllerian tumor (MMMT) which usually occurs after menopause and may have a previous history of radiation due to cancer cervix and present with PMB and mass per vagina.

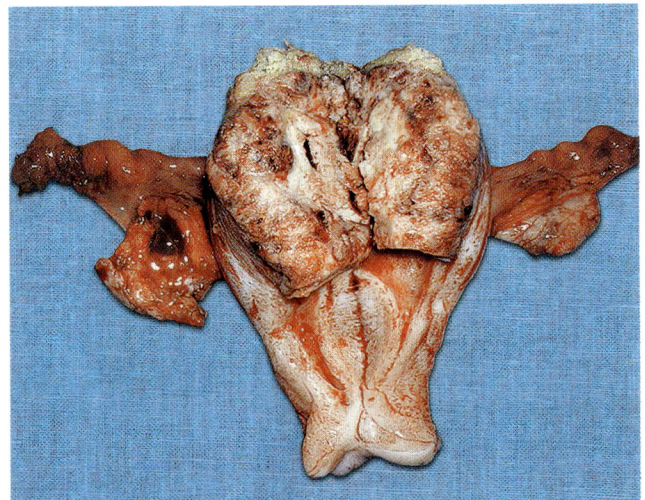

Fig. 17: Uterine sarcoma—hysterectomy specimen (TAH BSO done).
Courtesy: Professor Sukanta Misra, HOD, VIMS, Kolkata

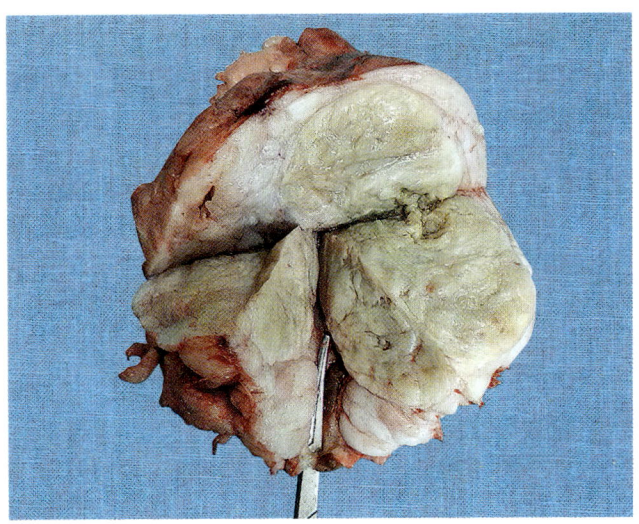

Fig. 18: Hysterectomy specimen showing uterine sarcoma in a 43 years multiparous woman who came with pain and lump abdomen, without any cycle disturbance.

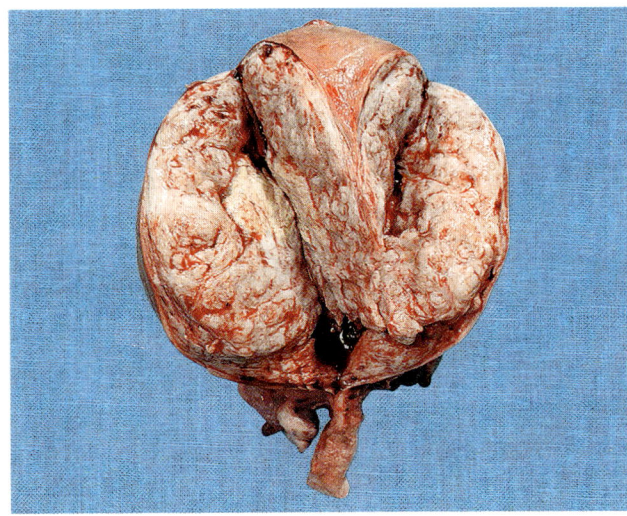

Fig. 19: Hysterectomy specimen showing leiomyosarcoma with multiple bleeding areas. 42 years P1+0, LI-1, LUCS 22 years back was admitted with lump abdomen, pain abdomen and heavy menstrual bleeding. CECT is suggestive of 22 cm, 20 cm, 15 cm heterogenous, highly vascular mass involving body and fundus with multiple pelvic lymph node involvement. TAH BSO with lymphadenectomy done.

- **Staging of uterine sarcoma:** FIGO staging leiomyosarcomas is given in the **Table 2** below and that of endometrial stromal sarcoma is little different. Staging of carcinosarcoma is like carcinoma of endometrium.

Treatment

Treatment of all varieties are surgery (TAH with BSO) **(Fig. 15)** followed by radiotherapy. If cervix is involved radical hysterectomy is done. In distal metastasis, chemotherapy is tried.

Table 2: FIGO staging of leiomyosarcomas.

Stage I: Tumor limited within uterus
IA: Size <5 cm
IB: Size >5 cm

Stage II: Tumor extends to the pelvis
IIA: Adnexa in involved
IIB: Tumor extends to extrauterine pelvic tissue

Stage III: Tumor involves abdominal tissues not just protruding into the abdomen
IIIA: One site involved
IIIB: More than one site involved
IIIC: Metastasis to pelvic and/or para-aortic lymph nodes

Stage IV
IVA: Tumor invades bladder and/or rectum
IVB: Distant metastasis

Survival Rate

Five-year survival rate largely depends on type of growth and extension, in general, the prognosis is poor and overall survival rate of leiomyosarcoma is about 40%. If it is confined to uterus at the time of treatment the survival rate is much higher. In earlier stages, five-year survival rate of endometrial stromal sarcoma is 90% and that of Mullerian adenocarcinoma is 70%.

A Case of Choriocarcinoma (Gestational Trophoblastic Neoplasia)

CHAPTER OUTLINE

Writing a case of choriocarcinoma and how to present the case?

- Classification of Gestational Trophoblastic Disease and Gestational Trophoblastic Neoplasia (GTN)
- Diagnosis of Choriocarcinoma, Placental Site Trophoblastic Tumor and Epithelioid Trophoblastic Tumor
- Treatment of Choriocarcinoma, Placental Site Trophoblastic Tumor and Epithelioid Trophoblastic Tumor
- Prognosis and Prognostic Scoring System

PATIENT'S PARTICULARS

1. Name: Gita Devi
2. Age: 39 years
3. Address: Central Kolkata
4. Occupation: Housewife
5. Married/unmarried: Married for one and half year
6. History of infertility: No such
7. Husband's occupation: Businessman
8. Socioeconomic status: Low
9. Religion: Hindu
10. Parous/nulliparous: P1+1

Bed No.: 25
Date of admission:
Date of examination:

HISTORY

- *Chief complaint/complaints:*
  - Irregular bleeding per vaginam (PV) since her last abortion 6 months back
  - Vague lower abdominal pain and uneasiness—2 months.
- *History of present illness:* The woman was admitted 2 days back for vaginal bleeding. She had a spontaneous abortion 6 months back at the period of gestation of 3 months. She was admitted in the hospital and dilatation and curettage (D&C) operation was done at that time. She was discharged after 1 day. But she was not recovered totally. She had irregular bleeding PV and persistent discomfort in the lower abdomen. As her bleeding per vagina continued repeat curettage was done one at 3 months back and another 10 days back but there is no cessation of bleeding per vagina. Now she is feeling severe weakness. On serum β-human chorionic gonadotropin (hCG) estimation, it is found to be very high.
- *Menstrual history:*
  - Last normal menstrual period: 8.03.2017 (6 months back)
  - Duration of menstruation: 4 days
  - Interval in days: 27± 2
  - Age of menarche: 12 years
  - Regularity of cycle: Regular
  - Pain during period/if pain relation with menstruation: No such
  - Amount of bleeding: Average
  - Clot: No such
    - Intermenstrual bleeding: No history
    - If amenorrhea: No amenorrhea now after abortion.

- *Obstetric history:*
  - Parity: P1+1
  - Living issue (LI): 1 (M), 9 years old, normal delivery
  - Last child birth (LCB): Had spontaneous abortion 2 months back. Write in tabular form as shown in Chapter 1.
- *Past history:*
  - Medical
  - Surgical: History of D&C operation 2 months back.
- *Family history:* Nothing suggestive
- *Sexual history:*
- *Functional history:*
  - Bowel
  - Bladder
  - Sleep: Decreased recently
  - Appetite: Reduced.
- *Personal history:*
  - Personal hygiene
  - Smoking/alcohol.
- *Contraceptive history:* Not practiced
- *Drug history:*
  - History of any drug allergy
  - History of intake of corticosteroids, antiepileptic or other drugs (previous or present)
- *Treatment history*: She has been undergone repeat curettage. Still she has bleeding and serum β-hCG is high in the range of 68,000/cmm.

PHYSICAL EXAMINATION

Patient—alert, conscious, and cooperative
- Build:
- Nutrition: Average
- Height: 5 feet 2 inch
- Weight/body mass index (BMI): 46 kg/m^2
- Edema: Nil
- Anemia: + +
- Cyanosis: Nil
- Jaundice: Nil
- Clubbing: Nil
- Tongue, teeth, gum, and tonsil
- Neck veins: Not engorged
- Neck glands: Not palpable
- Leg veins: Not engorged
- Pulse: 86 beats/min
- Respiration: Normal
- Temperature: Normal
- BP: 100/64 mm Hg.

Systemic Examination

- *Central nervous system:* No abnormality detected
- *Cardiovascular system*: No abnormality detected – Auscultation of heart S1/S2
- *Respiratory system*:
  - Auscultation of chest

- *Gastrointestinal system:*
  - Liver: Not palpable
  - Spleen: Not Palpable
- *Examination of other systems:*
  - Examination of back and spines skeletal system
  - Neurological
  - Ophthalmoscopic examination
  - Urinary system
- *Examination of breasts and nipple:*
  - Inspection
  - Palpation: No lump palpable.

GYNECOLOGICAL EXAMINATION

- *Abdominal examination:*
  - Inspection:
  - Palpation: No mass, no tenderness
  - Percussion:
  - Auscultation:
- *Vaginal examination:*
  - Inspection and palpation of external genitalia: No abnormality
  - Speculum examination: Mild fresh bleeding seen coming out through external os.
  - Bimanual examination: Uterus is uniformly enlarged, almost 10–12 week size, mild tenderness, and mobile.
  - Bilateral adnexa: Adnexae enlarged and cystics.
  - Examination of rectovaginal area and rectal examination: Same as bimanual findings.

SUMMARY OF THE CASE (SAMPLE)

A 39-year-old woman, P1+1 LI 1 LCB 9 years back, was admitted 2 days back with history spontaneous abortion 6 months back at 12 weeks of gestation for which D&C was done at that time. As the bleeding continued and did not respond to conservative treatment repeat D&C done twice one at 3 months back and another 10 days back but still the bleeding is continuing.

On examination, patient has moderate pallor, pulse rate is 86 beats/min, BP is 124/82 mm Hg per abdomen, no tenderness, and no lump. PV examination revealed enlarged uterus of 10 weeks size, bilateral enlarged adnexae, and presence of vaginal bleeding.

Her Hb level is 7 g%. Her serum β-hCG is high with a value of 68,000/cmm and uterus is enlarged of about 10 weeks and ovaries are also enlarged and cystic.

Histopathological (H/P) report is inconclusive.

INVESTIGATIONS SUPPLIED OR REQUIRED

- *Hb%*: 7 g%
- *Serum β hCG*: 68,000/cmm
- *H/P*: Inconclusive
- *USG*: Enlarged uterus with heterogeneous mass within, bilateral cystic enlarged ovaries

- *Color Doppler*: Shows increased vascularity in the uterine mass
- *Chest X-ray*: Within normal limit.

PROVISIONAL DIAGNOSIS

A 21-year-old woman with gestational trophoblastic neoplasia (GTN).

DIFFERENTIAL DIAGNOSIS

- Hydatidiform mole
- Invasive mole
- Trophoblastic tumors: Choriocarcinoma, placental site trophoblastic tumor (PSTT), and epithelioid trophoblastic tumor (ETT).

Q. Why are you saying this is a case of GTN?

- Patient has persistent bleeding PV with elevated serum β-hCG with a history of abortion not relieved with repeated curettage.
- Clinical examination
- USG: Uterus and adnexae are enlarged.

Q. What do you mean by gestational trophoblastic disease (GTD) and gestational trophoblastic neoplasia (GTN)?

- The *GTD* is a spectrum of tumors which arise from placenta which are interrelated but histologically distinct. GTD is characterized by elevation of serum β-hCG with a varied tendency to invade locally and to spread.
- GTD is comprised of molar pregnancy and trophoblastic tumor (*see* below).
- GTN is the subset of GTD with development of malignant sequelae. GTN develops either from molar pregnancy or from any other gestation (term, abortion, and ectopic).

Gestational Trophoblastic Neoplasia Includes

- Invasive mole
- Choriocarcinoma
- Placental site tropho blastic tumor
- Epithelioid trophoblastic tumor.

This classification of GTN is based on histological types, but in most of the cases tissue becomes not available for study and management is done on clinical basis and elevated serum β-hCG level.

Classification of GTD (Modified WHO, 2014)

Molar Pregnancies

- Hydatidiform mole
  - Complete **(Fig. 1A)**
  - Partial **(Fig. 1B)**
- Invasive mole **(Fig. 1C)**.

Trophoblastic Tumors

- Choriocarcinoma
- Placental site trophoblastic tumor
- Epithelioid trophoblastic tumor.

Q. How do invasive mole, choriocarcinoma, and PSTT and epithelioid trophoblastic tumor differ from hydatidiform mole?

These are all GTN or called malignant GTD and hydatidiform mole is a benign condition.

Q. Where from GTN develops?

Gestational trophoblastic neoplasia develops from any type of pregnancy—mostly from hydatidiform mole (50% cases), 25% after abortion, 23% after full-term normal pregnancy, and 20% after ectopic. In fact, many of the origin of GTN which are said to be abortion in origin are unrecognized early mole.

Q. What is the chance of GTN in complete mole and partial mole?

In complete mole, there is 20% chance of GTN. But in case of partial mole, the chance is less than 5%. Following

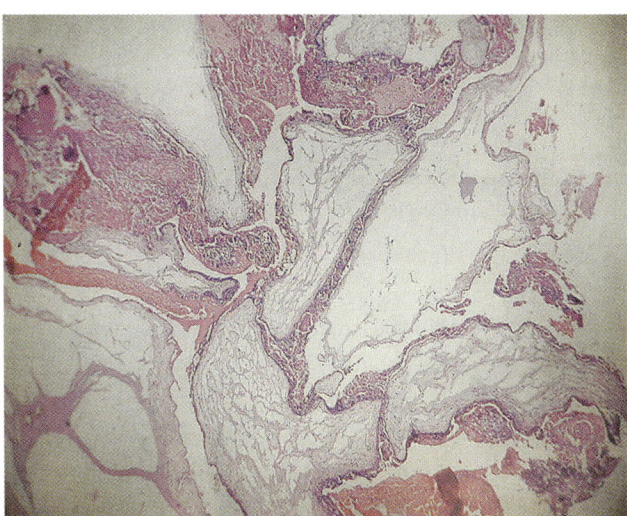

Fig. 1A: Microscopical features of hydatidiform mole—hydropic degeneration, proliferation of epithelial cells.
Courtesy: Dr Anup Boler, Associate Professor, Pathology

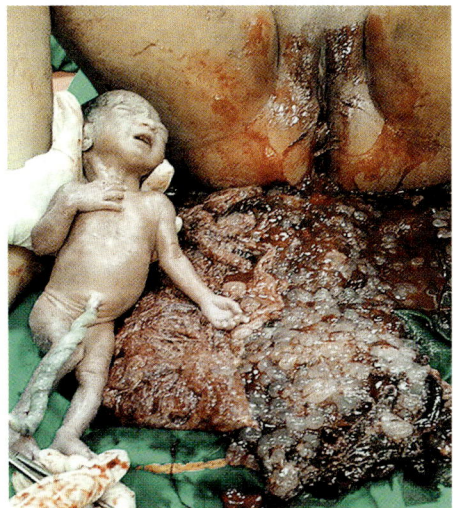

Fig. 1B: Partial hydatidiform mole with living baby.
Courtesy: Dr Keka Mondal

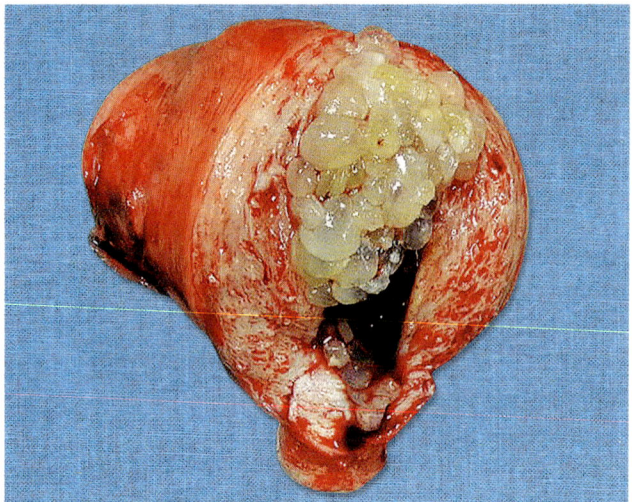

Fig. 1C: Hysterectomy specimen showing invasive mole. 41 years multigravida with living issue 3 presented with torrential hemorrhage with severe pallor.
Courtesy: Dr Rupali Modak, Assistant Professor, Obstetric and Gynecology, RG Kar Medical College

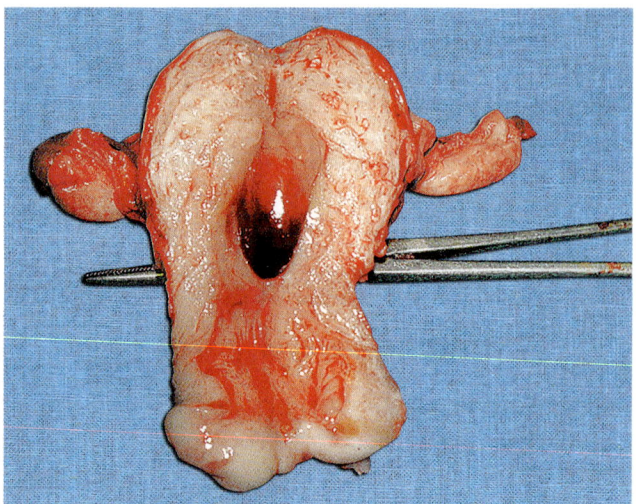

Fig. 2: Gestational choriocarcinoma.
Courtesy: Professor G Kamilya

normal pregnancy, chance of GTN is very less. The need for chemotherapy following a complete mole is 15% and that after a partial mole is 0.5%.

Q. How is GTN diagnosed?

- Primarily by the persistent elevated serum hCG.
- By histopathology. Usually, no tissue is available for pathological study in most of the cases.

Diagnostic Criteria of Post Molar GTN

- Plateau of serum β-hCG level (±10%) for four measurements during a period of 3 weeks or longer—days 1, 7, 14, 21.
- Rise of serum β-hCG >10% during three weekly consecutive measurements or longer during a period of 2 weeks or more—days 1, 7, 14.
- The serum β-hCG level remains detectable for 6 months or more.
- Histological criteria for choriocarcinoma.

Q. What are the features of invasive mole?

- In invasive mole, there are excessive trophoblastic overgrowth and extensive penetration by the trophoblastic cells including whole villi. These penetrate into the myometrium, sometimes involving the peritoneum, parametrium or vaginal vault.
- These are locally invasive and chance of wide spread metastasis is less.
- Invasive mole almost develops from mole—partial or complete variety.

Q. What are the features of gestational choriocarcinoma (Fig. 2)?

- This is an extremely malignant form GTN and carcinoma of chorionic epithelium.
- Mostly develops from molar pregnancy but may develop from nonmolar pregnancy. The incidence of development of gestational choriocarcinoma is 1 in 30,000 nonmolar pregnancy.
- Macroscopically, a large mass invades both myometrium and blood vessels. In case of involvement of the endometrium, sloughing and infection of the surface occur. The tumor is dark red or purple and ragged or friable.
- Microscopic features: Columns and seeds of trophoblastic cells penetrate the muscle and blood vessels, and cellular anaplasia may be present. Presence of intermediate trophoblast, multinucleate syncytiotrophoblast with hemorrhage and necrosis **(Fig. 3)**.
- *The important diagnostic feature of choriocarcinoma is absence of a villous pattern which is present in hydatidiform mole or invasive mole.*

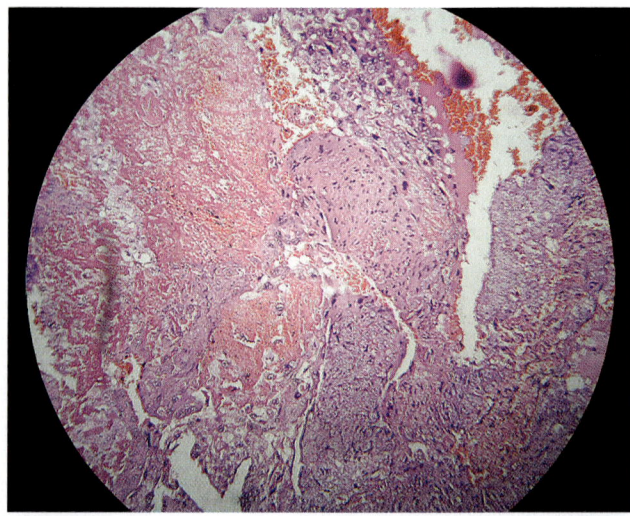

Fig. 3: Microscopical features of choriocarcinoma—intermediate trophoblast, multinucleated syncytiotrophoblast, large areas of necrosis, and hemorrhage.
Courtesy: Dr Anup Boler, Associate Professor, Pathology

- Metastasis occurs early and is usually blood borne. The common sites are lungs (75%) and vagina (50%). The other sites are vulva, kidneys, liver, ovaries, brain, and bowel. Direct spread to peritoneum, tubes, and ovaries.

Diagnosis of Choriocarcinoma

- Diagnosis of choriocarcinoma is done by possibility of this condition in mind.
- Unusual bleeding after term pregnancy or abortion, serum β-hCG measurement and chest X-ray. The most common symptom is vaginal bleeding.
- Prior history of pregnancy is also suggestive. Rarely occurs after 2 years.
- There may be lower abdominal pain, swellings, and pressure symptoms due to growth.
- There may be associated symptoms of metastasis (e.g., dyspnea and hemoptysis in lung metastasis).
- Per abdomen: Tenderness and uniformly enlarged uterus.
- Per speculum: Vaginal metastasis may appear as a bluish red vascular tumor which bleeds on touch.

Investigations

- Persistence or rising titer of *serum beta-hCG* in absence of pregnancy is indicative of GTN.
- Histopathology **(Fig. 3)** as above.
- Complete hemogram may show anemia due to bleeding and metastasis.
- Liver enzymes may be elevated if there is liver metastasis.
- Ultrasonography: Detects tumor **(Fig. 4)** cystic enlarged ovaries, and excludes remnants of conception.
- Doppler study shows increased vascularity in the uterine mass.
- Plain X-ray chest: It shows secondaries in lung; "Cannon balls" or "Snow storm" appearance.
- CT scan: It detects local extension and lung, liver, brain, and bone metastasis.

Role of Diagnostic Uterine Curettage

- Limited role in evaluation as intramural growth can remain be undetected.
- Prior chemotherapy and uterine curettage reduces the tumor bulk.
- Not used for routine histological diagnosis.
- Brisk hemorrhage can occur for which live saving hysterectomy may be needed.

Treatment of Choriocarcinoma

- Treatment is chemotherapy. Low risk—single agent chemotherapy; high risk—multiple agents chemotherapy. Hysterectomy reduces the total dose of chemotherapy.
- Sometimes, radiotherapy may be needed in condition like brain metastasis.
- Indication of hysterectomy—*see* below.

Q. How will you follow-up a case of choriocarcinoma?

Serum beta-hCG is measured weekly till it is undetectable for 3 consecutive week, thereafter monthly for 6 months and thereafter 6 monthly for whole life.

Death rate is 10–15%.

Placental Site Trophoblastic Tumor (PSTT)

Q. What are the features of PSTT?

- This trophoblastic neoplasia arises from the placental implantation site following term pregnancy, abortion, ectopic pregnancy or molar pregnancy. Uncommon (1–2% of all GTN) but important variant of choriocarcinoma. It occurs most commonly after term pregnancy.
- Histologically, there are predominantly cytotrophoblastic cells and arises from invasive intermediate trophoblast.
- Locally invasive. Primarily remain inside the uterus; rarely metastasize in very advanced cases to the lungs, liver or vagina **(Fig. 5)**.

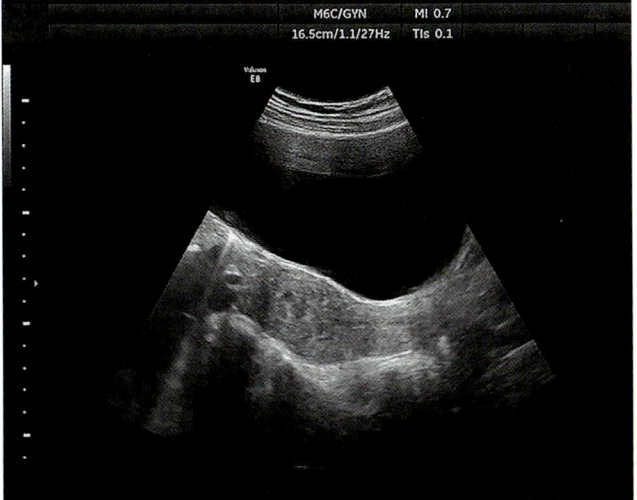

Fig. 4: Transabdominal sonography showing heterogenous opacity in uterine fundus in gestational trophoblastic neoplasia.
Courtesy: Professor Kamal Oswal

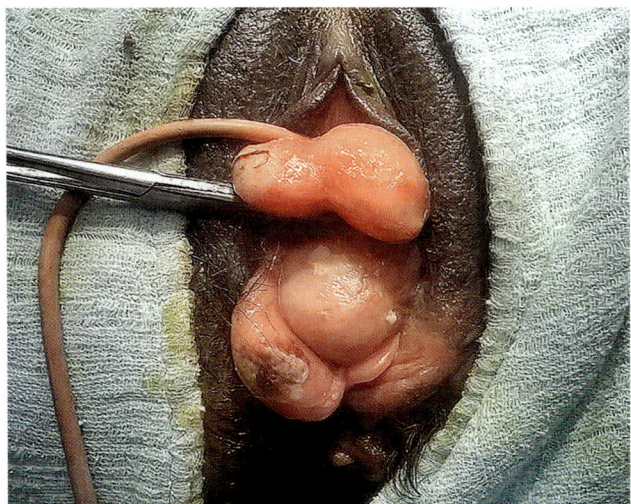

Fig. 5: Placental site trophoblastic tumor (PSTT) metastasis in vagina.
Courtesy: Professor Chandana Das, HOD, Obstetric and Gynecology, NRSMC, Kolkata

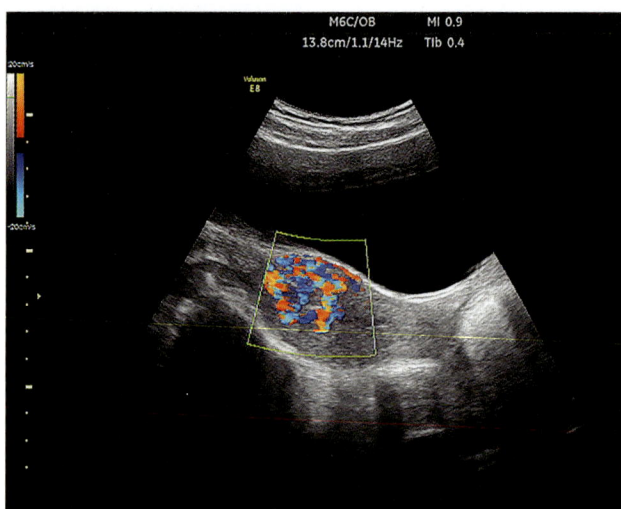

Fig. 6: Color Doppler study shows arteriovenous malformation in uterine fundus.
Courtesy: Professor Kamal Oswal

- Bleeding is the main symptom.
- Serum β-hCG level may be normal to elevated, produces small amount of hCG (<300) and human placental lactogen.
- Uterine arteriovenous fistula **(Fig. 6)** may be present.
- Hysterectomy is the most efficacious treatment for nonmetastatic variety as it is less sensitive to chemotherapy and if the ovaries are healthy these are not removed. Aggressive combined chemotherapy is given in metastatic variety. Radiation can also be given. 10-year survival is 70% but in advanced stage of IV it is much less.

Epithelioid Trophoblastic Tumor

- This is rare variety of trophoblastic tumor.
- It may develop many years after pregnancy.
- Usually reproductive age group patient presents with abnormal vaginal bleeding.
- It develops from chorionic type intermediate trophoblast by neoplastic transformation.
- Macroscopically presents as a discrete, hemorrhagic, solid, and cystic lesion located either in the fundus, lower uterine segment, or endocervix.
- Microscopically, uniform population of mononuclear intermediate trophoblastic cells forming nests and solid masses.
- Histologically, ETT is close to cervical squamous cell carcinoma (SCC). But ETT are positive for CK18 and human leukocyte antigen-G, cervical SCC is not.
- Metastasize in less than 25% cases, 10% became fatal.
- Diagnosis is done by endometrial biopsy.
- Hysterectomy is the treatment due to chemoresistance. Metastatic type is treated by multiagent therapy.

Q. What are the FIGO (International Federation of Gynecology and Obstetrics) criteria for diagnosis of post-molar GTN?

- Plateau of serum β-hCG level (±10%) for four measurements during a period of 3 weeks or longer—days 1, 7, 14, and 21.
- Rise of serum β-hCG more than 10% during 3 weekly consecutive measurements or longer during a period of 2 weeks or more—days 1, 7, and 14.
- The serum β-hCG level remains detectable for 6 months or more.
- Histological criteria for choriocarcinoma.

Q. How staging of GTN is done?

It is based on FIGO 2009 **(Table 1)**.

Table 1: FIGO anatomic staging of GTN (2009).	
Stage I	Disease confined to uterus
Stage II	Extends outside the uterus but limited to the genital structures
Stage III	Extends to the lung with/without genital tract involvement
Stage IV	All other metastatic sites

Abbreviations: FIGO, International Federation of Gynecology and Obstetrics; GTN, gestational trophoblastic neoplasia

Assessment of staging of choriocarcinoma is based on:
- Pelvic examination
- Chest X-ray
- CT of abdomen and pelvis for assessment of local extension
- CT/MRI of lungs, liver, and brain if metastasis is suspected.

Modified WHO Prognostic Scoring System as Adapted by FIGO

Modified WHO Prognostic Scoring System as adapted by FIGO is described in **Table 2**.

Q. How many patients are of low risk and how many are of high risk come in practice?

Ninety percent patients are of low risk and 10% belong to high risk.

Treatment of GTN

Primary treatment is *chemotherapy*, either by single agent therapy or multiagent therapy depending on the FIGO scoring system (2000).

Role of surgery: Hysterectomy is done in the following conditions:
- Primary treatment of PSTT, epithelioid trophoblastic tumor, and other chemoresistant cases
- In cases of uncontrolled vaginal or intra-abdominal bleeding as an emergency procedure
- Hysterectomy reduces the total dose of chemotherapy in low-risk cases.

Table 2: Modified WHO prognostic scoring system as adapted by FIGO.

Risk factor	0	1	2	4
Age	<40 years	≥40 years	–	–
Antecedent pregnancy	Mole	Abortion	Term	–
Interval months from index pregnancy	<4	4–6	7–12	>12
Pretreatment serum hCG* level	$<10^3$	10^3–10^4	10^4–10^5	$>10^5$
Largest tumor size (including uterus)	<3 cm	3–4 cm	≥5 cm	–
Site of metastases	–	Spleen, kidney	Gastrointestinal system	Liver, brain
Number of metastases	–	1–4	5–8	>8
Previous failed chemotherapy	–	–	1	≥2

*Scores of 0–6 are considered low risk. Scores of 7 and greater are considered high risk. The modified WHO prognostic scoring system is not applicable to patients with PSTT or ETT.
Abbreviations: FIGO, International Federation of Gynecology and Obstetrics; hCG, human chorionic gonadotropin; PSTT, placental site trophoblastic tumor; ETT, epithelioid trophoblastic tumor.

Disease Persistence after Hysterectomy in GTN

It is about 3–5%. Residual lung metastasis persists in 10–20% cases.

Chemotherapy for GTN Based on the FIGO 2000 Scoring System

- Women with score less than or equal to 6 are at low risk and treated with single-agent intramuscular methotrexate 50 mg on Day 1, 3, 5, 7 with tablet folinic acid 15 mg orally 24–30 hour after methotrexate on Day 2, 4, 6, 8. Repeat chemotherapy every 2 weekly. After hCG returned to normal, consolidation with 2–3 more cycle of chemotherapy needed to reduce chance of recurrence (FIGO-2015).
- Alternatively single agent actinomycin D can be used in low-risk group. If single agent fails combined regime is used.
- Women with score more than or equal to 7 are at high risk and are treated with multiagent chemotherapy which include methotrexate, actinomycin-D, etoposide, cyclophosphamide, and vincristine (**EMA–CO**).
- Bleomycine, etoposide, and cisplatin(BEP) regimen is also effective. Pembrolizumab, a passive immunotherapy agent, approved by FDA achieves good response.
- In high-risk cases, treatment is continued until the hCG level comes normal and then further 6 consecutive weeks.
- Cure rate is 100% in low-risk group and 95% in high-risk group.
- Adjuvant hysterectomy reduces total dose of chemotherapy.
- Radiotherapy is used for brain metastasis.

Dose of EMACO Regime (BAGSHWE Regime)

E = Etoposide (100 mg/m^2 IV infusion in saline over 30 minutes)

M = Methotrexate (100 mg/m^2 IV infusion over 12 hours)

A = Actinomycin D (0.5 mg IV stat)

C = Cyclophosphamide (600 mg IV in saline)

O = Vincristine (oncovin) (10 mg/IV stat).

Role of Radiotherapy

- Patient with brain metastasis: Whole brain radiation of 3,000 cGy over 10 days.
- High-dose intrathecal methotrexate used to prevent hemorrhage and for tumor shrinkage.
- Interventional radiotherapy (hepatic artery ligation or embolization) or whole liver radiation (2,000 cGy over 10 days) for liver metastasis.

Role of Surgery

Hysterectomy is considered in the following conditions:

When there is primary treatment failure of PSTT, epithelioid trophoblastic tumor, and other chemoresistant cases, in cases of uncontrolled vaginal or intra-abdominal bleeding (**Fig. 7**) as an emergency procedure. Hysterectomy reduces the total dose of chemotherapy in low-risk cases. Disease persistence after hysterectomy in GTN is about 3–5%. Residual lung metastasis persists in 10–20% cases.

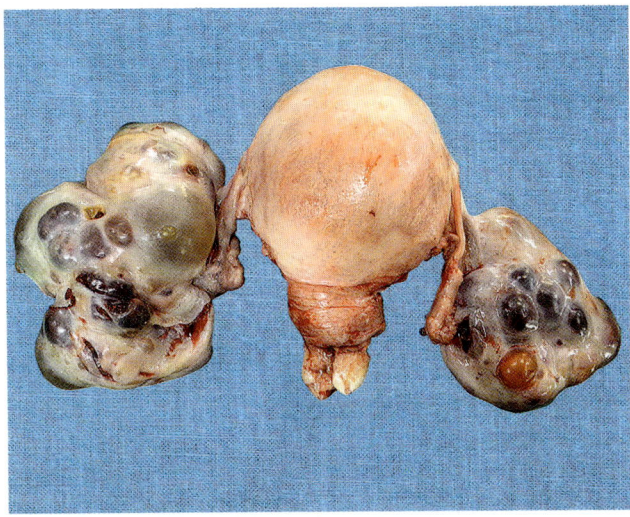

Fig. 7: Hysterectomy specimen showing bulky uterus and bilateral enlarged ovaries due to theca lutein cysts in a 38 years P2+0 patient, living issue 2 was admitted with recurrent excessive vaginal bleeding. Decision of hysterectomy was taken as there was uncontrolled bleeding. Initially, patient was tried with conservative treatment.
Courtesy: Dr Anirban Mondal, Associate Professor, Dr BC Kameswari, SR. BSMC

Other Surgery
Lung resection and craniotomy in lung and brain metastasis.

Survival Rate in GTN
In Stage I, II, and III survival rate is 100%.

Details of hydatidiform mole (complete and partial)—diagnosis, difference, complications, management and follow up—all are discussed in Author's Bedside Clinics in Obstetric, Fifth edition, Published by Academic Publishers.

A Case of Carcinoma Cervix and Premalignant Lesions of Cervix

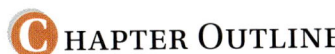

Writing a case of cancer cervix and how to present the case?

- Differential Diagnosis of Cancer Cervix
- Diagnosis and Stages of Cancer Cervix— Parameters of Staging
- Spread of Cancer Cervix
- Management of Cancer Cervix—Types of Hysterectomy
- Radical Hysterectomy and Trachelectomy
- Prognosis and Follow up
- Etiopathogenesis of Cancer Cervix—Role of HPV
- Premalignant Lesions of Cancer Cervix
- Comparison of Three Reporting System— Cervical Intraepithelial Neoplasia, Bethesda, Dysplasia/Carcinoma In situ
- Screening of Cervical Cancer
- Pap Test, Colposcopy—Illustrations
- Management Protocol of Premalignant Lesions—Ablative Procedures
- Human Papilloma Virus Vaccine

PATIENT'S PARTICULARS

1. Name: Bed No.:
2. Age: 39 years   Date of admission:
3. Address: Date of examination:
4. Occupation: ABC history of promiscuity
5. Married/unmarried: Almost invariably married
6. History of infertility:
7. Husband's occupation:
8. Socioeconomic status: Low
9. Religion:
10. Parous/nulliparous: Multiparous

HISTORY

- *Chief complaint or complaints:* Irregular vaginal bleeding (PV) for 6 months, history of postcoital bleeding, may be blood-stained white discharge.
- *History of present illness:* Elaborate the chief complaints. Try to assess the amount of bleeding as written in Chapter 1 of Section 1.

- ❖ *Menstrual history:*
  - Last menstrual period (LMP): Write when she had normal cyclical period
  - Duration of menstruation:
  - Interval in days:
  - Age of menarche:
  - Regularity of cycle:
  - Pain during period or if pain relation with menstruation:
  - Amount of bleeding:
  - Clot:
    - Intermenstrual bleeding—present during last 6 months
    - If any amenorrhea before this bleeding.
- ❖ *Obstetric history:*
  - Parity: Multiparous
  - Living issue (LI): Write "Nil" if patient is primi.
  - Last child birth (LCB)
  Detailed obstetric history is written in tabular form as written in Chapter 1 Section 1.
- ❖ *Past history:*
  - Medical: History of preinvasive lesion and their treatment

- Surgical: Any gynecological surgery for preinvasive lesion
- *Family history:* Nothing significant
- *Sexual history:* Multiple sexual partner, early age of coitus, early age of marriage, history of cervical cancer of previous spouse of husband
- *Functional history:*
  - Bowel: Rectal bleeding, constipation
  - Bladder: Dysuria, hematuria
  - Sleep
  - Appetite
- *Personal history:*
  - Personal hygiene
  - Smoking/alcohol
- *Contraceptive history:* Nonuse of barrier method and long use of combined oral contraceptives
- *Drug history:*
  - History of any drug allergy
  - History of intake of corticosteroids, antiepileptic or other drugs (previous or present)
- *Treatment history:* History of chemotherapy, radiotherapy.

PHYSICAL EXAMINATION

- Patient: Alert, conscious and cooperative
- Build
- Nutrition: Poor
- Height
- Weight or body mass index
- Edema
- Anemia: Present (degree of anemia reflects the severity of bleeding)
- Cyanosis
- Jaundice
- Clubbing
- Tongue, teeth, gum, tonsil
- Neck veins
- Neck glands
- Leg veins
- Pulse
- Respiration
- Temperature
- Blood pressure (BP).

Systemic Examination

- *Central nervous system*
- *Cardiovascular system:*
  - Auscultation of heart
- *Respiratory system:*
  - Auscultation of chest
- *Gastrointestinal system:*
  - Liver: May be palpable in case of metastasis
  - Spleen
- *Examination of other systems:*
  - Examination of back and spines skeletal system
  - Neurological
  - Ophthalmoscopic examination
  - Urinary system
- *Examination of breasts and nipple:*
  - Inspection
  - Palpation.

Gynecological Examination

- *Abdominal examination:*
  - Inspection: Lump, ascites in late cases
  - Palpation: Thoroughly palpated for any lump and other organs and any tenderness
  - Percussion: To detect fluid
  - Auscultation
- *Vaginal examination:*
  - Inspection and palpation of external genitalia
  - Speculum examination: A **fungating mass** protruding through the cervix is visualized which bleeds on touch **(Fig. 1)**.
  - Bimanual examination: Cervix is bulky and uterus is small, adnexa not palpable and pouch of Douglas (POD) is clear and growth is confined to cervix which bleeds on touch, no extent to vagina and no parametrial involvement.
  - Examination of rectovaginal area and rectal examination: Parametrium involvement. Extent of pelvic side wall involvement, rectal mucosa and uterosacral ligament involvement (as detailed below).

Summary of the Case (Sample Summary)

A 39-year-old multiparous with living issues 4 (last child birth 5 years), coming from low socioeconomic status, housewife

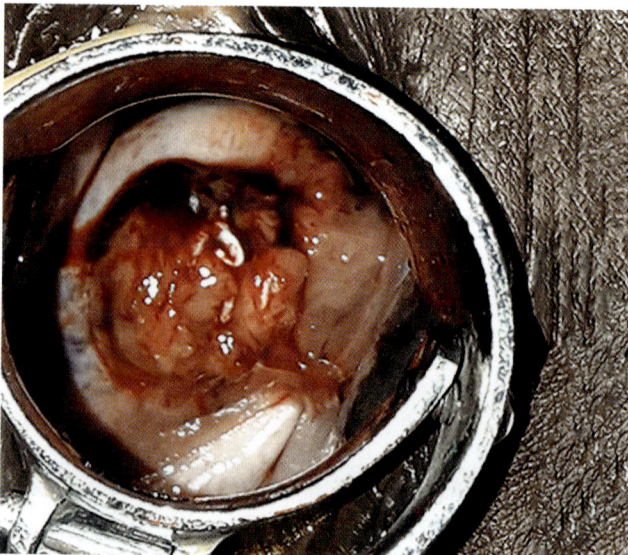

Fig. 1: A 39-year-old P3+0 woman complaining of heavy bleeding per vagina and watery discharge for last 10 months following 3 months of amenorrhea.

by occupation has been admitted with history of irregular vaginal bleeding for last 6 months. She also gives the history of bleeding during coitus. She has no other significant history.

- **On physical examination,** she has pallor, pulse, BP, edema present, no neck gland. Breast examination within normal limit.
- **On per abdominal examination,** abdomen is soft, nontender, no lump palpable, no organomegaly without any free fluid. On vaginal examination, vulva looks normal.
- **On speculum examination,** an ulcerative growth (3 cm in size) from the posterior lip of cervix is visualized which bleeds on touch.
- **On gentle bimanual examination,** cervix is bulky and uterus is small, adnexa not palpable and POD is clear and growth is confined to cervix and no vaginal and parametrial involvement.
- **Per rectal examination,** rectal mucosa freely mobile, cervix is bulky, parametrium is free in both side and there is free space between cervix and lateral vaginal wall and there is no rectal bleeding.
- **Histopathology** report shows squamous cell carcinoma of cervix.

Investigations Supplied or Required

Histopathological specimen shows squamous cell carcinoma of cervix.

Provisional Diagnosis

39 years women with irregular bleeding per vagina due to carcinoma cervix (early stage).

Differential Diagnosis (D/D)

Cervical polyp **(Fig. 2):** Red pedunculated mass arising from cervix or coming through os. Does not bleed on touch. Mass not friable. Biopsy confirms the diagnosis.

Cervical erosion **(Fig. 3):** Red velvety appearance, not indurated, no bleeding from surface or does not bleed on light touch. On rubbing, oozing may occur.

Cervical tuberculosis **(Fig. 4):** It may be vegetative, papillary or hypertrophic growth of cervix with or without ulceration giving a first impression of cancer and that may even bleed on touch. The lesion mostly ulcerative looking like an erosion. Ulcer margin is undermined. Diagnosis is confirmed by histology showing epithelioid granulomatous lesion with giant cells with or without caseation and presence of acid-fast bacilli in smear from cervix or from histological specimen or by culture of specimen. Result with treatment by multidrug regime of antitubercular (AT) drug for a long period is excellent with complete healing of cervix (*see* Chapter 33).

Cervical syphilitic ulcer: Ulcer is punched out (everted) with indurated base. History of exposure and venereal disease research laboratory positive. Biopsy confirms the diagnosis.

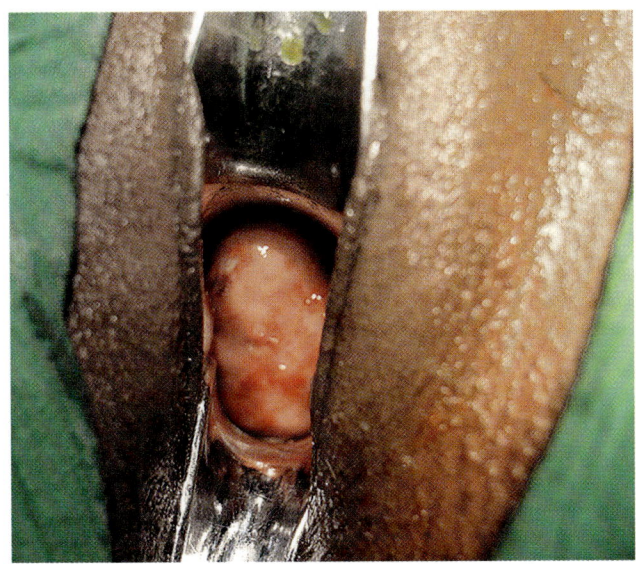

Fig. 2: Cervical polyp—a 38 year, P (2+0), presented with irregular and heavy menstrual bleeding for last 1 year. 4 cm-4 cm polypoidal mass felt coming out of external os (2).

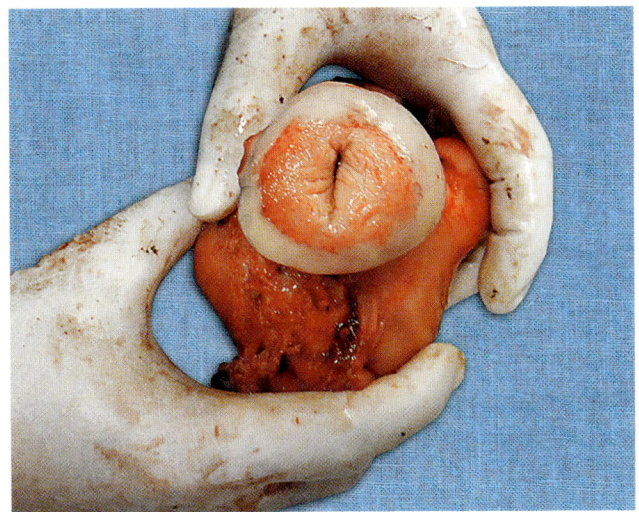

Fig. 3: Cervical erosion in a hysterectomy specimen.

Q. Why are you saying it as a cancer cervix?

Patient is young presented with irregular bleeding per vaginum with history of postcoital bleeding. On per speculum examination, there is a fungating growth arising from cervix, which bleeds on touch. Biopsy report shows squamous cell carcinoma.

Q. In which stage do you think and how did you determine?

Tell the stage on the basis of per vaginal and per rectal examinations and details of determining staging (*see* later).

Q. How would you diagnose a case of cancer cervix?

Diagnosis

- History
- Examination
- Investigations

SECTION 2: Clinical Cases

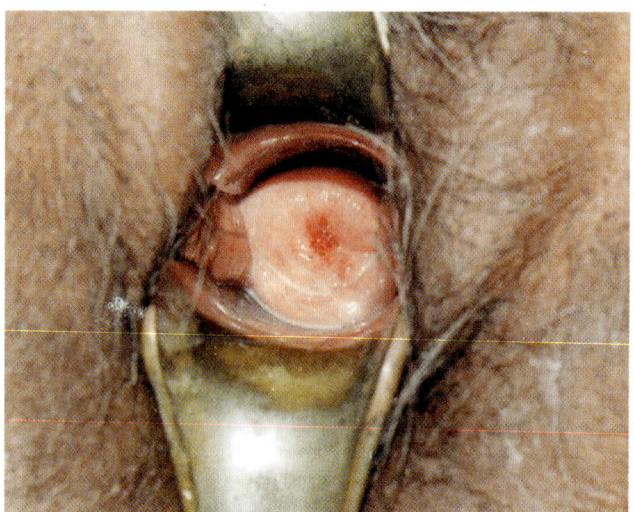

Fig. 4: Cervical tuberculosis—a 70 years parous woman presented with postmenopausal bleeding with suspected cancer cervix. She had past history of pulmonary tuberculosis 5 years back.

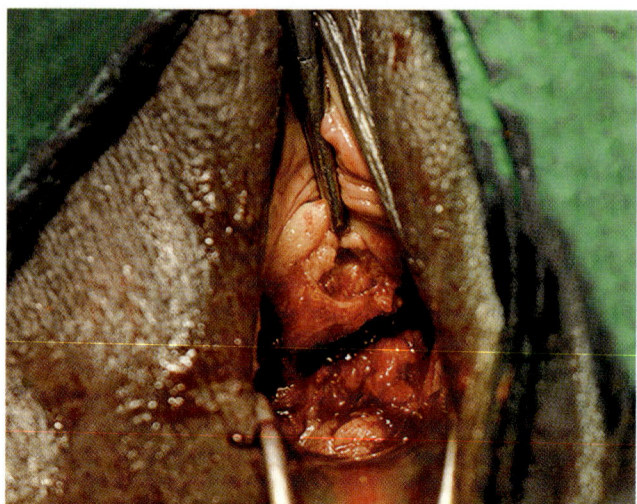

Fig. 5: Squamous cell carcinoma— friable growth.

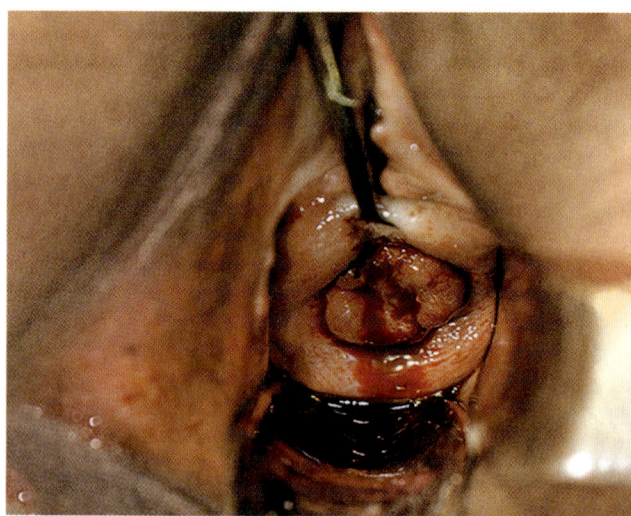

Fig. 6: Squamous cell carcinoma—a 60 years P 4+2 living issue 2 complaining of lower abdominal pain and 2 episodes of postmenopausal bleeding. Menopause 14 years back.

History

Symptoms and signs

- **Age:** Relatively younger—35–45 years in childbearing age
- **Parous:** Usually parous
- **History of vaginal bleeding:** Irregular, intermenstrual, postcoital bleeding, postmenopausal bleeding in menopausal women. First episode is usually following coitus or following straining at stool.
- Initially creamy or white discharge, blood-stained vaginal discharge, may be brown-stained, offensive discharge with characteristic odor.
- **In advanced stage:** Pain on back, rectal pain, deep pelvic pain, buttock due to spinal cord involvement, renal failure, incontinence of urine and stool (fistula), loss of weight, cachectic.
- May be asymptomatic in early stage, discovered during screening or loop biopsy in preinvasive carcinoma.

General Examination

- Edema
- Anemia, cachexia, neck gland and inguinal gland enlargement
- **Abdominal examination:** Usually nothing significant except advanced stage—hepatomegaly

Per Speculum Examination

In early stage, cervix looks hyperemic, eroded, later a growth is obvious or ulcerative lesion and bleeds on touch **(Figs. 5 and 6)**.

During speculum introduction in suspected cases, one must be very cautious as there may be torrential hemorrhage for which Sims' posterior vaginal speculum is better to be used and gently introduced instead of Cusco's bivalve speculum which may result sudden thrust on growth inflicting bleeding. Along with Sims' speculum, anterior vaginal wall retractor can be used for proper exposure. If such happens, tight vaginal pack is given immediately.

Bimanual Examination

Hardness, fixity and bleeding on examination are cardinal findings in established cases. In endocervical carcinoma, cervix becomes barrel shaped, feels broad and big, external os looks normal and diagnosis becomes difficult.

On vaginal examination, the followings things are noted:

- **Tumor:** Its size, character, papillary growth, ulcer or cauliflower growth, mobility and extension to vagina and parametrium
- **Uterus:** Size, position and mobility
- Adnexa.

On per rectal or rectovaginal examination, the following things are noted:
- Size of the cervix and uterus.
- Endocervical carcinoma is best evident by barrel-shaped cervix.
- Involvement of rectal mucosa
- Parametrium involvement and pelvic side wall involvement
- Induration of uterosacral ligaments

Rectovaginal examination under anesthesia (EUA) may be needed to see the size, fixity, parametrial, lateral wall involvement and vaginal involvement of growth. Parametrial involvement is best diagnosed by rectovaginal examination.

A central lesion as big as 8–10 cm size may not involve sidewall.

Complications of Cancer Cervix

- Uremia: Due to ureteral obstruction and infection
- Hydronephrosis
- Pyometra
- Vesicovaginal fistula and vesicocervical fistula and rarely rectovaginal fistula

Q. What are the causes of death in cancer cervix (in order of frequency)?
- Uremia: Most common cause of death
- Hemorrhage, infection and malnutrition
- Metastasis to vital organs
- Treatment complications.

Investigations for Diagnosis

- Pap smear in suspicious lesion
- Punch biopsy: Macroscopical growth **(Fig. 7)**
- Colposcopy and colposcopic directed biopsy (*see* **Fig. 25**)
- Endocervical curettage in suspected endocervical cancer
- Cone biopsy in microinvasive carcinoma.

Biopsy is ideal for diagnosis.

Pap smear cannot detect cervical cancer always. It is 53–80% sensitive for high-grade lesion in a single test. In stage I, only 30–50% is positive. For this, Pap smear alone in suspicious lesion is not favored and biopsy is taken.

Biopsy should be taken from *healthy and unhealthy zone,* not solely central zone which becomes often necrotic and deep to detect stromal invasion.

In Pap smear positive cases, colposcopy directed cervical and endocervical biopsy is performed. Cold knife conization is needed in some cases.

Cervical punch biopsy or conization specimens are best for invasion assessment. Other investigations for staging of carcinoma cervix are given later.

STAGES OF CANCER CERVIX (FIG. 8)

Q. What are the different stages of cancer cervix?

Staging system of cancer cervix has been revised by FIGO Oncology Committee in 2018 based on the recent development on imaging and use of minimally invasive surgery. Previously, FIGO staging was based on clinical examination with the addition of certain procedures. In the revised staging imaging and pathological findings, where available are allowed to determine the staging. Broadly, FIGO staging is categorized into four categories **(Table 1)** which are further subdivided **(Table 2)**.

Q. How would you determine staging?

Cancer cervix is staged clinically in contrast to endometrial cancer and ovarian cancer for both of which FIGO moved to surgicopathological staging. Staging of GTN is done on combined clinical and biological parameters.

Q. Parameters for assigning stage in cancer cervix in the revised FIGO staging system (2018).
- Clinical
- Pathological
- Any of the imaging modalities available—ultrasound, CT, MRI, positron emission tomography (PET)
- Needle aspiration or biopsy to exclude or diagnose lymph node metastasis in invasive disease
- X-ray chest, intravenous pyelography, renal USG in frank invasive carcinoma

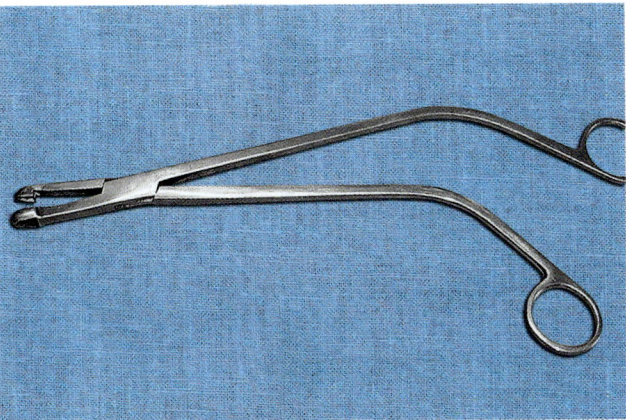

Fig. 7: Punch biopsy forceps.

Table 1: Staging of cancer cervix (FIGO 2018).	
Stage I	The carcinoma is strictly confined to the cervix (extension to the corpus is disregarded)
Stage II	The carcinoma invades beyond the uterus, but has not extended up to the lower third of the vagina or onto the pelvic wall
Stage III	The carcinoma extends onto the lower third of the vagina and/or extends up to the pelvic wall and/or hydronephrosis or nonfunctioning kidney due to tumor and/or involvement of pelvic and/or para-aortic lymph nodes
Stage IV	The carcinoma has extended beyond the true pelvis or has involved (proved by biopsy) the mucosa of the bladder or rectum. A bullous edema, as such, is not regarded to allot the case to stage IV

Table 2: Detailed FIGO staging of carcinoma of the cervix (2018).

Stage I: The carcinoma is strictly confined to the cervix (extension to the corpus is disregarded)
- **IA:** Invasive carcinoma which can be diagnosed only by microscopy, with maximum invasion in depth <5 mm[a]
  - **IA1:** Stromal invasion measurement <3 mm in depth
  - **IA2:** Stromal invasion measurement ≥3 mm and <5 mm in depth
- **IB:** Invasive carcinoma with deepest invasion ≥5 mm (more than stage IA), lesion confined to the cervix uteri[b]
  - **IB1:** Invasive carcinoma ≥5 mm in depth of stromal invasion and <2 cm invasion in greatest dimension
  - **IB2:** Invasive carcinoma ≥2 cm and <4 cm in maximum dimension
  - **IB3:** Invasive carcinoma ≥4 cm in maximum dimension

Stage II: The carcinoma invades beyond the uterus, but has not extended up to the lower third of the vagina or onto the pelvic wall
- **IIA:** Involvement limited to the upper two-thirds of the vagina without any parametrial involvement
  - **IIA1:** Invasive carcinoma which is <4 cm in greatest dimension
  - **IIA2:** Invasive carcinoma which is ≥4 cm in greatest dimension
- **IIB:** Parametrial involvement but not reaching up to the pelvic wall

Stage III: The carcinoma extends onto the lower third of the vagina and/or extends up to the pelvic wall and/or hydronephrosis or nonfunctioning kidney due to tumor and/or involvement to pelvic and/or para-aortic lymph nodes[c]
- **IIIA:** Involvement of the lower third of the vagina, but no extension to the pelvic wall
- **IIIB:** Extension to the pelvic wall and/or hydronephrosis or nonfunctioning kidney due to tumor
- **IIIC:** Involvement of pelvic and/or para-aortic lymph nodes, irrespective of the size and extent of tumor (notations with r and p)[c]
  - **IIIC1:** Metastasis of pelvic lymph node only
  - **IIIC2:** Metastasis of para-aortic lymph node

Stage IV: The carcinoma has extended beyond the true pelvis or has involved (proved by biopsy) the mucosa of the bladder or rectum. A bullous edema, as such, is not regarded to allot the case to stage IV
- **IVA:** Spread of growth to adjacent organs
- **IVB:** Spread to the distant organs

[a] Imaging and pathology can be used, when available, in addition to clinical findings with regards to tumor size and extent, in all stages
[b] Vascular/lymphatic spaces involvement does not change the staging. The lateral extent of the lesion is not considered in new staging system
[c] Notation of r for imaging and p for pathology are added to indicate the findings that are used for allocating the case to stage IIIC. For example, if pelvic lymph node metastasis is determined by imaging, the stage would be written stage IIIC1r and, if confirmed by pathological findings, it would be written as stage IIIc1p. The type of imaging modality or pathology technique used should always be recorded. If there is any doubt, the lower staging should be assigned

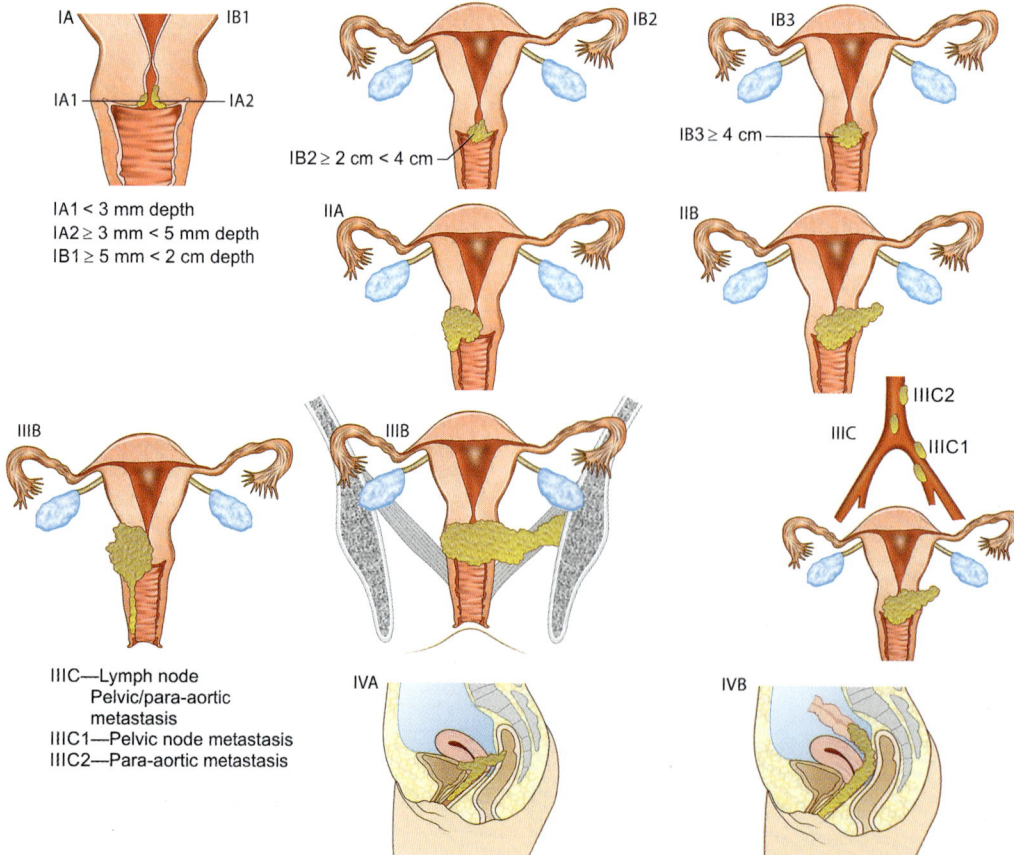

Fig. 8: Stages of cancer cervix.

❖ Cystoscopy, sigmoidoscopy not mandatory, but recommended on basis of on clinical findings (*see* below).

Q. Staging of microinvasive disease.

❖ Stage IA1 and IA2 is diagnosed on microscopical examination of a specimen obtained by loop electrosurgical method (LEEP) or cone biopsy (entire lesion) or trachelectomy or hysterectomy. The depth should be <3 mm (IA1) or <5 mm. Horizontal measurement is no longer considered due to artefactual errors. The margins should be negative, if positive it will be allocated to stage IB1.
❖ The lesions with larger dimensions or which are clinically visible are allocated in stage IB which is subdivided in IB1, IB2 and IB3 in revised staging depending on dimension.
❖ Lymphovascular space involvement must be noted as it helps to make treatment plan though it does not change the staging.
❖ For staging, extension to uterine corpus is not needed as it has neither effect on treatment nor on prognosis.

Q. Staging of invasive disease (Fig. 9).

❖ Clinical assessment is the primary step to allocate staging.
❖ In clinically visible lesions biopsy is taken by punch biopsy, if not satisfactory by small loop biopsy or by cone.
❖ Imaging assessment is done next as per availability—USG, CT, MRI and PET to evaluate tumor size, nodal status, and spread. MRI is the best in case of primary growth >10 mm. USG is also a good method in expert hands. Methods used are noted for future record. For detection of nodal metastasis >10 mm, PET scan is better than CT and MRI with few false negative results. Imaging is very useful to select the appropriate therapy, surgery or radiation to avoid dual therapy.
❖ In radical surgery pathological assessment is possible. Alternatively, needle aspiration cytology/biopsy can be done.
❖ In the revised staging system, all cases with lymph node involvement is assigned as stage IIIC irrespective of tumor size and extent, as lymph node involvement has a worse prognostic factor in cancer cervix, and para-aortic lymph node involvement is found in significant percentage of cases irrespective of the stages. Stage IIIC is further subdivided into IIIC1 (pelvic lymph nodes only) and IIIC2 (para-aortic lymph nodes). Notation of r (imaging) and p (pathology) is given depending upon which, the allocation of stage IIIC has been done.
❖ X-ray chest, intravenous pyelography and renal USG are done in frank invasive carcinoma.
❖ Other routine investigations, cystoscopy, sigmoidoscopy are not mandatory but done in clinically symptomatic cases. Cystoscopy is also recommended in barrel-shaped cervical growth and growth extended to the anterior vaginal wall.
❖ Bullous edema is not merely regarded as bladder involvement (stage IV) until and unless proved by biopsy.
❖ Pathological staging is done from surgical specimen or image-guided FNAC.

In revised system final staging is done after imaging and complete pathological reports are available. TNM classification is used for documenting nodal and metastatic disease status.

Q. Key changes in staging of cancer of cervix (FIGO 2018).

❖ Stage I: Definition of lesion size and microinvasion.
  ▪ Stage IA: Lateral dimension is removed

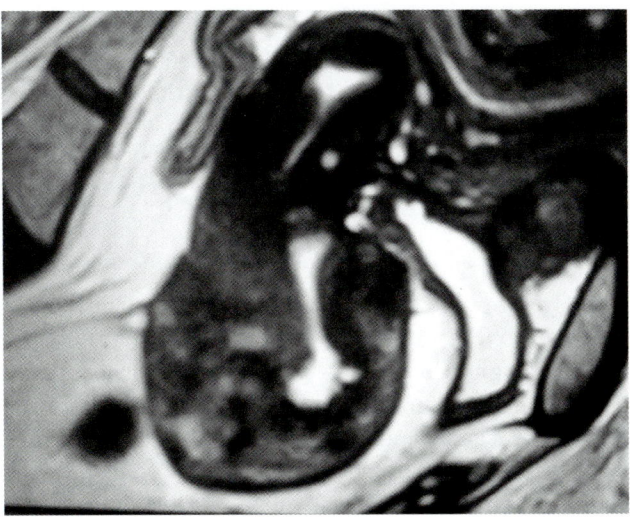

Fig. 9: MRI of cancer cervix. Large growth involving lower part of body of uterus.
Courtesy: Professor M Karmakar, Radiology, IPGMER, Kolkata

  ▪ Stage IB: Three subgroups instead of two subgroups—stage IB1: invasive carcinomas ≥5 mm and <2 cm in greatest diameter; stage IB2: tumors ≥2 cm and <4 cm; stage IB3: tumors ≥4 cm
❖ Stage IIIC has been added in metastatic cases; Stage III C1—only pelvic lymph nodes, Stage III C2—involvement of para-aortic lymph nodes. Notations r (imaging) and p (pathology) will indicate the method used to assign staging. Lymph node involvement did not change the stage in previous staging, but in new system in positive lymph node patient is upstaged to stage IIIC irrespective of tumor size and extent.
❖ Other than assessment of primary tumor by clinical evaluation, imaging (not specific) and pathology findings have been incorporated to assign new staging system.
❖ Use of any imaging modality and/or pathological findings for allocating the stage has been allowed, to assess the size of primary tumor, to assess the extent to the surrounding tissues and adjacent organs, and to assess the location and characteristics of the retroperitoneal lymph nodes.
❖ In stages I through III assessment of retroperitoneal lymph nodes by imaging and/or pathological findings is allowed.
❖ No recommendations for routine investigations and procedures, which are to be decided on the basis of clinical findings and standard of care.

Stages of Cervical Cancer at Diagnosis

❖ Stage I: 38%
❖ Stage II: 32%
❖ Stag III: 26%
❖ Stage IV: 4%

Q. What do you mean by early stage?
- *Early stage:* Stage IA, Stage B1, B2 and Stage IIA1 (except IB2) (where tumor size is <4 cm and primary operation can be done)
- *Advanced stage:* Stage B3 and IIA2 and higher

Pathology of Cervical Cancer
Macroscopic
- Of the total, 80% from ectocervix:
  - Hypertrophic or exophytic producing cauliflower-like growth **(Figs. 10A to C)**
  - Eroding and ulcerative—early growth simulates erosion
- Remaining 20% from endocervix: Papillary nodes appear in cervical canal and invades the cervix making it barrel shaped. Vaginal part looks healthy but becomes wide.

Microscopic (histological types)
- Squamous cell carcinoma—commonest: 70% **(Fig. 11)**—keratinizing, nonkeratinizing and papillary
- Adenocarcinoma: 25% **(Fig. 12)**
- Mucinous, endocervical, villoglandular, intestinal and minimal deviation, endometrioid
- Serous carcinoma
- Clear cell carcinoma
- Adenosquamous carcinoma
- Glassy cell
- Adenoid cystic carcinoma
- Adenoid basal carcinoma
- Small cell carcinoma
- Undifferentiated carcinoma

Squamous cell carcinoma arises from ectocervix and is declining for last 3 decades for screening of early squamous lesions. Adenocarcinoma arises from endocervical columnar cells and as it grows in endocervix, it is diagnosed in advanced stage and cervix becomes barrel shaped. From endocervix, both squamous cell and adenocarcinoma may arise.

Spread of Cervical Cancer
- Direct spread
- Lymphatic spread
- Hematogenous spread.

Direct spread: By continuity to stroma cervix, vagina, uterus, parametrium and by contiguity to urinary bladder (through vescicouterine ligaments) and rectum. Invasion of rectum occurs less due to the presence of intervening space, pouch of Douglas.

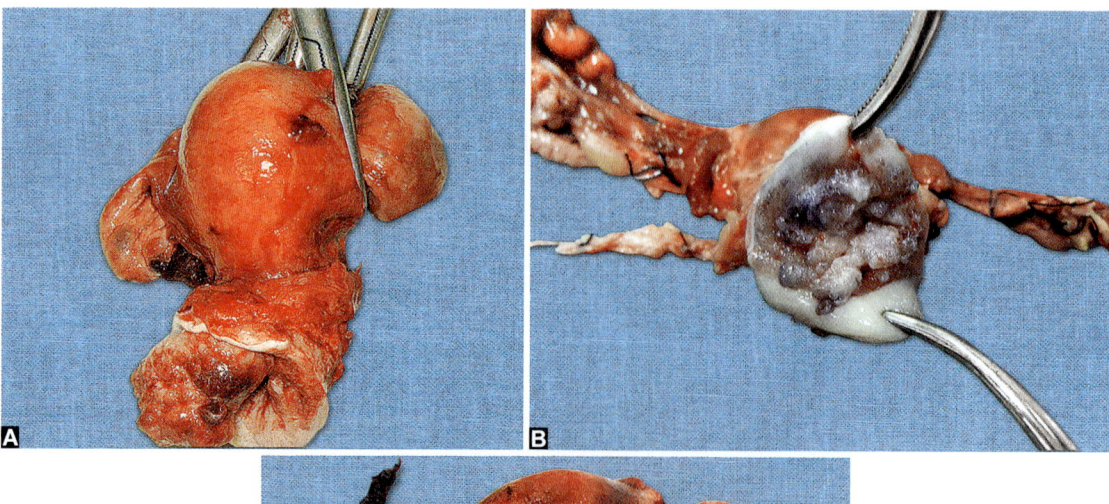

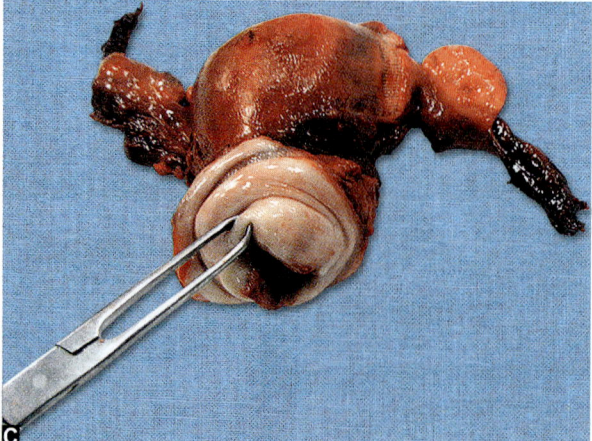

Figs. 10A to C: Hypertrophic or exophytic growth. (A) Radical hysterectomy specimen; (B) Cauliflower growth of cervix; (C) Ulcerative growth in one lip.

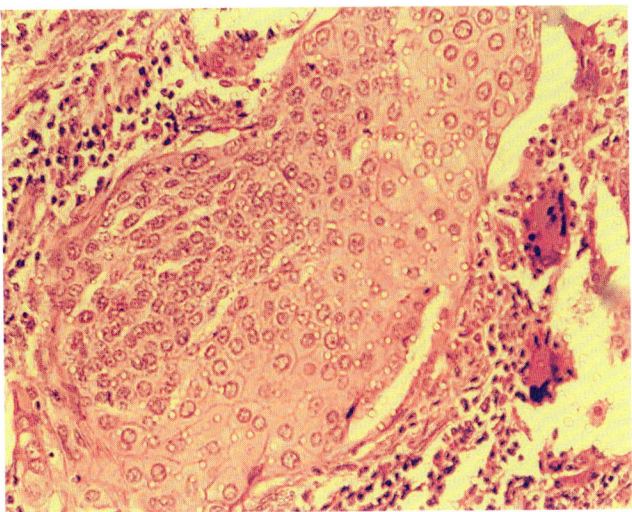

Fig. 11: Squamous cell carcinoma of cervix high power.
Courtesy: Dr Tripti Das

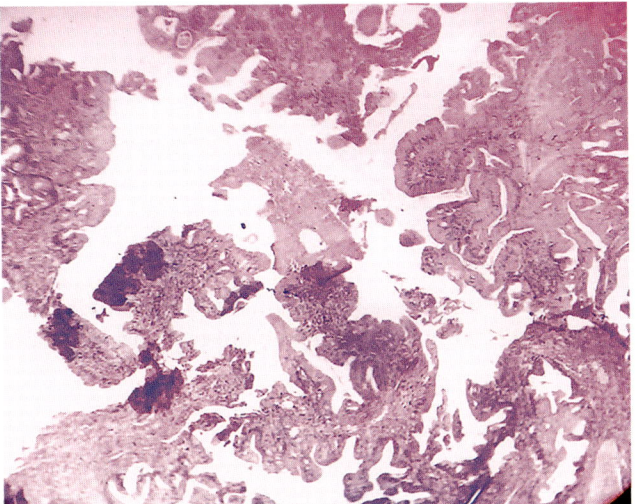

Fig. 12: Adenocarcinoma cervix.

Lymphatic spread: Pelvic lymph nodes—parametrial, paracervical, obturator, internal iliac, external iliac, common iliac, ultimately para-aortic (*see* below).

Hematogenous spread: Lungs, ovary, liver, bones, kidney and brain. Ovarian metastasis occurs 15% in squamous cell carcinoma and 19% in endocervical adenocarcinoma.

Intraperitoneal implantation

Q. What do you mean by lymphovascular space involvement?

Tumor invades into the blood capillaries and lymph channel, the presence of which indicates poor prognosis, particularly in early stage though it is not included in staging process.

Q. What is the percentage of lymph node involvement according to stage of carcinoma cervix? (Table 3).

Table 3: Lymph node involvement according to stage of carcinoma cervix.

Stage	Stage IA1 (3 mm)	Stage IA2 (>3–5 mm)	Stage IB	Stage IIA	Stage IIB	Stage III	Stage IVA
Pelvic node (%)	0.5	5	15	25	30	45	45
Para-aortic node (%)	0	<1	2	10	20	30	40

The overall stage-wise involvement of lymph nodes in cancer cervix is as follows:
Stage IA1: 0.5%
Stage IA2: 5%
Stage IB: 15%
Stage II: 30%
Stage III: 45%
Stage IV: 60%.

LYMPHATIC DRAINAGE OF CANCER CERVIX

Q. Discuss lymphatic drainage of cancer cervix and its clinical importance (Fig. 13).

The spread of the tumor typically occurs along cervical lymphatic drainage. Hence, knowledge of cervical lymphatics is very essential for proceedings of appropriate surgical steps for cancer surgery.

The cervix has an abundant network of lymphatics along the course of uterine artery.

The lymphatic channels drain principally into the *paracervical and parametrial lymph nodes* wherefrom the lymph passes to *obturator nodes* and to *internal, external, common iliac lymph nodes* and finally into *para-aortic lymph nodes*.

From the posterior part of cervix lymphatic channels pass through the rectal pillars and uterosacral ligaments to drain into the *rectal lymph nodes*.

Hence, it is very important that in radical hysterectomy:
* Paracervical and parametrial lymph nodes are removed by parametrial resection.
* All pelvic lymph nodes (obturator, internal iliac and external iliac)
* Common iliac lymph nodes with or without para-aortic lymph nodes up to the level of inferior mesenteric artery are traditionally removed.

Lymphovascular space involvement, as described above, indicates poor prognosis and often needs tailoring the planned surgical procedure and adjuvant radiotherapy.

Inguinal lymph nodes are involved occasionally either by retrograde flow through external iliac vessels or in late cases through involvement of vagina.

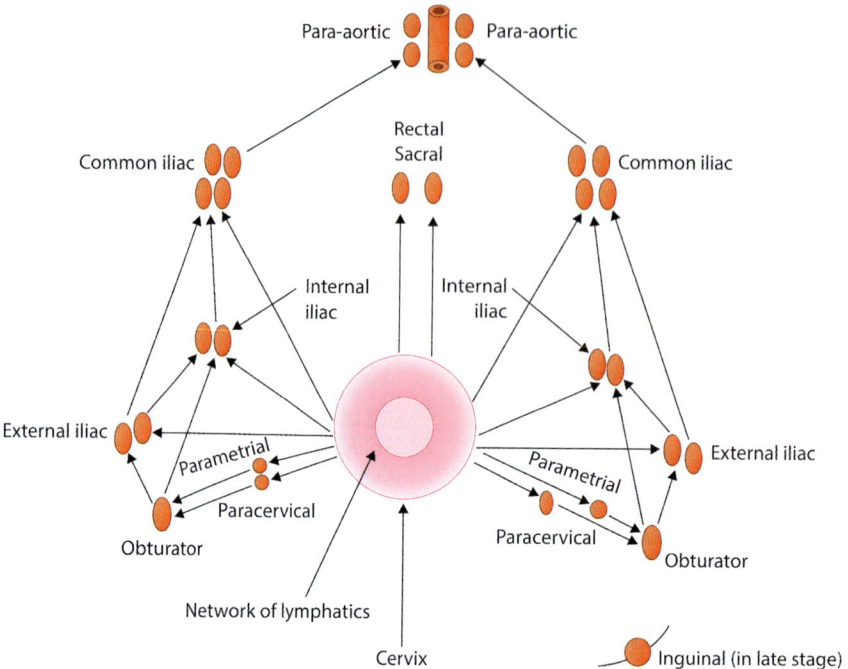

Fig. 13: Lymphatic drainage of cervix.

MANAGEMENT OF CANCER CERVIX

Q. How would you manage your case? Discuss the management of cancer cervix.

Treatment depends on the stage of the disease in cervical carcinoma.

- **Early stage** (stage I to stage IIA): Treatment is surgery and radiation therapy.
- **Advanced stage** (stage IIB to stage IV): Primarily radiation with or without chemotherapy (chemoradiation).

Treatment Modalities of Invasive Cancer Cervix are:

- **Surgery:** Mostly radical (Wertheim's operation) in younger age ovaries may be preserved. Fertility sparing surgery, trachelectomy, a novel development in surgical technique is done in early cases. *Conization* is done in very early cases (stage IA1).
- Radiation
- Chemotherapy
- Combined

Outline of stage-wise management of primary invasive cancer cervix is shown in **Table 4** and types are described in **Table 5**.

Types of Hysterectomy

It is classified into five types by Piver et al. (1974) and later revised by European Organization for Research and Treatment of Cancer (2004) depending on site of uterine artery ligation and extent of parametrial resection. Revised five types are described in **Table 5**.

Table 4: Stage-wise management of primary invasive cancer cervix.

Stage		Treatment	Pelvic lymphadenectomy
Stage IA1	No lymphovascular space involvement (LVSI)	Simple hysterectomy (type I) if family completed or Conization	No
	With LVSI	*Modified radical hysterectomy (type II) Or **Cervical conization/radical trachelectomy in patients desiring fertility	Yes Yes
Stage IA2		Radical hysterectomy (type III) or modified hysterectomy (type II) Or Radical trachelectomy or cervical conization in patients desiring fertility	Yes Yes
Stage IB1		Radical hysterectomy (type II or III) or Radical trachelectomy in patients desiring fertility	Yes

Contd...

CHAPTER 8: A Case of Carcinoma Cervix and Premalignant Lesions of Cervix

Contd...

Stage	Treatment	Pelvic lymphadenectomy
Stage IB2 IIA1	Radical hysterectomy (type III) or Chemoradiation	Yes
Stage IB3 IIA 2	Chemoradiation	
Stage IIB to IVA	Chemoradiation or rarely primary exenteration	
Stage IVB	Palliative chemotherapy and/or palliative radiation or supportive care	

*Surgery can be done abdominal route, vaginal route, laparoscopic or robotic
**In case of cervical conization where lymphadenectomy needed is done by laparoscopy or extraperitoneal pelvic lymphadenectomy

Table 5: Types of hysterectomy.

		Components of structures removed/tackled			
Type	Name	Parametrium and paracolpos tissue	Vagina	Uterine vessels	Uterosacral ligament
I A	Simple hysterectomy or extrafascial hysterectomy	Not removed	Not removed	Ligated at isthmus of uterus	Cut at junction with uterus
II B	Modified radical hysterectomy	Removed the tissue medial to ureter	Upper vagina 1–2 cm removed	Ligated at the site of crossing of ureter	Cut near rectum
III C	Radical hysterectomy	Entire parametrium from the origin of uterine artery	Upper third of vagina ≥2 cm	Ligated at the origin from internal iliac artery	Cut near rectum
IV	Extended radical hysterectomy	Entire parametrium from the origin of uterine artery	Upper 3/4th of vagina	Ligated at the origin from internal iliac artery, ligate superior vescical artery	Cut near rectum
V	Partial exenteration	Entire parametrium from the origin of uterine artery	Upper 3/4th of vagina, terminal ureter, segment of bladder or rectum is removed	Ligated at the origin from internal iliac artery, ligated superior vesical artery	Cut near rectum

RADICAL HYSTERECTOMY

Q. What do you mean by radical hysterectomy (Figs. 14 and 15)?

It includes:
- Total hysterectomy, bilateral salpingo-oophorectomy
- Parametrium
- Upper third of vagina
- Pelvic lymph nodes
- Uterine artery ligation at origin **(Fig. 15A)**
  See **Table 5** for detailed types

Q. In which route it is done?

Abdominal route: Open (Wertheim's operation), laparoscopic
Vaginal route: Schauta's operation, Mitra's operation

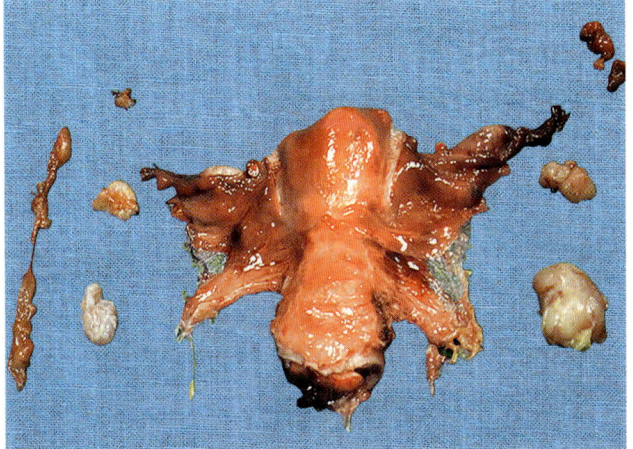

Fig. 14: Specimen following Wertheim operation including lymph nodes.
Courtesy: Professor RP Ganguly

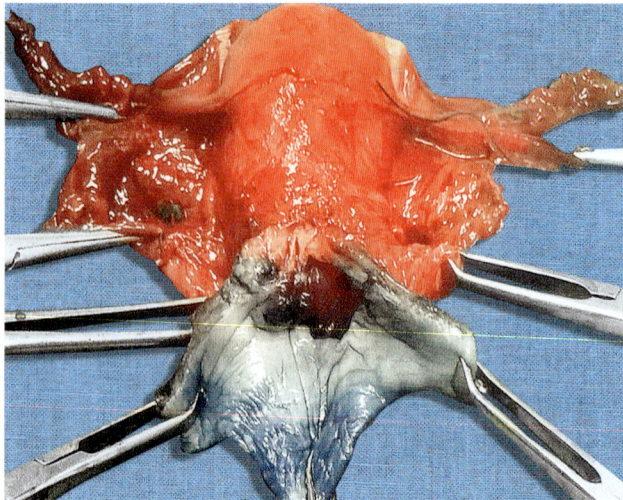

Fig. 15: Specimen following Wertheim operation—TAH with BSO with removal of parametrium and vaginal cuff. Lymph nodes are not shown here.

Courtesy: Professor Chandana Das, NRS Medical College, Kolkata

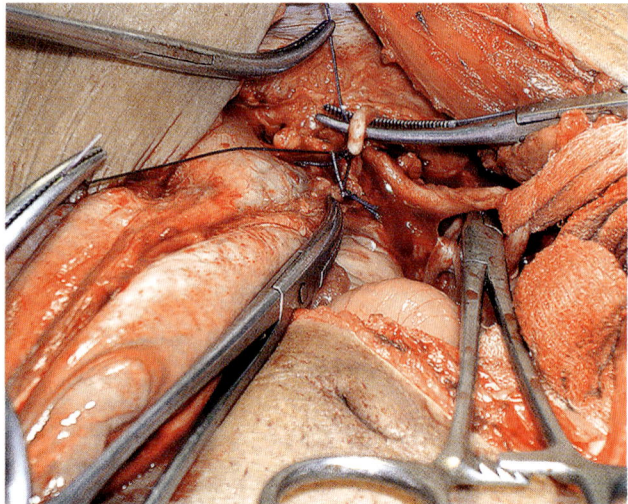

Fig. 15A: Uterine artery crossing ureter (left side). Uterine artery ligated in radical hysterectomy.

Courtesy: Professor Sukanta Mishra, Head, Obstetrics and Gynecology, VIMS, Kolkata

Wertheim's Operation

Abdominal—*Wertheim's (Ernst Wertheim 1864-1920) operation:* This may be:
- Bonney type (1941)—radical hysterectomy is done first followed by lymphadenectomy
- Meigs (1954) or Okabayashi—lymphadenectomy first followed by hysterectomy.

Main Steps of Radical Hysterectomy

- Cutting of round ligaments and dissecting the para vesical space
- Cutting of uterovesical fold of peritoneum and dissection of uterovesical space
- Clamping and cutting of infundibulopelvic ligament/tubo-ovarian ligament
- Identification of ureter, identification of uterine artery and ligation of uterine artery
- Dissection of ureter up to ureteric tunnel followed by dissection of ureteric tunnel and displacing the ureter laterally.
- Dissecting the pararectal spaces and rectovaginal space
- Excision of uterosacral—Mackendrot's ligament complex
- Excision of vaginal cuff
- Removal of pelvic lymph nodes (*see* below).

Lymph node involvement is determined by:
- Imaging—USG, CT and MRI mapping of lymph node involvement
- Identification of lymph nodes by injecting blue dye into cervical tissue before surgery
- Obturator gland is sentinel node, if not involved lymph node dissection is not necessary
- Image guided FNAC

Steps of lymph node dissection in radical hysterectomy—abdominal method (Fig. 15B)

- All visible lymph nodes should be removed through extent and techniques differ from surgeon to surgeon.
- Removal starts from bifurcation of common iliac artery and extended downwards. If any enlarged node is detected the dissection is extended cranially for search of common iliac and para-aortic nodes.
- With the help of retractors one above and medially displacing ureter and the other retracted below and laterally the area along the common iliac vessels and external iliac vessels are exposed. Using tooth dissecting forceps fascia over the iliopsoas muscle is incised along the artery up to the ingunal ligament from where lateral external iliac lymph nodes are drawn avoiding the injury of genitofemoral nerve. Individual lymphatic channels are diathermized very cautiously. Any torn small vessels

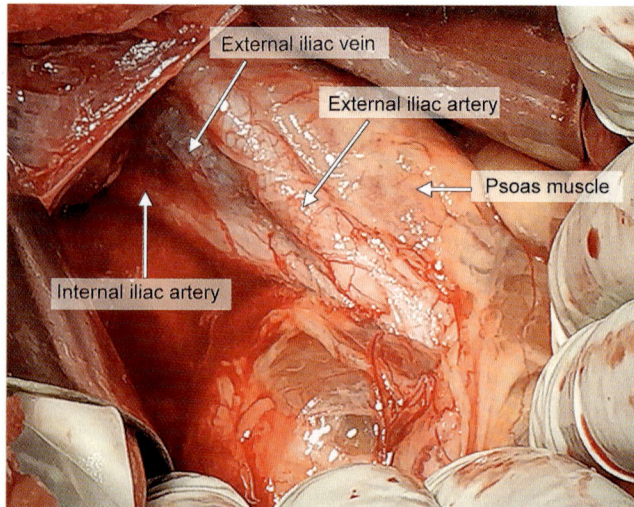

Fig. 15B: Lymphadenectomy in open abdominal approach showing the bifurcation of right common iliac artery along which lymph nodes are situated. External iliac artery lies over the psoas muscle. Medial to external iliac artery lies internal iliac artery and in between lies external iliac vein. Internal iliac vein lies medial and posterior to internal iliac artery (not visible here).

are ligated or diathermized. Dissection of the fascia and nodal tissue were done over the entire length of external artery, the procedure will make the vessel nude. All nodal tissue can be removed enbloc if the tissue is kept under tension with the forceps by left hand and dissection is done by scissor with the right hand.

- Then external iliac artery is retracted laterally to expose the external iliac vein, the fascia and nodal tissue over which is removed in the similar way but very gently.
- From the upper end of external iliac vessels the fascial tissue over the internal iliac artery is separated downwards.
- Dissection dipping below the external iliac vein will expose the obturator fossa which can be emptied of all nodal tissue in the final stage. Exposure of obturator fossa becomes easier by retracting the external vein and artery laterally. Following lifting of tissue bulk obturator nerve and vessels are visible. Any bleeding over the area is cauterized or pressed with gauze for hemostasis.

Vaginal (Radical Vaginal Hysterectomy)

Schauta's operation—the disadvantage is that there is no provision of lymphadenectomy.

Mitra's Operation

Q. What is Mitra's operation?

Hysterectomy through vaginal route and *lymphadenectomy* in extraperitoneal approach **(Fig. 15C)**. Mitra (1954) from India introduced bilateral lymphadenectomy through extraperitoneal approach with radical vaginal hysterectomy.

It is claimed that more parametrium removal is possible through vaginal route.

Laparoscopic radical hysterectomy and pelvic and para-aortic lymphadenectomy are novel approaches and have similar efficacy and similar recurrence to open method with advantages of less blood loss, wound complication and less hospital stay.

Robotic surgery is also coming into picture.

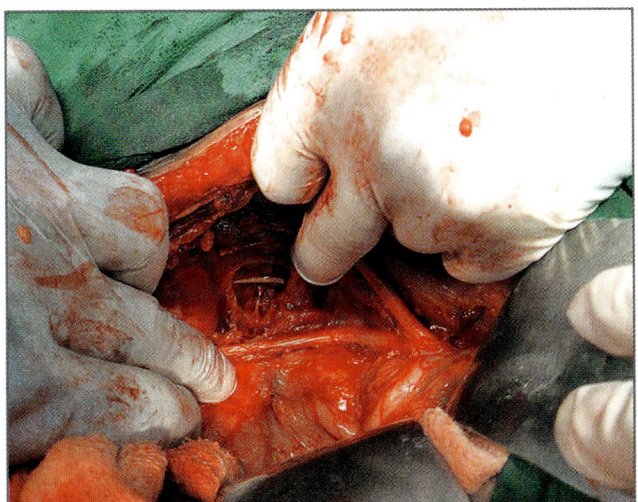

Fig. 15C: Lymphadenectomy in extraperitoneal approach showing obturator fossa.

Trachelectomy

Q. What is trachelectomy?

Radical vaginal trachelectomy (RVT) is fertility preserving operation for treatment of invasive cervical cancer.

Selection Criteria of Trachelectomy

- Desire of children
- Size of growth less than 2 cm
- Stage 1A and 1A2 cancer cervix with LVSI
- Stage 1B1
- Cervical cancer at least 1 cm away from internal cervical os in MRI
- No pelvic metastasis.

Procedure of Trachelectomy

It consists of 80% removal of cervix, upper vagina and transection of Mackenrodt's ligament on both side and removal of paracervical tissue.

It is done in two steps, firstly to exclude metastasis by laparoscopy and then radical resection of the cervix along with a vaginal cuff and the paracervical tissue.

Pregnancy Outcome

Chance of pregnancy 30–40% after 1 year, miscarriage 25%, preterm labor 20%, and recurrence 5%.

Chemoradiation

Chemoradiation should be completed within 56 days. If para-aortic node involvement is suspected, then it should be included along with pelvic field of radiation.

Both teletherapy and brachytherapy is used. Usually radiotherapy is given on D1–D5 of every week (teletherapy by either telecobalt-60 or linear accelerator or betatron). Mapping of teletherapy done by CT/MRI/PET CT.

Usually, total dose of radiation is 80 Gy at point A and 60 G at point B, of which 40–50 Gy is given by teletherapy and rest by brachytherapy.

Point A: 2 cm above lateral fornix and 2 cm lateral from uterine canal.

Point B: 3 cm lateral to point A. After 3 weeks of teletherapy, start brachytherapy (nowadays, high dose rate using Iridium 192 is preferred instead of low dose rate which uses cesium 137).

Chemotherapy

For chemotherapy, weekly Cisplatin 40 mg/m^2 is usually used (on D1).

In early stage, both mortality and survival rate is same in primary chemoradiation and surgery. But surgery is preferred in young patients, patients wish to preserve fertility, patients with irritable bowel syndrome and previous history of radiation.

Post-treatment Follow-up of Cervical Cancer

Every 3–4 months for first 2–3 years as most recurrence occurs within 3 years, then 6 monthly until 15 years, then annually for lifelong. In case of uterine preserving surgery—PAP smear 3 months for 2 years, 6 months for next 3 years.

Prognosis of Cancer Cervix

Overall 5 years survival of all stages of cervical cancer is 75% whereas those of uterine cancer is 85% and epithelial ovarian cancer is 45%.

Survival Rates According to Stage

- Stage IA: 100%
- Stage IB: 90%
- Stage IIA: 70%
- Stage IIB: 45%
- Stage III: 15–40%
- Stage IVA: 15–35%.

Q. How would you prevent cancer cervix?

See later (Page 182)

Q. What is the magnitude of problem of cancer cervix in India and developed country?

In India, cervical cancer is the most common (80%) genital malignancy in contrast to developed country where endometrial cancer is most common. Incidence is low in developed country due to regular screening and detection in very early or premalignant stage.

Each year 5 lakh of new cases are diagnosed of which India contributes 1.3 lakh. Death is 70,000 each year.

Reasons of High Incidence of Cancer Death in India

- Lack of screening
- Late diagnosis in advanced stage
- Early marriage, multiparity and presence of other risk factors are more.

Epidemiology, Etiology and Risk Factors of Cervical Cancer

Risk factors of CIN and invasive cancer are same. *See* later and discussed with CIN in Page 173.

PREMALIGNANT LESIONS OF CERVIX

Q. What is the natural history of the carcinogenesis of cervix?

Carcinoma cervix arises from a spectrum of pathway from normal cervix to cervical intraepithelial lesion to microinvasive lesion to invasive one. The main etiological agent is human papilloma virus (HPV) infection. There are other factors which play secondary role.

Terminologies Used for Preinvasive Lesions of Cervix

Q. What are the terminologies used for preinvasive lesions of cervix with historical importance (Fig. 16)?

The terminologies are:

- Dysplasia and carcinoma in situ (CIS)
- Cervical intraepithelial neoplasia (CIN) by WHO
- Bethesda system of cytology reporting
- Dyskaryosis by British Society of Clinical Cytology.

Dysplasia and Carcinoma In Situ (Fig. 16)

The term dysplasia was coined by Reagan et al. in 1956 and described as early precursor lesions with malignant potentiality.

Dysplasia was classified mild, moderate and severe depending upon cellular abnormality involving the depth of epithelium. In mild dysplasia, lower third of epithelium from basal layer is involved, in moderate dysplasia one half to two-third of thickness involved and in severe dysplasia, there is involvement of 75–90% of epithelial thickness.

Carcinoma in situ is meant for full thickness involvement. It is a very old term and was given by Rubin, 1910. Mild dysplasias to carcinoma in situ is considered a continuum of the neoplastic process and have potentiality to progress and is replaced by the term *cervical intraepithelial neoplasia*.

Cervical Intraepithelial Neoplasia (CIN): The concept of CIN was introduced by Richart in 1968 considering neoplastic process as a continuum progression.

Diagnostic criteria of intraepithelial neoplasia are based on the:

- Presence of cellular immaturity
- Cellular disorganization
- Nuclear abnormality
- Increased mitotic activity.

The **degree of neoplasia** is determined by the extent of immature cellular proliferation, mitotic activity and nuclear atypia. WHO (1975) categorized CIN in three grades—CIN1, CIN2, and CIN3 **(Fig. 16)**.

CIN1 means when the presence of immature cells and mitosis is confined to lower third of epithelium and corresponds to mild dysplasia.

CIN2 means involvement of middle third corresponding moderate dysplasia.

CIN3 refers to involvement of full thickness epithelium and corresponds to severe dysplasia and CIS.

Cervical intraepithelial neoplasia is truly an intraepithelial condition and more severe the grade more thickness of epithelium is involved and more atypia is found.

Invasive cancer is developed through a continuum of the neoplastic process of CIN and not suddenly from normal cervix. When the process breaks the basement membrane, cancer is diagnosed.

Normal epithelium → CIN1 → CIN2 → CIN3 → invasive cancer **(Fig. 17)**.

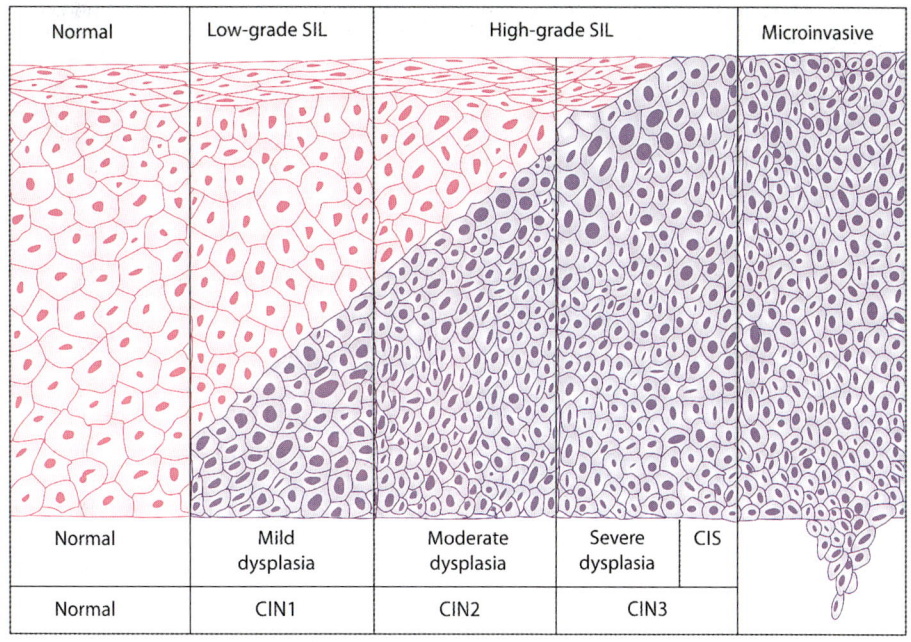

Fig. 16: Preinvasive and microinvasive lesions of carcinoma cervix with different nomenclature (reporting system).

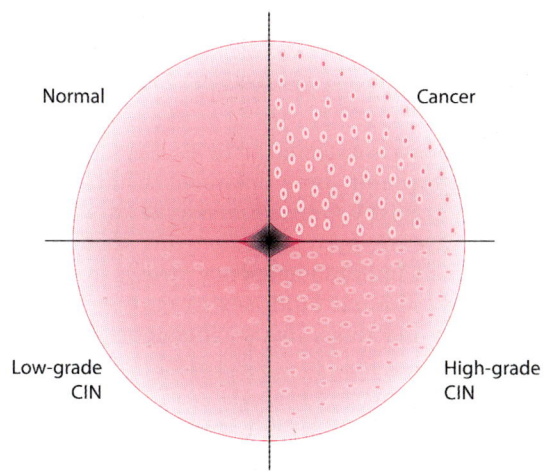

Fig. 17: Diagrammatic look of normal, cervical intraepithelial neoplasia and invasive cancer.

Later (1990), CIN was categorized as low grade (CIN1) and high grade (CIN2 and CIN3) disease.

It may persist, regress or progress. CIN1 mostly regresses spontaneously due to cell-mediated immunity for which follow up of low grade is sufficient. Some CIN2 and few CIN3 cases regress. As such, high grade CIN regresses less and may progress to cancer and if left untreated, 20% of patients of high grade may develop cancer.

Cervical intraepithelial neoplasia system is often used for histopathological reporting and others are for cytological reporting.

Q. What is Bethesda system?

Bethesda system is the recent development of uniform system of cytology reporting for clear guidance of clinical management. This system was first developed in 1988 in Bethesda, Maryland. In 2001, the terminology was refined in *Bethesda III system*. It is updated in 2014. The potentially premalignant lesions are categorized into the following broad groups.

Squamous Cell

1. Atypical squamous cells (ASC)
    a. Of undetermined significance [atypical squamous cells of undetermined significance (ASCUS)]
    b. Cannot exclude HSIL (ASC-H)
2. Low-grade squamous intraepithelial lesions (LSIL)
3. High-grade squamous intraepithelial lesions (HSIL)
4. Squamous cell carcinoma.

Glandular Cell

1. Atypical glandular cells (AGC): Endocervical, endometrial, not otherwise specified
2. Atypical glandular cells, favor neoplastic: Endocervical or not otherwise specified
3. Endocervical adenocarcinoma in situ (AIS)
4. Adenocarcinoma.

The Bethesda system on cervical cytology reporting which also includes non-neoplastic findings has been updated in 2014.

Comparison of Three Reporting Systems (*see* Fig. 16) (Table 6)

Q. What do you mean by dyskaryosis?

The term **dyskaryosis** is used by British Society of Clinical Cytology as abnormal cytology and is classified as mild, moderate and severe dyskaryosis and correspond to CIN1

Table 6: Comparison of three reporting system on cervical cytology.

Dysplasia/CIS	Mild	Moderate	Severe	CIS
CIN	CIN 1	CIN 2	CIN 3	
Involvement of epithelium	Lower third of epithelium from basal layer is involved	One half to two-third of thickness involved	Involvement of 75–90% of epithelial thickness	Full thickness epithelium involved
Bethesda	LSIL	HSIL		

Abbreviations: LSIL, low-grade squamous intraepithelial lesions; HSIL, high-grade squamous intraepithelial lesions; CIN, cervical intraepithelial neoplasia; CIS, carcinoma in situ

(mild dysplasia), CIN2 (moderate dysplasia) and CIN3 (severe dysplasia and CIS), respectively. Mild dyskaryosis corresponds to Bethesda system—LSIL, moderate HSIL and borderline corresponds to ASCUS.

Q. What do you mean by squamocolumnar junction and transformation zone (Fig. 18)?

In cervix, the **ectocervix** is lined by pink, smooth squamous epithelium and the endocervical canal is lined by red, velvety columnar epithelium. The **endocervix** contains many crypts which are lined by columnar epithelium.

The meeting of the two types of epithelia which lies throughout the circumference is called *squamocolumnar junction (SCJ)* **(Fig. 18)**.

* The position of SCJ varies with age (puberty, pregnancy, menopause) and hormonal status.
* In neonate, SCJ is located at ectocervix. At puberty, columnar epithelium of the area adjacent to SCJ is replaced by squamous epithelium due to physiological process of squamous metaplasia.
* Metaplasia advances from the original SCJ toward the external os. This process of metaplasia establishes an area known as *transformation zone (TZ)*. This TZ ranges from original SCJ to physiologically active SCJ or current SCJ **(Fig. 18)**. This squamous metaplasia of columnar cells occur due to the effect of estrogen which induces nonkeratinized squamous epithelium of vagina for glycogen synthesis. Lactobacilli acts on glycogen to form lactic acid resulting lowering of pH. This acidic pH stimulates squamous metaplasia.

Nabothian follicle or cyst: Mucous columnar epithelium is trapped occasionally under the squamous epithelium resulting retention of mucus called nabothian follicle or cyst. Martin Naboth (1675-1721) was a German anatomist and physician.

The TZ is the site of both squamous and columnar neoplasia. During adolescent and pregnancy, the metaplasia is most active which explains early ages of sexual activity and of first pregnancy as the risk factors for cervical cancer.

Locations of TZ and SCJ in different stages of life are shown in Figure 19A (normal), Figure 19B (nulliparous in reproductive age), Figure 19C (multiparous in reproductive age), Figure 19D (postmenopausal) (Figs. 19A to D).

Sites and Etiology of Development of Cervical Intraepithelial Neoplasia

Oncogenic process is triggered at the TZ due to the presence of HPV infection and some unknown factors. The main oncologic agent is HPV. Other secondary factors are sexually transmitted diseases—STDs (*Chlamydia*, syphilis, herpes simplex, human immunodeficiency virus), smoking, oral contraceptive, seminal fluid, sex in early age, multiple partners, early marriage, low socioeconomic status and under nutrition.

Role of Human Papilloma Virus in Cervical Neoplasia

* Human papilloma virus is a causative factor in nearly all cervical neoplasia and in significant proportion of cases of vulval, vaginal, and anal neoplasia.
* Human papilloma virus infection is the primary cause of cervical cancer. *90% of intraepithelial neoplasia is attributed* to HPV infection. HPV primarily infects squamous or metaplastic cells.
* It is a double-stranded deoxyribonucleic acid (DNA) virus. The cytological changes which occur due to HPV is called *koilocytosis* (Koss and Durfee, 1956) with irregular nuclear enlargement and a perinuclear halo.
* With increased severity of CIN, koilocytosis does not exist and the HPV DNA becomes integrated in host cells (basal cells) in persistent infections.
* DNA integration into the basal cells of cervical epithelium in the TZ results immortalization and rapid turnover of basal cells within the epithelium. This disordered immaturity within the epithelium is called *cervical*

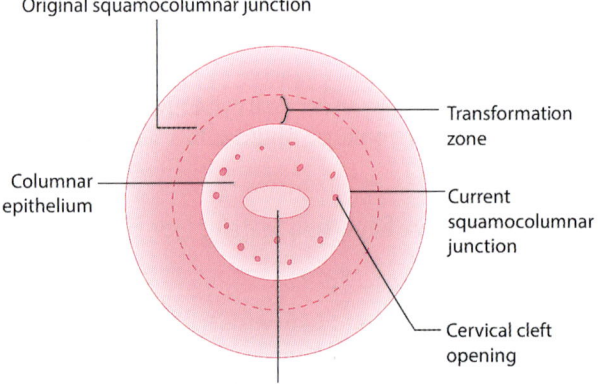

Fig. 18: Squamocolumnar junction and transformation zone.

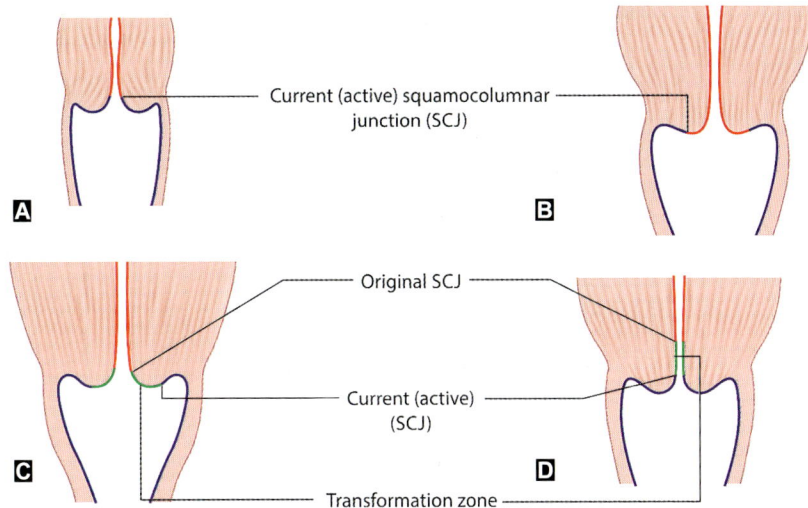

Figs. 19A to D: Squamocolumnar junction and transformation zone in different stages of life. (A) Normal; (B) Nulliparous in reproductive age; (C) Multiparous in reproductive age; (D) Postmenopausal age.

intraepithelial neoplasia. Expression of *E6* and *E7* HPV oncoproteins is required for malignant transformation.

Types of Human Papilloma Virus

Nearly 150 types of HPV have been identified and of them 40 are related with lower genital tract infection.

According to strength of association with cervical cancer, HPV types are classified as high risk (HR) or low risk (LR).

LR HPV types are 6 and 11 and responsible for genital warts and rarely oncogenic. HR types are 16, 18, 31, 33, 35, 45, 52 and 58. These HR HPV types and few other uncommon varieties are responsible for 95% of cervical cancer worldwide.

- *HPV 16 is most oncogenic* and the most common cause of CIN2, CIN3 and invasive cancers but nonspecific. *HPV 18* is most specific for CIN2, CIN3 and invasive cervical cancer.
- Type 16 is more associated with squamous cell carcinoma and type 18 is more with adenocarcinoma.
- Types 16 and 18 together account for 70% of cervical cancer.

Transmission of Human Papilloma Virus

Genital HPV is transmitted by direct, usually sexual contact by skin, mucous membrane or body fluid. Most HPV infection is subclinical.

Pathogenesis

In vast majority of cases of HPV infection, it will not persist and is cleared within 9–15 months in more than 90% cases. Those minor group which persists may progress to CIN with integration of HPV DNA.

High-risk HPVs, such as 16 and 18 persist and progress to invasive more. The risk of progression to high-grade neoplasia increases with the increased age of patient. Cell-mediated immunity plays a role in regression, persistence and progression of HPV infection **(Table 7)**.

Table 7: The reported regression, persistence and progression of untreated cervical intraepithelial neoplasia (CIN)- 1, 2 and 3.

	Regression	Persistence	Progress to carcinoma in situ	Progress to invasive carcinoma
CIN 1	60	30	10	1
CIN 2	40	35	20	5
CIN 3	32	<56	-	>12

Roughly 60% of CIN 1, 40% of CIN 2 and 30% CIN 3 regress, 10% and 20% of CIN 1 and CIN 2 progress to CIS and 1% of CIN 1, 5% of CIN 2 and 12% of CIN 3 progress to invasive carcinoma, respectively.

For invasion to occur, it takes 10–15 years. It takes 10 years to develop CIS. The risk of untreated CIN 3 for progression to invasive cancer is 30% in 30 years. CIN 3 is truly a cancer precursor.

The mean age for development of CIN 1 and CIN 2 are 24–27 years and that of CIN 3 is more than 10 years, i.e., 35–42 years and that of invasive carcinoma is after another 10 years, i.e., 49 years.

The development of invasive carcinoma can be shown in **Flowchart 1**.

CERVICAL CARCINOGENESIS

Risk Factors of Cervical Intraepithelial Neoplasia and Cervical Cancer

Risk factors of CIN and invasive cancer are same.

Demographic
- Increasing age
- Low socioeconomic status
- Undernutrition (vitamins A, C, E, beta carotene, folic acid)
- Lack of screening.

Flowchart 1: Development of invasive carcinoma.

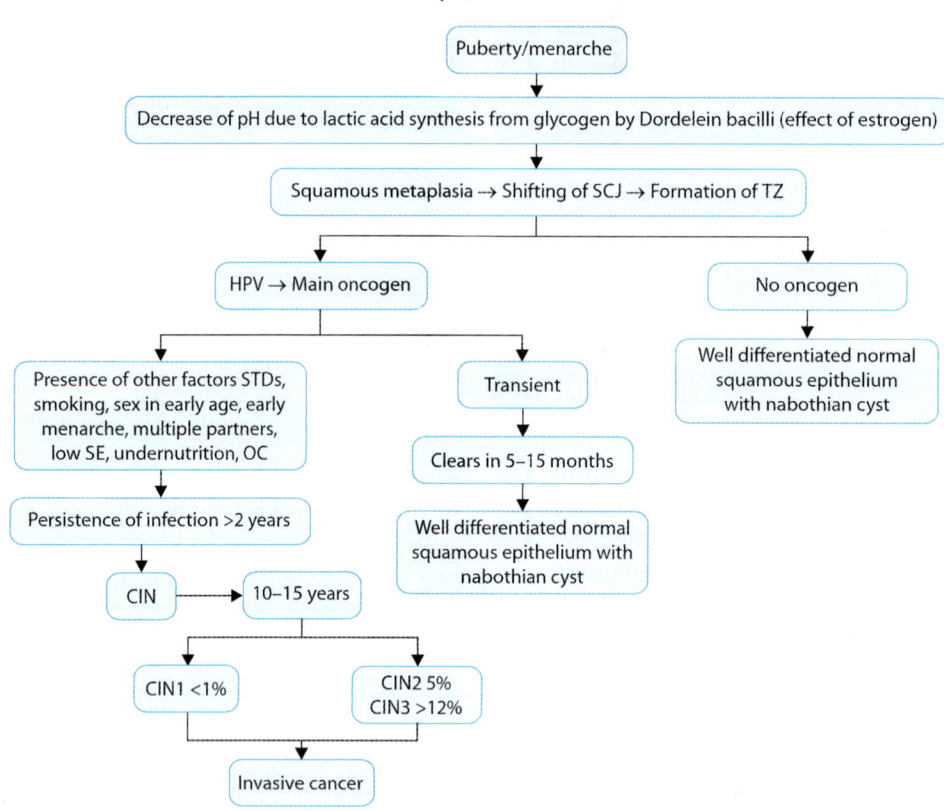

Abbreviations: SCJ, squamocolumnar junction; TZ, transformation zone; HPV, human papilloma virus, STDs, sexually transmitted diseases; SE, socioeconomic; OC, oral contraceptive; CIN, cervical intraepithelial neoplasia

Behavioral
- Early age of sex
- Early marriage
- Multiple partner
- Male partner who had prior multiple partner
- Smoking
- Multiparity

Medical-risk factors
- High risk HPV
- Combined pill (current user)
- Immunosuppression: Human immunodeficiency virus, immunosuppression drug
- Diethylstilbestrol exposure: Cervical and vaginal adenocarcinoma and high grade cervical disease

Cervical Cancer Screening

Q. What is cervical cancer screening? What is the basis of cervical cancer screening?

It is well recognized that cervical cancer does not develop suddenly but develops from a preinvasive process which takes a long time likely to be few decades to develop.

The **purpose** of screening is to detect the preinvasive lesions ideally or to detect early stage cervical cancer. The preinvasive lesions can be eradicated completely and the early-stage disease can be treated successfully.

Q. What are the advantages of cervical cancer screening?

Proper implementation of screening program has reduced the incidence of invasive cancer dramatically and cervical cancer death has been reduced up to 70% in developed country by detecting in preinvasive stage. In India, due to lack of proper screening strategy, the death toll from cancer cervix is very high.

Q. What are the different methods of screening?

Cytology and HPV testing are the two important tools for cervical cancer screening. As the preinvasive lesions of cervix is not visible, aided inspection is possible.
- Cytology
- HPV testing

Inspectory methods
- VIA: Visual inspection with acetic acid
- Schiller's test: VILI—visual inspection with Lugol's iodine
- VIAM: Visual inspection with acetic acid under magnification

Cervicography

Downstaging procedure devised for detecting invasive cancer in early stage for management in early stage is not strictly a screening procedure (*see* later Page 176).

CHAPTER 8: A Case of Carcinoma Cervix and Premalignant Lesions of Cervix

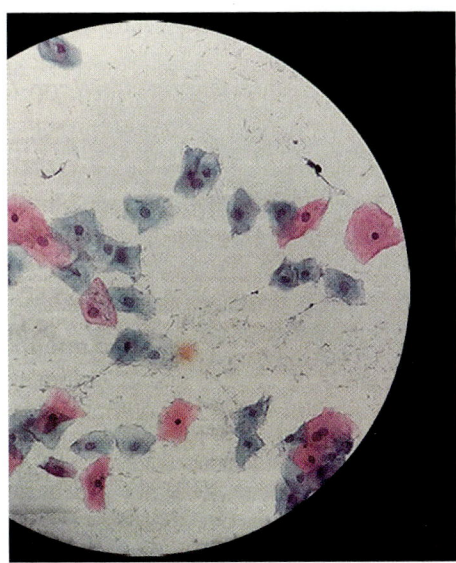

Fig. 20: Cervical cytology—normal cervical smear.
Courtesy: Dr Anup Boler, Associate Professor, Pathology

Cervical Cytology (Fig. 20)

Cytology was originally introduced by Papanicolaou in 1940 and traditionally called "Pap" smear. Later, liquid-based Pap smear was introduced.

So, there are two types:
1. Conventional glass slides method and
2. Liquid-based cytology. Both are equally acceptable.

Method of cervical cytology

The materials are collected from two sources:
- From squamocolumnar junction by wooden or plastic spatula: Ayre's or Aylesbury spatula **(Figs. 21, 22A and 23)**
- From endocervical canal by endocervical brush (Cytobrush) **(Figs. 21 and 22B)**.

Papanicolaou *slide method*

In Papanicolaou *slide method,* the materials collected are spread quickly over a glass slide, endocervical brush is firmly

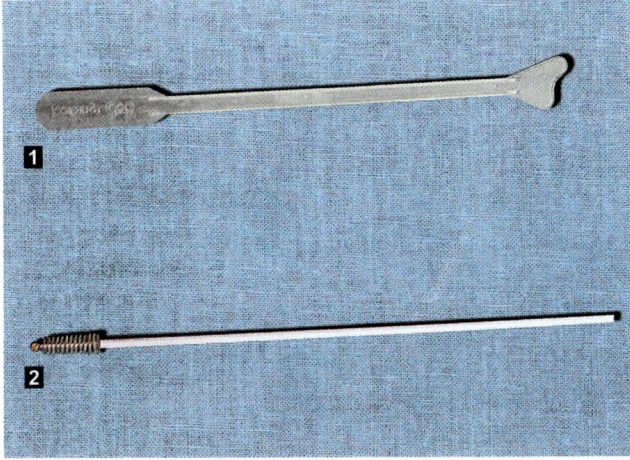

Fig. 21: (1) Ayer's spatula for external cervix and (2) cytobrush for endocervical canal.

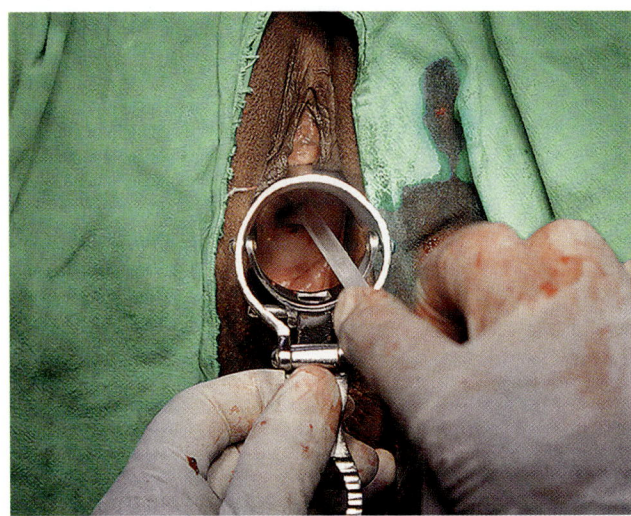

Fig. 22A: Pap smear from SCJ by Ayer's spatula.

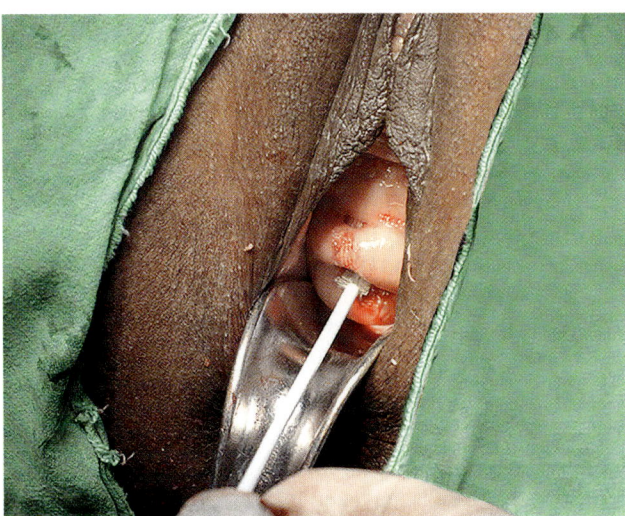

Fig. 22B: From endocervical canal by cryobrush.

rolled over the rest of the area of slide and fixed with 95% alcohol for at least 30 minutes and dried and stained with Papanicolaou stain and cellular abnormalities studied and reported (*see* below). Action is taken accordingly (*see* below).

Before the test, the patient should avoid coitus, douching, use of tampon and any vaginal drug or contraception for 24–48 hours. It should not be done during menstruation.

Three types of plastic devices are used:
1. Spatula **(Figs. 22A and 23)**
2. Cytobrush **(Figs. 21 and 22B)**
3. Broom **(Fig. 24)**.

A spatula is mainly for ectocervix, cytobrush for endocervical canal and a broom samples both endo- and ectocervical epithelia simultaneously.

Spatula may be wooden or plastic. Wooden spatula is now less popular, as cells stick to the micropore of wooden spatula. But it is still used in many countries. For broom, liquid base cytology is mandatory.

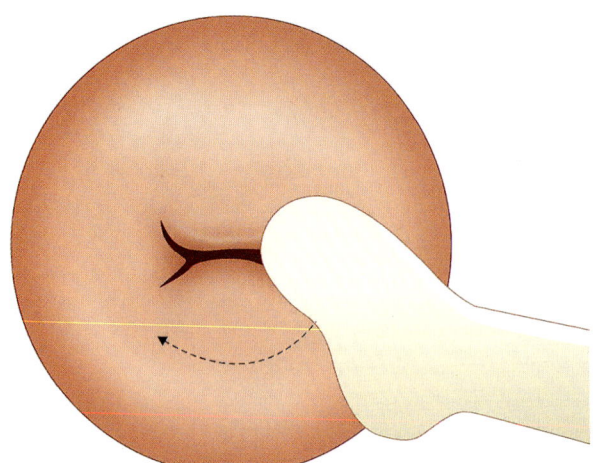

Fig. 23: Cervical cytology by Ayer's spatula.

With the spatula scraping is taken firmly from the cervical surface completing at least one rotation **(Fig. 23)**.

Cytobrush is inserted into the endocervical canal until the outermost bristles remain visible just near external os not to push inside near isthmus to avoid cells from cavity **(Fig. 22B)**. The brush is rotated only one-quarter to one-half turn and done after sampling from ectocervix by spatula.

With the broom devices, five rotations in the same direction is done with the longer central bristles inserting into endocervical canal **(Fig. 24)**. Broom devices are suitable for liquid-based pap staining.

Specificity of Pap test is very high about 98% and sensitivity of Pap test for CIN is about 70%.

Liquid-based Cytology

The smear plastic spatula is dipped into a liquid fixative which removes the blood, mucus and inflammatory cells. The suspended cells are taken into a filter membrane which pressed on glass slide to make a smear which is stained. The liquid may be used for HPV test.

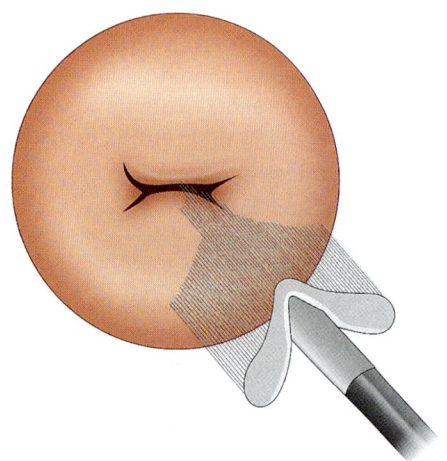

Fig. 24: Cervical cytology by plastic broom.

Human Papilloma Virus Testing (HPV Testing)

Human papilloma virus testing detects presence of HPVs 16 and 18 and also a group of 12 other oncogenic HPV. Testing is done only for HR-HPV types and there is no clinical role for low risk HPV testing.

Cotesting means combination of HR HPV with cytology. Food and Drug Administration (FDA) approved HPV test with cytology first in 2003 among women 30 years above. Cotesting increases the sensitivity for high-grade neoplasia to near 100%. Primary HPV testing was approved by FDA in 2014 in women 25 years and above.

VIA and VIAM

Cervix is applied with freshly prepared 3–5% acetic acid and after one minute, cervix is visualized. The areas of high nuclear density will look acetowhite as acetic acid is mucolytic and coagulates protein. It can be done by paramedics and treatment is possible in the same sitting. VIAM is visualization with magnification after application of acetic acid.

Schiller Test (VILI)

Cervix is painted with Lugol's iodine (Iodine in KI solution) and the unstained Schiller positive area indicates unhealthy, may be due to cervical erosion, atrophied epithelium, decubitus ulcer and CIN lesion (*see* **Fig. 33**).

The healthy portion takes mahogany brown color due to presence of glycogen and the dysplastic cells containing less glycogen looks pale. Schiller test is useful where colposcope is not available.

Both VIA and VILI positive cases are treated with cryotherapy.

Q. What do you mean by downstaging?

Due to high incidence of invasive cervical cancer and cervical cancer death in developing country like India, one strategy was taken to diagnose the invasive cancer cervix at earlier stage which can be cured to some extent. It can be done at primary healthcare level even by paramedics or nursing staff and the patient should be referred to higher center for definitive diagnosis and treatment. This is very useful in the regions where routine screening procedure is not possible.

Q. What is the interpretation of different grades of smear reporting of original Papanicolaou classification?

Originally, there were five grades with following interpretation **(Table 8)**.

Cytology Classification and Reporting System: Comparison of Three Systems

Traditionally, Pap smear was classified in five Papanicolaou grades (1954)—Grade I, Grade II, Grade III, Grade IV, Grade V

Table 8: Grades of original Papanicolaou classification.

Grade I	Grade II	Grade III	Grade IV	Grade V
Normal	Atypical cells as occurs in infection	Atypia due to dysplasia	Carcinoma in situ	Invasive carcinoma

Table 9: Comparison of three systems of cytology classification.

Papanicolaou system	Bethesda system	Dysplasia or cervical intraepithelial lesion (CIN) system
I	Within normal limit	Normal
II	Infection (organism should be mentioned)	Inflammatory atypia (organism)
	Reactive and reparative changes	
IIR	Squamous cell abnormalities Atypical squamous cells: (i) of undetermined significance (ASC-US), (ii) exclude high grade lesions (ASC-H)	• Squamous atypia • Human papilloma virus (HPV) atypia, exclude LSIL • Exclude HSIL • HPV atypia
III	Low-grade squamous intraepithelial lesion (LSIL)	Mild dysplasia CIN1
IV	High-grade squamous intraepithelial lesion (HSIL)	• Moderate dysplasia • CIN2 Severe dysplasia • CIN3 Carcinoma in situ
V	Squamous cell carcinoma	Squamous cell carcinoma

as above. Later, standard Bethesda system came into picture. The three systems are compared in **Table 9**.

Q. What is the plan of action in screen positive cases?

Cytology is reported as Bethesda system. The management is as follows:

- ASC-US positive → HPV-DNA testing → positive → colposcopy
- HPV-DNA-negative → Pap smear after one year
- ASC-H, LSIL, HSIL and squamous cell carcinoma → colposcopy and directed biopsy.

Loop electrosurgical excision procedure (LEEP) or colposcopy, both are acceptable for women with HSIL.

Q. What is the screening protocol for cancer cervix? (American Society for Colposcopy and Cervical Pathology, 2012)

- Screening is started at 21 years with Pap smear. Below 21 years of age, screening is not needed.
- 21–29 years: Every 3 years by cytology (HPV testing is not needed before 30 years)
- 30–65 years: Cytology every 3 years, if HPV not available. Primary choice is cotesting, both HPV and cytology every 5 years.
- After 65 years, screening is stopped provided no CIN2 lesion in last 20 years as chance of cancer cervix becomes less.
- In case of post-HPV vaccination, screening protocol is same.
- After hysterectomy, there is no role of screening.

WHO Policy (2013)

Every woman between 30 years and 49 years should have at least one cervical screening.

COLPOSCOPY (FIG. 25)

Colposcopy is a diagnostic procedure by which cervix is visualized through the optical instrument with 10x–40x magnification. It can also be used to see the vagina and vulva.

Advantages of Colposcopy

Premalignant and malignant lesions of cervix have characteristic features so far as look, color and vascular pattern are concerned, unhealthy areas are identified, specific diagnosis is possible under magnification from which biopsy can be taken.

The colposcope was introduced by Hans Hinselmann (Hamburg) in 1925.

Procedure

It is an outpatient procedure. Patient is put on lithotomy position and the cervix and vaginal vault is exposed by Cusco's speculum. If there is any discharge, it should be cleared with normal saline. Cervix is painted with 3–5% of acetic acid. The areas of high nuclear density (atypical cell) will look acetowhite as acetic acid is mucolytic and coagulates protein. Green filter is used to visualize the vascular pattern of the cervix. The TZ is identified and biopsy is taken.

Q. What do you mean by unsatisfactory colposcopy?

When the whole TZ, including the lesions is visible, satisfactory colposcopy is possible. When the SCJ is not

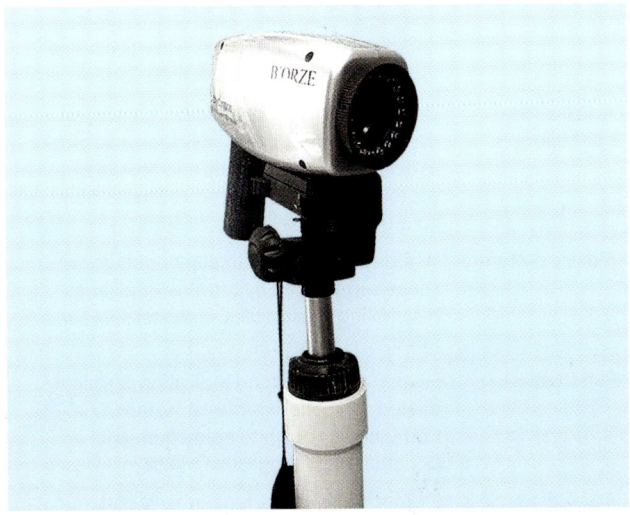

Fig. 25: Colposcopy.
Courtesy: Professor Arati Biswas, HOD, Calcutta National Medical College

visible and inside the endocervical canal beyond the vision, it is called unsatisfactory. Endocervical speculum can be used to see the extent of vision. Conization is suggested if it is still not visible.

Q. What are the different findings of cervix in colposcopy?

Findings may be normal or abnormal. Abnormal findings are leukoplakia, acetowhite epithelium, mosaic pattern, punctuation and atypical vascular pattern **(Table 10)**.

Colposcopic Findings in Cervical Intraepithelial Lesion

Characteristic features are:
- Acetowhite with acetic acid, pale with Schiller test. Margins are clear.
- Abnormal vascular pattern like mosaic and punctuation present. Coarse mosaic and punctuation indicate high-grade lesion. Fine mosaic and punctuation indicate low-grade lesion.

Appearance of Low-grade Squamous Intraepithelial Lesion, High-grade Squamous Intraepithelial Lesion and Invasive Cancer in Colposcopy (Table 11).

Q. Reid colposcopic index.

To improve the diagnostic accuracy several grading systems have been developed on the basis of colposcopic findings. Reid colposcopic index is one such popular system comprising of four colposcopic findings: **margin, color, vascular patterns and staining by Lugol solution.** Each type is scored from 0–2. Reid index is labeled as grade 1 (minor) when there is zero score in low grade lesions and as grade 2 (major) in higher grade lesions.

Various Colposcopy Findings are Illustrated with Description from Figures 26 to 35

The different colposcopic views are shown below in the Figures 26 to 35 with description.

Q. What is swede Score?

The score is determined based on five types of colposcopic findings; namely (1) aceto uptake, (2) margins/surface, (3) vessels, (4) lesion size and (5) iodine staining, each parameter having 0,1 and 2 scores as per severity of abnormality and maximum score is 10. Overall 0–4 Swede score is interpreted as low grade normal CIN1, Score 5–6 as high grade/noninvasive cancer CIN2+ and score 7–10 is regarded as high grade/suspected invasive cancer CIN2+.

Table 11: Appearances of different lesions and cancer in colposcopy.

Lesions	Low-grade squamous intraepithelial lesion	High-grade squamous intraepithelial lesion	Invasive cancer
Appearance	Multifocal and bright white with irregular borders with 5% acetic acid	Off-white dull color and coarse vascular pattern with 5% acetic acid	High-grade lesion with cuffed crypt openings and atypical vessels

Table 10: Different findings of cervix in colposcopy.

Colposcopic findings	Interpretation
Normal	Squamous epithelium—pink and smooth Columnar—grape like, columnar epithelium swells and become acetowhite on acetic acid application whether transformation zone is visualized or not
Leukoplakia	White epithelium without acetic acid. Usually caused by keratin deposition over epithelium. The most common caused is HPV infection. Keratinizing CIN, carcinoma may be similar looking. Biopsy should always be done
Acetowhite epithelium	On application of acetic acid high nuclear density (dysplastic cells) will look acetowhite as acetic acid is mucolytic and coagulates protein. Normal squamous cell looks pink, columnar cell may be acetowhite
Mosaic pattern	White epithelium of circular or polygonal shape surrounded by terminal capillaries resembling mosaic tiles. Indicates CIN2 and CIN3
Punctuation	Several dots are found indicating terminal dilated capillaries visible on surface. Combination of white epithelium and punctuation is suggestive of CIN
Atypical vascular pattern	If branching vessels, loop vessels and reticular vessels are seen, invasive cancer is likely

Abbreviations: HPV, human papilloma virus; CIN, cervical intraepithelial lesion

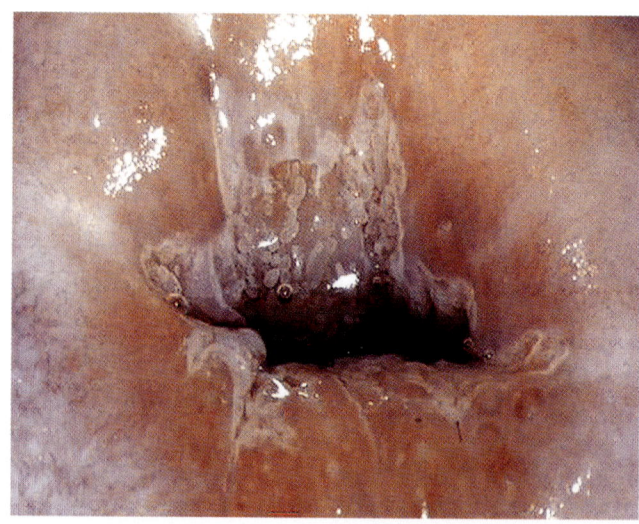

Fig. 26: Normal cervix: Note the smooth and uniformness between where the columnar epithelium ends centrally and the squamous epithelium starts peripherally, pink appearance of the outer squamous epithelium and the soft velvety inner columnar epithelium. The transformation zone is the area ally.

Courtesy: Dr Jaydip Bhaumik, Senior Consultant, Tata Medical Center, Kolkata

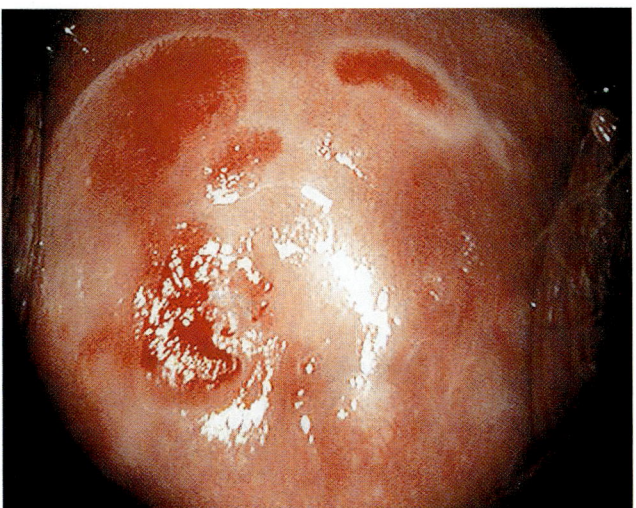

Fig. 27: Nulliparous cervix: Note the wide transformation zone in a nulliparous cervix. The external os is narrow like a pin hole. The squamous epithelium is peripherally placed.
Courtesy: Dr Jaydip Bhaumik, Senior Consultant, Tata Medical Center, Kolkata

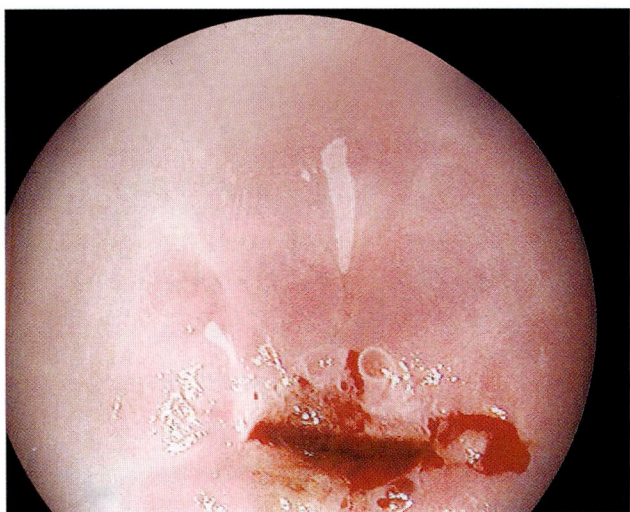

Fig. 29: Human papilloma virus (HPV) change: Note this geographic acetowhite lesion is toward the periphery of the transformation zone. This is lesion from an HPV infection, also called flat condyloma.
Courtesy: Dr Jaydip Bhaumik, Senior Consultant, Tata Medical Center, Kolkata

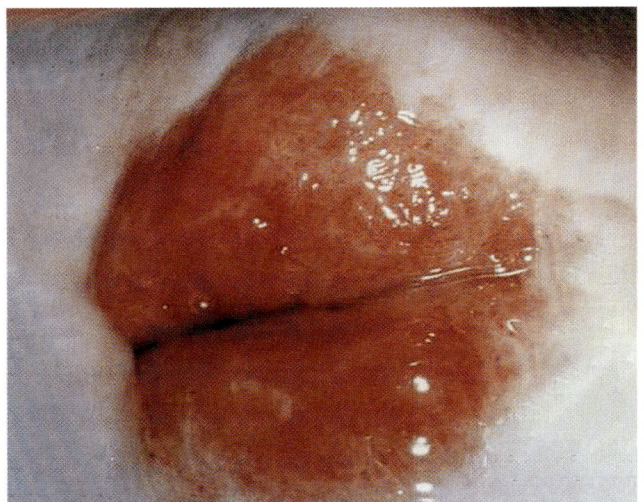

Fig. 28: Cervical ectopy: In some women, the soft velvety vascular columnar epithelium of the cervical canal extends outward in the portio vaginalis of the cervix, known as cervical ectopy. This is erroneously called cervical erosion. This is a physiological variation of the normal appearance of the cervix.
Courtesy: Dr Jaydip Bhaumik, Senior Consultant, Tata Medical Center, Kolkata

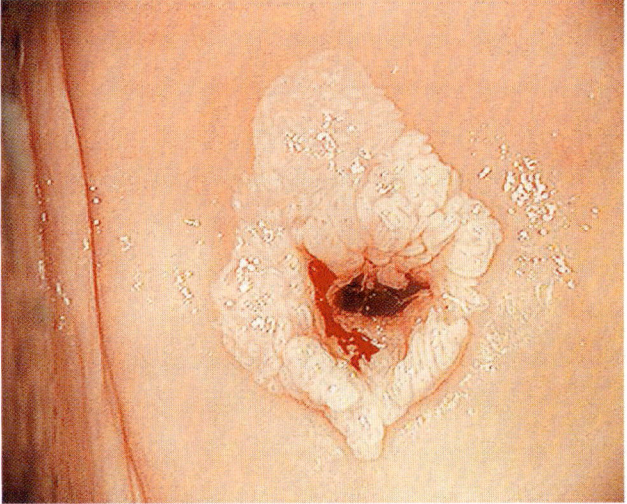

Fig. 30: Cervical condyloma: This is a typical condylomatous lesion. The finger-like projections are fragile and may bleed on touch. Most of these disappear without treatment over the next few weeks.

Diagnosis of Cervical Intraepithelial Lesion

Symptoms: It occurs 10 years earlier than invasive cancer. Many are asymptomatic. Few women may complain postcoital bleeding or discharge. Some women may present with postmenopausal bleeding.

Signs: Cervix may look normal or there may be features of cervicitis or erosion and bleeds on touch.

Cytology: Cervical cytological screening diagnoses cellular abnormality.

HPV testing: As given earlier

Visual detection: As given earlier

Colposcopy with directed biopsy: As given earlier.

Management of Cervical Intraepithelial Lesion

Management of CIN1 (Low-grade squamous intraepithelial lesions):

As majority regresses spontaneously, follow up after 6 months provided the diagnosis is correct and the patient will come on follow up. If after 12–18 months, lesion persists or progresses, treatment by ablation or excision is offered (*see* below). In case of noncompliant patient, treatment is given immediately after diagnosis.

Management of CIN 2 and 3 (High-grade squamous intraepithelial lesions): Treatment is necessary by ablation or excision:

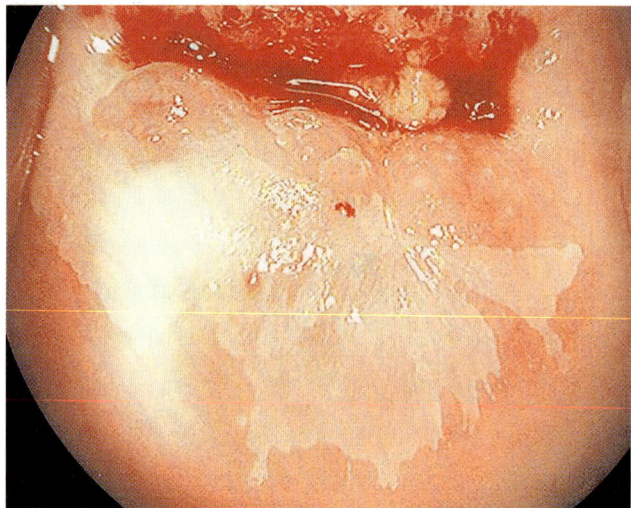

Fig. 31: Low-grade cervical intraepithelial neoplasia: The background is mild acetowhite epithelium; there are no abnormal vascular patterns and regular shaped, more or less symmetrical lesions with smooth, straight outlines.
Courtesy: Dr Jaydip Bhaumik, Senior Consultant, Tata Medical Center, Kolkata

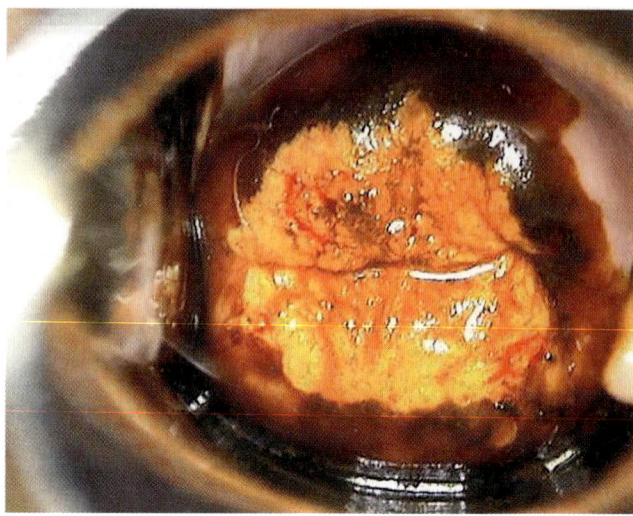

Fig. 33: After application of Lugol's iodine normal mahogany brown stain of glycophilic squamous epithelium, no iodine staining of columnar epithelium.
Courtesy: Dr Dipanwita Banerjee, Chittaranjan National Cancer Institute (CNCI), Kolkata

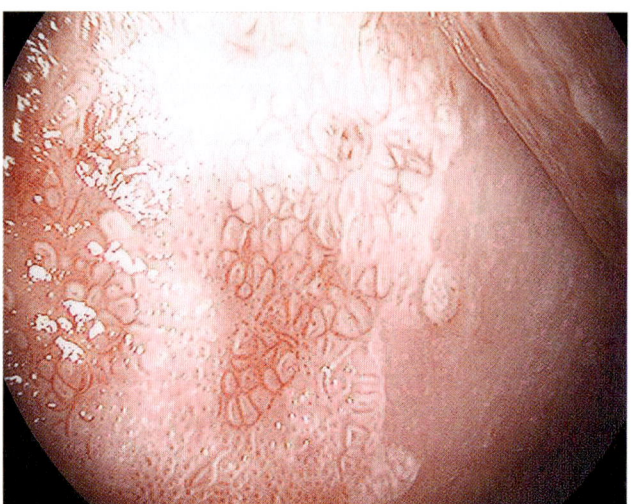

Fig. 32: High-grade cervical intraepithelial neoplasia: The hallmark of a high-grade cervical intraepithelial lesion on colposcopy is the presence of abnormal vascular pattern. On the background of dense acetowhite, the epithelium shows a mosaic pattern and punctation.
Courtesy: Dr Jaydip Bhaumik, Senior Consultant, Tata Medical Center, Kolkata

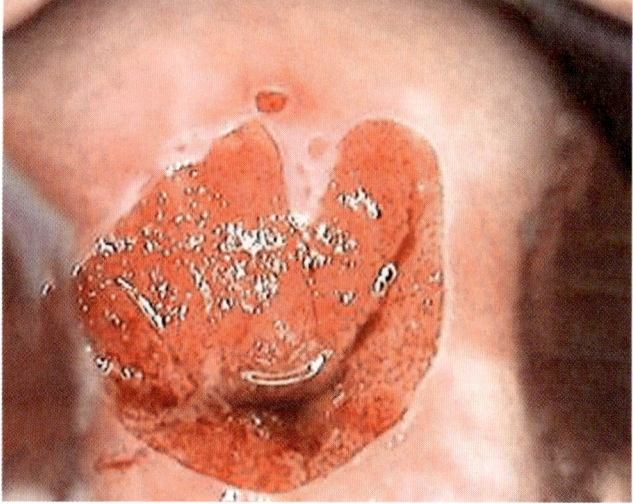

Fig. 34: Normal squamous metaplasia.
Courtesy: Dr Dipanwita Banerjee, Chittaranjan National Cancer Institute (CNCI), Kolkata

Role of Conservative Cryotherapy (Fig. 35A)

Principle is to destroy the surface epithelium of cervix by crystallizing the intracellular water, thus destroying the cells by cryocautery. It was introduced by Townsend.

The temperature needed is −20°–30° which is done by nitrous oxide (−80°), carbon dioxide (−60°) or freon (−60°). Nitrous oxide is said to be best of all. Freeze-thaw-freeze method for 9–10 minutes destroy the tissue up to 5 mm depth.

Lesion is identified by acetic acid, Lugol's iodine or best by colposcopic view.

In this method a cryoprobe **(Fig. 35A)**, made of silver or copper is pressed firmly over the cervix and cryogun trigger is squeezed, till frost is formed to cover the cryoprobe

Methods:

- *Local destruction*: Ablative procedure—cryotherapy, cold coagulation, electrocoagulation, laser ablation
- *Local excision*: Excisional where removal of TZ is done—LEEP, large loop excision of transformation zone (LLETZ), needle excision of transformation zone (NETZ), conization or cone biopsy—(a) cold knife, (b) loop, and (c) laser
- *Radical surgery*: Hysterectomy.

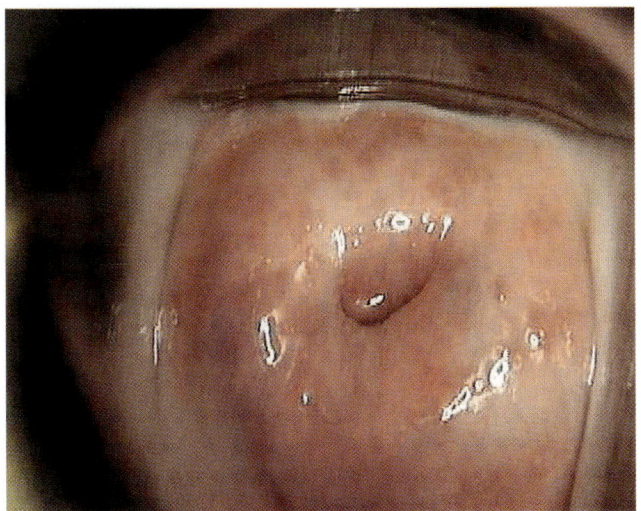

Fig. 35: Postmenopausal atrophic cervix.
Courtesy: Dr Dipanwita Banerjee, Chittaranjan National Cancer Institute (CNCI), Kolkata

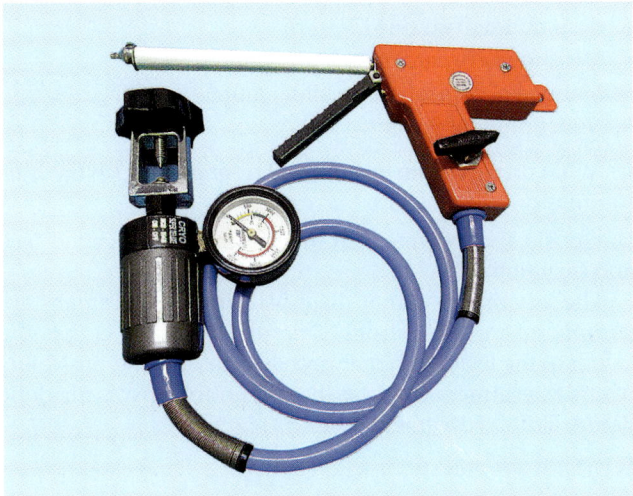

Fig. 35A: Cryoprobe with cryogun and connecting system used for cryotherapy.

Electrocoagulation

Laser Ablation

Laser steams and explodes the cell. It is also used for small lesions like cryotherapy. It is very expensive and special training is needed. Hence, it is not so popular, as there is good alternate option.

Loop Electrosurgical Excision Procedure (LEEP) (Figs. 36A and B)

- In LEEP, using radiofrequency electric current, a large loop excision of the TZ is done.
- Depending on the site of lesion varying sized loops are used. For etocervix, loops of 15–20 mm size are used and for endocervix **(Fig. 36A)**, 10 mm loops are appropriate.
- Tissue is cut in a single pass except in larger lesions. It can be done under colposcopic guidance.
- It is most commonly employed method for treatment of CIN. The advantage is that specimen can be retrieved for biopsy, procedure is simple and safe. It is done as OPD procedure with local anesthesia.
- Where colposcopy is satisfactory, it can be done in CIN2 and CIN3 cases.
- The success is 95%. It is better to do LEEP after getting biopsy report. See and treat policy is better avoided. LEEP is applicable anywhere in lower genital tract.
- Complications are reddish discharge for few weeks. There may be bleeding during surgery and postoperatively. Cervical stenosis, preterm labor and premature rupture of membranes are delayed complications.
- Following surgery, coitus and vaginal douching are avoided for 1 month.
- Follow-up with colposcopy is needed after 1 year.

Large Loop Excision of Transformation Zone

- In LLETZ, low-voltage diathermy is used **(Fig. 36B)**.
- Under local anesthesia, loop is advanced lateral to the lesion in cervix to reach the required depth and passed to the opposite side so that a chunk of conical tissue is removed.

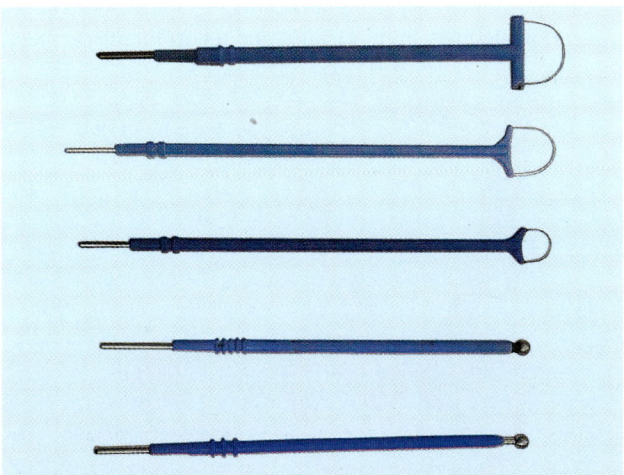

Fig. 36A: Varieties of loop electrosurgical excision procedure (LEEP) electrodes.
Courtesy: Department of Gynecological Oncology, CNCI, Kolkata

following a hissing sound. The cervical surface is cooled to form an iceball beneath the center of cryoprobe and expands circumferentially. It needs to keep after triggering for 3 minutes. It is only removed after completion of freezing, premature removal may cause patient's pain and bleeding.

It is good for small lesion (25%) not extending to endocervical canal, result is best with CIN1. CIN2 can also be treated, but not so effective for CIN3. Repeat cryocautery after 3 months may be needed in a few cases after follow-up.

Advantages are: It is OPD procedure, better tolerated by patient and, very little pain and it is cheap. *Disadvantage* is excessive discharge and drawing of SCJ.

Cold coagulation: It is misnomer as in this therapy a hot probe is placed on the cervix under local anesthesia as an outpatient procedure.

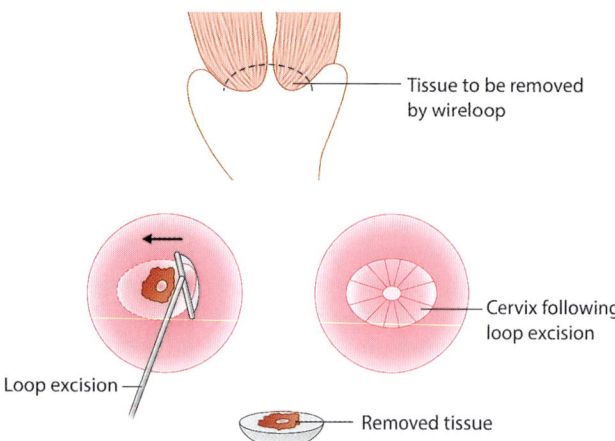

Fig. 36B: Loop electrosurgical excision procedure (LEEP).

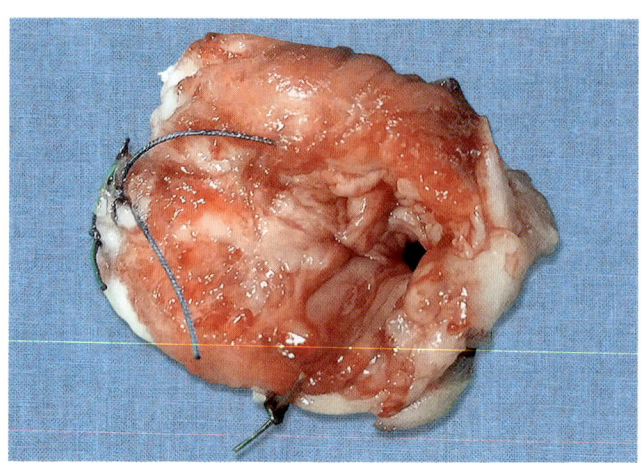

Fig. 38: Excised cervical tissue following conization.

- The advantage is that the cost of the instrument is low and not harmful to the user and takes short time.
- In NETZ, cervical tissue is removed in one piece.

Conization
- Conization or cone biopsy is performed using:
  - Cold knife
  - Electrosurgical loop (**Fig. 36**), or
  - Laser.
- It is both diagnostic and therapeutic.
- Indications are:
  - Unsatisfactory colposcopy—SCJ not visible
  - Limits of lesion not visible
  - Endocervical curettage positive for CIN2 or 3
  - Suspicious of microinvasive carcinoma in colposcopy, biopsy or cytology.
- **Procedure:** It is done under general anesthesia or local anesthesia in operation theater. With the help of a scalpel, entire TZ including the lesion (cone-shaped tissue) is removed (**Figs. 37 and 38**).
- Complications are preoperative and postoperative bleeding, cervical stenosis, preterm labor and recurrent miscarriage.

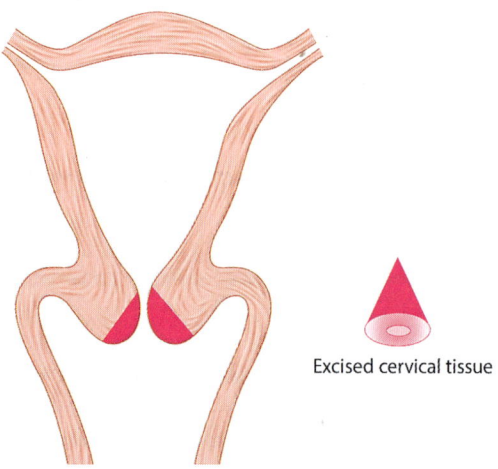

Fig. 37: Cone biopsy.

Hysterectomy
Indications of hysterectomy are:
- Parous elderly woman
- Associated with other uterine pathology like fibroid, dysfunctional uterine bleeding
- Microinvasive carcinoma
- Margins of conization specimen not free of CIN
- Noncompliant patient.

Q. What do you mean by "see and treat policy"? What is its rationality?

Diagnosis and treatment in the same sitting is called "see and treat policy".

The advantage is that diagnosis and management are completed in same sitting. The disadvantage is that the extent of the lesion is not always determined and possibility of under treatment is always there, if prior biopsy is not done before definite treatment.

WHO 2013 Policy
- Paradigm shift from screening–diagnosis–treatment to screen and treat at same sitting.
- According to WHO screen with HPV and VIA at the same sitting and treatment with cryotherapy (if not possible, then LEEP) is best till now.
- In low resource area screen with VIA and treatment is justified. In areas with previously existing proper Pap smear based testing facility, Pap smear with or without HPV DNA testing is reasonable.
- Every women between 30 years and 49 years should have at least one cervical screening.
- WHO recommended against cold knife conization.

Management Protocol of Preinvasive Lesions of Cervix (Flowchart 2)

Q. How would you prevent carcinoma cervix?

- Primary prevention:
  - Knowledge of high-risk cases and control of risk factors
  - Vaccination—HPV vaccine

Flowchart 2: Management protocol of preinvasive lesions of cervix.

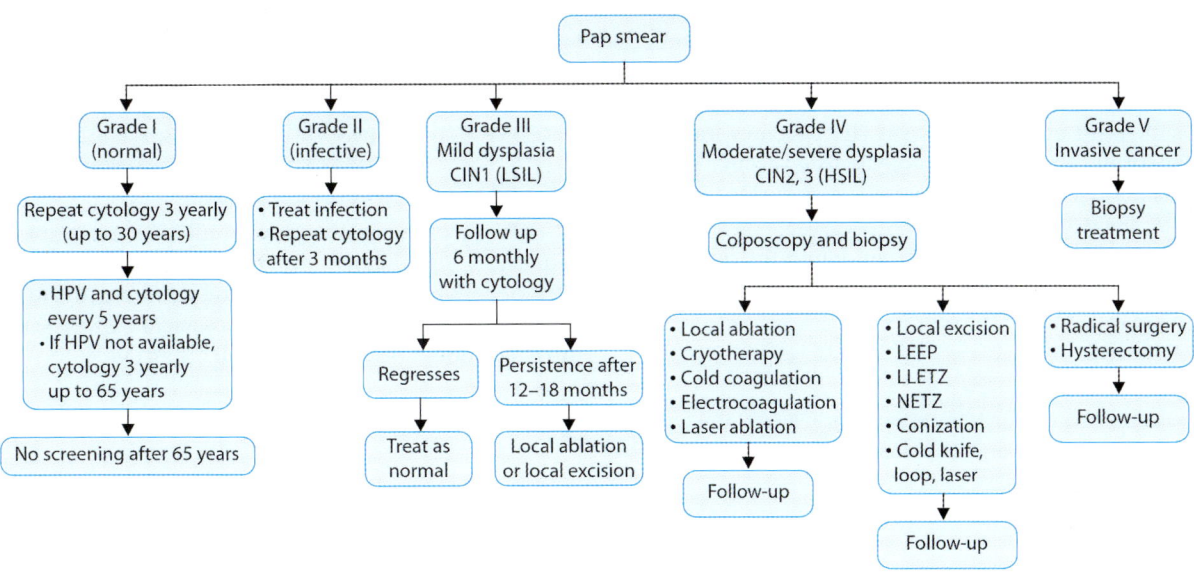

Abbreviations: HPV, human papilloma virus; LEEP, loop electrosurgical excision procedure; LLETZ, large loop excision of transformation zone; NETZ, needle excision of transformation zone

- Secondary prevention: Cervical cancer screening and treatment
- Tertiary prevention: Treatment of invasive cancer.

Change of Sexual Behavior

Delayed coitarche, sexual abstinence and avoiding the multiple sexual partners are the strategies that can be taken. Condom is completely protective but reduces the acquisition and transmission of HPV infection.

HUMAN PAPILLOMA VIRUS VACCINE

Human papilloma virus vaccines prevent the cancers at least six sites in the human body namely cervix, vagina, penis, anal canal and oropharynx.

Rationality of giving Human Papilloma Virus Vaccine

It is now well known that HPV causes anogenital disease in human being. An 80% of sexually active women acquire HPV infection within 50 years of age by sexual activity. In majority (80–90%) of the cases, the infection is cleared within 2 years with persistence in 10–20% cases. Persistence of high risk HPV infection in the cervix causes cervical cancer. However, it takes not less than 20 years to cause cervical cancer through a spectrum of intraepithelial neoplasia. A 90% of intraepithelial neoplasia is attributed to HPV infection.

High-risk HPV types are 16, 18, 31, 33, 35, 45, 52 and 58, and few uncommon varieties and are responsible for 95% of cervical cancer worldwide.

HPVs 16 and 18 together account for 70% of cervical cancer.

Vaccines Types

- Human papilloma virus vaccine has been developed by recombinant technologies and the resultant virus-like particles are highly immunogenic without infectivity due to lack of viral DNA.
- Three HPV vaccines are available and FDA approved. These are Cervarix (HPV2), Gardasil (HPV4) and Gardasil 9 (HPV9).
  - Cervarix (HPV2) is *bivalent vaccine* against HPV 16 and 18.
  - Gardasil (HPV4) is a *quadrivalent vaccine* against HPV 6, 11, 16 and 18. Gardasil (HPV4) vaccine is being replaced by Gardasil 9 (HPV9).
  - Gardasil 9 (HPV9) is *nonavaccine* which protects all four types of HPV 4 plus 31, 33, 45, 52, and 58.
- HPV vaccine is recommended for all females between 11 years and 26 years of age.
- FDA (2018) approves vaccination in 27–45 years also. A shared decision-making is recommended by ACOG (2019) for vaccination in aged 27–45 years who are at risk and not previously vaccinated for acquiring HPV infection. This is agreed by Advisory committee on immunization practices (ACIP).
- Vaccine should be given before sexual activity ideally to get maximum benefit. However, Sexual exposure, HPV infection and HPV positivity does not dissuade the vaccination. Before vaccination HPV test is not needed.

Doses and Route

- Women up to 15 years: 2 dose (0, 6 months) (Centers for Disease Control and Prevention 2016, WHO 2014)

- Women more than 15 years: 3 dose (for Cervarix 0, 1, 6 months; for Gardasil 0, 2, 6 months)
- Vaccines are given intramuscular in deltoid. Side effects are pain at site, headache, myalgia, rarely anaphylactic reaction and lymphadenopathy. It can be given with other vaccines but at separate sites. The vaccines have high safety profile and well tolerable. Before vaccination HPV test is not needed. *It is contraindicated during pregnancy can be given during lactation.*
- Government of India has no guideline for routine use of vaccine. Few countries like Australian Government provide vaccine free of cost.

Protection

All the vaccines are near 100% efficacious against the types of HPV related infection and neoplasia the types contained by the vaccine. Vaccines give maximum protection from HPV if vaccinated before sexual exposure. It gives protection 5–8 years after vaccination. The need of booster dose is not yet determined. HPV4 and HPV9 vaccines are also approved for genital wart prevention in both male and female. Genital wart is caused by type 6 and 11 (*see* Chapter 33).

Screening Program in the Era of Vaccine

As HPV vaccine cannot prevent all HPV related cervical cancers, a significant percentage of cases are found in HPV negative women and vaccine cannot prevent cancer in already infected women, the cervical cancer screening program should be continued with importance.

A Case of Carcinoma Vulva, Preinvasive Lesion of Vulva and Vaginal Cancer

Chapter Outline

Writing a case of cancer vulva and how to present the case?

- Diagnosis of Vulvar Cancer
- Etiology of Cancer Vulva
- Lymphatic Drainage and its Clinical Significance
- Staging of Cancer Vulva
- Management
- Simple Vulvectomy, Radical Vulvectomy with Operative Details with Illustrations
- Preinvasive Lesions of Vulva
- Vaginal Cancer

PATIENT'S PARTICULARS

1. Name:
2. Age: 65 years
3. Address:
4. Occupation:
5. Married/unmarried: Married
6. History of infertility:
7. Husband's occupation:
8. Socioeconomic status:
9. Religion:
10. Parous/nulliparous: Nulliparous

Bed No.:
Date of admission:
Date of examination:

HISTORY

- *Chief complaint(s):* Painful sore or swelling over the vulva, offensive discharge, and bleeding from the vulvar area for 3 months duration. There was pruritus vulva for prolonged period. There may be dysuria if lesion is close to urethra.
- *History of present illness:* Elaborate the chief complaint in chronological order. Whether there was any history of leukoplakia, it should be enquired. A biopsy was taken 10 days back.
- *Menstrual history:* Usually menopausal. If so write how many years. If not menopausal write the menstrual history as usual.
- *Obstetric history:* More common in nulliparous. Otherwise write the details of obstetric history.
    - Parity
    - *Living issue*—Write "Nil" if patient is primi.
    - Last child birth (LCB).
- *Past history:*
    - Medical
    - Surgical.
- *Family history*
- *Sexual history*
- *Functional history:*
    - Bowel
    - Bladder
    - Sleep
    - Appetite.

- *Personal history:*
  - Personal hygiene
  - Smoking/alcohol.
- Contraceptive history/hormone replacement therapy
- *Drug history:*
  - History of any drug allergy
  - History of intake of corticosteroids, antiepileptic, or other drugs (previous or present).
- Any treatment history of previous vulvar lesion.

PHYSICAL EXAMINATION

Patient—alert, conscious, and cooperative.
- Build
- Nutrition
- Height
- Weight/body mass index (BMI)
- Edema
- *Anemia*—mild
- Cyanosis
- Jaundice
- Clubbing
- Tongue, teeth, gum, and tonsil
- Neck veins
- *Neck glands*—any enlarged nodes
- Leg veins
- Pulse
- Respiration
- Temperature
- Blood pressure (BP).

SYSTEMIC EXAMINATION

- Central nervous system
- *Cardiovascular system:*
  - Auscultation of heart.
- *Respiratory system:*
  - Auscultation of chest.
- *Gastrointestinal system:*
  - Liver
  - Spleen.
- *Examination of other systems:*
  - Examination of back and spines and skeletal system
  - Neurological
  - Ophthalmoscopic examination
  - Urinary system.
- *Examination of breasts and nipple:*
  - Inspection
  - Palpation.

GYNECOLOGICAL EXAMINATION

- *Abdominal examination:*
  - Inspection

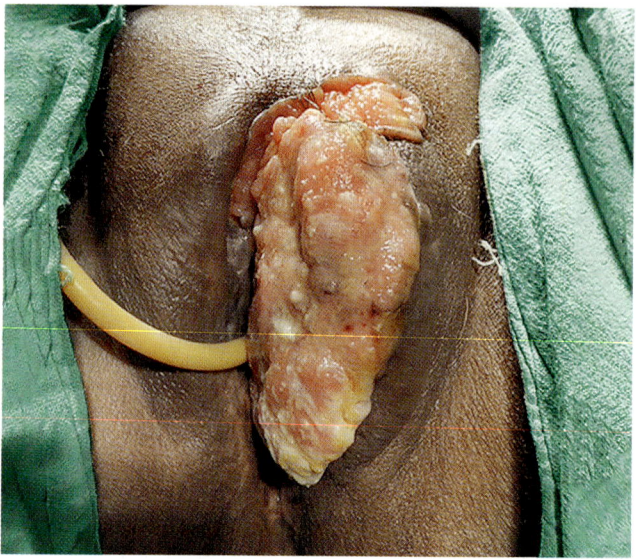

Fig. 1: A growth over vulva.

- *Palpation:* Any lump abdomen or enlargement of inguinal lymph nodes
- *Percussion*
- *Auscultation*.
- *Vaginal examination:*
  - Inspection and palpation of external genitalia **(Fig. 1)**. There may be nodule, ulcerated, or fungating mass with hard base over the vulva. Site, size, surface, bleeding from surface, fixity, and relation with the urethra are noted.
  - *Speculum examination:* Speculum examination is done to inspect the cervix and vagina for any growth or other pathology.
  - *Bimanual examination:* Done to palpate the cervix, uterus, and adnexal pathology.
  - Examination of rectovaginal area and rectal examination.

SUMMARY OF THE CASE (SAMPLE)

A 60-year-old widow nulliparous woman menopause for more than 12 years coming from low socioeconomic status was admitted with a fungating growth over the right side of vulva for about 3 months. There is occasional bleeding from the area and the inner garment stains frequently with the blood stained discharge and there is offensive discharge from the area. She has difficulty and painful micturition. She had history of itching around the vulva for more than 1 year.

On general examination, she has mild pallor, pulse 80/min, and normotensive (BP—110/ 70 mm of Hg), and weight with BMI. There was no enlarged neck glands, no mass on either breast.

Per abdominal examination shows no mass, no ascitic fluid, and no enlargement of inguinal lymph glands on either size.

Examination of vulva shows a large 7.5 cm × 3.5 cm elongated growth on left part of vulva over labium extending from external urethral meatus and the clitoris extending up to perineum. The mobility of the mass is restricted.

On vaginal examination, it has not extended inside the vagina and vagina is healthy except the introitus. Cervix is small and healthy. On bimanual examination, uterus was small, mobile, and there was no adnexal mass. On rectal examination, no abnormality was detected.

Histopathology report showed squamous cell carcinoma.

INVESTIGATIONS SUPPLIED OR REQUIRED

Biopsy report shows squamous cell carcinoma.

PROVISIONAL DIAGNOSIS

It is a case of vulvar squamous cell carcinoma in a 65-year-old nulliparous woman.

DIFFERENTIAL DIAGNOSIS (IF H/P NOT AVAILABLE)

- Vulvar cancer/vulvar intraepithelial neoplasia (VIN)
- Condyloma
- Any metastatic growth
- Vulvar tuberculosis
- Lymphogranuloma venereum
- Vulvar elephantiasis.

Q. What is your diagnosis?

It is a case of vulvar squamous cell carcinoma in a 65-year-old nulliparous woman.

Q. How would you diagnose?

- By symptoms
- Signs
- Vulvoscopy
- Biopsy of the lesion.

DIAGNOSIS OF VULVAR CARCINOMA

History

Age—Most commonly occurs in postmenopausal age between 50 years and 80 years with average 62 years. More than 50% occurs in older than 70 years, 20% women are less than 50 years of age.

Symptoms

Patient may have long history of pruritus vulva (itching) and history of white lesion of vulva. May present with:
- Pruritus
- Painful sore or swelling over the vulva
- Ulceration
- Offensive discharge and bleeding over the vulvar area
- There may be dysuria if lesion is close to urethra
- Swelling over the groin
- Pain appears late
- Patient may be asymptomatic, diagnosed on routine gynecological examination.

Signs (Figs. 2 and 3)

Lesions are raised, pigmented, or ulcerated with everted margin or warty. Lesions are commonly single, 98% in elderly but may be multifocal in younger. Surrounding area may look unhealthy with presence of fissure and leukoplakic patch.

Site, size, extent of lesion, and fixity with deeper structures and pubic bone. Involvement of urethra, vagina, bladder, and anus are assessed.

Vagina and cervix are examined for the presence of any growth which may be due to multifocal or extension.

Inguinal lymph nodes are palpated for enlargement.

Any fungating, ulcerative mass with inguinal lymph node enlargement is suggestive of vulvar carcinoma.

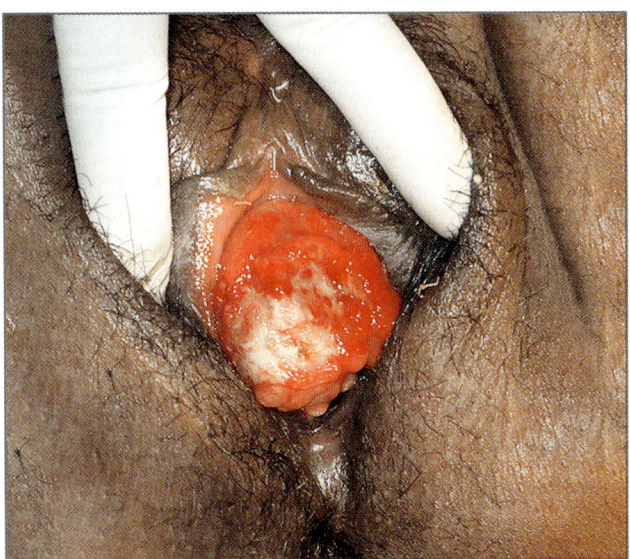

Fig. 2: Vulvar growth in a 30-year-old woman, swelling and ulcer with bleeding from external genitalia.

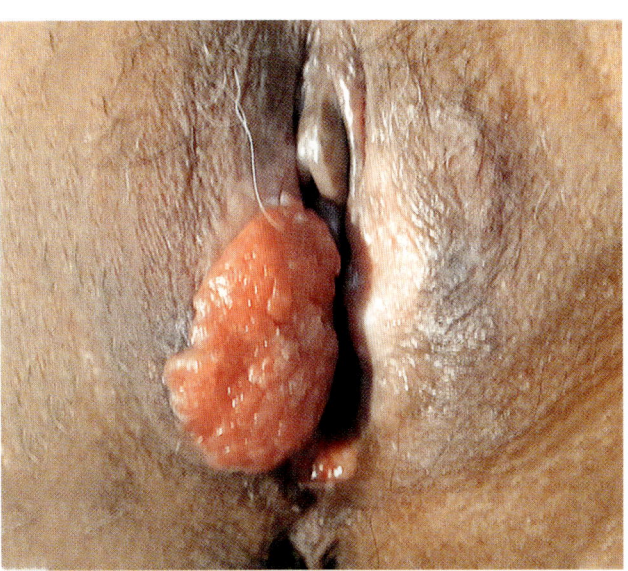

Fig. 3: Vulvar growth in a 75-year-old P6+0 woman; vulvar pruritus for last 3 months; swelling of external genitalia for 2 months and bleeding.

Q. What is kiss ulcer?

Presence of ulcer on both sides touching each other indicating spread by direct contact, the explanation of which is disputed **(Fig. 4)**.

Q. What are the different sites from where vulvar cancer develops? Which is the most common site? Which one is the most common side?

The vulvar cancer may develop from any of the vulvar structures namely mons pubis, labia majora, labia minora, clitoris, Bartholin glands, vestibule, vestibular bulbs, lesser vestibular glands, paraurethral glands, urethral meatus, and vaginal introitus. It develops from squamous epithelium.

Labia majora is the most common site (70%). Next are labia minora and clitoris. Anterior part of vulva is affected more. Right side is commonly involved. Squamous neoplasia develops predominantly from Hart line. Other gynecological pathology **(Fig. 4A)** may be associated with vulvar cancer.

Q. What is Hart line?

It is the demarcation between the skin and mucous membrane on the inner surface of labia minora. From this junction of keratinized stratified squamous epithelium and nonkeratinized squamous mucosa squamous neoplasia develops predominantly. There is no transformation zone (TZ) in vulva like cervix.

Q. How would you evaluate a vulvar cancer lesion?

Clinical examination—as earlier and biopsy.

Biopsy

When the tumor is clinically obvious, biopsy is performed.

Biopsy is usually taken as:

* Incisional biopsy from the lesion which should also include transition area to include the healthy tissue. Here all the tumor mass is not removed.
* *Excisional biopsy:* The whole tumor mass is removed but not like radical excision where surrounding 1 cm tumor free zone is removed.

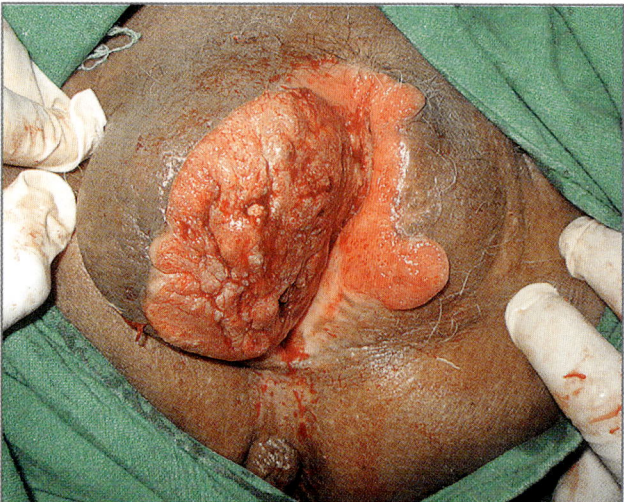

Fig. 4: Vulvar growth (kiss ulcer).

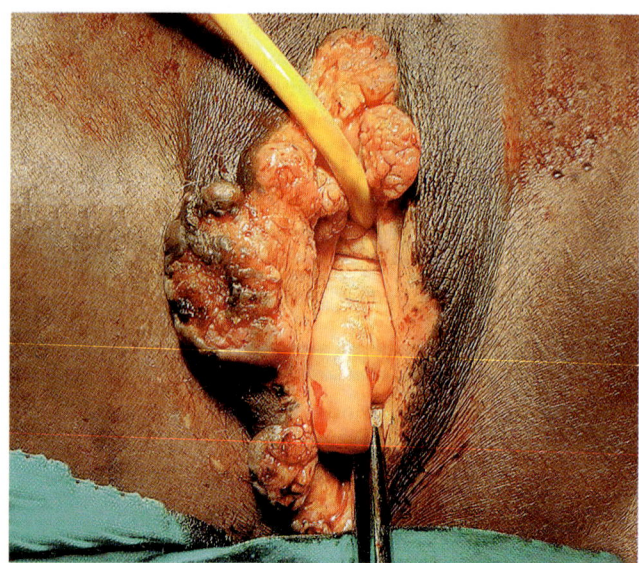

Fig. 4A: Vulvar growth along with pelvic organ prolapse.
Courtesy: Professor Abhijit Rakhsit, RG Medical College, Kolkata, India

* Radical excision includes removal of whole mass with surrounding 1 cm healthy zone. In radical vulvectomy lymph node dissection is done depending on the extent of disease.

Colposcopy (Vulvoscopy)

For early lesion or VIN colposcopy, directed biopsy is done. After painting the vulva with 3% acetic acid vulvoscopy is done after 5 minutes (here more time is needed for soaking keratin layer). Entire vulva is examined to find the acetowhite areas and abnormal vascular pattern where from the biopsy is taken. Deep tissue (4 mm) is taken by **Keyes punch biopsy** forceps to include epithelium and stroma. Multiple biopsies are taken. At the same time, vagina and cervix should also be examined by colposcopy to exclude any lesion.

Q. In which cases of vulvar lesion you want to do biopsy?

Other than the clinically evident malignancy any new lesion or change of epithelium in postmenopausal age should be biopsied. These are changes of color, appearance of surface irregularity, any polypoidal growth, and wart.

Q. What are the different histological varieties of vulvar cancer?

Most common is squamous cell carcinoma (90%). Second is malignant melanoma.

Types are:

* *Squamous cell carcinoma:* It also includes basal cell carcinoma* and verrucous carcinoma
* Malignant melanoma
* Bartholin's gland carcinoma
* Metastatic tumor.

*__Basal cell carcinoma or rodent ulcer__ is an invasive squamous cell growth which penetrates the dermis and deeper tissue, growth is slow and does not metastasize, and local excision is sufficient. Malignant melanoma is the second most cancer of vulva and commonly occurs on clitoris and labia minora.

Varieties of Vulvar Sarcoma
- Leiomyosarcoma
- Epithelial sarcoma
- Malignant fibrous histiocytoma
- Malignant rhabdoid tumor.

Q. What are the other investigations done in vulvar cancer?
- Cervical cytology
- *Cervix and vagina*—colposcopy
- Inguinal lymph node fine-needle aspiration cytology (FNAC).
- Computed tomography (CT) scan pelvis and inguinal regions
- X-ray chest and other bones for metastasis
- Complete hemogram, blood sugar, lipid profile, liver function test (LFT), and kidney function
- For detection of lymph node involvement CT scan, magnetic resonance imaging (MRI), and positron emission tomography (PET) scan are helpful.
  However, **lymphography** is superior to CT scan. Intradermal injection of blue dye overlying the tumor preoperatively, labeling tissue with radioactive tracer, and lymphoscintigraphy are the different methods.

Incidence of Vulvar Cancer

Vulvar cancer comprises 3-4% of all gynecological malignancies. Mostly diagnosed at early stage—Stage I and stage II. Advanced stages are mostly found in older women probably due to delayed presentation, especially in developing countries.

Q. What are the risk factors of vulvar cancer?
- Older women
- Nulliparity
- *High-risk human papilloma virus infection:* Human papilloma virus (HPV) deoxyribonucleic acid (DNA) is detected in 50-70% of invasive lesions and more than 90% in vulvar intraepithelial neoplasia (VIN). HPV vaccine reduces the vulvar cancer incidence.
- *Herpes simplex virus:* Not conclusive
- Smoking
- *Immunosuppression:* More in transplant patients. However, vulvar cancer is not considered as an acquired immunodeficiency syndrome (AIDS) defining malignancy.
- *Lichen sclerosus:* A chronic vulvar inflammatory disease
- Paget's disease
- Cancer cervix, cervical intraepithelial neoplasia (CIN)
- *Vulvar intraepithelial neoplasia:* Some cases of VIN3 may progress to invasive disease in 4 years.

Q. What are the two distinct etiologic entities of squamous cell carcinoma of vulva?
1. *Basaloid or warty types:* Generally occurs in younger patients, multifocal. These are related to human papilloma virus (HPV) infection, vulvar intraepithelial neoplasia (VIN), immunosuppression, and cigarette smoking. Risk factors are similar to those for cervical cancer.
2. *Keratinizing, differentiated, or simplex types:* It occurs in older age. These are not related to HPV and frequently found with lichen sclerosus and squamous hyperplasia (80% cases).

Q. Two age groups—two separate etiogenesis of vulvar cancer—explain.
1. *Younger women less than 55 years:* The cancers at this age group are related to human papilloma virus (HPV) origin in 50% cases like the other anogenital cancers and typically basaloid or warty on histology. This group is associated with smoking and immunosuppression. It is multifocal and multicentric. Its prognosis is good.
2. *Older age group:* Mostly keratinizing, no history of sexually transmitted disease (STD), they are associated with dermatological condition of vulva like lichen sclerosus, and genetic mutation. HPV prevalence is found only in less than 15% cases. They are nonsmoker. It is unifocal and unicentric. Its prognosis is bad.

Q. How does the vulvar cancer spread?
- *Direct spread* (25%)—to the adjacent organs, e.g. vagina, urethra, urinary bladder, anal canal. pelvic bone (2%).
- *Lymphatic spread:* Lymph node involvement in cancer vulva: Stage I—10%, stage II—30%, stage III—70%, and stage IV—100%.
- Hematogenous spread rarely occurs.

Q. Describe the lymphatics of vulva and its clinical importance (Fig. 5).

The *lymphatic spread* is based on Parry Jones description.

Vulvar dermis is abundant with lymphatic plexus which is connected with subcutaneous tissue plexus from where the lymphatics drain into the superficial inguinal lymph node, then → deep inguinal lymph nodes (deep femoral) and lastly → pelvic nodes (external iliac lymph nodes, obturator, common iliac, and para-aortic nodes).

Laterally, lymphatic spread is limited to labiocrural fold.

Nodes of superficial inguinal lymph group are numerous (10-15) and have two chains of transverse chain which lies just below the inguinal ligament and vertical chain of few nodes along the terminal part of saphenous vein. All the superficial nodes lie superficial to fascia lata in the membranous layer of subcutaneous tissue.

Deep inguinal nodes—1-3 in number lies deep to fascia lata in the femoral triangle in femoral canal, medial to femoral vein. The highest deep inguinal node is called Cloquet node or Rosenmuller's node which is situated deep to the inguinal ligament and may be absent in half of the cases and is said to have little clinical importance.

Normally, spread from vulva occurs to the **superficial inguinal lymph nodes, then → deep inguinal lymph nodes (deep femoral), then → pelvic nodes particularly external iliac lymph nodes.** Metastasis to deep femoral node without

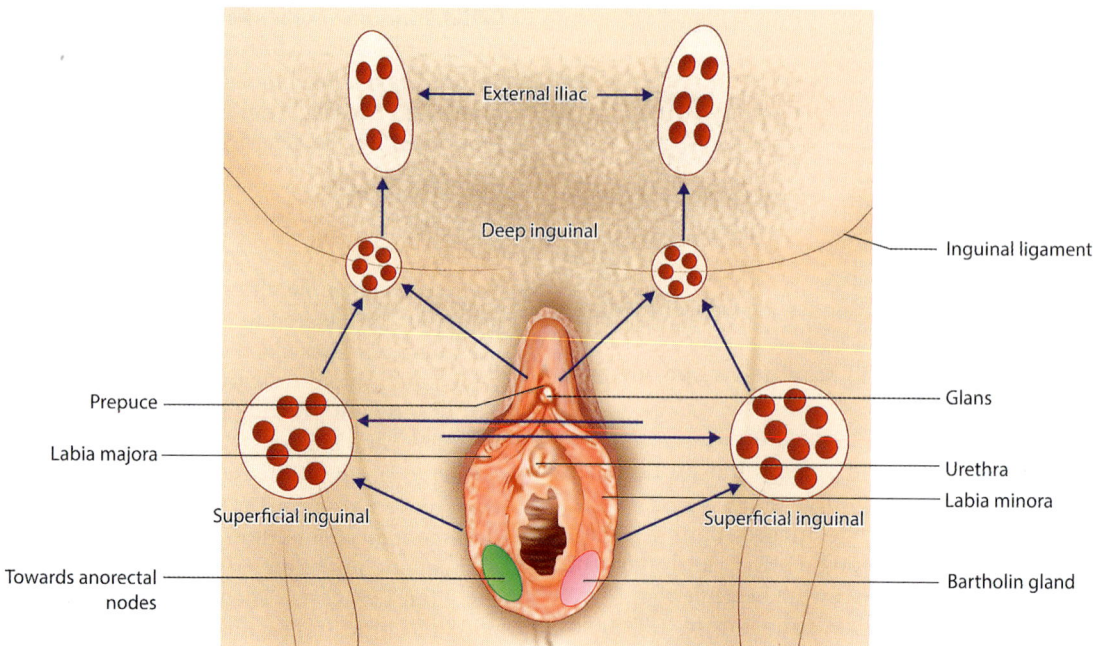

Fig. 5: Lymphatic drainage of vulva.

involvement of superficial inguinal lymph nodes has been reported.

Lymphatics from the skin of clitoris, labia majora, minora, and other areas of vulva drain into superficial lymph nodes.

The glans and corpora cavernosa of the clitoris directly drain into the deep inguinal lymph nodes.

For lateral lesions only ipsilateral nodes are involved and metastasis to contralateral side is very rare.

For midline lesions within 1 cm of midline both sided lymph nodes may be involved.

Lymphatic drainage of clitoris, anterior part of labia minora, and perineum is bilateral. Lymphatic drainage of anterior part of labia majora near the mons pubis is bilateral.

Pelvic nodes (iliac) are not involved without involvement of inguinal nodes. Occasionally, lymphatics from a tumor near the midline or from deep tissues of vulva may directly drain into internal iliac node along the internal pudendal vessels.

There may be metastasis in the absence of clinical suspicious of lymph nodes.

Clinical Importance of Vulvar Lymphatics

Knowledge of lymphatic drainage of vulva will guide the extent of vulvar surgery and the lymphadenectomy whether unilateral or bilateral and need of removal of pelvic nodes depending on the character of lesions—site, number, size, and depth.

Site, size, and depth of lesions determine the degree of lymph node involvement.

Overall involvement of inguinal nodes is 30% and that of iliac group of nodes is 12%.

Lymph node involvements in cancer vulva in:
Stage I—10%
Stage II—30%
Stage III—70%
Stage IV—100%.

Survival rate is more than 80% if no involvement, it becomes less than 50% if inguinal group of lymph nodes are involved and it comes down to 10% when iliac nodes are involved.

It is currently thought that sentinel lymph nodes are the first to be involved directly from the primary site. Prior detection of sentinel lymph node involvement may avoid unnecessary lymph node dissection. If intradermal injection of blue dye overlying the tumor or lymphoscintigraphy for mapping of lymph node shows no involvement of sentinel lymph node, lymph node dissection is not done and morbidity is avoided.

STAGING OF VULVAR CANCER

Q. How to stage vulvar cancer? Describe International Federation of Gynecology and Obstetrics (FIGO) staging of vulvar cancer.

FIGO Revised 2021 Staging of Vulvar Cancer

Until 2009 FIGO staging for vulvar cancer was clinicopathological staging. FIGO has introduced the revised 2021 staging considering the prognostic capability of staging.

In the 2021 new staging system, imaging (r), has been incorporated. Imaging plays a crucial role in the staging of the tumor, assessing the extent of the tumor, and planning the management. In addition, biopsy of the sentinel lymph node facilitates the histopathological staging of the draining lymph node, thus enabling detection of tumor metastases early and better survival rates.

MRI is excellent for soft-tissue resolution and helps local vulvar cancer staging by assessing the involvement of adjacent tissues. CT and PET/CT imaging aid are useful to determine the extent of the distant metastases. PET/CT is better in detecting lymph node metastases.

Table 1 shows gross staging. New (2021) FIGO staging for carcinoma vulva is given in **Table 2.**

KEY CHANGES IN FIGO STAGING FOR VULVAR CANCER 2021

- **Stage I (2021)**: No change in criteria; only methodology change for measuring depth of invasion.
- **Stage II (2021)**: No change.
- **Stage III (2021)**: Changed as below.
  - **IIIA:** Now includes—upper 2/3 urethra, upper 2/3 vagina, bladder mucosa or rectal mucosa (previously all stage IVA) and any number of lymph nodes as long as ≤5 mm.
    No longer includes - lymph node metastasis in a single node >5 mm (now stage IIIB).
  - **IIIB**: Now includes—any number of lymph nodes if size of metastasis >5 mm.
    Now excludes—3 or more lymph nodes if size is ≤ 5mm (now stage IIIA).
  - **IIIC**: No change.
- **Stage IV (2021):**
  - **IVA**: Now excludes—upper 2/3 urethra or upper 2/3 vagina, bladder mucosa or rectal mucosa (now stage IIIA).

Lymph nodes containing macro and/or micrometastases are considered involved. Isolated tumor cells do not change the stage but their presence should be noted.

MANAGEMENT OF VULVAR CANCER

Mode of Treatment

- The treatment of vulvar cancer is surgery. The traditional treatment is radical vulvectomy and bilateral inguinofemoral lymphadenectomy (Way and Taussig, 1935).
- Radiation is added in advanced stages—stage II to stage IV.
- Chemotherapy [cisplatin, bleomycin, and 5-fluorouracil (5FU)] may also be needed with/ without radiation in advanced disease especially in stage IV cases.

Recent Attitude of Treatment of Vulvar Cancer

- More conservative approach with less primary mortality with improved 5-years survival rate.
- Optimal surgery with avoiding the mutilating wide surgery and giving separate inguinal incision.
- Selection of the cases for lymph node dissection.

Types of Surgery (Table 3)

- Wide local excision (WLE) (also called simple partial vulvectomy) **(Figs. 6 to 8).**
- Radical partial vulvectomy **(Fig. 9)**.
- Radical total vulvectomy **(Figs. 10 and 11)**.

Inguinofemoral lymphadenectomy is accompanied with radical partial vulvectomy and radical total vulvectomy.

Radical vulvectomy itself means total vulvectomy and bilateral inguinofemoral lymphadenectomy.

In all cases of surgery removal of at least 1 cm marginal disease free area is removed to decrease the recurrence.

Stage-wise Treatment of Vulvar Cancer

The stage-wise treatment of vulvar cancer is illustrated in **Table 4**.

Table 1: Gross staging.	
Stage	Characteristics
I	Tumor confined to the vulva
II	Tumor of any size with extension to lower one-third of the urethra, lower one-third of the vagina, lower one-third of the anus with negative nodes
III	Tumor of any size with extension to upper part of adjacent perineal structures, or with any number of nonfixed, nonulcerated lymph node
IV	Tumor of any size fixed to bone, or fixed, ulcerated lymph node metastases, or distant metastases

Table 2: New (2021) FIGO staging for carcinoma of the vulva.	
Stage	Description
I	Tumor confined to the vulva
IA	Tumor size ≤2 cm and stromal invasion ≤1 mm[a]
IB	Tumor size >2 cm or stromal invasion >1 mm[a]
II	Tumor of any size with extension to lower one-third of the urethra, lower one-third of the vagina, lower one-third of the anus with negative nodes
III	Tumor of any size with extension to upper part of adjacent perineal structures, or with any number of nonfixed, nonulcerated lymph node
IIIA	Tumor of any size with disease extension to upper two-thirds of the urethra, upper two-thirds of the vagina, bladder mucosa, rectal mucosa, or regional lymph node metastases ≤5 mm
IIIB	Regional[b] lymph node metastases >5 mm
IIIC	Regional[b] lymph node metastases with extracapsular spread
IV	Tumor of any size fixed to bone, or fixed, ulcerated lymph node metastases, or distant metastases
IVA	Disease fixed to pelvic bone, or fixed or ulcerated regional[b] lymph node metastases
IVB	Distant metastases

[a]Depth of invasion is measured from the basement membrane of the deepest, adjacent, dysplastic, tumor-free rete ridge (or nearest dysplastic rete peg) to the deepest point of invasion.
[b]Regional refers to inguinal and femoral lymph nodes.

SECTION 2: Clinical Cases

Table 3: Types of surgery.

Surgery	What is done?	Where it is done?
Wide local excision (simple partial vulvectomy)	Tumor is excised with 1 cm margin and also 1 cm deep margin which corresponds to fascia of Colles	Microinvasive carcinoma (stage IA)
Radical partial vulvectomy	Only the tumor containing part of vulva with 1–2 cm margin and up to perineal membrane is removed with conservation of other part of vulva. Ipsilateral inguinofemoral lymphadenectomy is needed	Unifocal lesion confined to labia majora, minora, mons, vestibule, or perineum. No or limited involvement of vagina, urethra, and anus. Ipsilateral inguinofemoral lymphadenectomy done when vulvar lesion lies > 2 cm beyond the midline
Radical total vulvectomy	Complete dissection and removal of vulvar tissue with adequate margins in all sides deeply up to perineal membrane. Always associated with bilateral inguinofemoral lymphadenectomy. It is done by old butterfly or longhorn incision or vulvectomy with two separate inguinal incisions for lymphadenectomy. The butterfly or longhorn incision is abandoned due to severe morbidity	Stage IB–IVA. Bilateral is recommended for all lesions within 2 cm of midline

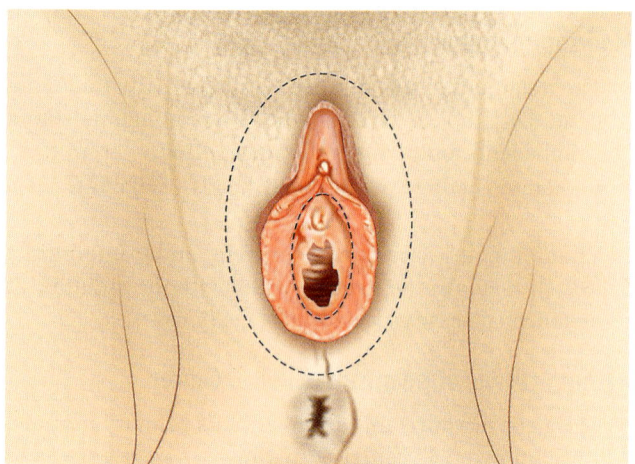

Fig. 6: Simple vulvectomy incision (*see* also Fig. 25).

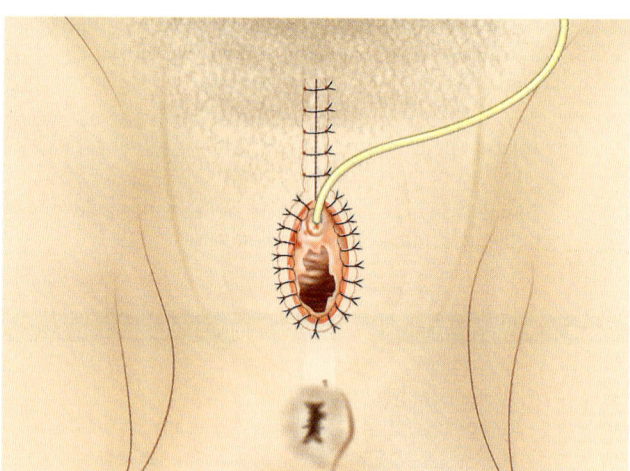

Fig. 8: Vulvar appearance after repair of simple vulvectomy.

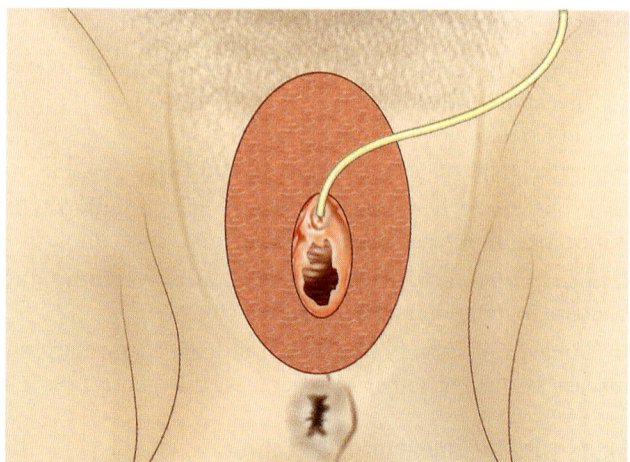

Fig. 7: Simple vulvectomy—after the excision of skin.

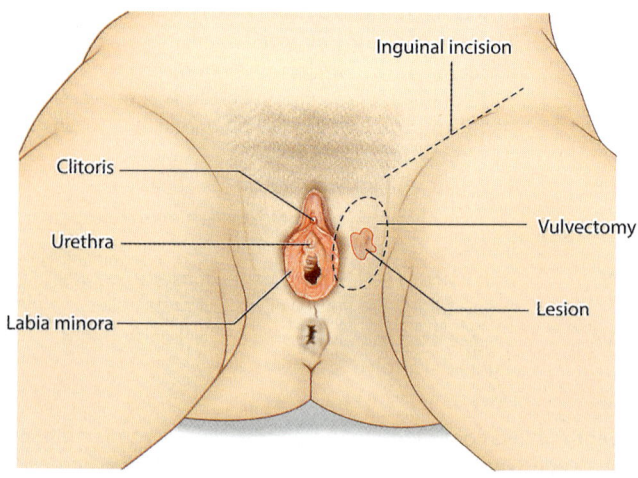

Fig. 9: Radical partial vulvectomy with ipsilateral inguinofemoral lymphadenectomy.

CHAPTER 9: A Case of Carcinoma Vulva, Preinvasive Lesion of Vulva and Vaginal Cancer

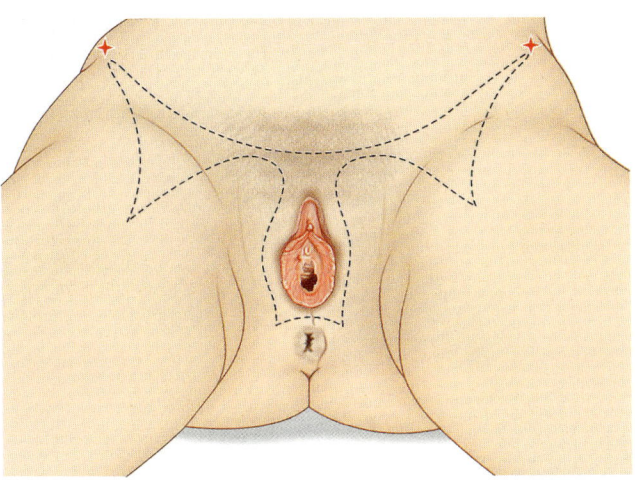

Fig. 10: Butterfly incision—en bloc radical vulvectomy with bilateral inguinofemoral lymphadenectomy (not favored nowadays).

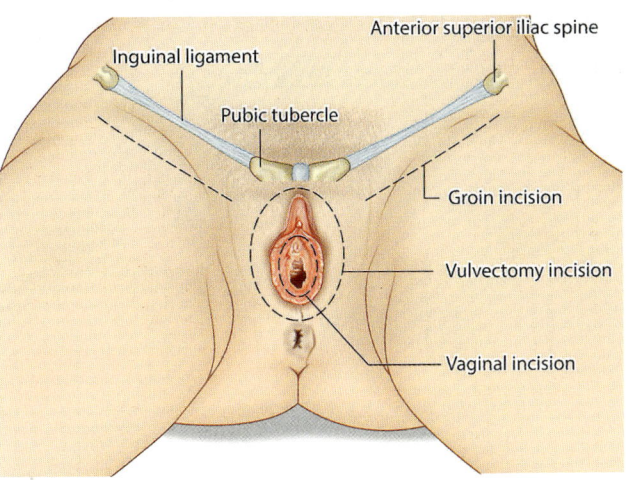

Fig. 11: Radical complete vulvectomy with bilateral inguinofemoral lymphadenectomy—separate incision (preferred incision).

Table 4: Stage-wise treatment of vulvar cancer.	
Stage	Treatment
Stage IA (microinvasive) ≤1 mm stromal invasion	Wide local excision (simple partial vulvectomy). No lymphadenectomy
Stage IA >1 mm stromal invasion	• Wide local excision and ipsilateral inguinofemoral lymphadenectomy • Bilateral inguinofemoral lymphadenectomy is needed when: (a) Labia minora involved, (b) If the lesion is within 1 cm of midline, or (c) Lymph node positive on that side
Stage II	• Larger radical partial excision and bilateral inguinofemoral lymphadenectomy with/ without radiotherapy • Occasionally radical complete vulvectomy may be required depending on size and location of tumor
Stage III	Primary radical surgery if possible or primary radiation followed by surgery after shrink- age of tumor over 5 weeks. Time and local excision instead of exenteration can be done
Stage IV	Primary radiotherapy or chemotherapy followed by excision of residual tumor

Steps of Radical Vulvectomy

❖ Radical vulvectomy—outline the steps **(Figs. 12 to 21)**
❖ Groin dissection **(Figs. 12 to 17)**
❖ An elliptical incision is made from 4 cm medial and 2 cm below the anterior superior iliac spine and pubic tubercle **(Fig. 12)**
❖ Dissection is done from the lateral side to remove subcutaneous tissue along with superficial lymph nodes that lie along the superficial circumflex artery, superficial epigastric artery, and external pudendal artery till the external oblique aponeurosis is reached **(Figs. 13 and 14)**.
❖ The above mentioned vessels are encountered from lateral to medial are ligated and cut.
❖ The saphenous vein is identified. The femoral vessels are identified. The common sheath enclosing the artery and vein is cut and any deep lymph node is noted for any enlargement. If any enlargement is noted then pelvic lymph nodes are also dissected **(Fig. 15)**.
❖ The common sheath is sutured **(Fig. 16)**.
❖ Drain is placed and skin is closed in layers **(Fig. 17)**.

Vulvectomy

❖ The 2 cm incision is given circumferentially along the growth **(Fig. 18)**.

❖ Lateral and medial flaps are raised to complete the dissection as deep as possible up to the perineal membrane **(Fig. 19)** and the specimen is removed as a whole **(Fig. 20)**.

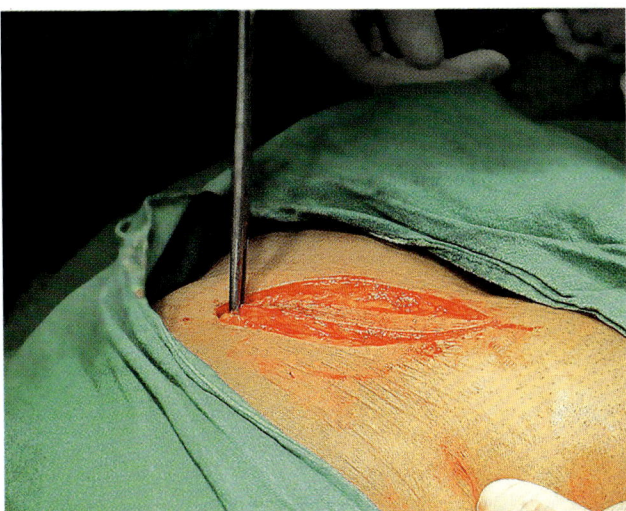

Fig. 12: Groin dissection (an elliptical incision is made from 4 cm medial and 2 cm below the anterior superior iliac spine and pubic tubercle).

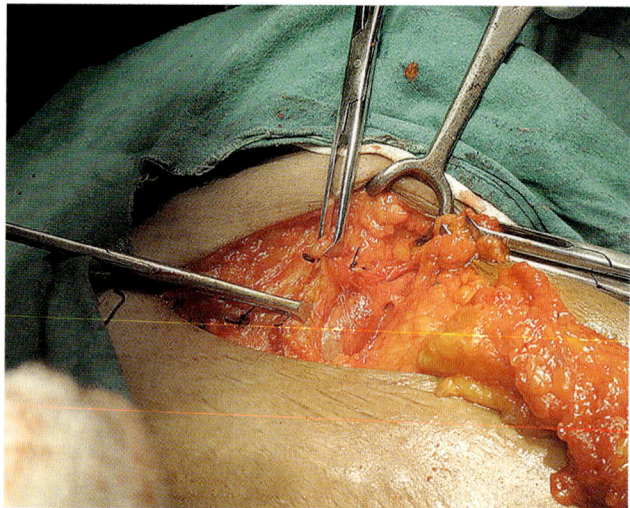

Fig. 13: Dissection is done from the lateral side to remove subcutaneous tissue along with superficial lymph nodes right side.

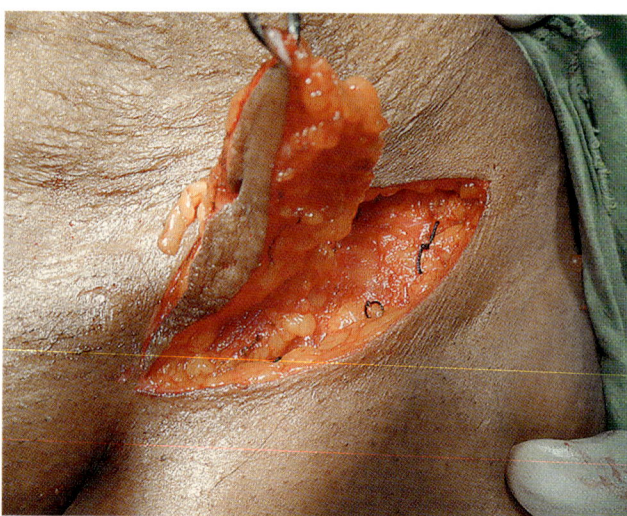

Fig. 14: Dissection is done from the lateral side to remove subcutaneous tissue along with superficial lymph nodes left side.

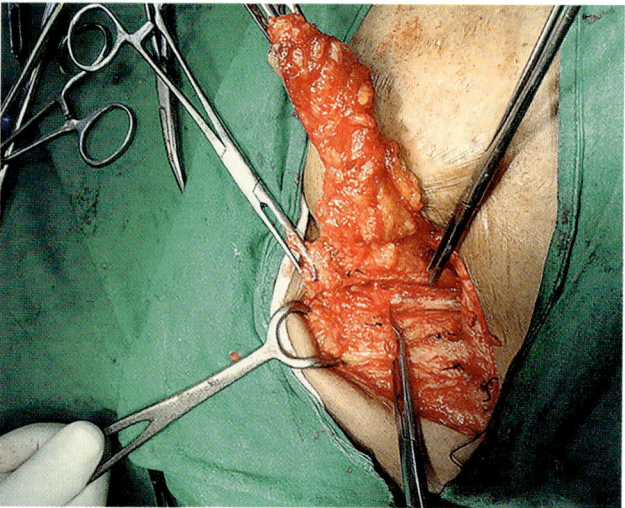

Fig. 15: Saphenous vein and the femoral vessels are identified. The common sheath enclosing the artery and vein is cut and any enlarged deep lymph node is dissected and removed.

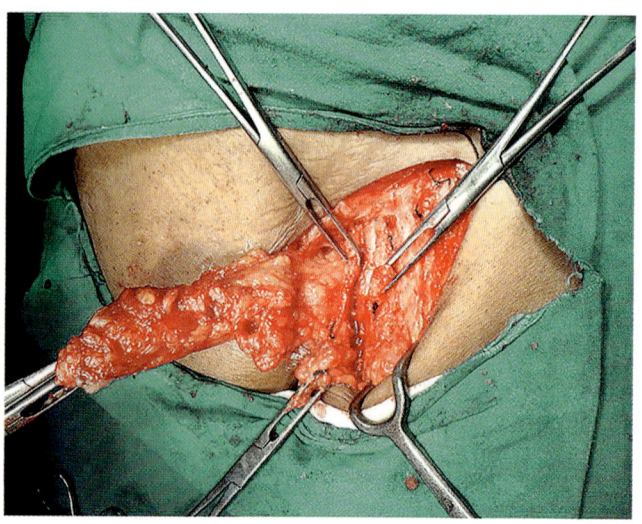

Fig. 16: Common sheath is sutured.

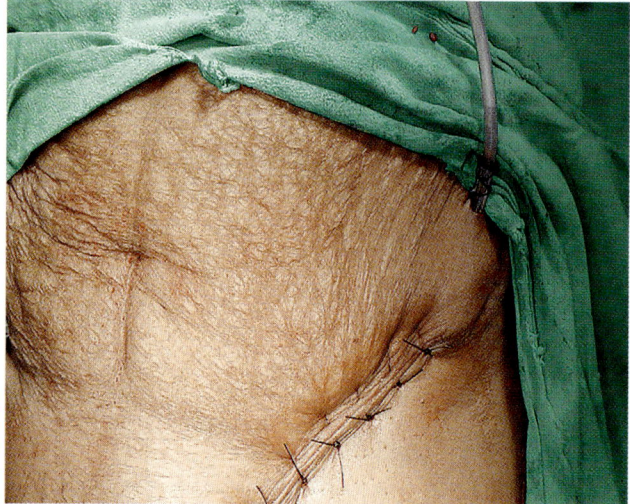

Fig. 17: After repair of inguinal incision left side.
Courtesy: Professor RP Ganguly

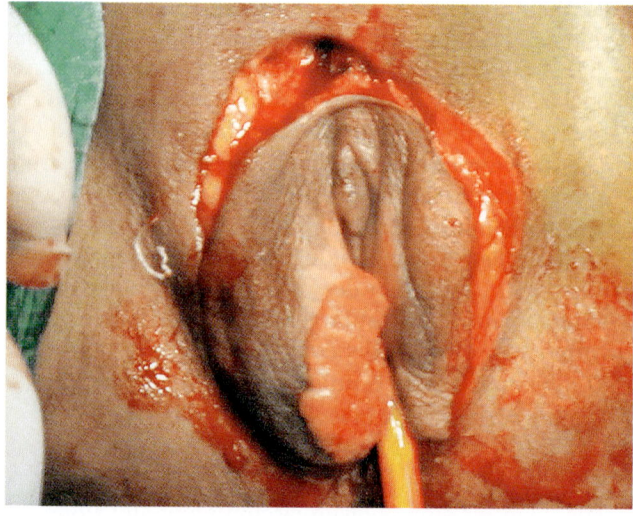

Fig. 18: The 2 cm incision is given circumferentially along the growth.

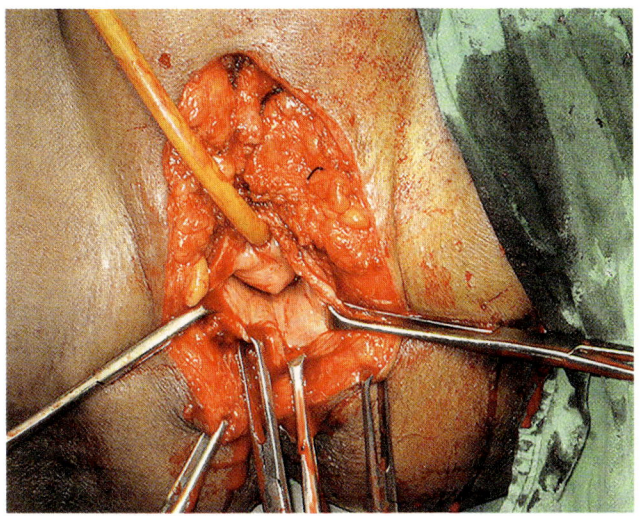

Fig. 19: Bare area after removal of vulvar tissue.

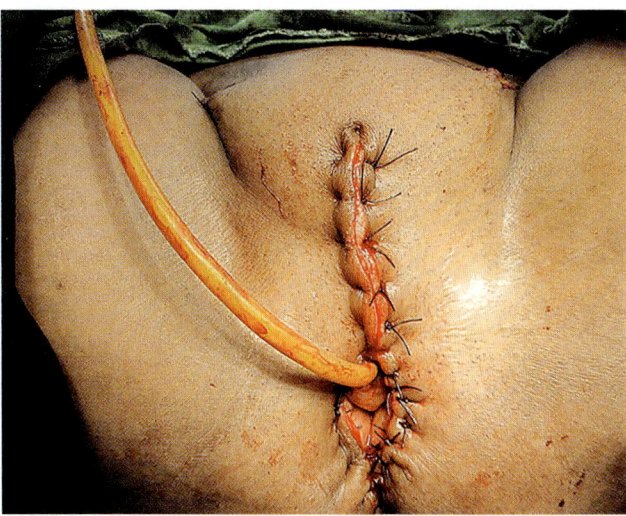

Fig. 21: Skin is closed.

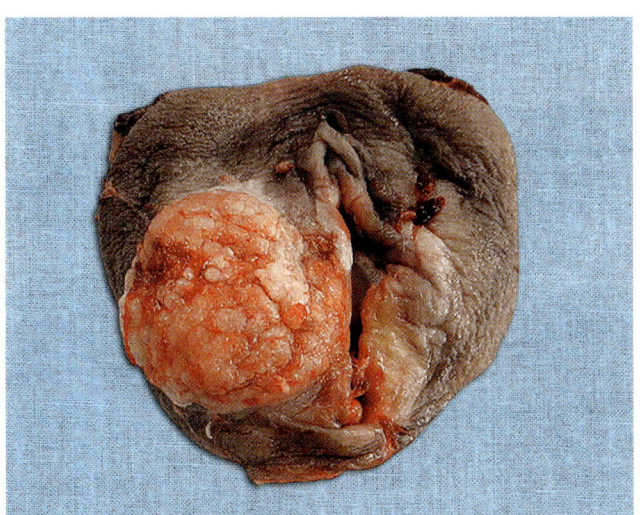

Fig. 20: Removed specimen. Look at the specimen with wide margin of healthy skin.

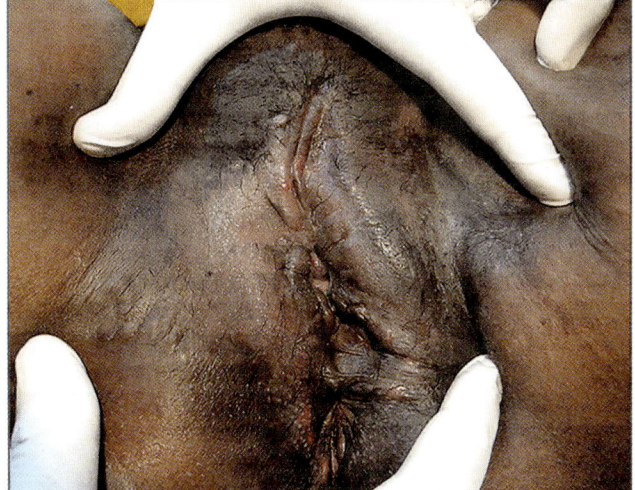

Fig. 22: Follow-up case of a 30-year-old woman after 2 months as in Figure 2.

- The artery supplying clitoris should be dealt carefully and if necessary it should be ligated.
- Skin is closed **(Fig. 21)**.

Complications of Radical Vulvectomy

Immediate

- *Wound dehiscence:* Three incisions technique has reduced the wound dehiscence
- Wound infection
- *Thromboembolic complications:* It can be reduced by heparin
- Secondary hemorrhage
- Ostitis
- Paresthesia of upper legs.

Late

- Disfigurement of vulva
- Vaginal introital stenosis

- Impaired sexual function, dyspareunia
- Leg edema/lymph edema (*see* **Fig. 24**)
- Fecal and urinary incontinence
- Complications of radiation
- All cases are followed-up regularly **(Figs. 22 to 24)**.

PROGNOSIS OF VULVAR CANCER

Overall prognosis of vulvar squamous cell carcinoma is very good from 75–90% in stage I and stage II. Stage-wise survival rate is as shown in **Table 5**.

Table 5: Stage-wise survival rate of vulvar cancer.				
International Federation of Gynecology and Obstetrics (FIGO) stage	Stage I	Stage II	Stage III	Stage IV
5-years survival rate	90%	75%	54%	16%

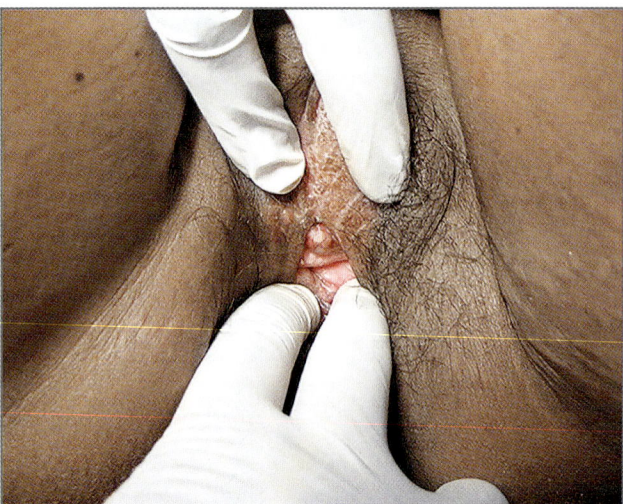

Fig. 23: Follow-up case of a 30-year-old woman after 5 years as in Figure 2, Patient can lead to sexual life.

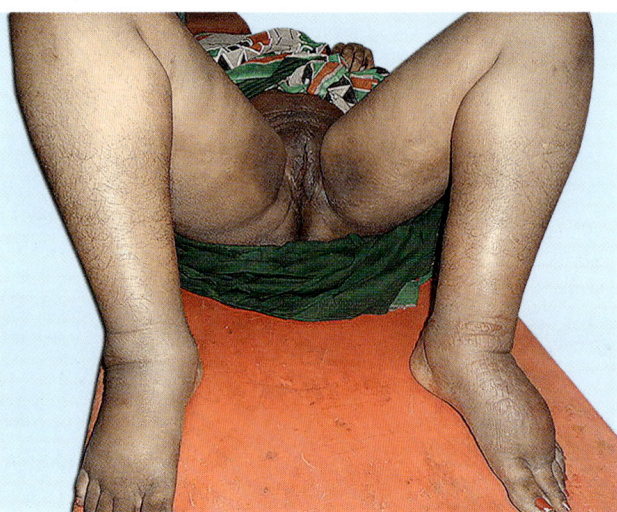

Fig. 24: Follow-up case of a 30-year-old woman after 5 years—edema of lower limbs and vulvar skin changes due to complication of radiotherapy as in Figure 2.

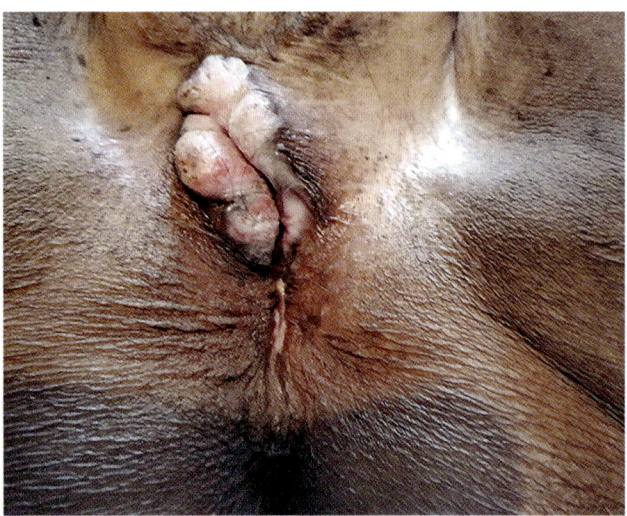

Fig. 24A: Recurrence of vulvar growth 3 years after radical vulvectomy.

Other than International Federation of Gynecology and Obstetrics (FIGO) staging the prognosis depends on many other factors.

Prognostic Factors of Vulvar Carcinoma

- Stage of the disease (*see* here).
- *Size of the tumor:* Survival rate is 90% when size is less than 1 cm, it comes down to 40% when size is more than 4 cm.
- *Depth of invasion**: Tumor depth of 1 mm has only 3% metastasis whereas more than or equal to 5 mm nodes become positive in 48% cases.
- *Lymph node involvement:* Single most important factor. Survival rate is more than 80% if no involvement, it becomes less than 50% if inguinal group of lymph nodes are involved, and it comes down to 10% when iliac nodes are involved. Site, size, and depth of lesions determine the degree of lymph node involvement.
- Lymphatic vascular space involvement.
- *Status of resected margin:* 1–2 cm tumor free margin is required to improve survival. There is no consensus value of tumor-free margin threshold for recurrence.
- Recurrence **(Fig. 24A)** is more common when tumor-free margin is within 8mm at final pathological analysis.

*Depth is defined as length of the tumor from stromal–epithelial junction of the adjacent most dermal papilla to the deepest point of infiltration.

PREINVASIVE LESIONS OF VULVA

Facts about Preinvasive Lesion and Vulvar Cancer

- Of all the vulvar cancers 90% are squamous cell carcinoma and in some cases they develop from VIN.
- Unlike cervical intraepithelial neoplasia (CIN) VIN progresses to invasive stage is less.
- But the incidence of vulvar carcinoma in situ has increased recently and presumed to be due to increase of sexually transmitted diseases (STDs) and human papilloma virus (HPV) infection and this trend is more evident in younger age group.
- The mean age of women suffering from VIN has come down to 39 years.

Q. What are the premalignant lesions of vulvar carcinoma?

These are:
- Vulvar intraepithelial neoplasia (VIN)
- Lichen sclerosus
- Paget's disease
- Squamous cell hyperplasia
- Condyloma acuminatum.

Vulvar Intraepithelial Neoplasia

Etiology

- Human papilloma virus deoxyribonucleic acid (DNA) in 80% cases of VIN mostly found in younger women (vulvar

carcinoma is associated with HPV in less—only 15–80% cases).
- Chronic inflammatory skin conditions or p53 mutations found in olderly women and responsible for VIN—only 2–10% cases.

Terminologies and Classification of Vulvar Intraepithelial Neoplasia

- The term VIN was introduced in 1986 by the International Society for the Study of Vulvovaginal Disease (ISSVD). Similar to CIN it was VIN I (mild atypia), VIN II (moderate atypia), and VIN III (severe atypia and carcinoma in situ).
- Later in 2004 by ISSVD VIN I was eliminated due to lack of evidence as it is precursor of cancer and VIN II and VIN III was combined under the term VIN as histological distinction is not reproducible and categorized in three groups (*see* here).
- Low-grade squamous intraepithelial lesion (LSIL) and high-grade squamous intraepithelial lesion (HSIL) terminology was recommended in 2012.
- Currently ACOG (2019) adopted ISSVD terminology of three groups namely vulvar low grade SIL, vulvar high grade SIL and differentiated VIN.

In the new classification and ISSVD terminology system vulvar intraepithelial neoplasia(VIN) is categorized into three groups: (a) vulvar low grade SIL, (b) vulvar high grade SIL and (c) differentiated VIN as given in **Table 6**.

Table 6: Current categorization of VIN and ISSVD terminology system (ACOG 2019).

Nomenclature	Previous name	Lesion characters and risk factors
Vulvar LSIL	VIN1	HPV effect, flat lesions consisting of basal atypia and koilocytic changes like condyloma, not precancerous and self-limited
Vulvar HSIL	VIN usual type (VIN2, VIN3, vulvar CIS)	• Multicentric and multifocal disease, common in oncogenic HPV infection, resembling high-grade CIN, young women. Associated with other STDs and in immunosuppression cases
Differentiated VIN	2–10% former VIN3 lesion	• Oncogenic HPV infection uncommon • Unicentric and unifocal • Commonly seen with dermatologic conditions like lichen sclerosus • Older postmenopausal (6th and 7th decades), nonsmoking • Probably precursor to all vulvar squamous cell carcinoma

Abbreviations: VIN, vulvar intraepithelial neoplasia; LSIL, low grade squamous lesion; HSIL, high grade squamous epithelial lesion; HPV, human papilloma virus; STD, sexually transmitted disease; ISSVD, International Society for the Study of Vulvar Disease

Diagnosis of Vulvar Intraepithelial Neoplasia
- Clinical
- Colposcopy (vulvoscopy)
- *Biopsy*—may be multiple.

Clinical presentation
- *Asymptomatic*—50%
- Pruritus (most common), burning, pain, and superficial dyspareunia—hampering sexual and day-to-day life
- *Vulvar swelling (unusual)*—raised areas like condylomata.

Signs

- Lesions vary widely—usually well-defined margins—white, hyperpigmented, keratotic plaques, erythematous, ulcerative, elevated, warty, or bulky lesions.
- Vulvar intraepithelial neoplasia lesions are usually visible without any aid in contrast to CIN or vaginal intraepithelial neoplasia (VaIN) where acetic acid is needed to visualize.
- dVIN is associated with lichen sclerosus or chronic lichen simplex.
- Large ulcerative lesions with palpable inguinal lymph nodes are suspicious of invasive nature.

Biopsy with/without colposcopy

Best done by colposcopic directed (vulvoscopy) with prior 3% acetic acid for 5 minutes. There may be pain or discomfort due to acetic acid. Lesions appear as acetowhite lesion, pigmented areas as dusky gray, and vascular pattern in high-grade lesions that may show coarse punctuation. Use of toluidine blue to select the area for biopsy is usually avoided due to high false positive and negative results.

Biopsy can be done as an outpatient procedure by **Keyes punch biopsy**, a 6 mm diameter skin tissue is taken under local anesthesia. Suturing may be needed in biopsied area.

Prevention

Prevention is done by immunization with quadrivalent human papilloma virus vaccine (HPV—6, 11, 16 and 18) vaccine to the target population to reduce vulvar cancer to one-third. Smoking cessation and optimization of immune status is another addressing areas.

Treatment

Principle: VIN1 is not treated, rather reassessed annually for high-grade lesion.

Treatment of high-grade lesion is mandatory. As progression is less (3–10%) local excision is sufficient with objectives of: (a) Prevention or exclusion of invasive disease, (b) Symptomatic cure, and (c) Preserving the normal vulvar configuration.

Treatment Modalities

- Excision: Simple and WLE **(Fig. 25)**
- Laser ablation
- Cavitational ultrasonic surgical aspiration (CUSA)
- Topical application: Many topical medicine is tried but there is no Food and Drug Administration (FDA) approval.

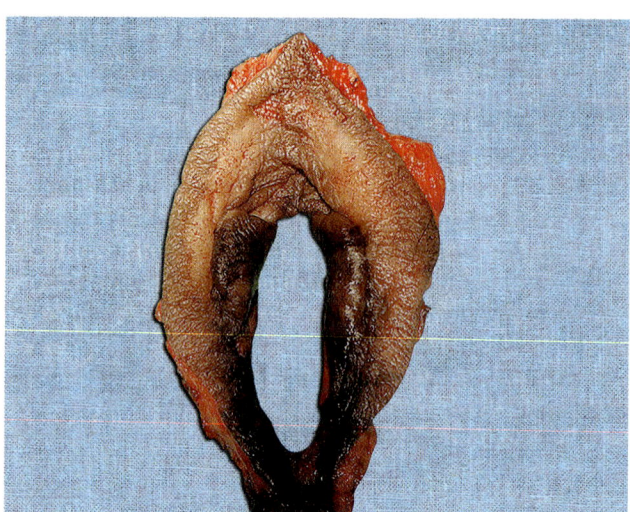

Fig. 25: Simple vulvectomy.
Courtesy: Professor Sukanta Misra

In the list topical imiquimod gathered interest with good response and is under trial.

Excision:
- For small single lesion local excision is sufficient.
- Wide local excision removal of tissue with at least 5 mm healthy margin is preferred for large VIN where invasive case cannot be excluded. Frozen section biopsy is preferred in these cases. Skin grafting may be needed in these cases.
- In case of extensive or large multifocal lesions simple or total vulvectomy may be needed with/without skin grafting.
- Older women with high-grade VIN should be treated by excision rather than ablation as chance of invasion and recurrence is more in this age group.

Laser ablation:
- Laser ablation provides good cosmetic result.
- Invasive lesion should be excluded with biopsy as tissue is not available for biopsy after treatment.
- Laser ablation is appropriate for multifocal lesions.
- However, recurrence rate is more common than that of WLE.

Cavitational ultrasonic surgical aspiration (CUSA)
In CUSA using ultrasound, cavitation and disruption of affected tissue is done following which tissue is aspirated and collected.

Treatment complications
Poor wound healing, infection, local discomfort, chronic pain, and scar formation.

Recurrence
In spite of treatment, 30% of cases of VIN recur and 5% may develop locally invasive cancer for which long-term follow-up is needed.

VULVAR INTRAEPITHELIAL DISEASE

Historical background of nomenclature of VID.

Terms used in the past for the epithelial growth disorders and differentiations:
- Leukoplakia
- Lichen sclerosis et atrophicus
- Primary atrophy
- Sclerotic dermatoses
- Atrophic and hyperplastic vulvitis
- Kraurosis vulvae.

Q. What do you mean by chronic vulvar dystrophy?

All the earlier terminologies were brought under the same umbrella *chronic vulvar dystrophy* by Jeffcoate (1966) as these terms did not refer to separate entities (due to lack of specific characteristic both macro, microscopic appearance, and frequent interchangeable findings).

Nonneoplastic Epithelial Disorders of Skin and Mucosa

In 1989, the *ISSVD 1989* recommended the replacement of term dystrophy by new classification as *nonneoplastic epithelial disorders of skin and mucosa* the malignant potentiality of which is low.

Old term for intraepithelial neoplasia was used as:
- Erythroplasia of Queyrat
- Bowen's diseases
- Carcinoma in situ simplex
- Paget's disease.

Squamous Cell Carcinoma in Situ (Stage 0)

In *1976, ISSVD* opined that earlier first three are variants of the same disease process and termed as *squamous cell carcinoma in situ (Stage 0)*.

Vulvar Intraepithelial Neoplasia

In 1986, ISSVD brought the term *VIN*.

Classification of Epithelial Vulvar Diseases

In *1989, a new nomenclature for epithelial vulvar disease* was introduced by *ISSVD* which is given below in the **Table 7**. This is based on whether it is neoplastic or nonneoplastic disorder.

In 2004, categorization of VIN was done by ISSVD: In 2004 by ISSVD VIN1 was eliminated due to lack of evidence as it is precursor of cancer and VIN2 and VIN3 was combined under the term *VIN* as histological distinction is not reproducible and categorized in three groups: *uVIN, usual type, dVIN, differentiated type, and VIN unspecified.*

In 2012 Low-grade squamous intraepithelial lesion (LSIL) and high-grade squamous intraepithelial lesion (HSIL) terminology was accepted.

Currently ACOG (2019) adopted ISSVD terminology of three groups namely vulvar low grade SIL, vulvar high grade SIL and differentiated VIN as described above.

Table 7: Classification of epithelial vulvar diseases.	
Non-neoplastic epithelial disorders of skin and mucosa	• Lichen sclerosis (lichen sclerosis et atrophicus) • Squamous hyperplasia (formerly hyperplastic dystrophy) • Other dermatoses
Mixed non-neoplastic and neoplastic epithelial disorders	
Intraepithelial neoplasia	• Squamous intraepithelial neoplasia • Vulvar intraepithelial neoplasia 1 (VIN1) • VIN2 • VIN3 (severe dysplasia or carcinoma in situ) • Nonsquamous intraepithelial neoplasia • Paget's disease • Tumors of melanocytes, noninvasive
Invasive tumors	

Q. What is Paget's disease?

Paget's disease is nonsquamous intraepithelial neoplasia of vulva and comparable to intraductal carcinoma of breasts.

Commonly occurs in postmenopausal women. Symptoms are itching, soreness, pain, and occasionally bleeding.

On examination, there is slightly elevated, well-demarcated areas with red, indurated, and eczematous lesion.

Biopsy shows characteristic Paget's cells in epidermis, cells are large pale vacuolated, and these are adenocarcinomatous mucus secreting cells with vesicular nuclei and mitotic figure is rare. Underlying adenocarcinoma of Bartholin's gland is found 20% of cases. Carcinoma of other organs like breasts, ovary, cervix, and intestines may be associated in 25% of cases.

As it is precancerous or may be associated with invasive disease treatment is local excision or vulvectomy followed by biopsy. Lymph node dissection depends on the biopsy report. Follow-up is mandatory as it recurs in 20% cases.

Lichen Sclerosus

Lichen sclerosus is the most common white lesion of vulva and an autoimmune-mediated dermatoses of anogenital area affecting the entire vulva. Incidence is 1 in 300.

Etiology is exactly not known and presumed to be autoimmune as it is may be associated with other autoimmune disorders like systemic lupus erythematosus (SLE), Grave's disease.

Commonly occurs in postmenopausal group, sometimes in prepubertal age.

Symptoms are pruritus, burning sensation, and dyspareunia and may be dysuria.

The skin over the affected area becomes thin, white, introitus becomes narrow, labium becomes shrinkage, and may be adhered of labium with other side. Urethral meatal may become stenosed with retention of urine. Vulvar skin becomes white parchment paper-like appearance. The lesion over vulva looks figure of eight. Subepithelial hemorrhage is due to constant scratching. Vagina, vestibule, and anal canal are not usually involved.

Diagnosis is done by biopsy with Keyes biopsy forceps as an outpatient procedure under local anesthesia. H/P shows thin hyperkeratotic epithelium with hyalinization, flattened rete pegs, and infiltration of lymphocytes and plasma cells.

Treatment

Surgery is usually not needed. Avoidance of irritants and topical steroid like clobetasol and emollients are the treatment. Immunosuppressions are rarely needed in case of resistance to steroids.

In advanced and neglected cases surgical correction of vaginal introitus and urethral meatus may be needed rarely.

Vulvodynia

Vulvodynia is a state of pain (chronic vulvar discomfort) over the vulva in absence of any disease or infection. It can occur at any age.

The incidence is as high as 15% among women. Woman suffers from psychosexual dysfunction, primary or secondary.

Patient described the pain as burning pain, aching, stinging, or rawness. It may be localized or diffuse. It may be provoked or unprovoked. The problem may have severe distress to woman and alters quality of life adversely.

Diagnosis is done by detailed history including sexual history and examination of the area to exclude any pathology including dermatitis.

Treatment—perineal massage, application of oil, and psychotherapy are the important treatment steps. Symptomatic treatment is the key of management. Though few women get relieved with neuromodulator but it has limited value.

VAGINAL CANCER

It is a rare cancer, incidence is less contributing 1–2% of all gynecological malignancy. Age—median age is 58 years. Chance increases with age. Peak age is more than or equal to 80 years.

Types

Majority of vaginal cancer is metastasis from endometrium and cervix.

Primary vaginal cancer is mostly squamous cell carcinoma and contributes 75–85% of vaginal cancers.

Other occasional tumors are clear cell adenocarcinoma and malignant melanoma. Malignant melanoma is very rare. Genital tract melanoma accounts for 3% of all melanomas and vagina contributes only 1%. Melanoma is most common in vulva (70%), then vagina (21%), and in cervix—3%.

Sarcoma botryoides (embryonal rhabdomyosarcoma) are vaginal tumor found in young girls (peak age—8 years). "Botrys" means bunch of grapes.

Risk Factors

- Vaginal intraepithelial neoplasia—a precursor of invasive cancer. 2–3% of VaIN will progress to invasive cancer.
- Previous malignant and premalignant disease of the cervix.
- About 60% of primary vaginal cancer is HPV associated—quadrivalent HPV vaccine can prevent VaIN 2 and 3 associated with HPV 16 or 18.

Diagnosis of Vaginal Cancer

Symptoms

- Vaginal bleeding or blood-stained vaginal discharge is the most common symptom.
- Pelvic pain, vaginal discharge, dysuria, urgency, hematuria, and constipation according to site of involvement.

Inspection and Speculum Examination

A mass or ulcer mostly found on upper third of vagina (**Figs. 26 to 28**).

Examination under Anesthesia

- *Biopsy:* Confirmation is done by biopsy— punch biopsy for a gross lesion. Tischler biopsy forceps may be used.
- *Cystoscopy and sigmoidoscopy* can detect local spread.
- *Magnetic resonance imaging (MRI)* to confirm local growth and extension/computed tomography (CT) scan of abdomen and thorax for distant metastasis.
- *Fluorodeoxyglucose positron emission tomography (FDG-PET)* is also useful.

FIGO Staging Classification of Vaginal Cancer Stage (2009)

International Federation of Gynecology and Obstetrics staging classification of vaginal cancer stage (2009) is described in **Table 8**. Staging of vaginal cancer is completely clinical. CT, MRI and FDG-PET help in treatment planning, but not used for staging purpose.

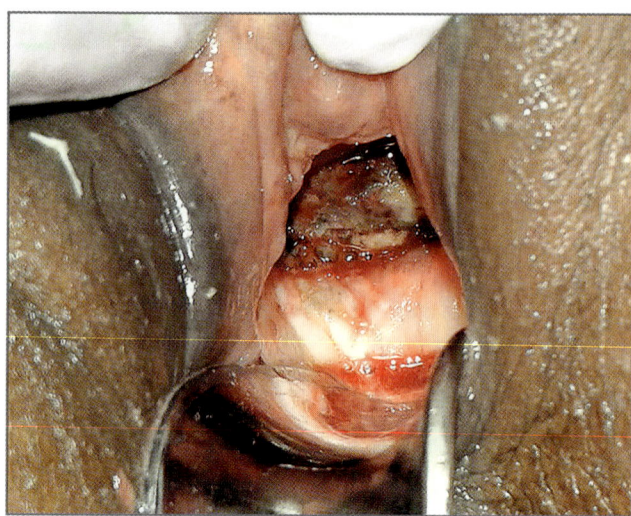

Fig. 27: Vaginal vault carcinoma 6 years after hysterectomy in a 60-year-old P2+0 woman. A fungating growth on anterior vaginal wall and vault which bleeds on touch.

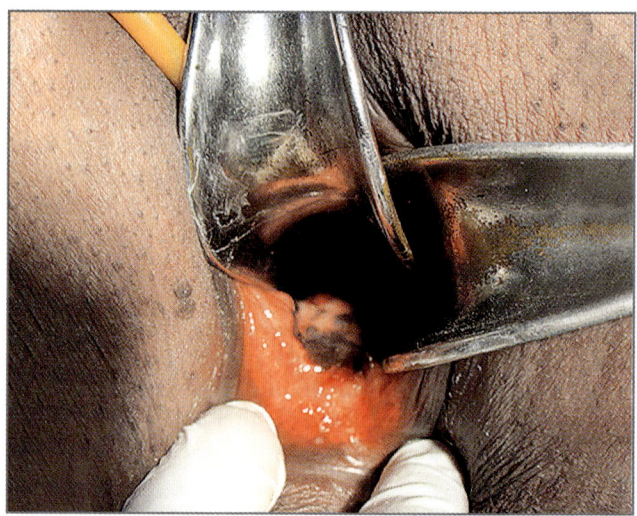

Fig. 28: Malignant melanoma vagina.

Treatment

Primary radiotherapy is treatment of choice of vaginal cancer. Surgery is done in early stages.

- *Stage I:* Surgery and radiotherapy both are options, surgery—radical vaginectomy, hysterectomy, and pelvic lymphadenectomy for tumor of upper third (**Figs. 29 and 30**).
- *Stage II:* Primary surgery or radiation.
- *Stage III and IVA:* Radiation with/without concurrent chemotherapy.
- *Stage IVB:* Not curable—systemic chemotherapy or supportive care.

Prognosis

Five-year survival rate ranges from 45-68% for all stage disease with 90% in first stage, 70% in stage II and 10 to 55% in stage III or IV. Older age, large tumor size, tobacco use and adenocarcinoma are poor prognostic factors.

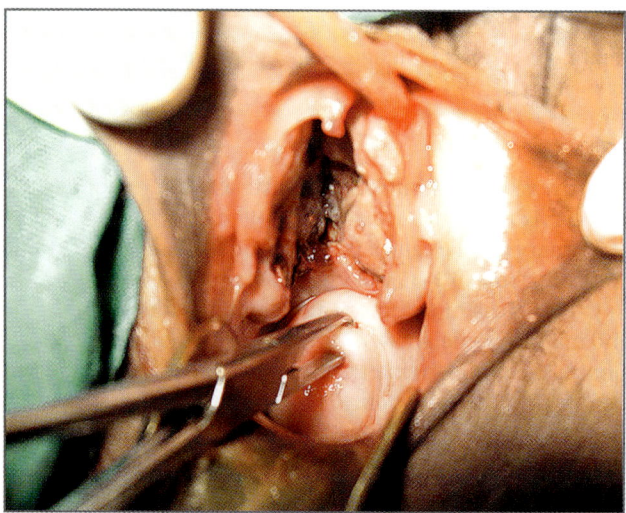

Fig. 26: Vaginal cancer—right anterolateral wall.

CHAPTER 9: A Case of Carcinoma Vulva, Preinvasive Lesion of Vulva and Vaginal Cancer

Table 8: International Federation of Gynecology and Obstetrics (FIGO) staging classification of vaginal cancer stage (2009).

Stage	Extent of lesion	Survival—5 years
I	The carcinoma is limited to the vaginal wall	75%
II	The carcinoma has involved the subvaginal tissue but has not extended to the pelvic wall	40%
III	The carcinoma has extended to the pelvic wall	30%
IV	The carcinoma has extended beyond the true pelvis or has involved the mucosa of the bladder or rectum; bullous edema as such does not permit a case to be allotted to stage IV	0–20%
IVA	Tumor invades bladder and/or rectal mucosa and/or direct extension beyond the true pelvis	
IVB	Spread to distant organs	

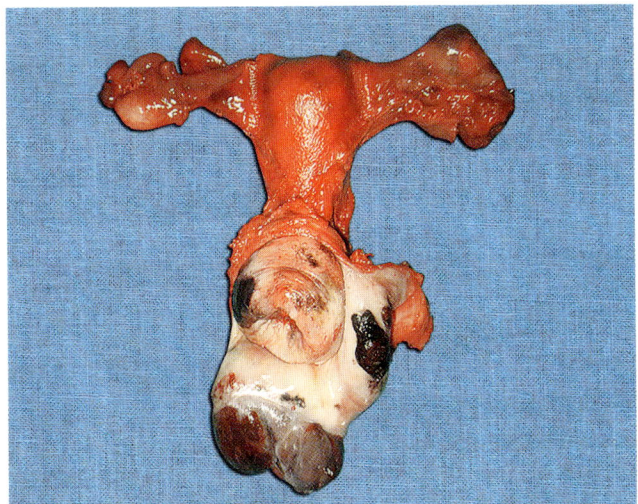

Fig. 29: Posterior aspect.

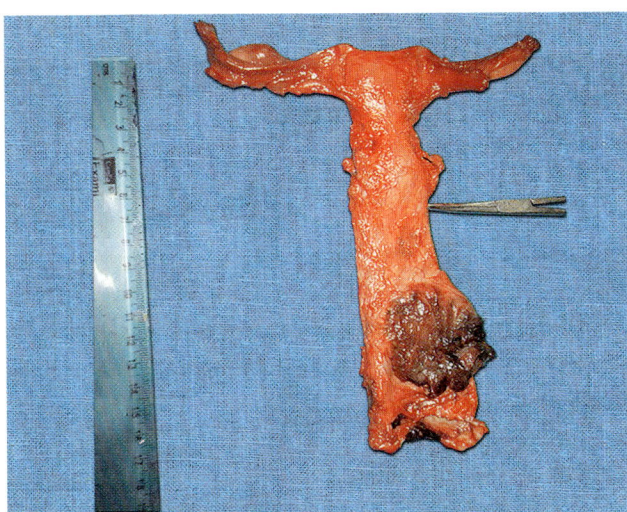

Fig. 30: Anterior aspect.

Figs. 29 and 30: Malignant melanoma vagina: Radical vaginectomy with total abdominal hysterectomy and bilateral salpingo-oophorectomy with pelvic lymphadenectomy done through abdomino-vaginal approach.
Courtesy: Professor RP Ganguly and Professor Debdutta Ghosh, RG Kar Medical College, Kolkata

CHAPTER 10

Pelvic Organ Prolapse (Genital Prolapse)

Chapter Outline

Writing a case of pelvic organ prolapse (genital prolapse) and how to present the case?

- Differential Diagnosis—Causes of Something Coming Down Per Vagina
- Anatomy of Pelvic Floor and Etiologies of Pelvic Organ Prolapse
- Anatomical Classification, Pathological Changes and Stages of Pelvic Organ Prolapse
- Symptoms, Signs and Diagnosis of Pelvic Organ Prolapse
- How to Examine and Demonstrate a Case of Pelvic Organ Prolapse?
- Prevention and Management of Pelvic Organ Prolapse
- Ring Pessary—Indication and Procedure of Application
- Surgery of Pelvic Organ Prolapse—All with Detailed Surgical Steps with Illustration:
  - Pelvic Floor Repair
  - Fothergill's Operation
  - Ward Mayo's Operation
  - Sacrocolpopexy, Sacrocolpohysteropexy
  - Sacrospinous Ligament Fixation
  - PIVS and McCall Culdoplasty

GENITAL PROLAPSE

While Dealing with a Case of Genital Prolapse You Must Know

- What are the causes of something coming down per vagina and their differential diagnosis?
- How will you classify genital prolapse, including the new pelvic organ prolapse (POP) Q classification?
- What are the varieties of symptoms, including bladder symptoms and what salient history you will take?
- Detailed local examination, including the presence of urinary incontinence and enterocele and how to demonstrate?
- Supports of pelvic organs, etiologies of genital prolapse and surgicopathological changes due to prolapse.
- Management depending on patients' profile—the classical and the newer surgical managements.

HISTORY TAKING

Patient's Particulars

- *Age*: More common in elderly.
- *Occupation*: History of (H/o) heavy weight lifting for a prolonged period.
- *Socioeconomic status*: Long-standing big prolapse is usually presented by the women of low socioeconomic status.
- *Occupation*: H/o weight lifting, work of labor.
- Multiparity is a high-risk factor for POP.

History

- *Chief complaint/complaints*: Patient usually complains of *something coming down per vagina or something falling out of vagina.* Sometimes, patient may complain pelvic pressure or heaviness **(Fig. 1)**.
- *History of present illness*: Elaborate the *chief complaints,* including the duration, whether the mass is spontaneously

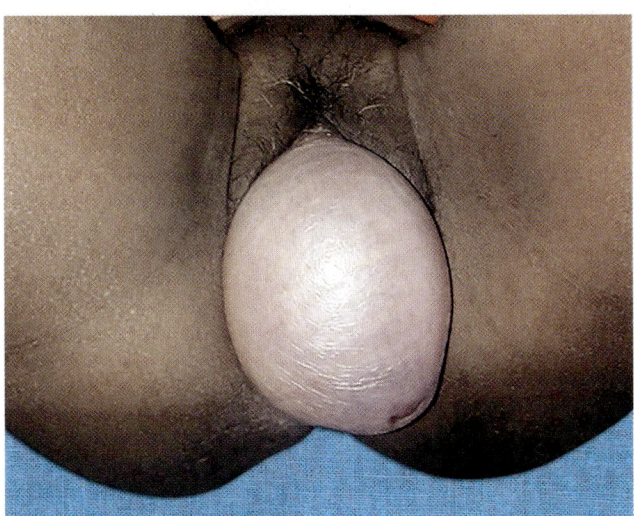

Fig. 1: Pelvic organ prolapse.

reduced during sitting or lying down posture or irreducible, and whether there is any difficulty in walking.
- You must enquire about the *urinary symptoms* like frequency, urgency, difficulty in micturition, incomplete micturition, and presence of stress incontinence. Daytime urinary frequency is more common in POP and nocturnal frequency is commonly seen in urinary infection. Sometimes, patient cannot evacuate her bladder completely, can only pass urine after reduction of the mass.
  If she has any *vaginal discharge*—white/or bloody. Whether there is any *constipation*.
  Patient may complain of backache.
- *Menstrual history*:
  - Routine history is taken.
  - If menopausal—duration of menopause, whether there is any postmenopausal bleeding?
  - Decubitus ulcer is one cause of excessive white discharge and postmenopausal bleeding and a cause of irregular bleeding per vagina in premenopausal women.
- *Obstetric history*:
  - *Parity*: Genital prolapse is common in multiparous woman but can also be found in nulliparous and low parity woman.
  - *LI (living issue)*: Write "Nil" if patient has no child.
  - *LCB* (last child birth).

It is taken in tabular form in usual manner.

Serial no.	Year and month	Pregnancy events	Labor events	Mode of delivery	Puerperium or postabortal period	Baby

Mode and quality of delivery has impact on pathogenesis of pelvic organ prolapse.

History of *prolonged labor, instrumental delivery in undilated cervix, unattended delivery,* and *repeated childbirth with short interval* favor pelvic organ prolapse.

Congenital prolapse in nulliparous woman accounts for 1% of all POP and usually occurs after menopause.

- *Past history*:
  - *Medical*: History of chronic bronchial asthma, chronic cough, chronic dysentery, chronic constipation, and other medical problems and neurological disorder.
  - *Surgical*: History of any type of previous surgery is taken. Whether the complaint is following abdominal or vaginal hysterectomy or there is any other vaginal operation. Hysterectomy itself is a predisposing factor for POP. Following hysterectomy vault prolapse may occur.
- *Family history*
- *Sexual history*: Difficulty in sexual intercourse. It should be enquired in details.
- *Functional history*: Bowel, bladder, sleep, and appetite—detailed H/o urinary problems and constipation as detailed above.
- *Personal history*:
  - Occupation history is important. Long-standing weight lifting job is a precipitating factor for genital prolapse.
- *Contraceptive history*
- *Drug history*: History of intake of corticosteroids for long period may predispose POP.

PHYSICAL EXAMINATION

Detailed general survey is recorded as the points written below. Undernutrition, obesity, and chronic anemia are predisposing factors for POP.
- Patient—alert, conscious, and cooperative
- Build
- Nutrition—undernutrition
- Height
- Weight or BMI
- Edema
- Anemia—present
- Cyanosis
- Jaundice
- Clubbing
- Tongue, teeth, gum, and tonsil
- Neck veins
- Neck glands
- Leg veins
- Pulse
- Respiration
- Temperature
- BP: High BP may be associated with fibroid.

Systemic Examination

- *Central nervous system*
- *Cardiovascular system*:
  - Auscultation of heart
- *Respiratory system*:
  - Auscultation of chest
- *Gastrointestinal system*:
  - Liver

- Spleen
- Kidney and renal angle tenderness.

Examination of Other Systems

- Examination of skeletal system—examination of back and spines is done.
- *Neurological*: Any gross neurological abnormality is looked for.
  - Whether there is any abnormal gait, joint hypermobility, and myopathy
  - Urinary system: Kidney and renal angle tenderness.
- *Examination of breasts and nipple*:
  - Inspection
  - Palpation

GYNECOLOGICAL EXAMINATION

Abdominal Examination

Routine inspection, palpation, and percussion are done to note any laxity, scar, other abnormality, lump, tenderness, and presence of free fluid (ascites). All other hernia sites are looked for.

Vaginal Examination

Details of vaginal examination is given later.
- Inspection, speculum examination and palpation, bimanual examination, examination of perineum and rectal and rectovaginal examination.
- See the local clinical (vaginal) examination for details. The relevant points are highlighted here.

Position of the Patient (see Page 216, Figs. 39 to 42)

Woman is examined commonly in dorsal position. But can be needed to examine in other positions also, standing position, lithotomy position, squatting position, and Sims' position. The following points are noted one by one.
(For undergraduate examination only inspection is allowed)

Inspection and Speculum Examination (Fig. 2)

Description of vulva and perineum, anterior vaginal wall prolapse, posterior wall prolapse, and uterine prolapse are written as written later.
- Grades and types are written during Valsalva maneuver and after coughing.
- Presence of thickening of vaginal mucosa, patchy pigmentation, and decubitus ulcer are looked for.
- Presence of stress incontinence (spurting of urine through urethra) is noted on coughing. For this examination, patient is asked not to evacuate of bladder before examination.

Palpation

By palpation findings of inspection are confirmed.
- Anteriorly, cystocele, and urethrocele are palpated.

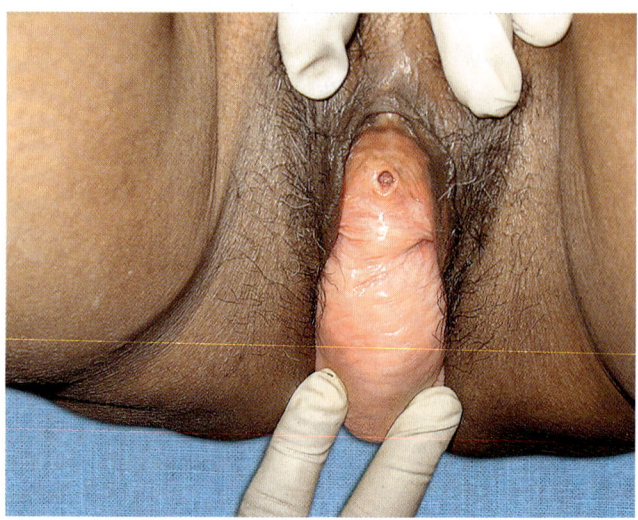

Fig. 2: Examination of genital prolapse.

- By palpation, exact degree of uterine prolapse is determined by grasping the protruding mass at the vaginal introitus between the thumb in front and the fingers behind.
- On bimanual examination after reducing the prolapse size of the uterus is measured, whether there is elongation of supravaginal portion of cervix is also noted and condition of adnexae is assessed.

Degree and grades are confirmed by inspection and palpation (*see* Page 220, **Figs. 48 to 54**). POPQ—staging is done. For measurement a Ayer's spatula graduated in cm, ruler, a graduated sponge holding forceps (if available) or any stick graduated from 1 to 10 cm is made ready and the measurements are taken one by one and put in the *three-by-three grid (make a grid)* and staging is done.

Paravaginal defect, apical, transverse, and midline defect if any are determined.
- Posteriorly, presence of rectocele and enterocele are searched for
- Examination of rectovaginal area and rectal examination is done.

Rectocele and enterocele can be differentiated by rectal or rectovaginal examination (*see* below).

Tone of perineal body and levator ani is assessed. Reflexes (sacral) are also noted down.
See the clinical examination for detailed examination procedure. Write the findings here.

SUMMARY OF THE CASE (SAMPLE SUMMARY)

Mrs XY 59 years P_{6+0} widow menopause for 10 years coming from low socioeconomic status was admitted on with H/o something coming down per vagina for 7 years. She has also white discharge per vagina and her inner garment sometimes becomes stained with bloody discharge. She has no urinary problems. She had to do hard physical work from early in her life. All were vaginal deliveries conducted at home. She has no chronic cough or constipation.

CHAPTER 10: Pelvic Organ Prolapse (Genital Prolapse)

- *On general examination*: Her weight is ----, pallor-mild, pulse/min, and normotensive.
- *Per abdominal examination*: Nothing abnormal.
- *On vaginal examination*:
    - Vaginal introitus widened, vulva atrophied, clitoris, labia normal, there is a mass protruding through the introitus.
    - Anterior part seems to be cystocele, in middle part there is uterine prolapse at least 2°, posterior wall of vagina was not visible as it is covered by prolapsed uterus (or write down if visible in case of 1° uterine prolapse).
    - There was some pigmented areas and decubitus ulcer over the mass (write if present). There was impulse on coughing over the mass.
    - And on straining and coughing there was no leakage of urine per urethra. (When palpation and speculum examination is allowed).

Write whether it is 2° or procidentia, POP-Q staging, describe the presence of rectocele, enterocele, and tone of perineal body and levator ani muscle and site specific defect.

INVESTIGATIONS SUPPLIED OR REQUIRED

- Hb%, routine blood count (TC, DC, and ESR)
- ABO, Rh factor, blood sugar, urea, and creatinine
- Urine examination report
- X-ray of chest
- ECG
- Urodynamic study report.

PROVISIONAL DIAGNOSIS

A 59-year-old P_{7+0} postmenopausal widow with POP at least 2° uterine prolapse.

DIFFERENTIAL DIAGNOSIS

In differential diagnosis the clinical conditions where the woman complains of something coming down per vagina will be considered.

These are:
- Gartner duct cyst
- Fibroid polyp
- Chronic inversion of uterus
- Hypertrophic elongation of cervix
- Large malignant growth of cervix.

Gartner Duct Cyst (Fig. 3)

It comes with the differential diagnosis of cystocele. It is usually situated at anterolateral wall of vagina, not reducible, well-defined margin, no vaginal rugosity over it, and wall is thin. When a metallic catheter is introduced through the external urinary meatus it does not go inside the gartner duct cyst.

There may be any other anterior vaginal wall cyst or tumor may mimic cystocele, e.g. vaginal wall cyst **(Fig. 4)** and vaginal wall fibroma **(Fig. 5)**.

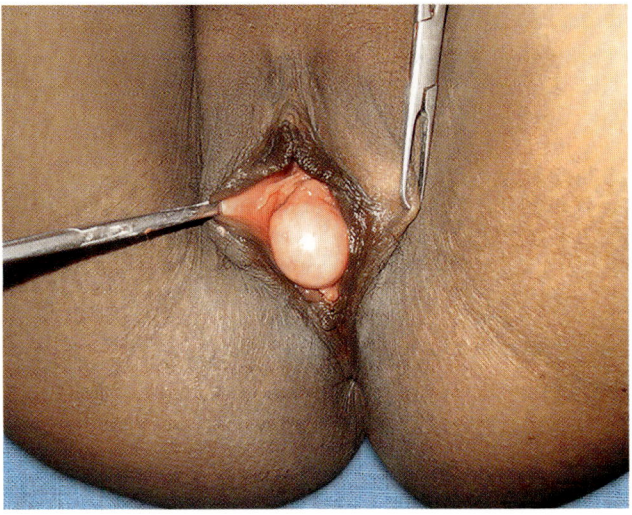

Fig. 3: Gartner duct cyst.

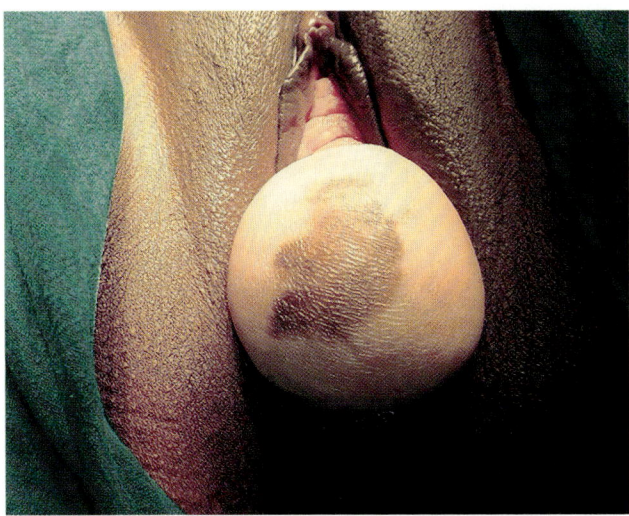

Fig. 4: Sebaceous cyst on anterior vaginal wall.

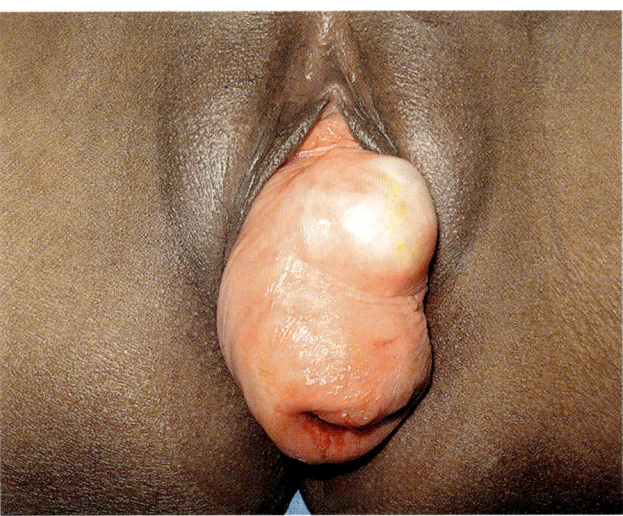

Fig. 5: Vaginal fibroma.

Fibroid Polyp (Fig. 6)

A fibroid may arise from the lips from cervix or arise from the body of uterus. The fibroid arising from the body of uterus may come through the cervical canal outside in vagina or even outside introitus connected by a pedunculated stalk. In the latter variety, a sound can be introduced in the cervical canal and all around the stalk and sides of stalk is free. In the cervical variety external os is found with difficulty above and lateral to mass. Sometimes a fibroid polyp may be associated with genital prolapse.

Chronic Inversion of Uterus (Figs. 7 to 9)

Pinkish mucosa of endometrium is seen covering the mass. External os is not visible. There is a rim (cervical) palpable over

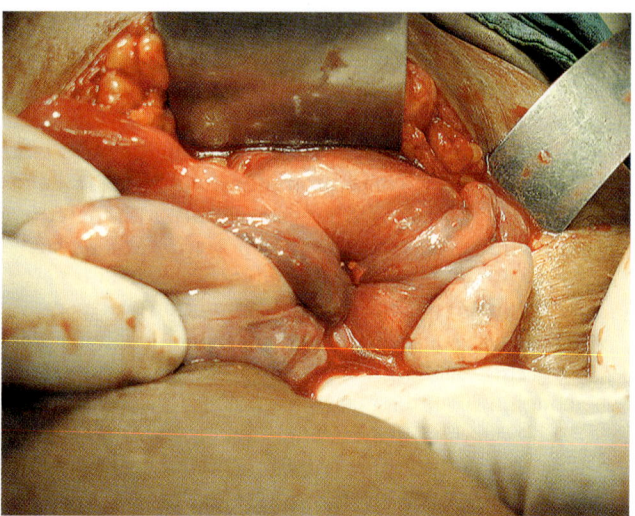

Fig. 8: Chronic inversion due to cervical fibroid—cupping of uterine fundus.

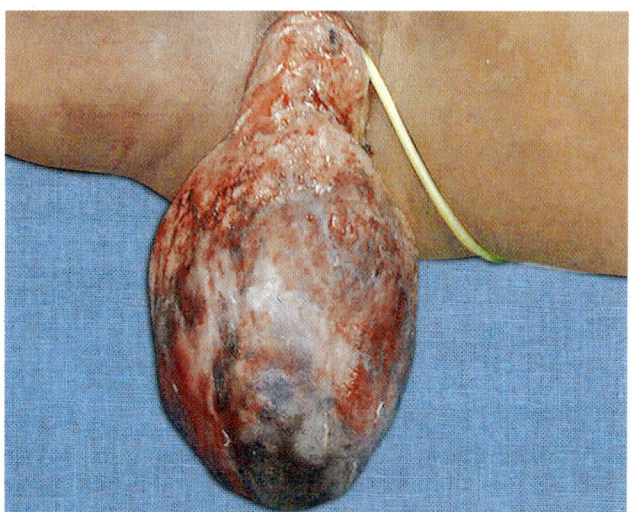

Fig. 6: Cervical fibroid polyp.

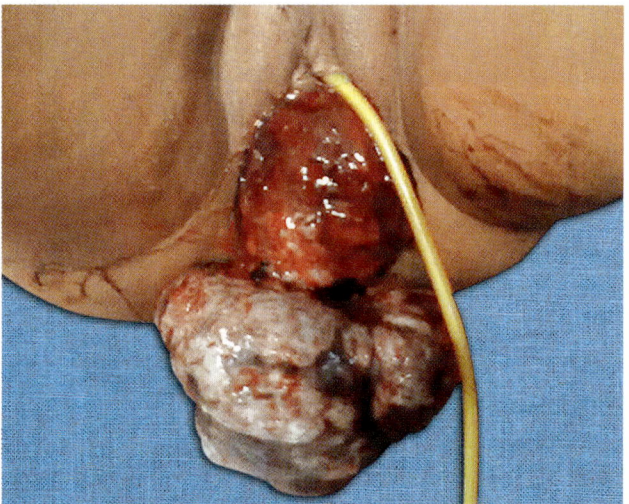

Fig. 7: Chronic inversion due to fibroid, 30 years P2+1, both normal delivery (ND) and last child birth (LCB) 6 years back, presented with something coming down per vagina, retention of urine, excessive menorrhagia. Per vaginal examination—uterus-bulky, a degenerated mass protruding outside introitus. Bimanual examination—cupping of fundus (Fig. 8). Polypectomy was done vaginally. In a later sitting, Haultain operation was done to repose the uterus (*see* Chapter 25).

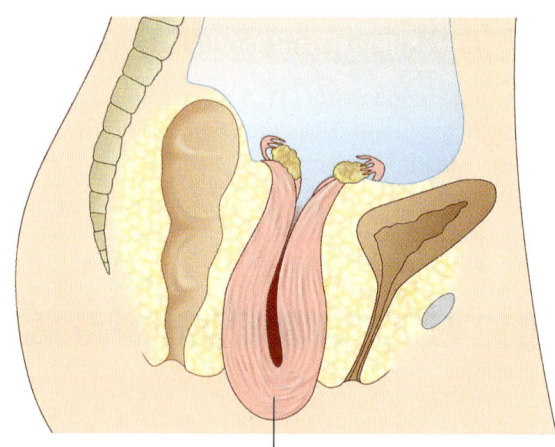

Chronic inversion of uterus
Fig. 9: Inversion of uterus.

and above the mass in incomplete variety and in complete variety no rim is palpable. Uterocervical canal is not found on attempting introduction of uterine sound in complete variety. There is cupping of fundus on bimanual examination.

Elongation of Cervix (Figs. 10 and 11)

Vagina is deep due to elongation of vaginal part of cervix and there is no impulse on coughing if not associated with prolapse. On bimanual examination uterus is in pelvic position and of normal size. Distance from bladder sulcus to tip of cervix is long. Uterocervical canal is enlarged (also in uterine prolapse).

Large Malignant Growth of Cervix (Figs. 12A and B)

Large cauliflower growth of cervix may sometimes present as something coming down per vagina. The growth usually bleeds and brisk hemorrhage occurs on palpation or on rubbing with a swab.

Q. What is your case?
Tell the summary of the case.

CHAPTER 10: Pelvic Organ Prolapse (Genital Prolapse)

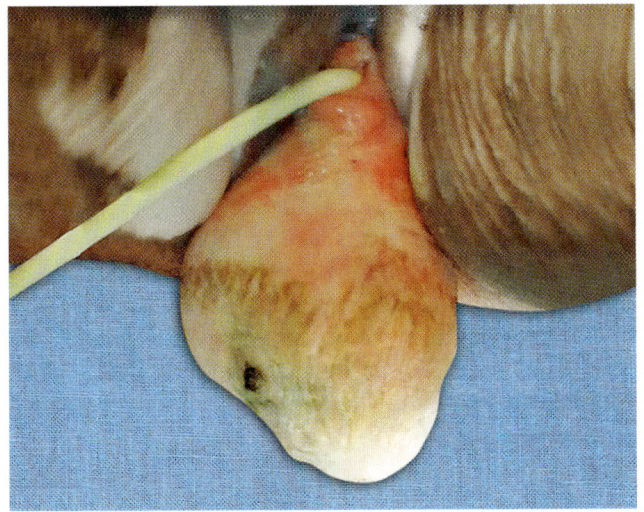

Fig. 10: Prolapse with hypertrophic cervix with leukoplakia.

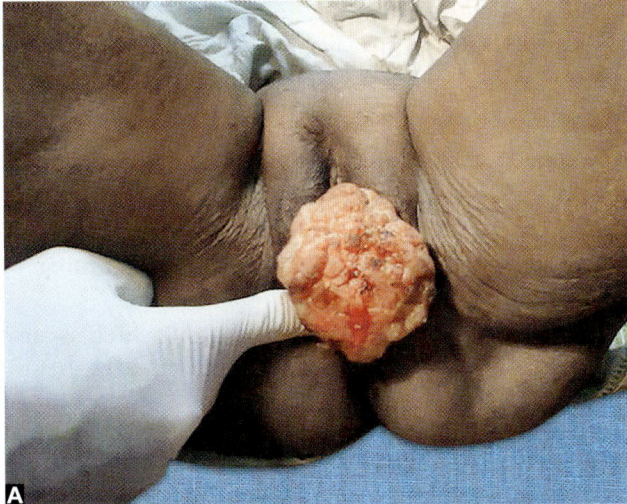

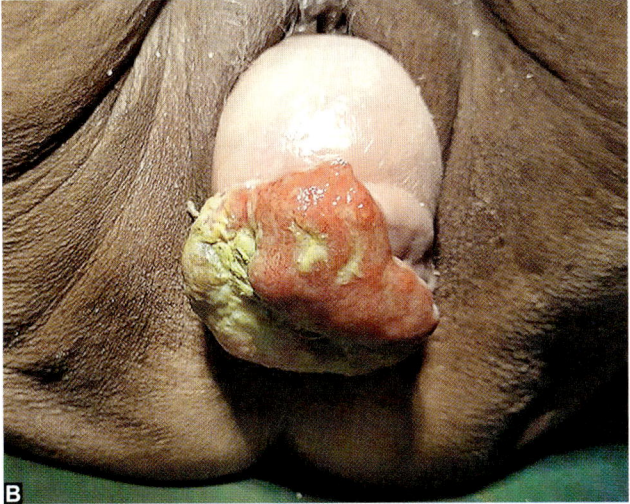

Figs. 12A and B: Pelvic organ prolapse with cancer cervix (rarely seen).

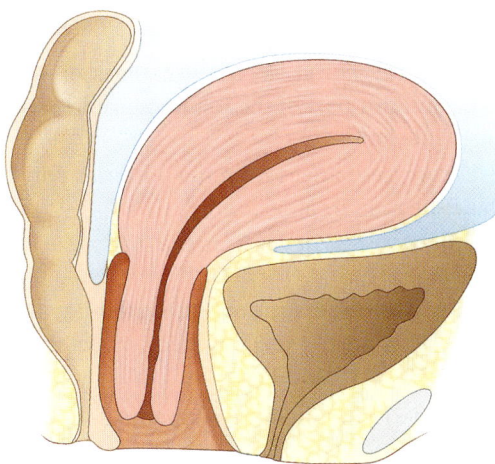

Fig. 11: Elongation of cervix.

Q. What is your diagnosis?

Tell the provisional diagnosis.

Q. What are the other causes of something coming down per vagina? And how will you differentiate?

The causes are:
- Gartner duct cyst
- Fibroid polyp
- Chronic inversion of uterus
- Elongation of cervix
- Large malignant growth of cervix.

They are differentiated on the basis as written above in differential diagnosis.

SUPPORTS OF UTERUS AND VAGINA

Q. What is the normal position of uterus? What is the normal position of external OS?
- It is anteverted and anteflexed (**Fig. 13**)

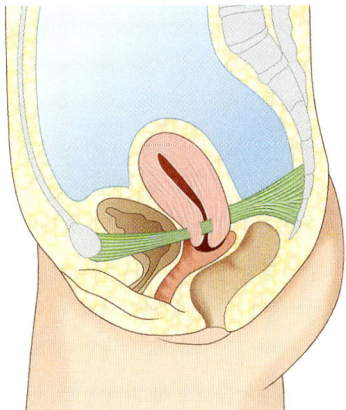

Sagittal view

Fig. 13: Sagittal view—posteriorly uterosacral ligaments and anteriorly pubocervical ligaments— normal position of uterus is anteflexed and anteverted.

- The long axis of uterus makes an angle of 90° with that of vagina (V for vagina) and it is called anteversion.

- The angle between the body and the cervix is 140°.
- The external os normally lies at the level of ischial spine.

Q. Outline the supports of uterus.

The uterus and vagina are kept in position by three important components. These are **(Figs. 14 and 15)**:

- Ligaments and fascia-suspension from walls of pelvis.
- Levator ani muscles—maintain the organs in position by their tone.
- The vagina—its posterior angulation which is also increased by increase of intra-abdominal pressure-results closure of *'flap valve'.*

Endopelvic Fascia (Figs. 14 to 16)

- This is the most important component of the support.
- It is derived from the paramesonephric ducts and not histologically similar to the fascia of levator ani muscle.
- This sheet extends from the symphysis pubis to ischial spines and laterally attaches to arcus tendineus and levator ani muscles and fills the space between the peritoneum and levator ani muscles surrounding the pelvic viscera.

This fascia thickens to form *uterosacral ligaments and cardinal ligaments* around the cervix and vagina like a cart wheel, the ligaments are like spokes and cervix and vault are like hub **(Fig. 14)**.

- The part of the fascia which lies between the bladder and vagina is called *pubocervical fascia* and supports the bladder. The part lying between the vagina and rectum is called *rectovaginal fascia* and prevents anterior rectal protrusion.

Levator Ani Muscle (Figs. 15 and 16)

This broad, flat muscles form the main muscular component of the pelvic floor and two muscles, one on either side constitute the pelvic diaphragm. It consists of three parts:

1. The *pubococcygeus* arises from the back of pubic bone and the anterior part of the tendinous arch of the pelvic fascia (white line).
2. The *iliococcygeus* arises from the posterior part of white line and the ischial spines, and
3. The *ischiococcygeus* arises from the medial surface of the ischial spine.

Describe **level wise supporting system** for the uterus and vagina. What are the specific effects on defect of each of these levels? **(Figs. 16 and 17)**.

DeLancey (1992) described the supports of vagina at three levels:

- *Level I support*: It consists of uterosacral and cardinal ligaments complex attached to the supracervix and upper part of vagina like that of a cartwheel and serve to maintain the vaginal length and horizontal axis.

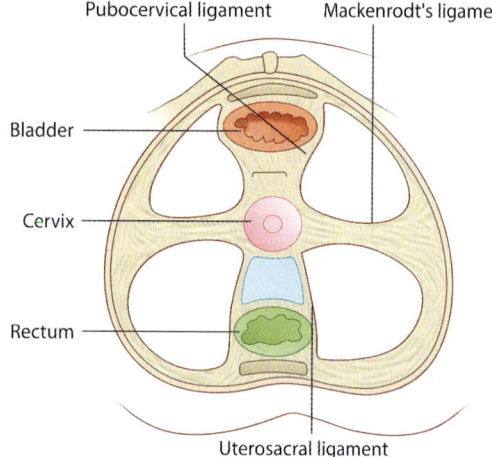

Fig. 14: Transverse view of pelvis showing the supports of fascia and ligaments like spokes of wheel—anteriorly pubocervical ligament laterally Mackenrodt's (cardinal) ligaments, and posteriorly uterosacral ligaments.

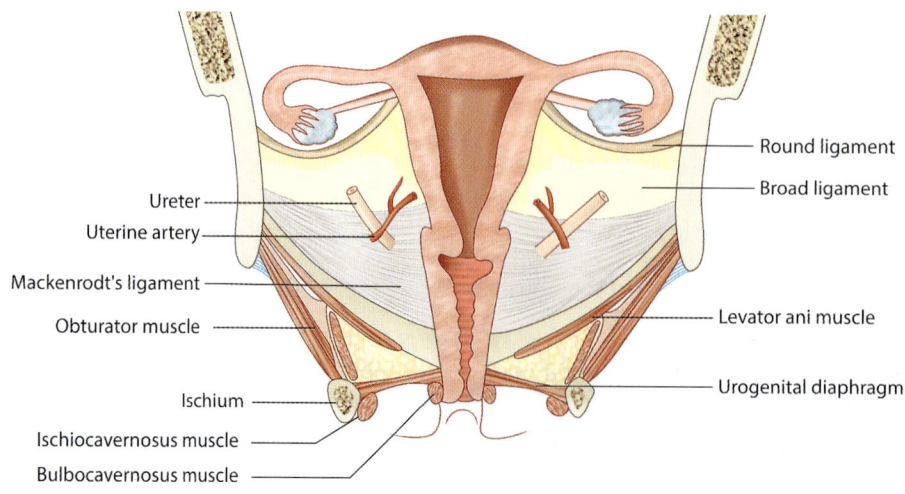

Fig. 15: Coronal view of pelvis showing supports of uterus and relation of pelvic structures.

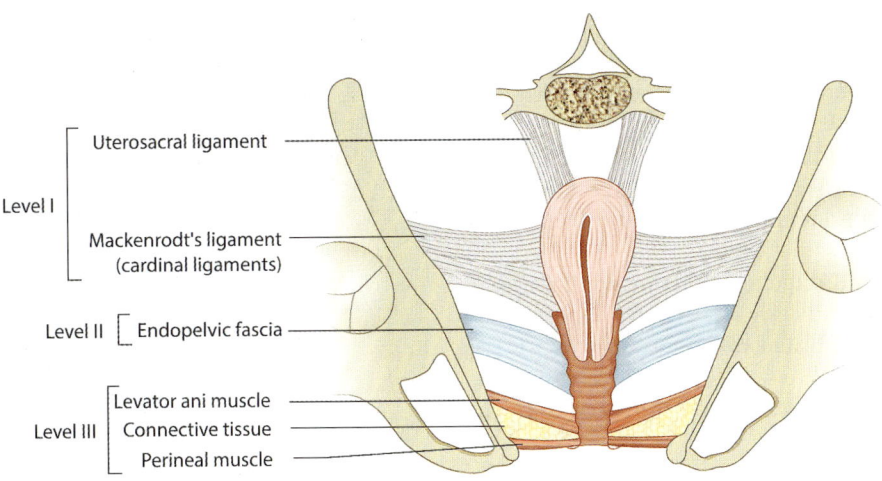

Fig. 16: Levels of supports of vagina and uterus as described by DeLancey (Level I, Level II, and Level III).

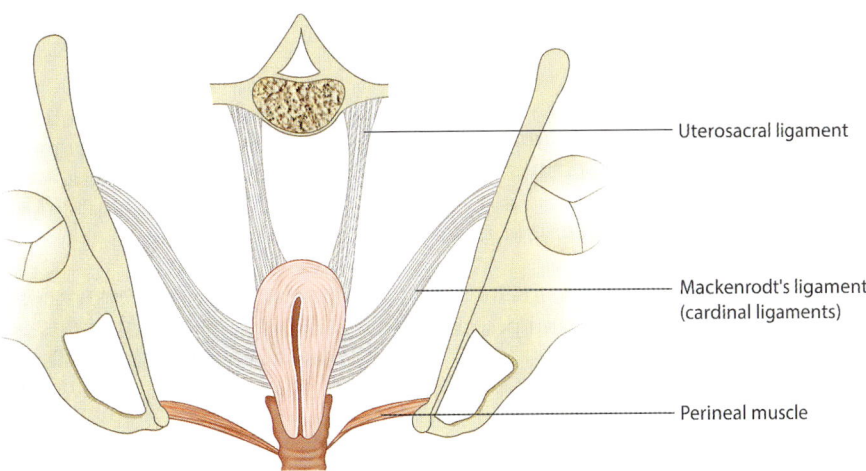

Fig. 17: Derangements of supports due to laxity of fascia and ligaments.

Cardinal ligament or Mackenrodt's ligament fans out laterally one on each side and attaches to fascia of obturator internus and piriformis muscle, anterior border of greater sciatic foramen, and ischial spines. Uterosacral ligaments are paired ligaments attaching from posterior surface of isthmus running on each side of rectum and inserted to the sacrum at the level of S2 through S4.

Defects in this level I support (*see* **Fig. 16**) cause apical prolapse—prolapse of vault, enterocele, and descent of cervix.

- *Level II support*: It consists of paravaginal attachment of lateral vagina and endopelvic fascia to the arcus tendineus (pubocervical fascia, rectovaginal fascia, and arcus tendineus fascia pelvis) and maintains midline position of the vagina by supporting the anterior and posterior vaginal walls.

Loss of level II support (*see* **Fig. 16**) results anterior vaginal wall prolapse (cystocele) and posterior wall prolapse (rectocele).

- *Level III support*: Made up of the perineal body, superficial and deep perineal muscles, and connective tissue around the distal vagina and perineum. This level supports the urethra, distal one-third of vagina, and introitus.

Damage to level III (*see* **Fig. 16**) results gaping of introitus, anteriorly urethral hypermobility, and posteriorly distal rectocele and lax perineum.

ETIOLOGIES OF PELVIC ORGAN PROLAPSE

Q. What are the etiologies of pelvic organ prolapse?

Pelvic organ prolapse occurs due to attenuation of the supportive structures by:
- "Tears" or "breaks"
- By neuromuscular dysfunction
- Both.

Factors resulting attenuation of supportive structures may be acquired or congenital or both precipitated by increased intra-abdominal pressure.

Q. What are the acquired causes?

Acquired causes are pregnancy and childbirth, menopause and aging, posthysterectomy or dragging of uterus by any mass-like cervical fibroid.

❖ *Pregnancy and childbirth*:
- Stretching and breaking of the endopelvic fascia, damage of levator ani muscle and nerve fibers occurs during childbirth.
- Prolonged second stage and forceps application in undilated cervix and early bearing down pain when the cervix is still undilated are important obstetric risk factors.
- Damage mostly occurs in first delivery than the subsequent deliveries.
- Repeated childbirth and short interpregnancy interval are contributory factors.

❖ *Menopause*: Atrophy of the supporting structure takes place in menopause due to estrogen deficiency resulting prolapse and urinary incontinence.

❖ *Age* is an independent risk factor for POP.

❖ *Undernutrition* and obesity both favors POP.

❖ Following *surgery* like hysterectomy, both abdominal and vaginal hysterectomy, surgery for prolapse and urinary incontinence.

❖ Dragging of uterus may occur by *cervical fibroid polyp* and vaginal prolapse **(Fig. 18)**.

❖ Increased *abdominal pressure* may occur due to chronic cough, constipation, chronic lung disease, and prolong weight lifting. The other risk factor is obesity.

Congenital Cause

❖ Congenital neuromuscular dysfunction may cause POP, especially in nulliparous prolapse **(Fig. 19)**.

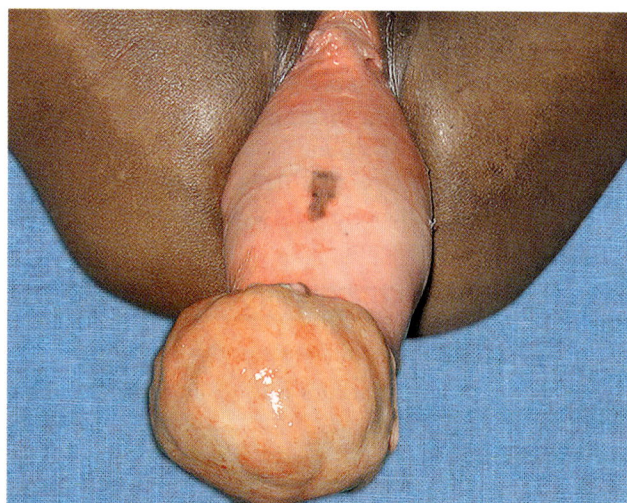

Fig. 18: Procidentia due to cervical fibroid. A 41-year-old nulliparous presented with sudden something coming down per vagina with offensive discharge. Her husband left her for this reason. Reposition tried manually but failed and it was reposited after cervical polypectomy (myomectomy).

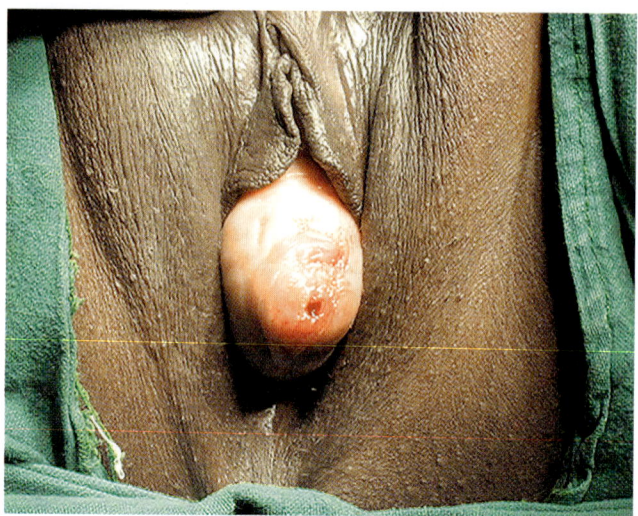

Fig. 19: Nulliparous prolapse—60 years, nulliparous, unmarried woman menopause for 10 years admitted with 4 months irregular bleeding. Vaginal hysterectomy done.

❖ Inherited disorders of collagen such as Marfan's syndrome. There is hypermobile joints and increase chance of recurrent prolapse.

❖ Nulliparous prolapse is more common following menopause **(Fig. 19)**.

ANATOMICAL CLASSIFICATION OF PELVIC ORGAN PROLAPSE

Q. How would you anatomically classify pelvic organ prolapse compartment wise?

❖ Anterior compartment (anterior vaginal wall prolapse)—most common:
- Upper two-thirds—cystocele **(Fig. 20A)**
- Lower one-third—urethrocele.

❖ Middle compartment or apical prolapse:
- Prolapse of uterus or vaginal vault **(Fig. 21)**

❖ Posterior compartment (posterior vaginal wall prolapse):
- Upper part—enterocele **(Figs. 22 and 23)**
- Middle part—rectocele **(Fig. 20B)**
- Lower part—lax perineum.

Q. What do you mean by uterovaginal prolapse and vaginouterine prolapse?

Uterovaginal (also called uterine prolapse) prolapse is one where descent of the uterus occurs primarily due to laxity of the uterine ligaments and then vagina is inverted secondarily. It may not be associated with cystocele or rectocele.

In vaginouterine prolapse (also called vaginal prolapse) primary defect lies in the supports of vagina and the vaginal prolapse drags the uterus in turn. It is associated with cystocele, rectocele, and lax perineum. This type is more common.

CHAPTER 10: Pelvic Organ Prolapse (Genital Prolapse)

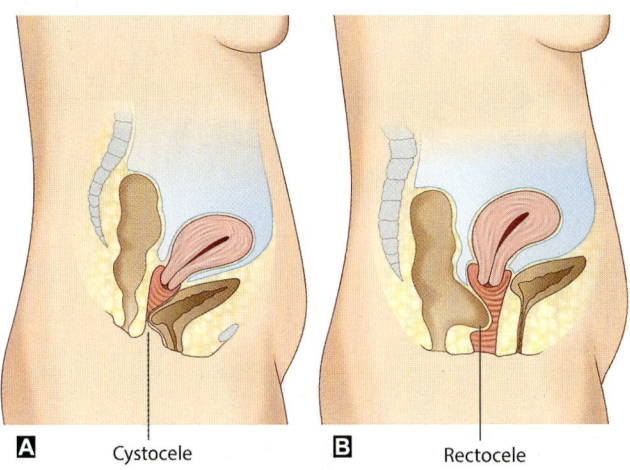

Figs. 20A and B: (A) Cystocele; (B) Rectocele.

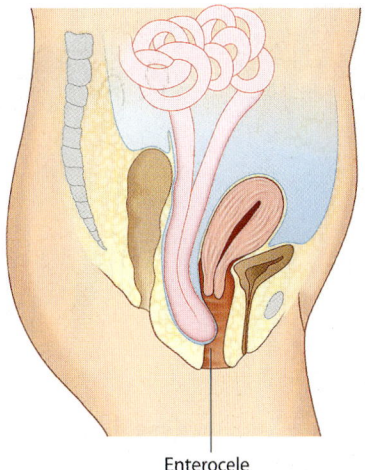

Fig. 23: Enterocele.

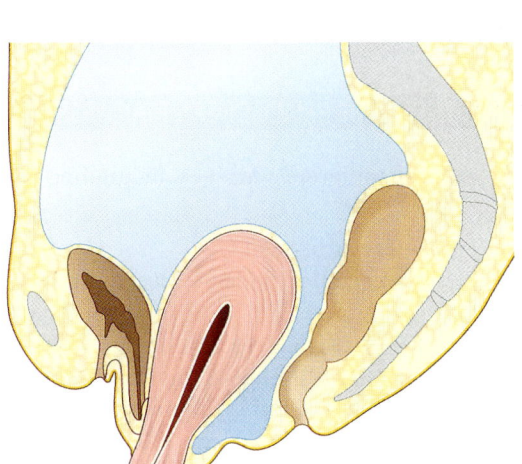

Fig. 21: Uterine descent.

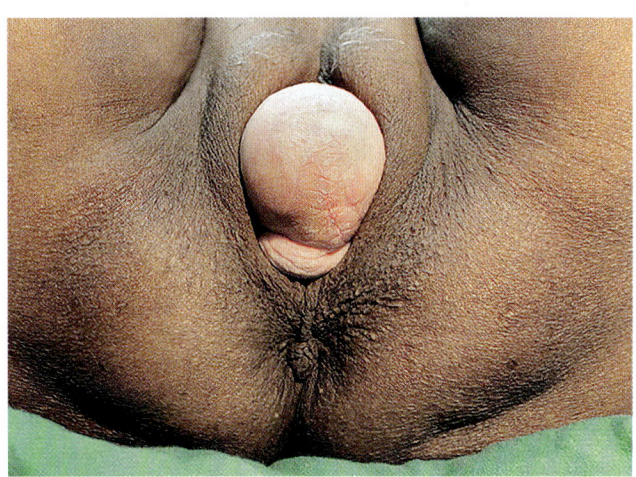

Fig. 24: Vault prolapse following hysterectomy.

Vault Prolapse

Q. What does vault prolapse mean?

In practice, the term vault prolapse is commonly used for prolapse of the vaginal vault following hysterectomy.

In wider sense vault prolapse means the prolapse of the vaginal vault. It encompasses:
- Enterocele **(Fig. 22)**
- Uterovaginal (uterine) prolapse.
- Vault prolapse following hysterectomy both abdominal and vaginal **(Fig. 24)**.

For degrees and management of vault prolapse (*see* later).

Distension Cystocele and Displacement Cystocele

Q. What is defect theory of pelvic organ prolapse? What do you mean by "distension" cystocele or rectocele and "displacement" cystocele or rectocele?

According to this theory herniation or prolapse may occur due to tear of endopelvic fascia either in the

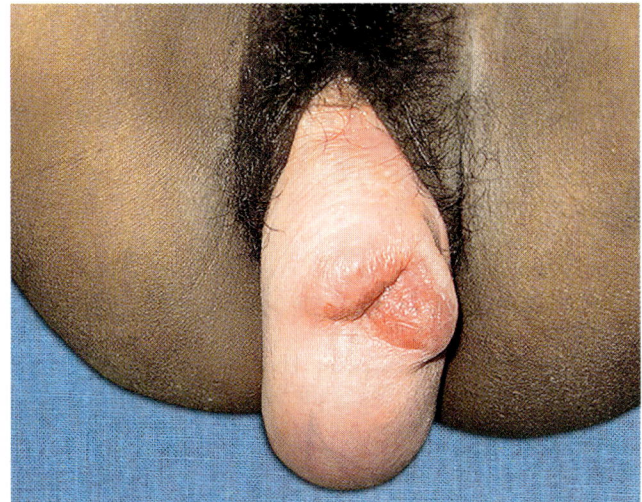

Fig. 22: Large enterocele—29 years P2+0 LI 2, LCB 8 years back, P1 FTND 11 years back, P2 FTND 8 years back, ligation 8 years back admitted with something coming down per vagina since after last childbirth. Small cystocele, large enterocele, and 2° uterine prolapse.

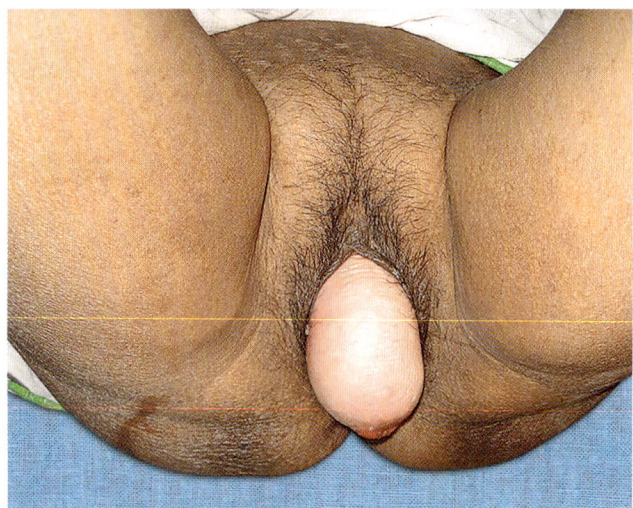

Fig. 25: Distension prolapse—midline cystocele. Loss of midline vaginal wall rugae.

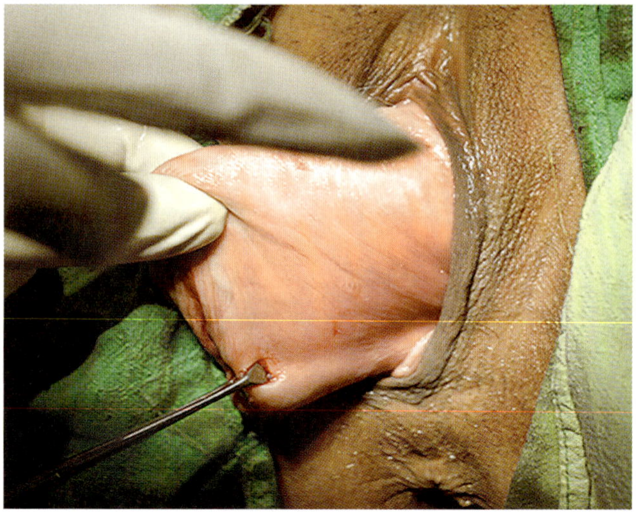

Fig. 27: Absence of lateral sulci indicating loss of lateral support.

form of attenuation of vaginal wall or due to tear of fascial attachment to the pelvic sidewall. When there is attenuation of vaginal wall without break of fascial attachment it is called *"distension" or midline cystocele* **(Fig. 25)** or rectocele. In distention type, vaginal rugae are lost and surface becomes smooth.

When anterior and posterior wall defects occur due to break of attachment of the lateral vaginal wall, it is called *"displacement"* cystocele (lateral or paravaginal cystocele) **(Figs. 26 and 27)** or rectocele. In displacement type, vaginal rugae are visible **(Fig. 26)**.

The importance of this concept is that if it is diagnosed which type of defect is there the specific repair can be done during surgery.

During second stage of labor both types of defect may occur.

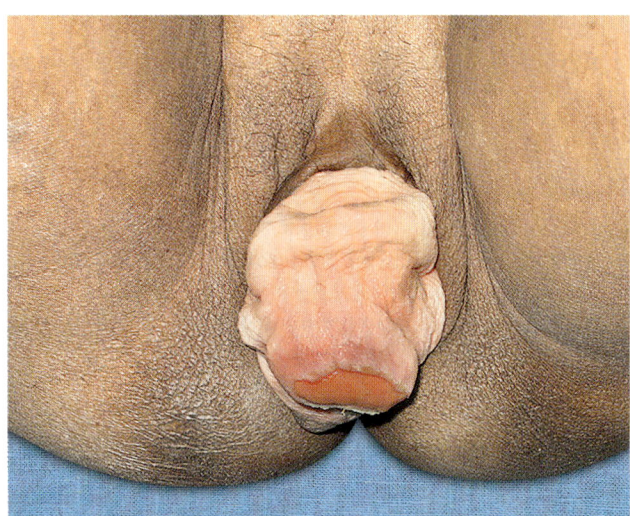

Fig. 26: Displacement cystocele (lateral). Rugae seen in midline indicating lateral defect not central.

GRADING SYSTEMS OF PELVIC ORGAN PROLAPSE

Q. What are the different varieties of grading systems (classification) of POP?

1. Porges 1963—three degrees
2. Baden 1972—four grades (Baden-Walker halfway system): Grade 0-4
3. Beecham 1980—three degrees
4. POP-Q (Pelvic Organ Prolapse Quantification system) 1996—current classification by international continence society: "Zero" to stage IV.

Three Degree Classification

Q. What are the different degrees or grades of pelvic organ prolapse?

The commonly used classifications in clinical practice are of three degrees (Beecham 1980) though four degrees (Baden 1972) are also used by many schools **(Figs. 28 and 29)**.

* *First degree*: The cervix and body of uterus descend from normal position but lies within the vagina. (This is clinically assessed by seeing the position of external os with the level of ischial spine, at the level of which external os lies normally).
* *Second degree*: The cervix comes down outside the introitus but the body of the uterus still is within the vagina.
* *Third degree or procidentia*: There is complete eversion of uterus and whole of the uterus lies outside the vaginal introitus. It is differentiated from 2° uterine prolapse by palpation.

Four Degree Classification

When four degree classification is considered basically first degree is subdivided into two separate degrees. In

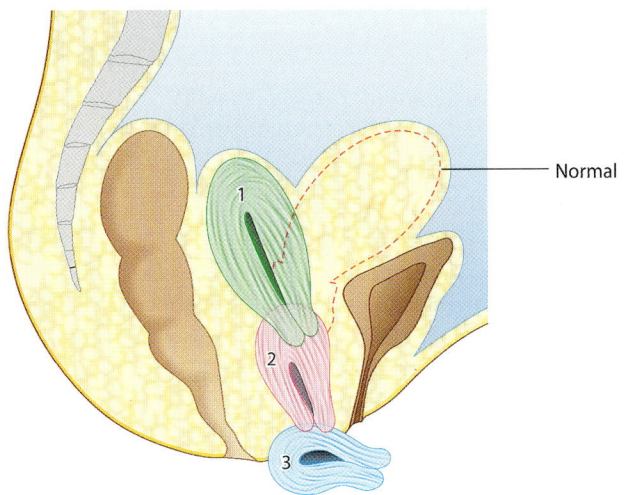

Fig. 28: Three degree of uterine prolapse.

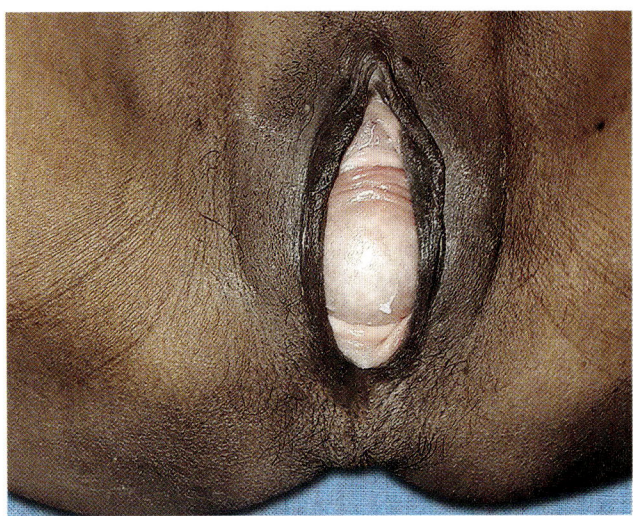

Fig. 30: Grade 2 genital prolapse (according to Baden four degree classification system).

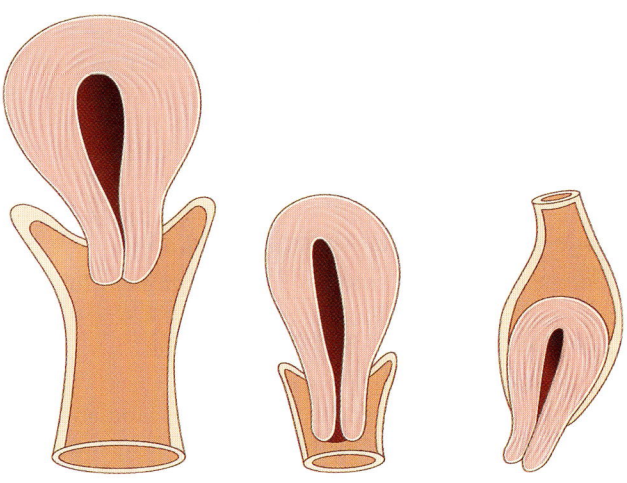

Fig. 29: Different degrees of prolapse.

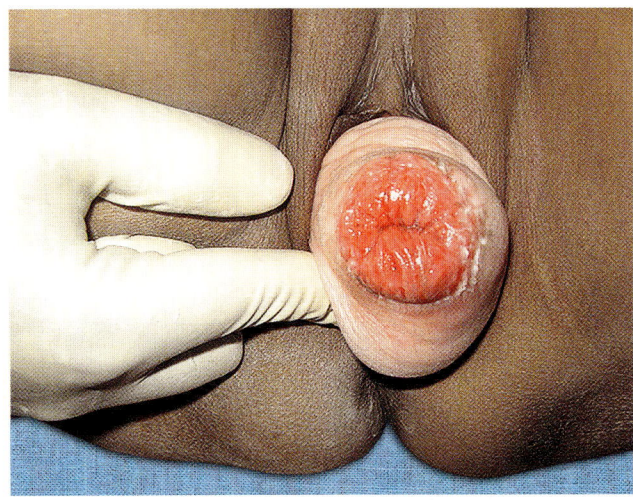

Fig. 31: Grade 3 prolapse (according to Baden four degree classification system).

Baden-Walker Halfway system, the term Grade is used not the stage and Grade 0 is used to denote normal position. Accordingly:

Grade 0—Normal position for each respective site
Grade 1—Descent is halfway to the hymen
Grade 2—Descent is up to the hymen **(Fig. 30)**
Grade 3—Descent is halfway after the hymen **(Fig. 31)**
Grade 4—Maximal possible descent for each site **(Fig. 32)**

Baden-Walker Halfway system is very useful in clinical practice encompassing all compartments, e.g. anterior, apical, and posterior though POP-Q system is more informative.

Not uncommonly pelvic organ prolapse is associated with other gynecological pathology **(Figs. 32A and B)**.

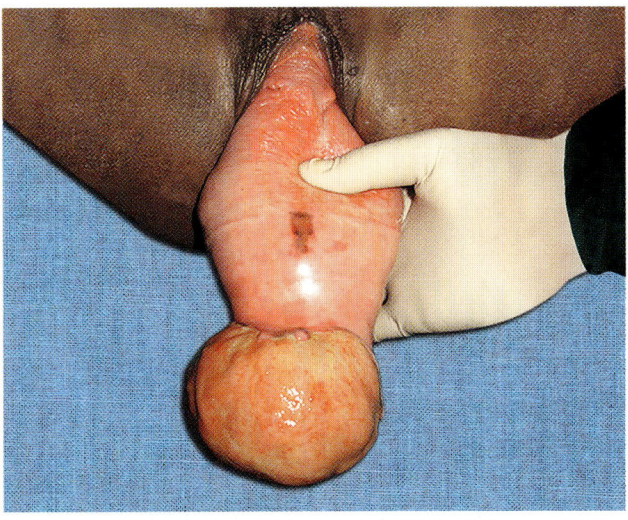

Fig. 32: Grade 4 prolapse with cervical fibroid.

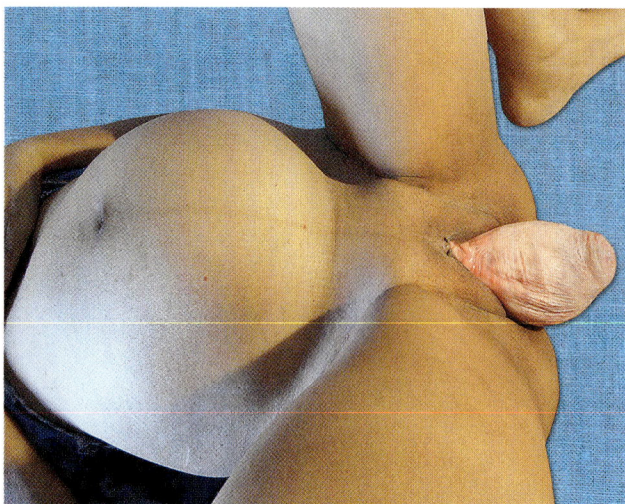

Fig. 32A: Pelvic organ prolapse with dermoid cyst.

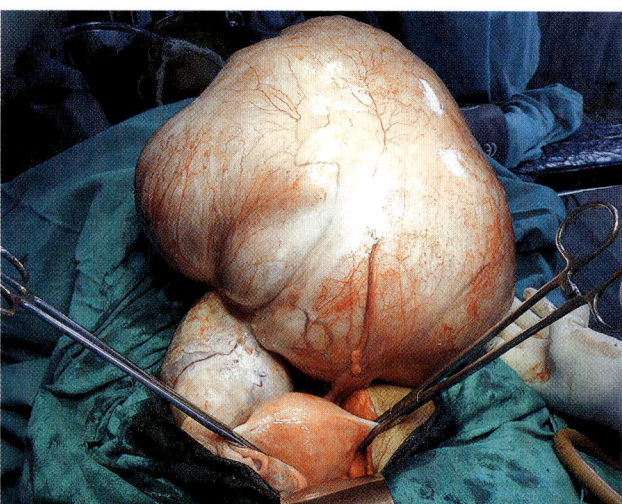

Fig. 32B: Large dermoid cyst on laparotomy in the patient as in Figure 32A.

PELVIC ORGAN PROLAPSE QUANTIFICATION SYSTEM (POP-Q)

By POP-Q classification "Zero" to stage IV are considered according to relation of distal portion with the level of hymen (*see* below).

Q. What is POP-Q?

It is one of the systems to stage POP.

Pelvic Organ Prolapse Quantification system has been approved by the International Continence Society (1996).

The POP-Q system references six vaginal points (two on the anterior vaginal wall—points Aa and Ba), (two at the apical vagina—points C and D), and (two on the posterior vaginal wall—points Ap and Bp) and three length namely genital hiatus (Gh), perineal body (Pb), and total vaginal length (TVL) **(Fig. 33)**. Aa and Ba measure the anterior compartment prolapse. Ap and Bp measure the posterior compartment prolapse. Point C and D measure middle compartment prolapse.

Considering hymen plane as zero the distance of these points from the hymen is measured in centimeters. Proximal or above the hymen the points are given negative number (-) and distal or below the hymen the points are considered as positive (+) number. All these points except TVL are measured during straining (Valsalva) resulting maximum protrusion.

Six Site-specific POP-Q Measurements (Fig. 33)

Six site-specific POP-Q measurements are given in **Table 1**.

Three Other Measurements of POP-Q (Fig. 33)

Other measurements are given in **Box 1**.

These nine measurement findings are tabulated in a three-by-three grid. The degree of prolapse is quantified by translating into an ordinal five staging system (from stage 0–IV). Most severe portion of the prolapse is taken into consideration during assignment of the stage.

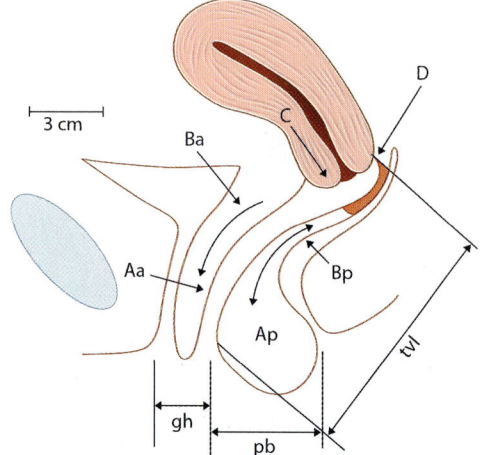

Anterior wall	Anterior wall	Cervix or cuff
Aa	Ba	C
Genital hiatus	Perineal body	Total vaginal length
gh	pb	tvl
Posterior wall	Posterior wall	Posterior fornix
Ap	Bp	D

Fig. 33: Points and measurements of pelvic organ prolapse quantification (POP-Q) system and three-by-three grid for recording.

CHAPTER 10: Pelvic Organ Prolapse (Genital Prolapse)

Table 1: Six site-specific POP-Q measurements.

Points	Description	Range and significance
Aa	Represents a point 3 cm proximal to external urethral meatus in the midline of anterior vaginal wall. It corresponds to proximal location of the urethrovesical crease	From −3 cm (normal) to +3 cm (maximal prolapse of Aa)
Ba	Represents the most distal portion of any part of the upper part of anterior vaginal wall cephalad to point Aa	From −3 cm (without prolapse) to a positive value measuring to the position of cuff from the hymen in posthysterectomy complete vaginal eversion (−3 cm to +TVL)
C	Cervix or vaginal cuff	A point that is either at the most distal edge of the cervix or the leading point of the vaginal cuff after total hysterectomy (±TVL)
D	A point at the location of posterior fornix if no hysterectomy. In absence of cervix the point is omitted	Represents the level of attachment of uterosacral ligament to proximal posterior cervix. It differentiates failure of uterosacral ligament from cervical elongation (±TVL or omitted)
Ap	Represents a point 3 cm proximal to hymen in the midline of posterior vaginal wall	From −3 cm (normal) to +3 cm (maximal prolapse of Ap)
Bp	Represents the most distal portion of any part of the upper part of posterior vaginal wall cephalad to point Ap	From −3 cm (without prolapse) to a positive value measuring to the position of cuff from the hymen in posthysterectomy complete vaginal eversion

Box 1: Other measurements of POP-Q.

Gh (genital hiatus)	Measured from the middle of the external urethral meatus to the midpoint of posterior hymenal ring
Pb (perineal body)	Measured from the posterior margin of genital hiatus to the midanal opening
TVL (total vaginal length)	Greatest depth of the vagina in cm when the vaginal apex (C or D) is reduced to its fullest normal position

Three-by-three Grid for Recording Quantitative Descent of Pelvic Organ Prolapse (Fig. 33)

For three-by-three grid for recording quantitative descent of pelvic organ prolapse, see **Box 2** and **Figure 33**.

Box 2: Three-by-three grid for recording quantitative descent of pelvic organ prolapse.

Aa Anterior wall	Ba Anterior wall	C Cervix or Cuff
Gh Genital hiatus	Pb Perineal body	TVL Total vaginal length
Ap Posterior wall	Bp Posterior wall	D Posterior fornix

Abbreviations: Gh, genital hiatus; Pb, perineal body; TVL, total vaginal length

Determination of Stages of Pelvic Organ Prolapse Following POP-Q Grid

Stages of pelvic organ prolapse following POP-Q grid have been listed in **Box 3**.

Box 3: Stages of pelvic organ prolapse following POP-Q grid.

Stage 0	No prolapse is demonstrated
Stage 1	The most distal portion of the prolapse is >1 cm above the level of hymen
Stage 2	The most distal portion of prolapse is within 1 cm (≤1 cm) proximal or distal to the plane of hymen
Stage 3	The most distal portion of the prolapse is >1 cm below the plane of hymen but < (TVL−2 cm)
Stage 4	Complete to nearly complete eversion of the vagina. The most distal portion of the prolapsed protrudes to ≥ + (TVL−2 cm)

Abbreviation: TVL, total vaginal length

Advantages of POP-Q System

- It allows the use of standardized technique with accurate measurements at straining relative to a constant point, the hymen.
- To assess prolapse at site specific points.
- This reliable, more objective, and site-specific descriptions of POP help to study research results uniformly and to compare more accurate assessment of postoperative outcome.

Q. How to demonstrate POP-Q staging during vaginal examination?

See in vaginal examination later on Page 220 **(Figs. 48 to 54)**.

Examples of POP-Q Grading (Figs. 34 and 35)

Example 1

Anterior vaginal wall prolapse (Fig. 34A): Complete diagram and grid of anterior vaginal wall prolapse.

Posterior vaginal wall prolapse (Fig. 34B): Complete diagram and grid of posterior vaginal wall prolapse.

Example 2

Complete eversion (Fig. 35A): Point Ba (most distal portion of anterior vaginal wall), Point C (the vaginal cuff scar) and Point Bp (most distal point of posterior wall) are all at the

SECTION 2: Clinical Cases

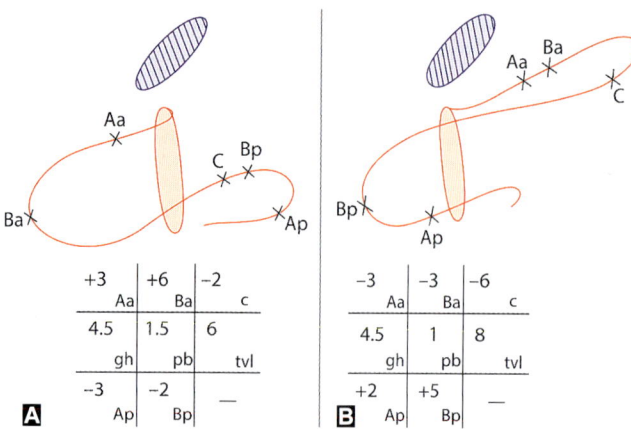

Figs. 34A and B: (A) Complete diagram and grid and of anterior vaginal wall prolapse; (B) Complete diagram grid of posterior vaginal wall prolapse.

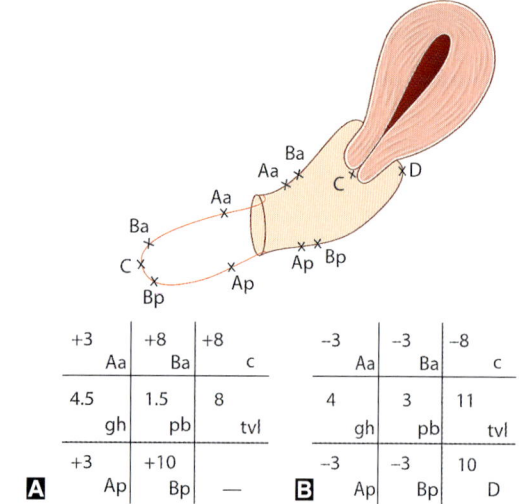

Figs. 35A and B: (A) Grid and complete diagram of complete eversion of vagina; (B) Normal with no prolapse.

same position (+8) and Point Aa and Ap are maximally distal (both at +3).

As TVL equals maximum protrusion this is stage 4 prolapse.

Normal (Fig. 35B): Aa and Bb and points Ap and Bp are all −3 as there is no anterior or posterior wall descent. Lowest point of cervix is 8 cm above hymen (−8). Posterior fornix (point D) is 2 cm above this (−10). Vaginal length (TVL) is 10 cm. Genital hiatus and Pb measure 2 cm and 3 cm, respectively. This is stage 0 support.

For demonstration of POP-Q, *see* **later.**

SURGICOPATHOLOGICAL CHANGES IN PELVIC ORGAN PROLAPSE

Q. What are the surgicopathological changes in genital prolapse?

- *Changes in vaginal mucous membrane:*
  - It becomes thickened and dry
  - Pigmentary changes **(Fig. 36)**
- Decubitus ulcer **(Figs. 37 and 38)**
- Infection—severe infection resulting adhesions may cause the protruding mass irreducible.

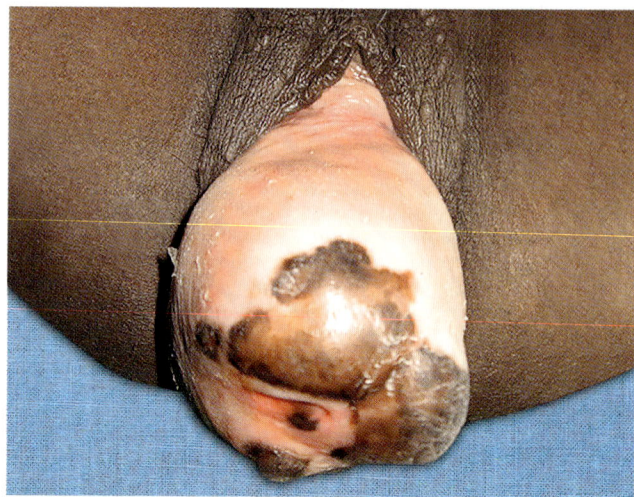

Fig. 36: 32 years P1+0 very low socioeconomic status married at 4 years of age—procidentia with pigmentary changes.

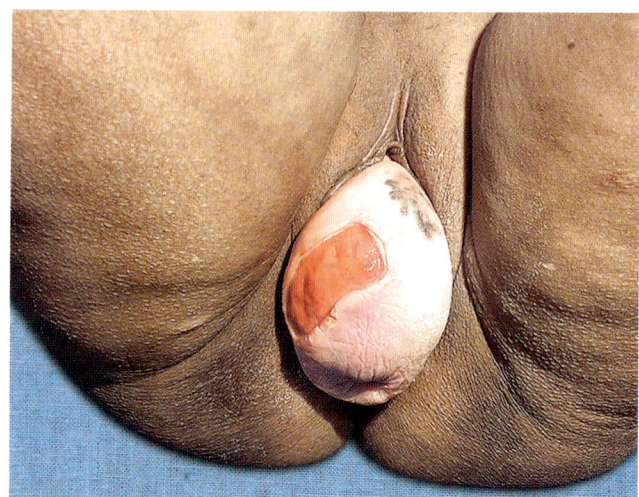

Fig. 37: Decubitus ulcer.

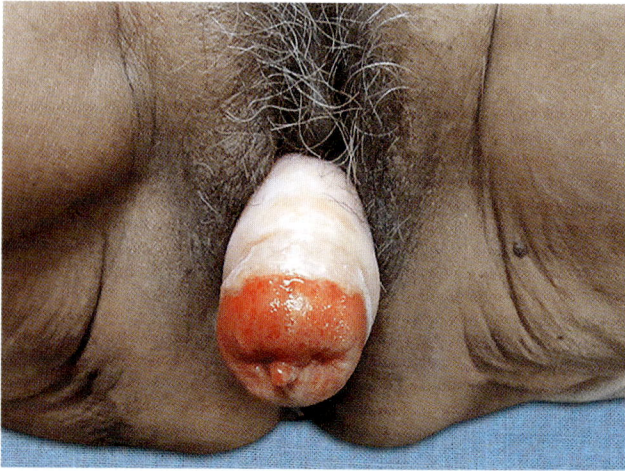

Fig. 38: Decubitus ulcer (erosion).

- *Changes in cervix*: Hypertrophic elongation of both supravaginal part and vaginal part (*see* **Fig. 10**)
- *Changes in uterus*
- *Changes in urinary system*: Hydroureter, hydronephrosis, and pyelonephritis.

DIAGNOSIS OF PELVIC ORGAN PROLAPSE

Q. What are the symptoms of pelvic organ prolapse? (written also in history taking)

History

- *Something coming down per vagina or something falling out of vagina (bulge symptoms)*: Sometimes patient may complain of pelvic pressure or heaviness; may complain of feeling of a ball in the vagina or sitting on a ball.
- Urinary symptoms like frequency, urgency, hesitancy, difficulty in micturition, feeling of incomplete emptying of bladder, retention of urine, and presence of *stress urinary incontinence* (SUI). Sometimes patient may complete the act of micturition after reduction of prolapse, with digitation or postural changes. She cannot evacuate her bladder completely and can only do after reduction of the mass.
- Daytime urinary frequency is more common in POP and nocturnal frequency is commonly seen in urinary infection. Recurrence of UTI is common.
- Bowel problems—constipation, incomplete emptying, incontinence of flatus or feces, fecal urgency, anal or vaginal digitation to defecate, and feeling of obstruction during passing of stool.
- Vaginal discharge—white or bloody.
- Patient may complain of backache.
- Sexual—sexual dysfunction—dissatisfaction.

Q. What do you mean by "bulge symptoms"?

Symptoms of sensation of vaginal protrusion, bulging or feeling or seeing a vaginal or perineal bulging. Important causes are POP, rectal prolapse or any cause of something coming down per vagina.

Q. What other history are important in pelvic organ prolapse (POP)?

- *Age*: More common in elderly.
- *Occupation*: History of heavy weight lifting for a prolonged period.
- *Obstetric history*: History of prolonged labor, instrumental delivery in undilated cervix, unattended delivery, and repeated childbirth with short interval; H/o delivery of large baby. Multiparity is a high-risk factor for POP.
- *Menstrual history*: History of menopause.
- *Medical*: History of chronic bronchial asthma, chronic cough, chronic dysentery, chronic con- stipation, and other medical problems, neurological disorder and connective tissue disorder.
- *Surgical*: History of any type of previous surgery is taken. Whether the complaint is following abdominal or vaginal hysterectomy or there is any other vaginal operation. Hysterectomy itself is a predisposing factor for POP. Following hysterectomy vault prolapse may occur.
- History of smoking.

Q. What are the different signs?

Physical findings in a case of pelvic organ prolapse.

General Examination

- Anemia and malnutrition
- Any neurological abnormality or myopathy and joint hypermobility
- Examination of spine and gait
- Cardiovascular, respiratory system, and renal function—which may alter the mode of treatment.

Per Abdomen

- Laxity of abdominal muscle
- Presence of any hernia
- Any lump or any abnormality
- Ascites
- All hernial sites.

Local Clinical Examination

It includes inspection, speculum examination and palpation, bimanual examination, examination of perineum, and rectal and rectovaginal examination.

- *Position of the patient:* Woman is examined commonly in dorsal position. But can be needed to examine in other positions also.
- *Dorsal supine position* (Fig. 39, also *see* Figs. 30 and 31 of Chapter 1): Thigh flexed and knee flexed making the head end of the table 45° elevated keeping the feet on extended footrests so that buttock comes to the margin

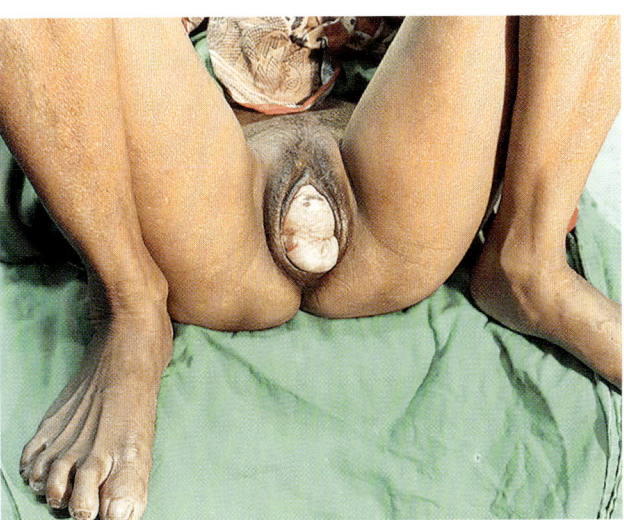

Fig. 39: Dorsal position (most common).

of table which facilitates the introduction of speculum. The degree and extent of prolapse is examined during *Valsalva maneuver* (which means maximum straining by increasing intra-abdominal pressure).

- **Other positions:**
  - *Standing position* **(Fig. 40)**: Genital prolapse examination sometimes needs *standing position* to visualize properly. It is essential when patient feels bulge, but prolapse is not evident in Valsalva.
  - *Lithotomy position*: Some schools prefer to do examination in *lithotomy position* routinely.
  - *Squatting position* **(Fig. 41)**: It is sometimes necessary for proper visualization of genital prolapse if not demonstrated in dorsal position.
  - *Sims' position* **(Fig. 42)**: It is very useful for inspection of lesions of anterior vaginal wall lesion. The following points are noted one by one.

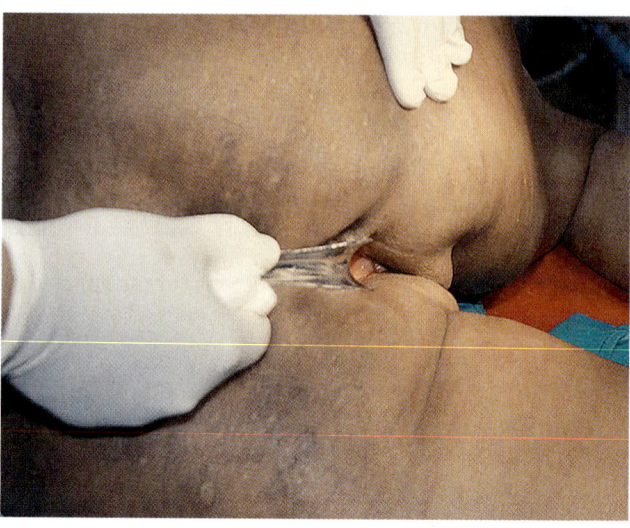

Fig. 42: Sims' position.

(For undergraduate examination only inspection is allowed).

Inspection and Speculum Examination

- Clitoris and labia are healthy, there is vulvar atrophy, vaginal introitus is widened and a mass is seen protruding through the vaginal introitus, well visible *when patient is asked to cough or to strain down (Valsalva)*.
- There is bulging of the anterior vaginal wall indicating cystocele and urethrocele and their degree is noted **(Figs. 43 and 44)**.
- Vaginal rugosity is looked for area wise whether present or not.
- There is three transverse sulcus, namely *submeatal sulcus*, *transverse sulcus*, and *bladder sulcus* **(Fig. 43)**. Submeatal sulcus is a small groove which lies immediately above the external meatus, transverse vaginal sulcus is situated 4 cm above the submeatal sulcus and it corresponds in position with the upper border of posturethral ligament.

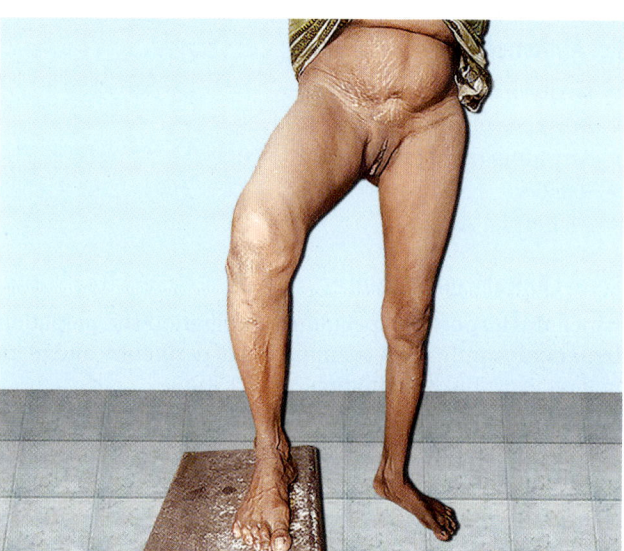

Fig. 40: Standing position.

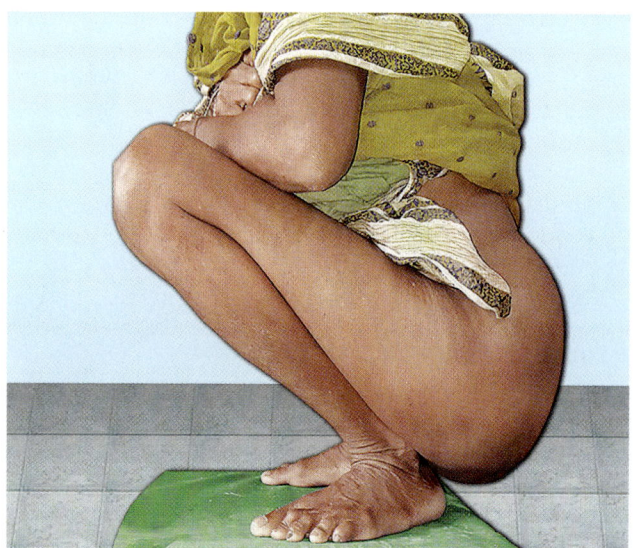

Fig. 41: Squatting position.

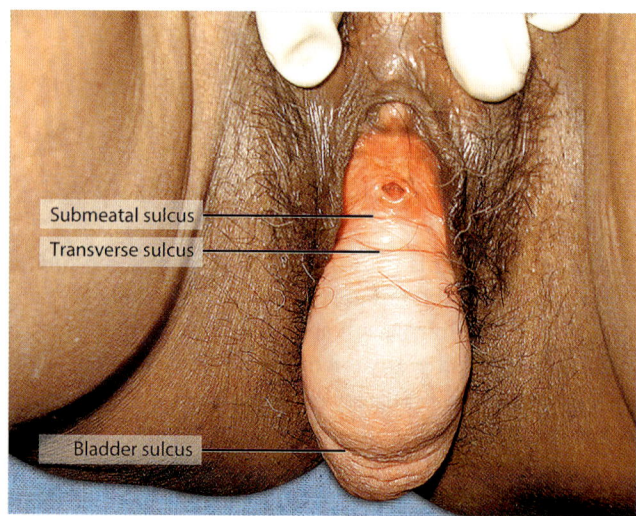

Fig. 43: Prolapse with large cystocele.

CHAPTER 10: Pelvic Organ Prolapse (Genital Prolapse)

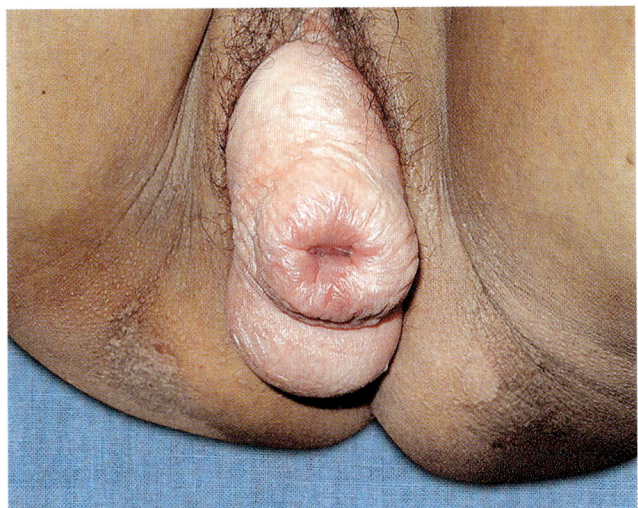

Fig. 44A: Cystocele, uterine descent and enterocele.

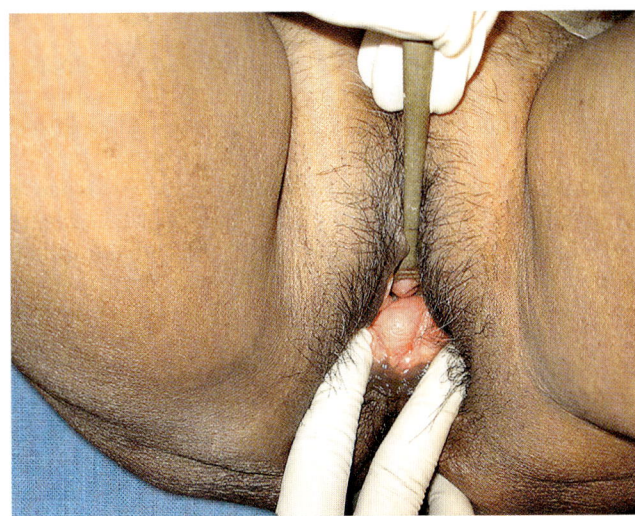

Fig. 45: Rectocele.

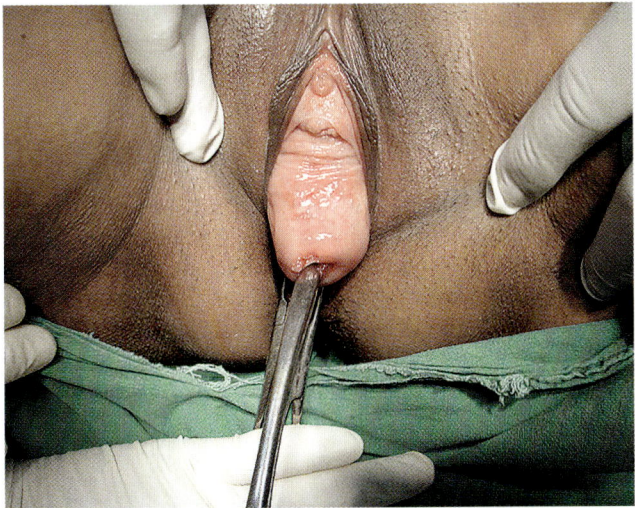

Fig. 44B: Uterine prolapse with no cystocele.

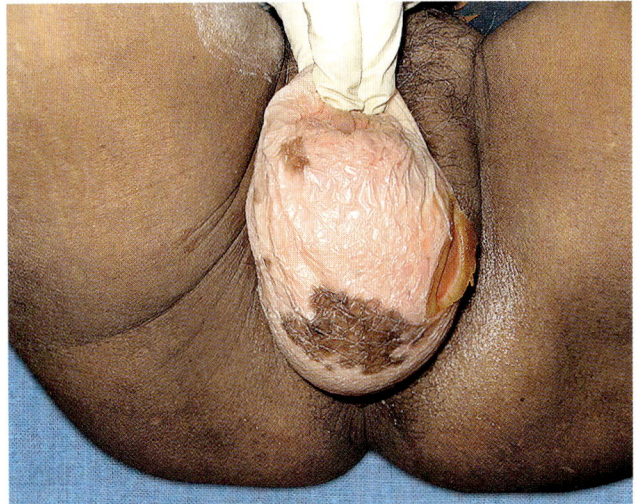

Fig. 46: Decubitus ulcer with pigmentation.

Bladder sulcus lies near cervix and indicates the junction of bladder and anterior vaginal wall. Cystocele is restricted in the space in between the transverse sulcus and bladder sulcus.
- Lateral vaginal sulcus which lies along the arcus tendineus fascia may be absent in paravaginal defect.
- In the middle part there is descent of uterus identified by the presence of external os of cervix which is the leading part of uterine prolapse.
- Posteriorly, perineum is lax, deficient and rugosity of anus is present in all its circumference.
- By retracting the posterior vaginal wall with the Sims' speculum anterior vaginal wall prolapse (cystocele and urethrocele) and descent of cervix are well visualized. In first degree uterine prolapse descent of cervix is seen above the introitus and in second or third degree prolapse cervix is seen at or outside the introitus.
- Bulging of posterior vaginal wall is seen by retracting cervix and anterior vaginal wall with the help of an anterior vaginal retractor or Sims' speculum. Bulging of upper part is enterocele and bulging of middle part is rectocele and is separated by a transverse sulcus. Lower part is lax perineum (How to demonstrate enterocele-for details *see* below) **(Fig. 45)**.
- During Valsalva maneuver the speculum is slowly withdrawn. The extent to which the cervix or the vaginal vault follows the speculum through and out of vagina is recorded.
- Presence of thickening of vaginal mucosa, patchy pigmentation, and decubitus ulcer are looked for **(Fig. 46)**.
- Presence of stress incontinence (spurting of urine trough urethra) is noted on coughing. For this examination, patient is not asked to evacuate of bladder before examination.
- "Occult" stress incontinence is a condition which is revealed after the prolapse is reduced and due to direct compressive effect or urethral kinking.

Palpation

- Anteriorly, cystocele and urethrocele are palpated. Catheter may be introduced through the urethra to confirm that it is cystocele, not other swelling like gartner duct cyst. Urethral hypermobility is also checked for.
- By palpation, exact degree of uterine prolapse is determined. The protruding mass is grasped at the vaginal introitus between the thumb in front and the fingers behind. If the fundus of uterus is felt below the grip (to get above the swelling) it is procidentia (complete eversion) and if the firm body is gripped it is second degree uterine prolapse **(Figs. 47A and B)**.
- On bimanual examination after reducing the prolapse size of the uterus is measured, whether there is elongation of supravaginal portion of cervix is also noted and condition of adnexae is assessed.
- Degree and grades are determined by inspection and palpation. POP-Q staging is done.
- Posteriorly, rectocele and enterocele are palpated.
- Examination of rectovaginal area and rectal examination
- Rectocele and enterocele can be differentiated by rectal or rectovaginal examination (*see* below).

Tone of perineal body and levator ani is assessed, presence of any hemorrhoids and rectal prolapse noted.

Pelvic floor muscle tone is assessed by introducing index finger 2–3 cm inside hymen at 4 and then 8 o'clock position. Tone and strength can be graded from 0 to 5 Oxford scales (5 indicates normal muscle tone).

Reflexes (Sacral)

- *Bulbocavernosus reflex*: On tapping or stroking on lateral side of clitoris contraction of the bulbocavernosus muscle on both sides indicates normal sacral pathway.
- *Anal wink reflex*: Elicitation of contraction of the anus on stroking on anus indicates intact anal sphincter innervations.

DEMONSTRATION OF POP-Q STAGING

Q. How to demonstrate POP-Q staging during vaginal examination? (*see* Fig. 33, Table 1 and Box 1)

Before demonstration read POP-Q classification as written before for easy understating.

- For measurement, Ayer's spatula **(Fig. 48)** graduated in cm, ruler, a graduated sponge holding forceps (if available) or any stick (e.g. plunger of Cu-T; **Fig. 49**) graduated from 1 to 10 cm is made ready and the measurements are taken one by one and put in the three-by-three grid.
- Measurement of Gh **(Fig. 50)** and Pb **(Fig. 51)** is taken during Valsalva maneuver and noted in the grid.

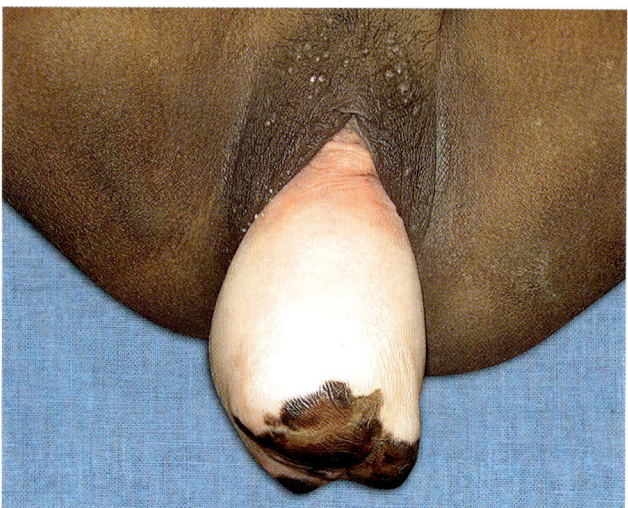

Fig. 47A: Procidentia with pigmentation.

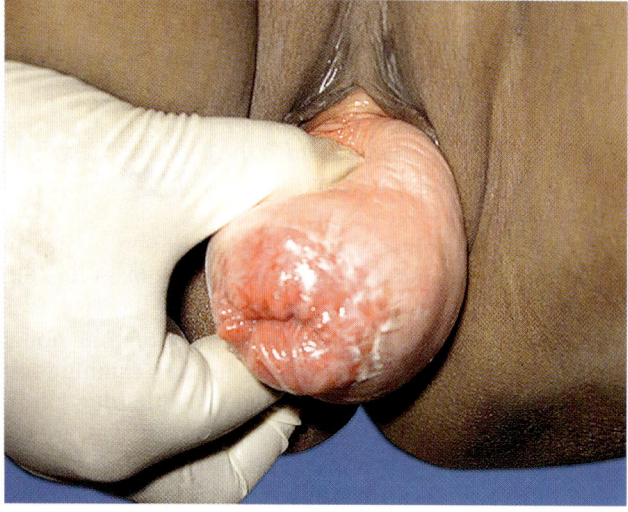

Fig. 47B: To get above the swelling.

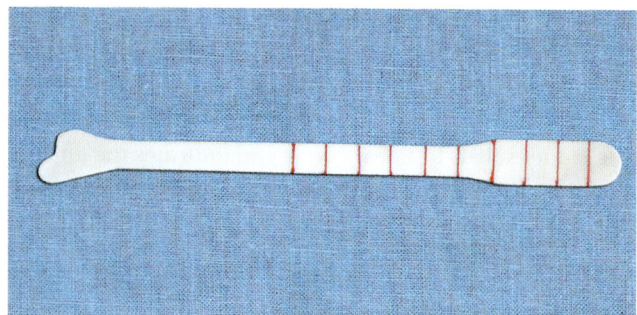

Fig. 48: Graduated Ayer's spatula.

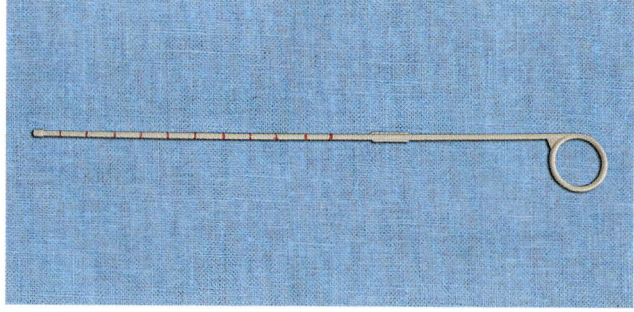

Fig. 49: Plunger of Cu-T (graduated by marking).

CHAPTER 10: Pelvic Organ Prolapse (Genital Prolapse)

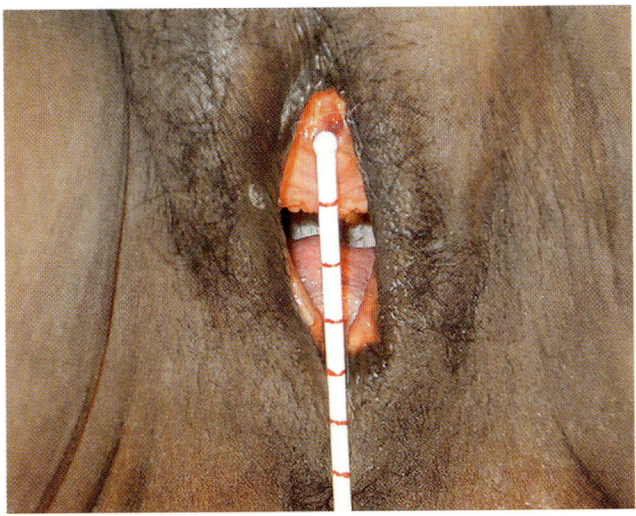

Fig. 50: Genital hiatus.

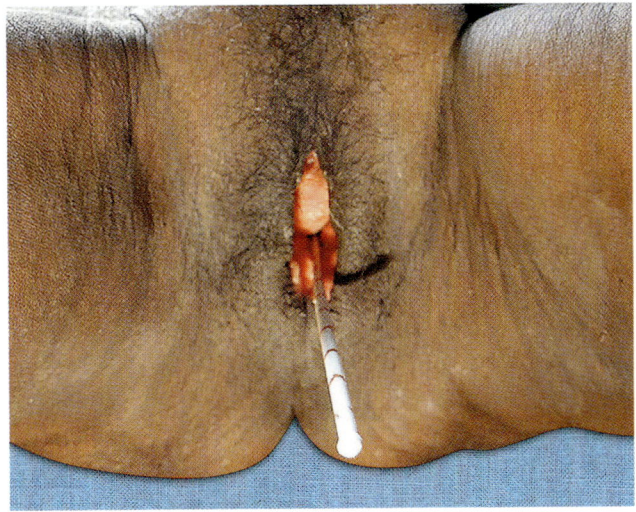

Fig. 52: Total vaginal length.

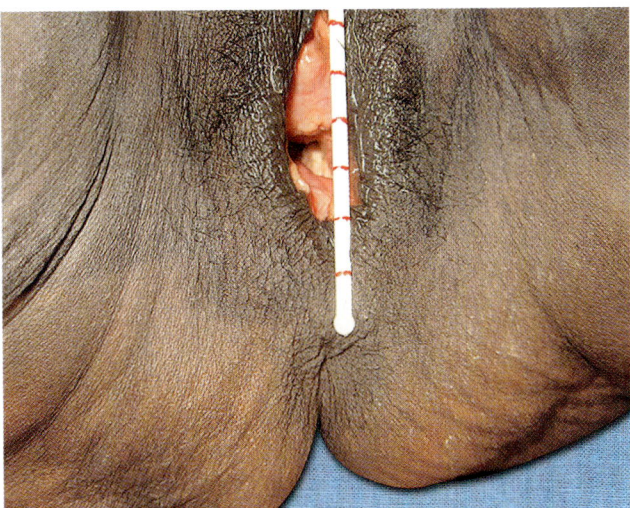

Fig. 51: Perineal body.

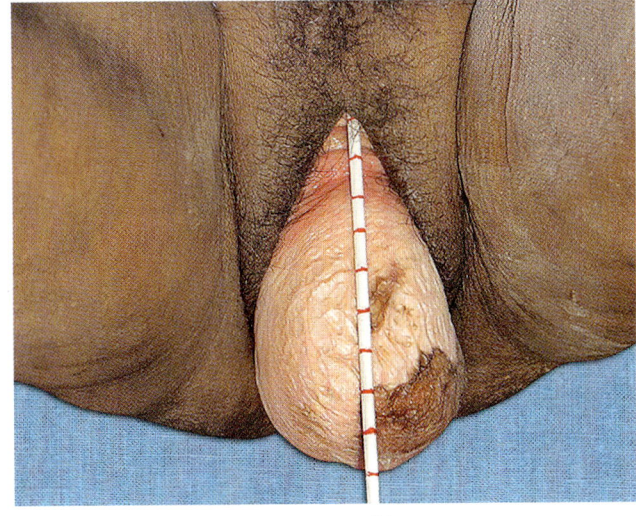

Fig. 53: Aa and Ba.

- Total vaginal length is measured from vaginal apex to the hymen after reduction **(Fig. 52)**.
- Point C and D are measured after inserting a Cusco's bivalve speculum. In posthysterectomy cases D point is omitted.
- Points Aa and Ba **(Fig. 53)** are marked after introduction of a Sims' speculum or Landon retractor to retract posterior vaginal wall and withdrawal during measurement. At this point any defect on anterior vaginal wall is detected. Downward traction of speculum is prohibited to avoid artificial descent of anterior vaginal wall which will give the wrong measurement.
- *Paravaginal defect*: Diagnosed by sagging of lateral vaginal sulcus (obliteration of lateral vaginal sulcus), but there is still presence of vaginal rugae in midline (displacement cystocele).
- *Midline or central defect*: There is central bulge and loss of vaginal wall rugae (distension prolapse).

- Anterior apical or transverse defect is detected by replacing the anterior apical segment and noting the descent of prolapse during Valsalva maneuver. Anterior defect arises due to loss of support of anterior vaginal wall's apical segment.
- During this examination Q-tip test can also be done to test urethral hypermobility (*see* Chapter 17).
- Points Ap and Bp **(Fig. 54)** are marked on examination of posterior vaginal wall after placing the Sims' speculum or Landon's retractor over anterior vaginal wall. Measurement is done after withdrawal of speculum. At this stage diagnosis of enterocele (bulging of apical segment of posterior wall) and rectocele (bulging of distal posterior wall) is done. For differentiation of the two, demonstration is shown below.
- Apical, midline, and lateral defects are also assessed for planning of surgery.

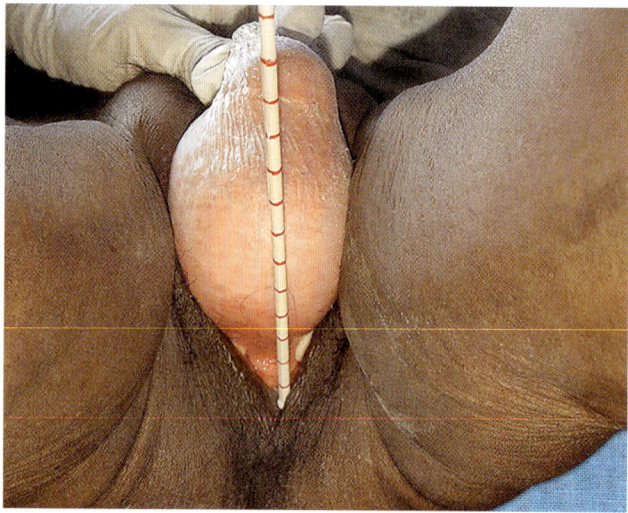

Fig. 54: Ap and Bp.

- Demonstration of presence of apical prolapse is very important as it is believed that anterior and posterior wall descent is due to the defect in apical region and if it is found that anterior and posterior support is restored after replacing the apical prolapse apex is thought to be the primary defect.

DEMONSTRATION OF ENTEROCELE

Q. How will you demonstrate enterocele? How rectocele and enterocele are differentiated?

Enterocele can be demonstrated by various methods:
- Patient is in supine position, thigh flexed and knee flexed. Uterus is pushed back and retracted by the anterior vaginal wall retractor. Sims' speculum is introduced up to the posterior fornix. Sims' speculum is gradually withdrawn and the patient is asked to cough. The enterocele sac will hang over the Sims' speculum **(Fig. 55A)**.
- Cervix and anterior vaginal wall are retraced with the help of an anterior vaginal retractor or Sims' speculum. Bulging of upper part is enterocele and bulging of middle part is rectocele and is separated by a transverse sulcus. Rectocele and enterocele can be differentiated by rectal or rectovaginal examination, the tip of examining finger bulges through the rectocele, while the finger cannot be pushed into enterocele.
- Right index finger is introduced into the rectum and left index finger inside the vagina. If small bowel is palpable in between the two fingers it is enterocele and in case of rectocele two fingers are felt each other.

DEMONSTRATION OF STRESS INCONTINENCE

Q. How will you demonstrate stress incontinence? What is occult or "hidden" stress incontinence?

- Presence of stress incontinence (spurting of urine through urethra) is noted on coughing. For this examination, patient is asked not to evacuate of bladder before examination.
- "Occult" or "hidden" stress incontinence is a condition which is revealed after the prolapse is reduced and supported by pessary or large cotton swab or ring forceps or speculum or by fingers **(Fig. 55B)**.
- In these cases due to direct compressive effect or urethral kinking there is no demonstrable stress incontinence normally.
- Urethra should not be overly straightened (showing false-positive test) or obstructed (showing false-negative test) or tension is not placed over puborectalis muscles by excessive posterior retraction during elicitation. If this test is not done preoperatively, occult incontinence may remain undetected, hence not corrected and patient may present with stress incontinence postoperatively.

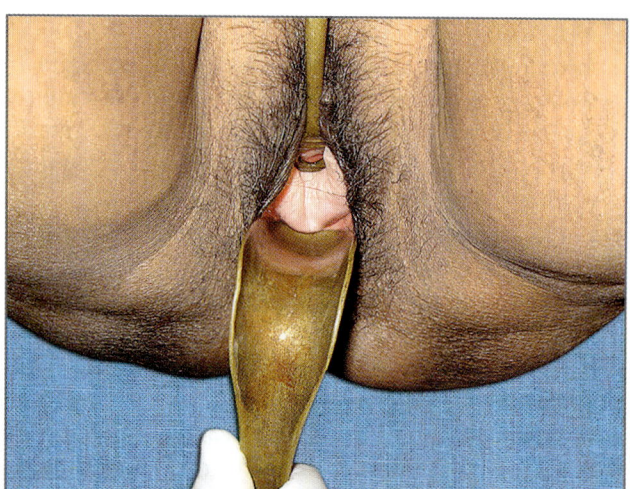

Fig. 55A: Enterocele demonstrated.

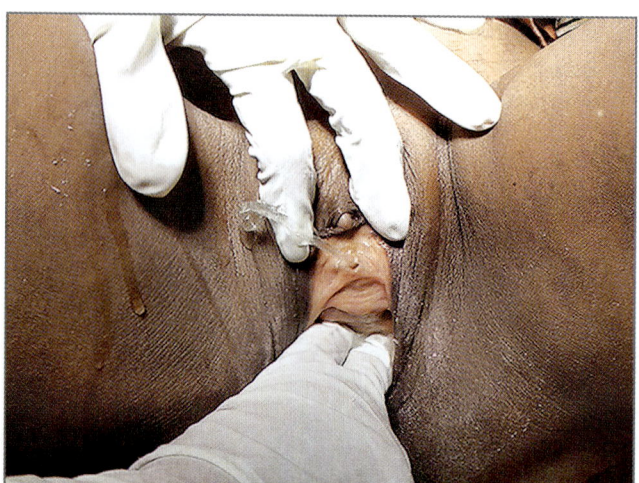

Fig. 55B: Demonstration of occult stress incontinence. Patient with pelvic organ prolapse was asked to cough with full bladder, there was no incontinence. When prolapse is reduced, supported with fingers and asked to cough there was spurting of urine as shown in the figure.

Q. What are the bladder function evaluations done in POP cases?

- A clean catch midstream urine sample is sent for culture.
- Postvoidal residual urine (PVR) volume is assessed either by USG scan or by catheterization. A PVR volume of 100 mL or less is quiet acceptable.
- Urodynamic study is valuable before surgery because this will help to determine the relationship between prolapse and urinary symptom and whether separate treatment for urinary symptom is needed or not.
- Various imaging techniques like dynamic MRI and transperineal ultrasound (TPUS) are also suggested, but their value in routine practice is questioned.

Q. Evaluation of bowel function.

In presence of rectocele and decision of surgery taken patient should be evaluated for defecatory dysfunction by symptoms and physical examination.

Pessary Test

Placing a pessary before surgical treatment and to observe the relieve of urinary symptoms may speculate the effect of surgery.

Decubitus Ulcer

Q. What are the sites of decubitus ulcer? Why does it occur? What is the management of decubitus ulcer?

- The sites are vagina and cervix.
- It occurs usually due to vascular impairment and friction with the thighs and garments and may be complicated with infection.
- The chance of malignancy is very rare.
- Management includes reduction of prolapse and keeping in position by rest, packing with roller gauze soaked with glycerin acriflavin solution or by pessary.
- Pap smear from the area is taken and estrogen is applied in postmenopausal women. In suspected cases, colposcopy-directed biopsy is done.

MANAGEMENT OF PELVIC ORGAN PROLAPSE

Q. What are the different options of management in genital prolapse? In your case how will you manage?

Conservative Management or Nonsurgical which Includes

- Weight reduction
- Alteration of lifestyle
- Pelvic floor exercise
- Pessary

Surgery

Q. What are the factors you will consider in planning of management in individual case of POP?

Age, parity and living issue, degree and type of prolapse, type of defect, associated symptoms and sign (presence of SI and enterocele), any previous surgery, and other uterine pathology.

CONSERVATIVE MANAGEMENT

Q. What will you do in asymptomatic woman?

Invasive therapy is not advocated in absence of other factors and pelvic floor muscle rehabilitation is offered.

Q. What are the indications of conservative (nonsurgical and no pessary) methods?

Women who have no complain, mild-to-moderate degree prolapse (leading point not extending beyond the hymen), where surgery is contraindicated, in very elderly women and in pregnancy with prolapse.

Lifestyle management includes weight loss and avoiding the works which increase intra-abdominal pressure.

Pelvic Floor Exercise

Pelvic floor muscle exercises may limit the progression of mild prolapse and related symptoms and also in stress incontinence but not in advanced prolapse. Exercise does not work if prolapse extends beyond introitus.

It was introduced by Arnold Kegel in 1948.

Kegel exercise is done by drawing up of anus and tightening the vagina for stopping or interrupting micturition.

Contraction is done against two fingers inside the vagina or against vaginal cone (20–100 g) avoiding contraction of gluteal muscles. Repeat 50–200 times/day, 5–10 sec/repetition.

The use of biofeedback and electrical stimulation are also effective treatment.

VAGINAL PESSARY

Q. What are the indications of vaginal pessary in POP?

Pessary is a palliative treatment not curative. It acts by stretching the vaginal wall and elevating the vagina.

- Women who decline surgery
- edically unfit for surgery
- During pregnancy
- Desires childbearing
- Pending for surgery

Vaginal Pessary: Types, Introduction, Follow up, and Complications

Q. What are the types of vaginal pessary?

Two types: Support pessary and space-filling pessary mostly made of silicone.

- Commonly used pessary is ring pessary (rubber or silicone) **(Figs. 56A and B)** which is a support pessary and permits sexual intercourse.
- Support pessary is placed under the symphysis pubis and sacrum, and elevate the vagina.

SECTION 2: Clinical Cases

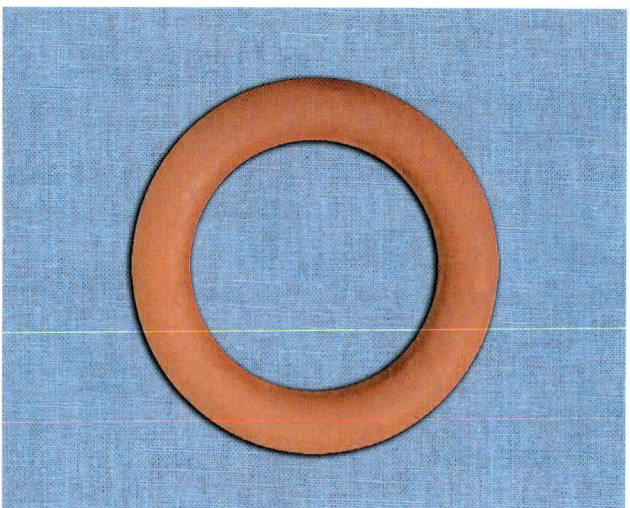

Fig. 56A: Ring pessary (rubber).

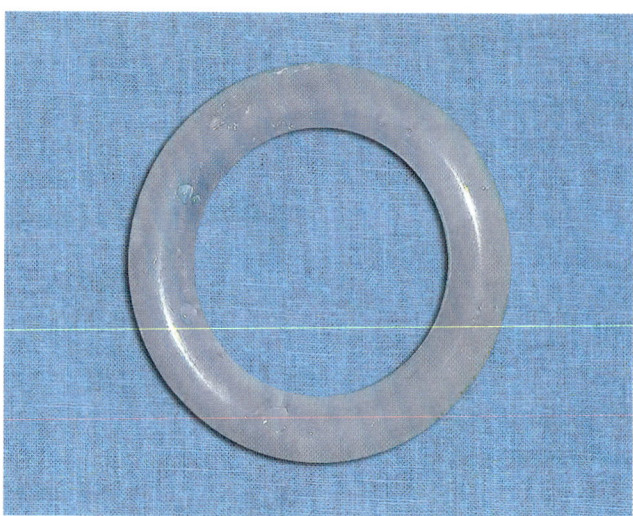

Fig. 56B: Ring pessary made of silicone.

- Gellhorn pessary (flexible made of silicone) **(Figs. 57A to F)** is commonly used space-filling pessary.
- Ring and other support pessaries are used for stage I and stage II and space-filling pessary for stage III and stage IV.
- Inflatable pessaries impair successful coitus.
- Different sizes are available and patient should be given the exact size by trial and error method. Usually patient is asked to bring three sizes after taking measurement as below.
- Measurement: By vaginal examination distance between the posterior vaginal fornix and external urinary meatus is measured and by deducting 1.25 cm the required size (diameter) is determined.

Steps of Pessary Introduction

Patient is asked to lie down on dorsal position with thigh and leg flexed and thigh abducted after passing of urine.

Manual reposition of prolapse is done first.

The posterior vaginal wall is pressed by left index and middle fingers.

The ring pessary is compressed by the right thumb and index finger and introduced in vertical position inside vagina

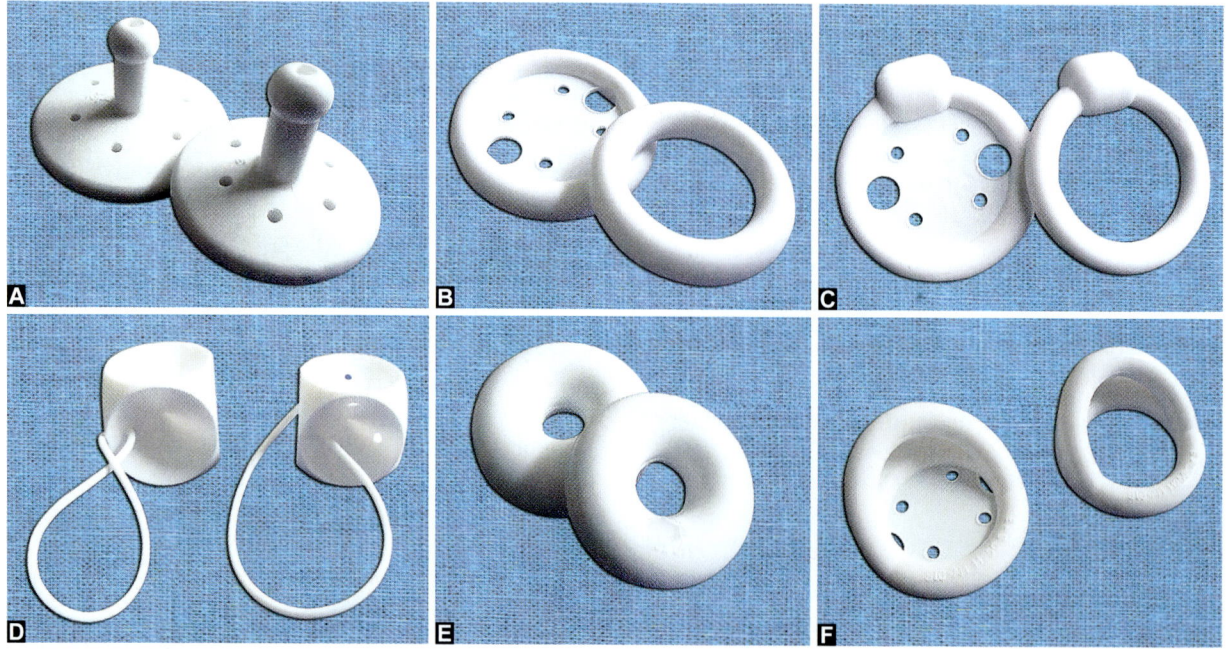

Figs. 57A to F: (A) Gellhorn; (B) Ring pessary; (C) Ring vs Knob pessary; (D) Cube pessary; (E) Donut pessary; (F) Marland pessary. Pessaries are of two types—support pessary and space filling pessary. Ring pessaries are support pessary. Gellhorn and cube pessaries are space-filling pessary. Today's pessaries are made of either silicone or inert plastic. Rubber ring pessary (*see* Fig. 56) is still popular and used. Ring pessary and Gellhorn pessaries are used mostly.

Source: With permission from Bioteque America

and rotated 90°. Posterior rim is placed in posterior fornix behind the cervix by the right index finger, then anterior rim is pushed behind the symphysis pubis at anterior fornix.

Follow-up

Pessary should be cleaned regularly with an interval of 3–4 days and the patient should be trained the procedure of insertion. After first insertion the woman should come for follow up after 2 weeks, then 3 monthly for 1 year, and then 6 month interval.

Complications

The important complications are vaginal discharge, infection, ulceration, offensive smell, incarceration, forgotten pessary, and rarely vesicovaginal fistula and rectovaginal fistula.

SURGERY IN PELVIC ORGAN PROLAPSE

Indication of Surgery

Patient is symptomatic, not relieved by conservative therapy or who does not desire conservative therapy and stage II or more with apparent progression.

Q. What counseling should be done before prolapse surgery?

Symptoms related to vaginal bulge and pelvic pressure symptoms are improved, but other symptoms like backache, urinary complains, bowel problems may not be relieved. Separate treatment maybe needed for urinary symptoms. There may be recurrence of prolapse in few cases.

Aim of Surgery

The purpose is to restore the anatomy and function and to make the patient symptom free.

Two types of surgery are done, namely reconstructive and obliterative.

SURGERIES DONE IN POP

Q. What are the different surgeries done in a case of POP? Which one is commonly done?

Surgery is the mainstay of treatment in POP.
- Anterior colporrhaphy with or without lateral repair
- Posterior colpoperineorrhaphy with or without perirectal fascial repair
- Pelvic floor repair (PFR): Anterior colporrhaphy and posterior colpoperineorrhaphy combinedly
- Fothergill's operation
- Ward-Mayo's operation—vaginal hysterectomy with PFR
- Repair of vault prolapse
- Repair of enterocele
- Sling operations
- Le Fort's operation (obliterative types).

Vaginal hysterectomy with PFR (Ward Mayo's operation) is commonly practiced procedure as mostly diagnosed in late reproductive or postmenopausal women.

Surgery may be:
- Vaginal
- Abdominal:
  - Laparoscopic
- Combination
- Surgery may be using mesh or fascia.

Anterior Vaginal Wall Prolapse

- *Anterior colporrhaphy*: Plication of pubovesicocervical fascia
- *Site-specific repair*: Paravaginal defect—pubocervical fascia to arcus tendineus (sutured with fascia covering obturator internus).

Posterior Vaginal Wall Prolapse

- Posterior colporrhaphy: Plication of prerectal fascia
- Perineorrhaphy: Repair of perineal body, approximation of superficial perineal muscle
- Site specific-repair of perirectal fascia
- McCall's culdoplasty: Plication of uterosacral ligament and fixation of uterosacral to vaginal vault.
- Moschcowitz operation—purse-string (concentric) sutures of pouch of Douglas (POD) peritoneum in abdominal approach.
- In Halban method, vertical row of suture is given in POD (uterosacral and peritoneum over rectosigmoid).

Management Preserving the Uterus

- Fothergill (by Manchester) operation
- *Sling operation*:
  - Purandare's sling—cervix to anterior abdominal wall by rectus strip.
  - Shirodkar's sling opn—cervix to sacrum with tape
  - Abdominal sacrohysteropexy—cervix to sacrum with mesh
  - Khanna—cervix to anterior superior iliac spine (fascia or tape).

Management of Vault Prolapse (Fig. 58)

Vault prolapse is also categorized as 1st, 2nd, and 3rd degree and commonly associated with cystocele and enterocele.

Vaginal Approach

- Sacrospinous colpopexy—vaginal vault to sacrospinous ligament.
- Iliococcygeus colpopexy—vaginal vault to iliococcygeus muscle.
- Infracoccygeus sacrocolpopexy—a permanent mesh tape is placed through the ischiorectal fossa as an inverted "U"

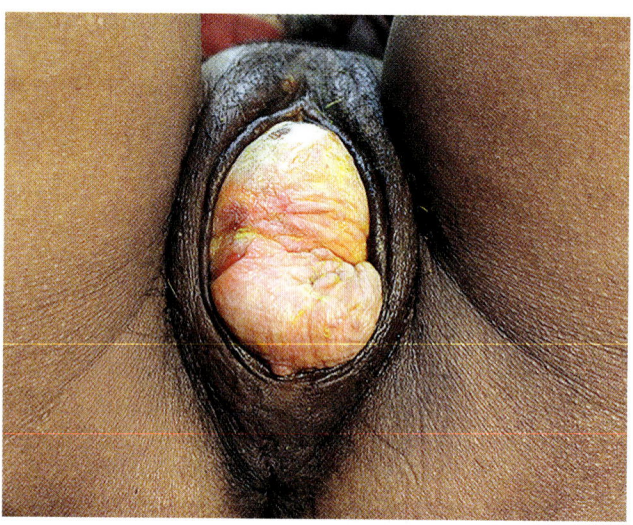

Fig. 58: Vault prolapse—transverse groove is well visible.

around the rectum and attached to the posterior vaginal wall.
- PIVS (posterior infracoccygeus vaginal sling)
- Uterosacral ligament suspension
- McCall's culdoplasty.

Abdominal Approach
- Abdominal sacrocolpopexy—vaginal vault to anterior longitudinal ligament
- Abdominal uterosacral suspension—vaginal vault to uterosacral ligament.

Laparoscopic Approach

Laparoscopic sacrocolpopexy—vaginal vault to anterior sacral ligaments.

Associated Stress Incontinence (see Chapter 17)
- Vaginal—tension free vaginal tape (TVT) or transobturator tape (TOT)
- Kelly's plasty—old classical surgery
- Abdominal—Burch suspension.

Q. WHICH TREATMENT WHEN?
- Younger woman with mild degree prolapse with insignificant symptom—pelvic floor exercise.
- Younger woman with anterior wall prolapse and posterior wall prolapse, no uterine descent—pelvic floor repair.
- Young woman, family completed 2° uterine prolapse or any woman who wants to preserve uterus with same degree prolapse—Fothergill's operation or sacrohysterocolpopexy. Sacrocolpopexy is the preferred and gold standard.
- Younger woman family not completed or nulliparous 1–2° uterine prolapse—abdominal sacrohysteropexy or any sling operation.
- Elderly women with symptomatic prolapse with completed family—vaginal hysterectomy with PFR.
- Elderly women with completed family with symptomatic prolapse and procidentia—vaginal hysterectomy with PFR combined with sacrospinous colpopexy.
- Vault prolapse following hysterectomy/abdominal or laparoscopic sacrocolpopexy/vaginal route—McCall's culdoplasty, sacrospinous colpopexy—vaginal vault to sacrospinous ligament (vaginal approach). Associated cystocele or rectocele is better dealt vaginally.
- Elderly woman unfit for surgery not desirous of sexual intercourse—Le Fort's operation (partial colpocleisis).
- Large paravaginal defect—better dealt abdominally or laparoscopically.
- Associated with stress incontinence—TVT, TOT or Kelly's plasty, and Burch suspension.

Parameters to be considered before planning of surgery
- Age
- Parity with or without desire of future child bearing
- Degree and type of prolapse
- History of previous surgery
- Associated pelvic or uterine pathology
- Presence of stress incontinence.

Preoperative Investigations
- Patient's surgical fitness by clinical evaluation and routine investigations as described in Chapter 1.
- Special emphasis is given on to exclude urinary tract infections.

OPERATIVE DETAILS OF PELVIC ORGAN PROLAPSE

ANTERIOR COLPORRHAPHY

Q. What do you mean by anterior colporrhaphy?

It is a repair procedure by which attenuated fibromuscular tissue between the vagina and urinary bladder are approximated to place the bladder in more anterior and normal position.

Q. What additional procedures may be done with anterior colporrhaphy?
- Along with anterior colporrhaphy posterior colpoperineorrhaphy is almost done as rectocele and perineal body relaxation are common association.
- Management of stress incontinence if it is there.
- In reproductive age group when family completed Fothergill's operation is done if there is uterine descent.

- In elderly vaginal hysterectomy is done when associated with uterine descent (Ward Mayo's operation) along with posterior colpoperineorrhaphy.
- Concurrent vaginal paravaginal defect repair (PVDR) and concurrent apical support surgeries.

Q. Is it mandatory to do vaginal hysterectomy along with anterior colporrhaphy?

It is not mandatory. However uterine descent is almost always common association and it is believed that removal of uterus may help the repair surgery better way.

Q. Describe the steps of anterior colporrhaphy (Figs. 59 to 78).

- Patient is in lithotomy position
- Anesthesia: Regional or general
- Antiseptic dressing, draping, and catheterization **(Fig. 59)**
- Vaginal examination and planning of surgery
- Sims' posterior vaginal speculum **(Fig. 60)** or Auvard weighted speculum is introduced to retract posterior vaginal wall. Anterior lip of the cervix is held by multiple teeth vulsellum or Allis tissue forceps and cervix is pulled.
- A female metal catheter is introduced to detect the lowest limit of bladder (vesicocervical junction)
- Now, a triangular area is selected and three Allis forceps are applied **(Fig. 60)**—one at the apex 1.5 cm below the external urethral opening in the midline, another two each on two lateral sides of cervicovaginal unction.
- A transverse incision **(Fig. 62)** is made from one Allis to other on two lateral ends with slight concavity of incision above and another vertical incision starting from midpoint of vertical incision to the Allis forceps at apex so that an inverted T-shaped incision is made **(Figs. 63 and 65)**.
- To make it technically easy, tips of a blunt pointed bent-on-flat scissors (Metzenbaum scissor) are introduced beneath the vaginal epithelium in the midpoint of

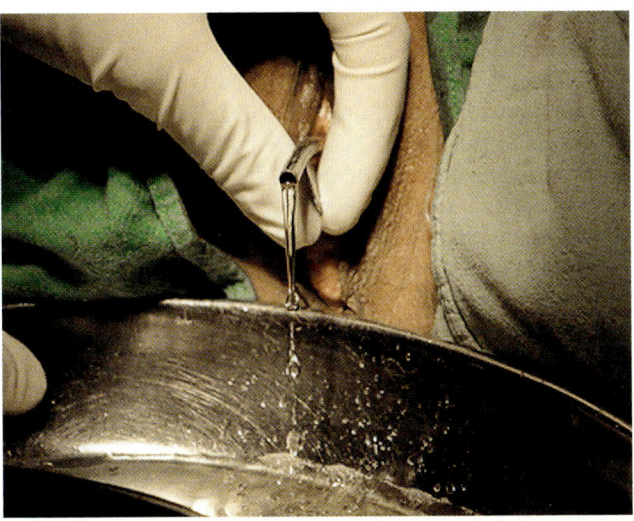

Fig. 59: Catheterization.

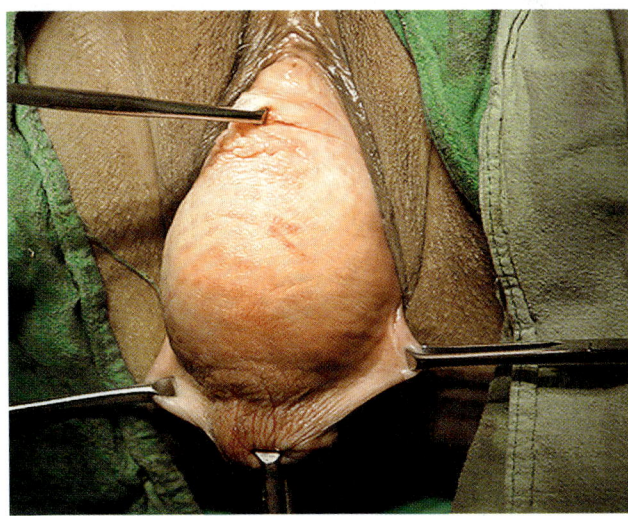

Fig. 61: Three Allis tissue forceps at three points.

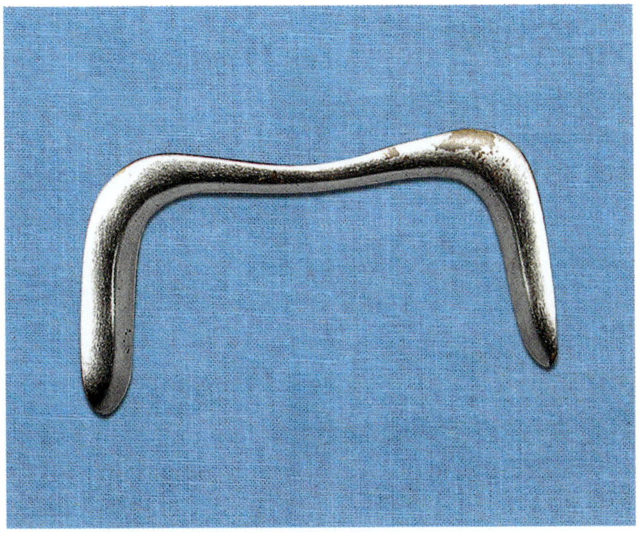

Fig. 60: Sims' speculum is introduced to retract posterior vaginal wall.

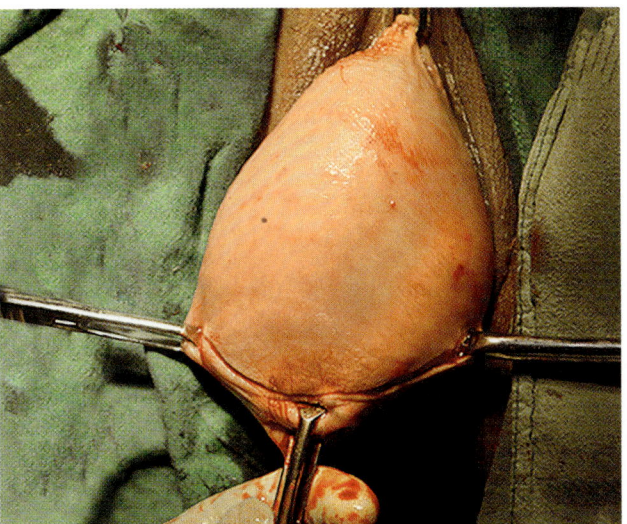

Fig. 62: Transverse incision below the cystocele.

transverse incision in a plane between the vaginal epithelium and the bladder vertically approaching toward the Allis forceps held at apex **(Figs. 63 and 64)**. The scissor blades are opened and closed beneath the vaginal mucosa with approaching to the apex so that a plane is already created and simultaneous vertical incision is given. The upper end of vertical incision extends up to 2–3 cm below the external urethral opening.

- Two triangular vaginal flaps are dissected laterally with the help of blades of scissors or finger covered with gauze (sharp and blunt dissection) laterally and providing simultaneous traction of the vaginal flaps holding with the help of more Allis forceps. Lateral dissection is extended to expose the bladder (cystocele) fully **(Figs. 66 to 68)**.
- Infiltration of normal saline with or without adrenaline (hydrodissection) makes the dissection easy. On infiltration of adrenaline anesthetist must be consulted. Instead of inverted T many surgeons like to give inverted V incision.

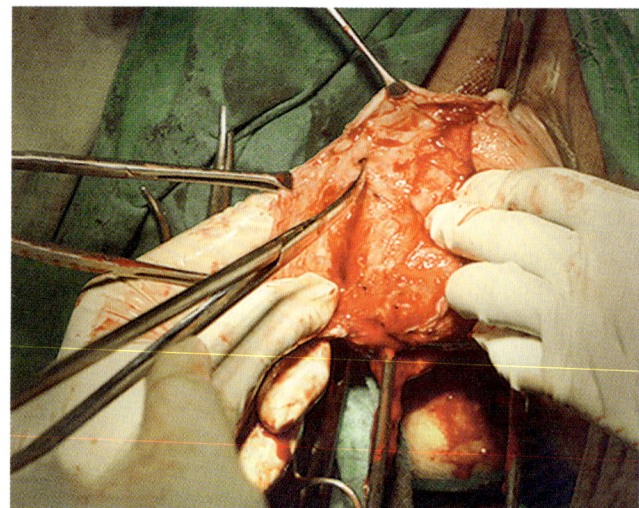

Fig. 65: After vertical incision vaginal mucosa is separated from bladder.

- The bladder is attached to cervix with vesicocervical fascia (ligament) which is cut and bladder is displaced upward with a gauze on the thumb **(Fig. 66)**.
- Next is to reduce the cystocele by tightening the fascial layer between the bladder and vagina. The layer is called pubocervical fascia, pubocervical ligaments or also Fascia of Denonvilliers. The two lateral masses of pubocervical fascia are sutured in the midline with interrupted stitches with 1-0 sutures **(Figs. 69 to 71 and 77)**.
- The lower suture is passed through the exposed cervix.
- If there is any site-specific defect like paravaginal or apical paravaginal defect repair (PVDR) **(Fig. 78)**, and/or apical support surgeries are done.
- Then redundant portion of vaginal mucosa is cut and sutured in the midline **(Figs. 72 to 76)**.
- The bladder is catheterized to check whether any injury of bladder wall has occurred.

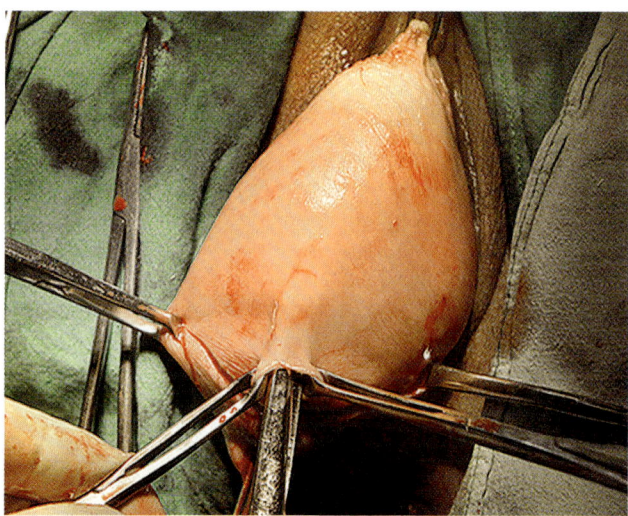

Fig. 63: Scissor is introduced vertically to separate vaginal mucosa from bladder.

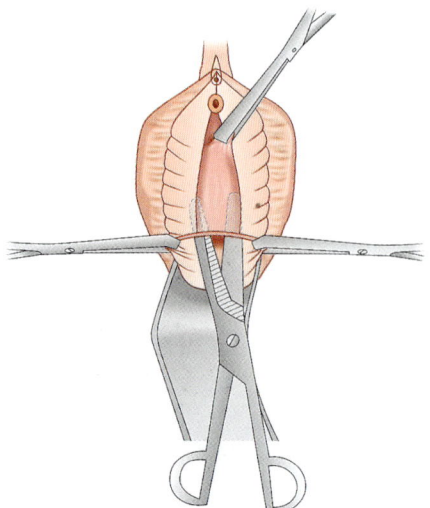

Fig. 64: Separation of vaginal mucosa from bladder by scissor in anterior colporrhaphy.

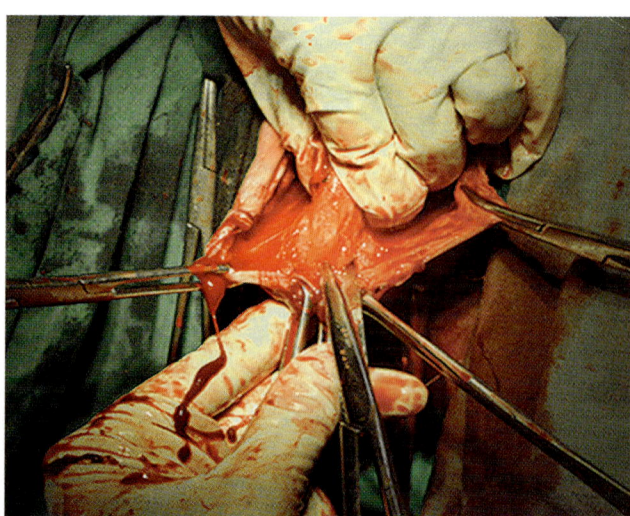

Fig. 66: Bladder is separated from cervix by cutting vesicocervical ligament.

CHAPTER 10: Pelvic Organ Prolapse (Genital Prolapse)

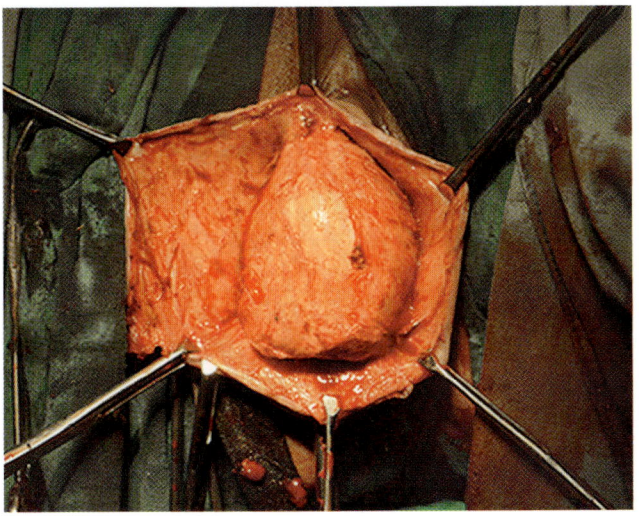

Fig. 67: Cystocele is dissected completely.

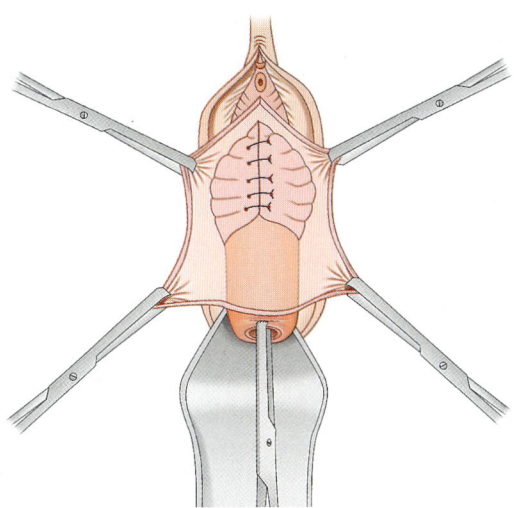

Fig. 70: Repair of pubocervical fascia in cystocele.

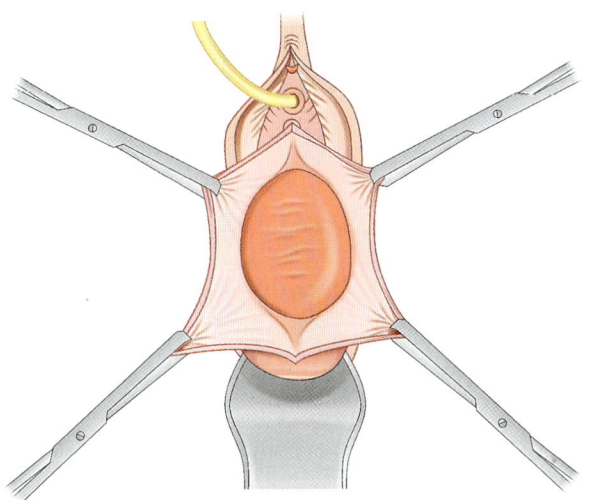

Fig. 68: Cystocele dissected completely.

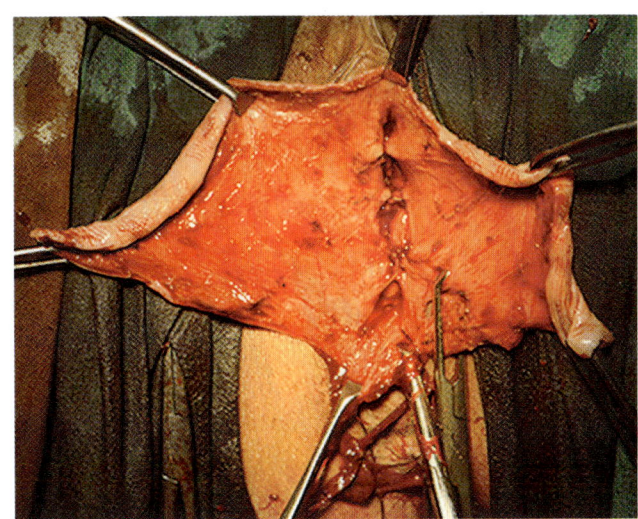

Fig. 71: Vaginal flaps from two sides brought in midline.

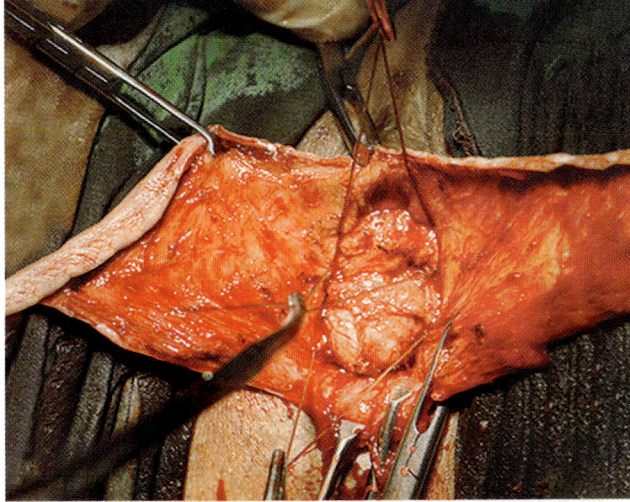

Fig. 69: Pubocervical fascia is repaired and sutured in midline.

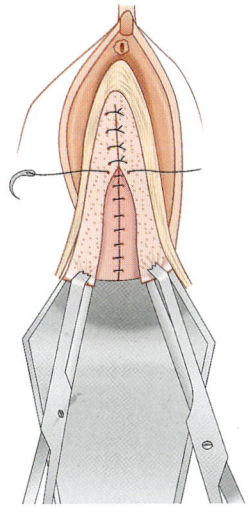

Fig. 72: Repair of vaginal mucosa.

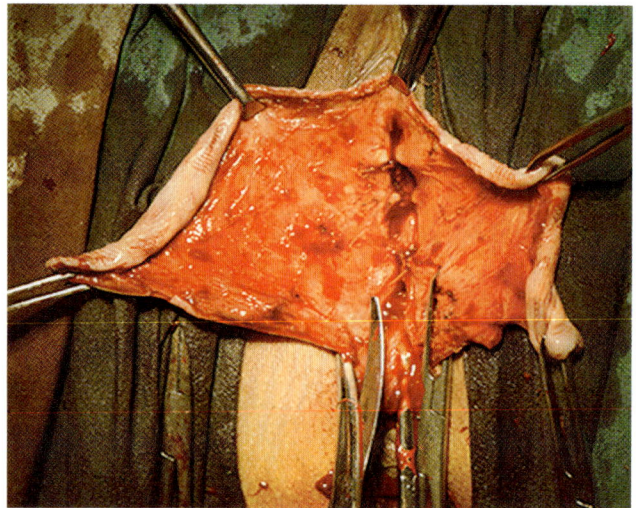

Fig. 73: Vaginal flaps cut.

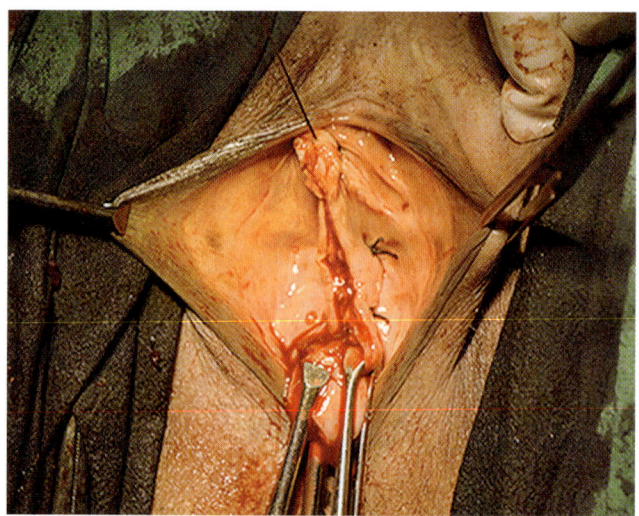

Fig. 76: Vaginal mucosa stitched in midline.

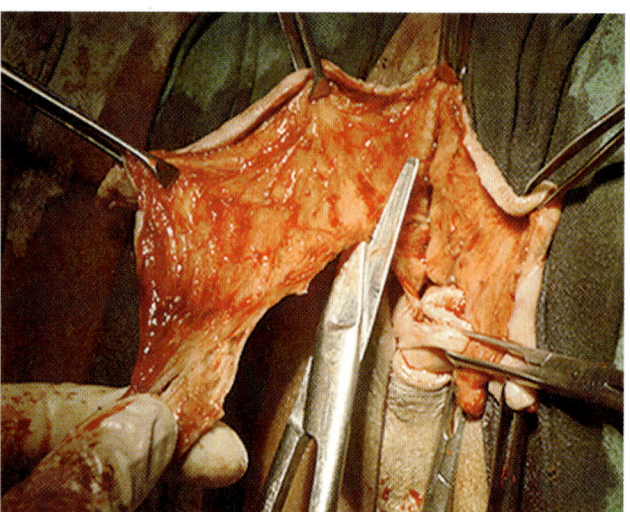

Fig. 74: Redundant part of vaginal mucosa cut.

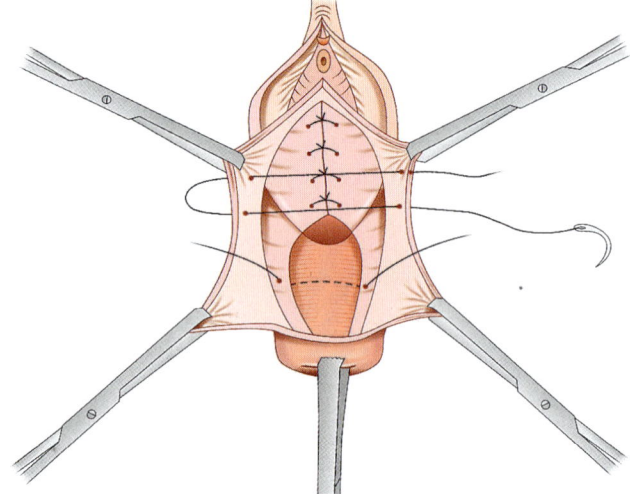

Fig. 77: Repair of cystocele—note only in anterior colporrhaphy last bite includes cervix.

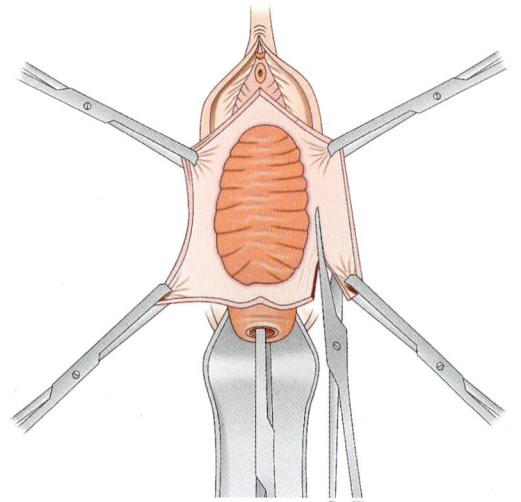

Fig. 75: Cutting the redundant portion of vaginal mucosa.

Q. How modification of anterior colporrhaphy is done in presence of other pathology?

The above description is for when only anterior colporrhaphy is done to correct cystocele. Modification is done in presence of other pathology, e.g.

- In case of *urethrocele*, vaginal wall is dissected further to correct urethrocele.
- In presence of *lateral defect* or break vaginal PVDR is performed. In that case lateral dissection is extended up to lateral pelvic walls at the level of arcus tendineus fascia pelvis (ATFP). Dissection is done from dorsal surface of pubic bones to ischial spines to reach the space of Retzius. Space is repaired by 4–6 2-0 sutures in the AFTP or obturator fascia to paravaginal tissue **(Fig. 78)**.
- In presence of *stress incontinence* either Kelly suture or TVT or TOT is performed during anterior colporrhaphy (described later in Chapter 17).

CHAPTER 10: Pelvic Organ Prolapse (Genital Prolapse)

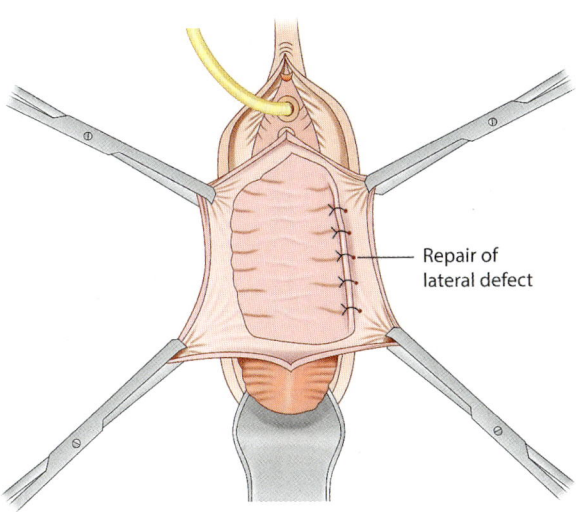

Fig. 78: Repair of lateral defect.

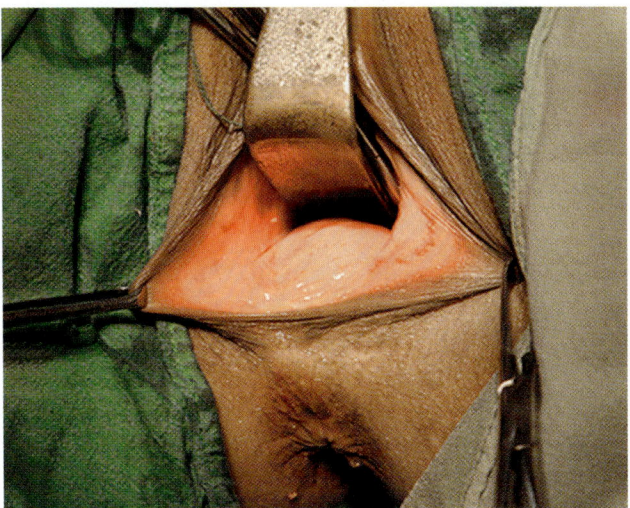

Fig. 79: Rectocele and lax perineum.

- For *Ward Mayo's operation*: After lateral dissection of bladder hysterectomy is done, followed by repair of whole vagina (*see* Page 236).
- In case of *Fothergill's operation*: After reduction of cystocele one circular incision is given behind the cervix lateral to two Allis tissue forceps as held previously, amputation of cervix is done. Mackenrodt's ligaments of both sides are cut and plicated anteriorly in front of cervix, posterior lip of cervix is covered by vaginal mucosa, followed by repair of anterior vaginal wall and the covering of the anterior lip of cervix by vaginal mucosa to form neocervix (*see* below).
- Synthetic or biologic mesh can be placed instead of or in addition to colporrhaphy.

Complications of Anterior Colporrhaphy

- *Perioperative*: Anesthetic complication, hemorrhage, and injury to bladder.
- *Postoperative*: Retention of urine—most common for which catheterization is done prophylactically; urinary tract infection and pelvic infection; secondary hemorrhage; stress incontinence; dyspareunia mostly due to posterior repair, and recurrence.

POSTERIOR COLPOPERINEORRHAPHY

Posterior colporrhaphy is the repair of rectocele and perineorrhaphy means the reinforcement of perineal body. Colpoperineorrhaphy is performed to correct rectocele and to repair perineal body.

Steps (Figs. 79 to 91)

- Usually done along with and after anterior colporrhaphy.
- Preliminary steps are like anterior colporrhaphy.
- Below the two ends of labia minora at the mucocutaneous junction two Allis tissue forceps are applied and another Allis tissue is applied above the highest point of rectocele at the midline (**Figs. 79 and 80**).

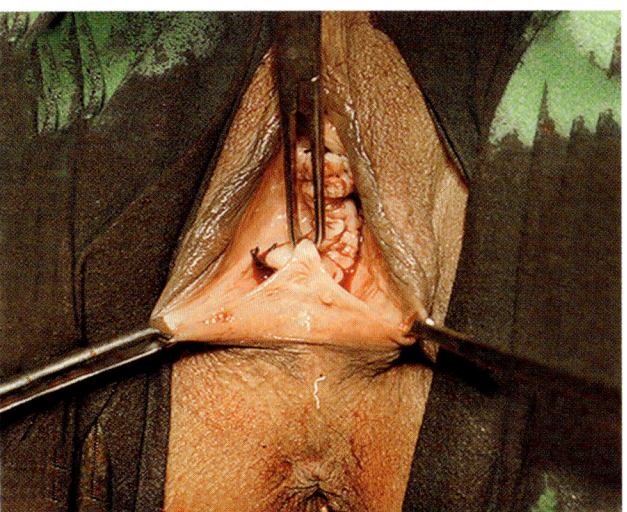

Fig. 80: Three Allis tissue forceps applied.

- First horizontal incision is given from one Allis tissue forceps to other at the mucocutaneous junction (**Figs. 81, 82 and 84**).
- At the midpoint of incision scissor blades are introduced beneath the vaginal mucosa and in front of the pelvic floor musculofascial tissues and rectum and a midline incision is given and triangular flaps are dissected laterally on both sides (**Figs. 83 and 85**).
- Prerectal fascia is plicated in case of rectocele (**Fig. 87**). Redundant part of both sided vaginal mucosa is excised (**Fig. 86**).
- Vaginal mucosa is repaired from apex to mucocutaneous junction by 1-0 or 2-0 Vicryl stitches (**Figs. 88 and 90**).
- *If there is any defect lateral, midline, apical or perineal is identified and closed by* interrupted 2-0 Vicryl stitches in single layer.
- The levator ani and perineal muscles are approximated at midline by 2 or 3 interrupted stitches (**Fig. 89**).

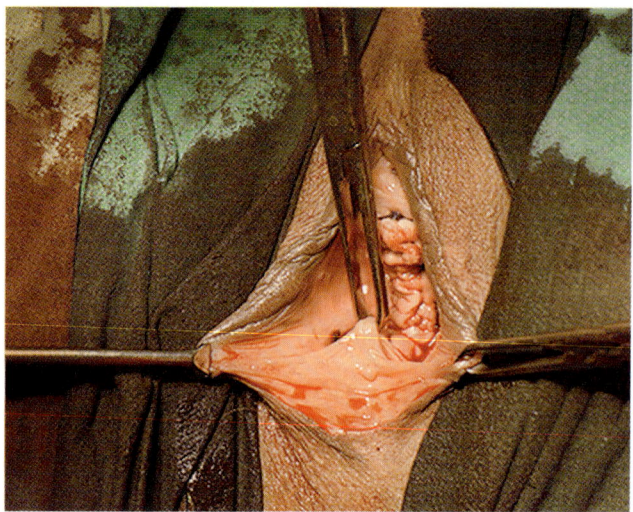

Fig. 81: Horizontal incision.

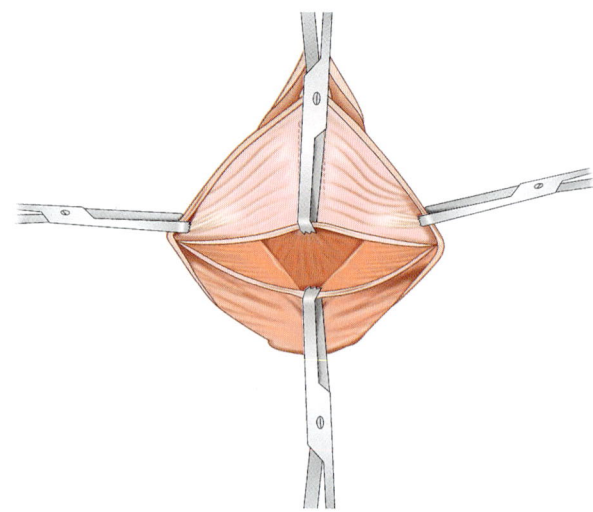

Fig. 84: Separation of vaginal mucosa.

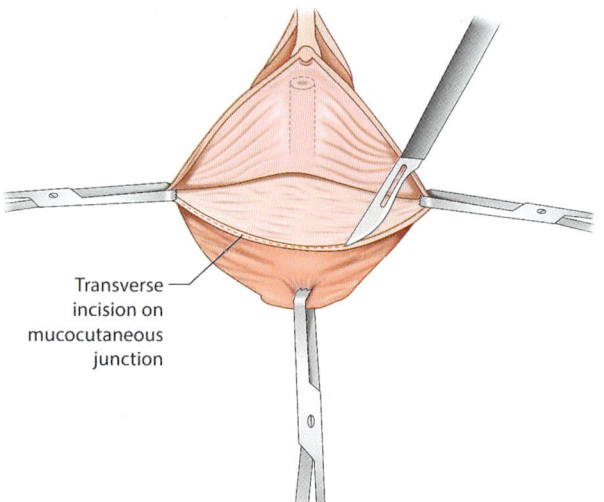

Fig. 82: Horizontal incision in mucocutaneous junction in posterior colpoperineorrhaphy.

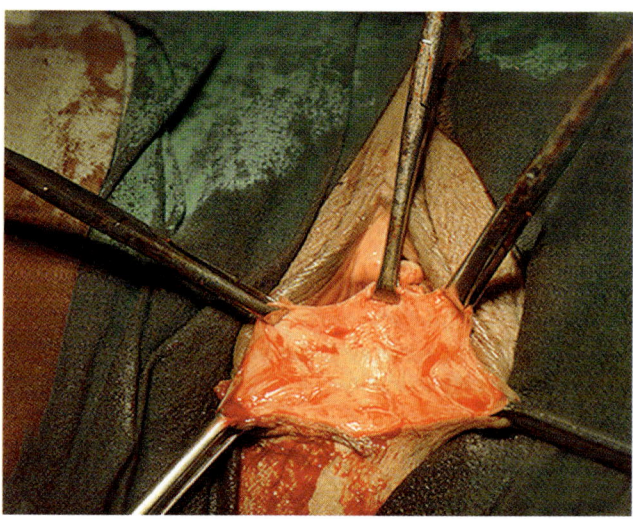

Fig. 85: Rectum and prerectal fascia is exposed.

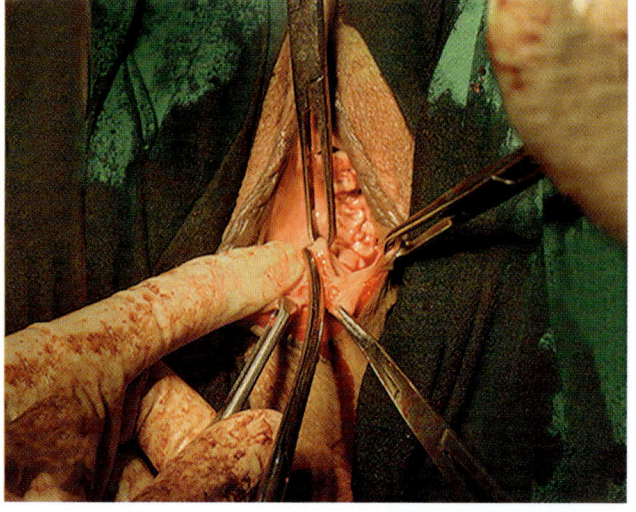

Fig. 83: Midline incision given to separate vaginal mucosa.

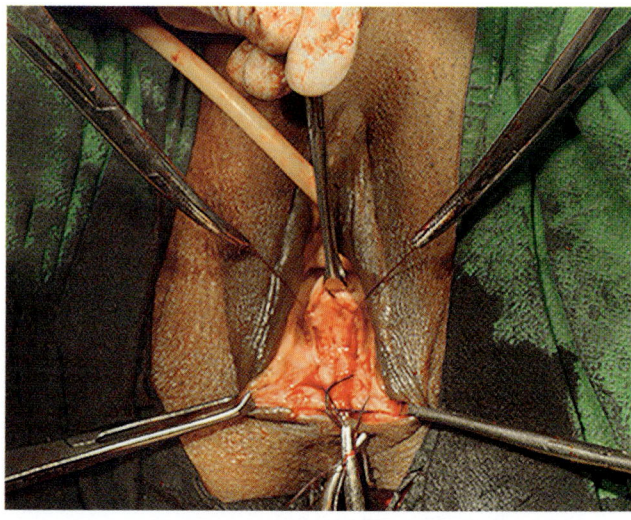

Fig. 86: Prerectal fascia plicated.

CHAPTER 10: Pelvic Organ Prolapse (Genital Prolapse)

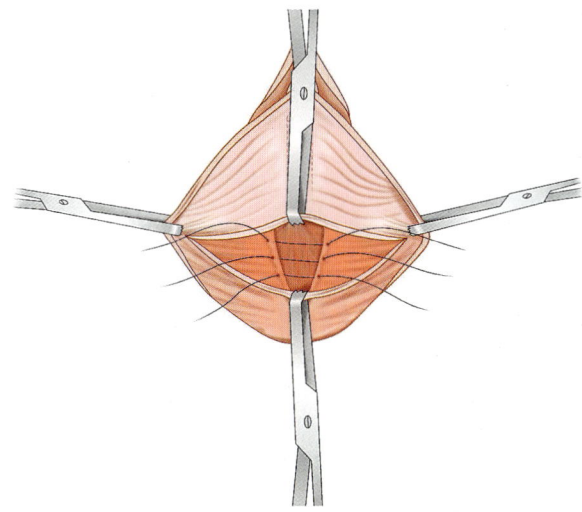

Fig. 87: Repair of rectocele by reinforcing prerectal fascia and perineal muscle.

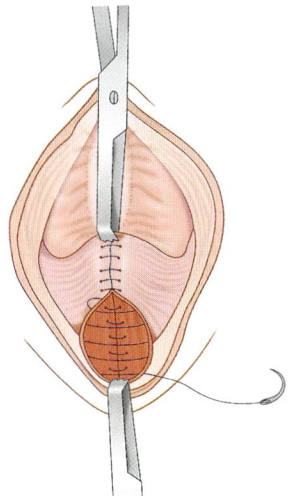

Fig. 90: Repair of vaginal and perineal skin at the end of posterior colpoperineorrhaphy.

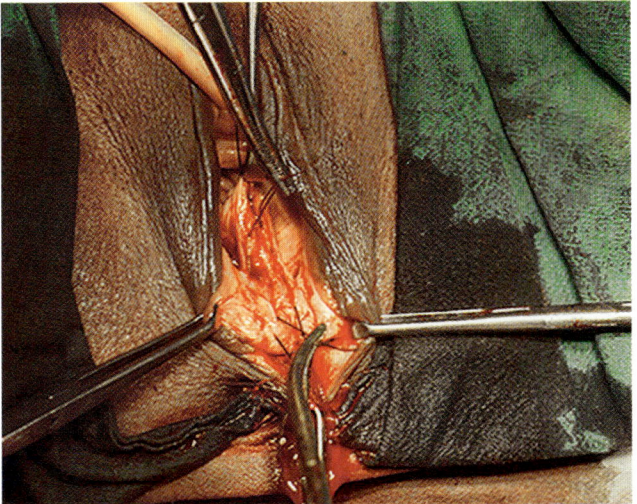

Fig. 88: Vaginal mucosa approximated.

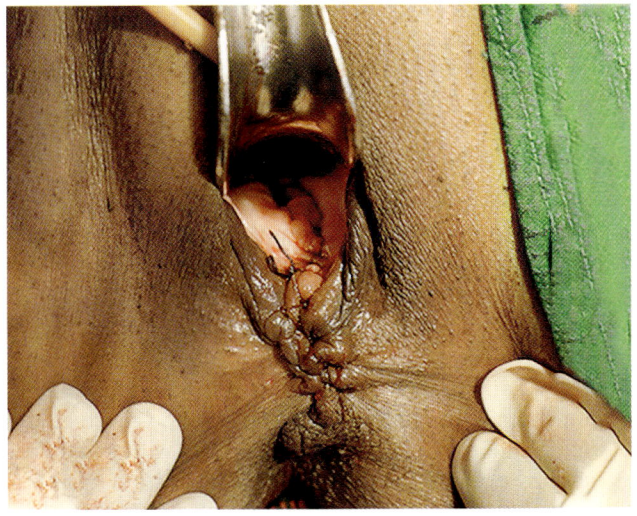

Fig. 91: Perineal skin is repaired.

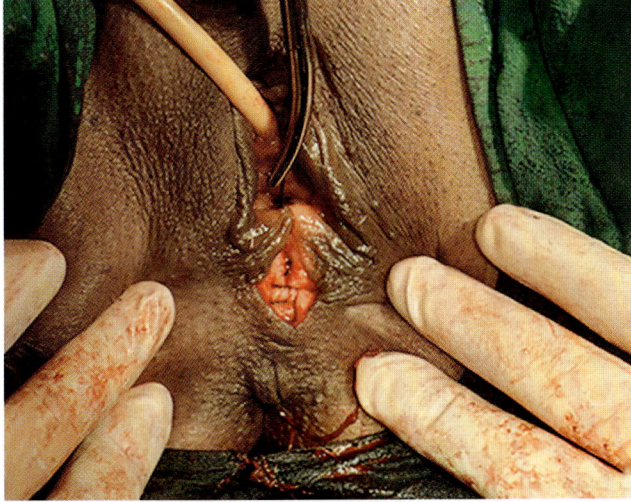

Fig. 89: Perineal muscles approximated.

- Finally, the perineal skin margins are sutured by interrupted or running delayed absorbable 2-0 sutures **(Fig. 91)**.

Complications of Posterior Colpoperineorrhaphy

- *Perioperative*: Anesthetic, hemorrhage, and rectal injury.
- *Delayed*: Infection, secondary hemorrhage, wound disruption and failure, rectovaginal fistula, and dyspareunia.

FOTHERGILL'S OPERATION (MANCHESTER OPERATION) (FIGS. 92 TO 102)

Fothergill's operation is done in POP where there is both uterine prolapse and vaginal prolapse but pelvic floor operation is done preserving the uterus.

Q. What are the components of Fothergill's operation?

- Dilatation and curettage (dilatation is mandatory but not the curettage)
- Anterior colporrhaphy
- Tightening of Mackenrodt's ligaments
- Amputation of cervix
- Formation of neocervix
- Posterior colpoperineorrhaphy
- Repair of enterocele in vaginal route if any.

Q. What are the indications of Fothergill's operation?

- It is an uterus preserving operation and done in reproductive age, not peri- or postmenopausal group.
- As fertility is impaired to some extent due to loss of original cervical mucosa and there is chance of abortion and/or preterm labor due to amputation of cervix it is done in woman who has completed the family.
- *Hence indication is young woman near 30 years or below and family is complete. Tubal ligation is suggested in the same sitting through the vaginal route.*
- After development of various sling operations recently the need of Fothergill's operation has been diminished particularly for its recurrence.

Steps of Fothergill's Operation (Figs. 92 to 102)

- Preliminary steps are like the steps of anterior colporrhaphy. Please read the steps of anterior colporrhaphy first to follow.
- Here, at the beginning before putting incision dilatation of cervix is done first. Length of uterine cavity is measured by uterine sound to determine how much length of cervix is to be amputated. Curettage is not mandatory but is done in case of abnormal uterine bleeding. Curettage also delays the menstruation not confusing with secondary hemorrhage. Dilatation helps for introduction of needle in cervical canal and also prevents future cervical stenosis.

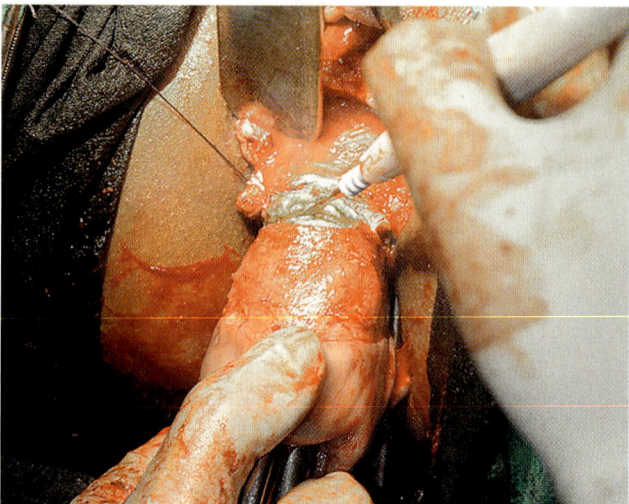

Fig. 93: Amputation of cervix: Look Mackenrodt's ligament cut and held with sutures.

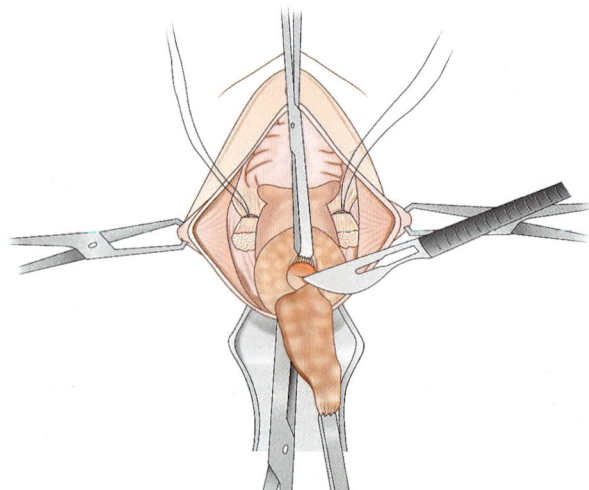

Fig. 94: Amputation of cervix in Fothergill's operation.

- Steps of anterior colporrhaphy are followed. Inverted V-shaped incision has some advantages over inverted T in Fothergill's operation. Rhomboid-shaped incision is one better option.
- After repair of cystocele redundant part of vaginal mucosa is cut.
- Now, instead of repair of vaginal wall extension of transverse incision is done laterally and posteriorly from one basal angle around the cervix along the posterior cervicovaginal junction to touch the opposite angle from behind.
- Posterior vaginal flap is raised and that will be necessary to cover the raw area of posterior lip of cervix.
- Mackenrodt's ligaments are exposed by dissection of vaginal wall laterally on both sides. Descending cervical artery is ligated on each side above the proposed level of amputation. Mackenrodt's ligaments on both sides are clamped and cut from the cervix and ligated with Vicryl

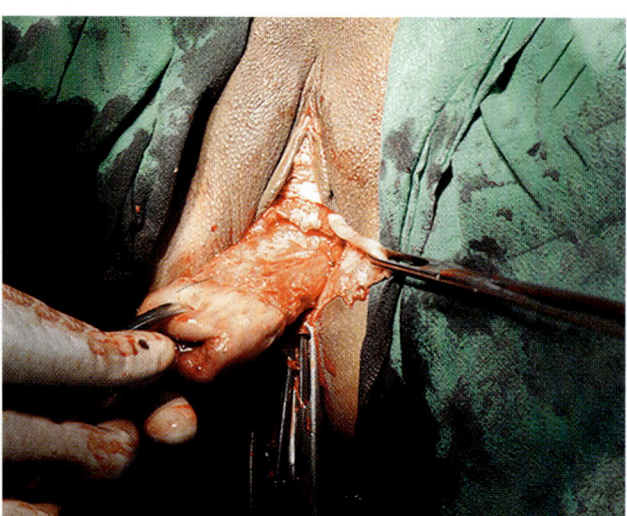

Fig. 92: Elongated cervix after dissection for anterior colporrhaphy.
Courtesy: Professor RP Ganguly

suture. Then these Mackenrodt's ligaments are tied in front of the cervix in the midline and with each other the ligaments become shortened and uterus is raised. This procedure tightens the Mackenrodt's ligaments and maintains anteversion of uterus by pulling the cervix upward and backward; it also lengthens the anterior vaginal wall. However, this is done after amputation of cervix.

- If there is enterocele POD is opened by reflecting posterior vaginal flap, redundant portion of peritoneal sac is excised after closing its base by purse-string suture followed by approximation of uterosacral ligaments.
- The cervix is amputated keeping the length of uterocervical canal at least 6.5 cm (as low as possible amputation should be done) **(Figs. 92 to 95)**.
- The uncovered cervix after amputation should always be held by single tooth vulsellum **(Fig. 96)** instead of multiple teeth.
- *Bonney's stitch*: The posterior lip of raw cervix is covered by posterior vaginal flap **(Fig. 97)**. A Vicryl stitch is fixed

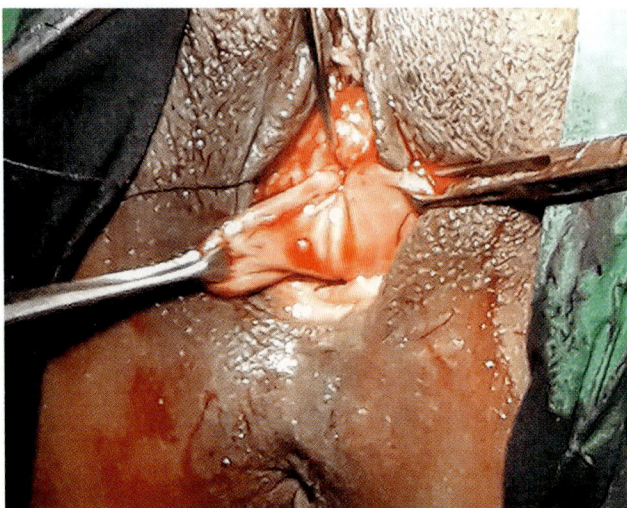

Fig. 97: Posterior lip is covered by vaginal flap—Bonney's stitch.

at the apex of the flap keeping reasonable lengths on both ends and the ends of the ligature are passed through the cervical canal brought out on the posterior surface of the cervix laterally one in each side of midline and tied in the midline posteriorly so that vaginal skin is snugly enfolded into the cervical canal. A series of radial stitch is given on cervix and vaginal skin on both sides to form new cervix which is covered by vaginal mucosa. The vaginal mucosa completely covers the posterior lip.

- Now the vaginal mucosa of anterior colporrhaphy over the reposed bladder is sutured in the midline **(Fig. 101)** and last portion of vaginal mucosa is used to cover the anterior lip of raw cervix by Bonney's like stitch as given posteriorly or Fothergill's suture as described below. Alternatively Stumdorf's stitch can be given.
- *Fothergill's stitch* **(Figs. 98 and 99)**: A suture is passed through the vaginal skin at 2 o'clock position, then left Mackenrodt's ligament, through the anterior lip of cervix

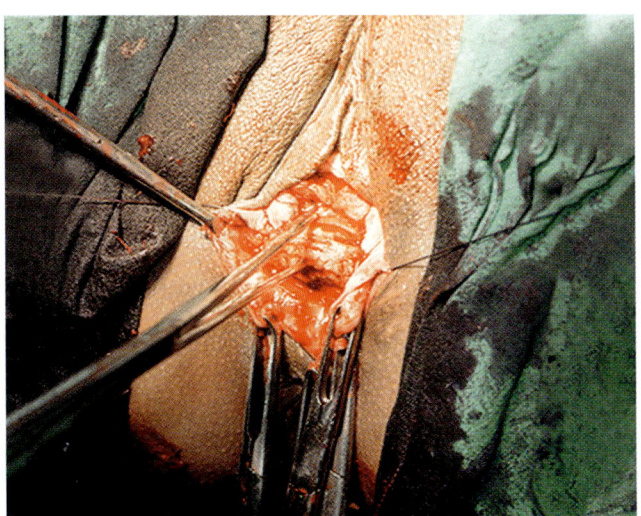

Fig. 95: After amputation of cervix, anterior lip is held by single tooth vulsellum.

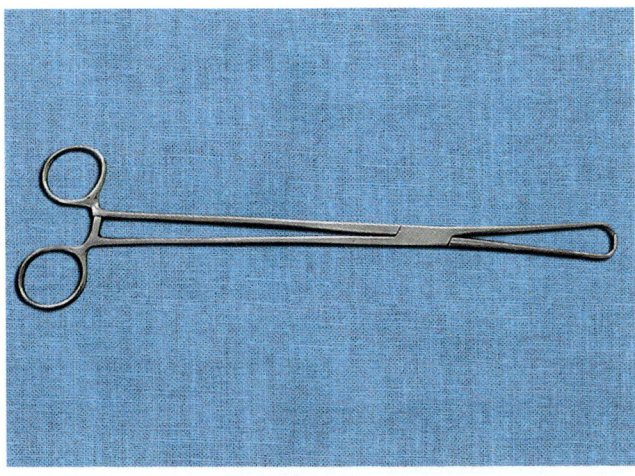

Fig. 96: Single tooth vulsellum.

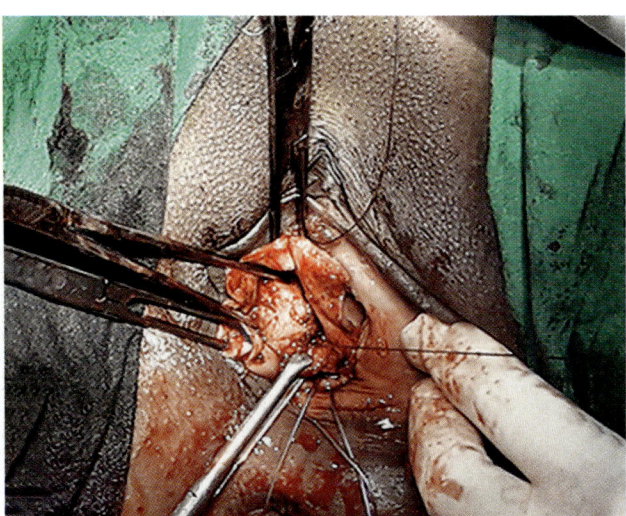

Fig. 98: Fothergill stitch is applied on anterior lip after completion of posterior lip.

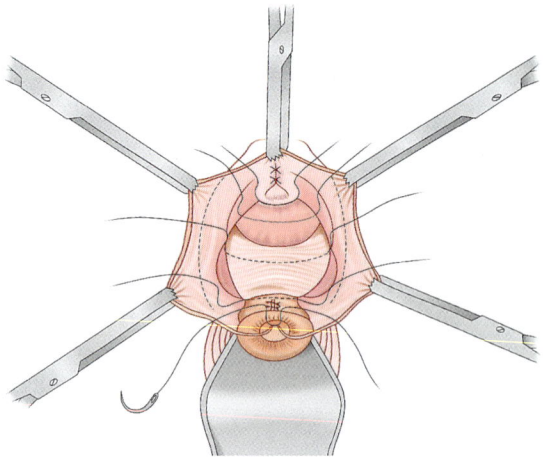

Fig. 99: Fothergill's stitch.

piercing the cervix to enter cervical canal, then piercing the cervix to outside cervical canal, then right-sided Mackenrodt's ligament and finally through vaginal flap at 10 o'clock position and then the two ends are tightened and the mucosa will cover anterior lip.

* The gap if any over the approximated mucosa is repaired **(Fig. 98)** with stitches and new cervix **(Fig. 99)** is formed.
* Posterior colpoperineorrhaphy is done as described.

Q. Who introduced Fothergill's operation?

A Donald from Manchester first reported (1908) the surgery by combining anterior and posterior colporrhaphy with cervical amputation which was the basis of Manchester operation. WE Fothergill (1914) who was junior to Donald popularized this operation adding tightening the cardinal ligaments. This surgery is also called Manchester operation.

Complications of Fothergill's Operation

Perioperative:

* Anesthetic complications

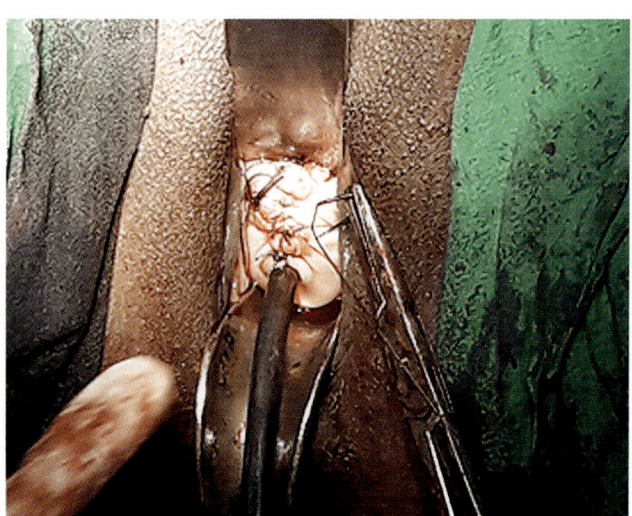

Fig. 100: Stitches are given in midline in vaginal mucosa after Fothergill stitch keeping dilator in cervix.

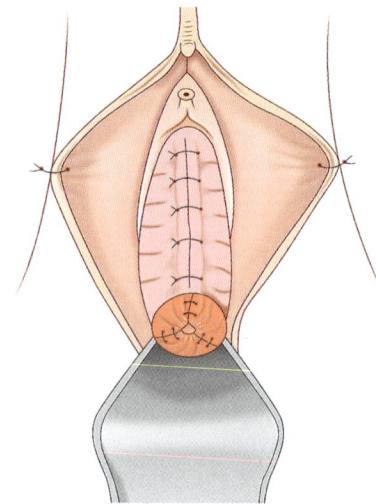

Fig. 101: Formation of neocervix at the end of Fothergill's operation.

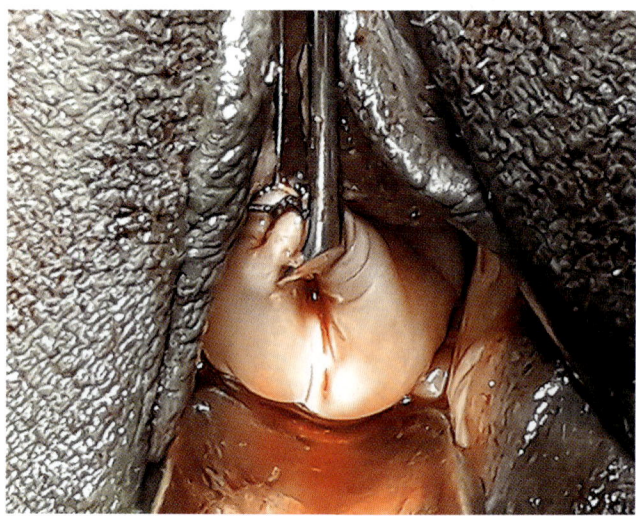

Fig. 102: Neocervix is formed.
Courtesy: Professor RP Ganguly

* Hemorrhage
* Injury to bladder, ureter, and rectum.

Postoperative:

* Retention of urine—most common complication
* Secondary hemorrhage—notorious in this operation
* Infection
* Cervical stenosis—hematometra and pyometra: For this, dilatation of cervix during surgery is mandatory.
* Recurrence of prolapse.

WARD MAYO'S OPERATION (VAGINAL HYSTERECTOMY WITH PELVIC FLOOR REPAIR)

This operation is named after CH Mayo (1915) and GG Ward (1919) from the United States of America.

Indications

* Pelvic organ prolapse in major degree prolapse in perimenopausal and postmenopausal women.
* Any degree with diseased uterus.

Components of the Operation

* Anterior colporrhaphy
* Vaginal hysterectomy
* Posterior colpoperineorrhaphy
* Suturing the pedicles of two sides one another
* Fixing the Mackenrodt and uterosacral ligaments with the vault
* Repair of enterocele vaginally if present.

Description of the Steps (Figs. 103 to 122)

* Patient is in lithotomy position
* Anesthesia—regional or general
* Antiseptic dressing, draping, and catheterization
* Vaginal examination and planning of surgery
* Sims' posterior vaginal speculum or Auvard weighted speculum is introduced to retract posterior vaginal wall. Anterior lip of the cervix is held by multiple teeth vulsellum or Allis tissue forceps and cervix is pulled.
* A female metal catheter is introduced to detect the lowest limit of bladder (vesicocervical junction).
* Now, a triangular area is selected and three Allis forceps are applied—one at the apex 1.5 cm below the external urethral opening in the midline, another two each on two lateral sides of cervicovaginal junction.
* A transverse incision is made from one Allis to other on two lateral ends with slight concavity of incision above and another vertical incision starting from midpoint of vertical incision to the Allis forceps at apex so that a inverted T-shaped incision is made.
* To make it technically easy, tips of a blunt pointed bent-on-flat scissors (Metzenbaum scissor) are introduced beneath the vaginal epithelium in the midpoint of transverse incision in a plane between the vaginal epithelium and the bladder vertically approaching toward the Allis forceps held at apex. The scissor blades are opened and closed beneath the vaginal mucosa with approaching to the apex so that a plane is already created and simultaneous vertical incision is given. The upper end of vertical incision extends up to 2–3 cm below the external urethral opening.
* Two triangular vaginal flaps are dissected laterally with the help of blades of scissors or finger covered with gauze (sharp and blunt dissection) laterally and providing simultaneous traction of the vaginal flaps holding with the help of more Allis forceps. Lateral dissection is extended to expose the bladder (cystocele) fully.
* Infiltration of normal saline with or without adrenaline (hydrodissection) makes the dissection easy. Instead of inverted T many surgeons like to give inverted V incision.

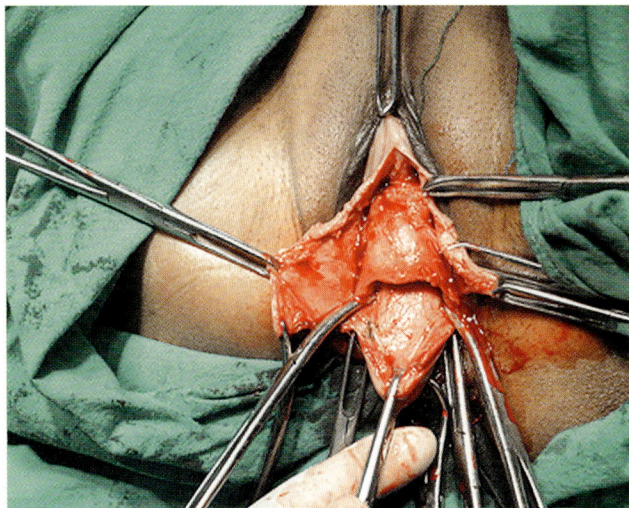

Fig. 103: Bladder is separated from cervix, bladder pillars are identified to cut.

* The bladder is attached to cervix with vesicocervical fascia (ligament) which is cut and bladder is displaced upward with a gauze on the thumb (Fig. 103).

Up to this, steps are exactly like anterior colporrhaphy.

* Now, posterior lip of cervix is held by multiple teeth vulsellum or Allis tissue forceps to retract cervix anteriorly.
* Posterior incision is given on posterior cervicovaginal junction starting from one lateral end of anterior incision to other posterior to cervix and pouch of Douglas is opened (Figs. 104 to 106).
* Now the anterior pouch (uterovesical pouch) is opened (Figs. 107 and 108) and bladder is retracted by Landon's retractor (Figs. 111 and 114).
* Now fundus of uterus is eventrated from anterior opening and traction is given by multiple teeth vulsellum holding at fundus. Then clamps are given from below above and cut one by one starting from Mackenrodt's and uterosacral

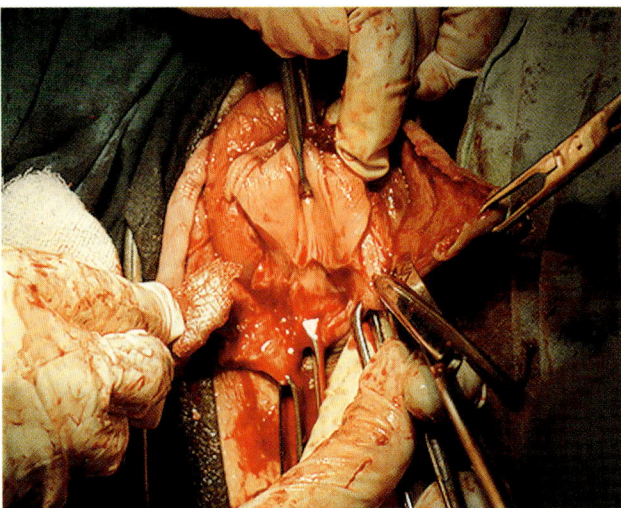

Fig. 104: Incision over cervicovaginal junction on posterior surface of cervix.

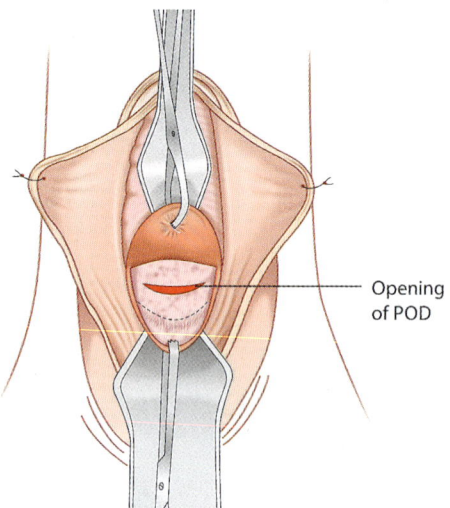

Fig. 105: Pouch of Douglas (POD) is opened by giving incision over posterior cervicovaginal junction.

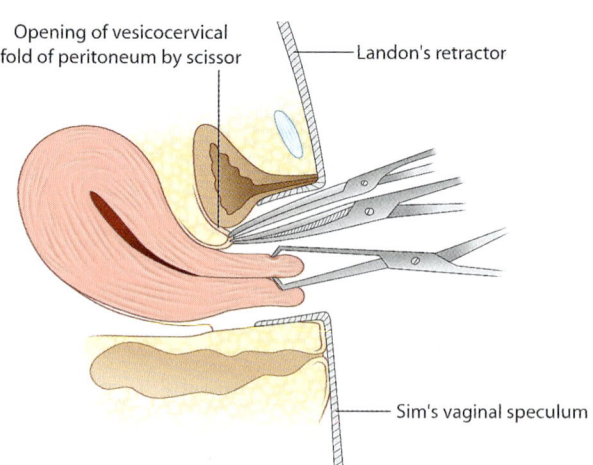

Fig. 108: Uterovesical fold of perineum is cut by scissor in Ward Mayo's operation.

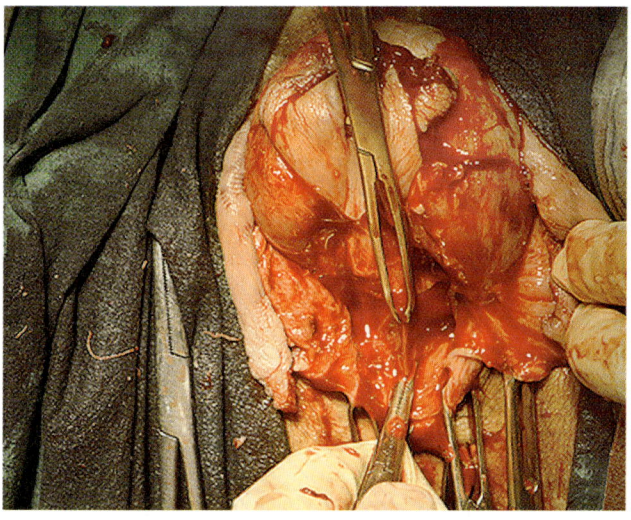

Fig. 106: Peritoneum in pouch of Douglas (POD) is visible to cut open POD.

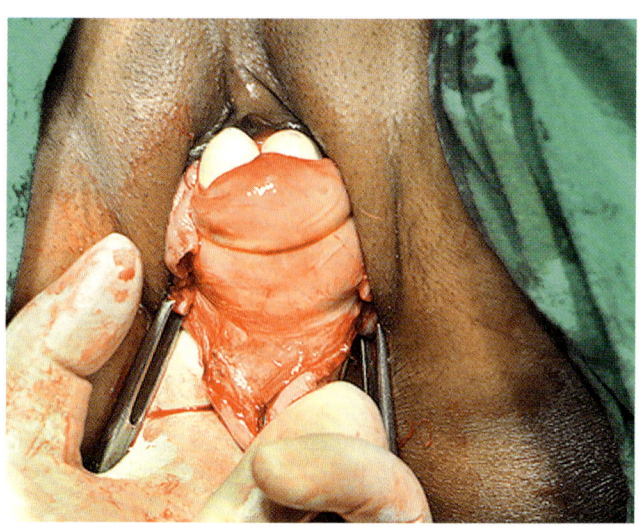

Fig. 109: Fundus of uterus brought out anteriorly.

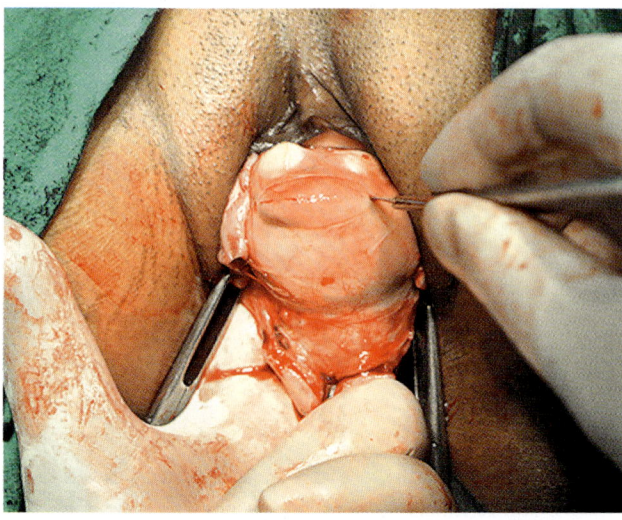

Fig. 107: Uterovesical fold of peritoneum is opened.

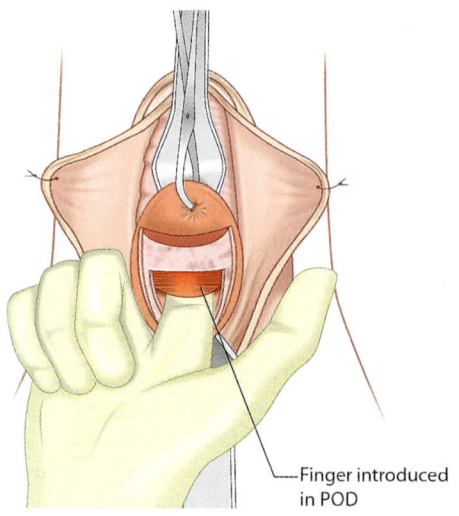

Fig. 110: Finger introduced in pouch of Douglas (POD).

CHAPTER 10: Pelvic Organ Prolapse (Genital Prolapse)

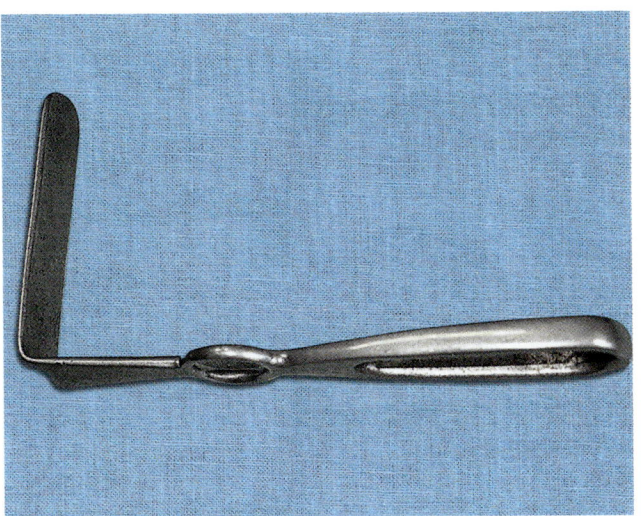

Fig. 111: Landon's retractor is used to retract bladder as shown in Figures 113 and 114.

together **(Figs. 112, 113 and 115 to 119)**. If eventration is not possible due to the large side of uterus, clamps are also applied.

- Usually three pairs of clamps are needed for each side **(Fig. 112)**.
- First pair of clamps is given on the pedicle containing Mackenrodt's and uterosacral ligaments, cut between clamps and transfixation suture is given. This is followed by the other side.
- Second pair of clamps is given on uterine vessels. Cut and ligated and so on opposite side.
- Third pair of clamps includes fallopian tube, round ligament, ovarian ligament, and mesosalpinx. The pedicle is cut and ligated with transfixation suture. Similarly opposite side is also done and uterus is removed **(Fig. 120)**.

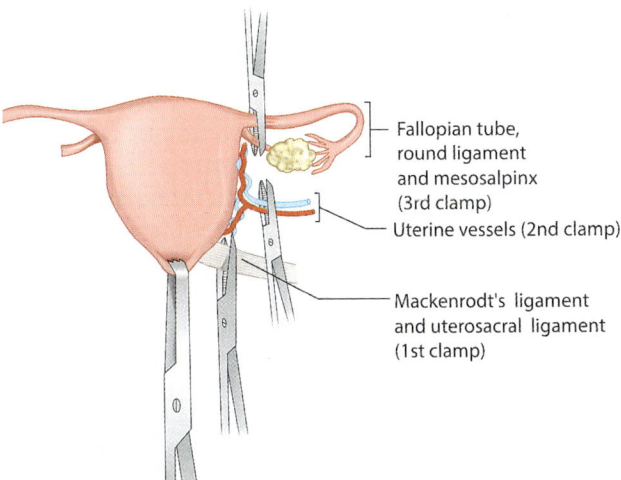

Fig. 112: Pedicles in Ward Mayo's operation. First pair of clamps are given on the pedicle containing Mackenrodt's and uterosacral ligaments; second pair of clamps are given on uterine vessels, and third pair of clamps includes fallopian tube, round ligament, ovarian ligament, and mesosalpinx.

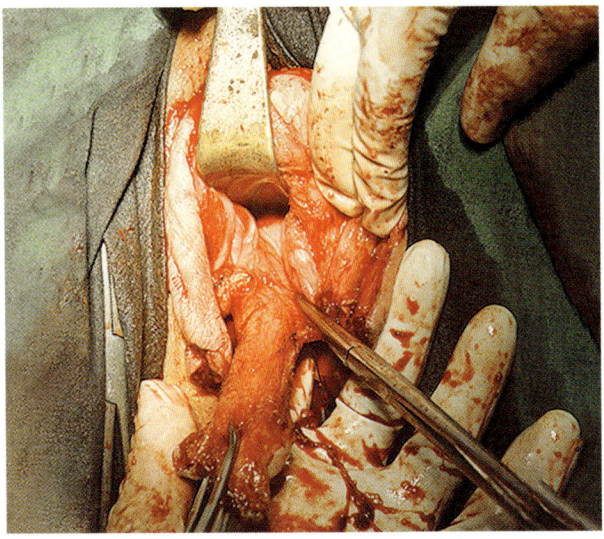

Fig. 113: Landon's retractor is used to retract the bladder.

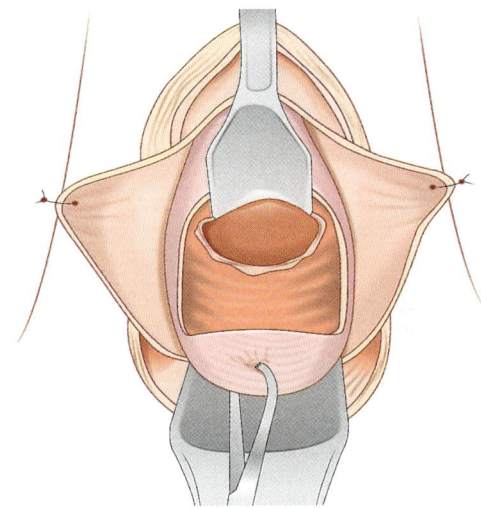

Fig. 114: Bladder is retracted by Landon retractor to prevent injury of bladder and ureter during clamping and cutting of stumps.

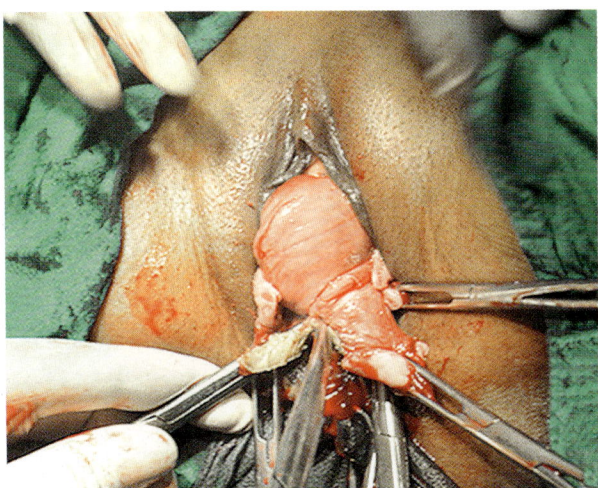

Fig. 115: Right Mackenrodt and uterosacral ligaments clamped and cut together.

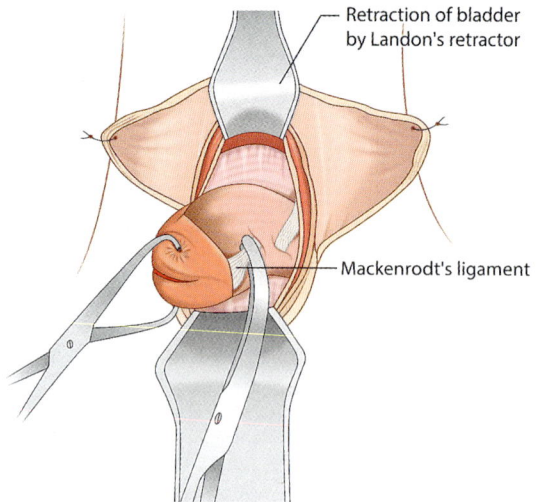

Fig. 116: Mackenrodt's ligament clamped to cut.

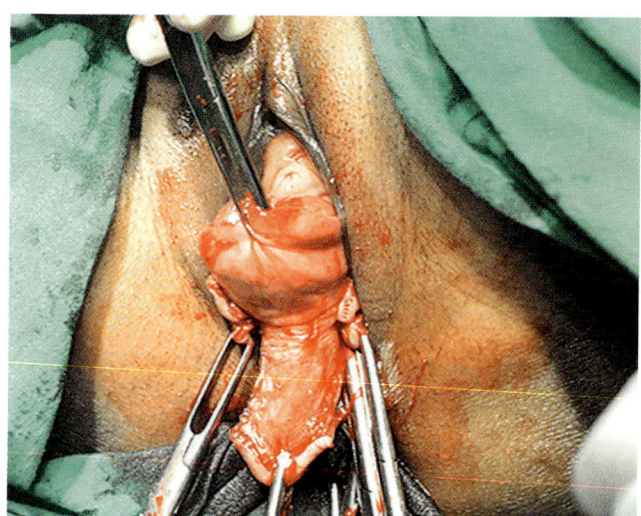

Fig. 119: Stumps are cut and ligated one by one on both sides.

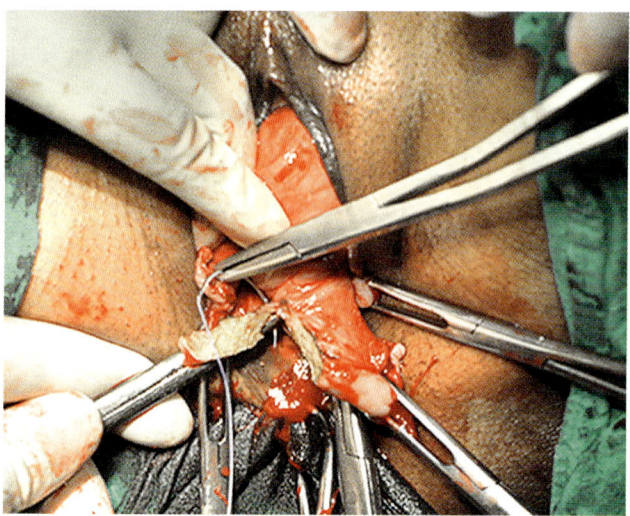

Fig. 117: Stump ligated.

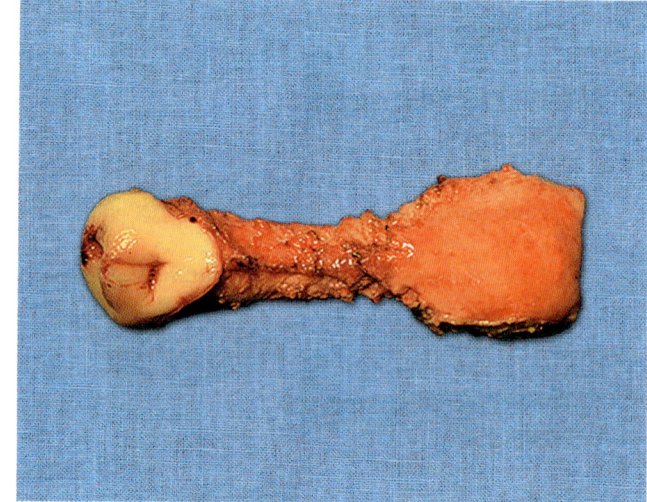

Fig. 120: Specimen of uterus after vaginal hysterectomy.

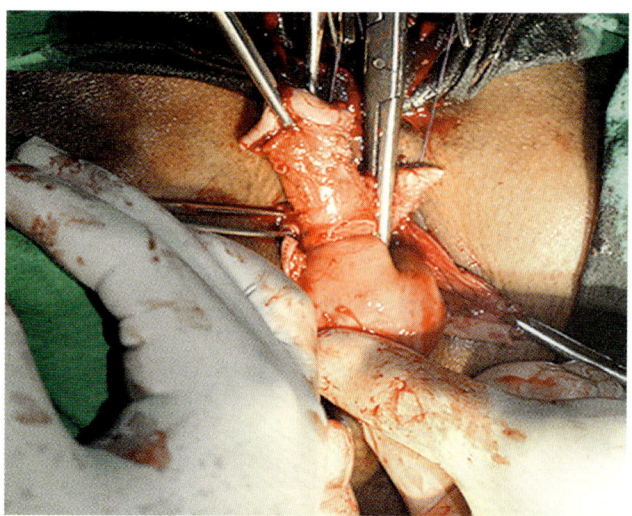

Fig. 118: Stump of right uterine vessels.

- Alternatively, after eventrating the uterus clamping is started from the fundus, so first pair includes fallopian tube, round ligament, ovarian ligament and mesosalpinx; second pair same, and third or last is Mackenrodt's and uterosacral ligaments and fundus can also be eventrated through POD.
- The ligated stump of the opposite sides is visible **(Fig. 121)** and fixed with each other in midline except the pedicle of uterine vessels.
- The ends of ligature of the first pedicles are passed through the corresponding sides of vaginal mucosa for fixing with the vault after closing the vaginal mucosa.
- Peritoneal cavity is closed with purse-string suture using 1-0 catgut suture.
- Now anterior colporrhaphy is completed by repairing cystocele, removal of redundant portion of vaginal mucosa and repair of vaginal mucosa. Vaginal mucosa

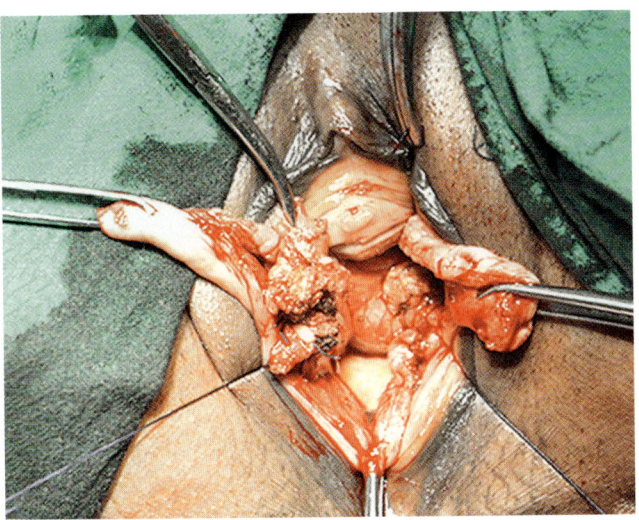

Fig. 121: Cut ends of stumps are visible after uterus is removed.

is apposed usually by few mattress stitches followed by continuous stitches.
- Finally ends of sutures of the pedicle of both sides are tied with each other to fix the Mackenrodt's and uterosacral stump with the vault.
- Posterior colpoperineorrhaphy is done in presence of posterior wall prolapse **(Fig. 122)**.
- A betadine-soaked vaginal pack is usually given and kept for 24 hours.
- Continuous catheterization is done for 48 hours.

Complications of Ward-Mayo's Operation

Perioperative: Anesthetic complication, hemorrhage, slipping of ligature and injury to ureter, bladder, and rectum.

Postoperative: Retention of urine—most common for which catheterization is done prophylactically; urinary tract infection, pelvic infection, pelvic abscess; abdominal distension; secondary hemorrhage; stress incontinence; dyspareunia mostly due to posterior repair; recurrence, and vault prolapse.

LE FORT'S OPERATION (COLPOCLEISIS)

This surgery is done in very aged menopausal women with major uterovaginal prolapse or unfit for major surgery.

Procedure

A central strip of vaginal mucosa of 1–2 cm is removed from both anterior and posterior wall and the cut edges are sewn together with catgut stitches after reducing the prolapse so that vagina is converted into a double-barreled channel thus preventing the uterine descent. The tunnels allow drainage of vaginal discharge.

It is contraindicated in women who are sexually active, who are menstruating where uterine cervix or uterus is diseased. Before surgery, a Pap stain is taken.

PURANDARE'S ABDOMINAL SLING OPERATION (1956)

In this surgery, rectal fascial strip is used as a sling. Abdomen is opened by low transverse incision (Pfannenstiel incision). Uterovesical fold of peritoneum is cut and bladder is pushed down slightly. Two strips of transverse fascia are fashioned from anterior rectus sheath making outer ends intact and medial ends free. Now the free end on each side is made entered through the inguinal ring and then through board ligament to fix on the anterior surface of cervix with the nonabsorbable stitch.

This is suitable for nulliparous prolapse or young woman with low parity. Recurrence after childbirth is common.

SHIRODKAR'S ABDOMINAL SLING OPERATION (1960)

This is also done for nulliparous prolapse.

By laparotomy a mersilene tape or a fascia lata is taken to stitch on the front of cervix and then fixed to the lumbosacral fascia between the fifth lumbar and first sacral vertebrae extraperitoneally. Thus cervix is drawn upward and backward. This is technically difficult operation.

KHANNA'S ABDOMINAL SLING OPERATION

In this technique, mersilene tape is first attached to posterior surface of isthmus of cervix and the two free ends are passed retroperitoneally lateral to rectus abdominis to fix to anterior superior iliac spines on both sides.

ABDOMINAL SACROCOLPOPEXY, SACROCOLPOHYSTEROPEXY (FIGS. 123 TO 127)

Indication is vault prolapse following hysterectomy (sacrocolpopexy) and also prolapses in young women in presence of uterus (sacrocolpohysteropexy) where fertility can be preserved. It is transabdominal approach by which vault of the vagina and also cervix and vagina where uterus

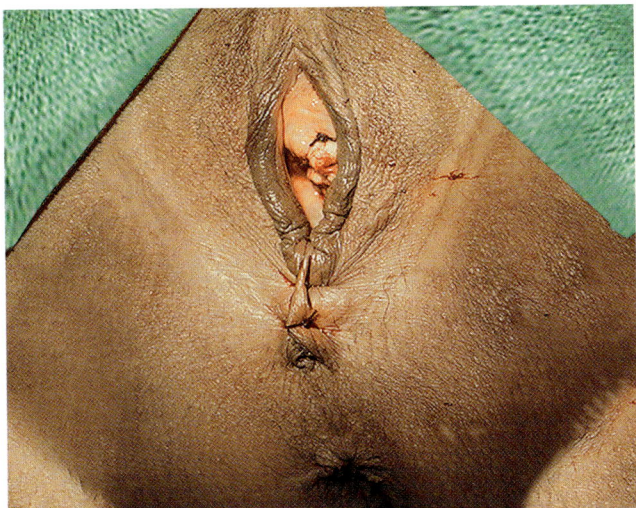

Fig. 122: At the end of posterior colporrhaphy.

SECTION 2: Clinical Cases

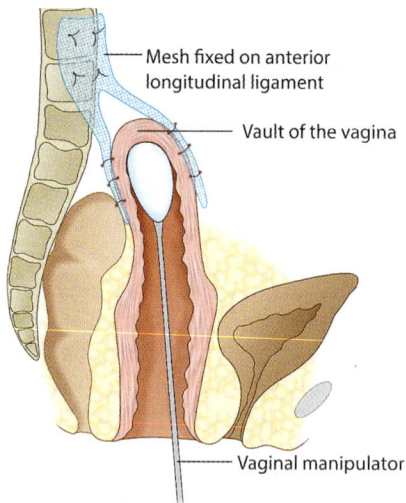

Fig. 123: Sacrocolpopexy.

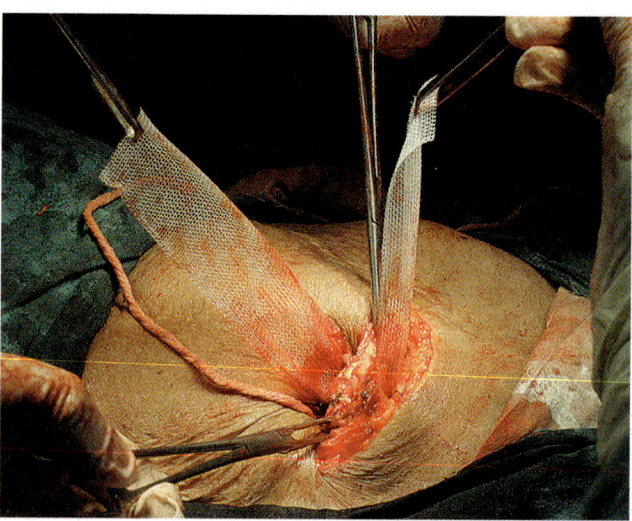

Fig. 126: Abdominal sacrocolpopexy—anterior wall and posterior wall of vagina is fixed with nylon mesh.

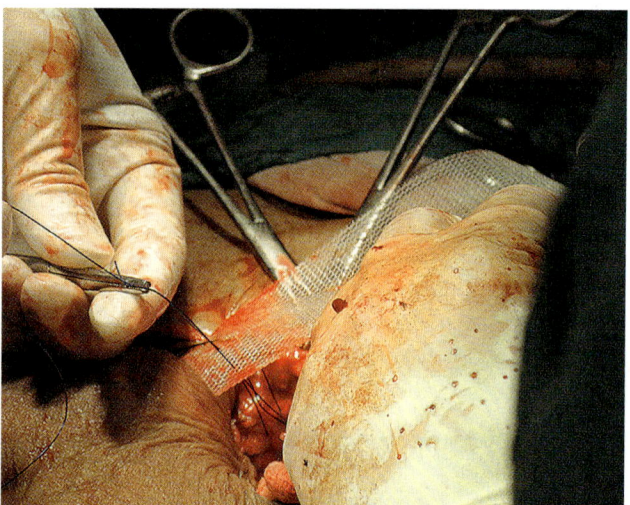

Fig. 124: Abdominal sacrocolpopexy—mesh is tied fixed with the vault of the vagina.

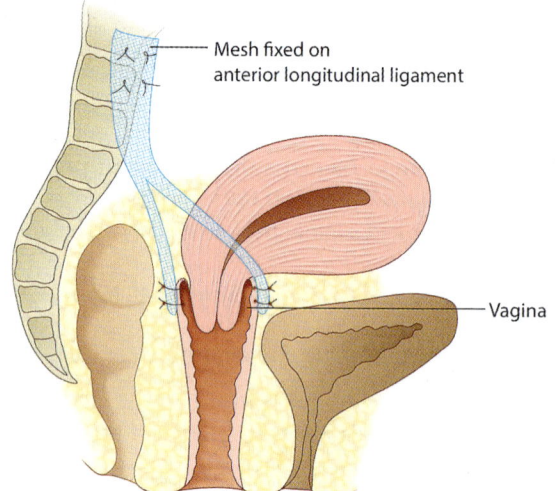

Fig. 127: Sacrocolpohysteropexy.

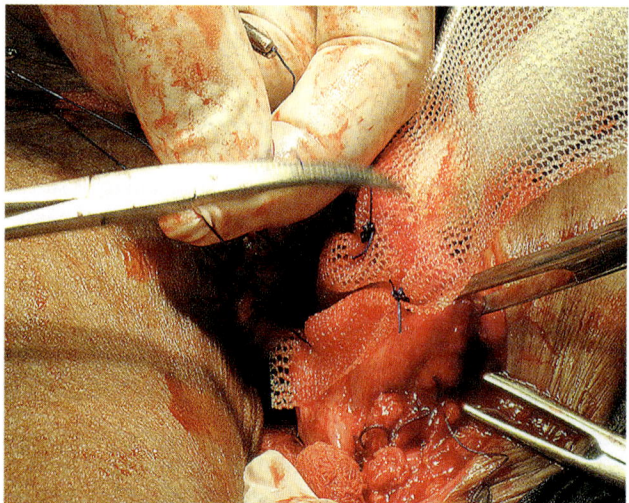

Fig. 125: Abdominal sacrocolpopexy—mesh is fixed with the posterior wall of the vagina with nylon stitches.

is present is fixed with anterior longitudinal ligament of sacrum at S1 and S2 level with synthetic mesh.

Abdominal sacrocolpopexy with graft is now widely accepted by transabdominal method of prolapse correction.

It has the advantages of correction of both anterior (apical or transverse cystocele) and posterior (enterocele or high rectocele) prolapse correction. In contrast to vaginal sacrospinous fixation, the length of vagina remains longer and dyspareunia becomes less. The success rate is high.

Steps of Abdominal Sacrocolpopexy (Fig. 123)

❖ General anesthesia or regional anesthesia.
❖ Position: Supine position with thighs parallel to ground and legs in booted stirrups (low lithotomy).
❖ Pfannenstiel incision is given to open the abdomen.
❖ After retracting the rectosigmoid colon to the left gently peritoneum over the sacral promontory is elevated and incised sharply taking care of the right ureter keeping it on right side and anterior longitudinal ligament is identified.

- The incision is extended caudally up to the vault of the vagina toward the posterior vaginal wall.
- A vaginal blunt manipulator is used to elevate the vault. In posthysterectomy vault prolapse, it is very difficult to separate the bladder from the vagina and one should be very cautious to avoid opening of bladder.
- Both anterior wall and posterior wall of vagina are dissected 4–5 cm each and vaginal vault is held with two Allis tissue forceps at two angles.
- Two or three nonabsorbable sutures (prolene) are taken through the ligament on each side one below the other with keeping the ends long and holding each with one artery forceps.
- A 15 cm length prolene mesh is taken either preformed Y-shaped mesh or two separate strips of self-cut mesh is used. The anterior arm of Y of prolene is sutured to anterior surface of anterior vaginal wall with 4–6 sutures and posterior arm with posterior surface of posterior wall of vagina with a similar number. The sutures are taken so that they do not pass through and through the vaginal wall **(Figs. 124 to 126)**.
- Now proximal part of the mesh is directed toward anterior longitudinal ligament over S1 and S2 vertebrae. If lower part of peritoneum is not incised completely, the mesh is passed behind the peritoneum.
- The mesh is fixed with the anterior longitudinal ligament with the sutures which were made ready earlier. The length of mesh is adjusted so that vault of the vagina is elevated sufficient at desired level **(Fig. 126)**.
- The incised peritoneum over the mesh sacrum is approximated and abdomen is closed in layers after proper hemostasis and counting.
- This procedure can also be done with concomitant hysterectomy and becomes easier than posthysterectomy vault prolapse cases.
- **Sacrocolpohysteropexy**: In case where it is done preserving uterus, anterior and posterior aspect of cervix are also included with the sutures in lower part so that both cervix and vagina are fixed with sacrum **(Fig. 127)**.
- This procedure can also be done laparoscopically.

Complications

- Hemorrhage from presacral vessels
- Injury to ureter, bladder, and gut
- Infection
- Stress incontinence
- Mesh erosion—3–5%
- Recurrence up to 10%.

SACROSPINOUS LIGAMENT FIXATION (FIG. 128)

The principle of this surgery is to fix the vaginal apex to the coccygeus-sacrospinous ligament complex. Apex fixation with the right ligament is often done due to the close proximity of rectosigmoid on left side.

Steps (Fig. 128)

In traditional approach, right sacrospinous ligament (SSL) is accessed through the posterior colporrhaphy incision in posterior vaginal wall via prerectal space and then creating a space in between the vagina and rectum (pararectal space) to reach the right sacrospinous ligament.

With the help of Miya hook a nonabsorbable thick suture material is pierced the right sacrospinous ligament approximately two finger breadths or 2–3 cm medial to ischial spine (corresponds to midportion of SSL). Placing of needle too close to ischial spine is a risk to the injury of pudendal vessels and nerve and fixed to the vaginal vault. Capio ligature carrier device is preferred to Miya hook recently. If there is enterocele, it is repaired before closure of vagina.

Success is 90%. But it is inferior to abdominal sacrocolpopexy so far as length of vagina and sexual satisfaction is concerned. However, other concurrent support defects can be repaired vaginally. Besides, it avoids abdominal surgery and it takes shorter operative time and quick recovery occurs, thus suitable for comorbid conditions.

Complications

- Bleeding
- Injury to pudendal vessels, nerve, and rectum
- Detrusor overactivity
- Gluteal pain
- Recurrence of prolapse.

Posterior Infracoccygeus Vaginal Sling (PIVS)

- A permanent mesh tape is placed through the ischiorectal fossa as an inverted "U" around the rectum and attached to the posterior vaginal wall.
- An incision in the posterior wall of vagina is given to open pararectal space.
- The needle fitted with tape is introduced through a point in perineum 4 cm lateral and 2 cm below the level

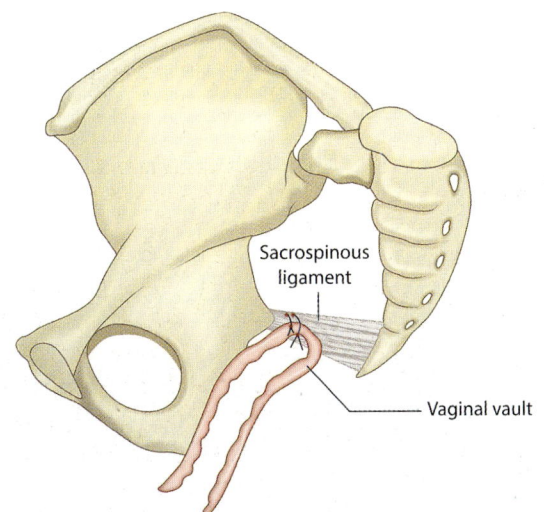

Fig. 128: Sacrospinous ligament fixation.

of anal canal after a small incision and pierced through sacrospinous ligament to bring inside the vaginal space.
- The other needle is introduced from the opposite side in the same manner and pierced through sacrospinous ligament and the tape is drawn.
- The transverse part of the tape is fixed with the vaginal vault.
- Tape on two sides is stretched and cut flushed with the skin surface **(Figs. 129 to 133)**.
- Rectal examination is done to rule out rectal injury.

MCCALL CULDOPLASTY

In culdoplasty techniques, POD is obliterated to prevent enterocele. McCall culdoplasty is performed during vaginal hysterectomy.

Two to three horizontal internal rows (not penetrating the vaginal lumen to bring outside) using nonabsorbable sutures are passed from one uterosacral ligaments to other

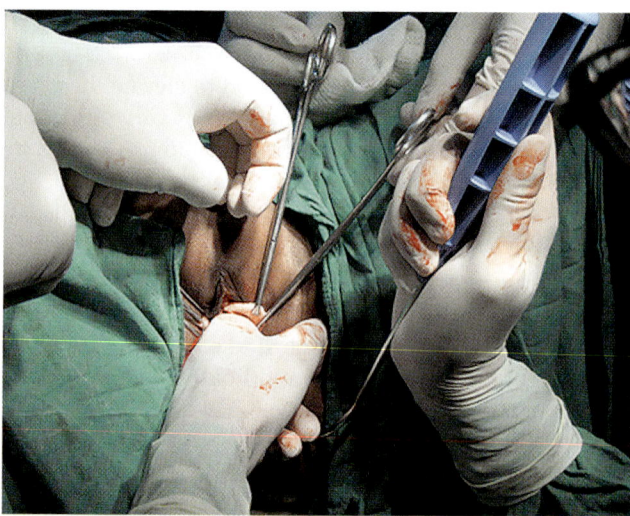

Fig. 131: Introduction of needle through perineum under guidance of vaginal finger.

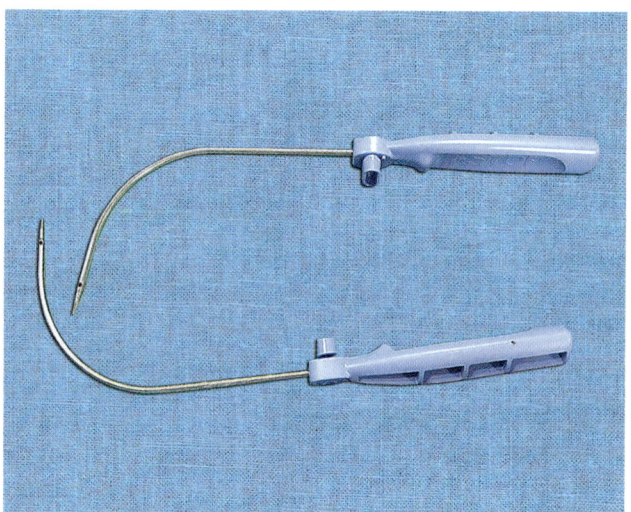

Fig. 129: Posterior infracoccygeus vaginal sling needle.

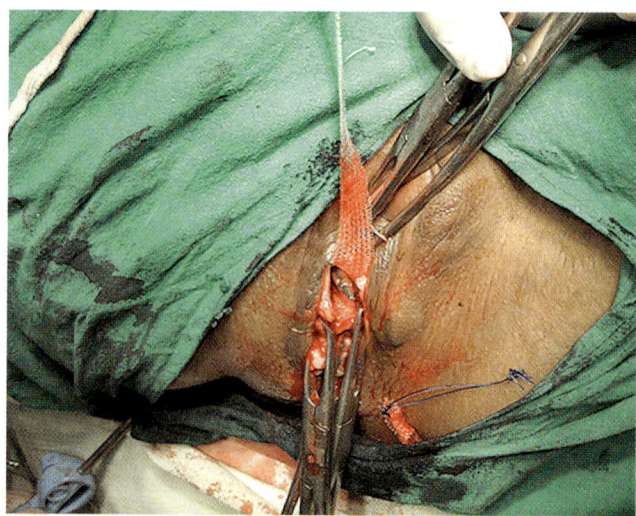

Fig. 132: Placing of mesh.

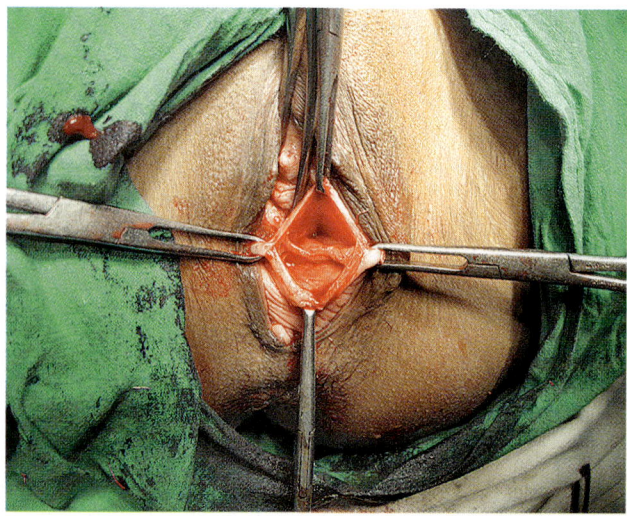

Fig. 130: Dissection for each pararectal space.

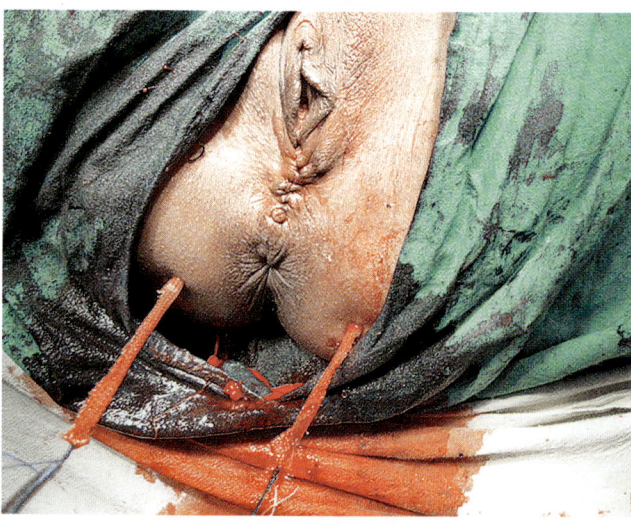

Fig. 133: Traction of mesh on both sides.
Courtesy: Professor Subrata Lall Seal

to obliterate posterior cul-de-sac. Additionally, one or two rows of absorbable sutures are placed externally through uterosacral ligaments which pass through the posterior vaginal cuff. Internal sutures are tied first. Initially tying of the most proximal sutures is followed by external suture of which most cephalad is dealt first. Ureteric kinking and obstruction is a risk though uncommon (10%).

Management of Enterocele

Types

Congenital and acquired—primary due to increased abdominal pressure (pulsion enterocele) or traction enterocele for vaginal and uterine prolapse.

Secondary following vaginal or abdominal hysterectomy and mostly due to failure to recognize the enterocele or faulty repair during hysterectomy.

During vaginal hysterectomy, redundant peritoneum in POD is excised after hysterectomy. After closing the enterocele sac, uterosacral ligaments and levator muscle ligaments are sutured midline to reinforce the sac.

During Fothergill's operation, POD is opened and sac is repaired and reinforce with uterosacral ligament.

In abdominal method, concentric purse-string suture is given to close the sac avoiding injury to ureter.

Q. Use of mesh and prolapse surgery—What is your opinion?

Principle

- Sheet or mesh is used to reinforce surgical repair to mimic the ligamentous support
- Usually done in recurrent prolapse.
- There are different types of mesh—I, II, III, and IV. Type I is preferred due to its big size pore.

Advantages

- Anatomical restoration is excellent.
- Recurrent is less.

Complications

- Mesh erosion through vagina, bladder, and or rectum (5%)
- Dyspareunia
- Chronic pelvic pain
- Excision of mesh is high
- American College of Obstetricians and Gynecologists (2014) discourages to use mesh as far as possible.

PREVENTION OF PELVIC ORGAN PROLAPSE

- Proper antenatal, intranatal, and postnatal care.
- Intranatal care: To avoid prolong labour (second stage), avoid bearing down pain before full dilatation, timely episiotomy, forceps delivery in second stage, not in undilated cervix.
- Spacing of childbirth.

Prevention of Posthysterectomy Vault Prolapse

- Identification of loss of pelvic floor support if any and their management during hysterectomy where indication is not prolapse.
- During abdominal hysterectomy, anatomical suturing of parametrium with angles of vaginal vault prevents vault prolapse.
- During vaginal hysterectomy, repair of enterocele and tightening of uterosacral and Mackenrodt's ligament with fixation of vaginal vault prevent vault prolapse.
- Fixing of uterosacral ligament with vaginal vault in McCall culdoplasty during vaginal approach is an effective method. Similar type of fixation can also be done when hysterectomy done in open or laparoscopical abdominal hysterectomy to prevent posthysterectomy vault prolapse.

PREGNANCY WITH PELVIC ORGAN PROLAPSE

Pregnancy may occur in a woman with pelvic organ prolapse. There may be cystocele, uterine descent, rectocele, and even enterocele depending upon the presence of which complication may occur in pregnancy and labor.

Prevalence

Pelvic organ prolapse is mostly found in developing countries in multiparous women and incidence varies from 1 in 200 to 500 labor.

Effect of Pregnancy over POP

The protruded cervix with prolapsed uterus usually ascends as the uterus becomes abdominal organ after 12 weeks of pregnancy and patient may relieve of symptoms. If uterus persists in prolapsed position, incarceration may occur at 12–14 weeks of pregnancy for which the uterus needs to be replaced sometimes in early pregnancy and suitable pessary is needed to keep the uterus in correct position as a preventive measure.

Effects of POP over the Course of Pregnancy and Labor

- In early pregnancy, POP causes distressing symptoms like something coming down sensation, white discharge, backache and bladder symptoms of frequency, incomplete evacuation and stress incontinence. Presence of cystocele may increase urinary stasis which predispose to urinary tract infection. Urinary stress incontinence becomes worsened as urethral closure pressure is not increased sufficient enough to compensate increased bladder pressure.
- Presence of large rectocele may cause constipation.
- Premature onset of labor occurs often.
- During labor, delayed dilatation, slow effacement, and edema of cervix may cause cervical dystocia and prolonged first stage. There is increase chance of early rupture of membranes. As the cervix descends in pelvic floor, there is early bearing down effort by mother and mother becomes

exhausted. Presence of cystocele, rectocele, and large enterocele may hinder the fetal descend and second stage becomes prolonged if they are not pushed out of the way.

Management

- Rest is given in early pregnancy. In large prolapse patient may be admitted in first trimester till uterus becomes abdominal organ. Ring pessary is needed sometimes (*see* above).
- During early labor if cervix looks edematous glycerin-acriflavine pack is given. In late first stage, if cervix is not dilated fully Duhrssen's incision (rarely) on cervical lip is given and delivery is accomplished by ventouse or forceps application. Sometimes lower uterine cesarean section is needed when the head is high up with edematous nondilating cervix.

CHAPTER 11

A Case of Infertility

Chapter Outline

Writing a case of infertility and how to present the case?

- How to Investigate a Case of Infertility
- Definition, Causes and Evaluation of Infertility—Female and Male
- Diagnosis of Ovulation—Spinnbarkeit Test, Fern Test, USG Folliculometry and Hormone Estimation
- Tubal Patency Test, Semen Analysis
- Management of Female Infertility
- Ovulation Induction and its Complications, Surgical Management for Ovulatory Dysfunction
- Tubal Factor Infertility—Causes, Diagnosis and Management
- Management of Male Factor Infertility
- Assisted Reproductive Technology—In Vitro Fertilization and Embryo Transfer, Intracytoplasmic Sperm Injection, Gamete Intrafallopian Transfer, Zygote Intrafallopian Transfer, Percutaneous Epididymal Sperm Aspiration, Microsurgical Epididymal Sperm Aspiration
- Intrauterine Insemination
- Erectile and Ejaculatory Dysfunction
- Azoospermia, Klinefelter Syndrome
- Unexplained infertility

PATIENT'S PARTICULAR

1. Name:
2. Age: 29 years
3. Address:
4. Occupation:
5. Married/unmarried: Married for 3 years
6. History of infertility: 3 years
7. Husband's occupation: School teacher
8. Socioeconomic status: Middle class
9. Religion: Hindu
10. Parous/nulliparous: Nulliparous

Bed No.:
Date of admission:
Date of examination:

HISTORY

- *Chief complaint/complaints*: Trying to have a baby for last two and half years but failure to conceive. Initial 6 months after marriage she used to barrier contraceptive following which she is trying for baby with regular intercourse.

- *History of present illness*: The woman states that initial 6 months after marriage her husband used condom. But she failed to conceive in spite of trying for last two and half years. Her period is regular with normal flow, only mild pelvic pain for initial 1–2 days during mens.

- *Menstrual history*:
  - Detailed menstrual history is taken
  - To diagnose oligomenorrhea, number of menstrual period would be eight or less in 1 year
  - Last menstrual period (LMP):
  - Duration of menstruation: 5–6 days
  - Interval in days: 28 ± 2 days
  - Age of menarche: 12 years
  - Regularity of cycle: Regular
  - Pain during period/if pain relation with menstruation: Lower abdominal mild pain present during first 2 days

- Amount of bleeding: Average; clot—occasional, and intermenstrual bleeding—absent
  - If amenorrhea—no.
- *Obstetric history*:
  - Parity: Nulliparous.

  If parous write in tabular form as written in Chapter 1. If there is any history of abortion, spontaneous or induced should be enquired in detail as it may cause tubal block by pelvic infection.

Serial no.	Year and month	Pregnancy events	Labor events	Mode of delivery	Puerperium or postabortal period	Baby

- *Past history*: Nothing significant.
  - Medical: Any endocrinopathy, thyroid disorder, diabetes, past history of polycystic ovarian syndrome (PCOS), past history of tuberculosis, pelvic infection, endometriosis, etc.
  - Surgical: Any surgery including gynecological surgery, pelvic surgery, and vaginal surgery.
- *Family history*
- *Sexual history*: Taken in detail—regularity and frequency of coitus, if there is dyspareunia and lack of complete penetration and if they use any lubricant which may be spermicidal. Whether the partners live together or separated for the job and meet weekend only, to be enquired.

  Any significant history of husband informed by the woman that may be related with subfertility must be noted.
- *History of galactorrhea*: If any spontaneous secretion of milk like liquid from breasts or on squeezing.
- *Functional history*:
  - Bowel
  - Bladder
  - Sleep
  - Appetite: Anorexia nervosa.
- *Personal history*:
  - Personal hygiene
  - Smoking/alcohol.
- *Contraceptive history*: Used barrier contraceptive for first 6 months after marriage but not now. History of sterilization.
- *Drug history*:
  - History of any drug allergy
  - History of intake of corticosteroids, antiepileptic or other drugs (previous or present), antipsychotic drug, any drug causing hyperprolactinemia and amenorrhea.
- *Treatment history in detail*: Medical/surgical—analgesics, hormones, etc. Many patients come with after treatment of infertility with ovulation induction and intrauterine insemination (IUI).

PHYSICAL EXAMINATION

Patient—alert, conscious, and cooperative, look anxious for not having child.
- Build
- Nutrition
- Height
- Weight/body mass index (BMI) obesity: If present, mention android or gynecoid type
- Edema
- Anemia: May be present due to menorrhagia
- Cyanosis
- Jaundice
- Secondary sexual character
- History of *galactorrhea*
- Hirsutism, acne, acanthosis nigricans, temporal balding, and enlargement of clitoris if any—not present
- Clubbing
- Tongue, teeth, gum, and tonsil
- Neck veins
- Neck glands
- Leg veins
- Pulse
- Respiration
- Temperature
- Blood pressure.

Systemic Examination
- *Central nervous system*
- *Cardiovascular system:*
  - Auscultation of heart.
- *Respiratory system:*
  - Auscultation of chest.
- *Gastrointestinal system:*
  - Liver
  - Spleen.
- *Examination of other systems:*
  - Examination of back and spines skeletal system
  - Neurological
  - Ophthalmoscopic examination
  - Urinary system.
- *Examination of breasts and nipple:*
  - Inspection
  - Presence of galactorrhea
  - Palpation.

GYNECOLOGICAL EXAMINATION

Abdominal Examination
- *Inspection:* Any scar mark, enlargement
- *Palpation:* Palpated all nine areas for any mass and tenderness
- *Percussion:* If needed
- *Auscultation:* Where needed.

Vaginal Examination

- Inspection and palpation of external genitalia—any abnormality, vaginal introitus. Digital examination gives the idea whether couple is accustomed with successful coitus.
- Speculum examination—any abnormal vaginal discharge.
- Bimanual examination: Uterus—adnexae, tenderness mobility, and pouch of Douglas (POD). Simple pelvic examination gives clue regarding cause infertility.
- Examination of rectovaginal septum and rectal examination—not mandatory as a routine in infertility case.

INVESTIGATIONS SUPPLIED OR REQUIRED

- Ultrasonography of pelvis
- Hysterosalpingography (HSG) report or sonosalpingography—for tubal factor
- Hormones—if any done like:
  - Thyroid-stimulating hormone (TSH)
  - Prolactin
  - Luteinizing hormone (LH) and follicle-stimulating hormone (FSH)
  - Anti-Mullerian hormone (AMH)
  - Other hormones.

Report of Husband's semen analysis: Within normal range.

SUMMARY OF THE CASE (SAMPLE)

A 29-year-old nulliparous woman married for 3 years attended outpatient department (OPD) with complain of inability to conceive in spite of trying for last two and half years. She states that they used barrier method of contraception for initial 6 months following which they are trying for conception. Since their marriage the couple always lives together. Her LMP was ..., menstruation regular, almost in monthly interval persisting for 4–6 days associated with mild pain for first 2 days of period and the flow is average. Her age of menarche was 12 year. She has no significant past or family history and no history of galactorrhea.

On examination, her height and weight with BMI ....., secondary sexual character well developed with no hirsutism. She has no pallor, pulse....../min, and normotensive. No abnormality in other systemic examination.

Per abdominally no tenderness and no mass palpable.

On vaginal examination—speculum examination shows normal cervix without any abnormal discharge. Bimanual examination revealed uterus normal size, anteverted, freely mobile, and no mass or tenderness on any fornix.

Her husband's semen analysis parameters are within normal range. No other report is available.

PROVISIONAL DIAGNOSIS

A 28-year-old woman with primary infertility.

DIFFERENTIAL DIAGNOSIS

No differential diagnosis (D/D) is needed to write here if she has no other problem.

Q. How will you define infertility?

Infertility is defined as inability to conceive after 1 year of regular unprotected intercourse.

Q. What are the types of infertility?

Primary: It means there is no previous conception.
Secondary: It means there is history of previous conception.

Q. What is fecundability and fecundity?

Fecundability means probability of conception within a single menstrual cycle which is 20–25%. Fecundity denotes probability of getting a live birth within one cycle.

In normal population half of the couples conceive within 3 months, three-fourths within 6 months and 85% becomes pregnant within 1 year of marriage. The peak age of fertility is 25 years. After 35 years of age one-fourth of women remain infertile and after 40 years it increases to one-third.

Q. What is the incidence of infertility?

About 10–15% among reproductive age couples.

Q. When to investigate an infertile couple?

After 1 year.

However, if the age of the woman is more than 35 years investigation should be started after 6 months. If there is obvious known cause like anovulation/amenorrhea or severe pelvic inflammatory disease (PID), there is no justification to delay.

CONTRIBUTION OF MALE AND FEMALE PARTNERS

Q. How do male and female partners contribute to the infertility?

Grossly, female contributes to one-third, male one-third and both one-third cases of all infertility cases.

However, etiology varies in different population and different studies. According to ASRM (2012):

- Male factor contributes to 25%
- Female: 58%
  - Ovulatory: 27%
  - Tubal/uterine: 22%
  - Other including endometriosis: 9%
- Unexplained: 17%. Prevalence may be high up to 30%

High incidence of tubal factor (up to 40%) is found in secondary infertility.

CAUSES OF FEMALE FACTOR INFERTILITY

Q. What are the causes of female factor infertility?

- Ovarian factors: 30–40%
- Tuboperitoneal factors: 40%
- Uterine factors: 10%

- Cervical factors: 5%
- Vaginal factors: 2–5%.

ETIOLOGIES OF MALE FACTOR INFERTILITY

Q. What are the etiologies of male factor infertility?

In large studies, it has been found that in near 50% cases no cause could be revealed in male subfertility and the treatable causes like infective (6–9%), varicocele (15%), and endocrinal cause (<1%) are few.

Important Causes of Male Infertility (Details are Given Later)

- *Endocrinal:* Hypogonadotropic hypogonadism, hypothyroidism, hyperprolactinemia, and diabetes
- *Genetic:* Klinefelter syndrome, Y chromosome deletion, and immotile cilia syndrome
- *Infective:* Orchitis, prostatitis, and epididymitis
- *Varicocele*
- *Obstructive:* Vasectomy and cystic fibrosis
- *Immunological*
- *Coital disorder.*

INVESTIGATION (EVALUATION) OF A CASE OF INFERTILITY

Q. How would you investigate (evaluate) a case of infertility?

In the first visit both partners should be present so that both are involved in the therapeutic process starting from acquiring the knowledge of normal process of conception.

The basic approach includes:
- *History taking* of male and female partner
- *Physical examination* of male and female partner
- *Basic investigations:*
  - Husband's semen analysis
  - Diagnosis of ovulation
  - Tubal patency test
  - Postcoital test.

Flowchart 1 shows the approach of a case of infertility with suggested outline of therapeutic option.

HISTORY AND EXAMINATION OF FEMALE PARTNER

History

- Age
- Duration of marriage and duration of infertility. Any previous history of marriage
- *Menstrual history:* Menarche, regularity, and dysmenorrheal
- *Past obstetric history:* History of miscarriage and medical termination of pregnancy (MTP) (in case of secondary infertility)
- *Past medical history:* History of pelvic pain, pelvic inflammatory disease, tuberculosis, diabetes, and hypertension. Past surgical history—pelvic surgery
- *Family history:* Genetic disorder and premature ovarian failure
- Contraceptive history
- Occupation history

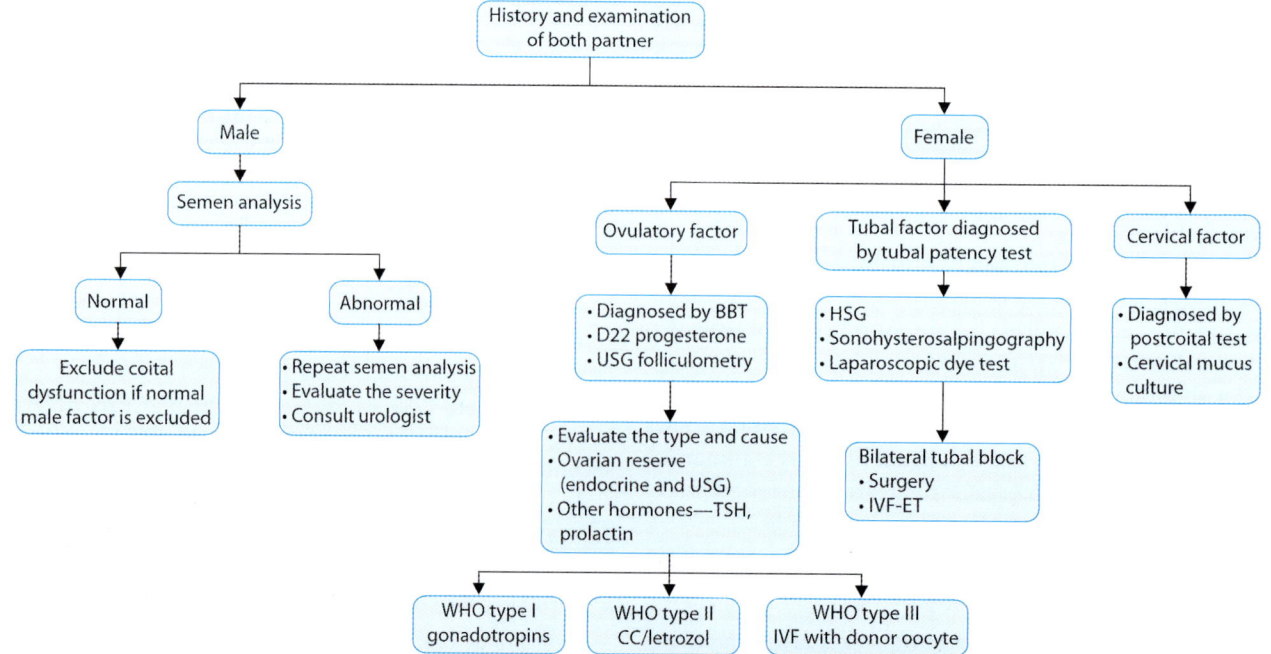

Flowchart 1: Approach of a case of infertility with suggested outline of therapeutic option.

Abbreviations: BBT, basal body temperature; HSG, hysterosalpingography; TSH, thyroid-stimulating hormone; IVF-ET, in vitro fertilization and embryo transfer; CC, clomiphene citrate

- Addiction history if any
- Sexual or coital history
- History of galactorrhea
- History of obesity and change of weight
- History of hirsutism.

Physical Examination
- Height, weight, BMI, and body habitus
- Secondary sexual character—breasts, pubic and axillary
- Galactorrhea
- Thyroid gland
- *Hair distribution*: Features of hyperandrogenism—hirsutism, acne, and balding
- Pulse, BP, and respiration

Systemic Examination
Cardiovascular system

Abdominal Examination
Any scar, tenderness, and any mass, liver, and spleen

Gynecological Examination
External genitalia and vaginal introitus.
- Inspection
- Per speculum examination: Presence of infection or narrow introitus
- Bimanual examination: Uterus—size, position, and mobility; adnexae—tenderness and any pelvic mass
- In digital examination: Vaginismus is diagnosed.

HISTORY AND EXAMINATION OF MALE PARTNER
See later (Page 262).

Q. How diagnosis or detection of ovulation is done?
- Menstrual history
- Basal body temperature (BBT)
- Vaginal cytology
- Cervical mucus study
- Endometrial biopsy
- Hormone estimation
- USG folliculometry—serial
- Laparoscopy.

Pregnancy is the surest sign of ovulation.

Methods of Tubal Patency Tests
There are several tubal patency tests; the important ones are:
- Hysterosalpingography
- Sonohysterosalpingography
- Laparoscopy chromopertubation test (dye test).

Tubal insufflation test (Rubin's test) where air was pushed by Rubin's cannula through the cervical canal and auscultation with the help of stethoscope over the iliac fossa to hear the hissing sound of passage of air through fallopian tube is obsolete now.

DIAGNOSIS OR DETECTION OF OVULATION
Today, diagnosis and detection of ovulation is done by serial USG folliculometry and by estimation of serum progesterone in luteal phase. Previously, in nonavailability of technology many methods were used to find the indirect method of ovulation diagnosis, now mostly are not used for this purpose. All are summarized here.

The parameters are given in details next.

Reader is requested to go through the "Physiology of Ovulation" in the Chapter 19 that will help to understand the procedure of diagnosis of ovulation easily (**Fig. 1**).

Menstrual History and Ovulation
Careful menstrual history gives clue regarding defective ovulation. A woman with cyclic menses at an interval of 25–35 days and duration of bleeding of 3–7 days is most likely ovulating. Regular cyclical menstruation indicates ovulation.

Mittelschmerz or midcycle pelvic pain is common at the time of ovulation. Ovulatory cycles are more likely to be associated with premenstrual spotting, premenstrual syndrome, and primary dysmenorrhea.

Basal Body Temperature (Fig. 2)
Progesterone is a thermogenic hormone. A postovulatory rise in progesterone levels increases basal temperature by approximately 0.4°F to 0.8°F. Morning oral temperature is taken.

Normal in follicular phase is 97.0°F to 98.0°F. Biphasic pattern is strongly predictive of ovulation (**Fig. 2**). Monophasic BBT pattern indicates anovulation.

But correlation of BBT with serum progesterone level is not always good and it has frequent false-negative results. It cannot predict ovulation prospectively; hence couple misses the maximal fertility period as temperature rises after ovulation. It is inexpensive.

Vaginal Cytology
Estrogenic (preovulatory) and progestogenic effects (postovulatory) are diagnosed by vaginal cytology.

In proliferative or preovulatory phase, the cells are large eosinophilic with pyknotic nuclei (cornified cells), with background clear and cells are discrete (**Fig. 3**).

In premenstrual or late secretory phase cells are basophilic (envelop cells) with vesicular nuclei, cells are in clusters and background dirty (**Fig. 4**). Cells are collected by Ayer's spatula.

Before ovulation the ratio of parabasal, intermediate, and superficial cells are 0/40/60 (estrogen increases superficial cells) and following ovulation it becomes 0/70/30 (shifting to left—progesterone increases intermediate cells).

Cervical Mucus Study
Just before ovulation (in the fertile window) due to the effect of estrogen cervical mucus becomes clear, thin, slippery, and copious. Volume of cervical mucus peaks 2–3 days prior to

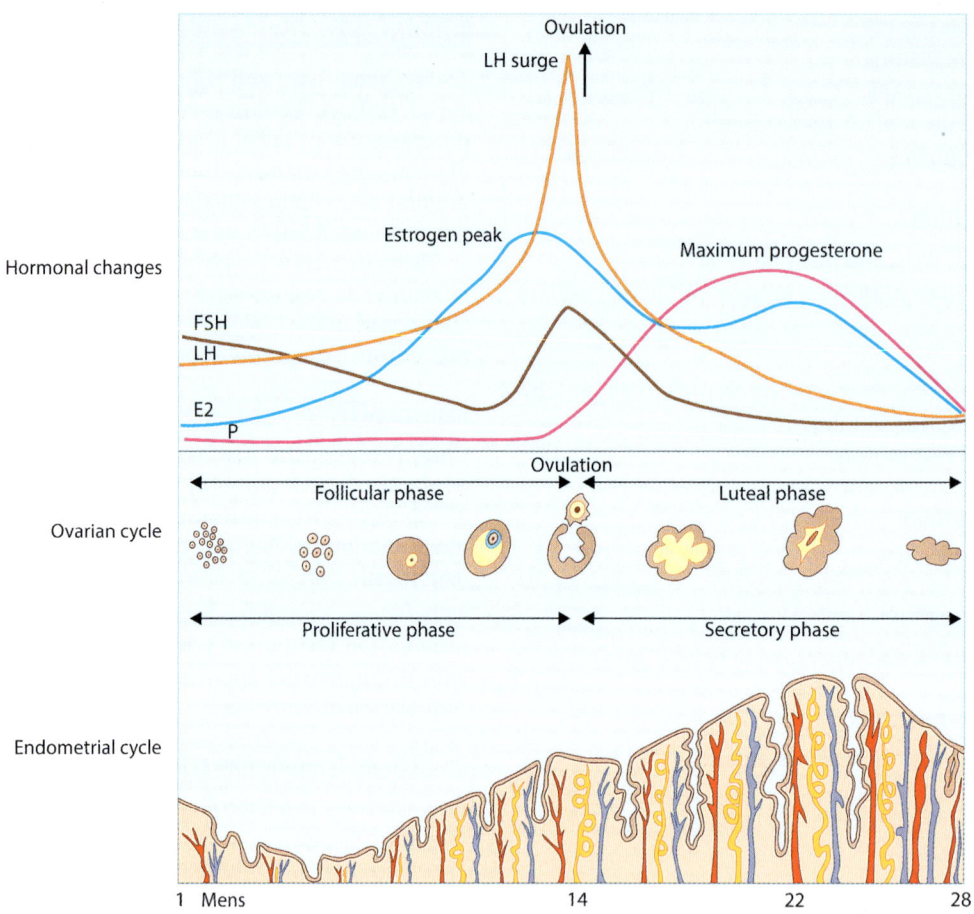

Fig. 1: Endometrial cycle, ovarian cycle, and cyclical changes of pituitary and ovarian hormones.
Abbreviations: LH, luteinizing hormone; FSH, follicle-stimulating hormone

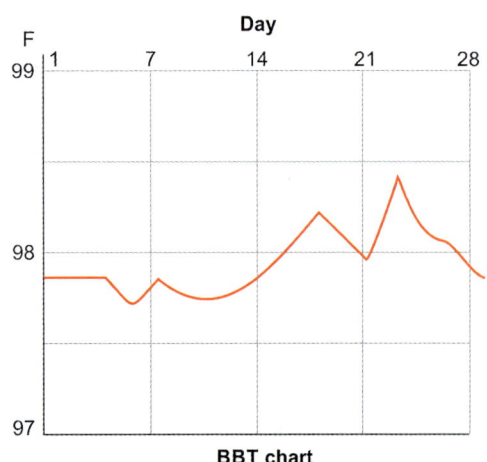

Fig. 2: Basal body temperature (BBT)—temperature rises after ovulation due to the effect of progesterone.

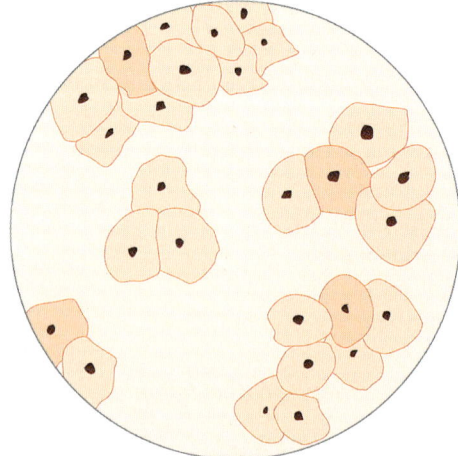

Fig. 3: Eosinophilic cells in vaginal cytology—estrogenic effect—before ovulation the cells are large eosinophilic with pyknotic nuclei (cornified cells), with background clear and cells are discrete.

ovulation, thus identifying higher day-specific probabilities of conception **(Fig. 5)**. *Spinnbarkeit test* (*see* below) becomes positive (>7 cm), there is *ferning* and cervical OS becomes open. Sperms can swim up easily in the lake of mucus as shown in **Figure 5**.

After ovulation, cervical mucus become scanty, thick, and sticky; spinnbarkeit test becomes negative, Fern test becomes negative, and cervical os becomes closed and sperms cannot swim easily **(Fig. 6)**.

CHAPTER 11: A Case of Infertility

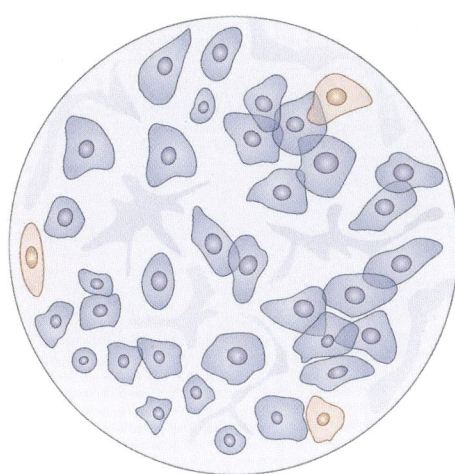

Fig. 4: Basophilic cells in vaginal cytology—progestogenic effect—basophilic (envelop cells) with vesicular nuclei, cells are in clusters and background dirty in late secretory phase.

Q. What is Insler score?

Insler score is based on the status of cervical mucus and condition of cervical os. The four parameters are considered:
1. Amount of cervical mucus
2. Spinnbarkeit test
3. Fern test
4. State of cervical os, each carrying maximum of four points. Insler score of 10–12 indicates full follicular maturation.

Spinnbarkeit Test (Thread Test) (Figs. 7 and 8)

This test is stretchability test of cervical mucus, based on the fact that cervical mucus becomes elastic, stretchable to thread up to 7.5–10 cm due to the effect of high estrogen which occurs just before ovulation.

It can be done by pulling the cover slip which is placed on drop of cervical mucus taken on glass slide **(Fig. 7)**. Simple way to demonstrate it with the help of artery forceps by drawing mucus from the os through the vagina after inserting

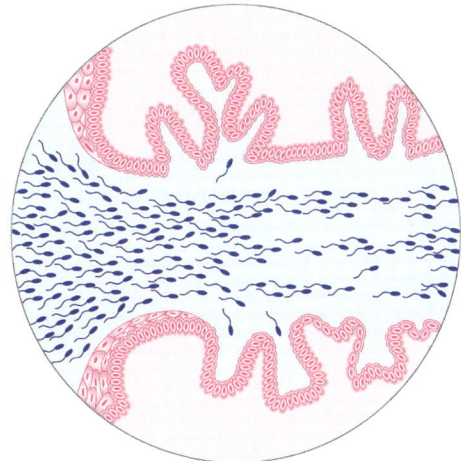

Fig. 5: Cervical mucus just before ovulation due to the effect of estrogen becomes clear, thin, slippery, and copious. Sperms can swim up easily in the lake of mucus.

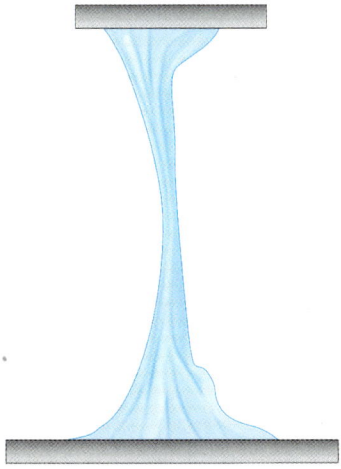

Fig. 7: Spinnbarkeit test (threadability test)—cervical mucus is taken on slide and covered with cover slip. On lifting the cover slip mucus becomes stretchable due to effect of estrogen.

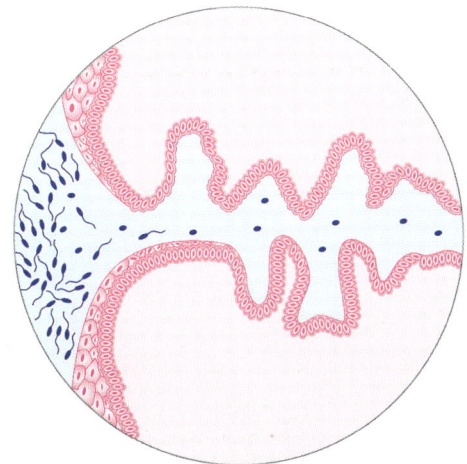

Fig. 6: After ovulation cervical mucus become scanty, thick, sticky and sperms cannot swim easily.

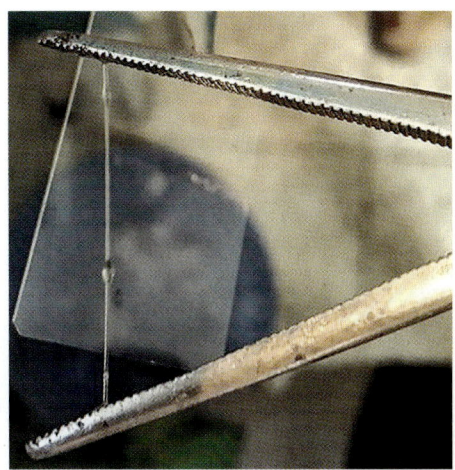

Fig. 8: Spinnbarkeit test.

a Cusco's speculum. Cervical mucus can be stretched up to the vaginal introitus extending whole vaginal length.

In the luteal phase after ovulation cervical mucus becomes thick and sticky and cannot be stretched.

Fern Test (Figs. 9 and 10)

Estrogenic cervical mucus when taken on glass slide, dried and seen under low power microscope ferning pattern is seen **(Figs. 9 and 10)**.

This palm leaf-like pattern is said to occur due to crystallization of sodium chloride in cervical mucus due to the effect of high estrogen in preovulatory stage. This is indirect method of diagnosis of ovulation.

Ferning pattern appears from 5th to 6th day of cycle, maximum at 24–48 hours before ovulation and disappears after ovulation. 1st degree, 2nd degree, 3rd degree and even more branching pattern is formed depending on the increase of estrogen level.

Ferning disappears with beaded cellular pattern after ovulation due to the effect of progesterone **(Fig. 11)**.

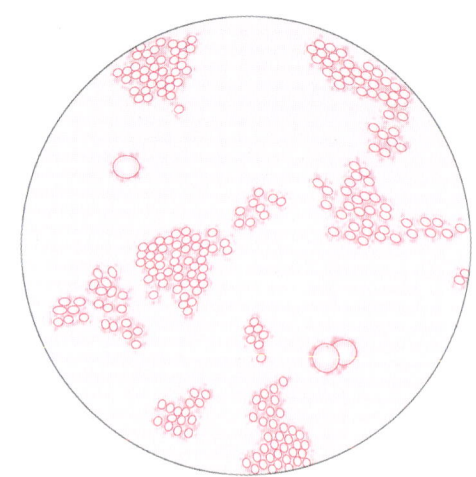

Fig. 11: Cervical mucus—ferning disappears with beaded cellular pattern after ovulation due to the effect of progesterone.

If on 21st or 22nd day of cycle ferning persists, it indicates anovulation. False negative result occurs due to blood contamination and false positive may result in presence of saline.

Endometrial Biopsy

The proliferative pattern **(Fig. 12)** of endometrium becomes secretory **(Fig. 13)** after ovulation due to the effect of progesterone. Earliest sign of ovulation on endometrial biopsy is subnuclear vacuolation which becomes evident on 16th day of 28 days regular cycle.

If on 22nd or 23rd day (midluteal phase) of cycle endometrial biopsy is taken, histology is expected to be secretory type in an ovulatory cycle and if proliferative type is seen on those days (mid luteal phase) it indicates *anovulation.*

This can be done as outpatient procedure with the help of biopsy curette (Sharman/Pipelle). The added advantage of endometrial biopsy is that presence of any pathology like tuberculous granuloma can be diagnosed.

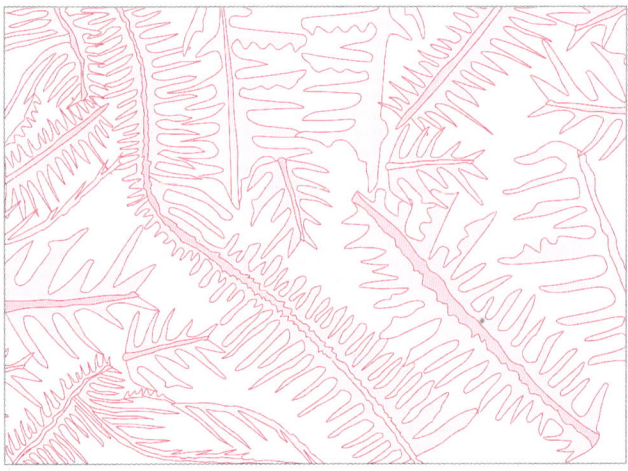

Fig. 9: Ferning of cervical mucosa—preovulatory cervical mucus due to effect of estrogen.

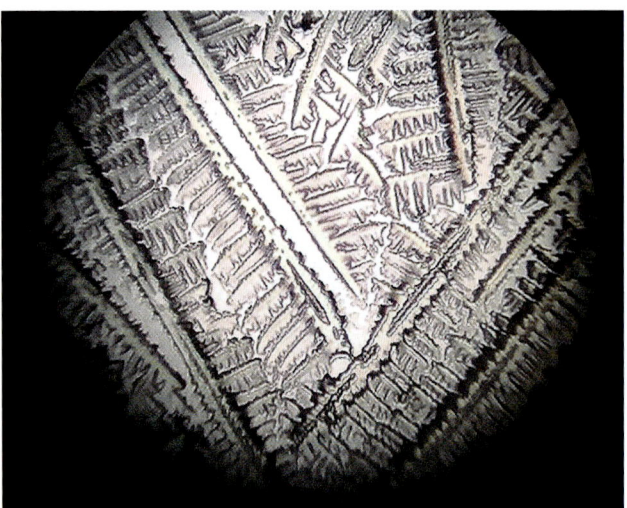

Fig. 10: Ferning of cervical mucus.

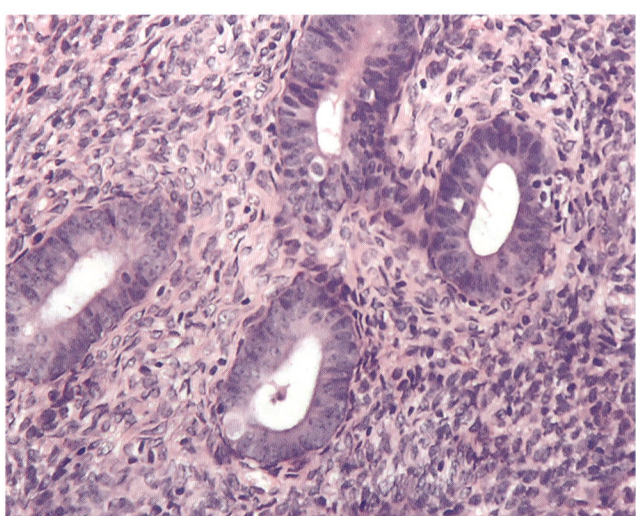

Fig. 12: Proliferative endometrium.

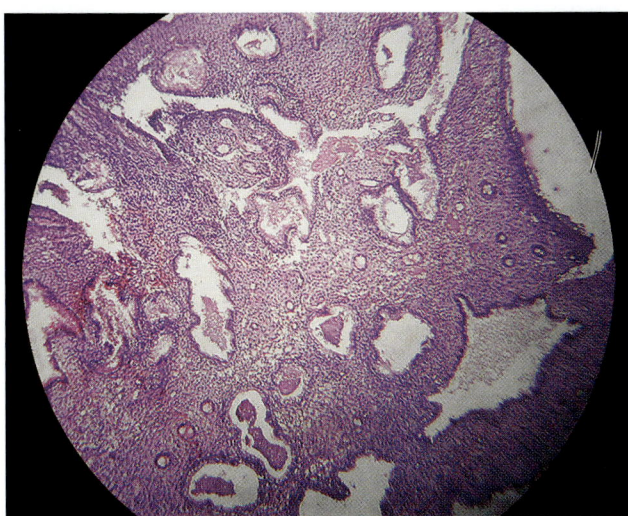

Fig. 13: Secretory endometrium.
Courtesy: Dr Anup Boler, Associate Professor, Pathology

Luteal Phase Defect—Diagnosis and Endometrial Biopsy

The diagnosis of *"out of phase biopsy"* is based on the concept of Noyes and associates (1975) who suggested the serial endometrial biopsy from early luteal phase and if there is lag of more than 2 days on endometrial histology relative to the actual day of the cycle determined retrospectively diagnosis of luteal phase defect (LPD) is reached.

However, this test is questionable due to the *intraobserver* and *interobserver* variations and similar findings in normal fertile women. Hence, out of phase biopsy to diagnose LPD is no longer considered a routine part of infertility evaluation.

Future of Endometrial Biopsy

Endometrial receptivity—potential markers of endometrial receptivity like cytokines, cell adhesive molecules (CAM—the integrins), and L-selectin ligand are thought to mediate embryo attachment. If expression patterns of these proteins prove to be predictive of endometrial receptivity endometrium study would have an immense future in infertility management.

Luteal Phase Defect—its Diagnosis and Management

When there is corpus luteal insufficiency resulting defective implantation or early miscarriage it is called LPD.

Diagnosis

Diagnosis is very difficult and not always evident:
- "Out of phase biopsy" in the serial endometrial biopsy from early luteal phase, i.e., there is lag of more than 2 days on endometrial histology relative to the actual day of the cycle determined retrospectively.
- Midluteal progesterone deficiency: A level above 3 ng/mL (10 nmol/L) indicates ovulation and value of above 10 ng/mL indicates good progestogenic effect.
- BBT: Biphasic but temperature in luteal phase is less and fluctuating.

Management

Progesterone—vaginal or injectable in luteal phase and human chorionic gonadotropin.

Luteinized Unruptured Follicle

Here follicle becomes luteinized without ovulation, but with normal menstrual cycle and infertility.

Luteinized unruptured follicle (LUF) is found in 10% normally fertile women and it is 25% in unexplained infertility where progesterone is secreted with corpus luteum formation without ovulation.

In vitro fertilization (IVF) after follicular aspiration is the treatment in persistent LUF cases.

Hormone Estimation in Infertility Workup

If only one hormone is considered for diagnosis of ovulation, it is the midluteal *progesterone* which is now recommended as routine.

Second hormone is the *LH* monitoring as preovulatory prediction marker.

Role of *d-3 FSH* measurement is reserved for ovarian reserve. FSH and LH are not measured routinely for diagnosis of ovulation.

Estradiol is measured in early part of cycle to (A) detect ovarian reserve and its measurement is invaluable in (B) monitoring of induced cycle especially to predict ovarian hyperstimulation syndrome (OHSS) complication. In follicular phase, normal level ranges from 30 pg/mL to 200 pg/mL, in ovulation phase 200–600 pg/mL, then after declining again rises on corpus luteum formation.

Midluteal Serum Progesterone

It is done on day 21–23 of an ideal 28-day cycle or 7 days following LH surge.

A level above 3 ng/mL (10 nmol/L) indicates ovulation and value of above 10 ng/mL indicates good progestogenic effect and good predictor of higher pregnancy rates.

Midluteal levels of progesterone are predictor of ovulation but not absolute indicator of adequate luteal function.

A single measurement lacks sensitivity as progesterone is secreted in pulses. There may be false positive in luteinized unruptured follicle.

Urinary LH Monitoring

Urinary LH monitoring is done by **ovulation prediction kit** which can detect LH as low as 35–50 mIU/mL. This enzyme-linked immunosorbent assay (ELISA) test is based on the fact that urinary LH can be detected 2 hours following the peak of the serum LH surge. Testing should begin 2–3 days prior to the predicted LH surge and done daily, even twice daily.

Following detection of LH surge ovulation is expected to occur within next 48 hours. This urinary kit test is convenient, quick, accurate, and useful.

Other Hormones in Infertility

Serum TSH and prolactin are frequently done in infertility workup to detect the *cause* of anovulation which can be treated easily with good outcome and hormones related to PCOS like *insulin and androgens*, etc., are estimated according to the indication.

Summary of Offer of Hormone Estimation in Infertility Workup

- *Progesterone*: The single most hormone for diagnosis of ovulation in midluteal phase.
- *LH*: Second hormone as preovulatory prediction marker.
- *d-3 FSH* estimation is reserved for ovarian reserve.
- *Estradiol*: In early part of cycle to detect ovarian reserve and monitoring to predict ovarian OHSS in induced cycle.
- *Serum TSH and prolactin* are frequently done in infertility workup to detect the *cause* of anovulation as treatment is easy with good outcome.
- *Anti-Mullerian hormone*: A good predictor of ovarian reserve independent of cycle stage.
- *Inhibin B* reflects the size of developing follicular cohort and no additional information is gained over FSH.
- Hormones related to PCOS like basal *FSH/LH ratio, insulin and androgens*, etc., are estimated according to indication.

USG Folliculometry

Serial transvaginal sonography is done to measure the size of Graafian follicle from day 10 onward.

Average mature follicular size is 17–19 mm in spontaneous cycles or 19–25 mm for clomiphene-induced cycles **(Figs. 14 and 15)**. Trilayered embryo thickness (ET) above 8 mm is favorable **(Fig. 16)**.

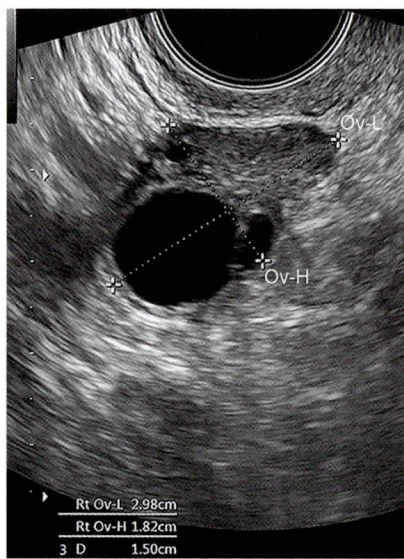

Fig. 14: Transvaginal sonography showing dominant follicle in ovary before ovulation.
Courtesy: Professor Kamal Oswal

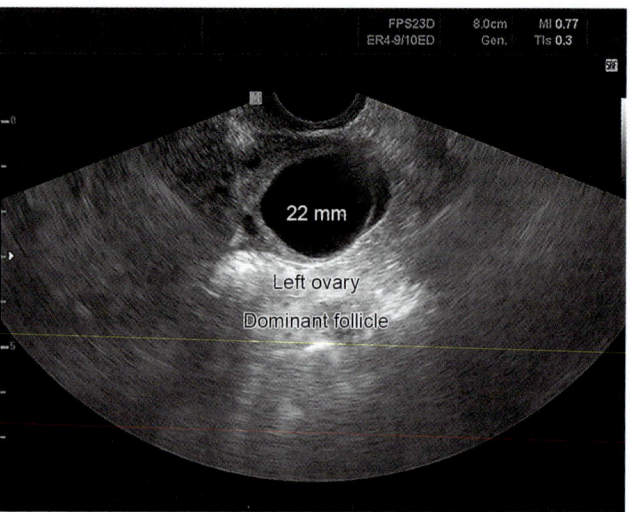

Fig. 15: Dominant follicle of 22 mm.
Courtesy: Dr Sanghamitra Ghosh, IRM, Kolkata

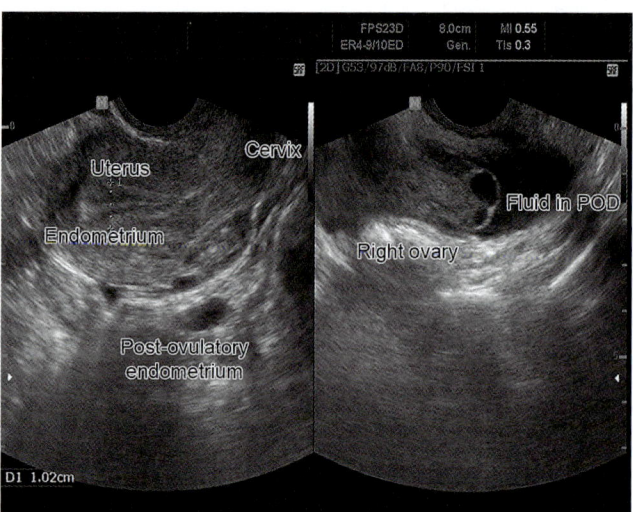

Fig. 16: Fluid in pouch of Douglas (POD) after ovulation.
Courtesy: Dr Sanghamitra Ghosh, IRM, Kolkata

Features of recent ovulation are collapsed follicle and fluid in POD. Endometrial thickness is measured to assess endometrial adequacy **(Fig. 17)**. Trilayered endometrial thickness (ET).

Though serial USG tracking is time consuming, inconvenient, and expensive, this is now the *standard definitive procedure* for diagnosis of ovulation.

Combination of ultrasonography and LH testing is also used for more accuracy. LH testing is started when follicular diameter becomes 14 mm.

Laparoscopy

If laparoscopy is done in premenstrual phase evidence of ovulation is seen by detecting ovarian stigma and formation of recent corpus luteum.

But solely for diagnosis of ovulation laparoscopy is not a preferred procedure.

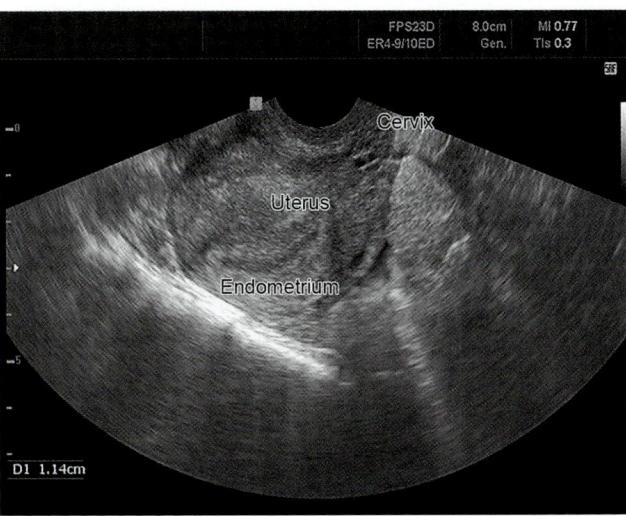

Fig. 17: Endometrial thickness (11.4 mm) when the follicle is matured.

The added advantages are that tubal patency test can be done, other pathology can be detected and minimal surgery can be performed if needed with prior counseling.

Laparoscopy is *the gold standard* for overall evaluation of female infertility.

OVARIAN RESERVE

Q. What is ovarian reserve?
- Ovarian reserve means the size and quality of the remaining ovarian follicular population at any given time.
- These are actually resting or nonmaturing primordial follicle pool present in the ovaries which are presumed to be growing and reflect the fertility potential of a woman.
- There are several tests to determine the ovarian reserve.
- Women's age is the most important predictor of ovarian reserve.

Markers of Ovarian Reserve

Markers of ovarian reserve are endocrine markers and ultrasound markers.
- *Endocrine markers*:
  - D-3 FSH level
  - Estradiol
  - Inhibin B
  - Anti-Mullerian hormone
  - Clomiphene citrate challenge test (CCCT).
- *Ultrasound markers:*
  - Antral follicle count (AFC)
  - Ovarian volume
  - Ovarian vascularity.

D-3 FSH Level

Cycle day 3 FSH level is a sensitive predictor of ovarian reserve. With loss of luteal inhibin, FSH levels rise in the early follicular phase. Inhibin is produced by granulosa cells and luteal cells. A value of *FSH above 10 mIU/mL* indicates significant loss of ovarian reserve and needs rapid evaluation and treatment.

Early Estradiol

Estrogen levels in older women will be elevated early in the cycle due to increased stimulation by elevated FSH levels. Day 3 estradiol level reflects follicular growth rather than number of antral follicles. *A cycle-day-3 estradiol level of above 80 pg/mL* is considered abnormal. Levels of both FSH and E2 are considered to diagnose ovarian reserve.

Serum AMH

Serum anti-Mullerian hormone, a glycoprotein, is a good predictor of ovarian reserve. AMH is produced by the granulosa cells of preantral and small antral follicles and possibly plays a role in recruitment of dominant follicle. It declines with age and undetectable after menopause.

Anti-Mullerian hormone level is independent of cycle stage and can be measured in any time of cycle unlike other hormones.

Level of AMH correlates with AFC more strongly than FSH or inhibin level. It is an earlier marker of ovarian function regression and its level decreases before the levels of FSH and estradiol drop.

Outcome is good when level is above *3.5 ng/mL* and poor when it is below 1 ng/mL. Anti-Mullerian hormone level is increased 2–3-folds in PCOS woman than normal.

Serum Inhibin B

A peptide hormone is produced principally by granulosa cells starting at preantral follicle stage and reflects the size of developing follicular cohort. A low level (<45 pg/mL) of early follicular phase may predict a poor ovarian response. This test is not so much preferred as no additional information is gained over FSH level and also due to its intercycle variability.

Clomiphene Citrate Challenge Test

Clomiphene citrate 100 mg daily orally is given from D5 to D9. Estradiol and FSH levels are measured on day 3, and FSH level on day10.

Follicle-stimulating hormone levels elevations at either time indicate poor ovarian reserve. CCCT is reported to be more sensitive than FSH alone to detect poor responder. CCCT is not practiced as day 3 FSH level is sufficient for initial screening.

Antral Follicle Count

Basal antral follicular count is the total number of follicles measuring 2–10 mm present in both ovaries.

It is most reliable USG predictor for subsequent response to ovulation induction.

The total AFC (2–10 mm size) is usually between *10 and 20* in a reproductive aged woman. A count *less than 4* is predictive of poor response to gonadotropin stimulation and higher cancellation rate in IVF.

Ovarian Volume and Ovarian Vascularity

Decreased ovarian volume of less than 3 cc and decreased stromal blood flow are implicated for poor response and poor treatment outcome.

Perifollicular vascularity is indicative of increase of mature oocytes and fertilizability. Follicles can be graded with degree of vascular perfusion.
- Grade 1 less than 25%
- Grade 2 less than 50%
- Grade 3 less than 75%
- Grade 4 more than 75%
- Vascularity more than 50% indicates good outcome.

Treatment of Poor Ovarian Reserve

Definite treatment is autologous IVF, use of donor oocytes, and embryo. Use of DHEA (dehydroepiandrosterone) (25 mg) thrice daily for 4–6 months has been tried to improve oocyte quality and IVF result.

TUBAL PATENCY TEST

Q. How would you do tubal patency tests?

There are several tubal patency tests; the important ones are:
- Hysterosalpingography
- Sonosalpingohysterography (HSG)
- Laparoscopy chromopertubation test (dye test).

Tubal insufflation test (Rubin's test) where air was pushed by Rubin's cannula through the cervical canal and auscultation with the help of stethoscope over the iliac fossa to hear the hissing sound of passage of air through fallopian tube is obsolete now.

Hysterosalpingography (Figs. 18 to 21) (*see* Also Page 579)

- The tubal patency test is commonly performed with HSG **(Figs. 18 to 20)**.
- It is done within 5–10 days of cycle after cessation of mens.
- Usually a water soluble radiopaque dye (Urografin or Conray 420) of about 5–10 mL is introduced slowly inside the uterine cavity transcervically with the help of HSG cannula **(Fig. 18)** or by hysterosalpingography catheter **(Fig. 23)** and seen through video monitor and X-ray is taken. Oil-based dye like ethiodol can also be used. Both types have advantages and disadvantages. Lipiodol is 40% iodine in poppy seed oil—oil soluble, less toxic and less viscous.
- Patency is determined by spillage of dye in pelvic cavity **(Figs. 19 and 20)**. Any uterine anomaly (bicornuate, unicornuate, septate, and subseptate), uterine synechiae, can also be diagnosed. However, whether is bicornuate or septate can be differentiated by laparoscopy by seeing the outer contour.
- It is done in radiology department with sedation and analgesics.
- Prophylactic antibiotic (doxycycline 100 mg bd) is given for 5 days to start 2 days before HSG.

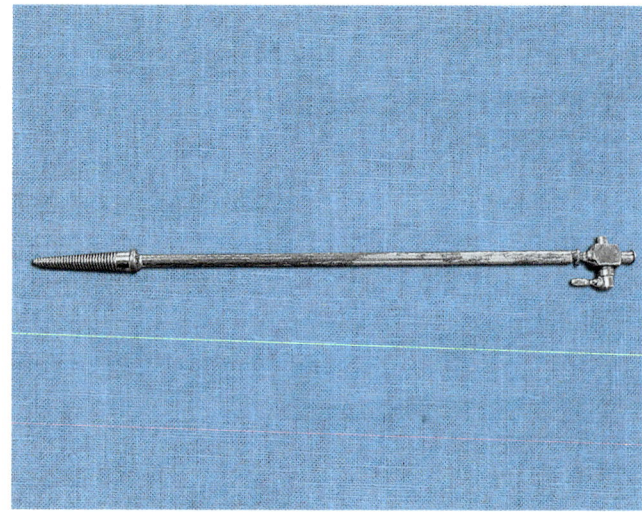

Fig. 18: Hysterosalpingography cannula (HSG cannula).

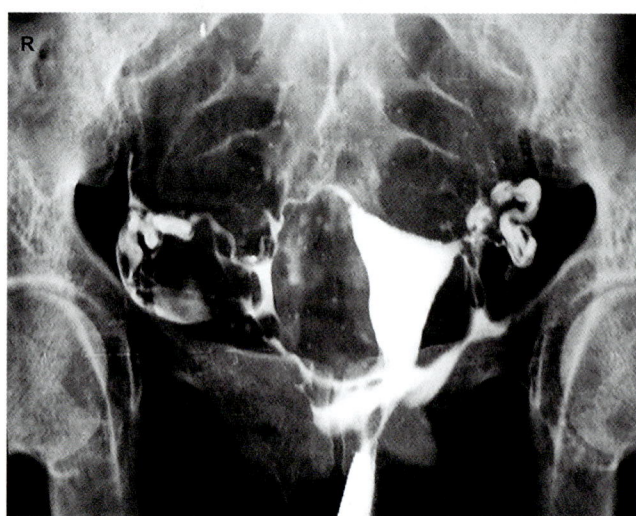

Fig. 19: Hysterosalpingography—bilateral patent tubes.

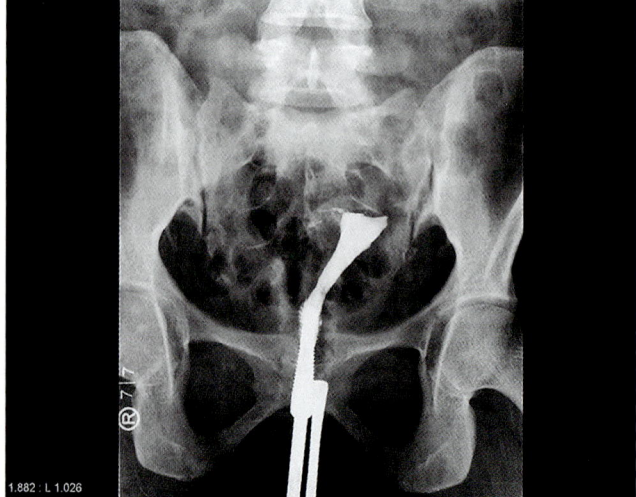

Fig. 20: Hysterosalpingography—bilateral tubal block suggestive of tuberculosis.
Courtesy: Professor Kamal Oswal

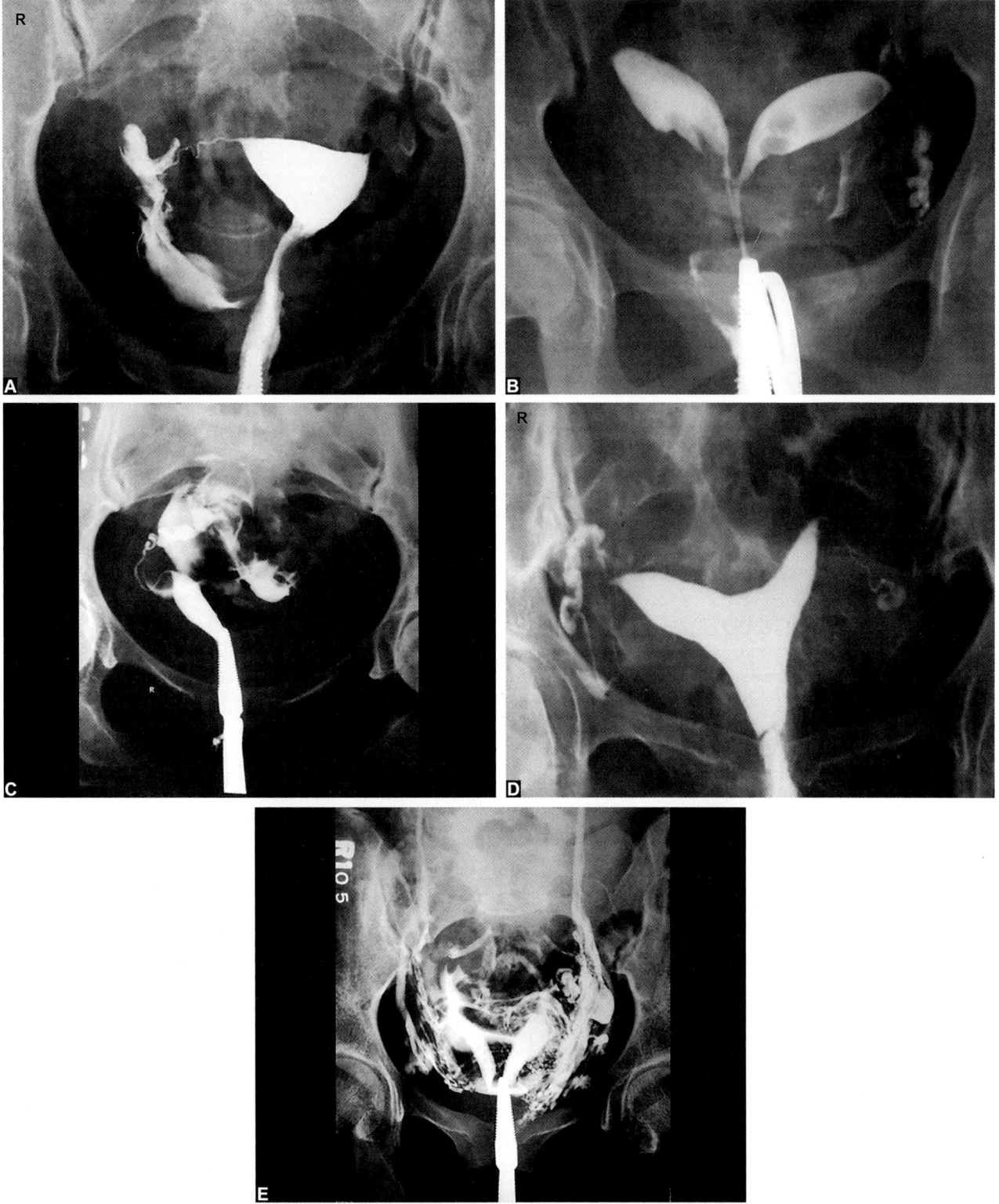

Figs. 21A to E: (A) Hysterosalpingography (HSG): Left side—ampullary block, right side—spillage present; (B) HSG bicornuate uterus; (C) HSG unicornuate uterus showing right horn with spillage; (D) HSG showing arcuate uterus; (E) Hysterosalpingography—extravasation of dye in venous and lymphatic route with bicornuate uterus.
Courtesy: Dr Subir Roy (Figures 21C and 21E)

- Usually three films are taken—first a preliminary view before injection, second showing the feeling of uterine cavity, and third spill of dye into peritoneal cavity.
- Average 1–2 rads of radiation to the ovaries.

Advantages

- It is an OPD procedure, a permanent record can be kept (X-ray plate), site and side of block is determined and any abnormality inside the uterine cavity like synechiae, septate or subseptate uterus, and unicornuate type can be diagnosed.
- It has also therapeutic effect.

Disadvantages

- Outer contour of uterus is not visualized.
- Chance of embolism and drug reaction, vasovagal attack, intravasation of dye through lymphatic or venous channel.
- Infection occurs rarely. Perforation of uterus and hemorrhage are other complications.
- There may be false negative test occasionally 50–60% of patients shown by HSG to have proximal tubal block occlusion were found to have patent tubes on subsequent laparoscopy.

Contraindication

- Hysterosalpingography should not be done in presence of hydrosalpinx and known or suspected cases of PID for fear of flaring up of infection, active uterine bleeding, and pregnancy.
- When block is detected or test is inconclusive diagnostic laparoscopy with chromopertubation test is advised.

Sonohysterosalpingogram

- Instead of radiopaque dye normal saline is pushed with the help of small balloon catheter (Foley catheter—size 8) inside the uterine cavity **(Fig. 22)**. Instead of Foley catheter especially designed hysterosalpingography catheter can be used **(Fig. 23)**.
- Fluid in the peritoneal cavity is seen by sonographic view **(Fig. 22)**.
- Presence of fluid in the POD confirms spillage.
- However, it is not always possible to determine whether both sides are open or not.
- Instead of saline, Echovist (an ultrasound contrast agent) can be injected and flow of fluid is seen through the fallopian tube. This is also called hysterosalpingo-contrast-sonography. This contrast media contains galactose granules.
- To fix the catheter and to prevent leakage bulb is inflated beforehand and slight traction is given. Before instillation of normal saline baseline USG is done.

Advantages

- It is noninvasive, abnormality of uterine cavity can also be diagnosed and there is no radiation exposure.

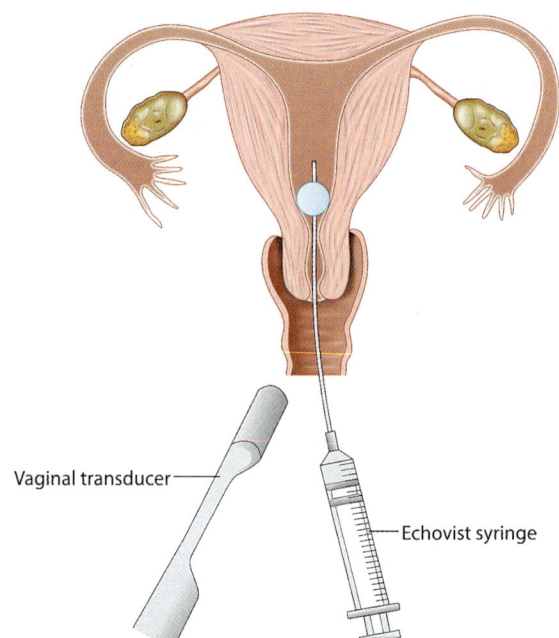

Fig. 22: Sonohysterosalpingography showing catheter and ultrasound probe.

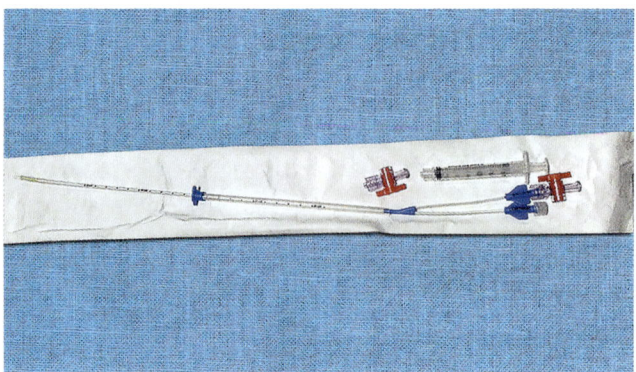

Fig. 23: Hysterosalpingography catheter.

- When saline is used the procedure is also recently called *saline infusion sonography (SIS)* by which uterine cavity is seen very well to diagnose any other pathology like polyp.

Laparoscopic Chromopertubation Test (Fig. 24)

- With the help of laparoscope abdominal cavity and pelvic structure are visualized.
- A color dye usually methylene blue is pushed transcervically with the help of HSG cannula.
- If the tubes are patent, dye is seen coming out through the fimbrial ends of tubes visualized through laparoscopy.
- It is usually done in premenstrual phase. Couple is asked to be abstinent or to use barrier contraceptive to avoid conception in that cycle which may be disturbed by the test.

Advantages

- Any pelvic pathology like endometriosis, PID, and polycystic ovary can be diagnosed

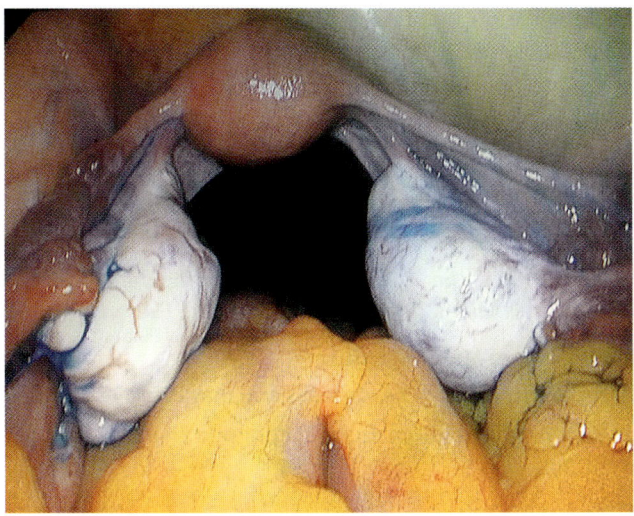

Fig. 24: Laparoscopic dye test—added advantage to diagnose polycystic ovaries in this case (blue dye is seen).

- Outer contour of the uterus—any abnormality can be seen which is not detected by HSG.
- False negative less. False negative cases of tubal patency in HSG can be diagnosed.
- Treatment can be done in the same sitting if prior planning and consent is taken.

Disadvantages

- It is more invasive procedure and uterine cavity could not be seen without hysteroscopy.
- Many advocate to do combinely with hysteroscopy (*hystero-laparoscope*) in the same sitting.

Falloposcopy

Falloposcopy can diagnose tubal patency in conjunction with *hysteroscope* but not used routinely due to fear of tubal perforation.

Salpingoscopy

During *laparoscopy* tubal patency can be seen through salpingoscopy through fimbrial end.

ANOVULATION

Q. What are the important causes of anovulation?

- Polycystic ovary syndrome (PCOS)
- Hyperprolactinemia
- Hypothyroidism
- Premature ovarian failure
- Primary ovarian failure.

Q. How would you classify anovulation according to WHO?

Anovulation: WHO classification on anovulation provides a basis for *therapeutic intervention* of the patients and categorized in three grades.

Grade 1—Hypogonadotropic hypogonadism:

- Low estradiol with low follicle-stimulating hormone (FSH) and low luteinizing hormone (LH).
- This is due to hypothalamo-pituitary failure. Examples are Kallmann syndrome, Sheehan's syndrome, stress or exercise-related amenorrhea, pituitary tumors, hyperprolactinemia, and hypothyroidism. It accounts for 10% cases of anovulation.
- These patients do not respond to most ovulation-inducing drugs and treated by gonadotropin *or* gonadotropin releasing hormone *(GnRH).*

Grade 2—Eugonadotropic eugonadal anovulation:

- Estradiol level and FSH level are normal and LH is either normal or elevated. *This is the most common type (75%) of anovulation and PCOS accounts for vast majority (90%).*
- These patients are ideal candidate for ovulation-inducing agents *like clomiphene or letrozole.*

Grade 3—Hypergonadotropic hypogonadism anovulation:

- There are high FSH, LH, and low estradiol level
  - Hypergonadotropic hypoestrogenic anovulation accounts for 10% cases of anovulation.
- The causes are primary ovarian insufficiency (previously called premature ovarian failure) (4–5%), gonadal dysgenesis (Turner syndrome), fragile X permutation carrier, and rarely ovarian resistance.
- These women are permanently amenorrheic and have near complete absence of follicle and no role of ovulation-inducing agent. With the donor oocyte IVF is the only way to get child.

CERVICAL FACTOR CAUSING INFERTILITY

Q. What are the causes of cervical factor causing infertility?

- Anatomical—spur
- Chronic cervicitis
- Mucosal damage by cautery
- Amputation
- Immunological.

Postcoital Test (Sims-Huhner Test)

- Postcoital test is performed to test the cervical hostility.
- Female partner is asked to come within 12 hours of coitus in preovulatory period.
- Cervical mucus drawn by pipette or by forceps is examined under microscope at high power.
- Inferences: Presence of more than or equal to 10 progressive motile sperms/hpf is normal and called positive. No sperm or all dead is abnormal and called negative. When the number of sperm is less than 10, it is inconclusive.
- Immotile sperm with normal sperm count in a good quality of cervical mucus indicates presence of antisperm antibody.

- A negative test could be due to improper timing, male factor, cervical factor, poor coital technique, or immunological factors.

Q. How would you diagnose cervical factor infertility?
- Clinical
- Postcoital test
- Sperm cervical mucus contact test (SCMCT)—in vitro is rarely done now. In vivo is the postcoital test.

Vaginal Factors Causing Infertility
- Congenital: Tough hymen, atresia, septum, and imperforate hymen.
- Functional: Vaginismus (details written later, Page 287).

Uterine Factors Causing Infertility
- Absent [Rokitansky-Küster-Hauser (RKH) syndrome]
- Congenital malformation
- Fibroid or polyp
- Synechiae
- Adenomyosis.

Q. How would you diagnose uterine factor?
- Clinical
- Imaging
- Karyotype
- Withdrawal bleeding.

CAUSES OF TUBAL BLOCK

Q. What are the causes of tubal block (tubal factor infertility)?

Details are written later (*see* Page 272)
- *Infection:* Tuberculosis, sexually transmitted disease (STD), and PID
- *Surgery:* Ectopic, tubectomy, and accidental injury
- *Endometriosis*
- *Congenital tubal defect.*

CAUSES OF INFERTILITY IN ENDOMETRIOSIS

Q. How does endometriosis cause infertility?
- Mechanical damage
- Increased prostaglandin
- Increased macrophages
- Anovulation, luteinized unruptured follicle (LUF), and luteal phase defect (LPD)
- Defect in ovum transport
- Altered tubal function
- Damage of the sperm
- Defective implantation and early fetal loss.

Causes of Male Infertility (in Details)

The causes can be categorized as pretesticular, testicular, and post-testicular. The details are given in **Table 1**.

Diabetes and Male Infertility

It impairs function of Leydig cells and may cause impotency.

Hyperprolactinemia causes hypogonadism and sexual dysfunction.

Cryptorchidism

Incidence is 8% at the age of 1 year. For spermatogenesis hypothermia is needed. If there is no spontaneous descent orchidopexy should be done before 2 years of age.

Varicocele is dilated internal spermatic veins. Hyperthermia causes seminopathy. Incidence in male population is 15%. In infertility clinic, it is 40%. It is one correctable cause.

Mumps and Infertility

When mumps occurs above the age of 10 years 25–30% cases testis become (orchitis) involved and seminiferous tubules are grossly damaged.

Immunological factor is involved in 3–13% cases of male infertility.

HISTORY AND EXAMINATION OF MALE PARTNER

History

- *Age:* Pregnancy rate decreases also with increase of paternal age particularly after 50s. However, age of man is not a bar to achieve a pregnancy. Men are reported to be father even into their 90s.
- *Duration of marriage*: History of previous marriage and history of any child
- *Occupation*: Working with pesticide, prolong bicycling, hyperthermia, and stress

Table 1: Causes of male infertility.

Pretesticular	Testicular	Post-testicular
• *Endocrinal:* Hypogonadotropic hypogonadism, hypothyroidism, hyperprolactinemia, diabetes • Coital dysfunction • Erectile dysfunction • Ejaculatory failure • Premature ejaculation • Retrograde ejaculation	• *Genetic:* Klinefelter syndrome, Y chromosome deletion, immotile cilia syndrome • *Congenital:* Cryptorchism • *Antispermatogenic agents:* Drugs, chemotherapy, drugs • *Infective:* Orchitis • *Vascular:* Torsion and varicocele • *Immunological*	Obstructive: • Epididymis-infective, congenital • Vas—cystic fibrosis and vasectomy • Ejaculatory duct—congenital • *Accessory gland infection:* Prostatitis and vesiculitis • *Immunological:* Postvasectomy and idiopathic

- *History of childhood problem*: Undescended testes and mumps orchitis
- *Past medical history*: Mumps, tuberculosis, leprosy, syphilis, renal failure, liver disease, hypertension, and multiple sclerosis
- *Chronic respiratory disease*: Young's syndrome—epididymal obstruction, cystic fibrosis—congenital absence of vas and in Kartagener syndrome sperms are immotile. In Kartagener syndrome, also called immotile cilia syndrome (autosomal recessive genetic disorder), the patient has situs inversus **(Figs. 25A and B)**, suffering from bronchiectasis with immotile sperm due to absence of protein, dynein which becomes normally present both in respiratory cilia, fallopian tube and tail of sperm, and responsible for ciliary movement and motility of sperm.
- *Endocrine disorder*: Diabetes, hypothyroidism, and hyperprolactinemia
- *Surgical and traumatic history*: Damage of vas—hernia, orchidopexy, vasectomy, trauma, torsion, and spinal cord injury.
- *Sexual history*: Timing, frequency, knowledge of conception window, and history of erectile and ejaculatory problem
- *Nocturnal penile tumescence (NPT) study*: The man who gets strong erection during sleep but no erection when he is with partner is likely to be suffered from psychological impotence. Morning stiffness and masturbatory erection is present in psychological impotence but not in organic type.
- *Family history*:
  - History of smoking, alcohol, radiation, heavy metals, and estrogen exposure
  - Drugs—antipsychotic, antihypertensives, cimetidine, anticonvulsants, sex steroids, environmental exposures. These factors cause male subfertility either by impairing spermatogenesis or by reducing libido or both.

Physical Examination

- *General:* Height, weight, and obesity
- *Secondary:* Sexual character, insufficient beard, and body habitus
- *Gynecomastia* (Klinefelter syndrome), thyroid gland, galactorrhea, visual field defect, and features of endocrinopathy
- *Per abdomen*: Scar of hernia and lymph node in groin region.

Local Examination

- *Scrotum*: Hernia, hydrocele, and varicocele. If varicocele is present, it is graded as I, II or III.
- *Testes*: Present or not (absent in undescended testes)
  - Size (normal—18 to 20 mL)—small in primary testicular failure (in Klinefelter syndrome it is less than or equal to 6 mL). Testicular volume is measured by Prader orchidometer.
  - Sensation: Lost in neuropathy or neoplasia, and tender in orchitis.
- *Penis*: Hypospadias and phimosis.
- *Epididymis and vas*: Presence, feel, and presence of cyst. Vas may be congenitally absent and in cystic fibrosis vas is virtually absent in all males. Epididymis becomes enlarged and tense in obstruction and irregular and tender in inflammation.
- *Rectal examination*: Done to palpate prostate and seminal vesicles. Prostate becomes tender, enlarged and irregular in prostatitis. By massaging prostate and seminal vesicle prostatic fluid is collected for examination of pus cells.

If history, clinical examination, and subsequent investigations suggest abnormality of male factor it is beneficial to refer him to urologist.

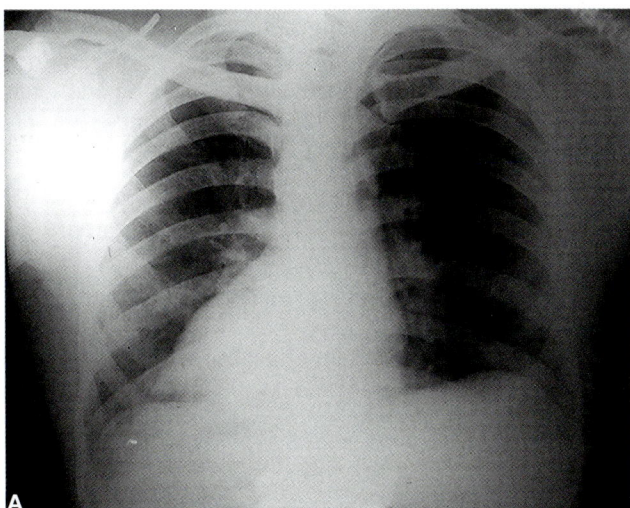

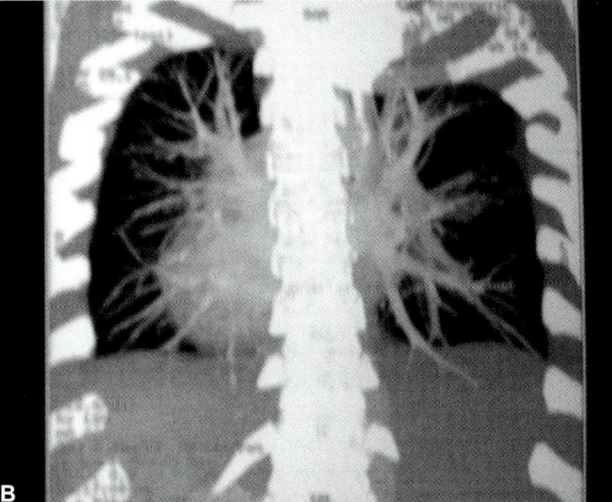

Figs. 25A and B: (A) Chest X-ray of male partner with all immotile sperms, sinusitis, and chronic respiratory disease—Kartagener syndrome (situs inversus); (B) Contrast CT in same patient with Kartagener syndrome as in Figure 25A.

Klinefelter Syndrome (see also Page 287)

* A male with fewer beards with gynecomastia, soft small testis, and azoospermia is most likely Klinefelter syndrome **(Figs. 26 and 27)**.
* The karyotype is 47 XXY.
* Klinefelter syndrome constitutes 14% cases of azoospermia. 10% cases of Klinefelter syndrome are mosaic and can achieve conception.
* For other causes of azoospermia, *see* later, Page 286.

SEMEN ANALYSIS

Semen analysis is the basic laboratory test and the time honored method of evaluating of male partner. Basic parameters of seminal report are semen volume, sperm concentration, sperm motility, and morphology.

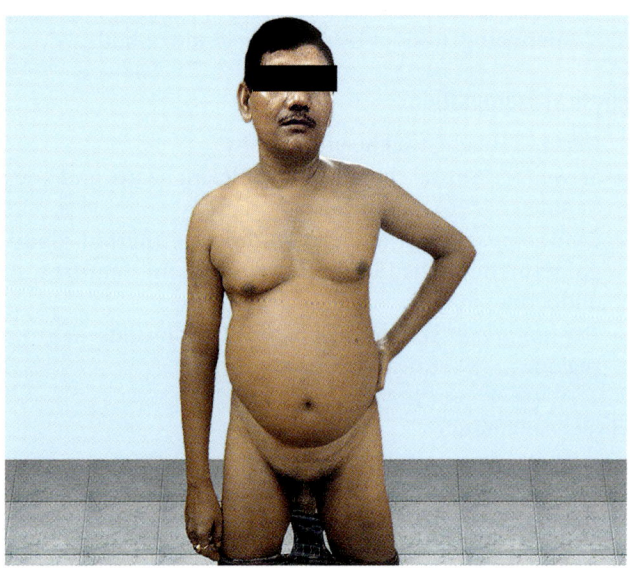

Fig. 26: Klinefelter syndrome. Patient came with azoospermia, gynecomastia with less beard.

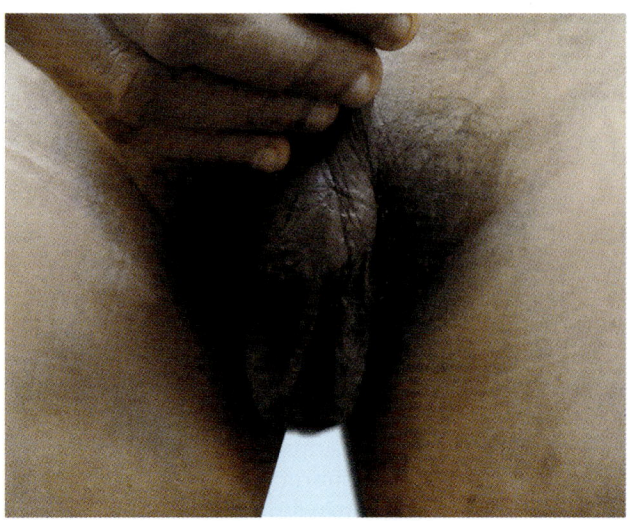

Fig. 27: Klinefelter syndrome—small, firm testis—same patient as in Figure 26.

Table 2: Semen parameters according to WHO 2010.

Parameter	Lower reference limit
Volume	1.5 mL
Sperm concentration/mL	15 million/mL
Total sperm concentration	39 million/ejaculate
Total motility (% motility)	40%
Progressive motility	32% (Grade a+b)
Vitality (% alive)	58%
Morphology	4% (Tygerberg criteria)
Leukocyte count	<1 million/mL

The normal values of the semen parameters as suggested by WHO in 2010 are given in **Table 2**. Normal composition of semen and spermatogenesis—description of sperm cells (*see* Page 421).

The sixth edition of the WHO laboratory manual for the examination and processing of human semen has been published in 2021 where the latest evidence-based information for the laboratory procedures of semen is described in detail. Reference value for sperm parameters according to sixth edition 2021: Semen volume is 1.4 mL, Sperm concentration 16 million/mL), total motility 42% and normal morphology is 4%.

Q. Semen analysis—manually or computer-assisted—which is preferred?

Semen is normally assessed manually, but computer-assisted semen analysis (CASA) is also performed.

Lack of standardization among laboratories, inability to differentiate between intact and nonintact sperms, possible biasness from artifacts limit wide use of CASA.

Q. How would you collect semen sample, and examine the sample?

Semen Collection and Analysis

Abstinence

Usually 2–3 days abstinence is advised. Prolong abstinence is avoided as there is impairment of motility. In very less abstinence, the quantity and concentration become less. Two semen samples should be examined in two occasions not less than 1 month and not more than 3 months interval.

Collection

* Specimen is collected in wide mouth clean glass or plastic container free of soap, detergents, and water by masturbation in the laboratory **(Fig. 28)**.
* Examination of the sample is started within 1 hour of collection. Man who cannot produce sample in the laboratory is asked to collect sample in residence or any nearby place and to deposit the same within 1 hour.
* Semen forms gel-like coagulum immediately after ejaculation due to presence of fibrinogen-like substance in seminal vesicles. *Liquefaction* occurs within 20–30 minutes due to the presence of proteolytic enzymes produced by prostate.

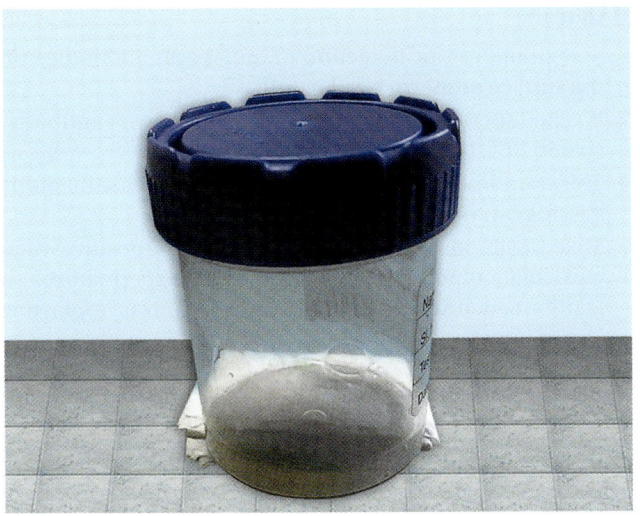

Fig. 28: Semen is collected in a wide mouth clean container.

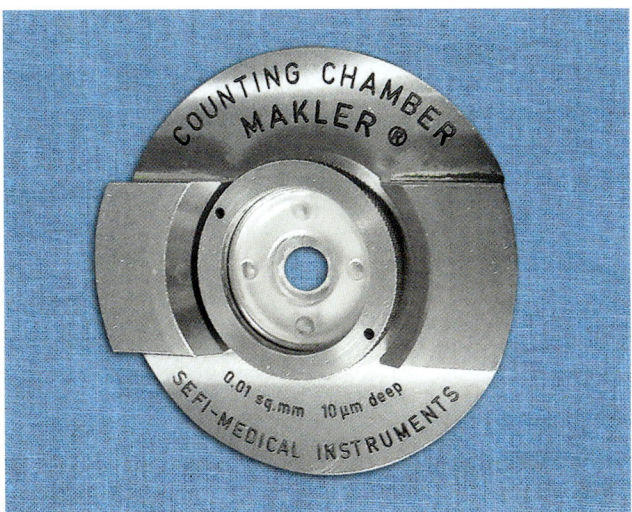

Fig. 29: Makler counting chamber.

Semen Volume

- Normal semen volume is 2–6 mL. Lowest limit according to WHO criteria is 1.5 mL.
- Low volume may be due to spillage during collection, retrograde ejaculation or testosterone deficiency. High volume may result from inflammation of accessory gland.
- Persistent low volume with pH less than 7 (normal 7.2–7.4) and absence of fructose is indicative of *ejaculatory duct obstruction or congenital absence of seminal vesicles* (secretion of seminal vesicle is alkaline and that of prostate is acidic).
  - In retrograde ejaculation, there is sense of orgasm but no ejaculatory fluid. Sperm can be retrieved by centrifuging the alkaline urine.

Sperm Concentration

- It is expressed as number of sperms per mL of ejaculate and normal lower limit is 15 million/mL. Hemocytometer with improved Naubauer ruling or Makler chamber **(Figs. 29 and 30)** is used for sperm counting. Only intact sperms are counted.
- Low count is called *oligospermia* and complete absence is called *azoospermia*.
- High FSH and low testosterone are due to testicular failure (nonobstructive azoospermia) and normal size testis with normal FSH indicates obstruction (obstructive azoospermia).

Sperm Motility

- It is percentage of progressive motile sperm in ejaculate.
- Progressive motility is the movement either linear or large circle regardless of speed.
- Progressive motility as per WHO criteria (2010) is 32% (Grade a+b).
- Nonprogressive means small movements or twitching and immotile refers to no movement. Grade of speed of progression like rapid (a) or slow (b) is not considered separately in 2010 WHO guideline because of observers' variation. Total a+b is taken.

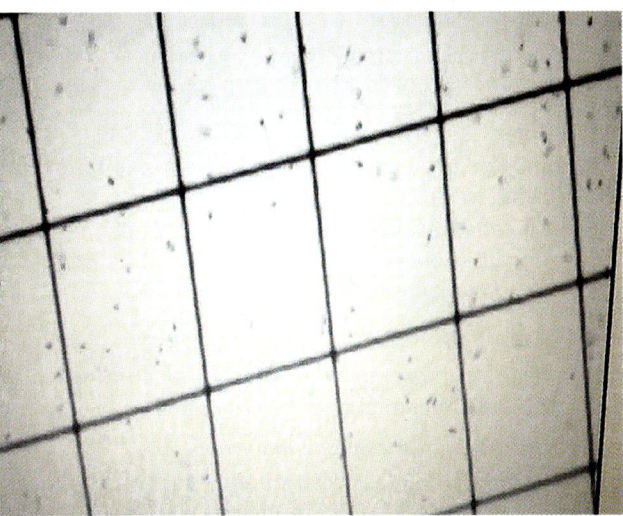

Fig. 30: Sperm seen in counting chamber under microscope.

- Sperm motility becomes poor (asthenospermia) in accessory gland infection, antibodies or intrinsic defect in sperm like Kartagener's syndrome. In cold semen sample motility may be reduced. In presence of large number of immotile sperms sperm viability test is performed as immotile sperm does not mean dead (necrozoospermia).
- Plasma membrane is intact in viable sperm and common test which is done to test viability is *hypo-osmotic swelling test (HOST)* where living sperm becomes swollen when immersed in hypo-osmotic saline. Other test is *eosin nigration test* where living sperm stains bluish white whereas dead sperm is colored with yellow.

Sperm Morphology

- Abnormal morphology means anatomical malformation of sperms.
- Normal morphology lower limit has been reduced to 4% according strict criteria in recent WHO guideline (strict Tygerberg criteria provided by Kruger et al. 1986).

- To assess morphology smear is prepared from semen, dried, stained with Papanicolau or sort stain after fixing with alcohol. Sperm is assessed for the normalcy of head, midpiece, and tail and the presence of cytoplasmic droplets in sperm head **(Fig. 31)**. At least 100 sperms are examined. Abnormality of sperm morphology is called teratozoospermia. It is claimed that sperm morphology is the best predictor of successful fertilization and pregnancy.

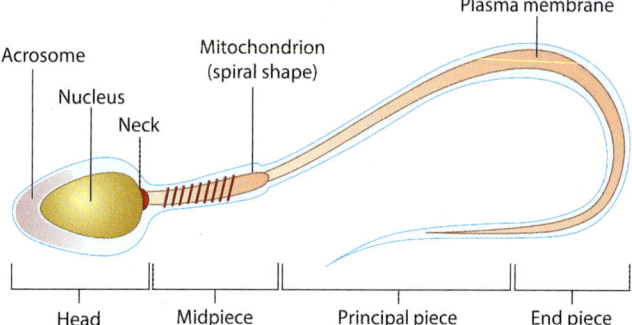

Fig. 31: Mature spermatozoa—it consists of head, neck and tail. Tail has three parts—midpiece, principal piece and end piece.

Round Cells

- Normal leukocyte count should be below 1 million/mL according to WHO criteria.
- Round cells in semen may be leukocytes or immature sperm cells. Leukocytes are differentiated by *Endtz test* (immunoperoxidase staining).

Q. Fructose in semen—what is its significance?

Absence of fructose may be due to ejaculatory duct obstruction or congenital absence of seminal vesicles.

Nomenclature related to sperm abnormalities:
- *Normozoospermia* means all parameters normal.
- *Oligozoospermia* when the sperm concentration is less than 15 million/mL, more than 5 mild to moderate, less than 5 million/mL severe oligospermia.
- *Teratozoospermia*: Increase number of abnormal sperms.
- *Asthenospermia*: Sperm motility is less.
- *Oligoasthenoteratozoospermia (OAT)*: All parameters are abnormal.
- *Azoospermia*: Absence of sperm in ejaculate.
- *Aspermia*: Absence of semen, i.e., no ejaculate. Hyposperm is—low volume semen.
- *Leukocytospermia*: High leukocyte count (pyospermia-increase pus cells).
- *Necrozoospermia*: All sperms are nonmotile.

Antisperm Antibody Test

- Two tests are employed:
    1. Immunobead test
    2. Mixed agglutination reaction (MAR) test.
- Indications are abnormal semen profile, abnormal cervical mucus sperm interaction, failed vasectomy reversal and marked agglutination (more than 10%).

MAR test

- Screening test for detection of antisperm antibodies on the surface of sperm head or tail.
- Washed sperms from the patient are mixed with antibody-coated RBC (sheep RBC + rabbit antibody).
- These antibodies will form mixed agglutinates with motile sperms carrying immunoglobulins.
- Mixed agglutination reaction test is said to be positive when particulate binding is found in over 10% spermatozoa. It is not needed when sperm is used for intracytoplasmic sperm injection (ICSI).

Q. What other additional investigations are done in male subfertility?

- Complete blood cell count (if infection suspected)
- Urine analysis
- Semen culture
- Sperm function tests
- Immunological tests
- Hormone assays
- Testicular biopsy
- Chromosomal analysis
- Vasography
- Scrotal ultrasound
- Transrectal ultrasound (TRU)
- MRI
- Measurement of reactive oxygen species (ROS)
- DNA integrity testing.

HORMONES PROFILE IN ASSESSMENT OF MALE INFERTILITY

Q. When and what hormones profile is done in assessment of male infertility?

- *Indication*: When sperm count is less than 10 million/mL
- *Hormones estimation which can be done*—FSH, LH, testosterone, estradiol, prolactin, and TSH.

Q. What are the interpretations in different hormonal levels?

Table 3 shows the interpretations in different hormonal levels.

Table 3: Hormone levels in different clinical conditions in male subfertility.

Findings	Diagnosis
Azoospermia or oligospermia Small testes FSH: High	Primary testicular failure (severe tubular damage)
Azoospermia Normal testicular volume FSH: Normal level	• Bilateral genital tract obstruction • Sertoli cell only syndrome
FSH: Lower or undetectable LH: Low Testosterone: Low Other evidences of androgen deficiency	Hypogonadism
LH: High Testosterone: High	Androgen receptor defect

Abbreviations: FSH, follicle-stimulating hormone; LH, luteinizing hormone

Q. What is the role of testicular biopsy?

- Biopsy is indicated to differentiate between obstructive and nonobstructive azoospermia.
- However, noninvasive technique like hormonal estimation (gonadotropin) can differentiate between the two.
- Recently in era of ICSI, it is also done in nonobstructive azoospermia to detect isolated areas containing sperm cells for TESE–ICSI (testicular sperm extraction and ICSI).

Q. What is the indication of genetic analysis/What genetic abnormalities may be in male factor infertility?

- *Indications* are azoospermia and severe oligozoospermia (<5 million)
- *Variety of genetic abnormalities are:*
    - Abnormal karyotype: Klinefelter syndrome (47 XXY) and sex reversal syndrome (46 XX male—translocation of SRY, i.e., testing determining factor of short arm of Y chromosome to the short arm of X) (*see* Page 287).
    - Deletion of a part of long arm of Y containing azoospermic factor (AZF) means azoospermia.
    - Mutation of specific gene like mutation of *CFTR* gene (cystic fibrosis transmembrane conductance regulator gene) in cystic fibrosis.

Sperm Function Test

- Sperm function test is one that evaluates one or more of the cellular processes exhibited by spermatozoa from the time of ejaculation to fertilization.
- Sperms have several functions from production to zygote formation like motility, capacitation, bind to zona pellucida (ZP) through separated cumulus, the acrosome reaction, zona pellucida penetration, and fusion with the oolemma **(Fig. 32)**. These functions are not reflected by the conventional semen analysis, for which several tests have been devised especially in the assisted reproductive technology (ART) centers.

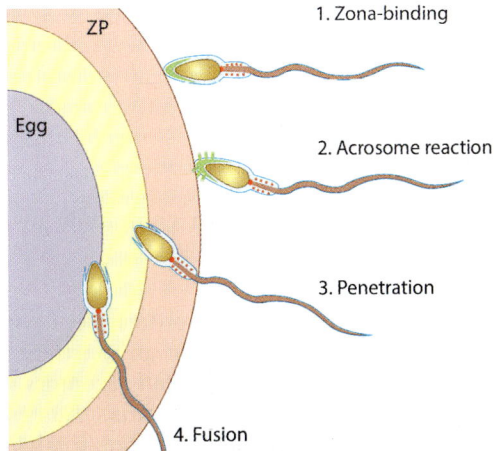

Fig. 32: Processes during fertilization—(1) Zona binding, (2) Acrosome reaction, (3) Penetration, (4) Sperm oocyte fusion.

- The purpose of sperm function tests is to diagnose a specific sperm dysfunction, prediction of fertilization or pregnancy rates and to formulate an appropriate therapy to alleviate the identified sperm dysfunction.

Few of the sperm function tests are:

- Sperm cervical mucus contact test—in vivo (postcoital test described later)
- Computer-assisted semen analysis
- Immunological test (MAR test)
- Sperm viability test (HOST)
- Sperm-zona pellucida binding tests
- Sperm penetration assay.

More advanced sperm function tests are:

- Acrosomal integrity test
- Tests of sperm DNA damage
- Assessment of ROS.

Q. How will you diagnose an immotile sperm—dead or live? (Sperm vitality test)

An immotile sperm can be assessed by HOST.

Hypo-osmotic swelling test (HOST):

- Sperms are placed in hypo-osmotic solution and incubated.
- "Swelling" and "coiling" of the mid piece or tail, indicates that sperms are living but immotile (vitality test).
- If more than 60% of sperms exhibit these changes sample is good and if less than 60%, such a sample cannot be used for IVF or ICSI.

Sperm DNA Integrity Test

- Sperm DNA damage [sperm chromatin structural assay (SCSA)] testing may be indicated in unexplained or idiopathic infertility, when a traditional semen analysis is normal and no evident female reproductive system pathologies can be revealed, and in selected cases of recurrent miscarriage.
- Tests for nuclear DNA fragmentation are TUNEL assay (terminal deoxynucleotidyl transferase dUTP nick end labeling), COMET assay, HALO sperm test, and DNA fragmentation index (DFI).
- DNA damage more than 20% indicates unsuitable for fertilization.

REACTIVE OXYGEN SPECIES

Q. What is reactive oxygen species and what is its importance in male subfertility?

- Reactive oxygen species are a group of highly reactive oxygen radicals that possess the ability to damage aerobic cellular systems impairing their functions and properties.
- These are superoxide anion ($.O_2$), hydroxyl radical (.OH) and hypochlorite radical (.OHCL). Spermatozoa are susceptible to be damaged by ROS.

- There is a negative correlation of seminal fluid ROS with sperm function, on the other hand minimal ROS is essential for normal sperm function.
- There is an equilibrium between ROS and antioxidants present in the system.
- Reactive oxygen species can be measured by luminometer.
- Recently, normal reference values for seminal ROS in fertile population have been developed and opened up a good therapeutic option using antioxidants.

Vasography
Vasography is done to detect obstruction in azoospermia where testicular biopsy is normal or suspected vas injury in inguinal surgery. Vas is cannulated near scrotum to inject dye.

Transrectal Ultrasound
Transrectal ultrasound is done to detect partial or complete block of ejaculatory ducts and seminal vesicles.

Scrotal USG with Color Doppler
It is indicated in testicular epididymal mass, loss of testicular sensation, and in postoperative resolution of varicocele.

MANAGEMENT OF FEMALE INFERTILITY

Management of female infertility includes:
- General management
- Specific management for the specific defects.

General management consists of:
- Counseling regarding the problems, various therapies, awareness about "conception window", involvement of husband, treatment cost, possible result, and side effects of therapy.
- Psychological support and assurance.
- Maintenance of BMI (between 25 kg/m^2 and 30 kg/m^2)
- Management of medical disorder if any like diabetes, thyroid disorder, and avoidance of antifertility drugs.

Specific management for the specific defects:
- Anovulation or oligoovulation
- Tubal factor infertility
- Cervical factor infertility
- Uterovaginal problems
- Immunological factors
- Unexplained.

Assisted reproductive technology has come in big way in management of infertility, both for female and male.

MANAGEMENT OF OVULATORY DYSFUNCTION

Ovulatory dysfunction is treated by:
- General: Weight loss in obesity and counseling
- Medical
- Surgical.

Exercise and Weight Loss
Modest reduction of body weight of at least 5–10% improves the fertility outcome substantially. Weight loss can be achieved by exercise, lifestyle modification, and change of diet habit.

Q. What do you mean by ovulation induction?

It is the procedure by which ovulation is induced by any agent usually by drugs.

Indication of Ovulation Induction
- Anovulation or oligoovulation
- In ovulatory women to induce more follicular development in cases of infertility.

Q. What do you mean by superovulation, ovulation enhancement, and controlled ovarian hyperstimulation (COH)?

- Superovulation and ovulation enhancement are synonymous where ovulation induction is done with medication even in ovulatory women to get more follicles.
- Controlled ovarian hyperstimulation—the term is usually applied in ART where follicles are stimulated to retrieve multiple eggs.

Medical Induction of Ovulation
- Selective estrogen receptor modulators (antiestrogens)—clomiphene citrate and tamoxifen
- Gonadotropins
- Gonadotropin-releasing hormones
- GnRH analogs
- Aromatase inhibitors—letrozole
- Adjuvant therapy:
  - Dopamine agonist
  - Insulin-sensitizing agents
  - Thyroxin
  - Dexamethasone.

Risks Associated with Ovulation Induction
- Multiple gestation
- Ovarian hyperstimulation syndrome (OHSS)
- Cancer risk.

Clomiphene Citrate
Clomiphene citrate is the most commonly ovulation-inducing drug. It is introduced in 1962.

Molecule and Mechanism
- Nonsteroidal triphenylethylene derivative with both estrogenic and antiestrogenic properties, mainly antiestrogenic. It binds to estrogen receptors on both hypothalamus and pituitary glands, thus blocking negative feedback of circulating estradiol. This will lead to increase FSH from pituitary which in turn, induces follicle maturation, estrogen production, and midcycle LH surge and finally ovulation.

- En-clomiphene is better than Zu-clomiphene due to shorter half-life.

Indication
- Most effective in *WHO class II* ovulation disorder, i.e., normogonadotropic, normoprolactinemic and euthyroid women. Patient may have oligo/amenorrhea with or without hyperandrogenism. This group includes *PCOS*.
- Clomiphene citrate has also been tried in *unexplained infertility*.

Dose, Regime and Duration
- Clomiphene citrate (CC) is given a daily dose of 50 mg for 5 days starting from day 2. However initiating on day 3, 4 or 5 outcome is not different and can be increased by 50 mg monthly if no ovulation occurs and maximum daily dose up to 250 mg. However, 250 mg dose is rarely used.
- If there is no ovulation in 150 mg dose some considers it as CC-resistant case and alternate agents like letrozole and gonadotropins are considered. Doses more than 100 mg are not approved by Food and Drug Administration (FDA).
- It should be given for 3–4 months after effective dose is achieved before considering failure.
- Monitoring with midluteal serum progesterone or TVS folliculometry should ideally be done to determine exact dose and to minimize complications. Standard duration is 6 cycles and should not be used more than 12 cycles as prolonged treatment may increase risk of ovarian malignancy.

Result
- Ovulation rate with CC is 60–85% with pregnancy rate of 30–40%.
- This discrepancy is explained by antiestrogenic effect on cervix and endometrium also due to the presence of other associated factors like tubal factor and endometriosis, etc.

Side effects and Risks of Clomiphene
- Risk of *multiple pregnancy* is as high as 10% and *OHSS* is 13% but severe OHSS is rare. Chance of miscarriage is 20% slightly higher than normal.
- Side effects are mild and up to 10%. These are hot flushes, nausea, vomiting, pain abdomen, headache, breast tenderness, and hair loss.

Tamoxifen
- It is triphenylethylene derivative structurally similar to clomiphene and widely used in breast cancer. It has no antiestrogenic effect on endometrium or vaginal mucosa and thought to be superior to CC.
- However, clinical reports do not show any better efficacy. It can be used as second line in women who exhibit side effects or nonresponsive to CC. Dose is 20–80 mg/day from day 2 to day 6 of cycle.

Aromatase Inhibitors (Letrozole)

Molecule and Mechanism of Action
- Letrozole is a third generation aromatase inhibitor (AI) and initially used for breast cancer. Now it is the most widely used aromatase inhibitor in female infertility. Experience with anastrozole, the other AI, used in breast cancer is limited.
- It decreases conversion of androgen to estrogen which in turn decreases negative feedback to hypothalamus and pituitary thus increases FSH secretion leading to follicle maturation and ovulation.
- It has no antiestrogenic effect on cervical mucus in contrast to CC.

Indication, Dose, and Duration
Letrozole can be used as effective agent in clomiphene-resistant cases and can also be used as first-line agent instead of CC. Daily dose is 2.5 mg from day 3 to day 7.

Result
It is claimed that it is superior to CC in ovulation induction in PCOS.

Limitation
Alleged increase congenital anomaly of offspring is not proved.

Gonadotropins
Used from late sixtys in ovulation induction.

Preparations of Gonadotropins
- Urinary human menopausal gonadotropin (hMG): It contains both FSH and LH (75 IU each).
- Urinary FSH: Purified FSH contains 75 IU FSH and less than 1 IU LH.
- Recombinant FSH: Developed by genetic engineering (1988).
- Urinary hCG: Extracted from placenta or urine of pregnant women. Used (5,000–10,000) for LH surge to trigger ovulation.
- Recombinant hCG 250 µg is equivalent to 5,000–10,000 IU urinary hCG recombinant.
- Recombinant LH: Recently developed.

Different gonadotropins are equally effective. Recombinants have certain advantages like unlimited supply, high purity, and less risk of allergy. Major drawback is high cost.

Indications of Gonadotropins
- WHO Group I anovulatory infertility (hypogonadotropic hypogonadism).
- WHO group II anovulatory infertility (including PCOS) not ovulated or conceived with CC/letrozole.
- For IUI in unexplained infertility or ovulatory women or mild male factor.
- Assisted reproductive technology (ART).

Regimens and Dose of Gonadotropins

"Step up" Protocol:
- In *"regular dose step-up protocol"* which is done in WHO group I.
  Usual starting dose is 150 IU daily subcutaneous (SC)/intramuscularly (IM), then increasing the dose by 75 IU after 4–5 days depending upon the response which is assessed by serum estradiol and TVS.

When one or two follicles attain a mean diameter of 18 mm, 5,000–10,000 hCG is administered to trigger ovulation. Ovulation is expected to occur 36–48 hours after hCG.

Couples are instructed to do intercourse on the day of injection and the next day.

❖ "*Chronic low-dose step-up protocol*" is followed in PCOS patients as PCOS ovaries are highly sensitive.

In this regime, low FSH dose (50–75 IU) is started and continued for longer period say about 14 days. Only small doses (25–37.5 IU every 5–7 days) may be increased.

"Step Down" Protocol:

In "*step down*" *protocol,* larger doses (150 IU) are started from day 2 or 3. When a dominant follicle is formed FSH is decreased by 37.5 IU and further decreased to 75 IU and continued. It has advantages of less duration of treatment.

"Sequential" Protocol:

In "*sequential protocol*" step up protocol is started first followed by step down when dominant follicle (≥14) mm is formed.

Risks of Gonadotropins

Ovarian hyperstimulation syndrome *and multiple gestation* are common for which counseling and monitoring by TVS folliculometry and serum estradiol is must. Multiple follicles are common in gonadotropin induction **(Fig. 33A)**. Chances of OHSS—mild: 20%, moderate: 6–7%, and severe type: 1–2%.

Monitoring of Ovarian Response

By serial USG—transverse diameter of follicle—1 mm/day at least 3 follicles more than 14 mm; ET—8 mm or more; E2—steady increase 200 pg/mL/follicle.

Results of Gonadotropins

WHO Group I: Pregnancy rate/cycle—25% cumulative pregnancy rate—90% after 6 cycles. In PCOS women, it is less—5–25% and 30–60%.

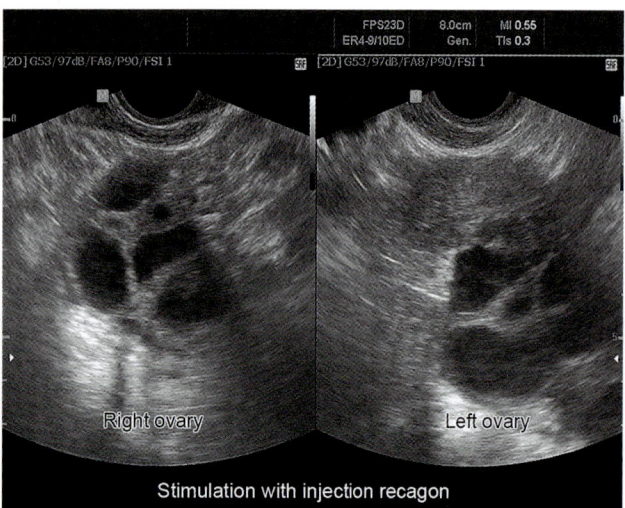

Fig. 33A: Maturing multiple follicles with gonadotropin stimulation.
Courtesy: Dr Sanghamitra Ghosh

Pulsatile GnRH

Mechanism

Administration of GnRH in pulses stimulates pituitary and releases FSH and LH.

Dose

Dose is 2.5–10 µg at 60–90 minutes interval mimicking normal pulse release by a portable mini pump either intravenous or subcutaneous.

Indication

WHO type I anovulation with intact pituitary.

Advantages

Multifollicular development and OHSS is less. Monitoring with pelvic USG and serum estradiol every 3–4 days interval.

Result

Per treatment cycle: Ovulation rate is 79–93% and pregnancy 18–29%. Recombinant LH recently developed.

Dopamine Agonists (Bromocriptine and Cabergoline)

Indication

Infertility with hyperprolactinemia. 30% PCOS patients are hyperprolactinemic.

Types

Bromocriptine and cabergoline: These two are commonly used. They are ergot alkaloids. Cabergoline inhibits only D2 receptor and is more effective with fewer side effects. Other new agent is *quinagolide*.

Mechanism

❖ They mimic dopamine and binds dopamine receptors. They enhance tonic suppression of prolactin synthesis and release from pituitary and cause euprolactinemia that *results ovulation in 80% cases.*

❖ Bromocriptine's half life is short and remains in circulation for 14 hours. Cabergoline is longer acting with higher affinity for receptor and inhibits prolactin secretion for 7 days.

Doses

❖ Bromocriptine is started with 1.25 mg daily at bed time for 1 week and then increased 1.25 twice daily for 1 month. Dose may be increased further if prolactin level does not become normal. Daily dose may be needed 7.5 mg.

❖ Cabergoline is started 0.25 mg twice a week for 2 months, if not normalized it can be increased thereafter.

Side effects

Side effects are more in bromocriptine than cabergoline; mainly gastrointestinal (GI) and cardiovascular. Others are headache and nasal congestion. No risk of OHSS, usually monofollicular ovulation.

Pregnancy Rate of Dopamine Agonists

❖ Cabergoline is superior to bromocriptine so far as euprolactinemia (80% vs. 55%), ovulation (72% vs. 52%) and conception (72% vs. 48%) is concerned.

- When pregnancy occurs in microprolactinoma bromocriptine is stopped as chance of growth is minimal (2%) but in macroprolactinemia chance of growth is high (25%) and needs continuation.
- If pregnancy is not achieved in spite of euprolactinemia CC or gonadotropin should be considered.

Metformin

Metformin is an insulin sensitizing drug, a biguanide, used for treatment of diabetes type 2.

Mode of Action

It is used for ovulation induction specially for PCOS patients and thought to induce ovulation by increasing SHBG and decreasing insulin resistance at target tissue and decrease glucose absorption in the intestine.

Indication

Polycystic ovarian syndrome patients who have not responded to CC and BMI more than 25 kg/m^2 are the ideal patient for metformin and it should not be offered as first-line agent.

Dose

500 mg thrice daily.

Side effects

Mainly GI side effects.

Dexamethasone

Glucocorticosteroids have been found to be beneficial for some CC-resistant cases.

The exact mechanism is not known and is believed to decrease adrenocorticotropic hormone peak which decreases adrenal androgens.

It is given 0.5 mg daily at bed time for 5 days starting on 1st day of CC, 0.5 mg for 6 weeks prior to start CC. It is given empirically or in elevated DHSO$_4$ cases.

MANAGEMENT OF DIMINISHED OVARIAN RESERVE

A basal level of FSH >15 IU/mL, even the woman menstruating spontaneously, gonadotropins therapy has little role. Though woman with AMH <1 ng/mL responds poorly with gonadotropins, still ART has beneficial effect.

OVARIAN HYPERSTIMULATION SYNDROME

Ovarian hyperstimulation syndrome (OHSS) is a clinical symptom complex potentially life-threatening rare complication of ovulation induction, occurs mostly due to exogenous gonadotropins.

Symptoms and Signs

Abdominal pain, distension, nausea, vomiting, ascites, pleural effusion, rarely pericardial effusion, hypovolemia, oliguria, and thromboembolism and respiratory distress.

It occurs in luteal phase or in early pregnancy.

Pathophysiology of OHSS

- Increased capillary permeability leads to shift of fluid from intravascular to extravascular space and accumulation of fluid, protein, and electrolyte in third space into peritoneal cavity.
- Permeability is due to the liberation of vasoactive agents by hyperstimulated ovaries.
- This causes intravascular dehydration and hemoconcentration leading to hypoalbuminemia, hypovolemia, oliguria, and electrolyte disturbance and hepatic or pulmonary end-organ failure if untreated. Vascular endothelial growth factor, angiotensin II, and high estrogen, etc., play major role in pathophysiology.

Diagnosis of OHSS

- Based on clinical findings with history of induction of ovulation.
- USG shows numerous follicular cysts with ascites (**Fig. 33B**). According to severity classified differently by different groups. In one classification, it is classified as mild, moderate, severe, and critical.
- *Differential diagnosis*: Ovarian cyst rupture, torsion, hemorrhage, and ectopic pregnancy should be kept in D/D.

Treatment of OHSS

- Mainly supportive
- Fluid balance by isotonic fluid and monitoring of fluid, electrolyte and output are crucial in management. Mild and moderate cases can be treated as outpatient.
- Severe cases onward are treated in critical care unit.
- Paracentesis transvaginally reduces abdominal and respiratory distress.
- Prevention and early diagnosis in early stage is very important. Death is rare with proper care.

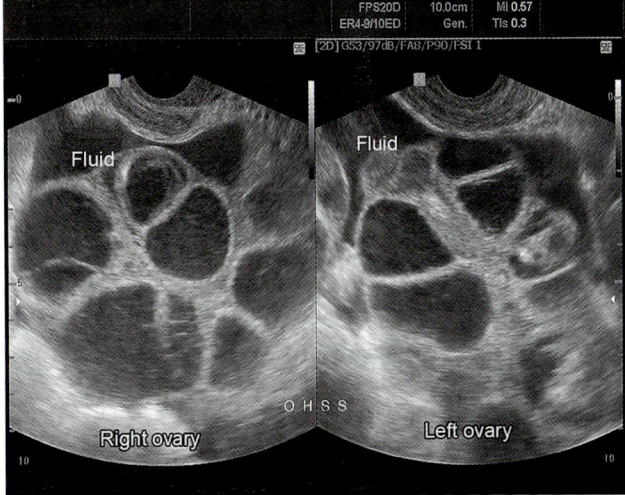

Fig. 33B: Ovarian hyperstimulated syndrome (OHSS): Right ovary—250.63 cc; Left ovary—287.77 cc; Estimated fluid in POD—1L.
Courtesy: Dr Sanghamitra Ghose, IRM, Kolkata

Q. Predisposing factors—where more chance of OHSS?
- Polycystic ovarian syndrome, young age, high estradiol levels during induction, pregnancy and types of ovulation-inducing drugs are the risk factors.
- Ovarian hyperstimulation syndrome mostly occurs with gonadotropins—mild: 20%, moderate: 6–7%, and severe: 1–2%. Increases with increase of doses. With CC OHSS is less, mostly mild form and is 13%, moderate and severe sporadically.
- Gonadotropin-releasing hormone agonist is associated with OHSS but GnRH antagonists do not increase OHSS.

Prevention
- All women undergoing ovulation induction must be counseled prior about the risks and to contact immediately with symptoms. Adaptations of ovulation regimen are adjusted according to risk factor present.
- Monitoring by USG and serum E2 may help in preventing OHSS.
- *Prediction of OHSS*: Rapidly increasing estradiol 4,000 pg/mL on the day of hCG in IVF cycle (range 1,900–6,000 pg/mL) and a total of 35 follicles (including small and intermediate size) are predictors of OHSS. Combination of E2 level more than 6,000 pg/mL on day of hCG and more than 30 oocytes retrieval is associated with 80% chance of developing severe OHSS.
- Reducing the dose of gonadotropins, withholding triggering by hCG or even cancellation of cycle in suspected OHSS may prevent OHSS. Couple is also advised to avoid intercourse. Use of low dose of GnRH agonist instead of hCG as triggering agent decreases the chance of OHSS.

SURGICAL MANAGEMENT IN ANOVULATION/OLIGOOVULATION
- Laparoscopic ovarian drilling (LOD)
- Wedge resection in PCOS
- Laparoscopic laser vaporization
- Surgery for ovarian or pelvic endometriosis.

Laparoscopic Ovarian Drilling
(*see* Page 294, Chapter 12, Fig. 7)
- Laparoscopic ovarian drilling is an option for selected group of patients who fail to respond to CC/AI or enhanced risk of gonadotropin-related sequelae (MP/OHSS) or cannot afford financial burden and it has an added advantage of long-term benefit for PCOS-related symptoms
- Five to ten punctures with monopolar needle, set between 20 and 30 W for 5 sec/puncture, are usually recommended
- For ovarian damage, adhesion formation and for less effectiveness it is not regarded as first-line treatment.

TUBAL FACTOR INFERTILITY
Tuboperitoneal factor constitutes 30–40% of female infertility.

Q. How does tubal factor cause infertility?
- Defective ovum pick up
- Impairing motility
- Loss of cilia
- Partial to complete obstruction.

Q. What are the causes of tubal block (tubal factor infertility)?

Causes of Tubal Block
The altered function may be due to peritubal adhesions following surgery, infection, and endometriosis.
- Infection: Tuberculosis, STD, PID—most common
- Surgery: Ectopic, tubectomy (voluntary sterilization), and accidental injury
- Endometriosis
- Congenital tubal defect—rare.

Pelvic inflammatory disease is said to be the most common cause of tubal infertility comprising more than half of the cases. PID is caused by endogenous (anaerobic and aerobic bacteria) or exogenous agents (*Neisseria gonorrhoeae, Chlamydia trachomatis,* and *Mycoplasma hominis*). Degree of endosalpingeal damage and pelvic adhesions vary widely. With the increase of size of hydrosalpinx (≥2 cm) the monthly fecundity rate following surgery decreases. Tubal pathology may alter the result of ART success, for example, in large hydrosalpinx salpingectomy is needed to improve outcome.

Pelvic tuberculosis is responsible for infertility in a significant number of patients especially in developing country. In tuberculosis, prognosis is worse so far as conception is concerned in both cases of surgery and ART, a little better in ART.

In *endometriosis,* tubal function is impaired by peritubal adhesions which distort tubal anatomy. Tubal lumen is rarely occluded by endometriotic deposits. Rupture of chocolate cyst may cause severe pelvic adhesions causing distortion of tubal anatomy.

About 20–30% of women *regret following tubal ligation.* Tubal block from *sterilization procedure* is reversed by surgery with good result if the length of the tube remains reasonable.

Classification of Tubal Disease
Tubal disease is classified in three stages mild, moderate, and severe depending upon thee presence, size, and severity of adhesions and hydrosalpinx.

Diagnosis and Assessment of Tubal Function
- History and clinical examination
- Tubal patency test as described before:
    - HSG
    - Sonohysterosalpingography

- Laparoscopy which is the gold standard method of assessment of tubal patency with added advantage of detecting other pelvic pathology.

Falloposcopy and salpingoscopy have added advantage to observe tubal lumen.

Treatment of Tubal Factor Infertility

Prevention
Early detection and management of pelvic infection. MTP should always be done in strict aseptic measure.

Definite management
- ❖ Medical: Antibiotics and antitubercular drugs
- ❖ Hydrotubation—little role
- ❖ Surgery:
  - Macroscopic (conventional)
  - Microscopic
  - Laparoscopy.
- ❖ ART: IVF-ET.

Surgery for Tubal Factor Infertility
- ❖ Adhesiolysis
- ❖ Fimbrioplasty: Lysis of fimbrial adhesion with dilatation of fimbrial phimosis
- ❖ Salpingostomy **(Fig. 34)**: Creation of tubal stroma with completely occluded distal including hydrosalpinx
- ❖ Tubotubal anastomosis **(Figs. 35 to 37)**

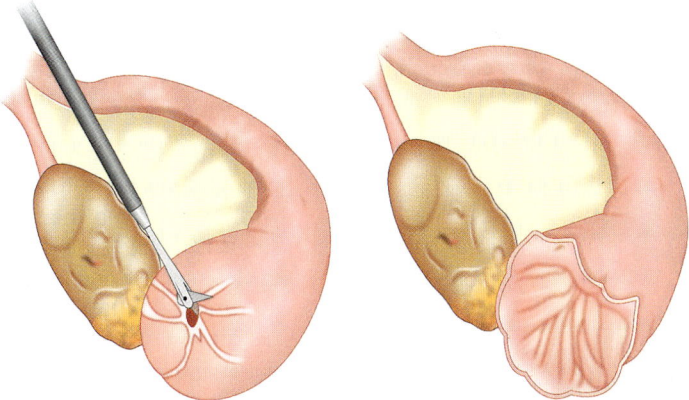

Fig. 34: Salpingostomy—creation of new ostium—an incision is given along the avascular line to open the stroma with multiple cut and the flaps are everted by giving 2-0 or 3-0 absorbable stitches.

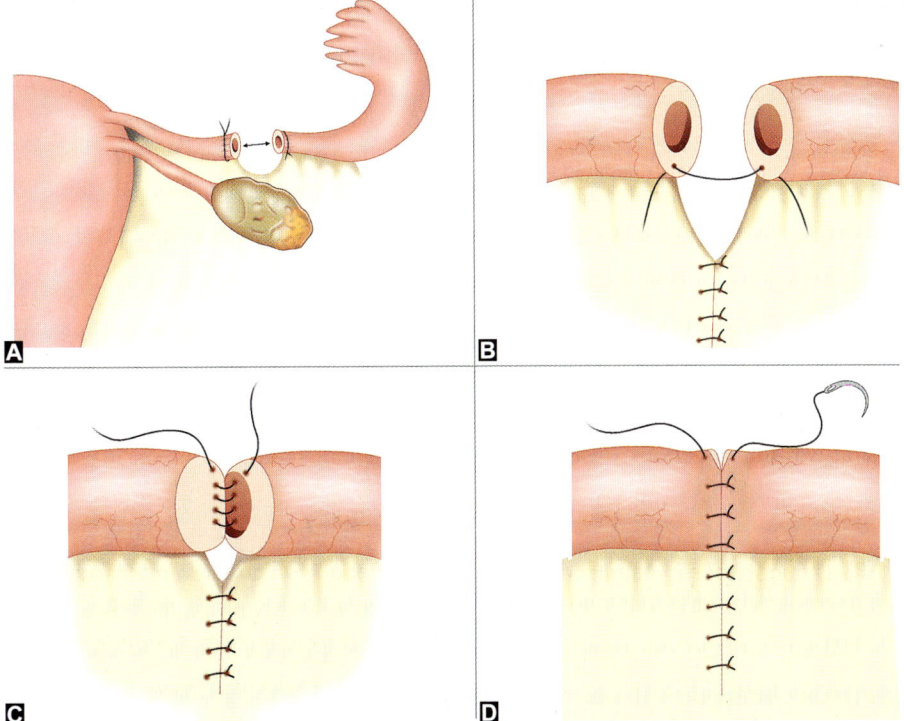

Figs. 35A to D: Tubotubal anastomosis—done in two layers musculo-muscularis avoiding the mucosa and serosal using average four interrupted nonabsorbable 6-0 or 7-0 stitches in each layer.

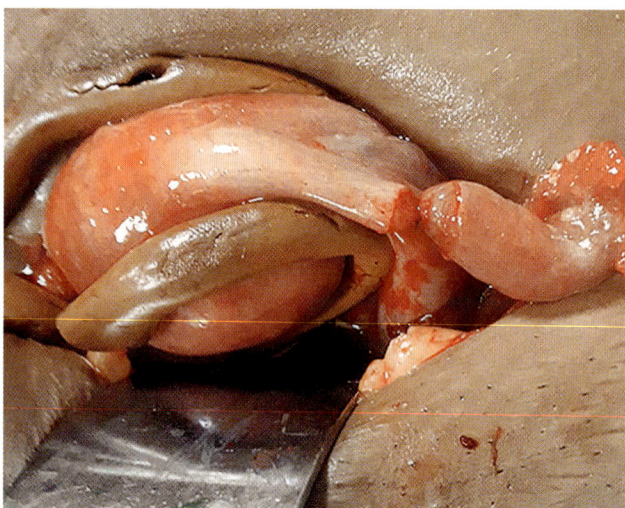

Fig. 36: Recanalization following tubectomy—after dissection, inner layer (musculo-muscularis) by 6-0 prolene.

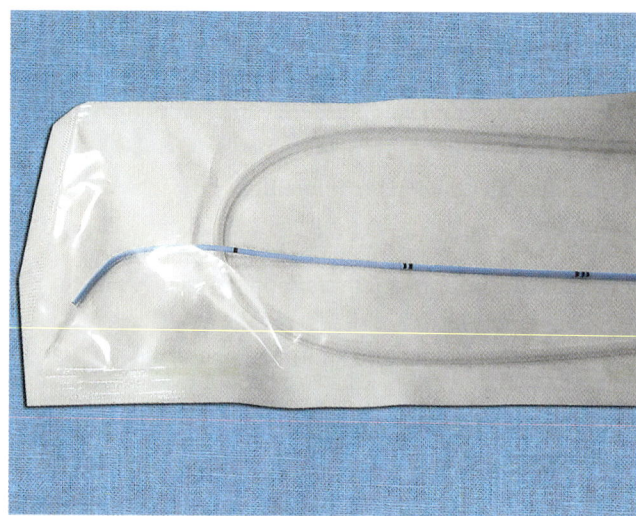

Fig. 38: Cannulation wire in tubal block—cannulation of tube done in hysteroscopic approach.

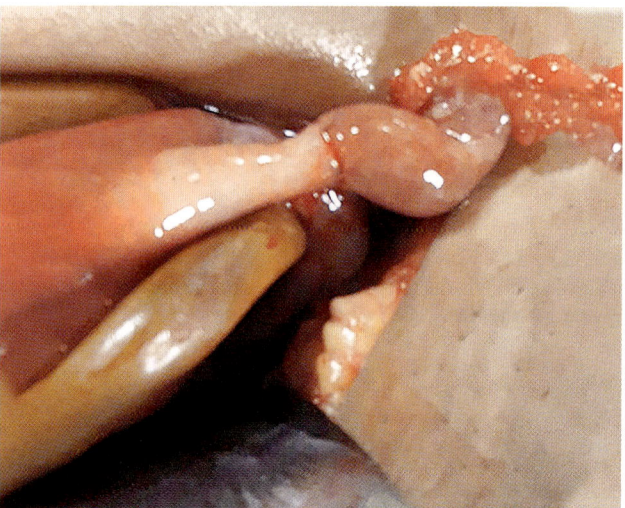

Fig. 37: Recanalization following tubectomy— repaired in two layers, outer layer (serosal) given by 6-0 prolene.

- Tubocornual anastomosis
- Cannulation and balloon tuboplasty (through hysteroscopy) in proximal tubal obstruction **(Fig. 38)**.

Conventional surgery has poor result and has been replaced by microsurgery. Laparoscopic surgery has come over microsurgery in a big way due to various advantages.

Q. ART (IVF and ET) vs. Surgery—which one is preferred in tubal factor infertility?

- The advantage of ART is that in grossly damaged or even absent tube where restorative surgery has no role, ART can bring a pregnancy.
- In vitro fertilization and ET is a procedure to achieve pregnancy bypassing the damaged or absent tube, but surgery does it by treating the abnormality, restoring anatomy of the tube to as normal as possible and maintaining the patency.
- After tubal reconstructive surgery, couples may have permanent ability to conceive in every cycle naturally without renewed therapy from a single intervention. A single IVF cycle gives only one chance to conceive. Several cycles may be needed to get one pregnancy. However, anatomical patency does not mean the functional restoration of the tube.
- Following reconstructive surgery, the overall risks are low, and include the known complications of surgery such as bleeding, infection, organ damage, and anesthesia. Chance of ectopic pregnancy is there in both cases.
- Assisted reproductive technology is associated with a number of potential complications—severe OHSS (0.25–2%) and multiple pregnancies (up to 25%).
- The average live birth rate per cycle of treatment following ART varies from 19% to 35%.
- In intrinsic tubal damage, surgery results pregnancy at the rate of 10–60% with ectopic pregnancy rate as high as 21%.

Q. For sterilization reversal, which is the treatment option?

The best result of surgery is achieved in *microsurgical reversal of sterilization* with pregnancy rates from 55% to 84%.

- For sterilization reversal in young woman with good tubal length surgical anastomosis is the treatment of choice by microsurgery.
- Laparoscopic recanalization is a good option with good pregnancy rate.

Microsurgery

Q. What do you mean by microsurgery?

Microsurgery means surgery requiring magnification either by operating microscope, loop or hoods.

Principle of Microsurgery

- Magnification
- Gentle operative techniques and delicate instruments using fine nonabsorbable microsuture

- Constant irrigation with heparinized solution
- Meticulous hemostasis with covering raw areas to prevent adhesion.

Tubotubal Anastomosis

Tubotubal anastomosis is done for sterilization reversal and pathological occlusion by using magnification.

Types of anastomosis are:
- Ampullary-ampullary
- Ampullary-isthmic
- Isthmic-isthmic
- Isthmic-cornual.

Steps in Sterilization Reversal (Tubotubal Anastomosis) (see Figs. 36 and 37)

- Both ends are cut vertically so that patency is recognized on both sides.
- Mesosalpinx is approximated by 5-0 catgut sutures.
- The anastomosis of tubes is done in two layers—musculo-muscularis avoiding the mucosa and serosal layer.
- In musculo-muscularis layer is done by four interrupted stitches using 6-0 or 7-0 nonabsorbable nylon or prolene stitches—starting from 6 o'clock and subsequently at 3, 12, and 9 o'clock position. Sutures are taken such a way that knot face the serosa.
- Afterwards serosal coat is repaired in four interrupted stitches. Lastly gap at mesosalpinx is closed with 5-0 catgut stitches.
- At the end tubal patency is tested.

Result of sterilization reversal depends on:
- Length of resultant tube—more than 4.5 cm should be minimal length
- Method of sterilization—diathermy sterilization is associated with poor reversal result
- Following fimbriectomy reversal is not suitable option
- Site of anastomosis—isthmo-isthmic anastomosis has the best prognosis
- Interval from tubectomy to reversal—prognosis inversely varies
- Associated pathology.

Fertility outcome following tubal surgery:
- Overall pregnancy rate—50%
- Ectopic pregnancy rate—10%.

Pregnancy rate following laparoscopic surgery:
- Salpingo-ovariolysis—60%
- Fimbrioplasty—32%
- Tubotubal anastomosis—75%
- Tubocornual anastomosis—55%

ASSISTED REPRODUCTIVE TECHNOLOGY

Conventionally, assisted reproductive technology (ART), by definition means the procedures where the extraction and manipulation of oocyte are done. ART involves the clinical and laboratory procedures to achieve a pregnancy in infertile couple where corrections of the etiology are not possible directly. In strict sense, intrauterine insemination (IUI) is not an ART technique, but the all principles are maintained like other ART procedures.

ART procedures include IVF&ET, ICSI, GIFT, ZIFT, gestational carrier surrogacy, oocyte donation and embryo donation, etc.

IN VITRO FERTILIZATION AND EMBRYO TRANSFER

Q. What is in vitro fertilization and embryo transfer (IVF-ET) (see Fig. 42, Page 277)?

- It is a procedure whereby eggs are removed from the ovaries.
- Fertilized in the laboratory with the male partner's sperm.
- The resulting embryos are then replaced back in the womb 3–7 days later.

Indications of IVF-ET in Female Infertility
- Tubal factor infertility
- Cervical hostility
- Infertility with endometriosis
- Unexplained infertility
- Failed ovulation induction.

Presence of hydrosalpinx increases implantation failure and abortion. In this case either it is removed surgically or interrupted proximally. Hydrosalpinx is diagnosed by sonography.

Basic Steps in IVF and ET (see Fig. 42, Page 277)
- Patient selection
- Downregulation by GnRH analog
- Controlled ovarian hyperstimulation
- Monitoring
- Oocyte retrieval transvaginally with sonographic guidance
- Sperm preparation
- Insemination: Sperm and ova are mixed in vitro for fertilization (IVF)
- Embryo transfer: Viable embryos are transferred transcervically into uterine cavity
- Luteal support.

Controlled Ovarian Hyperstimulation
- To get multiple number of oocytes superovulation is done by ovulation-inducing drugs
- Drugs used are clomiphene, gonadotropin, and GnRH.
- Gonadotropin-releasing hormone agonists are used for downregulation of hypothalamic-pituitary-ovarian axis to get multiple number of good quality oocytes expecting increase clinical pregnancy rate. GnRH prevents premature ovulation. hCG is given for final maturation and triggering ovulation which usually occurs 36 hours of hCG administration.

- The idea is to get multiple oocytes by aspiration, multiple embryo, multiple embryo transfer, and increase success rate.

Monitoring
- Monitoring is mandatory for fixing of time of hCG administration and to prevent and to detect OHSS (*see* OHSS above).
- Monitoring of ovarian response is done by serial folliculometry and measurements of serum estradiol.

Protocols of COH
There are several protocols for ovarian hyperstimulation, but basically three types for COH are followed depending upon the category of patients, normal responder, poor responder or hyper-responder.
- *Long protocol*—for normal responder
- *Short protocol* (flare protocol)—for poor responder
- *Gonadotropin-releasing hormone antagonist protocol* is increasingly used with several advantages.

Coasting is used for hyper-responder where gonadotropin is discontinued in last part to prevent OHSS.

Long protocol (Fig. 39)
- Gonadotropin-releasing hormone agonist is started from midluteal phase of previous cycle and continued throughout the follicular phase till hCG is given.
- Gonadotropins are administered after the onset of menses. Either leuprolide 0.1 mg SC daily or nafarelin 200 µg twice daily are usually used.
- Monitoring is done by serial folliculometry and measurements of serum estradiol. hCG is administered to trigger ovulation when three or more follicles of at least 17 mm diameter in USG.
- Ova are picked up 36 hours after hCG. Embryos are transferred to uterus 3–5 days after retrieval. Luteal support is given by progesterone either vaginal or injectable route.

Short protocol (Fig. 40)
In this regime, GnRH agonists usually leuprolide 20 pg SC twice daily is started from day 2 or 3 day of cycle followed by administration of gonadotropins after 2 days and continued through follicular phase.

Coasting
- Gonadotropin-releasing hormone agonist is started from third week of the previous cycle and gonadotropin in low dose (75 IU/day) is started after menstruation and if E2 is more than 3,000 pg/mL.
- Gonadotropin is discontinued irrespective of follicular diameter and GnRH is continued. After the fall of E2 less than 3,000 hCG is administered.
- This protocol is particularly useful for hyper-responders like PCOS to prevent hyperstimulation syndrome.

GnRH antagonist protocol (Fig. 41)
- Gonadotropin is started on day 2 or 3 of cycle followed by GnRH antagonist from day 6 (fixed) or in a flexible manner.
- The advantages are less duration of treatment cycle, OHSS less, overall less number of injection and less cost.

Oocyte Retrieval (Figs. 42 and 43)
- Under transvaginal sonographic guidance using transvaginal transducer mature oocytes are retrieved transvaginally puncturing through vagina and ovary.
- Oocyte with follicular fluid is aspirated. A washing media mixed with heparin is used and examined under microscope (Fig. 44).

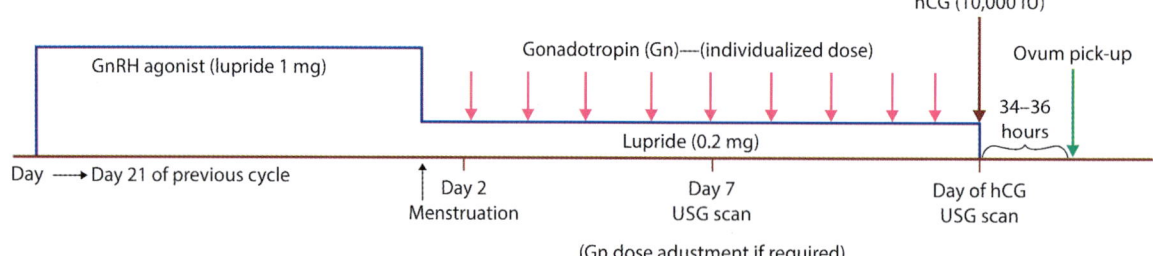

Fig. 39: Long agonist protocol.
Abbreviations: GnRH, gonadotropin-releasing hormone; hCG, human chorionic gonadotropin; USG, ultrasonography

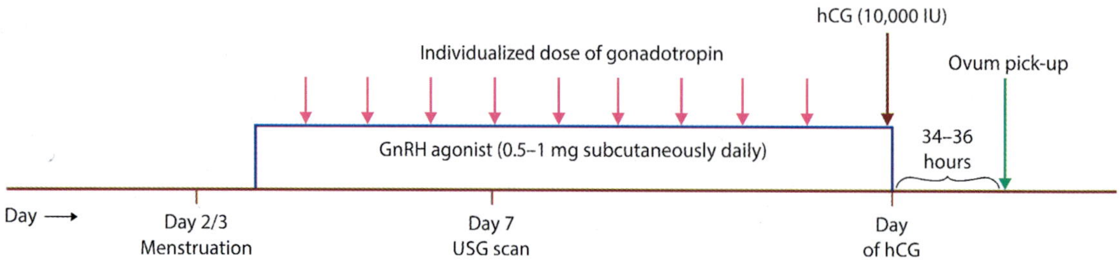

Fig. 40: Short agonist protocol.
Abbreviations: GnRH, gonadotropin-releasing hormone; hCG, human chorionic gonadotropin; USG, ultrasonography

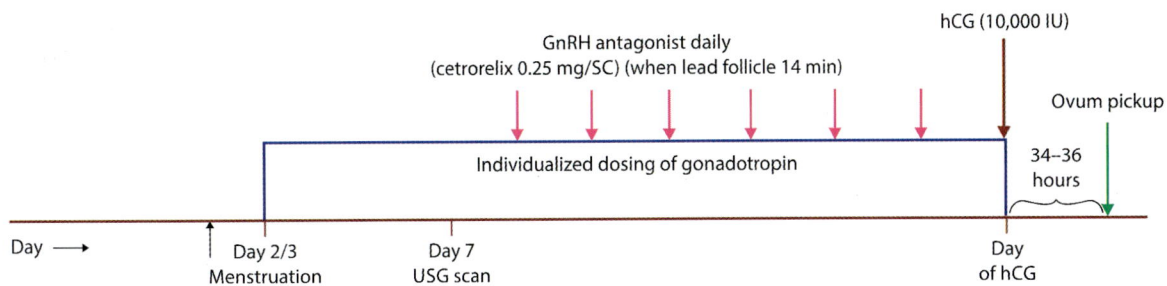

Fig. 41: Antagonist protocol.
Abbreviations: GnRH, gonadotropin-releasing hormone; hCG, human chorionic gonadotropin; USG, ultrasonography

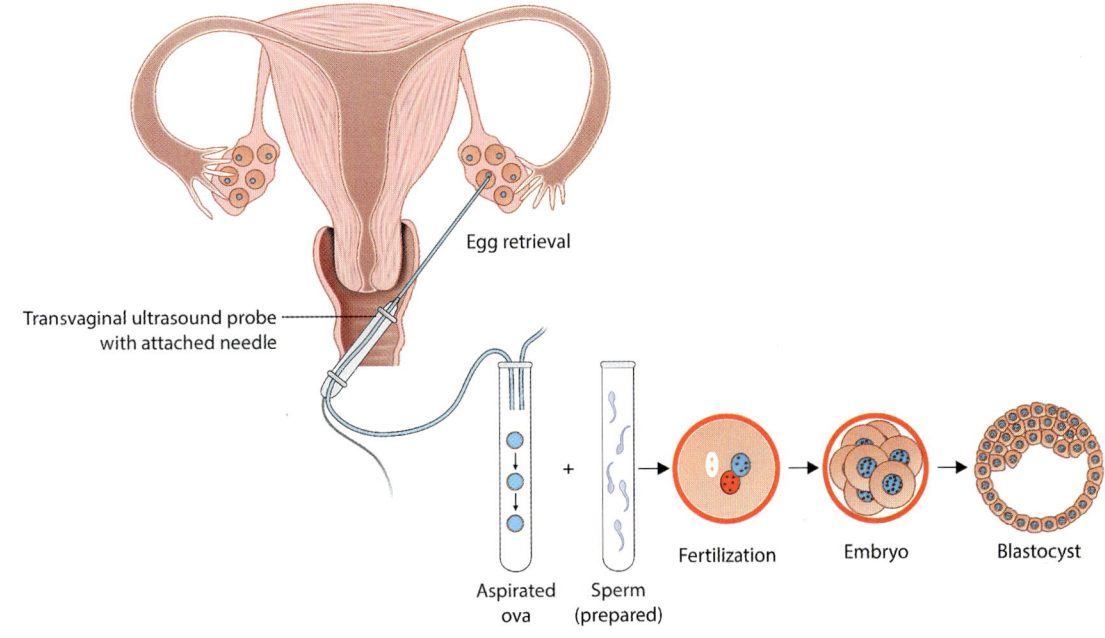

Fig. 42: Steps of in vitro fertilization.

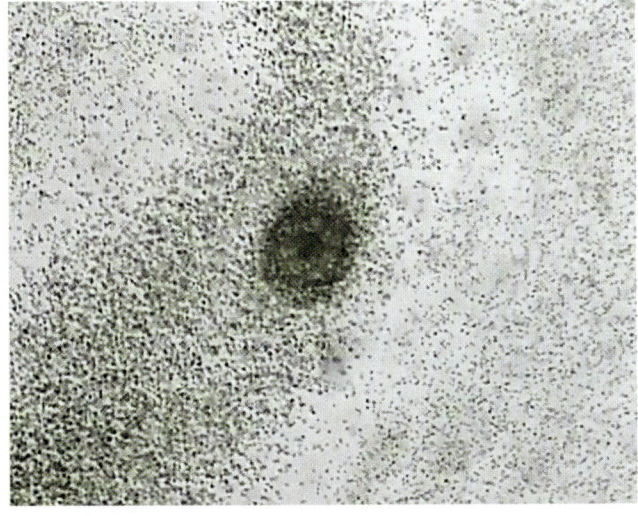

Fig. 43: Oocyte after retrieval and cumulus dispersal.
Courtesy: Dr Ratna Chattopadhyay, IRM, Kolkata

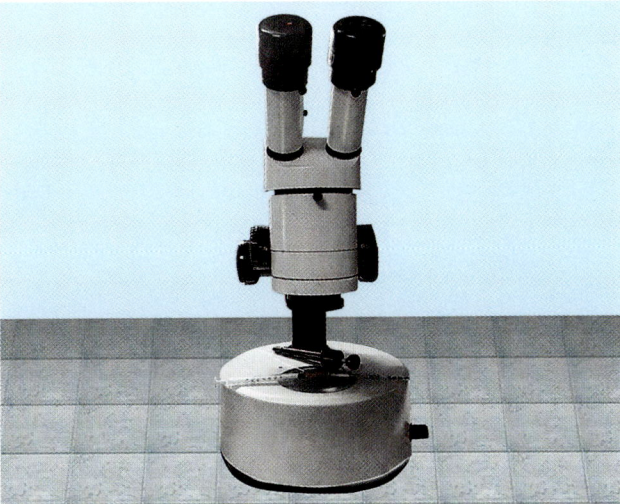

Fig. 44: Microscope.

SECTION 2: Clinical Cases

Mixing of Sperm and Ova, and In vitro Fertilization (Figs. 42 and 45 to 47)

- Sperm preparation is done as described later in IUI.
- The oocyte is inseminated by fresh or cryopreserved sperm. More than 50,000 sperms per egg are used.
- The mixture is incubated in the specialized incubator **(Fig. 45)**.
- Presence of formation of pronuclei after 18–20 hours indicates fertilization **(Fig. 46)** and allowed to cleave 2–4 cell stage when it is transferred into uterus **(Figs. 47 and 48)**.
- Transfer in the stage of blastocyst **(Fig. 49)** (which needs more time of culture outside) is also increasingly practiced in which less number of embryo is transferred to prevent

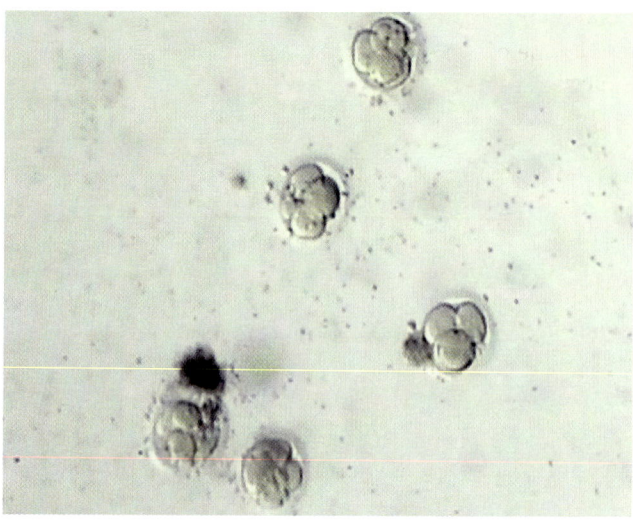

Fig. 47: Second day cleaved embryo—3 to 4 cells in each embryo.
Courtesy: Professor BN Chakravarty, IRM, Kolkata

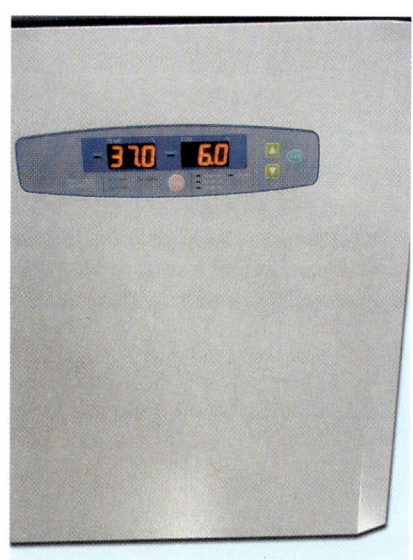

Fig. 45: Specialized incubator.

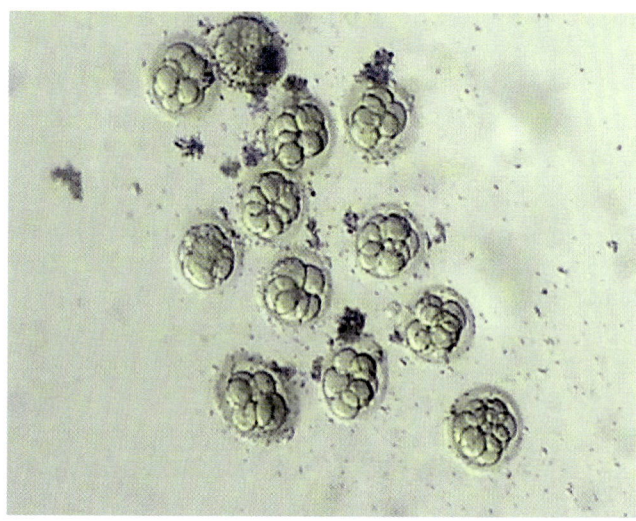

Fig. 48: Third day cleaved embryo (more than 4 cells).
Courtesy: IRM, Kolkata

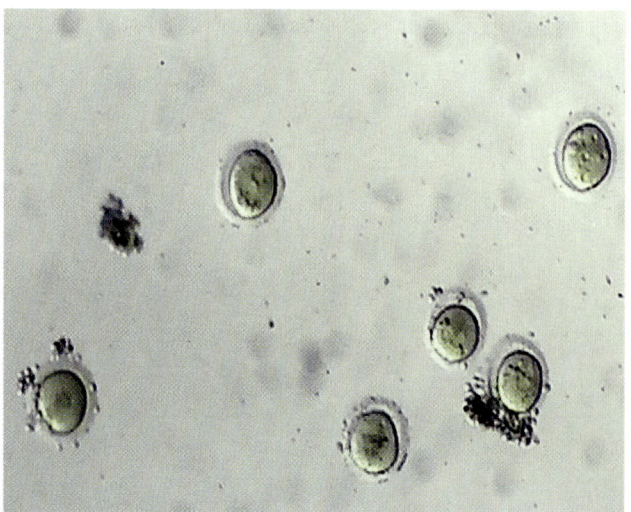

Fig. 46: Formation of pronucleus at 18–20 hours—multiple embryo (formation of pronuclei indicates fertilization).

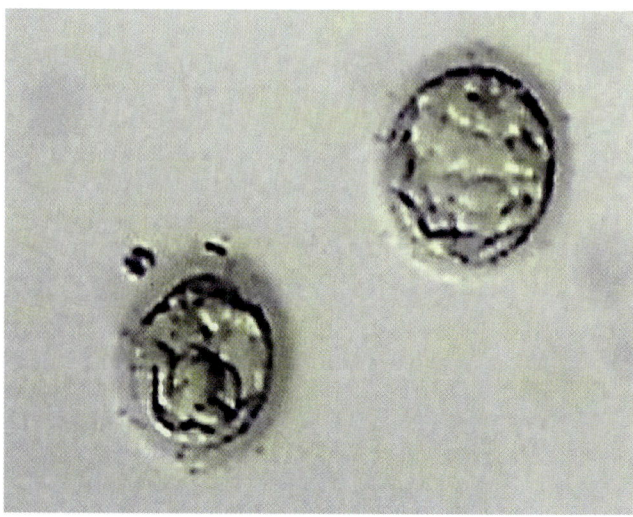

Fig. 49: Blastocyst (5–6 day).
Courtesy: IRM, Kolkata

multiple gestation and to make it more physiological as at the time of transfer synchronization of endometrial bed occurs.

Embryo Transfer (Figs. 50 to 52)

* With the help of an embryo transfer catheter **(Figs. 51 and 52)** 2–3 embryos in 0.15 to 0.3 mL of fluid are transferred after 46–48 hours of insemination little below (1 cm) the fundus.
* Abdominal sonographic guidance is very helpful during transfer.

Luteal Support

Luteal support is given by progesterone either in vaginal route or by intramuscular injection (50 mg IM/day). Injection hCG 2,000 IU biweekly used previously is not a good choice.

Results of IVF and ET

* Pregnancy rate: 25–30%
* Multiple pregnancy rate: 30%
* Take home baby: Less than 20%.

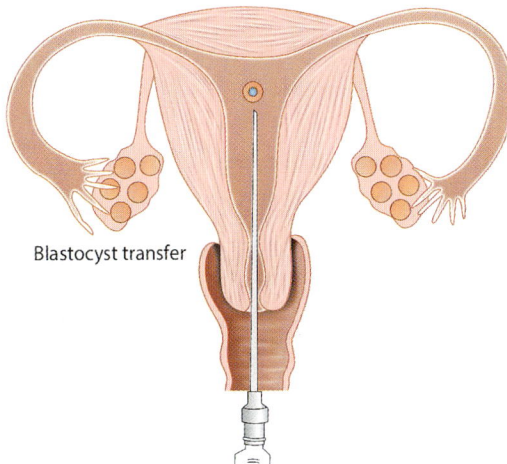
Blastocyst transfer

Fig. 50: Embryo transfer.

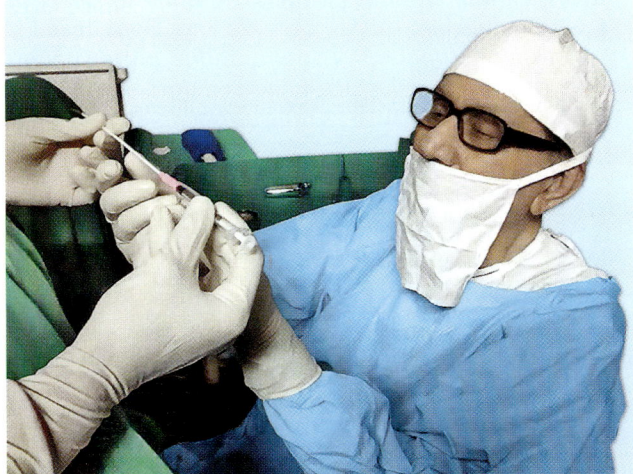

Fig. 51: Embryo transfer by Professor BN Chakravarty, Director, IRM, Kolkata, receiving the catheter containing embryo for transfer.

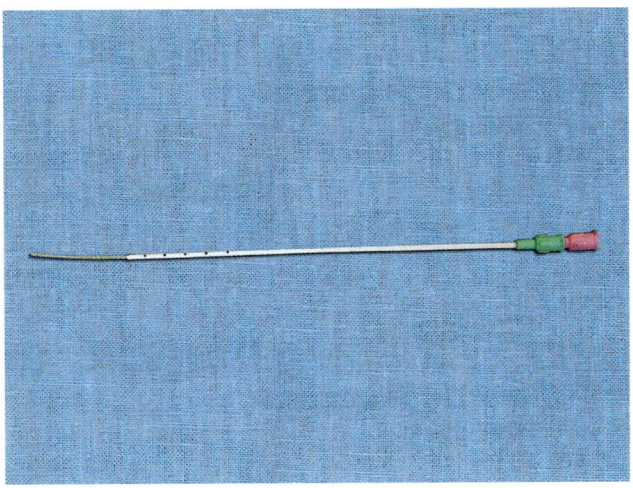

Fig. 52: Embryo transfer catheter.

World's first IVF-ET (test tube baby) Louise Brown was delivered in July 25, 1978 by Strepto and Edwards in Oldham.

First test tube baby of India, Durga (Kanupriya Agarwal) was born on 3rd October 1978 and was the second test tube baby of the world. Architect of first test tube baby of India is Dr Subhash Mukherjee who retrieved egg from the ovary after pulling down it through posterior colpotomy, fertilized outside and cryopreserved. He transferred the thawed embryo into the uterus in natural cycle.

Uterovaginal Surgery in Female Infertility

* Myomectomy in uterine fibroid
* Metroplasty in septate or subseptate uterus
* Adhesiolysis for uterine synechiae
* Fenton's operation in tight hymen/introitus (*see* later)
* Removal of vaginal septum
* Amputation of elongated cervix
* Gilliam's type operations for third degree retroversion of uterus if no other cause is found.

Treatment of Cervical Factor Infertility

* In chlamydia/microplasma infection—doxycycline (100 mg), bd × 2 weeks
* Intrauterine insemination (IUI)
* Assisted reproductive technology (ART): In vitro fertilization embryo transfer (IVF-ET), gamete intrafallopian transfer (GIFT), and zygote intrafallopian transfer (ZIFT).

SURROGACY (GESTATIONAL CARRIER SURROGACY)

Q. What is surrogacy?

This is one variant of IVF where fertilized egg (embryo) is transferred to the uterus of the surrogate, not to that of intended mother.

Indications

* Uterus absent like RKH, following hysterectomy, uncorrectable uterine defect

- Repeated unexplained miscarriage
- Carrying pregnancy is potential for severe health risk of woman.

Issues of Surrogacy

It involves psychological issues and various legal issues which will be guided by law of the concern state.

Uterine transplantation is an alternate to surrogacy. First pregnancy following uterine transplantation was reported by Brannstrom et al. (2014) from Sweden.

MANAGEMENT OF MALE FACTOR INFERTILITY

Different Modalities of Treatment for Male Subfertility

- General measures
- Medical management
- Surgical management: Vasovasostomy and epididymovasostomy:
  - Repair of varicocele, orchidopexy, surgery for hypospadias
- Artificial insemination: IUI
- Assisted reproductive technology: IVF and ET
- Intracytoplasmic sperm injection, percutaneous epididymal sperm aspiration (PESA), microsurgical epididymal sperm aspiration (MESA), and testicular sperm extraction (TESE)—ICSI, GIFT, and ZIFT
- Management of male sexual dysfunction.

General Measures

- Emotional support to reduce stress and sadness in both partners
- Change of lifestyle
- Ideal coital frequency, consisting of intercourse on multiple days during the "fertile window", which includes the 5 days preceding and the day of anticipated ovulation, should be reviewed with the couple
- Avoidance of alcohol, smoking, tobacco, and use of fertility—impairing medications.

Medical Management in Male Infertility—Very Little Role

- Hormonal—hCG, hMG, GnRH, testosterone, CC, thyroxin, bromocriptine, antibiotics, corticosteroids, and aromatase inhibitor
- Sperm vitalizing agents—pentoxifylline and kallikrein
- Empirical therapy
- Antioxidants—in increased ROS.

INTRAUTERINE INSEMINATION (IUI)

Washed sperms are injected inside the uterine cavity at the expected time of ovulation in stimulated cycle with proper monitoring of ovulation. Both fresh and frozen sperm can be used.

Indications of IUI

- *Male factor (mild and moderate)*:
  - Azoospermia with donor semen, oligospermia, asthenospermia, oligoasthenospermia, teratozoospermia, and delayed liquefaction
  - Primary count less than 10 million/mL has poor outcome
  - Other male factors are retrograde ejaculation and others like erectile dysfunction, ejaculatory dysfunction (severe hypospadias; retrograde ejaculation; impotence), neurological disorders—spinal cord injury, diabetic neuropathy, donor IUI in some cases of genetic defect.
- *Female factor*:
  - Unilateral tubal defect: Tubal excision as in ectopic and tubal occlusion as in endometriosis
  - Ovulatory dysfunction: PCOS and LPD
  - Others: Mild and moderate endometriosis with normal tubo-ovarian relationship, minimal endometriosis—unexplained and vaginismus
- Cervical factor: Abnormal PCT and cervical defect
- Immunological: Male and female
- Unexplained infertility.

Contraindications

- Cervical atresia
- Cervicitis
- Endometritis
- Bilateral tubal obstruction
- In most cases of amenorrhea or
- Severe seminopathy.

Basic Steps

Flowchart 2 shows the basic step of IUI

- Pretreatment counseling and screening
- Ovarian stimulation
- Monitoring of response to ovulation
- Semen collection
- Sperm preparation—commonly used method is "swim-up" technique and "density gradient" technique
- Insemination
- Postinsemination care—luteal support.

Pretreatment Counseling and Screening

- Detailed history taking, physical examination, and investigations of both partners are done to select for proper indication.

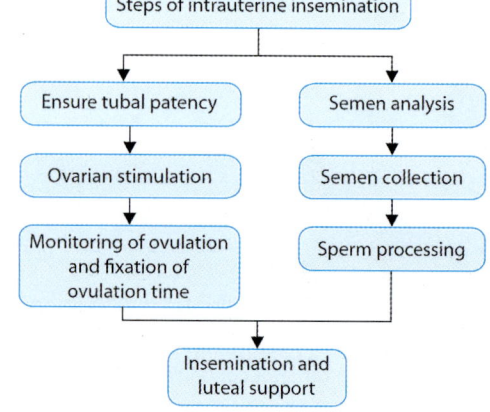

Flowchart 2: Basic steps of intrauterine insemination.

- Tubal patency is ensured.
- Serological screening (hepatitis B virus surface antigen, HIV, hepatitis C virus) is performed. Semen analysis and if necessary culture are done.
- Counseling is done for the treatment options and the probable results and informed consent taken.

Ovarian Stimulation

Intrauterine insemination is usually done in stimulated cycle mostly by clomiphene and sometimes gonadotropin is needed. One ampoule on day 3 and one ampoule on day 8 (soft protocol) is a good option instead of many ampoules as given in IVF cycle.

Monitoring

- Monitoring by clinical parameter (BBT and cervical mucus study) and serial ultrasound folliculometry are done from day 9/10.
- When follicular diameter becomes 18 mm and ET at least 7 mm (Serum E2 100–150 pg/one 18 mm follicle) exogenous hCG 5,000 IU is given IM which causes LH surge and ovulation is expected to occur 36 hours after hCG administration when insemination time is fixed up.

Semen Collection and Sperm Preparation

- Semen is collected in sterile container by masturbation. After liquefaction semen is processed by different methods. The purpose of all methods of sperm preparation is to eliminate seminal plasma containing abnormal sperms, antibody, prostaglandins, and other contaminants.
- Processed sperm will also contain large number of highly motile available sperms in concentrated form in small amount of media.
- Some chemical-like pentoxifylline sometimes added expecting to enhance motility.
- Unprocessed semen may cause prostaglandin-induced severe uterine contraction and there is chance of pelvic infection.

Sperm Preparation Techniques (Figs. 53 to 55)

There are several techniques. Commonly used techniques are:
- *"Swim-up technique"*
- *"Density Gradient Technique"*

Ham's F-10 media is widely used for sperm washing and colloidal suspension of silica particles are available as density gradient solution in different concentration.

Swip-up technique is sufficient for good semen sample. Density gradient is suitable for seminopathy.

Swim-up Technique (Fig. 56)

- Semen is collected by masturbation and allowed to liquefy which takes about 30 minutes (*see* **Fig. 28**).
- Liquid semen sample (**Fig. 53**) is mixed with equal amount of media and centrifuged at 1,000 rpm for 4–5 minutes.
- The supernatant fluid (**Fig. 54**) is decanted off and 2 mL media is added with the sperm pellet at the bottom of the tube and recentrifuged 1,000 rpm for 4–5 minutes.

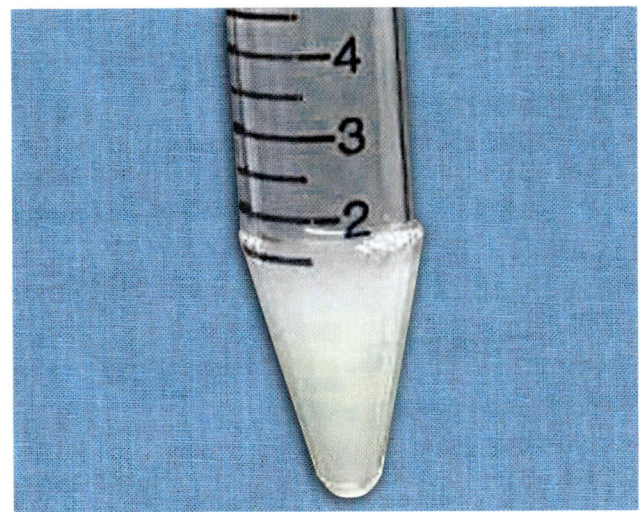

Fig. 53: Semen taken in test tube from the container after liquefaction.

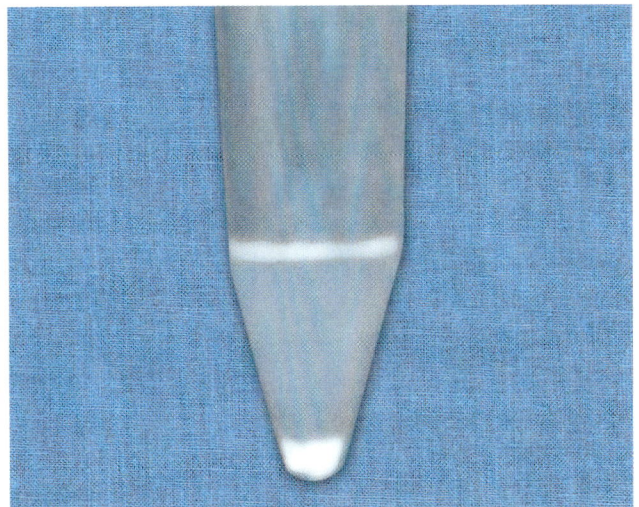

Fig. 54: Following centrifuge pellet is found at the bottom with supernatant fluid at upper part which is discarded.

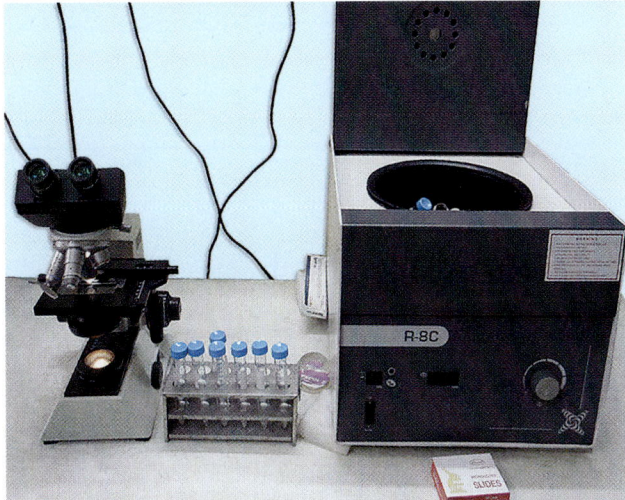

Fig. 55: Microscope and centrifuge machine in intrauterine insemination set-up.

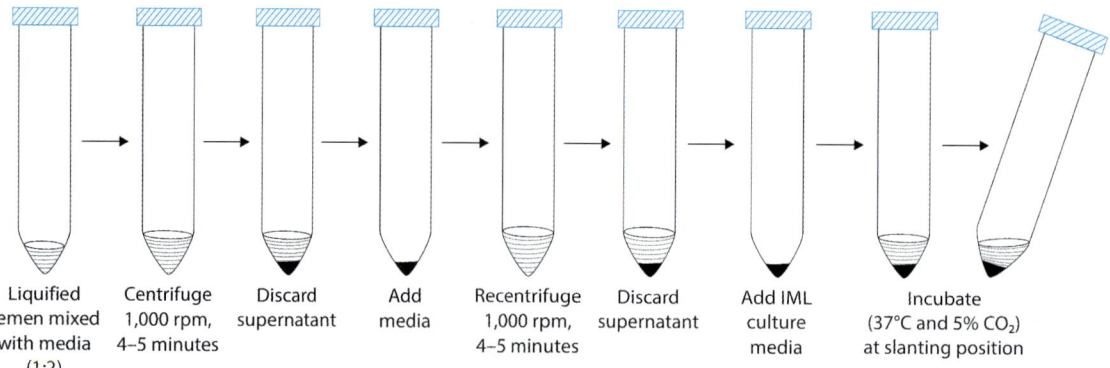

Fig. 56: Swim-up technique of semen preparation.
Courtesy: Dr Sunita Sharma, IRM, Kolkata

- Supernatant fluid is discarded and 1 mL of culture media is added incubated at 37°C and 5% CO_2 at 30° inclinations for 30–45 minutes when actively motile sperms swim up at the top of tube forming a cloud.
- Aspirate upper and middle part of cloud which contains maximum motile sperms with the help of IUI catheter fitted with syringe.
- Usually 0.3 to 0.5 mL of sperm suspension is taken for IUI.
- The percentage of motile sperm in final preparation should be 90%. Post wash motile sperm concentration should be 1 million/mL.

Layers Method of Density Gradient Centrifugation Technique (Fig. 57)

It can be done single-layer or double-layer method.

Double-layer Method

- Density gradient media is taken into the bottom of tube [in double layer first 80%, then 40% media **(Fig. 57)**], then about 2 mL liquid semen is poured gently over it.
- It is centrifuged at 1,500 rpm for 20 minutes and supernatant is discarded leaving pellet.
- Two mL of sperm wash media is added and mixed with pillet, then centrifuged at 1,000 rpm for 4–5 minutes, discard supernatant and leave pellet.
- Add 1 mL of sperm wash media and mixed well with pellet. Keep at 37° at 5% CO_2 for 10–15 minutes—sample ready for IUI.
- Alternatively at the last part sperm wash media is added gently without disturbing pellet and incubated for 30–45 minutes and upper part of suspension is aspirated (like swim up) for insemination.

In swim-up technique, speed should be restricted to 800–1,000/rpm and time should not exceed 5 minutes. In density gradient method, the optimum time of centrifugation is 1,500–2,000 rpm and should be completed within 20 minutes to protect the sperm from damage. High speed and longer time centrifugation damage the sperms.

Insemination (Figs. 58 and 59)

- 0.3 mL of processed sperm filled in IUI syringe fitted with catheter **(Fig. 58)** is introduced inside uterine cavity by

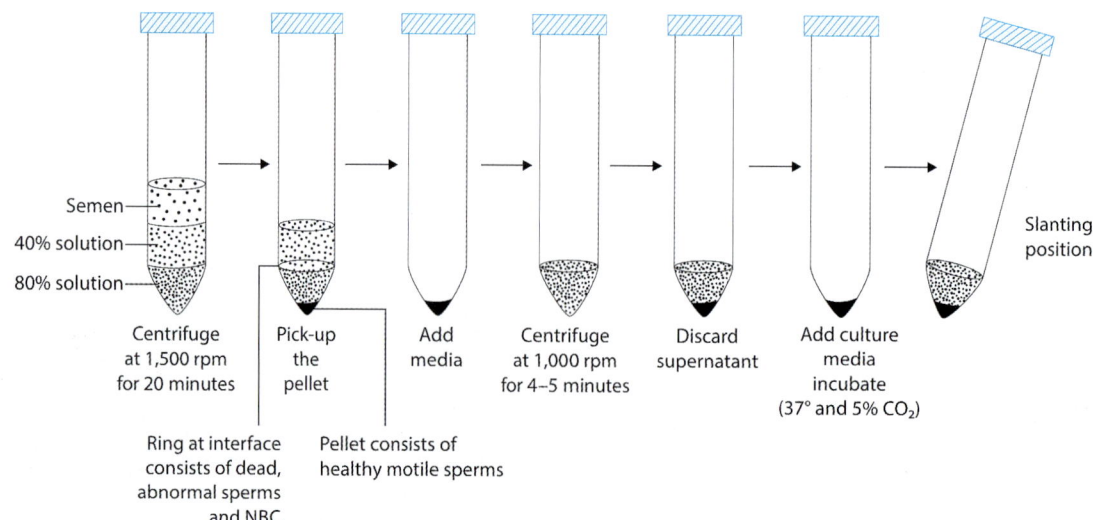

Fig. 57: Double layer density gradient centrifugation technique.
Courtesy: Dr Sunita Sharma, IRM, Kolkata

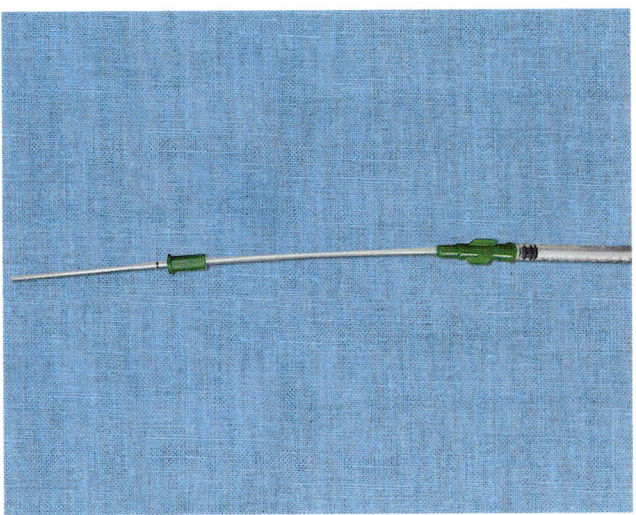

Fig. 58: Intrauterine insemination cannula.

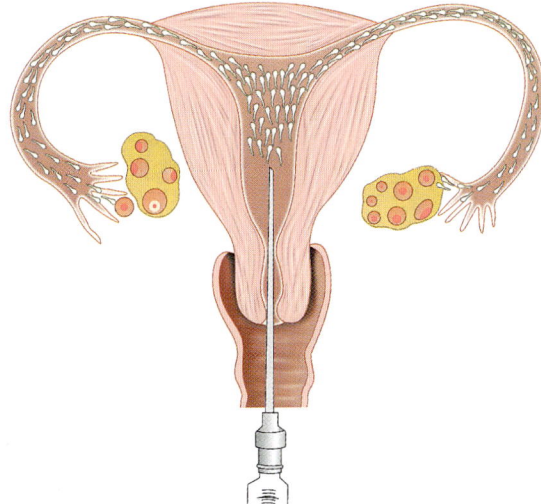

Fig. 59: Intrauterine insemination (schematic representation).

insemination cannula at the expected time of ovulation which is 32–36 hour following ovulation.
* Procedure should be atraumatic and bloodless.

Luteal Support
Luteal support is given by injection hCG or progesterone in natural cycle. In stimulated cycle natural progesterone in vaginal route is preferred.

Q. How many IUI should be attempted for the patient?
Maximum success occurs within 3 cycles. IUI should be switched off to other method after 6 cycles.

Complications
These are very few and rarely severe— cramping, spotting, infection, OHSS, and multiple pregnancy.

Results
Clinical pregnancy in IUI with husband's semen is 10–25% and with donor semen is 20–40%.

Result is expected to be good when in semen sample sperm motility is more than or equal to 30% and sperm count is more than 10 million total. In severe OAT, result is extremely poor.

Q. What are the different types of artificial inseminations?
* Intravaginal
* Intracervical and pericervical
* Intrauterine insemination
* Fallopian tube sperm perfusion
* Intraperitoneal insemination
* Intrafollicular insemination.

> **History of Artificial Insemination**
> Deposition of semen artificially into the genital tract is known from as early as third century. The first documented use of artificial insemination with husband's semen (AIH) was in 1770 by John Hunter who inseminated a woman using a quill with the semen of her husband who had hypospadias.
> First successful donor insemination was done by Joseph Pancoast in 1884.

INTRACYTOPLASMIC SPERM INJECTION

Intracytoplasmic sperm injection (ICSI) involves the direct insertion of a single sperm cell into the cytoplasm of a single oocyte by micropuncture **(Fig. 60)**.

Indications of ICSI
* Severe oligoasthenoteratozoospermia (OAT)
* Obstructive azoospermia by MESA, PESA, and TESA
* Nonobstructive azoospermia by TESE
* Unexplained infertility.

Procedure of ICSI (Figs. 60 to 63)
* In this method, the oocyte is stabilized with the micropipette, usually with the polar body at 6 or 12 o'clock position
* A microneedle containing a single sperm punctures the zona pellucida at 3 o'clock position from the opposite site and enters the ooplasmic membrane where a single sperm is injected directly into the ooplasm.

Sources of Sperm in ICSI
* Ejaculated sperm
* Microsurgical epididymal sperm aspiration (MESA)
* Percutaneous epididymal sperm aspiration (PESA) **(Fig. 64)**
* Testicular sperm extraction (TESE)
* Testicular sperm aspiration (TESA)

Epididymal Sperm Aspiration
In case of vasal block or very low count sperm is aspirated from the epididymis either macroscopically (PESA) or microscopically (MESA). **PESA** is a blind procedure and retrieval of sperm is less. In **MESA**, microscope and expertization are needed but sperm retrieval is good.

SECTION 2: Clinical Cases

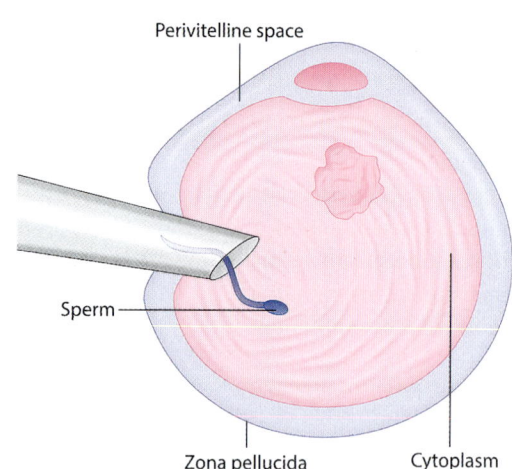

Fig. 60: Diagrammatic presentation of intracytoplasmic sperm injection.

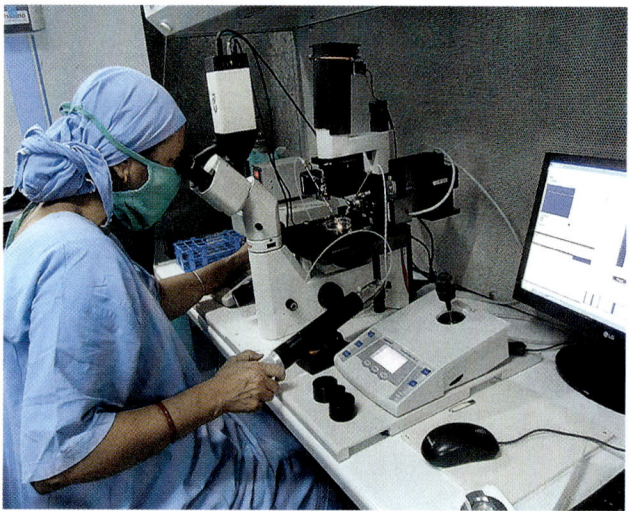

Fig. 61: Intracytoplasmic sperm injection procedure with microscope and monitor.
Courtesy: Dr Ratna Chattopadhyay, IRM, Kolkata

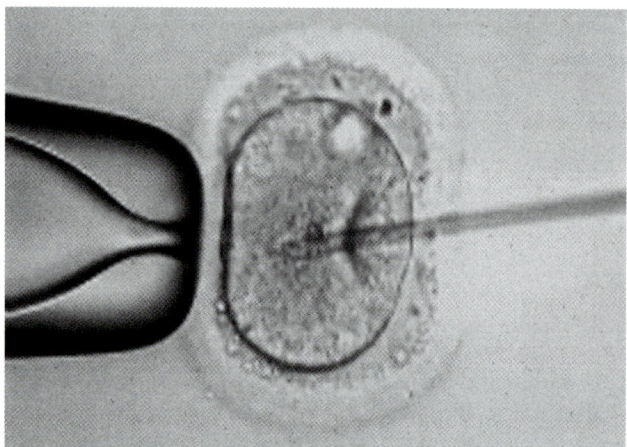

Fig. 62: ICSI oocyte is stabilized with the micropipette, microneedle containing a single sperm punctures—the zona pellucida and sperm is injected directly into ooplasm.

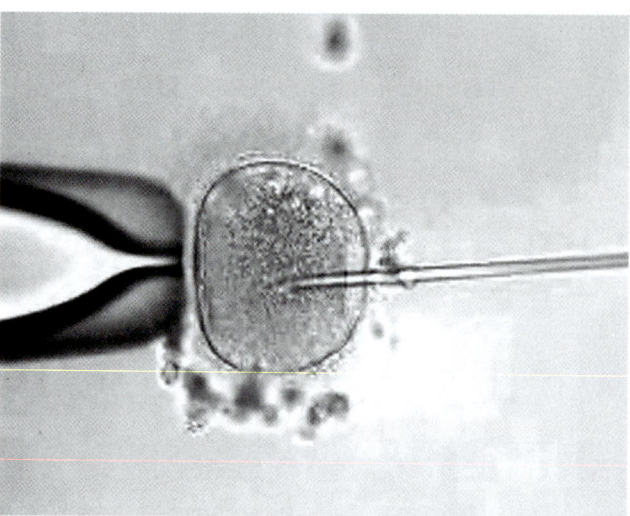

Fig. 63: Intracytoplasmic sperm injection.
Courtesy: Dr Ratna Chattopadhyay, IRM, Kolkata

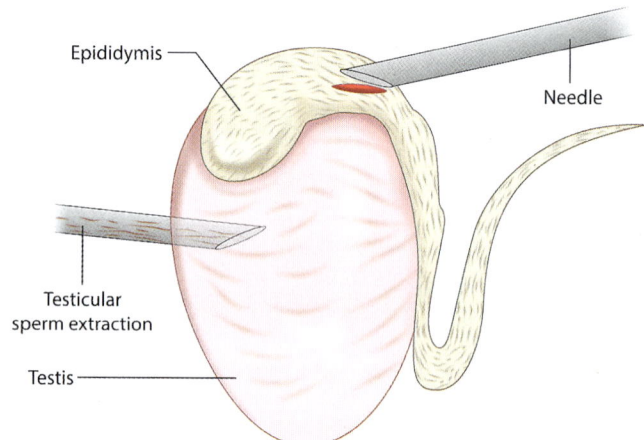

Fig. 64: Percutaneous epididymal sperm aspiration (PESA).

Advantages of ICSI

- Intracytoplasmic sperm injection has revolutionized in treatment of male infertility and more definitive procedure like tubal block in female infertility.
- In severe OAT, fertilization and pregnancy can be achieved by ICSI. Even an azoospermic man may become biological father by TESA and TESE-ICSI.
- Success rate is reasonably good.

Results of ICSI

- Fertilization rate: 60–70%
- Pregnancy rate: 20–40%/embryo transfer

Male partner having abnormal karyotype in Y-chromosome microdeletion should undergo genetic counseling before ICSI.

First pregnancy by ICSI was reported in 1992 by Palermo (Palermo G, Joris H, Devroey P, Van Stierteghem AC. Lancet. 1992)

Other ART Procedures (Micromanipulation)

- Gamete intrafallopian transfer (GIFT)
- Zygote intrafallopian transfer (ZIFT)
- Partial zona dissection (PZD)
- Subzonal sperm insertion (SUZI)

Gamete Intrafallopian Transfer (GIFT)

- It is a procedure where oocytes are retrieved like IVF under COH but instead of IVF mixture of oocytes (usually 2-3 oocytes) and processed sperm (50,000 to 100,000) are placed in the fallopian tube via fimbria by catheter through laparoscopic approach.
- Indication is unexplained infertility and seminopathy.
- At least one tube must be patent.
- It was popular in late 1980s but improve IVF technique has largely replaced it, only indication is ethical and religious ground.

Zygote Intrafallopian Transfer (ZIFT)

- It is like GIFT. Instead of transfer of oocyte, sperm mixture fertilized ova (zygote) is transferred to fallopian tube directly through laparoscopy.
- If zygote is cleaved, it is called tubal embryo transfer (TET)
- It is also rarely done except when very difficult transcervical transfer.

Oocyte Donation

- Oocyte donation has become now a treatment modality where the recipient lacks the competent oocyte.
- The indications are: (A) primary ovarian failure like Turner syndrome; (B) premature ovarian failure; (C) poor ovarian reserve; (D) poor quality oocyte or embryo especially in advanced age; (E) surgical removal of ovaries; (F) radiotherapy and chemotherapy.
- Donors are volunteer or known with previously sterilized or excess oocyte from IVF program.

Embryo Donation

It is done in some women in perimenopausal or menopausal age where husband is also subfertile.

Cryopreservation of Semen, Oocyte, Embryo, and Ovarian Tissue

- Use of cryopreserved semen is an old procedure and known for centuries with different indication.
- Cryopreservation of the excess embryo of IVF program has now almost routine as the embryos can be stored to utilize in later cycle if fresh embryo transfer fails or couple wants further child.
- The advantage of use of cryopreserved embryo is that superovulation is not needed and chance of OHSS is eliminated.
- Cryopreservation of oocyte and ovarian tissue is more challenging and needs ultrafreezing technique (vitrification).

In Vitro Maturation (IVM)

Antral follicle is aspirated from unstimulated cycle and the immature oocytes are cultured to achieve meiosis and maturity. This is very useful in PCOS where there is high risk of serious OHSS on stimulation.

Intravaginal Culture (IVC)

In IVC system fertilization and embryo maturation occur in vivo.

Peri-implantation Genetic Diagnosis (PGD) or Screening of Genetic Disorder (Fig. 65)

- In this process, genetic abnormalities of eggs or embryo are identified before transfer.
- Genuine indication is where there is risk of transmission of hereditary disease. Indications are recurrent miscarriage, repeated IVF failure, and advanced maternal age. Screening is also done to detect aneuploidy developed from gamete meiotic errors.
- During this technique, cells are extracted from developing embryo **(Fig. 65)** and tested for structural aberrations/or aneuploidy. Damage of good embryo is a concern.

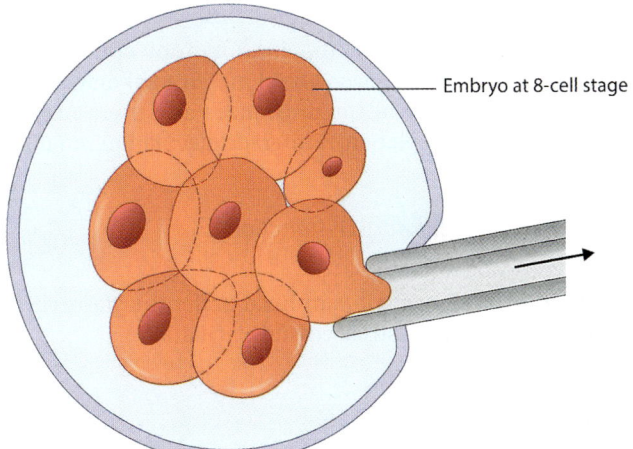

Fig. 65: Preimplantation genetic diagnosis (PGD)—cells are extracted from developing embryo for genetic aberration.

Q. What do you mean by assisted reproductive technology?

Assisted reproductive technology is a procedure which requires extraction and isolation of an *oocyte*. IUI in true sense is not an ART procedure where only sperm is handled.

TREATMENT OF ERECTILE AND EJACULATORY DYSFUNCTION

Erectile failure and ejaculatory failure are important causes of male infertility.

Erectile Dysfunction

- Impotency (erectile failure) refers to consistent inability to get and keep an erection suitable for coitus.
- The important causes of impotency are psychological (15%) and organic disease (85%) like diabetes, vascular

disease, neurological, some drugs, following trauma, and surgery. It may be genetic or endocrine origin.

Psychological impotence can be distinguished from organic by NPT (nocturnal penile tumescence) test (*see* Page 263).

Treatment is directed to the cause of impotence.

Treatment of Erectile Dysfunction

- Withdrawal of drugs.
- Treatment of underlying cause.
- Psychosexual therapy.
- Local injection: Injection alprostadil is better than papaverine. Priapism may be a problem.
- Vacuum pump.
- Transurethral pellet and penile implant.
- Sildenafil (Viagra), tadalafil, vardenafil—sildenafil citrate is called "anti-potency pill" and taken 1 hour before coitus and lasts for 1–4 hours. To act Viagra needs some degree of erection.

Ejaculatory Dysfunction

- An ejaculation is failure to ejaculate may be either situational or total.
- In situational ejaculation, man cannot ejaculate in certain situation or place like clinic. In total ejaculation does not occur in all circumstances and there may be anorgasm anejaculation, retrograde ejaculation or failure of emission.

Treatment of Ejaculatory Dysfunction

- Psychosexual therapy.
- Vibrator: Placing of vibrator head under the glans elicits ejaculatory reflex and successful ejaculation.
- Electroejaculation.

Retrograde Ejaculation

In this problem, semen instead of coming outside enters into the urinary bladder and patient feels sensation of orgasm.

Treatment Options of Retrograde Ejaculation

- Coitus in full bladder.
- Alpha adrenergic or cholinergic drugs.
- Insemination with post-voided urine after processing.

Treatment Options of Premature Ejaculation

- Use of condom
- Pelvic floor exercise
- Squeeze techniques
- Intrauterine insemination (IUI) with ejaculated sperm.

AZOOSPERMIA

Definition of Azoospermia

Absence of sperm in semen is called azoospermia.

Prevalence

About 1% of all male and 8% in infertile male.

Types

- *Obstructive azoospermia*: Congenital bilateral absence of vas deferens (CBAVD), vasectomy, and severe infection of vas and epididymis. In 80% of men with CBAVD mutation of *CFTR* gene (cystic fibrosis transmembrane conductance regular gene) is found. All male of cystic fibrosis essentially have CBAVD.
- *Nonobstructive azoospermia*: It is due to testicular failure; reasons are testicular damage due to any reason and genetic.
  Examples of genetic cause are Klinefelter syndrome where there is abnormality in karyotype (47 XXY).
  Other is microdeletion of AZF in the *long arm* of Y chromosome, here karyotype is normal. Presence of AZF is essential for normal spermatogenesis.
  Three nonoverlapping intervals within the AZF region (AZFa, AZFb, and AZFc) have been identified and microdeletions involving these regions are found in some infertile men. Viable sperms are not found in AZFa and AZFb microdeletion but found in AZFc microdeletion. Careful centrifugation and analysis of semen a small number of sperms can be identified and IVF can be done. Other rare example of abnormal karyotype is 46XX male. Here 'translocation' of SRY segment occurs from Y chromosome in 46XX individual. This accidental 'translocation' occurs at the time of fertilization from father's Y chromosome to nondisjuncted X chromosome of the developing zygote.

Diagnosis

- Diagnosis is done by repeated semen analysis. Before reaching diagnosis semen sample should be centrifuged and analysis done.
- To differentiate between obstructive and nonobstructive by clinical examination, palpation of testes, vas and epididymis, hormone assays, vasography, and testicular biopsy. Gonadotropin will be high in testicular failure and is normal in obstructive type.

Treatment

Artificial insemination with donor (AID) semen, also called TDI (therapeutic donor insemination). Other treatment options are:

- *Obstructive*: Surgery in the form of vasovasostomy and vasoepididymostomy is possible in vasectomy and ejaculatory duct obstruction cases. CBAVD is not treatable surgically. TESE and ICSI (TESE-ICSI) is performed to achieve pregnancy. PESA and MESA with ICSI is possible.
- *Nonobstructive*: In many cases isolated areas of sperm cells are found (47 XXY, AZFc) and TESE-ICSI is possible.

KLINEFELTER SYNDROME (47 XXY) (FIGS. 26, 27 AND 66)

Prevalence
It is 1 in 500 men in general population and accounts 1–2% of male infertility, 14% of all azoospermic male.
    Sex chromosome DSD

Phenotype
It is observed in male. Classically, these males are tall, undervirilized (less beard and mustache), gynecomastia and small, firm testes (*see* **Figs. 26 and 27**, Page 263).

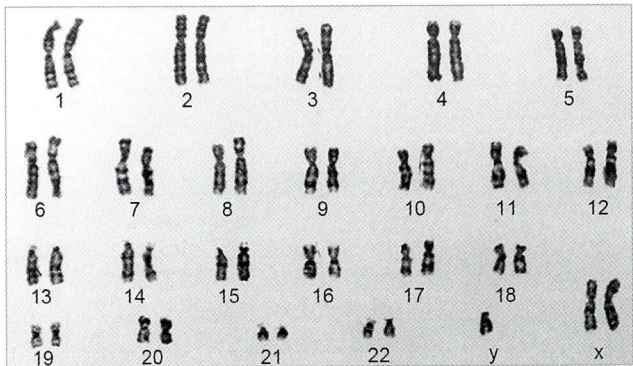

Fig. 66: 47 XXY karyotype.

Karyotype
Karyotype of Klinefelter syndrome is 47 XXY (**Fig. 66**). 10% mosaic and they can achieve natural conception.

Semen Analysis
Semen analysis shows azoospermia. On centrifugation of semen sample sperms can be retrieved.

Diagnosis
Clinical as above, semen analysis (azoospermia), karyotype (47 XXY), and high FSH.

Treatment
- In mosaic cases natural conception may occur
- TESE-ICSI if sperm cell is found in testicular biopsy
- Therapeutic donor insemination (TDI)-IUI with donor semen.

VAGINISMUS

Vaginismus is a condition where there is contraction of pelvic muscles including gluteal muscle associated with adduction of thighs during the attempt of coitus or even gynecological examination and successful intercourse is not possible.

Cause
It is mostly psychogenic. Newly married woman often becomes afraid of intercourse. There may be history of forceful coitus. There may be associated local pathology like tender fissure in hymen and vaginitis, etc.

Management
It can be managed by proper sex education and psychological reassurance. In mild cases, use of lubricant and local anesthesia may help. Tranquilizers, antispasmodic, and erotic love play may initiate gradual coitus. She may be cured following pregnancy and vaginal delivery.

In severe form, attempt of coitus is avoided initially. Use of dilators helping by the provider and later by self-introduction in front of mirror may regain her confidence, and apprehension gradually passes off. If there is tight hymenal ring, Fenton's operation is done.

Fenton's Operation
Indication: Done in tough hymen, not so useful in vaginismus.

Procedure: Under general anesthesia a transverse incision is given at the mucocutaneous junction of fourchette.

Posterior mucosa is dissected above the hymenal ring. The hymenal ring is longitudinally cut and perineal muscles are also incised vertically. The vaginal flap margins are repaired transversely.

Success is possible if there is no vaginismus of psychological origin.

UNEXPLAINED INFERTILITY

Prevalence of unexplained infertility may be as high as 30% among infertile couple. When the basic evaluation of infertility shows normal semen parameter, tubes are patent and there is evidence of ovulation with regular coitus and without any obvious cause of infertility this is called unexplained infertility.

The diagnosis of unexplained infertility is reached on the available diagnosed tests. The problem is that the tests may be incomplete and may not be reliable and there is also limitation of technology available to diagnose all cases of infertility.

The probable mechanism of unexplained infertility may be unexplored mechanisms of luteinized unruptured follicle syndrome, immunological factors, infection, undiagnosed pelvic pathology, occult seminal factor and oocyte factor.

Expectant management is considered in case of young woman and with short duration of marriage. Couple can be assured that there is 20% chance of pregnancy after one year, even they have attempted already for twelve months prior and there is chance of 50% couples to be conceived in next 36 months. As treatment is often sought for, superovulation, intrauterine insemination and even ART are attempted to achieve pregnancy.

CHAPTER 12

A Case of Polycystic Ovarian Syndrome and Hirsutism

Chapter Outline

Writing a case of PCOS and how to present the case?
- Diagnosis and Diagnostic Criteria of PCOS
- Short-term and Long-term Complications of PCOS
- Etiopathogenesis of PCOS
- Adolescent PCOS
- Management of PCOS Including Hirsutism, Acne and Infertility

Hirsutism
- Definition, Causes and Evaluation
- Androgens—Types and Sources
- Approach and Management in a Case of Hirsutism
- Physiology of Hair

A CASE OF POLYCYSTIC OVARY SYNDROME

A case of polycystic ovary syndrome (PCOS) may present with secondary amenorrhea, infertility, and hirsutism. So, one should be prepared to face the questions related to these topics.

PATIENT'S PARTICULAR

1. Name:
2. Age:
3. Address:
4. Occupation:
5. Married/unmarried:
6. History of infertility:
7. Husband's occupation:
8. Socioeconomic status:
9. Religion:
10. Parous/nulliparous:

Bed No.:
Date of admission:
Date of examination:

HISTORY

- *Chief complaint/complaints:* Patient usually complains of menstrual abnormality like oligomenorrhea, amenorrhea and/or there may be complain of excessive growth of hair over faces or other body surfaces.
- In married woman, presenting symptom may be infertility. If the presenting symptom is infertility, it is better to give the diagnosis of infertility as primary diagnosis the cause of which is polycystic ovary syndrome (PCOS).
- *History of present illness:* Chief complaints are elaborated. Duration of abnormality of menstrual period, mode of onset, and features of hyperandrogenism with onset and severity are noted.
  - History of alopecia, hoarseness of voice, and enlargement of clitoris are taken.
  - History of childhood problems, galactorrhea or any feature of hypothyroidism is recorded.
  Any increase in weight is also noted.
- *Menstrual history:* Detailed menstrual history is taken. To diagnose oligomenorrhea number of menstrual period would be *eight or less* in 1 year.
  - Last menstrual period (LMP)
  - Duration of menstruation

- Interval in days
- Age of menarche
- Regularity of cycle
- Pain during period/if pain relation with menstruation
- Amount of bleeding
- Clot
- Intermenstrual bleeding
- If amenorrhea—primary or secondary?

❖ *Obstetric history*: If parous parity, living issue and last child birth (LCB) are noted. Written in tabular form.
❖ *Past history*:
  - *Medical*: Hypertension, diabetes, and thyroid disorder
  - *Surgical*: If any, history of laparoscopy.
❖ *Family history*: Diabetes and hypertension
❖ *Sexual history*
❖ *Functional history*
❖ *Personal history*
❖ *Contraceptive history*
❖ *Drug history/treatment history:* Any medication particularly hormone, shaving or any mechanical method for treatment of hirsutism.

PHYSICAL EXAMINATION

Detailed general survey are done and noted. The points relevant to this case are:
❖ Height
❖ Weight
❖ Body mass index (BMI)
❖ Obesity: Android or gynecoid type
❖ Secondary sexual character and galactorrhea
❖ Acne, acanthosis nigricans, temporal balding, and enlargement of clitoris if any
❖ If there is hirsutism, scoring is done by Ferriman–Gallwey Scoring System (modified). Total nine body areas are examined. Score 0 to 4 for each area, 0 = no hirsutism; 4 = severe hirsutism. Total maximum score may be 36.
Total score 8 or more—hirsutism. Mild: 8–15; Moderate: 16–25; Severe hirsutism: >25 (*see* below).
❖ Pulse
❖ BP

Systemic Examination

Breasts examination—presence of galactorrhea searched for.

GYNECOLOGICAL EXAMINATION

Abdominal Examination

Any abdominal or abdominopelvic lump.

Per Vaginal Examination

❖ Inspection—clitorial enlargement.
❖ Speculum examination
❖ Palpation—to look for any congenital or acquired abnormality especially in secondary amenorrhea cases. Not done in unmarried virgin.

INVESTIGATIONS SUPPLIED OR REQUIRED

Ultrasonography of pelvis—12 or more antral follicles in either ovary ranging in size from 2 mm to 9 mm in diameter and/or increased ovarian volume (not less than 10 mm^3).

Hormones

❖ Increased luteinizing hormone (LH) and normal follicle-stimulating hormone (FSH) with elevated LH and FSH ratio (>2:1)
❖ Androgen (testosterone and $DHSO_4$) may be normal to twofold elevated
❖ Fasting insulin increased
❖ Abnormal glucose tolerance test (GTT)—fasting and 2 hours after 75 g of glucose
❖ Decreased sex hormone-binding globulin (SHBG)
❖ Abnormal lipid profile
❖ Prolactin may be mildly elevated in 10–25% cases
❖ Thyroid-stimulating hormone (TSH)
❖ Anti-Mullerian hormone (AMH)—usually elevated
❖ Other hormones to exclude other causes of hyperandrogenism, e.g., 17-hydroxyprogesterone (OHP) and adrenocorticotropic hormone (ACTH) stimulation test to exclude congenital adrenal hyperplasia (CAH) and dexamethasone suppression test and 24 hours urinary free cortisol level for Cushing syndrome, etc.

SUMMARY OF THE CASE (SAMPLE)

A 21-year-old unmarried woman has complaint of oligomenorrhea (<8 menses in last 1 year), amenorrhea for last 2 years and excessive growth of facial hair for 1 year.

On physical examination, her BMI is ......, BP ... with significant acne over facies......there is excessive growth of hair over facies and other body surface with Ferriman–Gallwey score of......... and presence of acanthosis nigricans over back of neck with normal secondary sex character. Her gynecological examination revealed no abnormality.

Ultrasonography of pelvis shows bilateral polycystic ovaries and LH:FSH ratio high with insulin level....., testosterone level and GTT is abnormal (give level if available).

Body areas	Upper lip	Chin	Chest	Upper abdomen	Lower abdomen	Upper arm	Thighs	Upper back	Lower back/buttock	Total score
Score										

Provisional Diagnosis

A 21-year-old woman with PCOS with hirsutism.

Differential Diagnosis

Q. Why are you saying this is a case of polycystic ovary syndrome?

As 21-year-old unmarried woman has the following features:
- Oligomenorrhea with occasional amenorrhea
- High BMI (......) indicating obesity
- Features of hyperandrogenism—acne and hirsutism
- Ultrasonography shows morphologically polycystic ovary.

Q. What is PCOS?

It is a complex disorder which is characterized by an array of clinical, endocrinal, and metabolic manifestations. It is a multifactorial endocrine disorder, usually involving peripheral insulin resistance.

Q. What are the diagnostic criteria of PCOS?

Polycystic ovary syndrome is diagnosed commonly by Rotterdam criteria 2003 (*see* below).
- Diagnostic criteria of PCOS was first reported by National Institute of Health (NIH) in 1990.
- It was revised by Rotterdam PCOS diagnostic criteria in 2003 which is most widely used.
- Further in 2006 Androgen Excess and PCOS Society (AE-PCOS S) defined in similar manner but viewed as a syndrome of androgen excess.

The diagnostic criteria given by three groups are given in **Table 1**. Of these three, Rotterdam criteria are widely practiced.

Other androgen excess or related disorders are CAH, androgen secreting tumors, and Cushing syndrome. PCOS is a diagnosis of exclusion.

DIAGNOSIS OF PCOS

- *Symptoms*: Menstrual irregularity
- *Signs*: Features of hyperandrogenism—hirsutism, acne, oily skin, any features of virilization (clitoromegaly, balding, deepening of voice, and reduced breasts size) the presence of which indicate probability of ovarian neoplasm.
  - Acanthosis nigricans
  - Obesity
  - External genitalia—clitoromegaly (clitoral length × width in mm >35 mm^2 is abnormal)
- Ovarian morphology on sonography (TVS)—multiple small hypoechoic cysts **(Fig. 1)**
- *Hormone levels*:
  - Changes in PCOS (as below)
  - To exclude other disorder.
- *Laparoscopy*: Typical picture enlarged ovary with white thick cortex with multiple small cysts without any mature follicle or no sign of ovulation **(Fig. 2)**.

Q. What types of menstrual abnormalities are found in PCOS?

The typical pattern is oligomenorrhea and amenorrhea followed by unpredictable heavy menstrual bleeding. It is due to unopposed estrogen action resulting thickened endometrium.

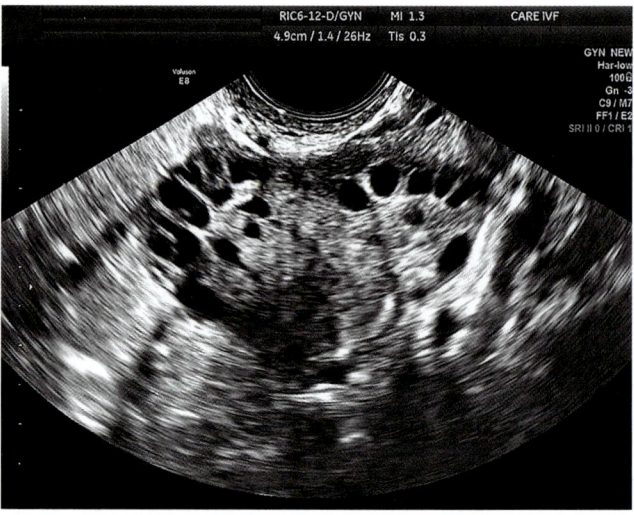

Fig. 1: Transvaginal sonography showing polycystic ovarian morphology with multiple small hypoechoic cysts.
Courtesy: Professor Kamal Oswal, VIMS, Kolkata

Table 1: Diagnostic criteria of PCOS.

NIH, 1990	Rotterdam, 2003	AE-PCOS Society, 2006
Both of the following*	At least two of the following*	Clinical and/or biochemical signs of hyperandrogenism and at least one of the following*
1. Chronic anovulation evident by oligo- or amenorrhea 2. Clinical and/or biochemical signs of hyperandrogenism (with exclusion of other etiologies, e.g., congenital adrenal hyperplasia) with or without polycystic ovaries on ultrasound	1. Chronic anovulation evident by oligo- or amenorrhea 2. Clinical and/or biochemical signs of hyperandrogenism 3. Polycystic ovaries (by ultra-sound)	1. Clinical and/or biochemical signs of hyperandrogenism and at least one of the following: – Ovarian dysfunction (oligo/anovulation and/or) – Polycystic ovarian morphology

*After exclusion of the diseases that produce a similar clinical picture.
Abbreviations: NIH, National Institute of Health; PCOS, polycystic ovary syndrome; AE-PCOS, Androgen excess and PCOS

CHAPTER 12: A Case of Polycystic Ovarian Syndrome and Hirsutism

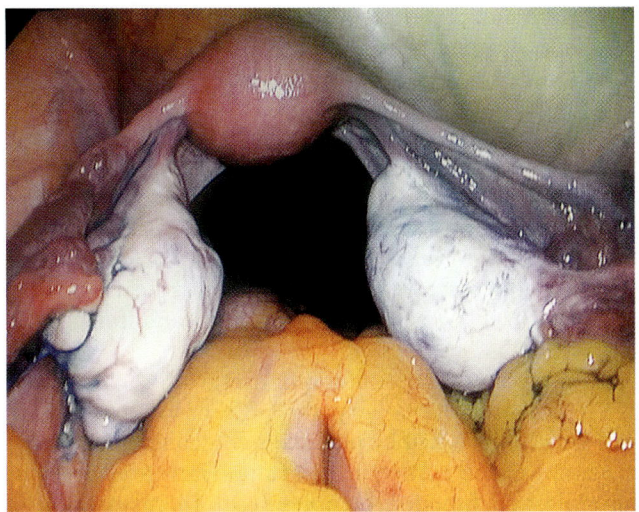

Fig. 2: Laparoscopic view of bilateral polycystic ovaries. Dye test showing bilateral patent tubes. Woman came with infertility.
Courtesy: Dr Subhas Halder

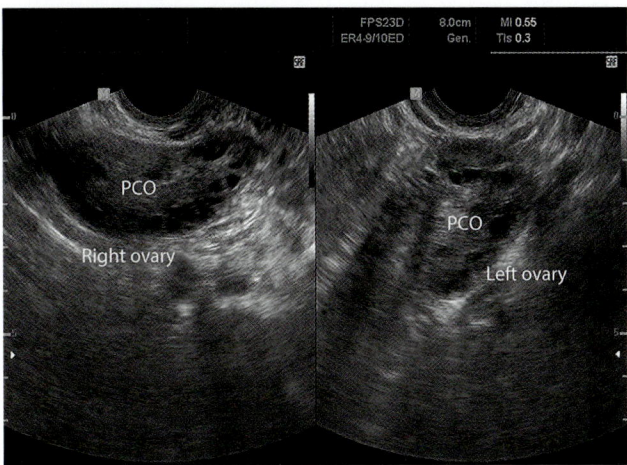

Fig. 3: Ovarian morphology in polycystic ovary syndrome (PCOS). Right side ovary—necklace looking 24 small hypoechoic cysts with volume 20.78 cc; left side ovary—18 small hypoechoic cysts volume 17.23 cc.
Courtesy: Dr Sanghamitra Ghosh, IRM, Kolkata

Q. What do you mean by oligomenorrhea?

Equal to or less than eight menses in a year.

Q. How will you define secondary amenorrhea?

The absence of menstruation for 6 months in a patient who had previously regular menses or absence for at least three previous cycles in a woman with previous irregular cycles.

Q. What are the causes of secondary amenorrhea in general?

- Hypothalamic (35%)—psychological stress, psychiatric illness, dieting, trauma, etc.
- Pituitary—hyperprolactinemia (19%) and Sheehan's syndrome
- Ovarian—PCOS (28%), POF, and arrhenoblastoma (1%)
- Uterine (1%)—tuberculosis and synechia
- Others—late onset CAH (0.5%), Cushing syndrome, hypothyroidism, and hyperthyroidism.

Q. How will you morphologically define polycystic ovary? (Figs. 1 to 3)

Sonographic findings are:

- Twelve or more antral follicles (multiple small hypoechoic cysts) in either ovary ranging in size from 2 mm to 9 mm in diameter and/or increased ovarian volume (not less than 10 mm^3) **(Fig. 3)**. Presence of these findings in one ovary is sufficient for diagnosis of PCOS. TVS is preferred except in virgins. Recently sonoAVC (sonography-based automated volume count), a new 3D technology has been introduced by which dimension of each individual follicle can be measured **(Fig. 4)**.
- However, these criteria exclude the women taking combined pill.
- Polycystic morphology of ovary can also be found in other androgen excess conditions like CAH, Cushing syndrome, and in exogenous intake of androgen.

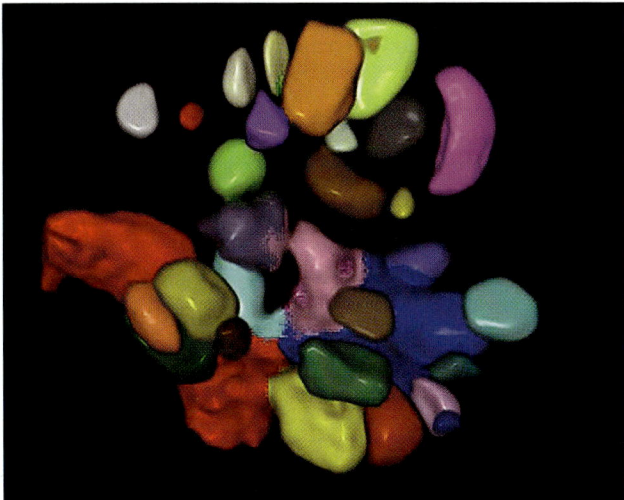

Fig. 4: SonoAVC (sonography-based automated volume count) 3D picture of polycystic ovary showing multiple follicles.
Courtesy: Professor Kamal Oswal, VIMS, Kolkata

Q. What are the different phenotypes of PCOS?

Classic PCOS which includes phenotype A and B which comprises 70% and the other two are ovulatory phenotype (C) and non-hyperandrogenic (D) comprising 30%. Using Rotterdam criteria one of four phenotypes A,B,C and D **(Table 2)** are identified (2012).

Types of Different Phenotypes of PCOS

Different phenotypes of PCOS have been listed in **Table 2**.

Q. What are the significances of different phenotypes?

- In classic PCOS (type A and B), there is higher prevalence of type 2 diabetes mellitus and cardiovascular risk factors.
- In type C (ovulatory), there is lower prevalence of metabolic syndrome and milder forms of dyslipidemia.

Table 2: Different phenotypes of PCOS.

Phenotype A	NIH PCOS: Hyperandrogenism and oligo/anovulation with PCO
Phenotype B	NIH PCOS: Hyperandrogenism and oligo/anovulation without PCO
Phenotype C	Non-NIH PCOS: Hyperandrogenism with PCO but with normal ovulation
Phenotype D	Non-NIH PCOS: No hyperandrogenism but with oligo/anovulation and with PCO

Abbreviations: PCOS, polycystic ovary syndrome; NIH, National Institute of Health

- In phenotype D (nonhyperandrogenic PCOS), metabolic profile is often similar to normal women.

CLINICAL PRESENTATIONS OF PCOS

Q. What are the clinical presentations of PCOS?
- Menstrual irregularities (most common)—oligomenorrhoea and amenorrhoea
- Features of androgen excess—hirsutism, oily skin, acne, and alopecia rarely male pattern balding
- Obesity is a common association
- Infertility
- Metabolic syndrome.

COMPLICATIONS OF PCOS

Q. What are the complications of PCOS?
- Menstrual irregularities.
- Features of hyperandrogenism—hirsutism, oily skin, acne, and rarely male pattern balding.
- Adverse reproductive outcome—infertility, miscarriage, maternal complications like gestational diabetes, pre-eclampsia, and fetal complications like fetal growth restriction (FGR), preterm labor, and fetal death.
- Metabolic syndrome (30–40%).
- Long-term risks:
  - Sequelae of metabolic syndrome—diabetes, hypertension, dyslipidemia, and cardiovascular diseases
  - Endometrial carcinoma
  - Depression and mood disorder.

Q. What is the incidence of PCOS?
It is the most common endocrine disorder in reproductive age of women. The incidence is 4–12%, may be as high as 15% depending on the criteria used for diagnosis.

ETIOLOGY OF PCOS

- Definite underlying cause is unknown.
- Polycystic ovary syndrome is a complex multigenetical disorder resulting from the interaction between multiple genetic, environmental and behavioral factors.
- Genes involving in the pathogenesis of PCOS are:
  - Insulin resistance-related genes
  - Genes that interfere with the biosynthesis and action of androgens
  - Genes that encode inflammatory cytokines
  - Other candidate genes.

Q. Who first described this syndrome?
Stein and Leventhal first described this syndrome comprising of amenorrhea with bilateral polycystic ovaries, popularly known as *Stein-Leventhal syndrome* from Michael Reese Hospital and Northwestern University Medical School in 1935. [Michael Leo Leventhal (1901–1971) and Irvingg stain (1878-1976)].

They reported a series of seven cases.

The diagnosis of ovarian pathology was done by clinically and greatly facilitated by pneumoroentgenography. Wedge resection of the cystic cortex of the ovaries restored the physiological function completely in all cases and two patients became pregnant.

Q. What is ovarian hyperthecosis?
It is more severe form of PCOS consisting of nest of luteinized theca cells throughout the ovarian stroma. There may be virilization due to severe hyperandrogenism.

HAIR-AN Syndrome

Q. What do you mean by HAIR-AN syndrome (Figs. 5 and 6)
It is hyperandrogenic-insulin-resistance acanthosis nigricans syndrome.
- HA—hyperandrogenism
- IR—insulin resistance
- AN—acanthosis nigricans.
- The etiology of this disorder is not clear. HAIR-AN syndrome is either a variant of PCOS or a separate genetic syndrome.
- *Acanthosis nigricans* is a marker in women with hirsutism. The skin becomes pigmented, thickened, and velvety and mostly found over the vulva. Other sites are over the nape of neck, axilla, below the breast, and inner side of thigh. The testosterone level is more than 100 ng/100 mL and

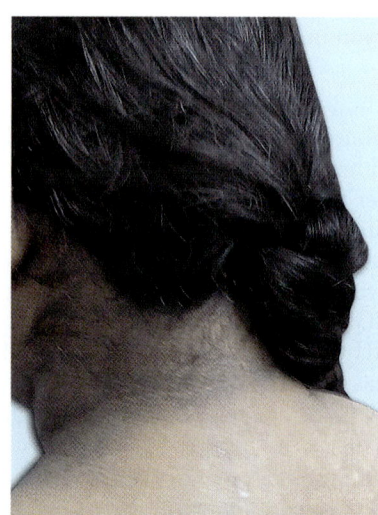

Fig. 5: Acanthosis nigricans in polycystic ovary syndrome.

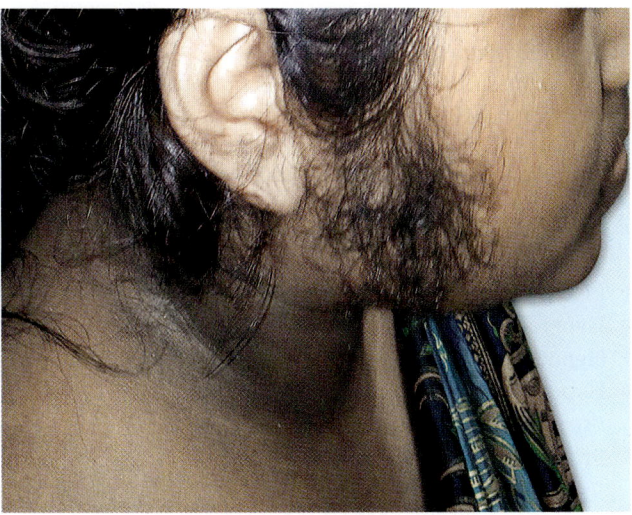

Fig. 6: Hirsutism and acanthosis nigricans in polycystic ovary syndrome—HAIR-AN syndrome.

fasting insulin is more than 25 µIU/mL (normal <20 µIU/mL). Maximal serum insulin responds to 2 hours post-glucose (75 g) load exceeds 300 µIU/mL (normal <160 µIU/mL).

❖ Treatment is to decrease insulin resistance and hyperinsulinemia with insulin sensitizers. Topical antibiotics, topical and systemic retinoids, keratolytics and topical corticosteroids have been tried but with little success.

Q. Is there any single biochemical marker to diagnose PCOS?
No.

ENDOCRINE PROFILE AND OTHER INVESTIGATIONS IN PCOS

Q. What are the endocrine profile and other investigations we do to diagnose PCOS?

❖ Increased LH and normal FSH with elevated LH and FSH ratio (>2:1)
❖ Androgen:
  ▪ Testosterone and $DHESO_4$ may be normal to twofold elevated—serum androgen levels are typically not more than twice the upper limit of normal in PCOS. In case of higher levels, other causes of hyperandrogenism should be searched for. Serum testosterone measurement is needed more to exclude ovarian neoplasm. Total testosterone value above 200 ng/dL warrants searching for ovarian lesion. Dehydroepiandrosterone sulfate (DHEA-S) above 700 µg/dL is mostly due to adrenal tumor.
❖ Fasting insulin increased (>20 µI U/mL)
❖ Abnormal GTT
❖ Decreased SHBG
❖ Abnormal lipid profile
❖ Prolactin may be mildly elevated in 10–20% cases.
❖ TSH—done as it one known cause of menstrual abnormality.
❖ AMH increases by 2–3 fold.
❖ Other hormones to exclude other causes of hyperandrogenism, e.g., 17-OHP and ACTH stimulation test to exclude CAH and dexamethasone suppression test and 24 hours urinary free cortisol level for Cushing syndrome, etc.

Testing of Hyperinsulinemia

❖ Standard 2-hour oral GTT gives an assessment on degrees of hyperinsulinemia and glucose tolerance.
❖ Fasting insulin—a peak level of >20 µU/mL.
❖ During 2-hour oral glucose test if insulin level is >55 µU/mL it indicates insulin resistance, if >100 µU/mL it indicates severe insulin resistance.
❖ Fasting glucose: Insulin values less than 4.5 indicate insulin resistance.

Values in Normal, Impaired GTT and Diabetes Mellitus

Values have been shown in **Table 3**.

Table 3: Values in normal, impaired GTT and diabetes mellitus.

	HbA1c	Fasting glucose	2-hour GTT
Normal	5.7%	100 mg/dL	<140 mg/dL
Impaired GTT	5.7–6.4%	100–125 mg/dL	140–199 mg/dL
Diabetes	≥6.5%	≥126 mg/dL	≥200 mg/dL

Abbreviation: GTT, glucose tolerance test

Q. When you will call insulin resistance?
Fasting glucose: Insulin values less than 4.5 indicate insulin resistance.

DIAGNOSIS OF ADOLESCENT PCOS

Q. How do you diagnose adolescent PCOS?

❖ Diagnosis is in the same line as adult PCOS.
❖ However as there is sometimes very difficult to differentiate the normal changes in adolescent from the diagnostic criteria of PCOS some authorities consider all three Rotterdam criteria instead of two to diagnose PCOS.
❖ Careful follow up is needed in incomplete criteria as PCOS may be diagnosed in late.

Q. Why there are difficulties in diagnosing adolescent PCOS?
In this age group:
❖ Normally, there is irregular menses for 2–4 years
❖ Acne is a common feature in this age group
❖ Instead of transvaginal route ovarian morphology is diagnosed by transabdominally which is not accurate.

Q. From management point of view, how do you categorize PCOS?

❖ Adolescent age group

- Adult with infertility
- Adult without infertility
- Pregnant women with PCOS
- PCOS in elderly.

MANAGEMENT OUTLINE IN A CASE OF PCOS

Depends on age, patient's desire of children, and severity of endocrinal abnormality:

- *Reduction of weight*—lifestyle modification, diet modification, and exercise
- *Medical management*—(1) hormonal suppression with EP; (2) insulin sensitizing agents; (3) dexamethasone; (4) thyroxin; (5) bromocriptine; (6) ovulation-inducing drug; (7) antiandrogen; and (8) spironolactone depending upon the indication.
- *Surgical*—wedge resection or laparoscopic ovarian drilling (LOD)
- Specific management in relation to *hirsutism* (*see* below)
- Specific management in case of *infertility* (*see* below)
- *Emerging therapies*—myo-inositol, treatment of hyperhomocysteinemia, treatment of oxidative stress, etc.

OUTLINE THE MANAGEMENT OF ADOLESCENT PCOS

Aim

- Regularization of menstrual cycle
- To reduce androgen excess
- Management of physical features of hyperandrogenism, e.g., hirsutism, acne, and acanthosis.

Treatment Options

- To reduce body weight—lifestyle management, diet modification, and exercises
- Combined oral contraceptive (COC) with less androgenic progestin like norgestimate, desogestrel or drospirenone. If amenorrhea withdrawal bleeding with MPA for 10 days prior to COC.
- Insulin sensitizing agents—Metformin 1,000 to 1,500 mg daily. Its side effects are nausea, bloating and diarrhea. To minimize side effects 500 mg extended-release form of tablet once daily is given, the dose can be increased gradually up to 1,500–2,000 mg daily
  Metformin increases insulin sensitivity, thus improves glucose tolerance. It increases ovulation rate, corrects menstrual abnormalities, and reduces serum androgen levels.
- Treatment of hirsutism—COC/EE+CA, antiandrogen, androgen blocking drugs, cosmetic—temporary and permanent hair removal (for details *see* later).

Q. What are the causes of infertility in PCOS?

- Anovulation/infrequent ovulation
- Poor oocyte quality
- Impaired fertilization
- Defective endometrium
- Implantation failure
- Blighted ovum/early pregnancy loss.

Anovulation or oligoovulation is not only the reason for infertility in PCOS as even after ovulation in 80% cases with ovulation induction successful pregnancy occurs in only 20% cases.

Q. In general, other than PCOS what are the other causes of oligoovulation or anovulation?

- PCOS: 80–90% cause of ovulation
- Hyperandrogenism
- Hypothyroidism
- Hyperprolactinemia
- Premature ovarian failure
- Primary ovarian failure.

Management Options of PCOS Women with Infertility

- Weight loss
- Ovulation induction: Clomiphene citrate (CC), insulin sensitizing agent, aromatase inhibitor (AI), gonadotropin (Gn), corticosteroid, and combination
- Surgical: Laparoscopic ovarian drilling (LOD)
- ART-IVF
- Emerging therapies as above.

Laparoscopic Ovarian Drilling (Fig. 7)

- Laparoscopic ovarian drilling (LOD) is a technique by which ovarian capsule is punctured with a electrosurgical needle or laser beam in laparoscopic approach. It can be done with monopolar, bipolar or laser with an aim to reduce the androgen-producing tissue in polycystic ovary.
- Five to ten punctures per ovary with monopolar needle, set between 20 and 30 W for 5 sec/puncture (2–4 mm wide and 4–10 mm deep) are usually recommended.
- For ovarian damage, adhesion formation and for less effectiveness it is not regarded as first-line treatment.

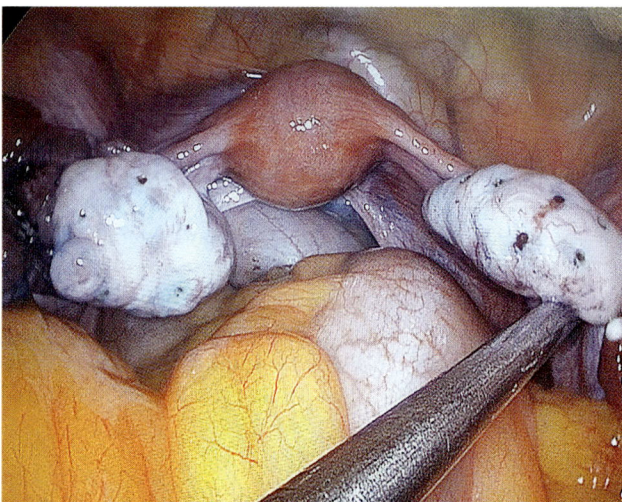

Fig. 7: Laparoscopic ovarian drilling in polycystic ovary syndrome.
Courtesy: Dr Subhas Halder

Q. Which treatment option when—in case of infertility?

- Clomiphene citrate is the first-line treatment for ovulation induction although AI is a promising alternative.
- Gonadotropin is second-line strategy with more risk of ovarian hyperstimulation syndrome (OHSS) and multiple pregnancy (MP).
- In vitro fertilization is a reasonable option to couple with additional factors (male/tubal).
- Laparoscopic ovarian drilling is an option for selected group of patients who fail to respond to CC/AI or enhanced risk of Gn-related sequelae (MP/OHSS) or cannot afford financial burden and it has an added advantage of long-term benefit for PCOS-related symptoms.

MANAGEMENT OF PCOS IN ELDERLY

In women more than 45 years with menstrual irregularity should always be evaluated by endometrial biopsy in addition to other management including the problems of metabolic syndrome.

In younger women without infertility should me managed in the same line including the serial monitoring of status of endometrium and hyperlipidemia.

DISCUSS THE PATHOPHYSIOLOGY OF PCOS

Abnormalities occur in four compartments, viz.
1. Hypothalamo-pituitary compartment
2. Ovaries
3. Adrenal glands
4. Periphery.

- In hypothalamo-pituitary compartment alteration of pulsatile gonadotropin-releasing hormone (GnRH) release may lead to increase LH:FSH secretion.
- Elevated LH increases ovarian androgen synthesis, but relative deficiency of FSH lead to decrease androgen conversion to E2 within the granulose cells.
- Increase intrafollicular level of androgen result follicular atresia and increase circulating level of androgen causes hyperlipidemia, acne, and hirsutism. Unopposed estrogen stimulation on endometrium leads to hyperplasia.
- Most women with PCOS inherit a genetic predisposition to insulin resistance which results in a compensatory hyperinsulinemia.
- Hyperinsulinemia in turn increases androgens at least by three mechanisms.
    - By decreasing SHBG production from the liver thus increasing the level of circulating free androgens
    - Stimulation of ovarian androgen production either through enhancing LH secretion or directly stimulating 17-hydroxylase/17,20-lyase activity at ovary and
    - Increasing adrenal androgen by augmenting 11-hydroxysteroid dehydrogenase activity.
- Peripheral fat contains aromatase enzyme which is responsible for conversion of androgens to estrogens (mainly estrone). This happens more in obese women.
- These enhanced androgenic and estrogenic condition leads to follicular atresia and anovulation.
- The increased androgens, acyclic estrogen production, and low progesterone give altered feedback to hypothalamus and pituitary gland leading to increased LH and diminished FSH which in turn increases further stromal androgen.
- Lack of ovulation causes oligoamenorrhea.
- Development of *noncyclic hormone pattern becomes the key factor in PCOS.*
- Presence of overweight or obesity makes the degree of insulin resistance much worse.
- Increased production of androgen alone in absence of hyperinsulinemia can also cause PCOS.

Altered Hypothalamo-pituitary Ovarian Relationship in PCOS

This relationship is shown in **Flowchart 1**.

The **Flowchart 2** showing the hyperinsulinemia and hyperandrogenemia leading to anovulation in PCOS.

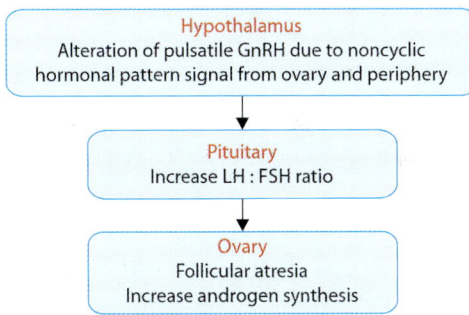

Flowchart 1: Alteration of hypothalamopituitary ovarian relationship in PCOS.

Abbreviations: PCOS, polycystic ovary syndrome; GnRH, gonadotropin-releasing hormone; FSH, follicle-stimulating hormone; LH, luteinizing hormone

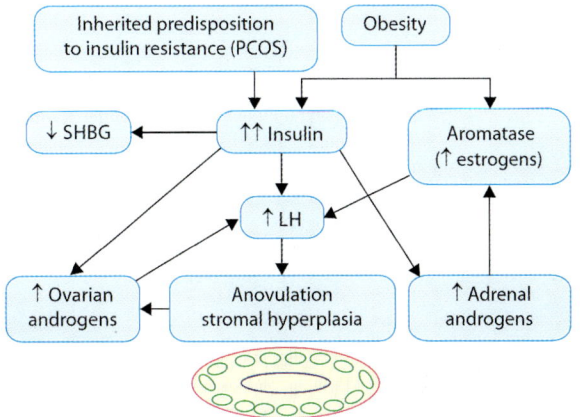

Flowchart 2: Hyperinsulinemia and hyperandrogenemia leading to anovulation in PCOS.

Abbreviations: PCOS, polycystic ovary syndrome; SHBG, sex hormone-binding globulin; LH, luteinizing hormone

Relation of PCOS and Obesity (Figs. 8A and B)

- About 65–74% of PCOS are obese. 25–35% are thin PCOS.
- Hyperinsulinemia in PCOS is not purely related to obesity because women with PCOS are more likely to have insulin resistance than weight-matched controls. Presence of obesity makes the condition worse.
- Most of the overweight/obese women are not hyperandrogenic and do not have PCOS as they have not inherited the genetic predisposition to PCOS and only mildly insulin resistance.
- Insulin resistance occurs in 30% of lean women with PCOS **(Fig. 8B)** and 95% of obese women with PCOS **(Fig. 8A)**.

Metabolic Syndrome and PCOS

- Prevalence of metabolic syndrome is 30–45% in women with PCOS in contrast to 4% in normal age-adjusted women

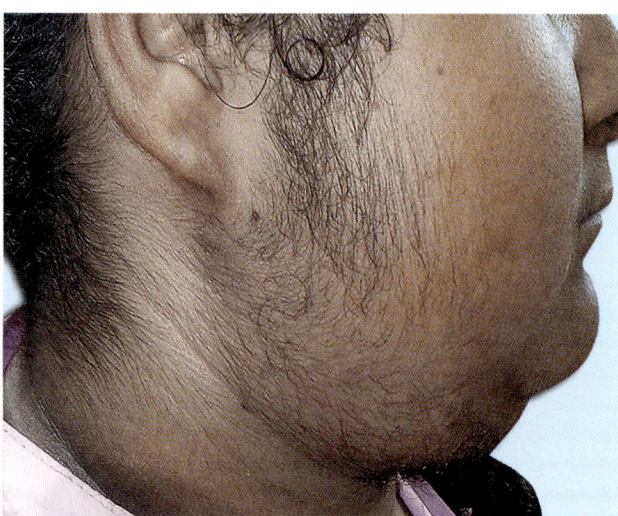

Fig. 8A: Hirsutism in obese polycystic ovary syndrome girl.

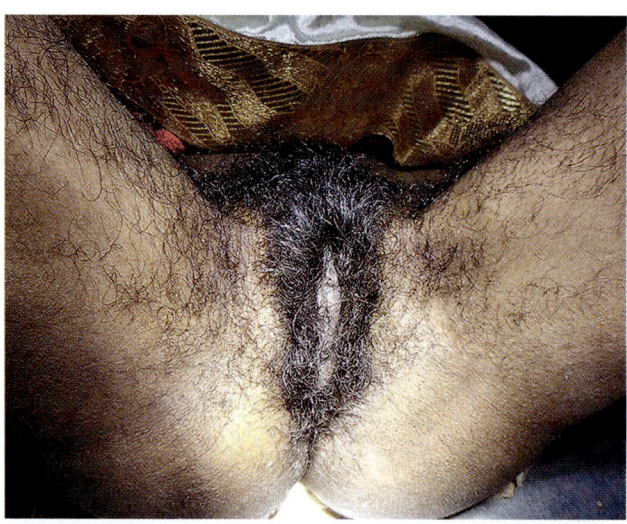

Fig. 8B: Hirsutism in lean polycystic ovary syndrome girl.

- Metabolic syndrome is a syndrome of medical disorders the presence of which increases the individual risks of developing cardiovascular disease and diabetes. It is also known as syndrome X.
- Many of the metabolic manifestations in PCOS are attributed to hyperinsulinemia and hyperandrogenemia.
- Obesity exacerbates the metabolic syndrome and reproductive disorder.
- Obese PCOS women also have a 10-fold increase in their risk of suffering from diabetes mellitus 2 and a seven fold increase of impaired glucose tolerance compared with normal weight (BMI <25 kg/m^2) PCOS women.

Q. What are characteristic features of metabolic syndrome?

Metabolic syndrome is characterized by:
- Central obesity
- Insulin resistance and hyperandrogenemia
- Impaired glucose tolerance
- Type 2 diabetes mellitus
- Dyslipidemia
- Hypertension
- Subclinical atherosclerosis.

Diagnostic Criteria of Metabolic Syndrome

Any three of five (Rotterdam/ESHREE/ASRM 2003):
- Female waist more than 35 inches
- Triglyceride more than 150 mg/dL
- HDL less than 50 mg/dL
- Blood pressure above 130/85 mm Hg
- Fasting glucose 110–126 mg/dL or 2 hour glucose (75 g) 140–199 mg/dL.

Monitoring for Metabolic Syndrome

- Waist, BMI, and BP measurement every year
- Lipid profile every 2 years
- 2 hour 75-g GTT in PCOS women with BMI above 30 kg/m^2 or lean patient with age above 40 years or having risk factors
- Impaired GTT-tested annually
- Endometrial cancer monitoring by USG/histopathology in obesity and menstrual abnormality.

Management of Metabolic Syndrome

- Physical activity, diet manipulation, and exercise
- Insulin sensitizing agents—metformin
- Specific management for obesity, hypertension, diabetes, and dyslipidemia.

Management in Overweight and Obese Women with PCOS (AE-PCOS Society)

- Lifestyle management
- Dietary management
- Structured exercise

- Behavior modification (reduction of psychological stressors)
- Antiobesity drug: Orlistat is the only FDA approved drug for obesity. Dose is 60/120 mg thrice daily. Very rare complication is severe liver injury. Sibutramine was voluntarily removed in 2010 for increased cardiovascular adverse events.
- Bariatric surgery is considered when BMI is above 40 kg/m^2 or above 35 kg/m^2 with comorbid condition.

Dietary Management and Exercise in Overweight and Obese Women

- About 500–1,000 kcal/day dietary energy reduction helps to reduce body weight by 7–10% in 6–12 months.
- The diet should contain less than 30% of calories from fat, less than 10% of calories from saturated fat, with increased consumption of fiber, whole-grain breads, cereals, fruit and vegetables.
- More than 30 minute of structured exercise per day is minimally required.

Weight reduction is more important than dietary manipulation.

Acne

Q. What is the incidence of acne among PCOS women?

Acne vulgaris is common in adolescent. In PCOS girl, there is persistent and late onset acne. Moderate acne is found in 50% PCOS women. In women with severe acne, 80% are associated with hyperandrogenemia.

Q. How does acne occur (pathogenesis)?

- Due to excessive stimulation of androgen receptors in pilosebaceous unit in androgen excess women sebum is produced in excess amount.
- Acne is characterized by blockage of hair follicle due to hyperkeratosis, excessive production of sebum, growth of *Propionibacterium acnes (P. acnes)* associated with inflammation. Scarring may occur due to long standing inflammation.

Q. How would you treat acne?

- Treatment consists of reducing androgen level to reduce sebum production, to minimize keratinization, to prevent inflammation and to reduce colonization of *P. acnes*.
- Lowering of androgen excess can be achieved by—(1) COC, (2) antiandrogens like spironolactone or flutamide or (3) 5α-reductase inhibitors like finasteride.
- Topical retinoids (tretinoin) is used to regulate keratinocyte function and to prevent inflammation.
- In mild degree local retinoid and benzoyl peroxide is used.
- In moderate variety other than local treatment oral antibiotic and/or COC is added.
- In severe variety additionally oral isotretinoin is administered. Dermatologist is always consulted.

Specific Management for Hirsutism in PCOS Women

- Pharmacologic therapy: Androgen suppression agent and androgen blocking agent (antiandrogen) → *see* below
- Physical methods of hair removal (as described next).

HIRSUTISM

Q. What do you mean by hirsutism?

- Hirsutism is the presence of prominent facial and body (excessive terminal hair) hair in female caused by excessive androgen effect.
- Hirsutism is not an increase in the number of hair follicle but an alteration in their character— *vellus* hair to *terminal* hair. The number of hair follicles is determined by 22 weeks of intrauterine life, after which no follicle is developed de novo.

Q. What is hirsutism, virilism, and hypertrichosis?

- *Hirsutism* is an increase in the transformation of vellus to terminal hair.
- *Virilism*: Extreme hyperandrogenism (usually due to tumor and may be due to CAH and androgenic drugs). Other than hirsutism it includes acne, amenorrhea, androgenic alopecia, decreased breasts sizes, deepening of voice, and increased muscle mass and enlarged clitoris (length >10 mm and diameter > 7 mm at proximitly) **(Fig. 9)**. Virilization occurs in less than 1% of patients with hirsutism.
- *Hypertrichosis*—a diffuse increase in vellus hair growth and not androgen dependent.

Q. What are the causes of hirsutism?

Basic factors responsible for hirsutism: Hirsutism is due to increase in level of androgen or increase in androgen sensitivity.
- ↑androgen production or exogenous androgen
- ↑sensitivity of androgen receptor

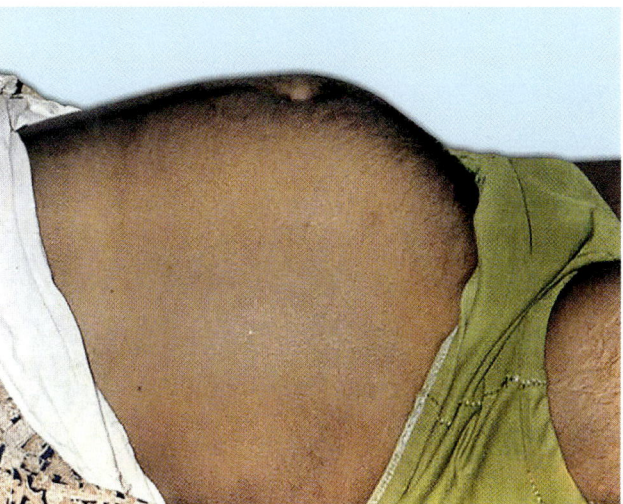

Fig. 9: Virilization in arrhenoblastoma—excessive course hair, reduced breasts sizes, masculine figure and she had hoarseness of voice.

- ↑activity of 5α-reductase
- ↓sex hormone-binding globulin.

Decrease of SHBG production increases free testosterone.

SHBG is *reduced by* increase of insulin, prolactin, and androgen itself. SHBG is *increased* by estrogen and thyroid hormones.

Causes of hirsutism are:
- Ovarian cause: PCOS and tumor
- Adrenal cause: Cushing syndrome, CAH, and tumor
- Exogenous pharmacological agents as described below
- Familial
- Idiopathic hirsutism.

Q. What are the common causes of hirsutism?
- PCOS (70–80%)
- Idiopathic hirsutism (5–15%)
- CAH (2–8%)
- Cushing syndrome and neoplasm (0.1–0.3%).

Q. How does hyperandrogenemia occur in PCOS?
Described above in **Flowchart 2** (*see* Page 295).

Q. How does hyperandrogenemia occur in congenital adrenal hyperplasia? (Figs. 10 to 13)

- Congenital adrenal hyperplasia is a spectrum of inherited disorders of adrenal steroidogenesis.
- With decreased cortisol production negative feedback for ACTH is withdrawal resulting stimulation of ACTH which in turn results adrenal hyperplasia to produce steroid and also simulates androgen production resulting virilization of female fetus (showing in the **Fig. 13**).
- Severe form is usually congenital. Milder form is late onset, partial, nonclassical and acquired and comes in differential diagnosis.

- Most common enzyme deficiency is 21-hydroxylase. Others are 11β-hydroxylase and 3β-hydroxysteroid dehydrogenase.
- Hirsutism, acne, menstrual disorders, and infertility may be presenting symptoms during adolescence or adulthood. Degree of masculinization of external genitalia varies according to the severity. There may be excessive growth of hair all over the body with enlarged clitoris and fusion of labia **(Figs. 10 to 12)**.
- Diagnosis is important, because therapy must be long-term, needs genetic counseling and in stress, there may be cortisol deficiency.
- *Diagnosis is done by elevated levels of 17-OHP, dramatic increase after ACTH stimulation* **(Fig. 13)**.

Cushing's Syndrome
- Although rare, it should be considered in the differential diagnosis.

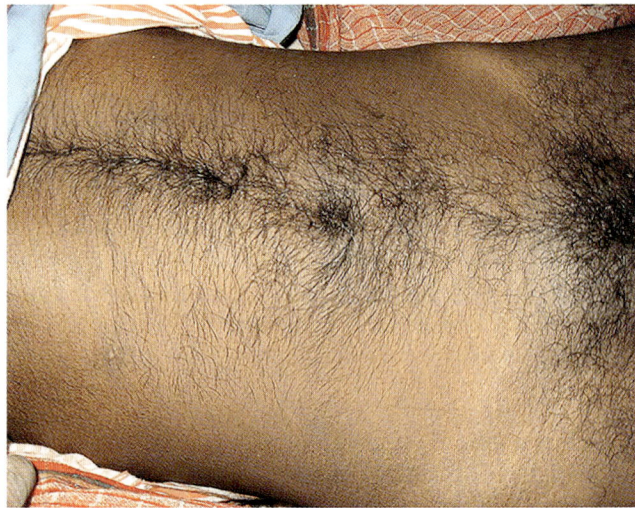

Fig. 11: Male hair pattern in congenital adrenal hyperplasia.

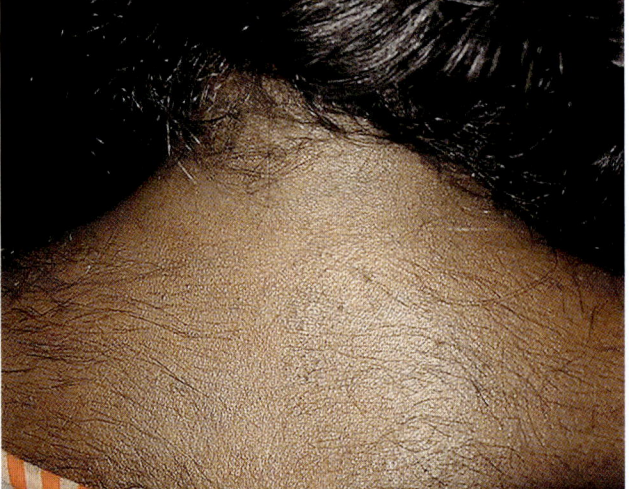

Fig. 10: Hirsutism—in congenital adrenal hyperplasia. Note that here, there is no acanthosis nigricans as found in polycystic ovary syndrome due to hyperinsulinemia—compare with Figures 5 and 6.

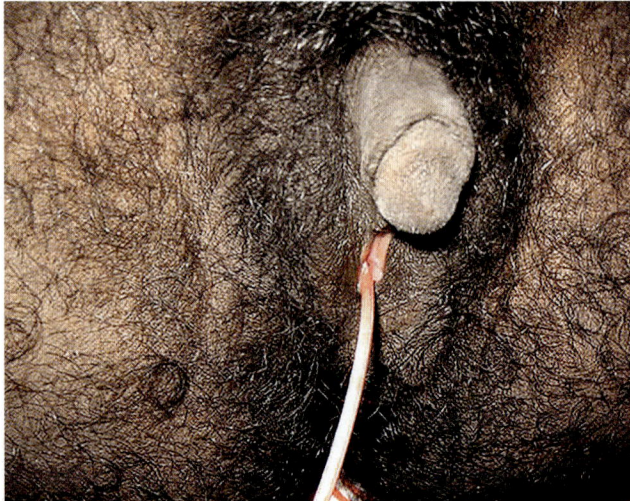

Fig. 12: Clitoromegaly and labial fusion in congenital adrenal hyperplasia.

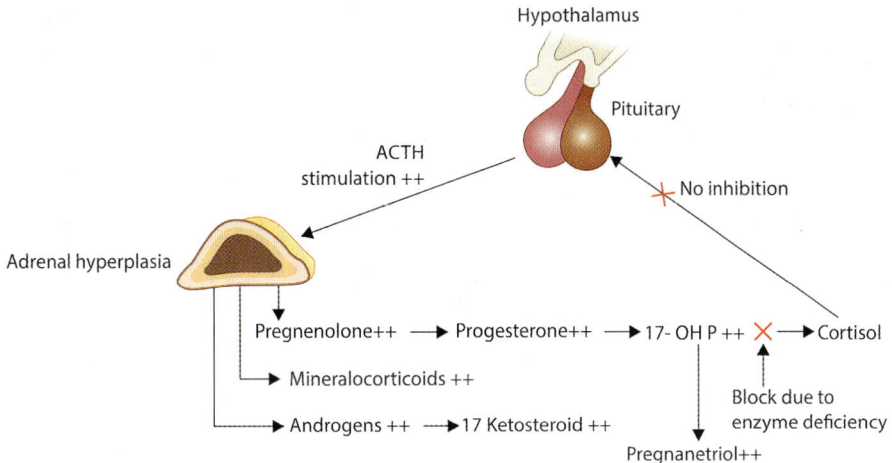

Fig. 13: Hormone synthesis in congenital adrenal hyperplasia.
Abbreviations: ACTH, adrenocorticotropic hormone; OHP, hydroxyprogesterone

- It may be caused by increased production of adrenocorticotropic hormone (ACTH) by the pituitary, adrenal carcinoma or adenoma, or secretion of ectopic ACTH resulting increase cortisol and sex steroid production.
- Profound hirsutism is seen most commonly in patients with macronodular hyperplasia, and clinical signs of Cushing's syndrome characterized by central obesity, "moon" facies, striae, ecchymosis on skin, and amenorrhea are apparent.
- It is screened by *dexamethasone suppression test and confirmed by 24-hour urinary free cortisol level.*

Androgen-secreting Tumors of the Ovary or Adrenal Gland (Figs. 14 to 17)

- These are relatively rare affecting 0.1 to 0.3% hirsute patients.

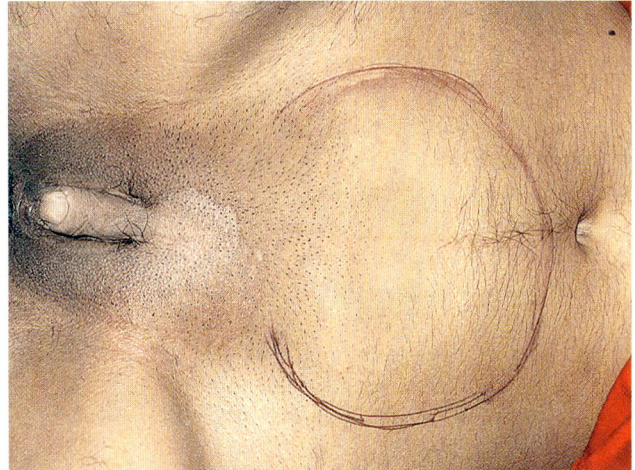

Fig. 15: Ovarian tumor with enlarged clitoris. Her pubic hairs have been shaved before surgery— woman as shown in Figure 14.

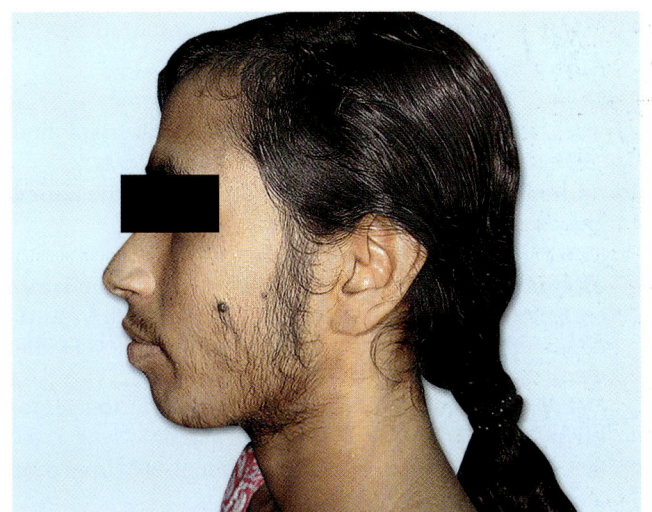

Fig. 14: Hirsutism in arrhenoblastoma.

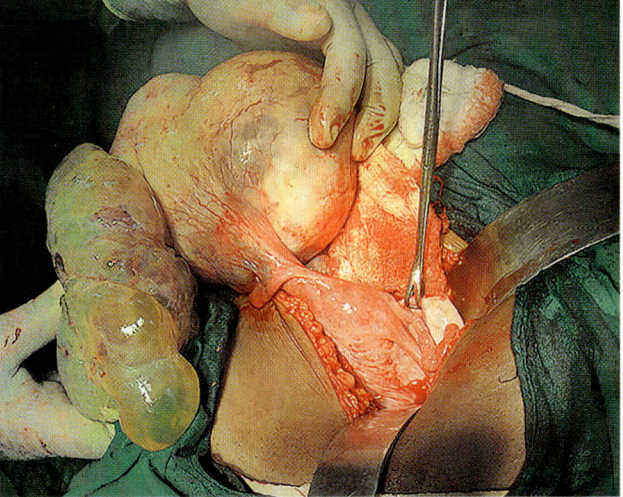

Fig. 16: Arrhenoblastoma—right-sided salpingo-oophorectomy in patient as shown in Figures 14 and 15.
Courtesy: Dr Subir Bhattacharya

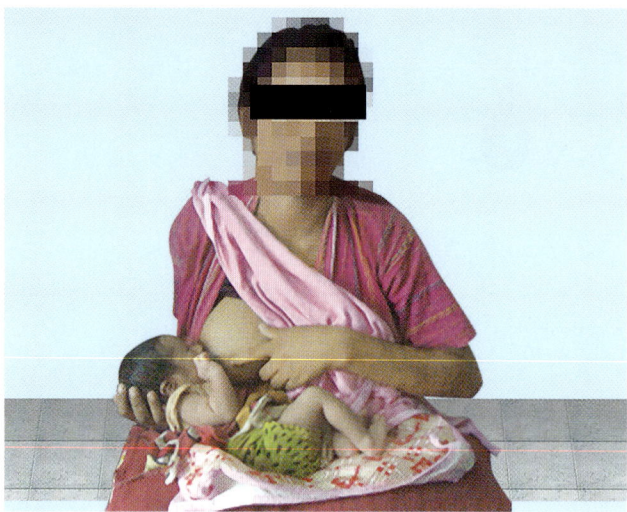

Fig. 17: Pregnancy following oophorectomy in arrhenoblastoma (same patient as in Figure 14).
Courtesy: Professor Anita Roy

- Neoplasm is suspected in rapid progression of hirsutism with virilization, enlarged clitoris, and masculinization, cessation of menses, and swelling abdomen (**L13, L14**).
- Virilization occurs in less than 1% of patients with hirsutism.
- Arrhenoblastoma is the most common ovarian tumor
- *Diagnosed* by unilateral adnexal mass, imaging with TVS, CT or MRI.
- *Serum testosterone levels above 200 ng/dL* are highly suspicious of androgen secreting tumor.
- Androgen-secreting adrenal tumors are less common and are a life-threatening cause of hirsutism.
- Usually large at the time of diagnosis, these adrenal tumors are associated with a poor prognosis.

EXOGENOUS PHARMACOLOGICAL AGENTS CAUSING HIRSUTISM

- Danazol, anabolic steroids, and testosterone may cause hirsutism. Medications that cause hyperprolactinemia may also cause hirsutism. Metoclopramide, methyldopa, reserpine and phenothiazines, and some progestins cause hirsutism.
- Oral contraceptives containing levonorgestrel, norethindrone, and norgestrel tend to have stronger androgenic effects, while those with ethynodiol diacetate, norgestimate, and desogestrel are less androgenic. Drospirenone has less androgenic effect.

MEDICATIONS CAUSING HIRSUTISM AND HYPERTRICHOSIS

Medications causing hirsutism and hypertrichosis are listed in **Table 4**.

Table 4: Medications causing hirsutism and hypertrichosis.

Hirsutism	Hypertrichosis
• Testosterone	• Cyclosporine
• Anabolic steroids	• Diazoxide
• Danazol	• Hydrocortisone
• Metoclopramide	• Minoxidil
• Phenothiazines	• Penicillamine
• Progestogens	• Phenytoin
• Reserpine	• Streptomycin
• Methyldopa	• Psoraleas

IDIOPATHIC HIRSUTISM

- Diagnosis of exclusion
- Common and often familial
- Probably related to disorder in peripheral androgen activity
- Onset shortly after puberty and slow progress
- Menses normal
- Serum T, 17α-OHP, and DHEA-S normal.

ANDROGEN SYNTHESIS IN FEMALE

- In female androgens and the precursors are synthesized in ovary and adrenal glands stimulated by ACTH and LH respectively.
- Conversion of cholesterol to pregnenolone is the first step.
- Pregnenolone, thereafter is converted to 17-ketosteroid DHEA by two step along the Δ-5 steroid pathway by the enzyme CYP17, with 17α-hydroxylase and 17,20-lyase activities.
- In the Δ-4 steroid pathway progesterone is transformed to androstenedione parallelly.
- Δ-5-isomerase, 3β-hydroxysteroid dehydrogenase (3β-HSD) accomplish the metabolism of Δ-5 to Δ-4 intermediates.

DIFFERENT ANDROGENS AND THEIR SOURCES

Q. What are the different androgens and what are the sources (Fig. 18)?

Different androgens are testosterone, dehydroepiandrosterone sulfate (DHEA-S), DHEA, androstenedione and Dihydrotestosterone (DHT)

- Androgens are produced by the ovaries and the adrenal glands and peripheral conversion.
- 50% of *testosterone* is derived from peripheral conversion of androstenedione, whereas the adrenal gland and ovary contributes approximately equal amount (25%) to the circulating levels of testosterone, except at midcycle when ovarian contribution increases by 10–15%.
- *Dehydroepiandrosterone sulfate (DHEA-S)* arises almost exclusively (100%) from the adrenal gland.
- 50% of the *DHEA* is derived from adrenal, 20% from ovary and rest 30% from DHEA-S.
- 50% of *androstenedione* is derived from the ovary and another 50% from adrenal gland.

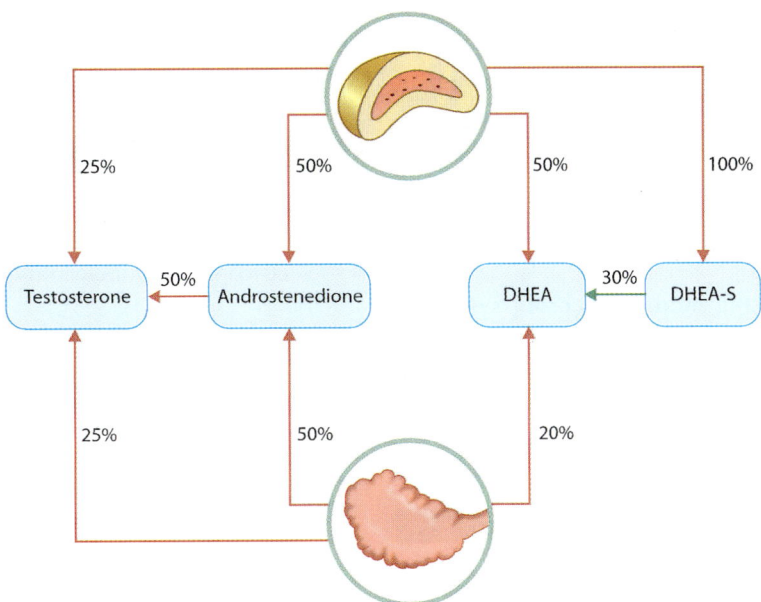

Fig. 18: Androgen synthesis with their sources.

- *Dihydrotestosterone (DHT)*, the most potent and active androgen, is derived from conversion of testosterone in the target tissue (hair follicle) by the enzyme, 5α-reductase.
- The most potent androgen is dihydrotestosterone (300) which is followed by testosterone (100), then androstenedione (10) and DHEA-S (5) with decreasing potency.

Evaluation of Androgen Excess

Androgen excess is evaluated by measurement of *testosterone, DHEA-S and* 3α-androstanediol glucuronide *(3α-AG)*. 3α-AG is the peripheral tissue metabolite of DHT.

However, 3α-AG is not a part of routine clinical approach, because the ultimate diagnosis and therapy of the problem are not affected by this test.

Factors Determining the Androgenicity

- Androgenicity depends mainly on *unbound testosterone and partly upon the fraction associated with albumin.*
- In addition, the androgen effect depends on the level of SHBG. *When SHBG level becomes low free testosterone rises resulting increase androgenicity and vice versa.* SHBG is reduced by increase of insulin, prolactin, and androgen itself. SHBG is *increased by estrogen and thyroid hormones.*
- Androgenicity is also increased with increased 5-α *reductase activity.*
- In normal women, 80% of testosterone is bound to SHBG, 19% is loosely bound to albumen, and 1% circulates free in the bloodstream. In men, 78% is bound to SHBG, 19% is bound to albumen, and 3% circulates free. In hirsute women, 79% is bound to SHBG, 19% is bound to albumen, and 2% circulates free depending upon the causes.
- Free testosterone assay at present lacks uniform standard, for which total testosterone is measured for suspected tumor. *Total serum testosterone level above 200 ng/mL warrants ovarian neoplasm.*

EVALUATION OF HIRSUTISM

Evaluation of hirsutism consists of:
- Thorough history taking
- Physical examination
- Initial investigation to exclude life-threatening condition
- Further investigations to pinpoint the diagnosis.

History

- Age of onset and progression of symptoms and weight gain
- History of abdominal swelling
- Symptoms of virilization
- Menstrual history
- History of galactorrhea
- Family history
- History of medication
- Use of hair removal method.

Physical Examination

- Quantification of sexual hair
- Height, weight (BMI), and BP
- Acne, acanthosis nigricans, galactorrhea
- Signs of Cushing syndrome
- Signs of virilization—temporal balding and clitoromegaly
- Abdominal and pelvic examination to exclude palpable tumor.

HAIR-AN syndrome is characterized by hyperandrogenemia (HA), insulin resistance (IR), and acanthosis nigricans (AN) and is encountered in a subset of patients of PCOS.

Q. How would you quantify hirsutism? What is the drawback of Ferriman–Gallwey scoring system?

Quantification scoring is done by *Ferriman–Gallwey Scoring System (modified)* **(Fig. 19)**.

Total nine body areas are examined. Score 0 to 4 for each area, 0 = no hirsutism; 4 = severe hirsutism. Total maximum score may be 36.

Total score 8 or more—hirsutism. Mild: 8–15; Moderate: 16–25; Severe hirsutism: >25.

A score of ≥4 to 6 using modified scoring system is regarded as hirsutism by some investigators. AE-PCOS society considers ≥3 as hirsutism for Far East Asians.

It is subjective and hence differs among investigators. Moreover, substantial hirsutism may exist in one or two areas without yielding a high score.

LABORATORY INVESTIGATIONS

Initial screening (to exclude life-threatening conditions):
- Serum testosterone assay—normal 20–80 ng/dL
- 17-OHP (morning level)
- DHEA-S normal 100–350 µg/dL

As adrenal gland produces both testosterone and DHEA-S, initial evaluation of adrenal tumor measurement of DHEA-S level is not mandatory, because in adrenal tumor testosterone levels become significantly elevated.

FURTHER INVESTIGATIONS

- TSH
- Prolactin
- Insulin
- FSH and LH
- 24-hour urinary cortisol or dexamethasone suppression test to exclude Cushing syndrome
- ACTH stimulation test to confirm CAH.

IMAGING

- Sonography of pelvis
- CT scan or MRI
- Selective venous catheterization.

Approach following Initial Screening

- If basal levels of 17-OHP is elevated, ACTH stimulation test is performed to confirm adrenal hyperplasia. A morning level of 17-OHP below 200 ng/dL are usually found in normal women. Values greater than 800 ng/dL are often associated with an enzyme deficiency. Values between 200 ng/dL and 800 ng/dL should be evaluated by ACTH stimulation test.
- If 17-OH is more than or equal to 1,000 ng/dL by ACTH stimulation test, it is late-onset adrenal hyperplasia or 21-hydroxylase deficiency. If it is less than or equal to 1,000 ng/dL, it is likely to be heterozygous carriers of 21-hydroxylase deficiency.
- Levels of serum total testosterone greater than 200 ng/dL (6.94 nmol/L) and/or DHEA-S greater than 700 µg/dL (24.3 nmol/L) are strongly indicative of virilizing tumors. It is evaluated by abdominopelvic clinical examination and imaging.
- Levels of serum DHEA-S and urinary 17-KS run parallel. Upper limit of DHEA-S is 350 µg/mL. Moderate elevation is also seen in chronic anovulation. DHEA-S above 700 µg/dL or greater is a marker of abnormal adrenal function and is rarely found.

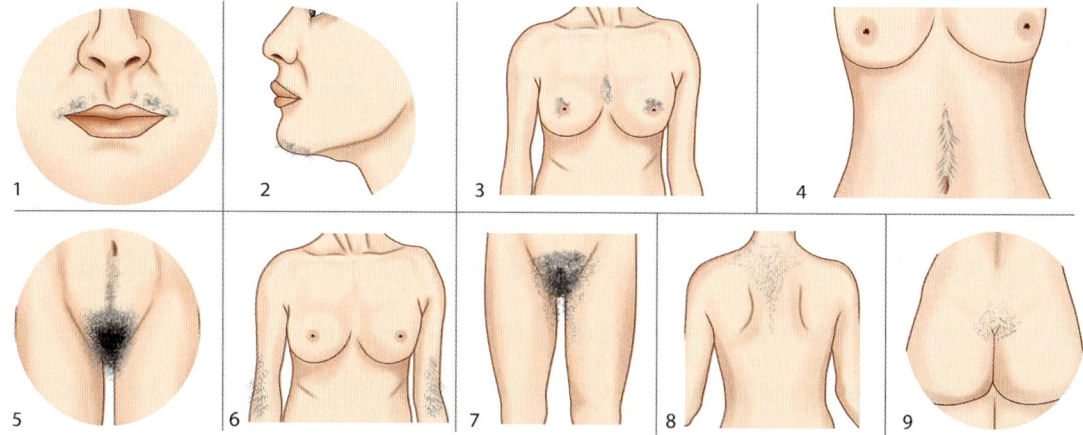

Fig. 19: Ferriman–Gallwey scoring system (modified). There are total nine body areas: (1) Upper lip; (2) Chin; (3) Chest; (4) Upper abdomen; (5) Lower abdomen; (6) Upper arm; (7) Thighs; (8) Upper back; and (9) Lower back/buttock.

Body areas	Upper lip	Chin	Chest	Upper abdomen	Lower abdomen	Upper arm	Thighs	Upper back	Lower back/buttock	Total score
Score										

CHAPTER 12: A Case of Polycystic Ovarian Syndrome and Hirsutism

- 3α-androstanediol is the peripheral tissue metabolite of DHT, and its glucuronide, 3α-AG, is a good marker of 5α-reductase and is not routinely done.
- Measurement of serum level of basal FSH and LH, fasting insulin and glucose estimation may help for evaluation of PCOS.
- *Imaging*: In case of clinical suspicion of neoplasm and or very high level of androgens imaging like sonography, CT scan, and MRI are done to arrive at diagnosis. Selective venous catheterization is reserved whenever a tumor has not been identified by imaging but strong clinical suspicion remains.

SUMMARY OF RECOMMENDATION FOR EVALUATION OF HIRSUTISM

- *Initial test*: Serum testosterone and 17-OHP measurement.
  - TSH screen if alopecia present
- Single dose overnight *dexamethasone* test is done to screen Cushing syndrome. Abnormal result confirmed by 24-hour urinary free cortisol.
- Always consider hyperinsulinemia.
- Rapidly developing virilization—think of neoplasm.

OUTLINE THE MANAGEMENT OF HIRSUTISM

Specific therapy is addressed to serious disorders like neoplasia, etc., where treatment of pathology is the primary concern rather than attention to hirsutism. Use of androgenic drug is withdrawn if any.

- Once life-threatening disorder is excluded and proper diagnosis is made a therapeutic approach is designed. Majority are either PCOS (70–80%), idiopathic (5–15%) or familial.

Management of hirsutism consists of:
- Counseling
- Therapy.

Counseling

- Counseling is very important for these patients giving stress on psychological aspect, response of therapy, duration of therapy which may be for many years, chance of recurrence, future fertility outcome, and long-term effects of hyperandrogenism like hyperlipidemia, type 2 diabetes and cardiovascular effects.

- Patient should be informed that the medications are contraindicated during pregnancy.

Therapy

Therapy for hirsutism **(Table 5)** can be classified broadly into two categories:
1. Pharmacologic therapy: (A) Hormonal suppression; (B) Antiandrogens (androgen blocking agents). Hormone suppression drugs act by reducing androgen production. Antiandrogens block androgen action at hair follicles.
2. Local management at site of hair follicle: (A) Physical methods of hair removal and (B) Topical treatment.

Reduction of weight and avoidance of androgenic agents are the general measures to be taken. Surgery is reserved as last resort to reduce hormone production.

Pharmacologic Therapy

Role of Pharmacologic Therapy in Hirsutism

- Once terminalization of hair has occurred, it cannot be reversed back completely.
- No agent is capable to reverse the terminalization of vellus hairs already transformed, i.e., physical and cosmetic measures are the cornerstone of care for hirsutism.
- Permanent removal of the already androgenized hair follicles will require electrolysis or laser hair removal.
- However, there is definite role of pharmacologic agents in the improvement of hirsutism.
- These agents can help—(1) to stop new hairs from growing; (2) to potentially slow the growth of terminal hairs already present, and (3) to produce a thinning and loss of pigmentation of terminal hairs to some extent.
- Response to pharmacologic agents is slow. At least 6 months are necessary to see the success of medical therapy and even may take up to 1–2 years. Following withdrawal of drug recurrence of hair growth is common.
- Almost all medications are contraindicated during pregnancy.

All these aspects should be discussed during counseling. Hence, combination treatment is the rule. However, combination treatment with electrolysis and laser is more effective following hormonal suppression at least for 6 months.

Oral Contraceptives

- Oral contraceptives are most common means of hormonal suppression. OCs containing less androgenic progestins,

Table 5: Therapy for hirsutism.

Hormonal suppression	Antiandrogens	Physical and cosmetic methods	Topical treatment	General measures
• Oral contraceptive • Dexamethasone • Gonadotropin-releasing hormone agonist • Bromocriptine Ketoconazole • Insulin sensitizing agents	Spironolactone Cyproterone acetate Flutamide Finasteride	• *Temporary depilation*: Shaving and chemical depilatories • *Temporary epilation*: Plucking and waxing • *Permanent hair removal*: Electrolysis and laser hair removal	Eflornithine hydro-chloride (Vaniqa) cream application	• Weight reduction • Avoidance of androgenic agents

such as norgestimate, gestodene, and desogestrel and drospirenone, are preferred. Cyclically one tablet daily 28 days with 7 days gap.
- They act in several ways. OCs suppress LH production thus reduces ovarian androgen production. It also decreases DHAS from adrenal. Estrogen increases SHBG thus decreases free testosterone. Progestin antagonises 5α-reductase and the androgen receptor.
- Women with idiopathic hirsutism, PCOS, or late-onset CAH should be started with low dose OCs.

No antiandrogens are approved by the US FDA for the treatment of hirsutism.

Antiandrogens

The commonly used antiandrogens are spironolactone, finasteride and flutamide. However, due to its hepatotoxicity flutamide is not recommended routinely.

Spironolactone

- Spironolactone is most commonly used because of its safety, availability, and low cost.
- It is aldosterone-antagonist diuretic. It inhibits ovarian and adrenal production of androgen. It also acts as receptor blocker and inhibits 5α-reductase activity.
- The dose is 50–200 mg daily. It is better in COC resistant cases.
- The important side effects are diuresis, fatigue, dysfunctional uterine bleeding (DUB), and hyperkalemia.

Cyproterone acetate:
- Cyproterone acetate (CA) is a potent progestational agent. It acts by inhibiting gonadotropin secretion and blocking androgen receptor.
- It is used by combining with ethinylestradiol (EE). 35 µg EE is combined with 2 mg CA (Diane 35, Krimson 35) and given cyclically. Reverse sequential EE for 21 days CA (50–100 mg daily) for first 10 days.
- Side effects are fatigue, edema, loss of libido, weight gain, and mastalgia.
- The drug is as effective as combination of spironolactone and OC.
- Improvement of facial hirsutism is seen from third month onward.

Flutamide:
- Flutamide is a nonsteroidal antiandrogen approved by the FDA as adjuvant treatment of prostatic cancer, not for hirsutism. It acts at receptor level. It directly inhibits hair growth.
- Dose is 250 mg 2–3 times daily.
- Flutamide has been shown to be as effective as spironolactone.
- Marked improvement is observed within 6 months. It is best choice for alopecia in comparison to others.
- However, it is *hepatotoxic* and makes skin dry and there may be greenish colored urine. During its use hepatic function must be monitored.

Finasteride:
- Finasteride (Fincar, Finax), a competitive inhibitor of 5α-reductase, approved by the FDA for use in benign prostate hyperplasia has been shown to be effective in treating hirsutism. Dose is 5 mg/day.
- It is somewhat less effective than the androgen receptor blocker. It has the least side effects of all the drugs used for treating hirsutism. It should not be used in pregnancy.

Gonadotropin-releasing Hormone

Gonadotropin-releasing hormone analogs should be reserved for severe case of ovarian hyperandrogenism and also in women who do not respond to combination hormonal therapy or those who cannot tolerate OCs. In prolong use (>6 months) add back therapy is recommended. It has advantage of prolong remission period. After completion of course treatment is maintained by OC or antiandrogen.

Insulin-sensitizing agents (metformin and troglitazone):
- Several insulin-sensitizing agents (metformin and troglitazone) have been shown to improve insulin sensitivity and decrease testosterone levels in patients with PCOS.
- Hyperandrogenism features have shown improvement after metformin therapy.
- Troglitazone is a better insulin-sensitizer than metformin; however, it should used with cautiously due to its alleged idiosyncratic hepatotoxicity.

Corticosteroids (dexamethasone and prednisolone):
- Dexamethasone suppresses androgen production from nonspecific hypersecretion or adult-onset adrenal hyperplasia. Standard dose is 0.25–0.5 mg every. Equivalent dose of prednisolone is 5–7.5 mg.
- In patients with uncomplicated adrenal hyperplasia glucocorticoid therapy usually results in normal menstrual cycles and improvement in hirsutism or acne.
- Combination with E-P, antiandrogen or GnRH gives maximum effect.
- Due to side effects, long-term use of glucocorticoids should be discouraged.

Ketoconazole

Ketoconazole, an antifungal agent, decreases androgen production by inhibiting enzymes necessary for androgen synthesis. Due to its severe side effects, including alopecia, dry skin, abdominal pain, vaginal spotting and it is reserved only for patients with severe hirsutism that has not responded to other drugs.

Cimetidine

Cimetidine can be used to treat hirsutism. It acts by blocking androgen receptor. Response to treatment is disappointing.

Topical Cream

- *Eflornithine*
- Eflornithine (Vaniqa), 13.9% topical cream has been approved by FDA for treatment of unwanted facial hair growth.

CHAPTER 12: A Case of Polycystic Ovarian Syndrome and Hirsutism

- It inhibits L-ornithine decarboxylase, an enzyme of dermal papilla, essential for controlling hair growth and proliferation. It is used twice daily. It does not remove hair, but slows and miniaturizes the hairs that are present and they become much less visible and coarse.
- Improvement of unwanted facial hair occurs significantly in almost 60% cases within 8 weeks.
- It worsens acne by obstructing pilosebaceous unit. On discontinuation recurrence is common.

Physical Methods of Hair Removal

- Physical and cosmetic measures are the cornerstone of care for hirsutism. Physical methods can be temporary or permanent.
- Depilation and epilations are temporary methods. Temporary depilations are shaving and chemical depilatories. In depilation part of hair is removed. Epilation removes the entire hair and consists of plucking and waxing.
- For permanent hair removal, the dermal papilla needs to be destroyed which is done either by electrolysis or laser.

Physical methods are:
- Temporary *depilation* (shaving and chemical depilatories)
- Temporary *epilation* (plucking and waxing)
- *Permanent hair* removal: Electrolysis and photoepilation therapy (laser, pulsed light)
- Eflornithine hydrochloride (Vaniqa) cream application.

Q. Which physical methods?
- Shaving—easiest and safest method
- Bleaching may be ineffective for dark hair
- Plucking and/or waxing kill the hair follicles, and induces folliculitis
- Depilating agents may result chronic skin irritation and worsen hair growth
- Electrolysis is the very effective and permanent method of hair removal and adjunct to medical therapy but time consuming, costly and has other disadvantages like pain, scarring, and pigmentation. Electrolysis has been largely replaced by use of laser techniques.
- Laser-assisted hair removal is a promising and rapid method of hair removal. Laser selectively causes thermal damage without damaging adjacent tissues, a process known as photothermolysis. Several lasers are available, among those pulsed diode lasers are generally less expensive and more reliable than other laser sources for hair removal.
- 13.9% topical application of eflornithine hydrochloride (Vaniqa) cream is very effective.

Surgery

Surgery in the form of wedge resection of ovary and LOD should be reserved as a last resort for hormonal suppression usually done when associated with infertility.

SUMMARY OF RECOMMENDATION OF TREATMENT

- Initial choice is low dose OC in anovulatory woman. Less androgenic progestogen is preferred. Combination of CA and EE is claimed to be a good choice—at least 6 months are required to demonstrate the impact.
- Not responding well with OC antiandrogen is added, spironolactone or finasteride (in order). Flutamide is best choice for alopecia but hepatotoxic and makes skin dry. Finasteride is safe but less effective.
- Polycystic ovary syndrome-associated hirsutism may improve modestly with insulin sensitizer.
- Gonadotropin-releasing hormone agonist should be reserved for resistant to initial therapy.
- Combination medical therapy is given in nonresponding to single drug.
- Combination treatment with electrolysis and photoepilation therapy (laser, pulsed light) is not recommended until hormonal suppression for 6 months.
- A trial of eflornithine chloride cream might be tried initially for facial hirsutism, although cost is a consideration. One should always be encouraged to control weight.
- Therapy can be continued for 2 years and then re-evaluation.
- No agent is superior to other. Choice is governed by cost, availability, and side effect.

PHYSIOLOGY OF HAIR

Structure of Hair (Fig. 20)

- The hair follicle is a member of the pilosebaceous unit the other components of which are sebaceous glands and the arrector pili muscle.
- The hair follicle consists of hair shaft, bulb, and the dermal papilla.
- Dermal papilla is surrounded by the bulb. It is composed of connective tissue and is the active part of hair follicle. Growth and regeneration of hair depends on its survival.
- Permanent hair loss is due to destruction of dermal papilla. Sufficient electrolysis and laser treatment are needed to destroy dermal papilla and to remove hair permanently.
- Epilation can remove the hair temporarily and dermal papilla remains intact. By depilation part of hair is removed.
- Ornithine decarboxylase, an enzyme which is present in dermal papilla, is essential for growth of hair. Eflornithine (Vaniqa), a topical cream, when applied inhibits this enzyme and retards hair growth with improvement of hirsutism significantly.

Types of Hair

There are three general types of hair namely—(1) lanugo hair, (2) vellus hair, and (3) terminal hair.
- *Lanugo hair* is lightly pigmented and covers the fetus and is shed sometimes late in gestation or early postpartum.

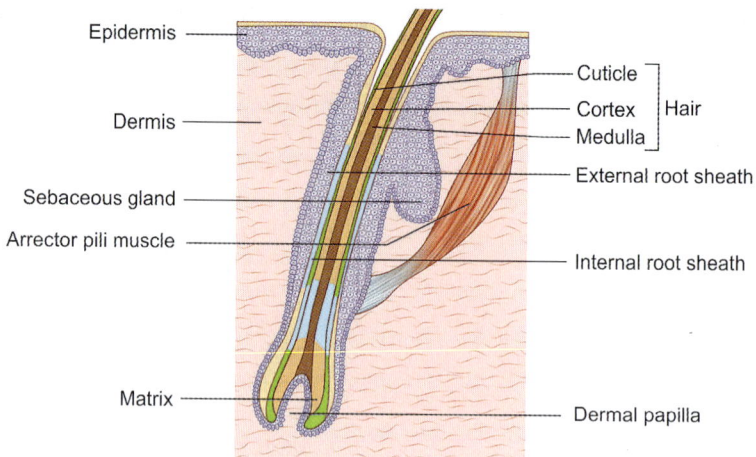

Fig. 20: Structure of a hair follicle.

- *Vellus hair* is soft, usually nonpigmented, and gradually replaces lanugo hair. They cover the apparently hairless areas of the body.
- *Terminal hair* is longer, coarser, darkly pigmented and arises from vellus hair. This hair makes up the eyelashes, eyebrows, the scalp hair, pubic, axillary hair, etc.

Androgens convert lanugo hair and vellus hair into terminal hair. *Once the pattern is established it will persist despite withdrawal of androgen which is the major problem of getting treatment response in hirsutism.*

Phases of Hair

Each hair follicle perpetually goes through three phases (**Fig. 21**):
1. *Anagen* (growth)
2. *Catagen* (involution)
3. *Telogen* (resting) phases.

Length and Duration of Survival of Hair

The overall length of hair is determined primarily by the duration of the anagen phase. Longer the anagen phase larger is the hair. Long hair like scalp hair and male beard have longer anagen phase of 2–5 years with short resting phase. Shorter hair like forearm hair has longer telogen phase but shorter anagen phase of only few months.

Asynchronization of Scalp Hair is a Rule

Scalp hair is *asynchronous* and always seems to be growing. If marked synchrony is achieved, then most of the hairs go to telogen phase at the same time resulting shedding of hairs called, *telogen effluvium*. In puerperium due to fall of estrogen level excess hairs of anagen phase will return to telogen phase with excessive shedding of hair follicles at one time followed by onset of new anagen phase. This is the reason why most women complain of fall of hair during puerperium.

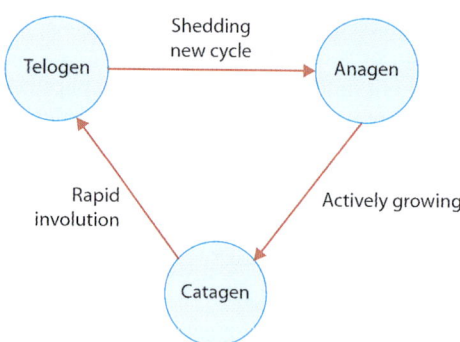

Fig. 21: Phases of hair.

Q. How hairs can be categorized according to the sensitivity of androgens?

Nonsexual hairs are independent of androgen and present over eye lashes, eyebrows, and lateral and occipital aspects of scalp.

Sexual hairs respond only to high levels of androgen and are predominantly located in the midline areas of the body-face, chest, breasts, axillae, lower abdomen, pubic area and thigh.

Ambosexual hairs are those which are quite sensitive to low androgen level and present over lower pubic triangle and axillary region.

Alopecia (Baldness)

Alopecia (baldness) is a vexing problem for both, patient and clinician. It is very conflicting that a hirsute girl who has come for excess growth of hair over body and faces frequently complains of loss of hair over scalp.

Alopecia, in most instances, is a temporary phenomenon and is due to synchronous hair growth and loss.

Thus, *telogen effluvium* often occurs in late pregnancy and puerperium. With time, following asynchronization of hair growth, hair density becomes normal. Alopecia may be due to acute, stressful events or consequences of aging process, beginning at the age of about 50 years in both sexes or, may be hereditary.

It is worthwhile to rule out thyroid disease in alopecia by measuring TSH.

Alopecia may not be associated with hirsutism or menstrual dysfunction. However, patients with alopecia need evaluation for hyperandrogenism, because significant number of cases may be successfully treated.

As alopecia reflects increased scalp 5α-reductase activity antiandrogens like flutamide, etc., act very well to treat the cases.

DIFFERENTIAL DIAGNOSIS OF PCOS

All cases of secondary amenorrhea. All cases of hirsutism.

CHAPTER 13

A Case of Primary Amenorrhea and Disorder of Sexual Development

Chapter Outline

Writing a case of primary amenorrhea and how to present the case?

- Description of Six Types of Commonly Encountered Primary Amenorrhea Cases
- Causes and Classification
- Diagnostic Approach
- Management and Discussion of Individual Cases
- Tanner Staging of Breasts and Pubic Hair Development
- Physiology of Sexual Differentiation
- DSD (Intersex)—Definition and Recent Classification
- Diagnosis and Approach to DSD Cases
- Sex of Rearing
- Medical and Surgical Management of DSD

INTRODUCTION

The following common cases are kept in mind while dealing with a case of primary amenorrhea:

- Constitutional delay (delayed puberty)
- Turner syndrome
- Mayer-Rokitansky-Küster-Hauser (MRKH) syndrome
- Androgen insensitivity syndrome (AIS) (testicular feminization syndrome)
- Congenital adrenal hyperplasia (CAH) (adrenogenital syndrome)
- Hypogonadotropic hypogonadism.

Everyone must be aware about the diagnosis and management of those above common cases. Majority (80%) of primary amenorrhea cases can be diagnosed from the history and clinical examination findings. Investigative procedures are needed to confirm the diagnosis and planning the treatment of the cases and to diagnose the other rare cases.

For management of every primary amenorrhea case, the following points are to be addressed.

- To manage the health problem, if any
- To address secondary sexual character
- Restoration of menstrual function, coital function, and reproduction as much as possible
- In case of ambiguous genitalia, rearing of sex is the important issue.

In evaluation of primary amenorrhea all causes of secondary amenorrhea should be considered. All causes of secondary amenorrhea can also present as primary amenorrhea.

The examples of above six cases of primary amenorrhea with their salient features are depicted below with photographs.

Delayed Puberty (Constitutional Delay)

- 16-year-old girl developed secondary sexual characters by 14 years
- It has not had menarche
- Family history (mother) of delayed menarche
- Other investigations within normal limit.

Turner Syndrome (Figs. 1 and 2)

- Age 17 years
- Height 4 feet 9 inches

CHAPTER 13: A Case of Primary Amenorrhea and Disorder of Sexual Development

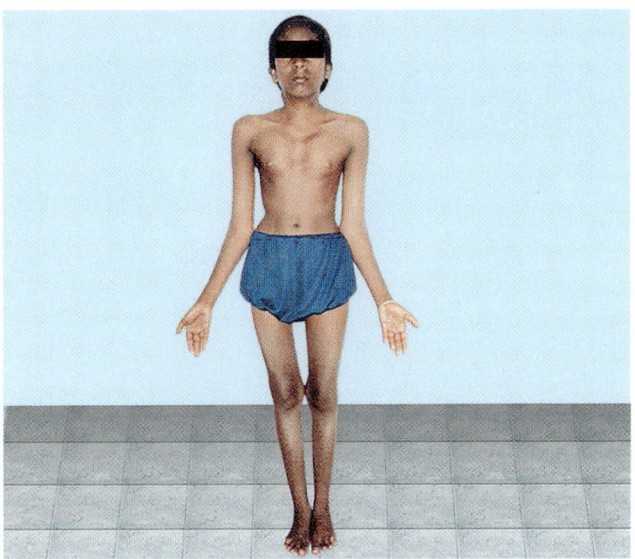

Fig. 1: Turner syndrome—short stature, webbing of neck, cubitus valgus, shield chest, and small fourth metatarsals.

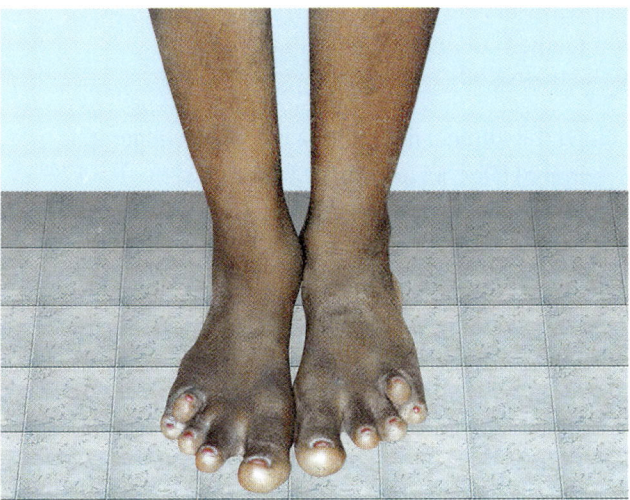

Fig. 2: Turner syndrome—bilateral small fourth metatarsals (the same patient as in Figure 1).

- No onset of menses, withdrawal bleeding +
- Cubitus valgus
- Small 4th metatarsal
- Pubic hair/axillary hair scanty
- Breasts—Tanner 1
- Vagina patent
- Karyotyping—45 XO
- Laparoscope/ultrasonography (USG)—small uterus, streak ovaries

Mayer–Rokitansky–Küster–Hauser (MRKH) Syndrome (Fig. 3)

- 18 years
- Primary amenorrhea
- Secondary sexual characters—normal, breasts, and pubic hair-like female

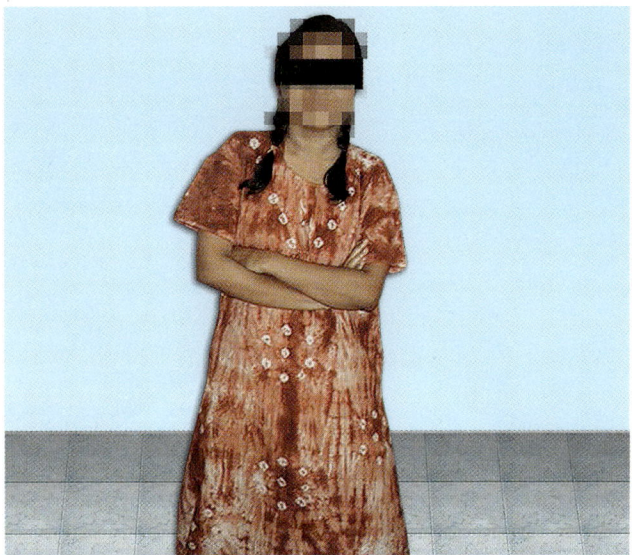

Fig. 3: Mayer–Rokitansky–Küster–Hauser (MRKH) syndrome.

- Vagina blind
- USG—uterus—absent, ovaries present, follicle present
- Karyotype—46 XX
- Serum testosterone—normal (female range)

Androgen Insensitivity Syndrome (AIS) (Testicular Feminization Syndrome) (Figs. 4 and 5)

- 22-year-old female
- Case of no onset of periods
- Cardiovascular system (CVS)—normal

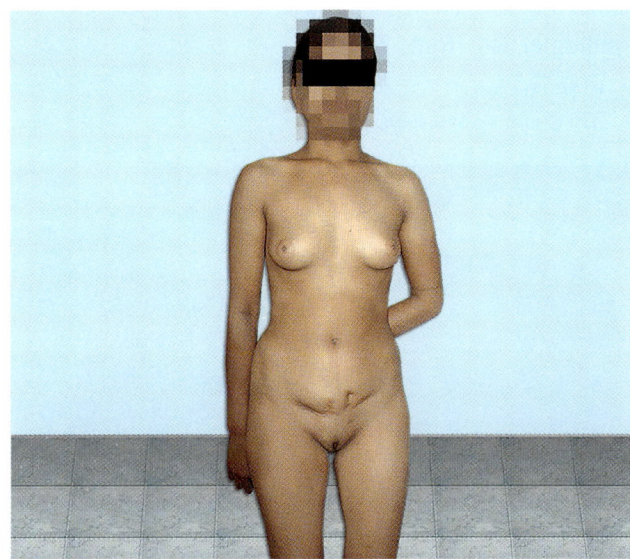

Fig. 4: Androgen insensitivity syndrome (AIS)—this patient had surgery for inguinal hernia at 9 years of age and surgery for hernia was done. Patient again came at the age of 22 years after marriage, karyotype showed 46XY and after counseling gonadectomy performed.

Courtesy: Professor Asok Biswas, Dr Ranjan Basu, Associate Professor, Obstetrics and Gynecology

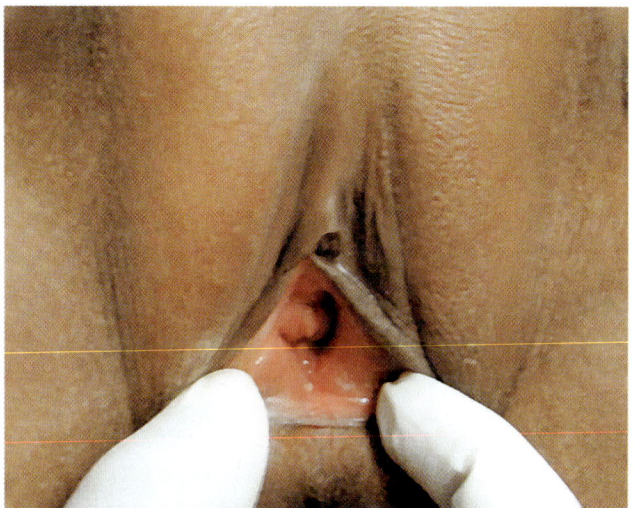

Fig. 5: Showing vaginal introitus in androgen insensitivity syndrome (AIS).

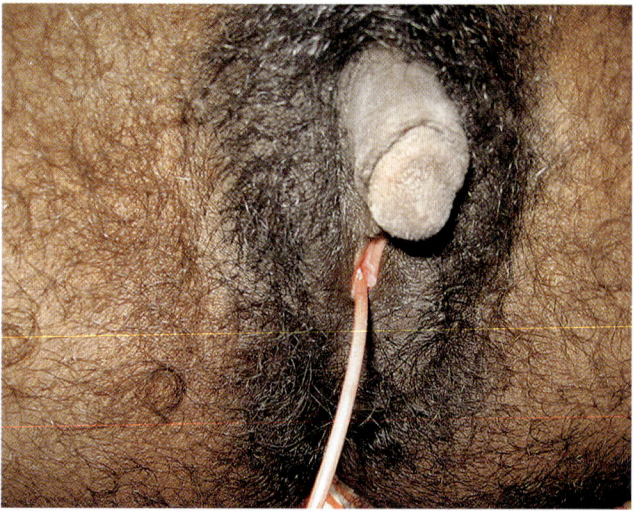

Fig. 7: Adrenogenital syndrome.

- *Secondary sexual character*:
  - Breast—Tanner 3
  - Axillary and pubic hair—absent
- Presence of gonads on inguinal region or at labia
- Vagina—blind vagina, approximately 3 cm
- USG—absence of uterus and ovaries in pelvis, gonads in inguinal region
- Karyotype—46 XY
- Serum testosterone—level like male
- Family history—2 daughters of the patient's aunt (mother's younger sister) presented with primary amenorrhea to have similar picture with karyotyping 46 XY.

Congenital Adrenal Hyperplasia (CAH) (Adrenogenital Syndrome) (Figs. 6 and 7)

- 15 years
- Hirsutism—severe type
- Hoarseness of voice—present
- Breasts not developed
- Enlarged clitoris, fusion of labia
- Increase 17KS

Congenital Adrenal Hyperplasia (CAH)(Adrenogenital Syndrome) (Figs. 8A and 8B) in a Newborn (Text Described Later)

Hypogonadotropic Hypogonadism (Fig. 9):
- 26 years
- No onset of menstruation, withdrawal bleeding +
- Height—5 feet 6 inches
- Breasts—Tanner 2
- Axillary hair/pubic hair—present
- Vagina present
- Laparoscope/USG—small uterus and gonads

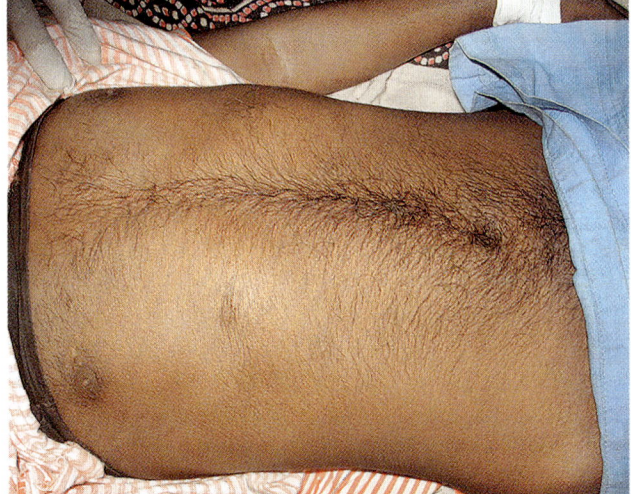

Fig. 6: Congenital adrenal hyperplasia—virilization, male pattern hair over abdomen, breast atrophy.

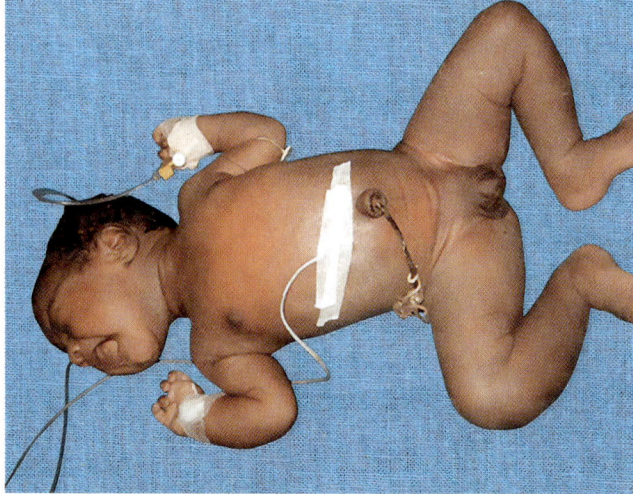

Fig. 8A: Congenital adrenal hyperplasia (CAH): 3rd day newborn developing hyponatremia and hypoglycemia.

CHAPTER 13: A Case of Primary Amenorrhea and Disorder of Sexual Development

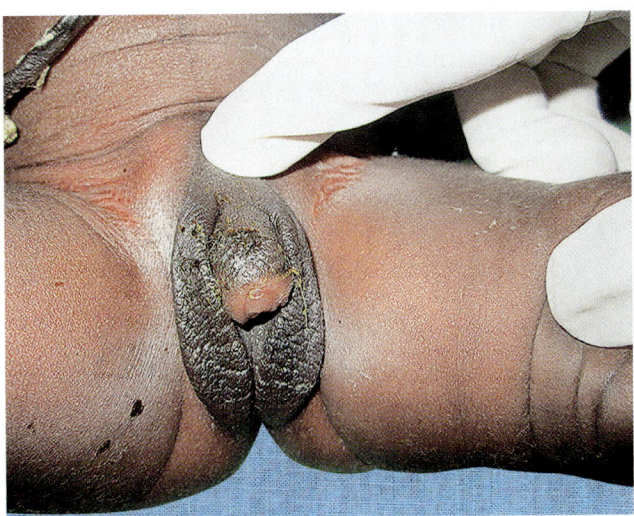

Fig. 8B: External genitalia-enlarged clitoris, fused labioscrotal folds and penile urethra.

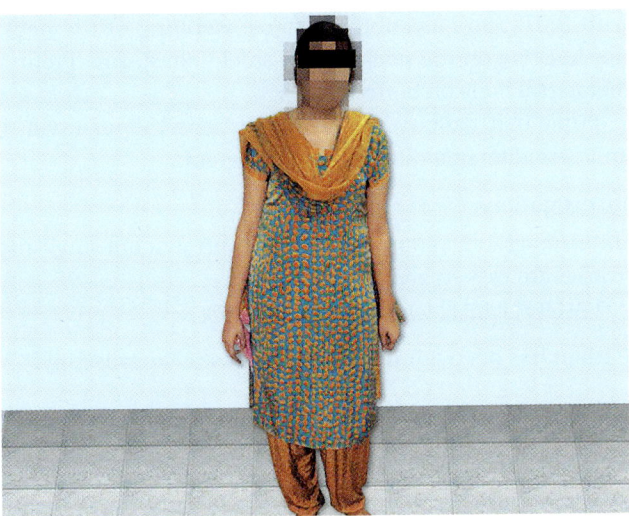

Fig. 9: Hypogonadotropic hypogonadism.

- Follicle-stimulating hormone (FSH)—low 0.01, luteinizing hormone (LH) low 17 mIU
- Karyotype 46 XX

WRITING A CASE OF PRIMARY AMENORRHEA

History Taking and Examination

Patient's particular

1. Name: Miss XY
2. Age: 17 years
3. Address:
4. Occupation:
5. Married/unmarried: Unmarried
6. History of infertility:
7. Husband's occupation:

Bed No.:
Date of admission:
Date of examination:

8. Socioeconomic status:
9. Religion:
10. Parous/nulliparous: Nulliparous

History

1. *Chief complaint:* Usually comes with no onset of menstruation in normal age with or without development of secondary sexual character.
2. *History of present illness:* Chief complaints are elaborated. Headache, visual defect [pituitary adenoma and central nervous system (CNS) tumor], and history of galactorrhea are enquired. Age of development of secondary character/thelarche, rate of growth- growth charts available or not, history of abdominal pain, lump, retention of urine (cryptomenorrhea), anosmia (Kallmann syndrome), weight loss, poor nutrition, vigorous exercise, psychological stress, dieting, and vasomotor symptoms.
   - History of hirsutism, acne [polycystic ovary syndrome (PCOS), CAH, ovarian or adrenal tumor, Cushing syndrome].
3. *Menstrual history:* Cyclical pain abdomen indicates cryptomenorrhea
4. *Obstetric history:* Not applicable
5. *Past history:*
   - *Medical*—childhood meningitis/encephalitis, tuberculosis (TB), hypothyroidism, and history of radiotherapy/chemotherapy
   - *Surgical*—history of surgery (abdominal/inguinal).
6. *Family history:* Diabetes, hypertension, history of PCOS, same incidence in family (sibling), testicular feminizing syndrome, and history of delayed menarche of mother.
7. *Sexual history:* Coital difficulty, vaginal dryness due to estrogen deficiency.
8. *Functional history:* Anorexia
9. *Personal history:* Vigorous exercise, stress, and psychological problem
10. *Contraceptive history*
11. *Drug history/treatment history*—any medication particularly hormone, shaving or any mechanical method for hirsutism. Other medication causing hyperprolactinemia like antipsychotic, metchlorpropamide, phenothiazine. History of radiation and chemotherapy.

Physical Examination

Detailed general survey are done and noted. The points relevant to this case are:
- *Height:*
  - *Short*: Turner's and pituitary dwarfism
  - *Abnormally tall*: Primary ovarian failure and gigantic acromegaly
  - *Normal*: Hypogonadotropic hypogonadism, RKH syndrome, and mosaic Turner.

- *Weight/body mass index (BMI):*
  - *Obese*: PCOS, hypothyroidism, Cushing's, pituitary, and hypothalamic obesity.
  - *Abnormally thin*: TB and anorexia nervosa.
- *Hirsutism, acne, male-balding pattern:* PCOS, Cushing's, CAH, ovarian neoplasm.
  If there is hirsutism, scoring is done by Ferriman and Gallwey scoring system (modified):
  - Total nine body areas are examined. Score 0–4 for each area, 0 = no hirsutism, and 4 = severe hirsutism. Total maximum may be 36.
  - Total score 8 or more—hirsutism.
- *Stigma of Turner:* Webbing of neck, shield chest, and cubitus valgus.
- Buffalo hump, central obesity, striae, hypertension—Cushing syndrome.
- *Secondary sexual character:*
  - Breasts examination (Do Tanner staging, *see* Page 318, **Fig. 19A**):
    - Absent or ill-developed breast—Turner's, CAH, cretinism
  - Pubic and axillary hair (Do Tanner staging of pubic hair, *see* Page 318, **Fig. 19B**):
    - Turner's—scanty
    - Androgen insensitive syndrome—absent or less.
- Blood pressure—both arms
- Pulse—all limbs.

Systemic Examination

- *Cardiovascular system*—for presence of coarctation of aorta.
- *Breasts examination*—presence of galactorrhea searched for.

Gynecological Examination

Abdominal Examination
Any abdominopelvic lump.

Pelvic/Per Vaginal Examination

- *Absence or abnormalities of uterus and cervix:* RKH syndrome, hematometra, and cervical atresia
- *Ambiguous genitalia*
- *Enlarged clitoris:* CAH, testicular-feminizing syndrome (incomplete variety), androgen-secreting tumor
- *Absence of vaginal opening:* CAH, imperforate hymen, and RKH syndrome
- *Closure of upper part of vagina:* Transverse vaginal septum, vaginal agenesis, and testicular-feminizing syndrome.

Investigations Supplied or Required

- *Pregnancy test*—pregnancy should always be excluded in any type of amenorrhea.
- *Serum FSH and LH*—high
- *Thyroid-stimulating hormone (TSH)*—normal
- *Prolactin*—normal
- *Testosterone (free and total) and dehydroepiandrosterone sulfate (DHEA-SO$_4^-$)*
- *Karyotype*—45 XO
- *USG pelvis*—small ovary and no follicle
- Magnetic resonance imaging (MRI) of brain
- *Diagnostic laparoscopy*—streak gonad and small uterus.

Summary of the Case (Sample)

A 17-year unmarried girl attended gynecological outpatient department (GOPD) with no onset of menstruation and no development of breasts. She has no cyclical pain abdomen or any other significant complain. She has no significant past history. She has one elder sister but without such abnormality. She had occasional vaginal bleeding only after taking of some hormone tablets.

On examination her height is 4 feet 9 inches, thin built with BMI. She has cubitus valgus, webbing of the neck, low hairline on the neck, broad-shield chest, small fourth metatarsal bone on both side.

Pubic hair/axillary hair scanty, breasts Tanner 1, vulva, and perineum infantile, and vagina patent.

Investigations
Ultrasonography report shows uterus present but small and ovaries are very small with no follicle.
- FSH/LH—high, with karyotype 45 XO.

Patient has been admitted for diagnostic laparoscopy.

Provisional Diagnosis
A case of Turner syndrome.

Differential Diagnosis
Differential diagnosis (D/D) as above.

Q. What is your case?
Tell the summary.

Q. So, what is your diagnosis?
A case of primary amenorrhea probably Turner syndrome.

DEFINITION

Q. How would you define primary amenorrhea?

- Absence of menses by 14 years of age with no visible secondary sexual characteristic development.
  Or
- Absence of menses by 16 years of age in the presence of normal secondary sexual characteristics.

In other opinion—the ages are 13 years and 15 years, respectively.

Q. When to start investigations in case of primary amenorrhea?

Absence of menses by 13 years of age with no visible secondary sexual characters or by 15 years with normal secondary sexual characters.

- *Exception*: Patient presenting with typical features, e.g., Turner syndrome, absent vagina, etc., need to be investigated immediately.

ETIOLOGIES OF PRIMARY AMENORRHEA

Q. What are the etiologies of primary amenorrhea?

Menstruation is an end result of coordinated activity of hypothalamic pituitary ovarian uterine axis with normal outflow tract with normal thyroid, adrenal, and metabolic function. Karyotyping and environment also have great influence in normal menstruation. This can be schematically diagrammed in **Flowchart 1**.

Abnormality/abnormalities on any point may cause amenorrhea.

Compartment-wise Causes

Compartment-wise the causes are:
- *Hypothalamus/CNS cause (compartment 4):* Idiopathic, Kallmann syndrome, functional, weight loss, anorexia, stress, psychological, and damage by tumor.
- *Pituitary cause (compartment 3):* Hyperprolactinemia, damage by radiation, surgery, compression by tumor, hypoplasia, infarction (Sheehan), and empty sella syndrome.
- *Ovarian cause (compartment 2):* Gonadal dysgenesis (Turner syndrome, mosaic Turner), PCOS in early age before menarche.
- *Uterovaginal cause (compartment 1):* RKH syndrome, cervical atresia, transverse vaginal septum, imperforate hymen, and endometrial receptor defect.
- *Adrenal:* CAH and tumor.
- *Thyroid:* Juvenile hypothyroidism.
- *Miscellaneous:* 5α-reductase deficiency, testicular feminization syndrome, liver disease, kidney disease, etc.

In **hypogonadotropic hypogonadism amenorrhea**, primary defect is in hypothalamus or pituitary (*see* **Table 1**), gonadotropins are low and estrogen is low.

In **hypergonadotropic hypogonadism**, primary defect is in ovary, gonadotropins are high and estrogen low.

Whereas, in **eugonadotropic hypogonadism**, site is variable, gonadotropins and estrogen level are generally normal.

Primary amenorrhea can also be classified as:

1. Delayed puberty
2. Anatomical defect
3. Chromosomal abnormalities
4. Endocrine abnormality.

- *Delayed puberty:* Nutritional and familial
- *Anatomical defects:* (1) Outflow tract obstruction—imperforate hymen, transvaginal septum, isolated vaginal atresia, cervical atresia or stenosis, and labial agglutination. (2) Absent of endometrium—complete Mullerian agenesis (absent uterus, cervix, and vagina) and uterine synechia (Asherman syndrome).
- *Chromosomal abnormalities:* Turner (XO), mosaic Turner (XO/XY), and XY(AIS).
- *Endocrine abnormality:* Hypogonadotropic hypogonadism, ovarian failure, hyperprolactinemia, hypothyroidism, PCOS, androgen-secreting tumor of ovary and adrenal.

COMMON CAUSES OF PRIMARY AMENORRHEA

Q. What are the common causes of primary amenorrhea?

Primary amenorrhea is mostly due to chromosomal abnormality or anatomical defect, but not always. The important causes are:
- Chromosomal abnormality—50%
- Hypogonadotropic hypogonadism—20%
- Mullerian agenesis—15%
- Transverse vaginal septum or imperforate hymen—5%
- Pituitary disease—5%
- Others (AIS, CAH, and PCOS)—5%.

Q. How will you clinically classify primary amenorrhea?

- Primary amenorrhea with normal breast development
- Primary amenorrhea with absent breast development, which is further subdivided according to level of FSH (**Table 1**).

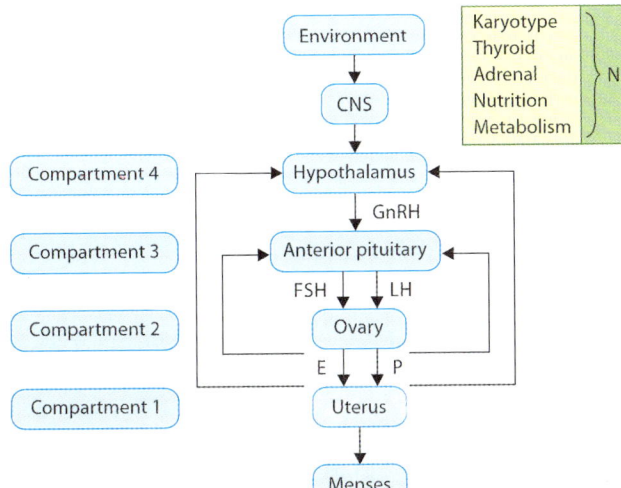

Flowchart 1: Control of menstruation.

Abbreviations: CNS, central nervous system; FSH, follicle-stimulating hormone; LH, luteinizing hormone

Table 1: Clinical classification of primary amenorrhea.

Normal breast development (30%)	Absent breast development with high FSH (40%)	Absent breast development with low FSH (30%)
• Müllerian agenesis—10% • Androgen insensitivity—9% • Vaginal septum—2% • Imperforate hymen—1% • Constitutional delay—8%	• 46 XX (ovarian failure)—15% • 46 XY (gonadal failure)—5% • Abnormal Karyotype (most common 45 XO)—20%	• Constitutional delay—10% • Prolactinomas—5% • Kallmann syndrome—2% • Other CNS—3% • Stress, weight loss, anorexia—3% • PCOS—3% • Congenital adrenal hyperplasia—3% • Other—1%

Abbreviations: FSH, follicle stimulating hormone; CNS, central nervous system; PCOS, polycystic ovary syndrome
Courtesy: ASRM, Practice Committee. Amenorrhoea, FerilSteril. 2008.

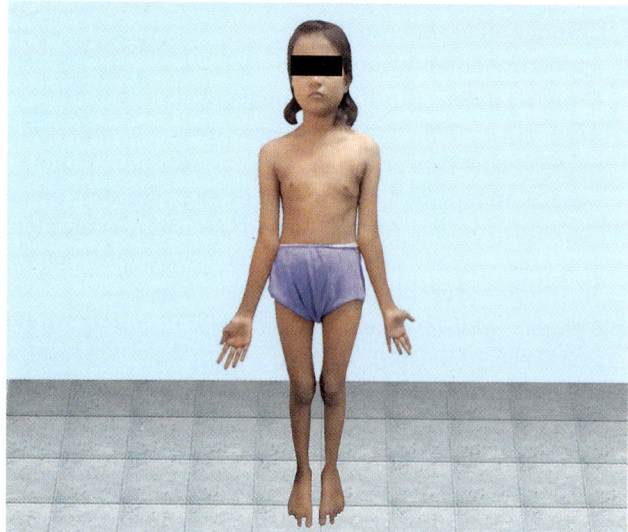

Fig. 9A: Turner syndrome: 19 years, short stature (4 feet 1 inch), short length of some toes.

Classification according to height:

- *Short stature:* Turner syndrome (classical) (**Fig. 9A**), hypothalamic lesions, and pituitary lesions.
- *Normal height:* Physiological delay is the most common. Others are CNS tumors, hypothalamic or pituitary tumors, severe systemic diseases, e.g., TB, hypogonadotropic hypogonadism, Kallmann syndrome, gonadal dysgenesis, Mosaic Turner syndrome.

DIAGNOSIS A CASE OF PRIMARY AMENORRHEA

Q. How would you diagnose a case of primary amenorrhea?

- History
- Physical examination
- *Investigations:* Pregnancy test, serum FSH, LH, TSH, and prolactin, USG pelvis/MRI, karyotyping, laparoscopy, and other laboratory tests as required.

History

- Age
- Age of development of secondary character/thelarche
- Rate of growth—growth charts available or not
- Abdominal pain
- Retention of urine
- Anosmia
- Weight loss, poor nutrition, vigorous exercise, psychological stress, and dieting
- Headache/visual defect—empty sella syndrome and CNS tumor
- Vasomotor symptoms—premature ovarian failure (POF)
- History of hirsutism; acne—PCOS, CAH, ovarian or adrenal tumor; and Cushing syndrome
- Galactorrhea (pituitary tumor—hyperprolactinemia)
- Palpitations, cold intolerance, diarrhea, constipation—thyroid disorder
- *Past history*:
  - *Medical*—childhood meningitis/encephalitis, TB, hypothyroidism, history of radiotherapy/chemotherapy
  - *Surgical*—history of surgery (abdominal/inguinal)
- *Family history*: Similar type of incidence in family (sibling), testicular feminizing syndrome, history of delayed menarche of mother.
- *Drug history*: Steroids, metoclopramide, cimetidine, TCA, reserpine.

Physical Examination

- Height
- Short—Turner's, pituitary dwarfism
- Abnormally tall—primary ovarian failure
- Gigantic—acromegaly
- Normal—hypogonadotropic hypogonadism, RKH syndrome, and mosaic Turner
- *Built/weight/BMI*:
  - *Obese*—PCOS, hypothyroidism, Cushing's, pituitary, and hypothalamic obesity
  - *Abnormally thin*—TB and anorexia nervosa
- *Thyroid gland examination*: To detect thyroid disorder
- *Hirsutism*, *acne*, and *male-balding pattern*: PCOS, Cushing's, CAH (**Fig. 10**), ovarian neoplasm
- *Stigma of Turner*—webbing of neck, shield chest, and cubitus valgus
- Buffalo hump, central obesity, striae, hypertension—Cushing syndrome

Systemic Examination

Cardiovascular system: *Coarctation of aorta* in Turner syndrome.

Per Abdominal Examination

- *Lower abdominal lump*: Hematometra (**Fig. 11**), displaced kidney, and ovarian neoplasm.
- Any swelling over inguinal region or over labia (testis in androgen insensitivity syndrome).

CHAPTER 13: A Case of Primary Amenorrhea and Disorder of Sexual Development

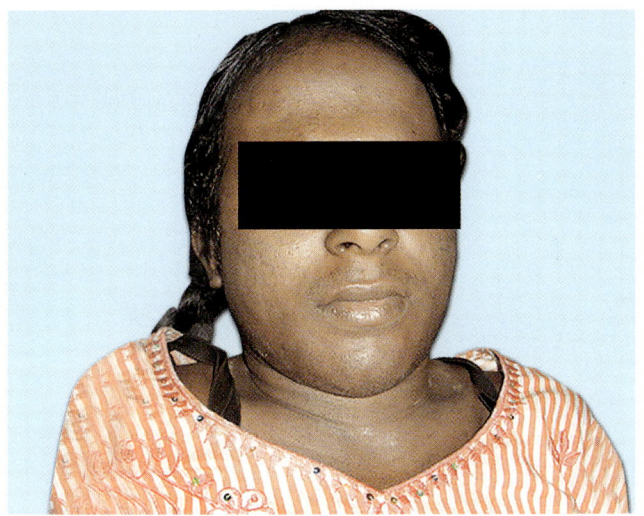

Fig. 10: Congenital adrenal hyperplasia (CAH)—balding loss of hair, hirsutism (shaved beard)

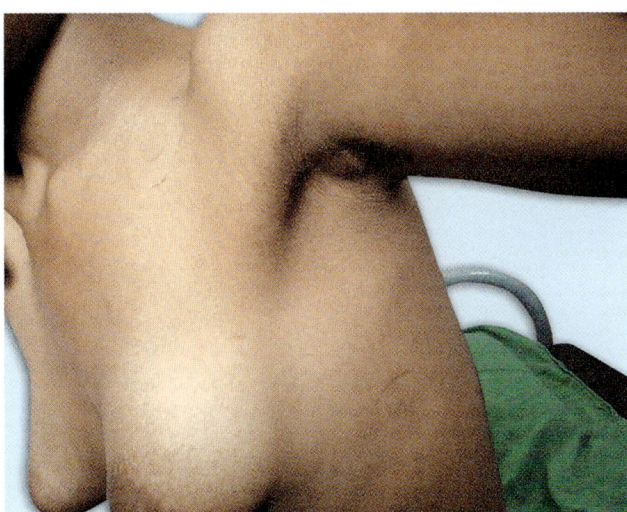

Fig. 12: Androgen insensitivity syndrome (AIS) (less axillary hair).

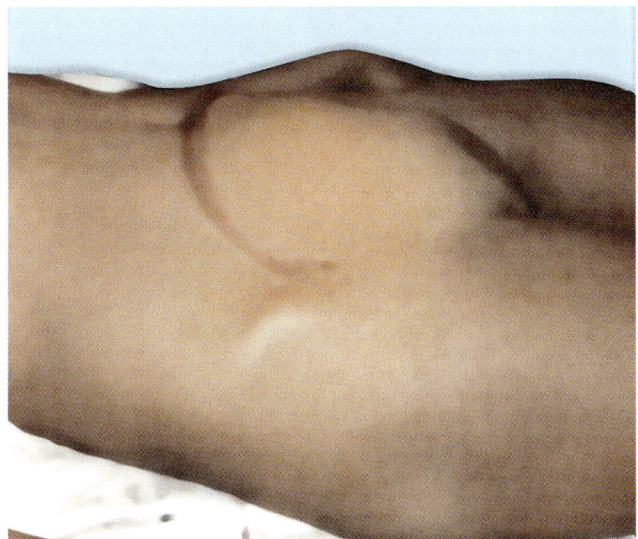

Fig. 11: Hematometra (cryptomenorrhea in imperforate hymen).

Secondary Sexual Character

- *Breasts examination* (Do Tanner staging, *see* Page 318, **Fig. 19A**):
  - Absent or ill-developed breast—Turner's, CAH, and cretinism.
- *Pubic and axillary hair* (Do Tanner staging of pubic hair, *see* Page 318, **Fig. 19B**):
  - Turner's—scanty
  - Androgen insensitivity syndrome (ASI)—absent (**Fig. 12**).

Pelvic/External Genitalia Examination

- *Absence or abnormalities of uterus and cervix*: RKH syndrome, hematometra, and cervical atresia.
- *Enlarged clitoris*: CAH, testicular-feminizing syndrome (incomplete variety), androgen-secreting tumor.
- *Absence of vaginal opening*: CAH, imperforate hymen, and RKH syndrome.
- *Closure of upper part of vagina*: Transverse vaginal septum, agenesis, and testicular-feminizing syndrome.

Q. What are the causes of blind vagina?

The causes are:

- MRKH syndrome (**Fig. 13**)
- Androgen-insensitivity syndrome (**Fig. 14**)
- Transverse vaginal septum (**Fig. 15**)
- Imperforate hymen (**Fig. 16**).

Investigations

- *Pregnancy test*—pregnancy should always be excluded in any type of amenorrhea
- *Serum FSH and LH*—see below (**Table 2**).
- *TSH:* High-hypothyroidism and low-hyperthyroidism
- Prolactin is raised in pituitary adenoma, drugs, hypothyroidism, and other tumor.
- Testosterone (free and total), $DHEA\text{-}SO_4^-$ is raised in PCOS, ovarian, and adrenal neoplasm, CAH, Cushing syndrome.
- *Karyotype:* Abnormal in Turner syndrome and other rare conditions.
- *USG pelvis:* Small ovaries without follicle in Turner, ovarian enlargement, hematometra (**Fig. 17**).
- *MRI of brain:* Adenoma, MRI pelvis—hematometra (**Fig. 18**).
- *Diagnostic laparoscopy:* Müllerian agenesis in RKH, streak gonad in Turner, sometimes testes in parieties in AIS and also for diagnosis of pelvic TB.
- Hysteroscopy has value in diagnosing synechiae.

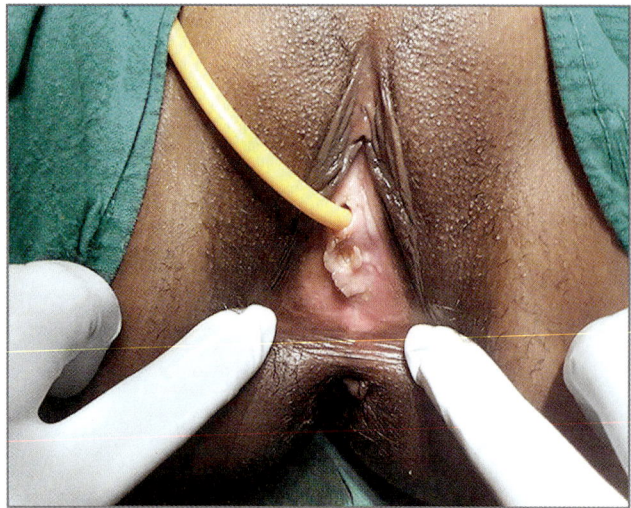

Fig. 13: Vaginal atresia in Rokitansky–Küster–Hauser (RKH) syndrome (concave appearance).

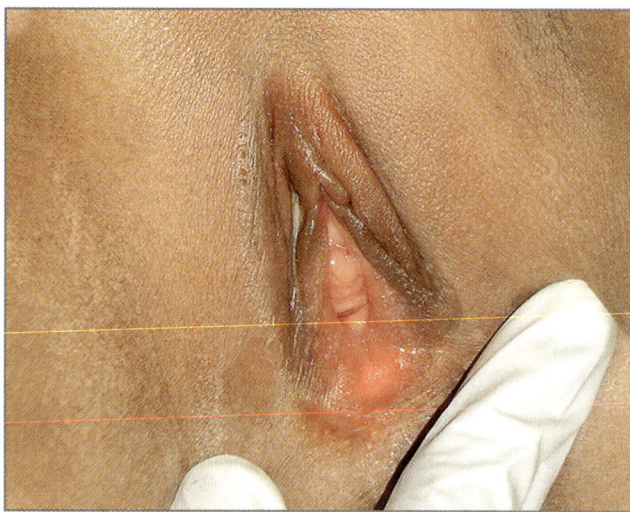

Fig. 14: Vagina in androgen insensitivity syndrome (AIS).
Courtesy: Dr Subir Bhattacharyya

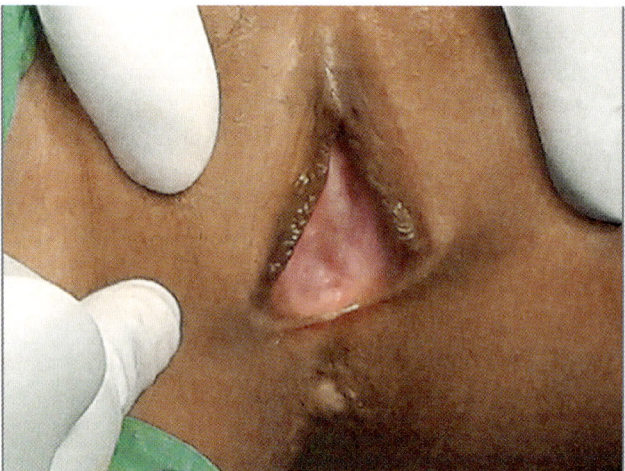

Fig. 15: Vaginal agenesis—lower third—presented with hematometra—ultrasonography (USG) (as in Figure 17), magnetic resonance imaging (MRI) (as in Figure 18).

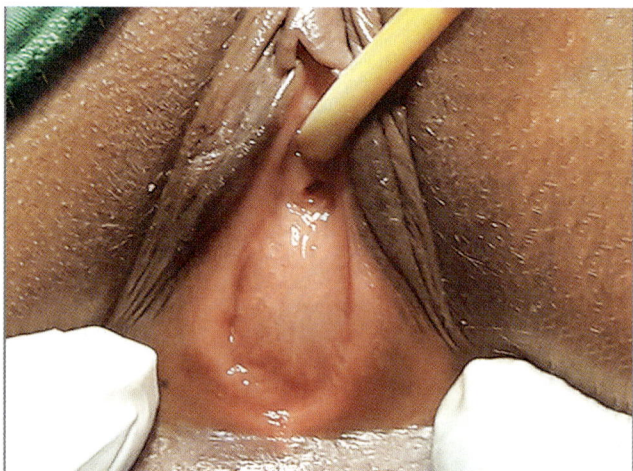

Fig. 16: Imperforate hymen (bulging—convex—compare with Figure 13).

Figs. 13 to 16: Four important causes of blind vagina (Note the differences).

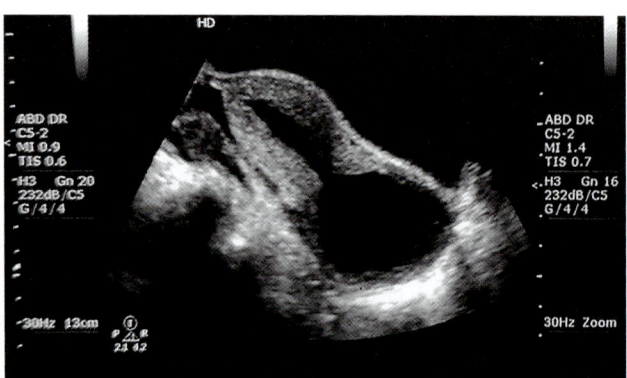

Fig. 17: Ultrasonography (USG)—hematometra.

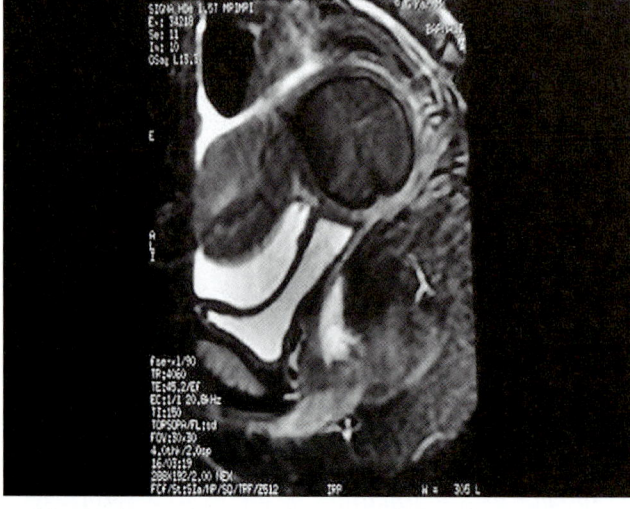

Fig. 18: Magnetic resonance imaging (MRI)— hematometra (cryptomenorrhea).

Q. What are the different clinical conditions of primary amenorrhea depending on the levels of gonadotropins?

See **Table 2**.

Table 2: Primary amenorrhea cases according to gonadotropin level.

Gonadotropin	Normal	High	Low
FSH	5–20 IU/L	>20 IU/L	>5 IU/L
LH	5–20 IU/L	>40 IU/L	>5 IU/L
Clinical conditions	• Normal adult female • PCOS • Asherman syndrome	• Hypergonadotropic hypogonadism • Primary ovarian insufficiency • Turner syndrome	• Hypogonadotropic hypogonadism • Functional hypothalamic amenorrhea

Abbreviations: FSH, follicle-stimulating hormone; LH, luteinizing hormone; PCOS, polycystic ovary syndrome

Diagnostic Approach in a Case of Primary Amenorrhea

See **Flowchart 2**

Sequence of development of puberty

- Breast budding (thelarche) is the first sign, which occurs at 10–12.5 years of age.
- Beginning of growth spurt starts 1 year after thelarche.
- Then pubic and axillary hair growth (adrenarche) occurs.
- Following which growth peak in height.
- Menstruation (menarche) starts at 10–15 years corresponding to breast and pubic hair stage 4.
- The last event is adult mature breast and pubic hair stage 5. From onset of puberty to menarche, it usually takes about 2 years.

Tanner staging of development of breasts (Fig. 19A):

- *Stage 1*: At the beginning, only papilla are elevated.
- *Stage 2*: In this stage breast bud and papilla are elevated with a small mound and areola diameter is enlarged.
- *Stage 3*: Further enlargement of breast mound and there is increase of palpable glandular tissue.
- *Stage 4*: A second mound is formed with the elevation of areola and papilla above the level of the rest of the breast looking almost adult-type.
- *Stage 5*: Final maturation occurs to form adult breast with recession of areola to the mound of breast tissue with rounding of the breast mound. Only the projection of papilla is evident.

Tanner staging of growth of pubic hair (Fig. 19B):

- *Stage 1*: In this stage, there is vellus hair only. Truly, there is no pubic hair.
- *Stage 2*: Long, slightly pigmented, downy hair grows sparsely or only slightly curled hair, and appears along labia.
- *Stage 3*: Hairs become darker, coarser, more curled, and spreads to the pubic area.
- *Stage 4*: Adult-type hair but there is no spread to the medial surface of thighs.
- *Stage 5*: Hairs spread to medial surface of thighs; distribution looks like an inverse triangle.

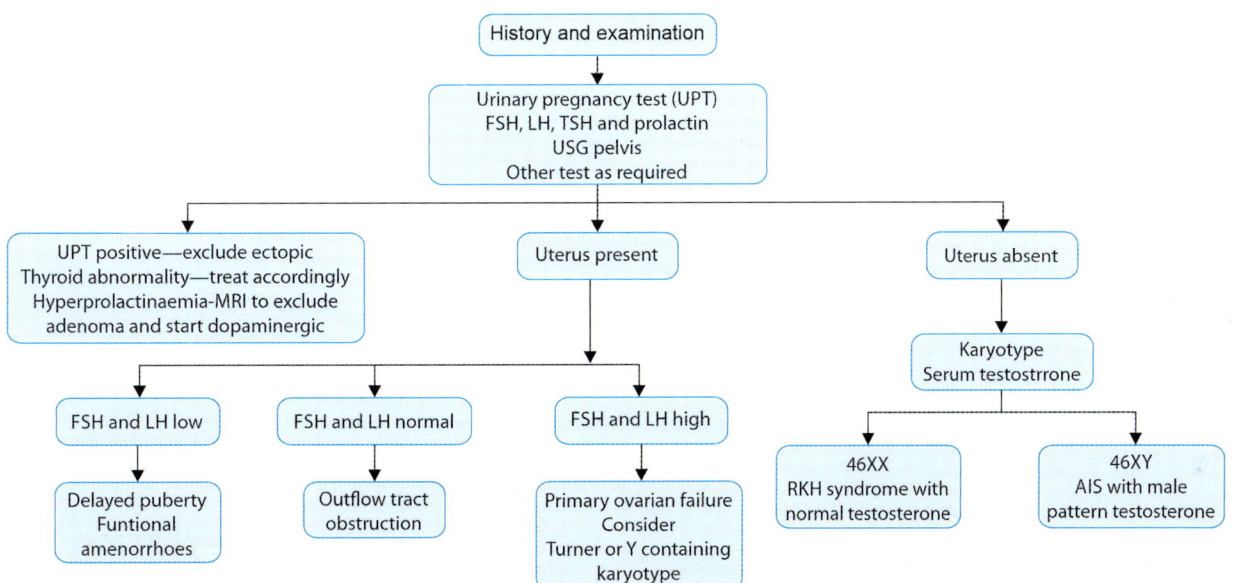

Flowchart 2: Diagnostic approach in a case of primary amenorrhea.

Abbreviations: FSH, follicle-stimulating hormone; LH, luteinizing hormone; ASI, androgen insensitivity syndrome; USG, ultrasonography; MRI, magnetic resonance imaging; TSH, thyroid-stimulating hormone

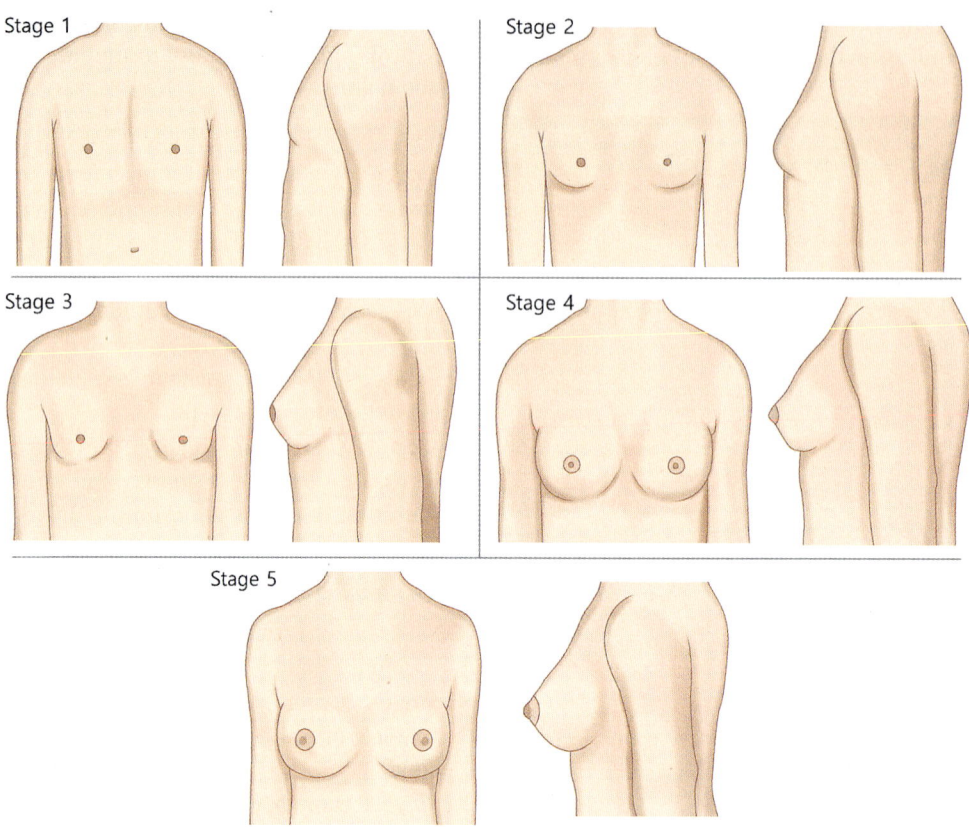

Fig. 19A: Sequence of breast development (Tanner staging).

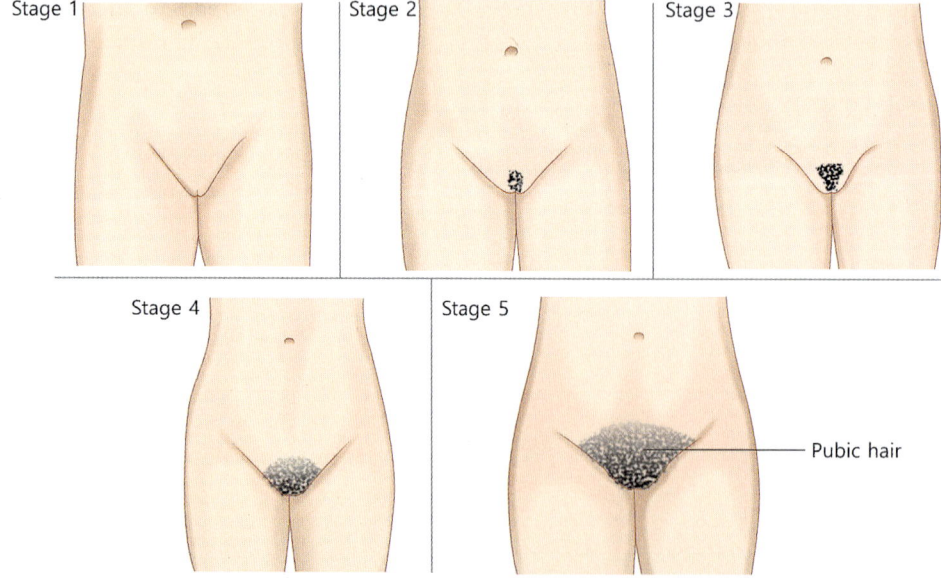

Fig. 19B: Sequence of pubic hair development (Tanner staging).

Management of Case of Primary Amenorrhea

Q. How would you manage a case of primary amenorrhea?

The basic principles of management are:
- ❖ Counseling and psychological support
- ❖ General health management
- ❖ Development of secondary sexual character in cases where it is not present
- ❖ Restoration of **genital tract function**:
  - ▪ *Menstrual function*

- Coital function
- Reproductive function
- If it is a variety of intersex, rearing of sex is an important part
- Treatment is individualized depending on diagnosis.

DISCUSSION OF INDIVIDUAL CASES

Delayed Puberty—Constitutional Delay

- Failure to develop secondary sexual characters by 13 years, which is more than two standard deviations from the mean age or, have not had menarche by age 16 years is called delayed puberty. The incidence is 3% among adolescents.
- *Cause*—constitutional delay is the most common. Other causes are malabsorption syndrome, underweight, chronic anovulation, anatomical abnormality, hypergonadotropic hypogonadism, and hypogonadotropic hypogonadism.
- The probable cause of constitutional delay is delay in gonadotropin-releasing hormone (GnRH) pulse generator reactivation. Often, there is family history of late puberty. Girls are otherwise healthy.
- *Investigations* are done to exclude other causes. History of impaired olfaction and marked weight loss are taken. Investigations like brain imaging, and FSH, prolactin, TSH measurement and other investigations are done. All investigations are within normal limit in constitutional delay and the diagnosis is confirmed retrospectively when spontaneous activation of H-P axis occurs.
- *Management:* It is very difficult to differentiate hypogonadotropic hypogonadism from constitutional delay in puberty, for which it is wise to commence treatment and revisit the diagnosis in later date. Treatment is started with low-dose estrogen until puberty progresses when estrogen is stopped. Progesterone withdrawal is not needed during low-dose estrogen treatment as in normal puberty similar long period of unopposed estrogen is found before ovulatory cycles.

TURNER SYNDROME

Turner syndrome is described in 1938 and was named after Henry Hubert Turner (1892–1970) who was born in Harrisburg, Illinois.

- **Turner syndrome** is the most common variety (50–60%) of gonadal dysgenesis with karyotype of 45 XO. Incidence is 1 in 2,500 women. In dysgenesis disorder in early fetal ovary, a normal complement of germ cells lies, but later due to accelerated atresia of ovary, ovary is replaced by fibrous streak, which is called streak gonad.
- **Gonadal dysgenesis** is broadly divided into two groups one of normal karyotype (46 XX, 46 XY) and the other abnormal. Among the abnormal karyotypes, Turner syndrome (45 XO) is the most common with classical multiple stigma.

Other patients with gonadal dysgenesis may have mosaic karyotype, or structural abnormality of second X chromosome and the most common form of mosaicism is 45 XO/46 XX.

Mosaic Turner is found in one-fourths cases. *Dysgenetic gonad with Y chromosome material should be removed as in 25% cases they will develop malignant germ cell tumor.*

Spontaneous menstruation with some degree of sexual maturation and pregnancy may occur in case of mosaicism, but POF usually occurs.

- Dysgenetic patients with normal karyotype are called **"pure" gonadal dysgenesis.** *Patients with gonadal dysgenesis having karyotype 46 XY are phenotypically female (called "Swyer syndrome") due to deficient testosterone and* anti-Müllerian hormone (AMH) secretion by dysgenetic gonad, as there is no development of testis due to absence of SRY or other testis determining factors on the Y chromosome. These patients have normal Müllerian system due to lack of AMH.

Clinical Presentation of Turner Syndrome

They usually present with:
- Short stature **(Fig. 20)**
- Absent breast development
- Prepubertal external genitalia **(Fig. 21)**
- Primary amenorrhea

However, they can be recognized even in early childhood with other physical stigma.

Classic Stigma of Turner Syndrome

- Short stature
- Low-set ears
- Epicanthal folds
- High-arch palate **(Fig. 22)**
- Cubitus valgus
- Nevi
- Webbing of the neck **(Fig. 23)**

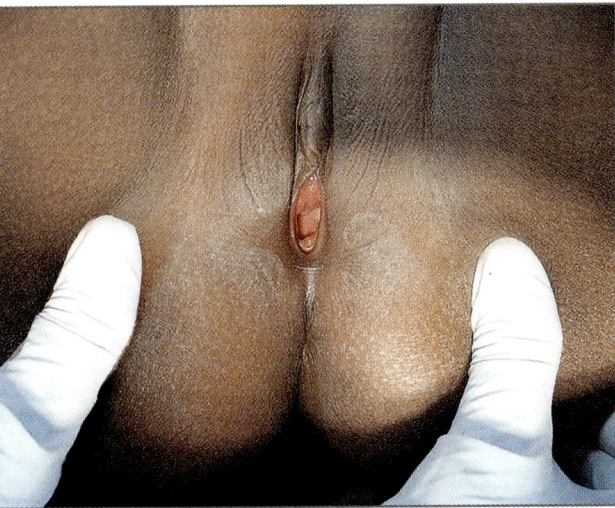

Fig. 20: Turner syndrome—prepubertal external genitalia—16-year-old girl as in Figure 21.

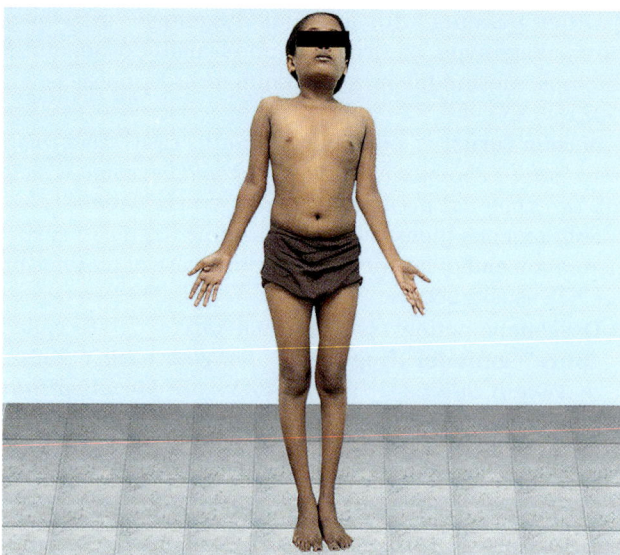

Fig. 21: Turner syndrome—16-year-old girl short stature (3 feet 11 inches).

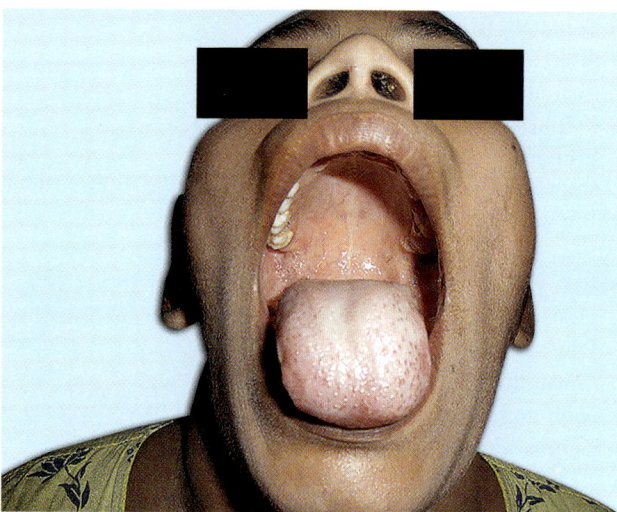

Fig. 22: Turner—high-arch palate.

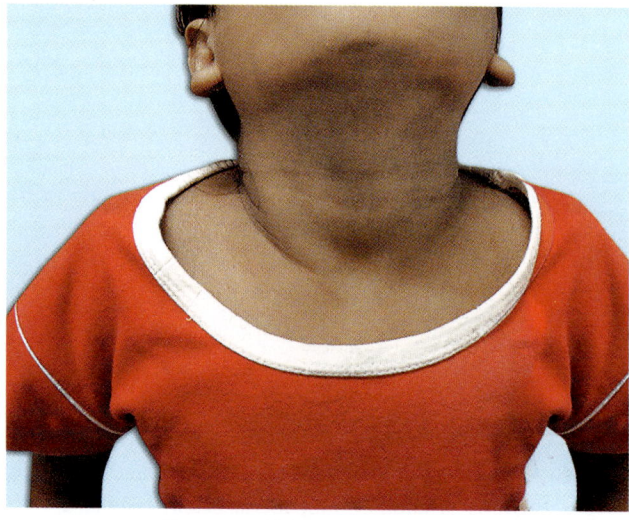

Fig. 23: Webbing of neck in Turner.

- Broad-shield chest
- No breast development
- Hypoplastic nipple
- Coarctation of aorta
- Horse-shoe kidney
- Streak ovaries
- Short fourth metatarsal
- Medical problems—one-third manifest one or more cardiovascular abnormalities in the form of bicuspid aortic valve, coarctation of aorta, mitral valve prolapse and aortic aneurism and spontaneous aortic dissection. *Aortic dissection is real danger which is aggravated in pregnancy with high risk of mortality.* Renal anomalies are also common. These are horse-shaped kidney, single kidney, pelvic kidney and duplication of collecting systems. Other problems may be hearing impairment, otitis, mastoiditis, and increase incidence of hypertension, Type I diabetes, autoimmune disorder, autoimmune hepatitis, thrombocytopenia and Hashimoto thyroiditis.

Q. Why short stature and somatic abnormality and amenorrhea in Turner?

Short stature and somatic abnormality are linked to the deletion in the short arm of the X chromosome (Xp); while loss of long arm is linked to amenorrhea, which is result of estrogen deficiency due to streak gonad.

One X chromosome is completely absent in Turner (45 XO).

External genitalia, uterus, and fallopian tube develop normally in Turner till puberty at the point of time maturation is not achieved due to deficient estrogen production by ovary, which is streak.

Q. What do you mean by long Turner?

- Deletion of the long arm of X chromosome have normal stature even may have eunuchoid look.
- Delayed closure of epiphysis of long bones occurs due to less estrogen.
- This results in long arms and legs and called eunuchoid habitus.
- Girls are tall (>63 inches), absence of secondary sexual characters, streak gonads, and 46 XX.
- Absent ovarian estrogen—unopposed GH action—delayed epiphyseal fusion.

Investigations in Turner Syndrome

- Sex chromatin—negative.
- Karyotype—45 XO, At least 30 cells to be examined due to possibility of mosaicism. Cytogenetic analysis should be performed to detect any fragments of Y when gonads should need removal due to chance of malignancy.
- Serum E2—very low, FSH, and LH—high, autoantibodies may be present.
- USG and laparoscopy—uterus, fallopian tube, and vagina are present. Gonads are streak.

Management of Turner Syndrome

- *Secondary sex character* is developed by estrogen administration
- *Menstrual function* is achieved by cyclical estrogen or E/P combination
- *Coital function*—vagina is present, so no problem
- *Pregnancy* is achieved by donor oocyte (*see* below)
- *Associated cardiovascular anomaly* (coarctation of aorta) and renal anomaly, if any, etc., should be taken care of.

Therapy is initiated with estrogen—conjugated estrogen 0.625 mg/day or estradiol 1 mg/day may be continued *alone for 12-24 months without progesterone* and then to add progesterone 12-14 days in a month for withdrawal (200 mg micronized progesterone at night or 5-10 mg MP daily for 12-14 days in a month). Initially estrogon therapy is started with low dose (.25-0.5 mg micronized progesterone), then gradually increased in 3-6 months interval according to response (secondary sexual character) with an aim to achieve sexual maturity over 2-3 years. Progesterone is started when vaginal bleeding first occurs or after 12-24 months which one is earlier. Estrogen should not be started not later than 15 years of age and not before 12 years of age when growth is priority.

Pregnancy in Turner syndrome is achieved by donor oocyte, but considered as high risk due to increased cardiovascular problems with life-threatening risk. The mortality rate is increased by 100% due to aortic dissection or rupture for which attempt of pregnancy should be seriously considered.

Q. Can you do something for the height in Turner syndrome?

Exogenous growth hormone starting from 2-8 years of age and continued treatment for 7 years (GH dose is .375 mg/kg/week). Final height can be achieved greater than 150 cm in most of the patients in early diagnosis and treatment.

Q. Any other management?

- Management of coarctation of aorta
- Periodic medical evaluation is essential with Echo, USG of kidney, thyroid profile, complete blood count, fasting blood sugar, lipid profile, renal function test and LFT and audiometry.
- Gonadectomy, if there is any Y chromosome containing gonad.

ANATOMICAL DEFECTS LEADING TO AMENORRHEA

Q. What are the anatomical defects that may lead to amenorrhea?

- *Outflow tract obstruction:* Imperforate hymen, transvaginal septum, isolated vaginal atresia, cervical atresia or stenosis, and labial agglutination.
- *Absence of endometrium:* Complete Müllerian agenesis (absent uterus, cervix, and vagina) and uterine synechia (Asherman syndrome).

Mayer–Rokitansky–Küster–Hauser Syndrome (Figs. 24 and 25A)

It results from complete Müllerian agenesis where uterus, cervix, and upper part of vagina are absent and only a small vaginal pouch measuring 1-2 inches deep is present. Distal part of fallopian tubes is present and ovaries are normal **(Figs. 24 and 25A)**.

Incidence is 1 in 5,000 newborn girls second to gonadal dysgenesis as a cause of primary amenorrhea.

A transverse Müllerian ridge (knob) is present in between urinary bladder and sigmoid colon. Mostly, Müllerian knob is devoid of any active endometrium.

Rarely (2-7%) active endometrium may be present resulting accumulation of menstrual blood and causing cyclical lower abdominal pain. In these cases, excision of rudimentary knob is needed.

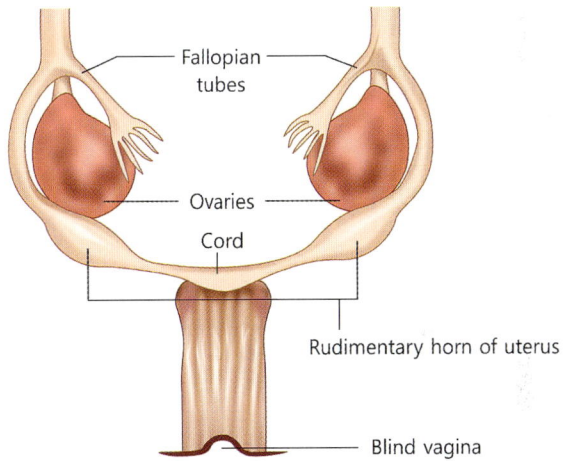

Fig. 24: Mayer-Rokitansky-Küster-Hauser (MRKH) syndrome—complete absence of uterus and vagina—both-sided tubes and ovaries are normal.

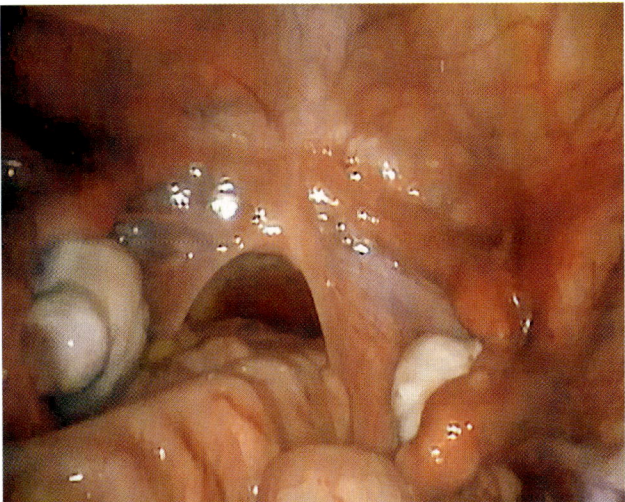

Fig. 25A: Transverse ridge with normal bilateral tubes and ovaries in Rokitansky–Küster–Hauser (RKH) syndrome.

Courtesy: Dr Alok De, Associate Professor

Associated Abnormalities

Renal (15–40%) and skeletal abnormalities (12%) may be present in this syndrome. Renal abnormalities may be in the form of absent kidney, pelvic kidney, horseshoe-shaped kidney, or double urinary collective system.

Scoliosis, spina bifida, sacralization of lumbar vertebra, lumbarization of sacral vertebra, and cervical vertebra malformation are the skeletal abnormalities.

Müllerian, renal, cervicothoracic somite (MURCS) syndrome includes Müllerian duct aplasia, renal aplasia, and cervicothoracic somatic dysplasia.

Karyotype is typical female 46 XX with normal secondary sexual character.

Clinical Presentation

- Primary amenorrhea with developed secondary sexual character. Patients typically present in late adolescent or as young adults well after onset of menstruation is expected, as there is no other complaint.
- There may be cyclical pain in 10% cases due to functional amenorrhea and hematometra.

On Examination

- Looking like female.
- All secondary sexual characters are present with well-developed breasts.
- Labia well developed
- Vagina is blind (*see* Fig. 13) and only lower part of vagina is present.

Investigations

- USG—uterus absent. Renal abnormalities may be detected. Pelvic USG and MRI can also detect functional uterine remnant.
- Karyotype—46 XX. Karyotype helps to differentiate from androgen insensitivity syndrome (AIS) where it is 46 XY. Testosterone in AIS is male pattern, whereas in RKH it is normal female level.
- Laparoscopy—tubes present, ovaries normal, a transverse ridge representing Müllerian knob
- Intravenous pyelogram (IVP) is done to exclude urinary tract abnormalities.
- X-ray may be needed for skeletal abnormality.

Treatment Plan

- Restoration of genital tract function—of the three functions—(1) menstrual function, (2) coital function, and (3) reproductive function.
  - Menstruation not possible
  - Coitus by vaginoplasty
  - Reproduction by gestational surrogacy. Pregnancy following uterine transplantation is a new hope. IVF and ET is mandatory for achievement of pregnancy in uterine transplantation. Branstrom M, et. al., reported first in 2015.
- Usually, no need of general health management except to take care of any renal and skeletal abnormality.

CREATION OF NEOVAGINA

Vaginoplasty (*see* also Chapter 21—Müllerian Anomaly, Page 452)

Goal is to create a functional vagina. It may be achieved by surgery or conservative surgery. Postoperative dilatation is important after vaginoplasty either regular intercourse or manual dilatation.

Different methods of vaginoplasty are:

- Progressive vaginal dilatation is the first choice. *Frank (1938) and Ingram (1981):* Conservative method by using graduated hard dilators, modified by Ingram affixing the dilators over bicycle—0.5–2 hour per day.
- McIndoe-Reed operation—using skin graft over a solid mold (*see* Chapter 21, **Figs. 35 to 37**, Page 454).
- William's vulvovaginoplasty (*see* Chapter 21, **Fig. 40**, Page 455).
- Vaginoplasty using amnion (Chakravarty) (*see* Chapter 21, **Figs. 38 and 39**, Page 455), peritoneal graft (Davydov, et al.), bladder mucosa, or sigmoid colon (Freund, et al.).
- Vecchietti technique (sphere connected to two metal wires and guided through potential vaginal space) using laparoscope.
- Laparoscopic vaginoplasty with peritoneum (Davydov, et al.).

Q. How to differentiate between MRKH from AIS (TFS) (both present with developed breasts and blind vagina)?

See **Table 3**.

Table 3: The difference between Mayer–Rokitansky–Kuster–Hauser (MRKH) from androgen insensitivity syndrome (AIS) [testicular feminization syndrome (TFS)].

	AIS (TFS)	MRKH
Breast	Developed	Developed
Pubic and axillary hair	Absent/less sparse	Normal
Vagina	Blind	Blind
Uterus	Absent	Absent
Gonad	Testis (location-variable)	Ovary in normal site
Testosterone	Male range	Female range
Karyotype	46 XY	46 XX
Inheritance	Recessive X-linked	None

Management of Other Müllerian Anomaly causing Primary Amenorrhea

- Hypoplasia or absent cervix with functioning uterus—recently various techniques attempted. In many cases, hysterectomy needed.

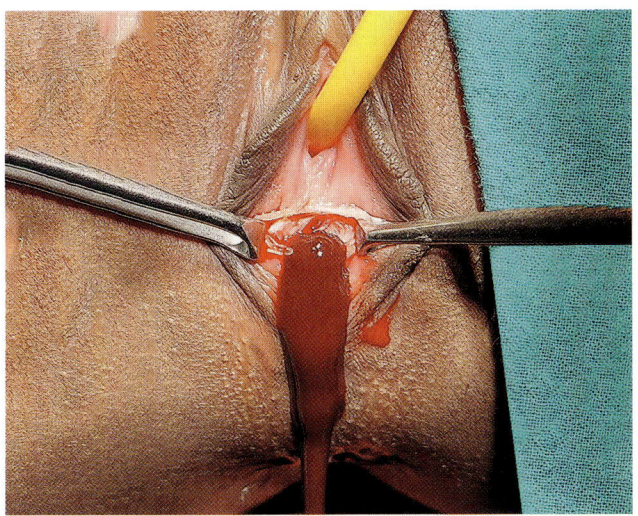

Fig. 25B: In imperforate hymen—blood is drained following incision.
Courtesy: Dr Abhisek Bhadra, Assistant Professor, Medical College, Kolkata

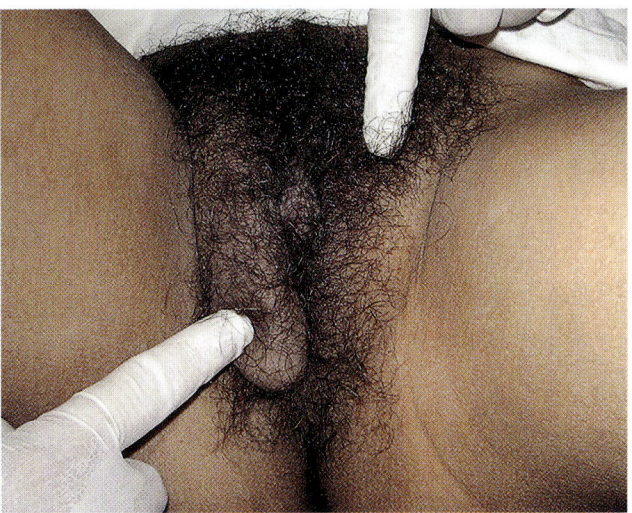

Fig. 26: Partial androgen sensitivity syndrome— showing right testes in labia, enlarged clitoris.

- Transverse vaginal septum—septum resection and vaginoplasty, if required.
- Imperforate hymen—hymenotomy and drainage of collected menstrual blood (cryptomenorrhea) **(Fig. 25B)**—a crisscross incision is given by the scalpel and four vaginal flaps are cut. Hemostasis is done on the cut margin with 1–0 interrupted catgut stitches. Collected blood is allowed to drain spontaneously.

Androgen Insensitivity Syndrome (Testicular Feminization Syndrome)

Androgen insensitivity syndrome is also called testicular feminization syndrome. The term testicular feminization syndrome is no longer favored.

It is one type of male pseudohermaphroditism where karyotype is 46 XY, but due to androgen receptor defect, in complete variety, patients phenotypically present as normal female at birth. The incidence of AIS ranges from 1 in 12,000 to 40,000 live birth.

It is X-linked recessive disorder. Androgen receptor lies on the short arm of X chromosome.

Complete androgen insensitivity syndrome was first described by Morris, at Yale who gave the nomenclature "Testicular feminization syndrome".

Pathology

Patients have functioning testis with production of normal male testosterone level. But androgen receptors mutations prevent normal testosterone binding, formation of ductal system, and virilization. Presence of AMH prevents development of internal Müllerian structure. Estrogen derived from peripheral conversion, unopposed by androgen is responsible for breasts development.

Varieties

- Complete variety (CAIS)
- Incomplete variety in 10% cases and called partial androgen insensitivity syndrome (PAIS), where there may be ambiguous external genitalia, labioscrotal fusion and there is virilization **(Fig. 26)**.
- 5α-reductase deficiency, which results failure of conversion of testosterone to DHT.

Clinical Presentation

Clinical presentation of complete variety **(Table 4)** of AIS **(Fig. 27)**:

- At puberty present with a hernia mass or/and primary amenorrhea with sparse or absent pubic and axillary hair. AIS patient may present with inguinal hernia at childhood.

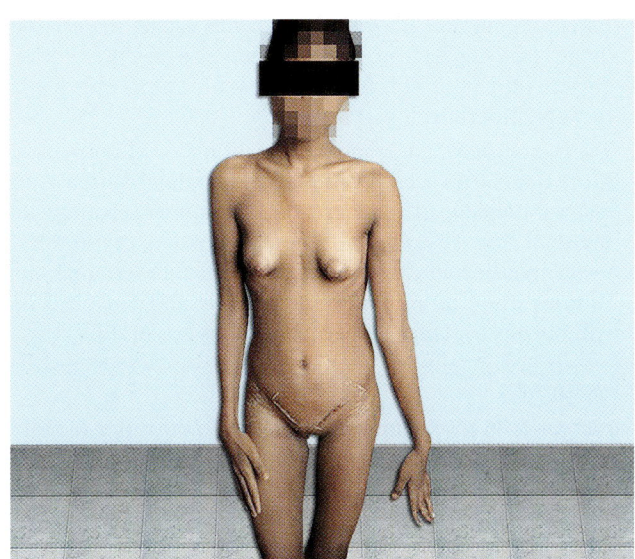

Fig. 27: Androgen insensitivity syndrome after gonadectomy, which lied on inguinal region.
Courtesy: Professor RP Ganguly

Table 4: Different varieties of androgen insensitivity syndrome (AIS).			
Type of androgen sensitivity	Complete androgen insensitivity (CAIS)	Partial androgen insensitivity (PAIS)	5α-reductase deficiency
Inheritance	X-linked recessive	X-linked recessive	Autosomal recessive
Defect	Androgen receptors mutations—lacking or inactive receptors	Androgen receptors mutations—lacking or inactive receptors	Failure of conversion of T to DHT
External genitalia	Female	Ambiguous	Female or ambiguous
Internal genitalia	Male	Male	Male
Gonad	Testis	Testis	Testis
Presentation	At puberty, present with primary amenorrhea with or without hernia mass	Most common presentation at infancy is hypospadias with urethral opening at base of phallus, may be cryptorchidism with ambiguous genitalia with small phallus or of normal size penis (**Fig. 32**). Testis azoospermic	At infancy—a small phallus, little hypospadias, bifid scrotum, and blind vaginal pouch. Testes either in inguinal canal or at labioscrotal fold
Phenotype at puberty	Female and developed breast	Partial masculine and partly developed breasts (gynecomastia) (**Fig. 33**)	Masculine
Management	• Reared as female • Gonadectomy followed by estrogen therapy • Vaginal dilation may be needed, rarely vaginoplasty	• Depends on degree of ambiguity and subsequent choice of rearing • If reared as female gonadectomy and estrogen therapy	• Diagnosis is important • At birth to assign sex of rearing, which should be based on potential for normal sexual function in adult life. • If reared as female gonadectomy and estrogen therapy

❖ Breasts are well developed due to presence of estrogen available from conversion of androgen to estrogen. Nipples are small with pale areola. There is eunuchoidal tendency (long arm, big arm, and feet). Breasts are relatively large and have little glandular tissue, due to deficiency of progesterone.

❖ External genitalia are well formed with vagina of variable length (see **Fig. 5**) from short to adequate and the uterus, cervix, and fallopian tube are absent. Labia minora is usually underdeveloped.

❖ Testes are present at labia, parities, or inside abdomen. In more than 50% cases in CAIS there is inguinal hernia. And testes is palpable in inguinal canal, commonly at superficial inguinal ring. Histologically gonads look like cryptorchid testes, may be nodular. After puberty immature seminiferous tubules lined by immature germ cells and Sertoli cells without any evidence of spermatogenesis are found.

Investigation

Karyotype is 46 XY, serum testosterone is in the range of male level and LH is elevated due to androgen insensitivity at H-P level.

USG—upper two-thirds of vagina, uterus, and FT absent.

Gonadal Biopsy

❖ Seminiferous tubules small and hylanized, spermatogenesis absent, Leydig cells, and Sertoli cells are normal.

Management

❖ Patient should be reared as female and psychological counseling is very important. Individual's psychology is usually like female.

❖ Testes are surgically excised after puberty (at 16–18 years of age) as there is chance of malignancy in 25% cases. In complete AIS surgery is delayed awaiting for smooth pubertal development and chance of tumor is less before puberty. Surgery can be done by open method (**Figs. 28 and 29**) or by laparoscopy (**Figs. 30 and 31**). In partial AIS gonadectomy is done earlier, the one reason is to prevent further virilization.

❖ *Following orchidectomy estrogen therapy is done* to maintain breast development to avoid vasomotor symptom and to prevent osteoporosis.

❖ Initially E/P is given till pubic and axillary hair develop and later changed to premarin (equine estrogen) 0.625 mg daily orally or 0.5–1 mg oral estradiol and continued till age of 50 years.

❖ Coitus is possible, if required, progressive dilatation of vagina or reconstruction (vaginoplasty) is needed rarely like MRKH syndrome.

❖ There is no possibility of menstruation. Reproduction is not possible, neither by donor oocyte (Turner) nor by surrogacy (MRKH syndrome). Only way to get a child is adoption.

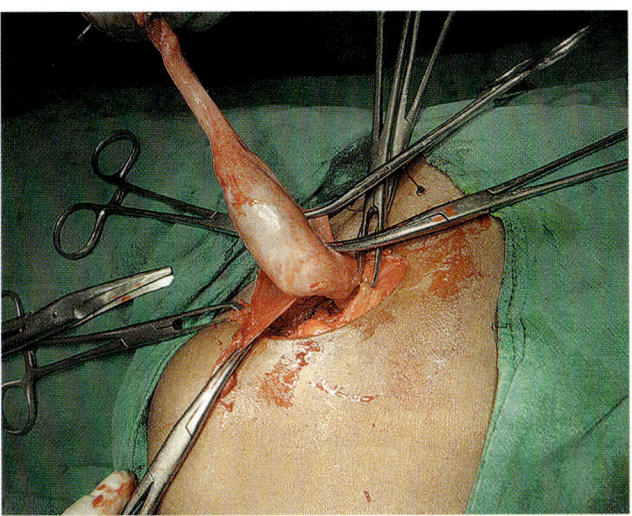

Fig. 28: Androgen insensitivity syndrome (AIS)— removal of testes from inguinal region—open method.

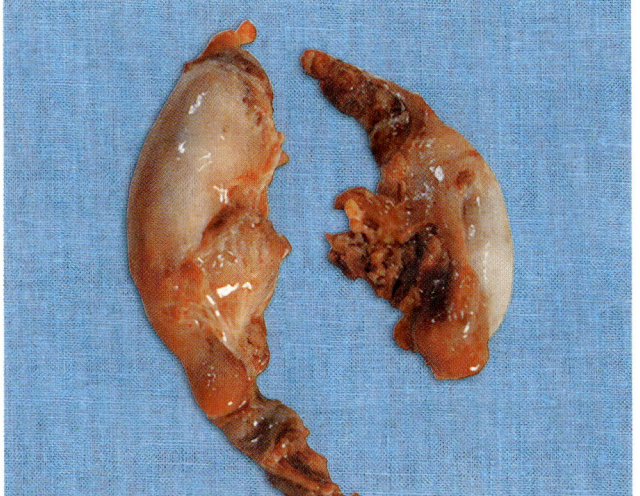

Fig. 29: Androgen insensitivity syndrome (AIS)— removal of testis in open method.

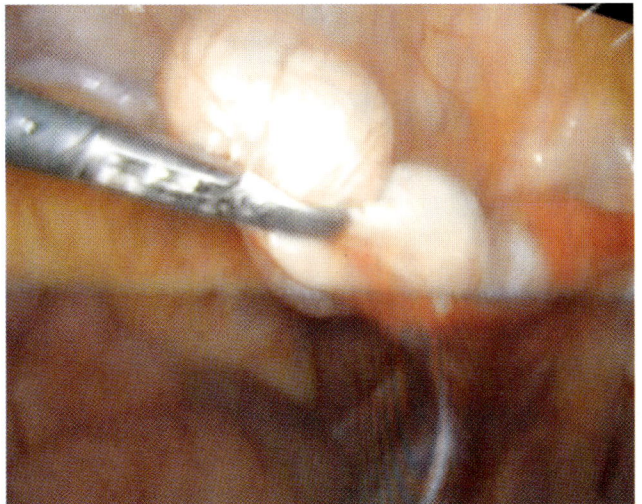

Fig. 30: Androgen insensitivity syndrome (AIS)— testes in parietis—laparoscopic removal.

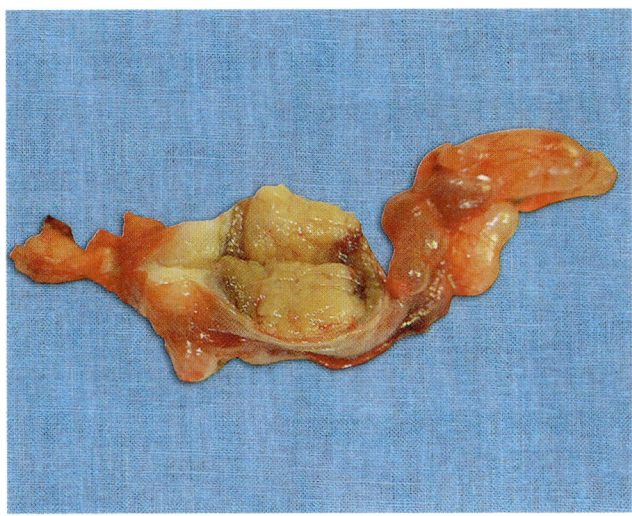

Fig. 31: Cut section of testes after laparoscopic removal.

Quality of Life in Complete versus Partial Androgen Insensitivity Syndrome (AIS)

So far, as quality of life is concerned in complete AIS (CAIS) is far better than partial AIS (PAIS), as in complete variety there is no alternative of sex of rearing other than female and individual's psychology is like female, spends life as female, and even married with normal sexual activity, obviously without capability of reproduction.

But in PAIS, sex of rearing is a problem due to the presence of partial androgenic activity, ambiguous external genitalia (phallus is not completely developed) and possibility of male psychology. Life sometimes becomes miserable in PAIS. Continuous psychological counseling is needed for them.

The differences of different varieties of AIS is given in **Table 4**.

REIFENSTEIN SYNDROME

It is one variety of partial androgen insensitivity syndrome where the phenotype is predominantly male but undervirilized. They mostly present as infertile male with bifid scrotum and hypospadias. External genitalia varies widely but internal genitalia is incompletely developed male. Mullerian structure and prostate are absent. Testes may be undescended or normally descended, and there is a maturation arrest in spermatogenesis. No chest or facial hair but axillary and pubic hair normal, and may have gynecomastia. Sexual dysfunction is common and gender identity depends on the sex of rearing.

SWYER SYNDROME

Swyer syndrome as described above is complete variety or pure gonadal dysgenesis characterized by a 46 XY karyotype.

Phenotype is female in spite of presence of Y chromosome as the dysgenetic (streak) gonads neither produce androgen nor AMH.

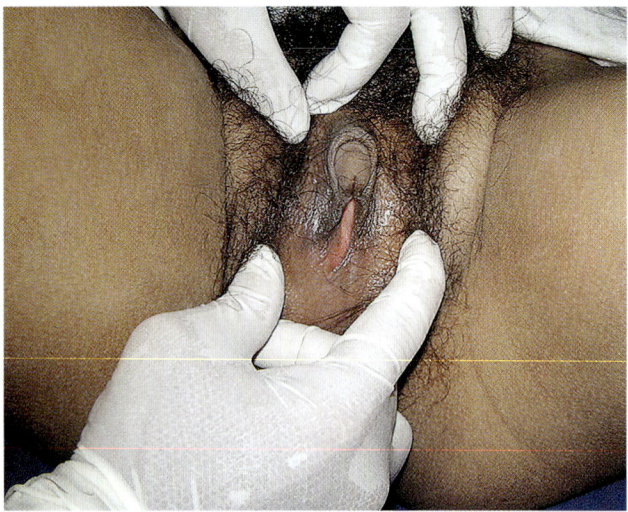

Fig. 32: Enlarged clitoris, hypospadias, and labioscrotal fusion in partial androgen insensitivity syndrome as the patient in Figure 33.

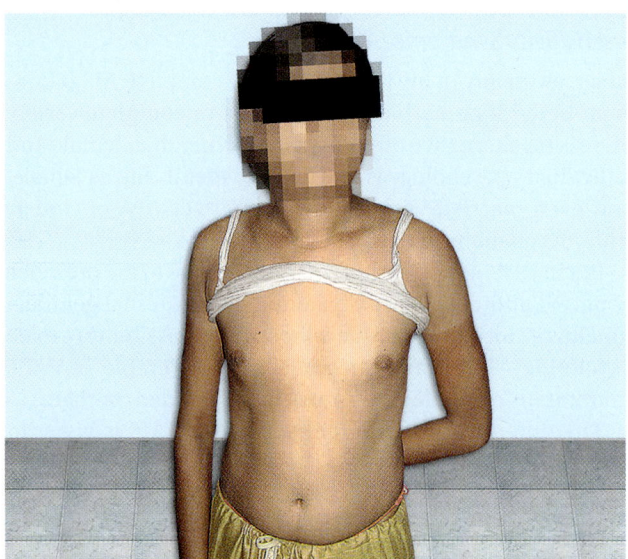

Fig. 33: Partial androgen insensitivity syndrome—breasts poorly developed.
Courtesy: Dr Debmalya Maity

There is no development of testis due to absence of SRY or other testis determining factors on the Y chromosome. Consequently uterus, cervix, vagina, and fallopian tubes develop normally and there is no masculinization of external genitalia. The incidence is 1:80,000 birth.

Presentation

Usually presents after expected time of puberty with primary amenorrhea, normal stature, delayed sexual maturation with normal pubic hair, normal external and internal genitalia like female.

Investigation

Features of hypergonadotropic hypogonadism, karyotype XY, and presence of uterus on USG.

Management

Sex of rearing and assignment is unequivocally female. Estrogen therapy is needed for breast development followed by cyclical estrogen and progesterone therapy to maintain sexual maturation and menstruation. Pregnancy is possible by in vitro fertilization and embryo transfer (IVF and ET) with donor oocyte without any specific risk or complication. Gonadectomy is done soon after diagnosis due to the potential risk (30%) of germ cell tumor.

Give Examples of Two Cases Where Both Cases are Phenotypically Female but Karyotype XY

The two examples of phenotypically female but karyotype XY are:
1. Complete androgen insensitivity syndrome (AIS)
2. Swyer syndrome

In AIS, the primary defect is at receptor level and in spite of normal testosterone production there is no feature of masculinization. In Swyer syndrome, the gonad is complete dysgenetic (*see* details above). Differences are described in **Table 5**.

Table 5: Difference between androgen insensitivity syndrome and Swyer syndrome.

	AIS (TFS)	Swyer syndrome
Primary defect	Defect on androgen receptor	Complete gonadal dysgenesis (absence of SRY or other TDF on Y-chromosome—no testes)
Karyotype	XY	XY
Phenotype	Female	Female
Breast	Developed	Poorly developed
Pubic and axillary hair	Absent/less	Present
Vagina	Blind	Normal
Uterus	Absent	Present
Gonad	Testis (location-variable)	Streak gonad in pelvis
Testosterone	Male range	Female range
Sex of rearing	Female	Female
Treatment	Testis is surgically excised after puberty. E/P therapy followed by estrogen	Gonadectomy as soon as diagnosed. Estrogen therapy followed by E/P
Reproductive function	Coitus possible, no menstruation, pregnancy not possible	Coitus possible, menstruation with withdrawal by hormones, pregnancy possible by donor oocyte

CONGENITAL ADRENAL HYPERPLASIA (ADRENOGENITAL SYNDROME) (*SEE* FIGS. 6, 7, 8A AND 8B AND 10)

Congenital adrenal hyperplasia (CAH), an autosomal recessive disorder, is due to complete or partial deficiency of enzyme, which is essential for cortisol or aldosterone synthesis in adrenal gland.

It is the most common cause of female pseudohermaphroditism and accounts for 50% of ambiguous genitalia.

Congenital adrenal hyperplasia contributes 1% of all primary amenorrhea cases and late onset CAH contributes to 0.5% of all secondary amenorrhea.

Pathophysiology

Cortisol is produced in adrenal under the control of adrenocorticotropic hormone (ACTH), which also influences the adrenal androgen production.

Lack of any enzyme in the pathway results in deficient synthesis of cortisol and due to absent negative feedback ACTH level increases, which in turn causes adrenal hyperplasia to produce steroid and also simulates androgen production resulting virilization of female fetus (*see* the diagram—hormone synthesis in CAH in Chapter 12—PCOS).

The most common enzyme involved is 21-hydroxylase (21-H) the deficiency of which occurs in 90% cases the incidence of which is one in 10,000 to 15,000 births and the other two enzymes involved are 11-hydroxylase (5–8%) and 3β-hydroxysteroid dehydrogenase (rare).

Failure of conversion of progesterone to 11-deoxycorticosterone due to lack of 21-H results aldosterone deficiency and may result "salt-losing" type of CAH and occurs in two-thirds cases.

There is increase production of 17-hydroxy progesterone and in urine pregnentriol and 17-KS increases. In the milder form or nonclassic form, it presents as late onset or adult onset CAH where features of hyperandrogenemia does not develop until puberty when it is manifested by hirsutism, acne, anovulation, and amenorrhea primary or secondary mimicking PCOS.

The incidence of late onset is much commoner, which is about 1 in 300.

Clinical Presentation of CAH

Depending on the severity of enzyme deficiency, clinical presentation varies.

Congenital adrenal hyperplasia may be manifested in newborn female enlarged clitoris, fused labioscrotal folds, and penile urethra (*see* **Figs. 8A and B**, Page 310).

Degree of masculinization of external genitalia varies according to the severity.

In severe enzyme deficiency there may be "salt-losing" type of CAH and the infant may suffer from dehydration, hypotension, and hyponatremia between 1st and 4th weeks of age called *salt-losing crisis*, which may be fatal, if not treated by steroid. There is less masculinization in nonsalt-losing variety. There may be hyperpigmentation of the skin due to ↑↑ACTH in CAH.

Investigation

* Elevated level of serum 17-OH progesterone (>800 ng/mL) is the diagnostic screening marker of CAH. It should be done in follicular phase to avoid false positive in luteal phase. Level of 17-OHP less than 200 ng/dL (<2ng/mL)in follicular phase excludes CAH whereas value >1,000 ng/dL (>10 ng/mL) is almost diagnostic for 21-hydroxylase deficiency. If value lies in between 200 ng/dL and 800 ng/dL it should be confirmed by ACTH stimulation test.
* CAH is confirmed by ACTH stimulation test in which 250 μg of synthetic ACTH is injected IV after 1 hour of which 17 OH is measured which becomes more than 1,500 ng/dL (>15 ng/mL) in CAH.
* 24-hour urinary excretion of pregnanetriol and alpha ketosteroid, which are also increased.
* Serum Na^+ and K^+ are done in suspected cases of salt-losing variety.
* USG—uterus, fallopian tube, ovary, and vagina present.
* Sex chromatin study—positive bar body.
* Karyotype—46 XX.

Prenatal detection and management of CAH

It is possible to detect CAH antenatally and antenatal treatment with steroid has been successfully used to prevent masculinization. If parents are heterozygous carriers of 21-hydroxylase deficiency there is 1:4 chance of fetus to be affected. Prenatal diagnosis by amniocentesis to measure 17-OH progesterone, human leukocyte antigen (HLA) typing of amniotic cell and by CVS is possible.

Treatment of CAH

* Salt-losing crisis—correction of fluid-electrolyte balance, e.g., hyponatremia, hypoglycemia by glucose and isotonic solution and deoxycorticosterone to replace cortisol deficiency, when severe, fludrocortisone is given.
* Maintenance of cortisol replacement therapy for lifelong.
* Rearing of sex is established usually within 1.5 year as female.
* Clitoroplasty (reduction clitoridectomy) done after sex of rearing, if clitoris is enlarged.
* Vaginal reconstruction—simple posterior incision, if labial folds are thin—at age of 3–4 years. Flap vaginoplasty at puberty when the girl is mature mentally, physically, and sexually.
* Coital function possible
* Menstruation occurs
* Pregnancy possible.

Hypogonadotropic Hypogonadism

Causes of hypogonadotropic hypogonadism are described in **Table 6**.

Table 6: Causes of hypogonadotropic hypogonadism and sites of defect.

Site of defect	Congenital causes	Acquired causes
Hypothalamus	Idiopathic hypogonadotropic hypogonadism, Kallmann syndrome	Anorexia nervosa, vigorous exercise, stress, pseudocyesis tumor (most common—craniopharyngioma, others are glioma, meningioma, endodermal sinus tumor), radiation, and infection
Pituitary	Hypoplasia	• Mostly secondary amenorrhea • Adenoma (prolactinoma), damage by radiation, surgery, compression by tumor • Infarction (Sheehan), empty sella syndrome
Others		Kidney disease, liver disease, malignancy, AIDS

Abbreviation: AIDS, acquired immunodeficiency syndrome

Salient features of a case of idiopathic hypogonadotropic hypogonadism (IHH) presenting with primary amenorrhea:

- No onset of menstruation, withdrawal bleeding+
- *Height*—normal
- *Breasts*—less developed Tanner 2
- *Axillary hair/pubic hair*—present
- *Vagina present*
- *Laparoscope/USG*—small uterus and gonads
- *FSH or LH*—very low
- *Karyotype 46 X*
- *Treatment*: Logically, patient should be treated with long-term administration of pulsatile GnRH. However, it is impractical to use an indwelling catheter and portable ports for long periods.

Kallmann Syndrome

- It is one example of hypogonadotropic hypogonadism and can be differentiated from IHH by olfactory testing (presence of hyposmia or anosmia).
- Incidence is one in 50,000
- It can be inherited as X-linked, autosomal dominant or autosomal recessive.
- Women with this problem present with primary amenorrhea with poor growth of secondary sexual character and impairment of olfactory function and infertility. Failure of activation of pulsatile GnRH secretion results gonadotropic deficiency. It is associated with midline facial defects like cleft palate, cleft lip, ataxia, epilepsy, and synkinesis.
- Cyclical estrogen and progesterone restore menstruation. Ovulation induction with exogenous FSH and LH may achieve pregnancy.

DISORDER OF SEXUAL DEVELOPMENT (INTERSEX)

DEFINITION OF DSD

Q. What do you mean by disorder of sexual development (DSD)?

DSDs are congenital conditions, which are characterized by atypical chromosomal, gonadal, or anatomical sex and may be incongruent with each other.

The term *disorder of sexual differentiation* (DSD), a new taxonomy has been accepted recently in a consensus opinion (2006) avoiding the controversial/confusing old terms *intersex, hermaphrodite, sex reversal*, etc., to bring these types of disorder under one umbrella term, "DSD" which is classified on etiological basis.

[The Lawson Wilkins Pediatric Endocrine Society (LWPES) and the European Society for Pediatric Endocrinology (ESPE) consensus group proposed the classification of DSDs (2006)].

Incidence: 1 in 5,500

GENDER IDENTITY

Q. How gender identity of an individual is determined?

It depends on the following factors:
- Chromosomal sex/genetic sex
- Gonadal sex
- Phenotypic sex and anatomical sex (internal and external)
- Psychological sex—gender identity, gender role, and sexual orientation (*see* later)
- *Sex of rearing*

Genetic sex: Genetic sex means chromosomal sex like XX and XY.

Gonadal sex: Defined by the differentiation of gonad either testes or ovary.

Phenotypic sex: Defined by the external genitalia and secondary sexual character at puberty.

SEXUAL DIFFERENTIATION: MECHANISM

Q. How does sexual differentiation occur?

Sexual differentiation occurs in *three* stages:

1. *First stage*—*determination of chromosomal sex*. Chromosomal sex or genetic sex is determined at *the time of fertilization and conception* whether the ovum is fertilized by a sperm containing X or Y.
2. *Second stage*—*gonadal differentiation*. It occurs at 6–7 weeks of differentiation and depends of *SRY* (sex-determining region on Y) gene of Y chromosome. It is the Y chromosome, which will determine the development of testes by virtue of presence of a gene, *SRY* gene and other testes-determining factor (TDF) on its short arm

and the undifferentiated gonad will be differentiated into testicular tissue.

3. *Third stage—phenotype sex determination.* It occurs at 8-12 weeks of gestation and depends upon hormones like testosterone and Müllerian inhibiting factor (MIF/AMH) secreted by the different cells of testes and are follows:
   - Testosterone produced by the Leydig cells influences the formation of epididymis, vas deferens, and seminal vesicles from Wolffian structure. AMH secreted by Sertoli cells will regress the Müllerian structures.
   - Dihydrotestosterone, a potent androgen, is produced by testosterone at periphery is responsible for the virilization of the external genitalia and appearance of masculine body habitus.
   - Ovarian structures are developed passively due to absence of *SRY* gene and other testes determining factor (TDFs) and facilitated by the antitesticular action of the genes *DAX1*, *Rspo1*, and *WNT4*.
   - In absence of Y chromosome, genitalia are developed as female, which is independent of hormonal influence. During fetal life ovaries do not produce any hormone.
   - At the end of first trimester from the external genitalia, fetal gender is identifiable by sonography.

Alteration of any event in this complex pathway may lead to genotypic, phenotypic, and anatomic discordancy resulting disorder of sex development.

CLASSIFICATION OF DISORDER OF SEXUAL DIFFERENTIATION

Q. How would you classify disorder of sexual differentiation (DSD)?

According to 2006 consensus conference classification, DSDs are basically categorized into three groups based on chromosome component, which are further subdivided *etiologically* into subcategories **(Table 7)**. The three categories are:

1. Sex chromosome DSDs—45 X Turner and variants, 47 XXY Klinefelter and variants, 45 X/46 XY mixed gonadal dysgenesis (MGD) and chromosomal ovotesticular DSD "46 XX/46 XY chimeric type or mosaic type").
2. 46 XY DSDs (disorders of testicular development or disorders in androgen synthesis/action).
3. 46 XX DSDs (disorders of ovarian development, androgen excess or others).

1. **Sex chromosome DSDs**—45 X Turner and variants (*see* Page 319), 47 XXY Klinefelter and variants (Page 264 and 287), 45 X/46 XY mixed gonadal dysgenesis (MGD) and chromosomal ovotesticular DSD "46 XX/46 XY chimeric type or mosaic type".
   - Numerical sex chromosomal abnormality leads to abnormal gonadal development. Sex chromosomal DSDs were previously called gonadal dysgenesis. A poorly formed testis is called *dysgenetic testis* and poorly developed ovary is called *streak ovary*.
   - A Y chromosome containing streak or dysgenetic gonad is at higher risk of malignancy.

Table 7: Disorder of sexual development.

Disorder of sexual development (DSD)—Based on new classification and nomenclature

Sex chromosome DSDs	46 XY DSDs		46 XX DSDs		
	Disorder in development of testes	Disorder of androgen production or its action	Disorder of development of ovary	Androgen excess	Others
45 Turner and its variants	• Complete gonadal dysgenesis (Swyer syndrome)	• Androgen synthesis defect	• Ovotesticular DSD	• Fetal androgen excess (CAH)	• Cloacal extrophy
47 XXY Klinefelter and variants	• Partial gonadal dysgenesis	• LH receptor defect	• Testicular DSD, e.g., SRY+, duplicate SOX9 (46 XX sex reversal)	– 21-OH deficiency	• Mullerian agenesis (MRKH)
45 X/46 XY mixed gonadal dysgenesis	• Gonadal regression	• Androgen insensitivity (AIS)	• Gonadal dysgenesis	– 11-OH deficiency	• MURCS (Mullerian, renal, cervicothoracic somatic dysplasia)
Chromosomal ovotesticular DSD	• Ovotesticular DSD	• 5α-reductase deficiency		• Fetoplacental origin	
		• Disorder of AMH or its receptor		– Aromatase deficiency	
				– POR gene defect	
				• Maternal origin	
				– Luteoma	
				– Exogenous	

Abbreviations: CAH, congenital adrenal hyperplasia; POR, p450 oxidoreductase deficiency; MRKH, Mayer-Rokitansky-Kuster-Hauser syndrome

- *Turner and Klinefelter syndromes are most common sex chromosomal DSDs.*
  - In 45 X/46 XY, MGD clinical pictures are highly variable. It may range from partial virilization and ambiguous genitalia to complete male or female phenotype. In MGD asymmetrical development of the testes, usually dysgenetic testes in one side and streak gonad on the other is a common feature with asymmetrical external and internal genitalia.
  - In chromosomal ovotesticular DSD, the ovarian and testicular tissue are found in either the same or opposite gonad, so also found in 46 XX and 46 XY ovotesticular DSD.

2. **46 XY DSDs** (disorders of testicular development or disorders in androgen synthesis/action). Theses case are basically "male pseudohermaphrodite" previously termed.
   Disorders of testicular development are due to abnormalities of gene expression for testicular development. In this group lies the complete and partial gonadal dysgenesis, testicular regression syndrome (gonadal regression) and ovotesticular DSD.
   - In complete gonadal dysgenesis in 46 XY (**Swyer syndrome,** previously called **XY sex reversal,** *see* Page 325) phenotypically type is female, there is fully developed unambiguous female genitalia, streak gonad and normal Mullerian structure due to absence of SRY or other testis determining factors on the Y chromosome. Streak gonads are removed due to chance of gonadoblastoma.
   - In 46 XY partial gonadal dysgenesis there is ambiguous genitalia and partial testicular differentiation found at birth. **Frasier syndrome** (with uterus) and **Denys-Drash** syndrome (without uterus) with renal dysfunction are the example of partial gonadal dysgenesis.
   - In gonadal regression (vanishing testes syndrome, testicular regression) agonadism occurs but had testicular function in fetal life and present with normal male genitalia with bilateral anorchia.

   Disorders of androgen synthesis/or its action: Defects in hormone, their receptors and improper timing of exposure may be due to various abnormalities.
   - Androgen synthesis defect may be due to Leydig cell aplasia/hypoplasia caused by LH receptor defect and biosynthesis defects.
   - Disorders of AMH or its receptors may cause persistent Mullerian duct syndrome (PMDS).
   - Complete/partial forms of androgen insensitivity—AIS and Reifenstein syndrome (*see* Pages 323–325).
   - 5α-reductase result deficient androgen action

3. **46 XX DSDs**: These were previously termed as "female pseudohermaphrodite". Karyotype is 46 XX with musculinized external genitalia. These disorders result either from disorders of ovarian development or fetal androgen excess.
   Disorders of ovarian development: Testis-like formation within the ovary (streak gonad, dysgenetic testis or ovotestis) may occur due to SRY positivity, WNT4, RSPo1, β-carotene gene defects and duplication of SOX9 gene in the 46 XX patients.
   In 46 XX SRY + testicular DSD translocation of SRY genes occur to an X-chromosome and *female to male sex reversal (46 XX male)* occurs and phenotypically male (*see* Page 286). Testicular volumes are usually small (<5 mL), no ovary or uterus and testicular morphology is normal in infancy, but hyalinization of seminiferous tubules in early childhood result azoospermia. 46 XX testicular DSD was previously called XX male or XX sex reversal.
   SERKAL syndrome is due to the absence of both copies of WNT4 gene and female shows male sex with **female to male sex reversal**, renal, adrenal and lung dysgenesis.
   Fetal androgen excess: Virilized 46 XX infants are mostly due to CAH (*see* Page 327) commonly 21-OH deficiency, 11-OH deficiency or rarely 3β hydroxysteroid dehydrogenase deficiencies. Non CAH is rare but may occur either **fetoplacental or maternal origin androgen excess**. Aromatase deficiency is rare in human.

HERMAPHRODITE

Q. What do you mean by true hermaphrodite, male pseudohermaphrodite, and female pseudohermaphrodite?

These are the traditional terms, which used to mean:
- **True hermaphrodite**—contains both testicular and ovarian tissue
- **Male pseudohermaphrodite**—contains testes but phenotypically female
- **Female pseudohermaphrodite**—contains ovary but phenotypically male.

TRANSGENDER

Q. What is transgender?

According to World Professional Association for transgender Health, 2012 an individual is called "transgender" whose gender identity, expression, and behavior differ from those typically associated with their gender assigned at birth.

NEW NOMENCLATURE

Q. What is the new nomenclature of old terms?

These are given in the following **Table 8**.

Table 8: New nomenclature of old terms.	
Previous	Currently accepted
Intersex	Disorder of sexual development (DSD)
Male pseudohermaphrodite	46 XY DSD
Undervirilization of an XY male	46 XY DSD
Undermasculinization of an XY male	46 XY DSD
Female pseudohermaphrodite	46 XX DSD

Contd...

Contd...

Previous	Currently accepted
Overvirilization of an XX female	46 XX DSD
True hermaphrodite	Ovotesticular DSD
XX male or XX sex reversal	46 XX testicular DSD
XY sex reversal	46 XY complete gonadal dysgenesis

Q. What are the different "ovotesticular DSD" (formerly true hermaphroditism) in new DSD nomenclature?

- 46 XY ovotesticular DSD
- 46 XX ovotesticular DSD
- Chromosomal ovotesticular DSD ("46 XX/46 XY" chimerism or "45 X/46 XY" mosaic type).

In ovotesticular DSDs, the most common karyotype is 46 XY followed by 46 XX/46 XY chimerism or mosaicism and 46 XY.

Cloacal extrophy: In this rare malformation the rectum, vagina and urinary tract open in a common everted orifice and is associated with omphalocele and imperforate anus.

Chimerism: Chimerism means one body derived from the cells of both twins of a dizygotic twins. They are mosaics derived from two distinct zygotes not from single zygote.

Mixed gonadal dysgenesis (MGD—45 X/46 XY): It is asymmetric gonadal dysgenesis with one gonad a testes and other is streak or absent. Phenotype depends on the proportions of 45 X and 46 XY cells, mostly ambiguous genitalia, but may be male or female.

Q. When do the cases of DSD present to clinician?

- Mostly at birth with ambiguous genitalia
- As precocious puberty
- Puberty—late—primary amenorrhea.

GONADS IN DIFFERENT DSDs

Q. What may be the gonads in different DSDs?

These are given in **Table 9**.

Table 9: The gonads in different disorder of sexual developments (DSDs).

Gonads on two sides	DSDs
Ovary–ovary	46 XX DSD (fetal androgen excess)
Testis–testis (both normal testis)	46 XY DSD (disorder of androgen synthesis/action)
Testis–testis (both small)	46 XX 46 XX testicular DSD
Ovotestis	46 XX or 46 XY or chromosomal ovotesticular DSD
Streak–testis	45 X/46 XY Mixed gonadal dysgenesis (MGD)
Streak–streak	46 XX complete gonadal dysgenesis 46 XY complete gonadal dysgenesis
No gonadal tissue	46 XY agonadism (testicular regression)

Q. Which is the most common cause of ambiguous genitalia at birth?

CAH, which contributes 50% of all ambiguous genitalia (*see* **Figs. 8A and B**, Page 310). Incidence is 1:14,500 and potentially life-threatening for which biochemical screening should be done in any suspected 46 XX DSD newborn.

APPROACH IN A CASE OF AMBIGUOUS GENITALIA

Q. How would you approach in a case of ambiguous genitalia?

- Parents must be informed at the first opportunity.
- Need for diagnostic studies to announce sex is informed.
- Multidisciplinary team (MDT)—consisting of pediatric endocrinologist, psychologists, urologists, geneticists, radiologists, and child's primary care physicians.
- Psychological assessment and support of the family are essential in newborn period.
- Delay *registration* of birth.
- No guarantees should be made about fertility.
- Circumcision is contraindicated until decision about surgical reconstruction is made.

DIAGNOSIS OF A CASE OF AMBIGUOUS GENITALIA

Q. How would you diagnose DSD?

- History
- Physical examination
- Investigations.

History

- *Antenatal history:* Symptoms of maternal virilization or maternal medication (androgen) in pregnancy. Antenatal karyotype report, if chorionic villus sampling or amniocentesis is done. Abnormality of genital anatomy in second trimester USG.
- *Family history of DSDs:* Siblings or relatives with ambiguous genitalia, e.g., X-linked disorder in androgen insensitivity syndrome, CAH-autosomal recessive, early neonatal death in a male sibling may be due to CAH of salt loosing variety. Consanguinity increases autosomal recessive pattern diseases.
- Time of development of ambiguity.
- *History of maternal medication:* Progestins, danazole, androgens, cimetidine, spironolactone.

Physical Examination

Overall assessment:

- Abnormal facial appearance or other dysmorphic features suggesting a multiple malformation syndrome.
- Evidence of salt wasting—↓↓skin turgor, poor tone, dehydration, low BP, vomiting, poor feeding. Salt-loosing crisis with CAH generally occurs between 4th and 15th day of neonatal period.

- ❖ Hyperpigmentation of the skin due to ACTH in CAH
- ❖ Abdominal masses—virilizing tumor
- ❖ In adolescent—evidence of hirsutism/virilization.

Gonadal examination:
- ❖ Palpate gonad in labioscrotal region or inguinal canal.
- ❖ Note number of gonads, size, symmetry, and position.
- ❖ Palpable gonads below the inguinal canal are almost always testicles—excluding gonadal female, e.g., CAH. Gonads that are bilaterally palpable are generally testes, they may be dysgenetic.

External genitalia examination:
- ❖ Phallus size—(clitoral size in term infant is 2–8.5 mm in length with width of 2–6 mm). Full term newborn penis is at least 2 cm, usually more than 3.5 cm ± 0.4 cm. Less than 2 cm is consistent with micropenis.
- ❖ **Degree of virilization (Prader staging):** Prader scale ranges from 1 to 5 reflecting progressive virilization of external genitalia and the urogenital sinus.
- ❖ Fusion of labioscrotal folds—rugosity.
- ❖ Presence of persistent urogenital sinus—single perineal opening.
- ❖ Vaginal opening
- ❖ Position of urethral meatus
- ❖ Hyperpigmentation of genitalia and nipple due to ACTH.

In preterm infant, there is chance of overdiagnosis of DSD, as clitoris is prominent in preterm baby and descend of testis may not occur before 34 weeks in male preterm baby.

Rectal examination: To palpate for the presence or absence of the uterus.

Q. What investigations are done to diagnose DSD?

Initial investigations to be done in all DSDs:
- ❖ Karyotype [DX1 for X and sex determining Y (SRY) for Y]. Details to be done to detect any mosaicism.
- ❖ Imaging of internal genitalia—USG, MRI, and genitogram for urogenital sinus.
- ❖ *Laboratory*: Gonadotropin, androgens (testosterone, DHESO$_4$, and androstenedione).

Other specific testing based on earlier tests report and physical examination:
- ❖ AMH—to detect presence of testicular tissue especially Sertoli cells
- ❖ Human chorionic gonadotropin (hCG) simulation test to detect defects in testosterone biosynthesis.
- ❖ ACTH stimulation test—to rule out CAH
- ❖ GnRH stimulation test
- ❖ Gonadal skin biopsy to determine mosaicism, androgen receptor binding assay, and 5α-reductase activity.
- ❖ Molecular genetic DNA mutation analysis to detect genes involved in sex development—*CYP21A2* for CAH, androgen receptor gene for AIS, *SRY* gene for XY dysgenesis, etc.

In some patients:
- ❖ Gonadal biopsy
- ❖ Laparoscopy.

Rule out CAH, if any suspicious as it is the most common cause of ambiguous genitalia at birth—17-hydroxyprogesterone, 11-deoxycrotisol, ACTH, renin, aldosterone, electrolytes (serum, urine-hyponatremia, hyperkalemia, and dehydration), ACTH stimulation test.

In spite of all investigations, a definite diagnosis cannot be reached in newborn in 50% cases.

MANAGEMENT OF A CASE OF DSD

Q. How will you manage a case of DSD?

The basic management of these cases should be addressed to the two most important aspects, namely:
- ❖ **General health management**
- ❖ **Gender assignment,** which will be based on three components of psychological development, namely—gender identity, gender role, and sexual orientation.
- ❖ **Gender identity**—it refers intrinsic sense of oneself as female or male.
- ❖ **Gender role**—it is the set of behavior typical of one gender or another that vary with surrounding culture.
- ❖ **Sexual orientation**—it refers to an individual's erotic response to gender or genders to whom one is attracted (homosexual, heterosexual, or bisexual).

The management should be done with multidisciplinary team consisting of pediatric endocrinologist, psychologists, urologists, geneticists, radiologists, and child's primary care physicians. Parent must be involved in decision-making discussion (**Flowchart 3**).

Q. What are the different components of management of DSD?
- ❖ Gender issue and assignment
- ❖ Medical management
- ❖ Surgical management
- ❖ Conveyance of information
- ❖ Disclosure
- ❖ Psychological issue.

GENDER ASSIGNMENT

Q. What are the points to consider before gender assignment?
- ❖ Karyotype
- ❖ Gonadal function
- ❖ Phenotype
- ❖ Internal genitalia
- ❖ Potential for fertility and sexuality
- ❖ Risk of future malignancy
- ❖ Prenatal androgen influence on target tissue
- ❖ Information regarding long-term studies.

CHAPTER 13: A Case of Primary Amenorrhea and Disorder of Sexual Development

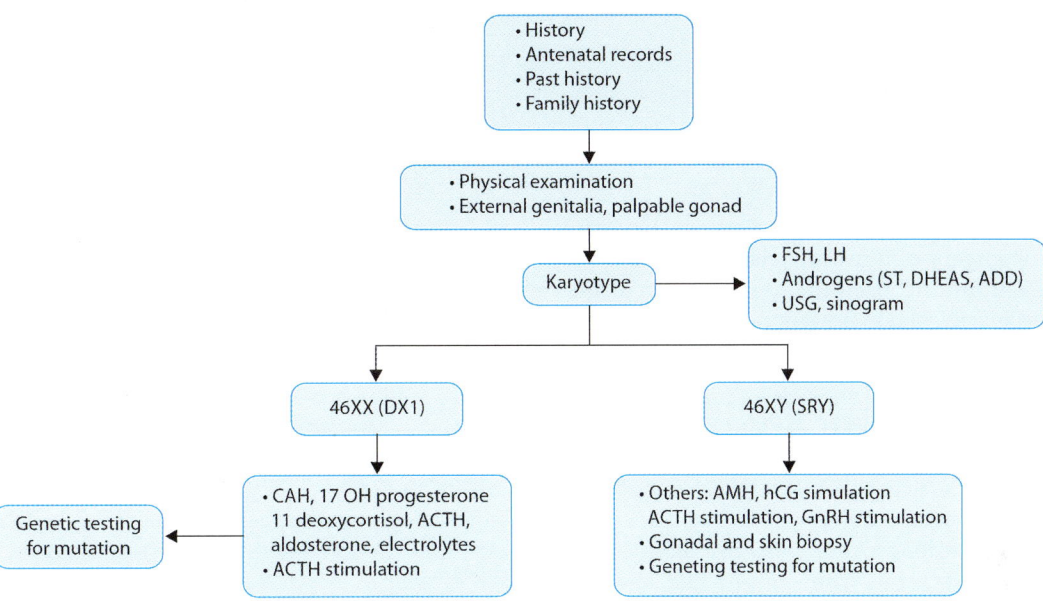

Flowchart 3: Diagnosis of disorder of sexual differentiation (DSDs).

Abbreviations: FSH, follicle-stimulating hormone; LH, luteinizing hormone; ACTH, adrenocorticotropic hormone; GnRH, gonadotropin-releasing hormone; AMH, anti-Müllerian hormone; hCG, human chorionic gonadotropin

Although gender assignment should be based on the expected gender identity that an individual will develop his/her lifetime, society has also influenced. Cultural, religious, and family values are additional considerations for the team before gender assignment.

The traditional gender assignment for some medical conditions resulting DSDs is given below and also discussed in **Table 10**.

Table 10: Gender assignment in disorder of sexual differentiation (DSD).

Diagnosis	Traditional gender assignment
46 XX CAH (congenital adrenal hyperplasia)	Female
Complete androgen insensitivity syndrome (AIS)	Female
XY cloacal extrophy	Male
Partial androgen insensitivity (PAIS)	Male/female
Mixed gonadal dysgenesis (MGD9)	Male/female
Ovotesticular DSD	Male/female

Assignment of Female Gender is Done in Case

- 46 XX DSDs resulting from fetal androgen exposure
- Complete AIS
- 46 XY complete gonadal dysgenesis (Swyer syndrome).

Assignment of Male Gender

46 XY cloacal extrophy

Assignment of Male or Female Gender

- PAIS, 5α-reductase deficiency, ketoreductase deficiency, 46 XY partial gonadal dysgenesis, MGD, and ovotesticular DSD.
- Patients with PAIS, 5α-reductase deficiency, ketoreductase deficiency, 46 XY partial gonadal dysgenesis, and MGD are reared as female, but at puberty they change their social sex as male. Sex assignment is very problematic in this group (ambiguous genitalia, testicular differentiation disorder and Y chromosome). Sex of rearing in ovotesticular DSD is based on gonadal and internal ductal formation.

In most cases, there is endocrine disturbance and medication is needed.

Q. What is the current recommendation of sex of assignment in 46 XX CAH?

- To rear the individual as female and to perform feminizing genitoplasty depending on severity of masculinization.
- But in CAH, where diagnosis is not made earlier and virilization is severe in nature in 46 XX CAH male sex assignment is mandatory.

SURGERIES IN DSDs

Q. What are the surgeries may be needed in DSDs?

- *Feminizing genital surgery*:
  - Clitorial surgery for hypertrophy—clitoral resection, clitoroplasty. Clitoral recession is done nowadays instead of resection due to impact of resection on sexuality.
  - Urogenital sinus mobilization

- Labiaplasty
- Neovaginal construction
- Gonadectomy in Y-containing gonad.

Q. What is the aim of feminizing surgery?

Surgery is done for three aims:
1. To reduce the size of masculinized clitoris
2. To reconstruct the female labia
3. To increase opening and the length of vagina, if possible.

The goal of surgery is to restore anatomy like female to preserve sensation and promote sexuality, to preserve reproductive capacity, and to prevent urologic sequelae and to promote better psychosocial and psychosexual outcomes.

Decision of feminizing genital surgery:
- In Prader I and II stages, surgery is deferred to adolescents or adulthood when the individual can take decision.
- In Prader III and IV, there is dilemma in decision regarding time of surgery. Early surgery is considered.
- Most surgeries are done within 1 year of infancy.
- Consent must be taken from parent and should be discussed about the genital function later in life, risks of gender self-assignment, and future need of further surgery.

Q. Why gonadectomy is needed? It is needed for two main reasons:

1. Risk of malignancy
2. Risk of ongoing virilization:
   - Highest risk of malignancy—dysgenetic intra-abdominal gonad and PAIS—15–50%
   - Lowest risk—CAIS and ovotesticular DSD—2–3%
   - Intermediate risk—dysgenetic or PAIS intrascrotal gonad
   - Mosaic Turner—risk is 12%.

Q. Timing of gonadectomy—in which age it should be done?

- *Complete AIS*: In CAIS, gonadectomy is done after the natural process of pubertal development (16–18 years of age). This will avoid need of estrogen for induction of secondary sexual character and the candidate can give the consent. Risk of malignancy is very low within 20 years of life in CAIS. However, it can be done at diagnosis or at the time of hernia repair, then hormone therapy is given for secondary sexual character.
- *PAIS*: Gonadectomy is done in PAIS in early neonatal period.
- In 5α-reductase deficiency, it is performed before puberty and this will prevent further masculinization. Recommended timing is given in **Table 11**.

Table 11: Recommended time of gonadectomy.

DSD	Age of gonadectomy
PAIS (female gender)	In 1st 6 months/at diagnosis earliest (chance of malignancy/virilization)
Gonadal dysgenesis with Y chromosome (intra-abdominal gonad)	Childhood (chance of malignancy)
Androgen biosynthesis defect 5 α-reductase deficiency (female gender assignment)	Prepuberty (virilization at puberty)
CAIS	At diagnosis or at the time of hernia repair or may be deferred up to puberty for spontaneous pubertal development as chance of malignancy is low
Gonadal dysgenesis (scrotal testis) (assigned as male gender assignment)	Biopsy at puberty, sperm banking is option

Abbreviations: PAIS, partial androgen insensitivity syndrome; CAIS, complete androgen insensitivity syndrome

MEDICAL MANAGEMENT IN DSDs

- Steroid in CAH
- Hormone therapy.

Indications of Hormone Therapy

- Postgonadectomy
- Turner's syndrome
- Premature ovarian failure.

In CAIS, who had not gonadectomy spontaneous pubertal development of puberty will occur due to aromatization of androgens to estradiol, though pubic and axillary hair will not develop due to androgen resistance.

Goals of Hormone Therapy in DSD

- Initiate and maintenance of secondary sexual characters including uterine growth
- Psychosexual development
- To protect bone.

The presence of Müllerian structure (uterus) will determine whether estrogen alone or E-P both are needed.

The maintenance dose of hormone therapy for oral conjugated equine estrogen is 1.25 mg, oral estradiol 2 mg and transdermal patch 100 μg daily and those for medroxyprogesterone acetate (MPA) and micronized progesterone are 10 mg and 200 mg daily both from 10–14 days cyclically in a month.

CHAPTER 14

A Case of Secondary Amenorrhea

Chapter Outline

Writing a case of secondary amenorrhea and how to present the case?

- Definition
- Causes of Secondary Amenorrhea
- Diagnostic Approach
- Galactorrhea
- Hyperprolactinemia—Causes, Evaluation and Treatment
- Hypothyroidism
- Asherman Syndrome
- Premature Ovarian Failure
- Late Onset Congenital Adrenal Hyperplasia
- Management

INTRODUCTION

When you are given a case of secondary amenorrhea following clinical situations are kept in mind:
- A case of polycystic ovarian syndrome (PCOS)
- Premature ovarian failure (POF); Synonym—primary ovarian insufficiency (POI)
- Hypothalamic amenorrhea
- Hyperprolactinemia
- Hypothyroidism
- Uterine synechia.

CASE TAKING IN A CASE OF SECONDARY AMENORRHEA

PATIENT'S PARTICULAR

1. Name:
2. Age: 33 years
3. Address:
4. Occupation:
5. Married/unmarried: Married

Bed No.:
Date of admission:
Date of examination:

6. History of infertility: No
7. Husband's occupation:
8. Socioeconomic status:
9. Religion:
10. Parous/nulliparous: Parous

HISTORY

- *Chief complaint/complaints*: Woman usually comes with complaint of amenorrhea for certain duration. There may be previous history of prolonged amenorrhea followed by heavy menstrual bleeding or there may be permanent cessation of bleeding in young age group. The patient may have infertility or may present with excessive growth of hair (hirsutism in PCOS).

- *History of present illness*: Chief complaints are elaborated. The duration of problem of amenorrhea is enquired in details, whether is permanent amenorrhea or occasional is to be noted. History of headache and visual defect [pituitary adenoma and central nervous system (CNS) tumor]. History of galactorrhea and presence of excessive growth of hair all over the body.

- *Menstrual history*:
    - Detailed menstrual history is taken
    - Last menstrual period (LMP)
    - Duration of menstruation
    - Interval in days
    - Age of menarche
    - Regularity of cycle
    - Pain during period/if pain relation with menstruation
    - Amount of bleeding
    - Clot
    - Intermenstrual bleeding
    - Duration of amenorrhea.
- *Obstetric history*: If parous parity, living issue and last childbirth (LCB) are noted. It should be written in tabular form. If there is any history of postpartum hemorrhage (PPH), lactation failure (Sheehan syndrome), lactation—lactational amenorrhea, and abortion (synechia) puerperal sepsis should be enquired in detail.
- *Past history*:
    - *Medical*: Hypertension, diabetes, history of eating disorder, heat or cold intolerance, sleep disorder in thyroid disease, psychiatric illness, pelvic infection, and tuberculosis (endometritis).
    - *Surgical*: If any history of laparoscopy, history of dilatation and curettage (D and C), and medical termination of pregnancy (MTP).
- *Family history*: Diabetes, hypertension, premature menopause, and history of PCOS
- *Sexual history*: Hot flash, loss of libido, and vaginal dryness due to either menopause or POF.
- *Functional history*: Anorexia
- *Personal history*: Vigorous exercise
- *Contraceptive history*: Postpill amenorrhea, injectable contraceptive, if any to be taken.
- *Drug history/treatment history*: Any medication particularly hormones, other medication causing hyperprolactinemia like antipsychotic, metoclopramide, phenothiazine, shaving or any mechanical method for hirsutism. History of radiation and chemotherapy.

PHYSICAL EXAMINATION

Detailed general survey are done and noted. The points relevant to this case are:
- Height
- Weight
- BMI
- Obesity: Android or gynecoid type
- Build/nutrition
- Pallor
- Neck glands: Enlargement of thyroid glands
- Secondary sexual character
- Galactorrhea
- Features of hirsutism: Acne, acanthosis nigricans, temporal balding, and enlargement of clitoris, if any.
- If there is hirsutism, scoring is done by Ferriman–Gallwey Scoring System (modified) as detailed in Chapter 12; A Case of Polycystic Ovary Syndrome and Hirsutism (**Fig. 19** of Chapter 12)
- Pulse
- Respiration
- Temperature
- Blood pressure.

Systemic Examination

As described in Chapter 1.
Examination of breasts—regression of breasts and presence of galactorrhea

GYNECOLOGICAL EXAMINATION

Abdominal Examination

Any abdominopelvic lump—always exclude pregnancy, any androgen-producing tumor.

Per Vaginal Examination

- *Inspection*:
    - Clitoral enlargement
    - Labial fusion in congenital adrenal hyperplasia (CAH)
- *Speculum examination*: Cervical stenosis and vaginal stenosis
- *Palpation*: To look for any congenital or acquired abnormality
- Not done in unmarried virgin
- Per rectal examination can be done in virgin.

INVESTIGATIONS SUPPLIED OR REQUIRED

- Urinary pregnancy test report [beta-human chorionic gonadotropin (β-hCG)]
- Ultrasonography of pelvis
- Investigations: Hematological, hormone levels, and karyotyping
- Hormones relevant to this case: Follicle-stimulating hormone (FSH), luteinizing hormone (LH), thyroid-stimulating hormone (TSH), prolactin, and anti-Mullerian hormone.

SUMMARY OF THE CASE (SAMPLE SUMMARY)

A 33-year-old married woman has complaint of amenorrhea for last 10 months. She has history of hot flash, loss of libido, and vaginal dryness. She had regular period before cessation of menstruation. She has two children both vaginal delivery; last child birth 6 years back. Her mother has history of premature menopause at the age of 36 years. She has no galactorrhea and no history hormonal intake. Her food habit is normal.

On physical examination, her BMI is ......, BP....... Her breasts examinations showed no galactorrhea; per abdominal examination showed no lump; bimanual examination revealed uterus normal size with no palpable adnexa.

Urinary pregnancy test is negative. USG of pelvis shows normal size uterus, no abnormality of adnexae, and FSH level is 40 IU/L and LH level is 37 IU/L; serum TSH and prolactin are within normal limit.

PROVISIONAL DIAGNOSIS

A 33-year-old woman with premature ovarian failure (POF).

DIFFERENTIAL DIAGNOSIS

- PCOS
- Infertility.

Q. What is your case?

Tell the summary.

Q. So, what is your diagnosis?

A case of secondary amenorrhea due to premature ovarian failure (POF).

DEFINITION OF SECONDARY AMENORRHEA

Q. How would you define secondary amenorrhea?

No menstruation for an interval of time equivalent to a total of at least three previous cycles or no menstruation over a six-month period in women who have menstruated previously.

CAUSES OF SECONDARY AMENORRHEA

Q. What are the common causes of secondary amenorrhea encountered in clinical practice (Fig. 1)?

- Ovarian (PCOS and POF): 40%
- Hypothalamus: 35%
- Pituitary (hyperprolactinemia): 19%
- Uterine: 5% including Asherman syndrome
- Others: 1% (late-onset CAH, ovarian tumor, undiagnosed).

Q. In general, what are the causes of secondary amenorrhea?

Menstruation is an end result of coordinated activity of hypothalamo-pituitary-ovarian uterine axis with normal outflow tract with normal thyroid, adrenal, and metabolic function.

Karyotyping and environment also have great influence in normal menstruation.

The control of menstruation has been schematically diagrammed in Flowchart 1, Chapter 13 of Primary Amenorrhea.

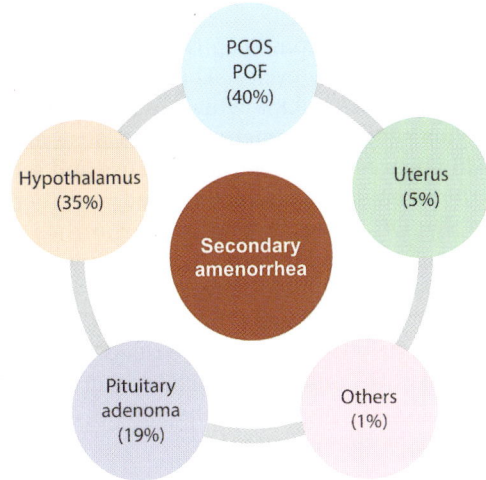

Fig. 1: Common causes of secondary amenorrhea encountered in clinical practice.
Abbreviations: PCOS, polycystic ovarian syndrome; POF, premature ovarian failure

Important Pathological Causes According to Anatomical Sites:

- Hypothalamic (35%)—psychological stress, psychiatric illness (pseudocyesis), loss of weight (dieting, athlete, anorexia), weight gain (increase BMI—obesity), trauma, chronic illness, encephalitic, tuberculosis, sarcoidosis, VVF, drugs like postpill amenorrhea, phenothiazine, metoclopramide, etc.
- Pituitary—hyperprolactinemia (19%, macroadenoma and microadenoma), Sheehan's syndrome, and pituitary adenoma.
- Ovarian—PCOS (28%), POF, and arrhenoblastoma (1%).
- Uterine (1%)—tuberculosis and synechiae.
- Others—late-onset CAH (0.5%), Cushing syndrome, Addison's disease, adrenal tumor hypothyroidism, and hyperthyroidism.

Etiologies According to Gonadotropin Level (ASRM, 2009)

- Low or normal FSH level: 67.5%
    - Eating disorders, exercise, stress: 15.5%
    - Nonspecific hypothalamic: 18%
    - Chronic anovulation (PCOS): 28%
    - Hypothyroidism: 1.5%
    - Cushing syndrome: 1%
    - Pituitary tumor/empty sella: 2%
    - Sheehan syndrome: 1.5%.
- High FSH level—gonadal failure: 10.5%
    - 46 XX: 10%
    - Abnormal karyotype: 0.5%

Physiological Causes of Secondary Amenorrhea

- Lactation
- Pregnancy
- Menopause.

Postpill Amenorrhea

After stoppage of oral contraceptives, it takes few months for return of ovulatory cycles. The incidence of postpill amenorrhoea is 0.7%–0.8% which is near incidence of spontaneous secondary amenorrhoea. Cause-and-effect relationship between oral contraceptive use and secondary amenorrhea could not be documented and there is no evidence that OC causes secondary amenorrhea. Women who have amenorrhea for more than six months following discontinuation of OC should be evaluated like other patients with secondary amenorrhea. The presence for prolactin-producing pituitary tumor should be ruled out. This is not related to use of OC rather to probability that slow growing tumor was already present. Management is advocated depending on the cause revealed.

Q. When would you start investigation in case of secondary amenorrhea?

- Missed period for 1 week in women with regular menstrual cycles may require the exclusion of pregnancy.
- Secondary amenorrhea lasting for 3 months and oligomenorrhea involving less than nine cycles a year require investigation.

DIAGNOSIS OF SECONDARY AMENORRHEA

Q. How would you reach diagnosis in a case of secondary amenorrhea?

- From history taking
- Clinical examination
- Investigation report.

History

- *Age*: Near menopause or not
- *Menstrual history*: Details of menstruation—LMP, duration of amenorrhea, whether period was regular or irregular before amenorrhea?
- Hot flash, loss of libido, and vaginal dryness due to either menopause or POF
- Excessive growth of hair (hirsutism), acne and alopecia in PCOS, and adult onset congenital adrenal hyperplasia (AOCAH)
- Headache and visual defect (pituitary adenoma and CNS tumor)
- History of weight gain (PCOS), weight loss, anorexia, and vigorous exercise
- History of galactorrhea (hyperprolactinemia)
- *Obstetric history*: PPH, lactation failure (Sheehan syndrome), lactation (LAM), and abortion (synechiae)
- *Past history*:
  - **Medical**: Heat or cold intolerance, sleep disorder in thyroid disorder, psychiatric illness, pelvic infection, and tuberculosis (endometritis)
  - **Surgical**: History of D and C
- *Family history*: POF and PCOS
- *Drug history*: Antipsychotic, metoclopramide, and phenothiazine causing hyperprolactinemia
- History of radiation and chemotherapy
- *Contraceptive history*: Postpill amenorrhea and injectable contraceptive.

Physical Examination

- Height
- Weight
- BMI: Low—less than 18.5% may have amenorrhea. Low BMI with tooth enamel erosion with repeated vomiting suggests eating disorder. High BMI—in obesity with or without PCOS.
- Hirsutism, acne, acanthosis nigricans **(Fig. 2)**, balding in PCOS or any hyperinsulinemia and hyperandrogenemia
- Enlarged thyroid gland, delayed reflexes, and bradycardia in hypothyroidism
- Bilateral galactorrhea in hyperprolactinemia
- Supraclavicular fat, abdominal striae, and hypertension—Cushing syndrome.

Per Abdomen

Any lump—ovarian mass and cryptomenorrhea.

Vulva and Vagina

Stenosis of vagina, cervix, features of estrogen deficiency, and enlarged clitoris—virilization.

Digital Vaginal Examination

Uterine size and adnexal mass.

Rectal Examination Especially for Virgin

Uterine size and adnexal mass.

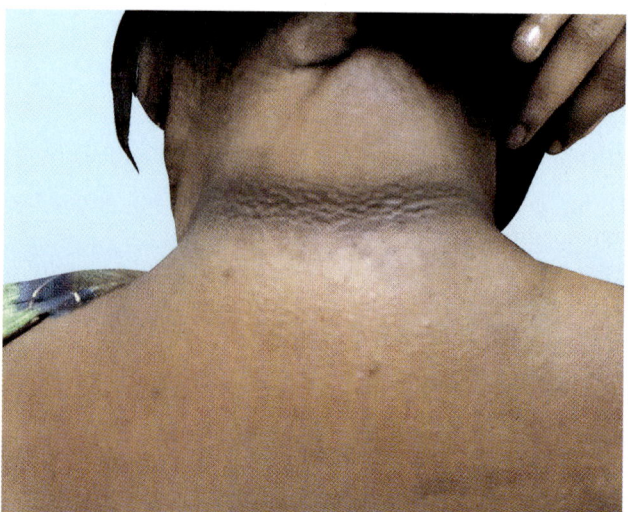

Fig. 2: HAIR-AN syndrome in polycystic ovarian syndrome woman who came with amenorrhea and oligomenorrhea.

Q. What investigations would you do in case of secondary amenorrhea?

- *Urinary pregnancy test*: Pregnancy should be thought of in any case of amenorrhea in reproductive age women until proved otherwise.
- Thyroid-stimulating hormone, prolactin, and FSH and LH to rule out hypothyroidism, hyperprolactinemia, hypergonadotropic, and hypogonadotropic hypogonadism, respectively.
- Assessment of estrogen status—serum estradiol, progesterone challenge test (PCT), endometrial thickness, and cervical mucus.
- Serum testosterone, dehydroepiandrosterone sulfate (DHEAS), and 17-hydroxyprogesterone:
    - Mild elevation of serum testosterone levels is consistent with PCOS, testosterone level more than 200 ng/dL is suggestive of ovarian neoplasm and needs USG to confirm the same.
    - High normal or mild elevation of DHEAS is found in PCOS, level above 700 µg/dL suggests adrenal tumor and needs CT/MRI.
    - 17-hydroxyprogesterone is high in adult onset congenital adrenal hyperplasia (AO CAH) (*see* details in Chapter 12, Page 298 and Chapter 13, Page 327)
- USG of pelvis and abdomen: Typical ovarian morphology (multiple small hypoechoic cysts in ovary) in PCOS **(Fig. 3)** or any androgen secreting ovarian tumor.
- CT and MRI of brain and pituitary gland to exclude tumor or infiltrative diseases.
- Chromosome analysis for POF.
- Investigation to diagnose tuberculosis.

APPROACH TO DIAGNOSE A CASE OF SECONDARY AMENORRHEA

Q. How to approach a case of secondary amenorrhea?

Flowchart 1 shows how to approach to diagnose a case of secondary amenorrhea.

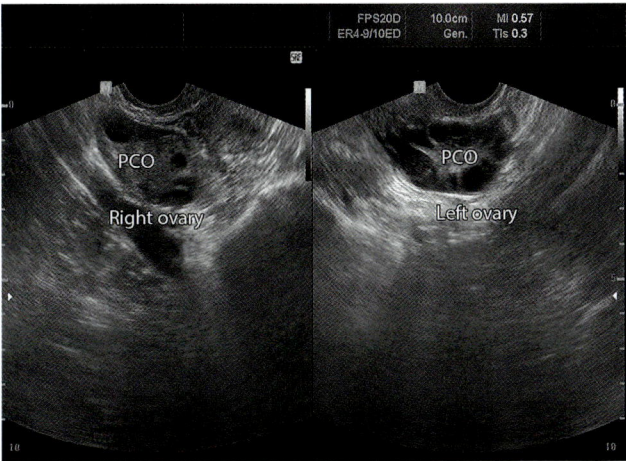

Fig. 3: Multiple small follicles in polycystic ovarian syndrome.
Courtesy: Dr Sanghamitra Ghosh, IRM, Kolkata

Q. How would you assess estrogen status?

- Serum estradiol level
- Progesterone challenge test (PCT)
- Endometrial thickness
- Cervical mucus.

Serum Estradiol Level

A random E2 level of more than 40 pg/mL suggests presence of functional ovarian follicles. Low level suggests ovarian failure, hypothalamic amenorrhea or normal woman in early follicular phase.

Progesterone Challenge Test

- Progesterone challenge test is done to confirm functional anatomy and presence of adequate estrogen.
- Medroxyprogesterone acetate (MPA) 10 mg orally or progesterone in oil 200 mg IM daily for 7–10 days is given with anticipation of a withdrawal bleeding.
- Positive test means normal estrogen production with patent outflow tract with normal endometrium. Negative suggests hypogonadism or defect in outflow tract.
- If bleeding does not follow with progesterone then estrogen—progesterone combination is given and failing to bleed indicates anatomical abnormality (uterine synechia, defective endometrial receptivity, etc.)
- *Limitation*: Withdrawal bleeding correlates poorly with estrogen status. False-positive rate and false negative rate both are high. In 40–50% of women with amenorrhea related to exercise, stress, loss of weight, hyperprolactinemia or ovarian failure shows withdrawal bleeding in spite of low estrogen level. Up to 20% women with high estrogen level fail to bleed due to high androgen-related atrophic endometrium in PCOS and CAH cases. Hence, many experts defer this testing.

Cervical Mucus

Clear, watery, and relatively abundant mucus in preovulatory stage suggests normal estrogen production.

Endometrial Thickness

Endometrial thickness measuring 6.0 mm or greater by TVS predicts withdrawal bleeding with 95% accuracy.

HYPERPROLACTINEMIA AND AMENORRHEA

Incidence of Hyperprolactinemia

- Less than 1% among general population
- In secondary amenorrhea cases as high as 30% cases
- In infertile women 30%
- With galactorrhea and amenorrhea 75%.

Q. How does amenorrhea occur in hyperprolactinemia?

Amenorrhea occurs in hyperprolactinemia by **two mechanisms:**

1. Reflex increase of central dopamine. Stimulation of dopaminergic receptors on gonadotropin-releasing hormone (GnRH) neurons alters GnRH pulsatility, decreases GnRH, decreases gonadotropin, thus hampers

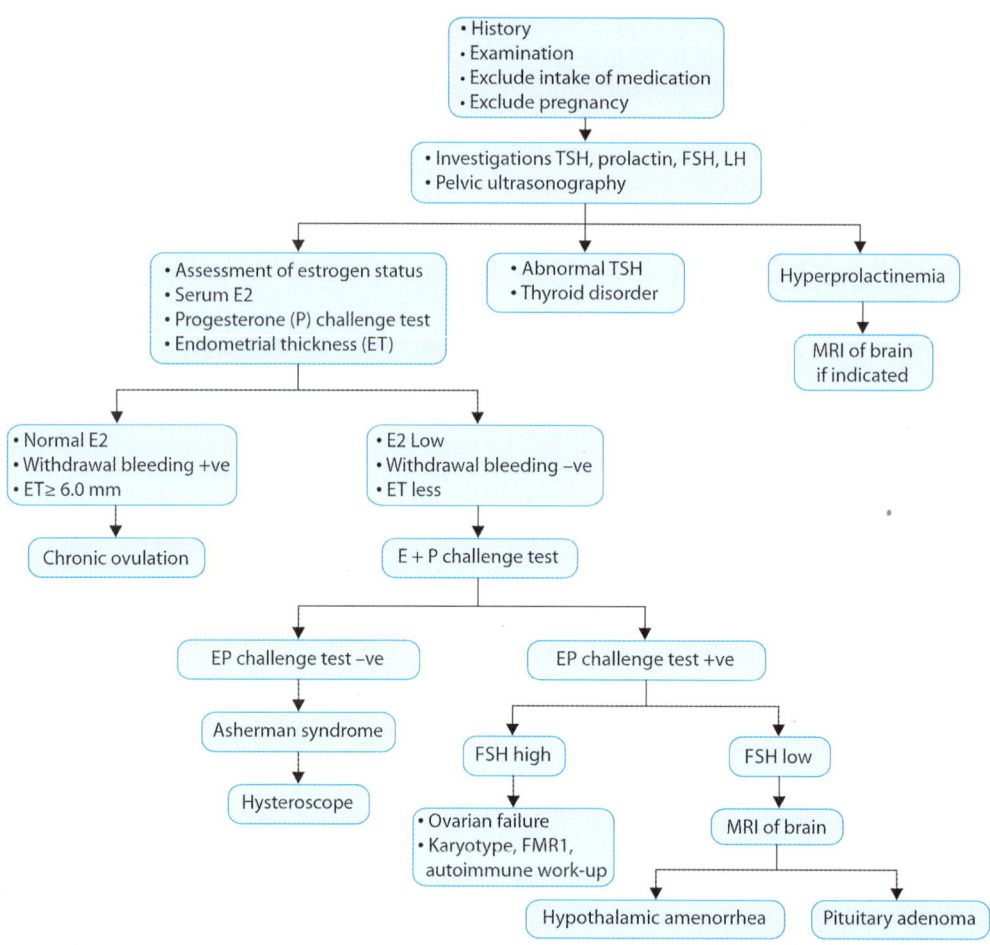

Flowchart 1: Approach to diagnose a case of secondary amenorrhea.

Abbreviations: TSH, thyroid-stimulating hormone; FSH, follicle-stimulating hormone; LH, luteinizing hormone

folliculogenesis resulting low estradiol, amenorrhea and oligomenorrhea.
2. Disruption of folliculogenesis also occurs due to presence of dopamine receptors in ovaries.

Hyperprolactinemia and Galactorrhea

- 50% patients of hyperprolactinemia are associated with galactorrhea and 50% patients of galactorrhea have normal prolactin.
- Association of amenorrhea and galactorrhea is called *"galactorrhea-amenorrhea syndrome"*.

In all cases of hyperprolactinemia, galactorrhea does not occur because that normal estrogen level is essential for milk formation which is not seen all cases of hyperprolactinemia. Hyperprolactinemia often causes anovulation, hypogonadotropic hypogonadism, and low estrogen level.

Known Causes of Galactorrhea without Prolactinemia

- There may be "Hook effect" in estimation of serum prolactin due to very high prolactin level. In that suspected case diluted sample is used. Hook effect is a phenomenon where the very high level is not shown due to prozone phenomenon. This type of phenomenon is also found in case of β-hCG, ferritin, prostate specific antigen, CA-125, and thyrotropin.
- Galactorrhea may be due to local cause of breasts without hyperprolactinemia.

Known Causes of Hyperprolactinemia without Galactorrhea

- Presence of macroprolactin which is biologically inactive. Elevated prolactin level is seen without clinical features of hyperprolactinemia due to *macroprolactin* which is multimer of native prolactin but physiologically inactive (*see* Page 341).
- Due to significant hypoestrogenemia as estrogen is essential for milk synthesis as described above.

Causes of Hyperprolactinemia

- *Physiological*: Pregnancy, lactation, stress, and nipple stimulation
- *Pathological*:
    - Prolactinoma (50–60% of cases)
    - Drugs—1-2%—phenothiazines, haloperidol, metoclopramide, cimetidine, reserpine, methyldopa, antipsychotic drugs (most common)

- Hypothyroidism 3–5% cases
- Others: Ectopic production by pituitary tissue in pharynx, chronic renal failure, breast or chest wall injury, cervical spine lesions by activating afferent sensory neural pathway.

Source and Structure of Prolactin

Prolactin is secreted from 'lactotrophs'; cells of anterior pituitary. It is single chain polypeptide hormone with three intramolecular disulfide bonds.

Types of Prolactin

- Monomeric (molecular weight—23 kDa)—most common (80–90%)
- Dimmers or trimmers called big prolactin (molecular weight 50–60 kDa)
- Macroprolactin (>100 kDa) is larger variety.

Monomeric is more biologically active than larger prolactins.

Q. What is the normal level of serum prolactin and what is its physiological variation?

- Normal serum prolactin level is less than 10–20 ng/mL. Half-life is 50 minutes.
- Level rises after onset of sleep, nocturnal peak up to 30 ng/mL and may be double of daytime (between 4 AM and 6 AM).

Measurement of Prolactin

Serum prolactin level is done in morning at the time of prolactin nadir. Prior to testing breast examination and any stress are avoided. In mild prolactin elevation repeat testing is done as it varies throughout the day.

Effects of Hyperprolactinemia

- Mild hyperprolactinemia (20–50 ng/mL) levels may cause short luteal phase.
- Moderate (50–100 ng/mL) causes oligomenorrhea and amenorrhea.
- Severe type (>100 ng/mL) result typical hypogonadism with low estrogen.

Q. What is macroadenoma and microadenoma?

- Macroadenoma: When the tumor diameter is greater than or equal to 10 mm and/or may extend beyond pituitary fossa.
- Microadenoma when the tumor diameter is less than 10 mm and it does not distort or extend beyond pituitary fossa.
- Microadenoma rarely progresses to macroadenoma.
- Microadenoma is rarely associated with 200 ng/mL, in macroadenoma prolactin level becomes usually more than 200 ng/mL.

MRI and Hyperprolactinemia

The poor correlation between tumor presence and prolactin level indicates that MRI should be performed whenever prolactin level is *persistently* elevated.

- To diagnose macroadenoma
- Mild prolactin level may be associated with other organic CNS lesion.

Treatment of Hyperprolactinemia

- *General*: Elimination and treatment of specific etiological factors like drugs, nipple stimulation, and use of thyroxin in hypothyroidism.
- *Medical*: In general, *first line of therapy is medical* in both micro- and macroadenoma.
    - Both type of dopamine agonists, bromocriptine a nonspecific dopamine-receptor agonist (both type 2 and type 1 agonist) and cabergoline, a selective dopamine receptor type 2 agonist, are used.
    - Bromocriptine is associated with side effects like nausea, headache, postural hypotension, blurred vision, and leg cramps. Due to its short half-life, it is taken once or twice daily. It is started at a low dose, i.e., 1.25 mg orally at bed time and then gradually increased to 2–3 times daily as per tolerability.
    - Cabergoline is found to be more effective having fewer side effects than dopamine, with greater potency, longer duration of action, and less frequently needed (0.25 mg orally twice weekly). However, it is associated with hypertrophic valvular heart disease on long-term use.
- *Indication of surgery*:
    - In lactotrophs adenomas in case of intolerance or resistant to dopamine agonists or in acutely worsening symptoms of visual field defect or severe headache surgery through transsphenoidal approach is indicated.
    - In case of very large macroadenoma (>3 cm), if patients want to be conceived surgery is considered even it responds to medical therapy.
- *Radiation* is given surgically nonresectable or persistent tumors.

THYROID DISORDER AND AMENORRHEA (FIG. 4)

Hypo- and hyperthyroidism both may cause amenorrhea but hypothyroidism commonly causes oligomenorrhea and amenorrhea while hyperthyroidism causes menorrhagia.

Mechanism of Amenorrhea in Hypothyroidism

- Decreased thyroid hormones by compensatory mechanism increase thyrotropin-releasing hormone which in turn increases TSH as well as increases prolactin secretion by binding pituitary lactotrophs.
- Increase of prolactin increases central dopamine, primary inhibitor of prolactin. This dopamine inhibits GnRH secretion which in turn disrupts gonadotropin secretion and inhibits folliculogenesis leading to anovulation and amenorrhea.
- In hypothyroidism, prolactin levels usually lies below 100 ng/mL
- *Treatment of secondary hyperprolactinemia is thyroid hormones not the dopamine agonist.*

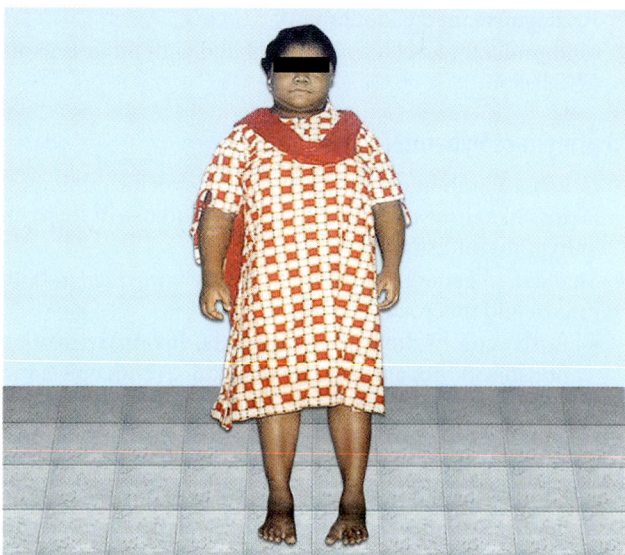

Fig. 4: Hypothyroidism in a 16-year-old obese (BMI 32 kg/m²) girl presented with secondary amenorrhea followed by heavy menstrual bleeding—recurrent episodes. She responded well with thyroxin.

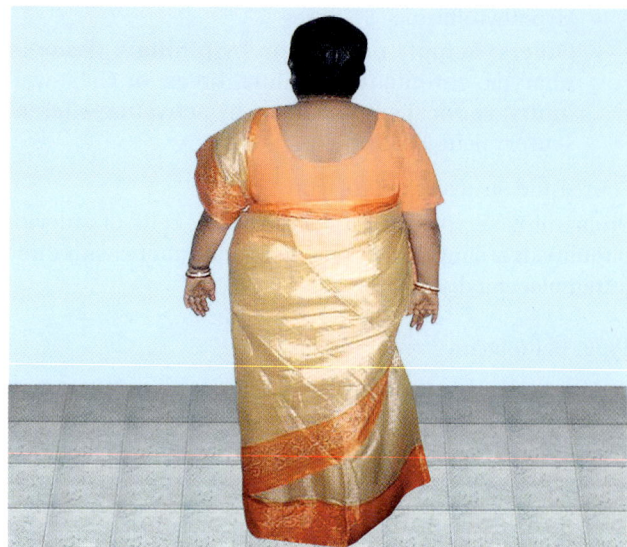

Fig. 5: Secondary amenorrhea in obese woman (BMI 31 kg/m²) who came for infertility for 3 years associated with polycystic ovarian syndrome.

POLYCYSTIC OVARIAN SYNDROME

It is the most common cause of amenorrhea as a single entity contributing about 28% of all secondary amenorrhea.

Details are given in Chapter 12; A Case of Polycystic Ovary Syndrome. The subject is to be reviewed on the following points:
- Define PCOS
- Diagnostic criteria of PCOS
- Diagnosis of PCOS
- Endocrinal changes in PCOS
- Clinical presentation
- Complications of PCOS
- Obesity and PCOS
- Hirsutism, acne, metabolic syndrome, HAIR-AN syndrome
- Management of PCOS.

OBESITY AND MENSTRUAL ABNORMALITY (FIG. 5)

- In obesity, there is oligomenorrhea, amenorrhea, and dysfunctional uterine bleeding (DUB).
- Abnormalities are due to obesity resulting from anovulation, hyperestrogenemia and increased free biologically active portion of estradiol due to much lower level of sex hormone-binding globulin. Circulating androgen is converted to estrogen more on abundant peripheral fat in obesity.
- Excess adipose tissue is associated with more inflammation of adipose tissue which is linked to increase insulin resistance and cardiovascular disease.
- Menstrual abnormalities are more common when obesity is associated with PCOS **(Fig. 5)**. Weight loss can improve menstrual abnormality up to 80% cases.

ASHERMAN SYNDROME (UTERINE SYNECHIAE)

Causes
- Vigorous curettage in PPH, miscarriage, and MTP
- Endometritis stage in PPH and miscarriage
- Following metroplasty, myomectomy, and cesarean section.

Diagnosis
USG, saline sonography, hysterosalpingography, and hysteroscope.

Treatment
- Hysteroscopic lysis, Cu-T placement, and cyclical high dose estrogen
- Antitubercular drug in tuberculosis.

PREMATURE OVARIAN FAILURE (ALSO CALLED PRIMARY OVARIAN INSUFFICIENCY)

- About 1–5% of women may experience POF (in age <30 years 1 in 1,000 and in age <40 years 1 in 100 women).
- Amenorrhea, persistent estrogen deficiency, and elevated FSH levels *prior to the age of 40 years.*

Causes
- The most common cause is a premature ovarian depletion leading to a continuum of impaired ovarian function. (A) Chromosomal, (B) other genetic, and (C) autoimmune disease must be excluded as those have health implications. In majority cases, cause is not determined.

Diagnosis

- **Two serum FSH levels** more than a threshold range of 30–40 mIU/mL at least 1 month apart.
- **Karyotype** is done to rule out sex chromosome translocation, short-arm deletion, or the presence of an occult Y chromosome.
- *Family history:* To rule out autosomal disorders as up to 40% there may be autoimmune abnormalities.
- Patient is screened for other abnormalities by means of TSH, thyroid autoantibodies, fasting glucose, etc., as autoimmune POF could be a part of polyglandular syndrome.
- Testing of *FMR1* (fragile X mental retardation 1 gene) gene as it is associated with POF and confers risk of *fragile X syndrome* in offspring.
- There is no specific antibody marker to confirm autoimmune POF.
- Ovarian biopsy is not indicated in clinical practice.
- Premature ovarian failure due to chemotherapy and radiation has a potential for recovery.

Therapy

- No therapy for infertile patients with autoimmune ovarian failure has been proven effective.
- Estrogen–progesterone treatment is offered to maintain secondary sexual characteristics and to reduce the risk of osteoporosis.
- Rarely spontaneous ovulation and conception occur due to presence of some follicles.
- Inconsistent GnRH drive.
- E2 is low, may be normal.
- Hormone therapy with either 100 μg transdermal estradiol or 0.625 mg conjugated equine estrogen daily on days 1–26 of menstrual cycle and 10 mg of MPA for 12 days (from 14–26) until average age of natural menopause is usually given to prevent osteoporosis, ischemic heart disease, and vasomotor symptoms. Conventional oral contraceptive is avoided for risk of thromboembolism.
- Patient is advised for weight bearing exercise, calcium (1,200 mg), and vitamin D3 (800 IU daily).
- If pregnancy is desired, good nutrition, optimal body weight, and ovulation induction with assisted reproductive technology are indicated. Donor eggs are considered.

LATE-ONSET CONGENITAL ADRENAL HYPERPLASIA

(*See* Also Chapter 13; Primary Amenorrhea)

- Presents with features of hyperandrogenism and irregular menstrual function like PCOS.
- Late-onset congenital adrenal hyperplasia (LOCAH) is mostly due to a mutation in the *CYP21* and in mild mutation patient becomes asymptomatic till adrenarche.
- Progesterone to cortisol and aldosterone is not converted adequately due to deficiency of 21-hydroxylase, thus progesterone precursor is converted to the androgen and increased androgen levels (*see* **Fig. 13** in Chapter 12; A Case of Polycystic Ovary Syndrome, Page 299) disrupt follicular maturation resulting anovulation and amenorrhea.
- Diagnosis is made by estimation of serum 17-hydroxyprogesterone which becomes elevated above 800 ng/mL and positive adrenocorticotropic hormone stimulation test. Bilateral adrenal hyperplasia may be seen on USG. Urinary excretion of pregnanetriol and alpha ketosteroid are increased.
- Management is done by hydrocortisone replacement therapy.

FUNCTIONAL HYPOTHALAMIC AMENORRHEA

- It occurs when the hypothalamic-pituitary-ovarian axis is suppressed due to deficiency of energy resulting from stress, weight loss, vigorous exercise, or eating disorder.
- There is low estrogen without any organic or structural disorder. Serum FSH, LH, and estradiol levels are low.
- Treatment includes:
  - Nutritional rehabilitation
  - Reductions in stress and exercise
  - Bone density evaluation is done and bone loss is best treated by reversal of the underlying disorder, and intake of calcium and vitamin D supplementation.

AMENORRHEA IN ANDROGEN-PRODUCING TUMOR (FIGS. 6 TO 9)

- Sertoli–Leydig cell tumor (arrhenoblastoma or androblastoma) is a male hormone producing tumor with an incidence of less than 0.2% of ovarian cancer.
- About 70–85% women may present with abdominal mass **(Fig. 7)** with features of virilization, breast atrophy, acne, hirsutism **(Fig. 6)**, clitoromegaly, deepening of voice

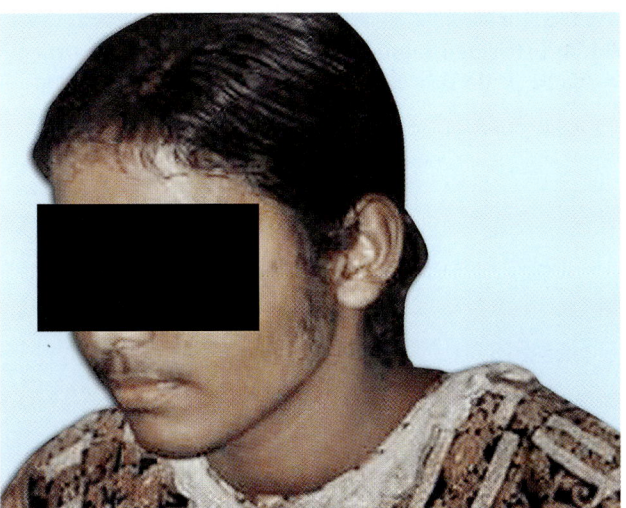

Fig. 6: Hirsutism in a 16-year-old girl with arrhenoblastoma (Sertoli–Leydig cell tumor) who presented with amenorrhea, lump abdomen, and regression of breasts, features of virilization, and high serum testosterone level.

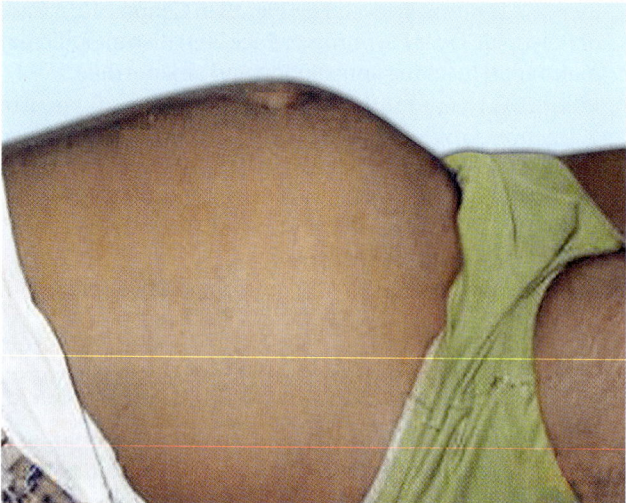

Fig. 7: Lump abdomen with growth of excessive hair over body—arrhenoblastoma in 16-year-old girl as shown in Figure 6.

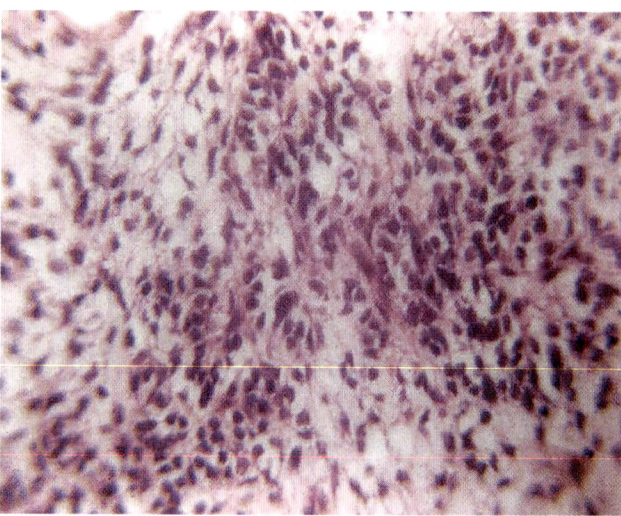

Fig. 9: Undifferentiated arrhenoblastoma (Sertoli–Leydig cell tumor) in specimen shown in Figure 8.
Courtesy: Professor Tamal Ghosh, Pathology

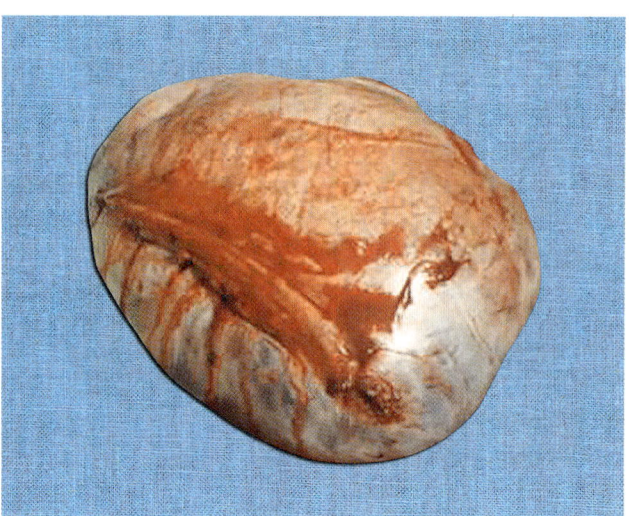

Fig. 8: Left-sided salpingo-oophorectomy done in arrhenoblastoma—in the patient as in Figure 7. It was diagnosed in stage IA.

and a receding hairline and oligomenorrhea followed by amenorrhea in reproductive age woman. Serum testosterone becomes high.

❖ They are rarely bilateral (<1%). 90% cases are diagnosed in stage I and in young age unilateral salpingo-oophorectomy is done **(Fig. 8)**.

CHAPTER 15

A Case of Precocious Puberty (Pediatrics and Adolescent Gynecological Problem)

CHAPTER OUTLINE

Writing a case of precocious puberty and how to present the case?

- Etiologies of Precocious Puberty
- Diagnosis of Different Types of Precocious Puberty
- Central Precocious Puberty
- McCune-Albright Syndrome
- Management of Precocious Puberty
- Van Wyk and Grumbach Syndrome

- Gynecological Problems in Pediatric and Adolescent Age Group (PAG)
  - Labial Adhesion
  - Primary Amenorrhea, Disorders of Sexual Development
  - Vulvovaginitis, Vaginal Bleeding
  - Ovarian Neoplasm and Endometriosis
  - Adolescent Polycystic Ovarian Syndrome

A CASE OF PRECOCIOUS PUBERTY

PATIENT'S PARTICULARS

1. Name:
2. Age:
3. Address:
4. Occupation:
5. Married/unmarried: Usually unmarried
6. History of infertility:
7. Husband's occupation:
8. Socioeconomic status:
9. Religion:
10. Parous/nulliparous: Nulliparous

Bed No.:
Date of admission:
Date of examination:

HISTORY

- *Chief complaint/complaints:* Patient usually brought by parent with complains of development of breasts and other secondary character and may or may not be onset of menstruation.

- *History of present illness:*
  - Chief complaints are elaborated.
  - Sequence of development of secondary sexual character is noted.
  - Breasts development, development of pubic hairs and axillary hairs with sequences, whether associated with increase growth.
  - History of childhood problems, galactorrhea or any feature of hypothyroidism are recorded. Any increase of weight gain is noted.
- *Menstrual history:* Whether menstruation is started. If started what is the duration? It is regular or irregular, associated with pain or not? Whether there is breasts development and if so sequences with the menstruation.
- *Obstetric history:* Mostly irrelevant
- *Past history:*
  - Medical—brain tumor, any headache, history of seizure (laughing seizure)
  - Surgical—if any.
- *Family history*
- *Sexual history*

SECTION 2: Clinical Cases

- *Functional history*
- *Personal history*
- *Contraceptive history:* Does not arise
- *Drug history/treatment history:* Any history of exposure to exogenous estrogens or androgens or any treatment already initiated for precocious puberty.

DETAILED GENERAL SURVEY ARE DONE AND NOTED

The points relevant to this case are:
- Height
- Weight
- Body mass index (BMI)—obesity
- Skin examination—McCune-Albright: Large café-au-lait spots with irregular borders (coast of Maine), acne, hirsutism in hyperandrogenicity
- Secondary sexual character, development of breasts, pubic and axillary hair—Tanner staging presence of galactorrhea
- Pulse
- Blood pressure
- Respiration
- Temperature.

SYSTEMIC EXAMINATION

- As a routine.
- Funduscopic examination, visual fields.

GYNECOLOGICAL EXAMINATION

- *Abdominal examination:* Any abdominopelvic lump
- *Per vaginal examination:* Inspection—whether labia are well developed or not
- *Rectal examination*—if needed.

INVESTIGATIONS SUPPLIED OR REQUIRED

- Ultrasonography of pelvis
- Magnetic resonance imaging (MRI) of brain, abdominal CT or MRI (adrenal and ovarian pathology)
- X-ray elbow and wrist to determine bone age
- Hormones—serum follicle-stimulating hormone (FSH), luteinizing hormone (LH), testosterone, estradiol, thyroid profile, 17-hydroxyprogesterone, dihydroepiandrosterone (DHEA), human chorionic gonadotropin (hCG)
- Gonadotropin-releasing hormone (GnRH) stimulation test to differentiate premature thelarche from true central and peripheral precocious puberty.

SUMMARY OF THE CASE

A 7-year-old girl attended in gynecology outpatient department (OPD) by her parent with complain of development of breasts during last 6 months and there is also development of axillary and pubic hair and her height is also increasing quickly for which she is teased by her friends in school. If she gives history of onset of menstrual period.
- On examination her height is....., weight....., no breasts—Tanner stage 3, pubic hair and axillary hair—Tanner stage 2, no pallor, thyroid gland not enlarged.
- Per abdominal examination—no lump abdomen.
- On inspection of vagina, labia are developed and not infantile.

PROVISIONAL DIAGNOSIS

A 7-year-old girl with precocious puberty.

DIFFERENTIAL DIAGNOSIS (D/D)

Q. What is your diagnosis?

Tell the provisional diagnosis—a 7-year-old girl with precocious puberty.

Q. What is your case?

Tell the summary of the case.

Q. Why are you saying this is a precocious puberty?

There is development of breasts in an 8-year-old girl. She has also started menstruation (if so).

Q. Define precocious puberty.

Onset of puberty (development of secondary sexual characteristics) before the age of 8 years in girls or menarche before the age of 10 years.

Incidence is 29/100,000 girls per year.

Q. What is puberty?

Puberty is a process leading to physical, sexual and psychosocial maturation.

Q. How would you classify precocious puberty?

- *Central or true [GnRH-dependent] precocious puberty (GDPP)—80%]*—early but otherwise normal activation of hypothalamic-pituitary-gonadal function (always isosexual) or due to pathology of central origin.
- *Peripheral or GnRH-independent precocious puberty (GIPP)*—excess peripheral secretion of sex steroids—any estrogen secreting tumor.
- *Incomplete*—premature thelarche, adrenarche and menarche.
- It may be isosexual (excess estrogen) or heterosexual (excess production of androgen).

Etiologies of Central Precocious Puberty (GnRH-dependent)

- Constitutional: 80–90% are idiopathic **(Fig. 1)**—most common
- Central nervous system (CNS) tumors:
  - Hamartomas of the tuber cinereum (hypothalamus) **(Fig. 2)** can present as *gelastic* (laughing) seizures with precocious puberty.
  - Gonadotropin-secreting tumor astrocytomas

CHAPTER 15: A Case of Precocious Puberty (Pediatrics and Adolescent Gynecological Problem)

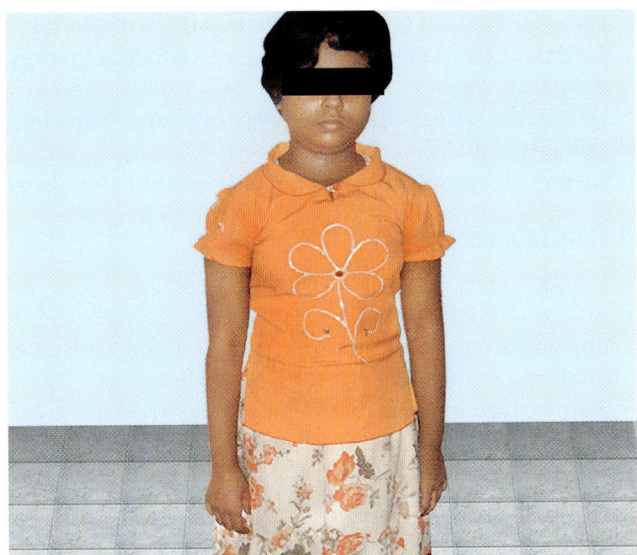

Fig. 1: Idiopathic precocious puberty in a 8 years 9 months girl, menarche at 7 years 6 months age, secondary sexual character developed 6 months before menarche, on examination (O/E) no other abnormality, USG abdomen and MRI brain normal.

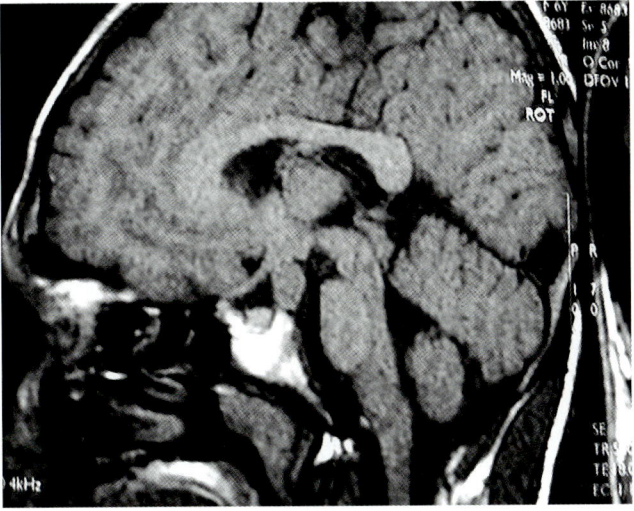

Fig. 2: MRI showing hypothalamic hamartoma—the girl presented with laughing seizure and precocious puberty.

- Ependymomas, pineal tumors, optic gliomas [neurofibromatosis 1 (NF1)], hypothalamic gliomas
❖ Acquired CNS injury: Inflammation, surgery, trauma, radiation therapy, abscess
❖ Congenital anomalies: Hydrocephalus, arachnoid cysts, suprasellar cysts, midline defects
❖ Autoimmune hypothyroidism
❖ Genetic causes (*GPR54 and KiSS-1* mutations)
❖ Sexual abuse

Diagnosis of Central Precocious Puberty

GnRH stimulation positive, and LH less than FSH (*see* below).

Problems of Central Precocious Puberty

❖ Psychosocial stress
❖ Short stature: Paradox of short adult stature despite being tall childhood stature
❖ Taller in lower class, shorter in upper class
❖ Increase in sex steroids causes increase in height velocity and rate of skeletal maturation, leading to premature epiphyseal fusion.

Etiologies of GnRH and Gonadotropin-independent Precocious Puberty

❖ Autoimmune functional ovarian cysts are the most common cause gonadotropin independent precocious puberty
❖ Sex steroid-secreting tumor (adrenal, ovarian)
❖ McCune-Albright syndrome
❖ Liver—hepatoblastoma
❖ Congenital adrenal hyperplasia (CAH)
❖ Cushing's disease
❖ Exogenous estrogen administration
❖ Aromatase excess syndrome
❖ Severe primary hypothyroidism (Van Wyk and Grumbach syndrome) (*see* later)

Problems of Gonadotropin-independent Precocious Puberty

❖ Psychosocial stress
❖ Short adult stature
❖ Also depend on etiologies.

McCune-Albright Syndrome

❖ Sexual precocity
❖ Multiple cystic bone lesions (polyostotic fibrous dysplasia)
❖ Large café-au-lait spots on skin (coast of Maine)
❖ Genetic mutation of G-protein alpha (α) subunit
❖ Early and excessive production of estrogen from ovaries due to spontaneous activation gonadotropin receptors
❖ Diagnosis is done by skin biopsy to identify genetic mutation
❖ Treatment includes medical and orthopedic management [aromatase inhibitor or estrogen receptor blocker (fulvestrant)].

Premature Thelarche (Fig. 2A)

❖ Isolated breast development in girls before 8 years usually between 2 years and 4 years of age. One or both may be enlarged.
❖ Breast tissue increases minimally over time, can even decrease.
❖ Elevated FSH not LH.
❖ Bone age is not advanced.
❖ Nipple development is absent.
❖ No treatment is needed.

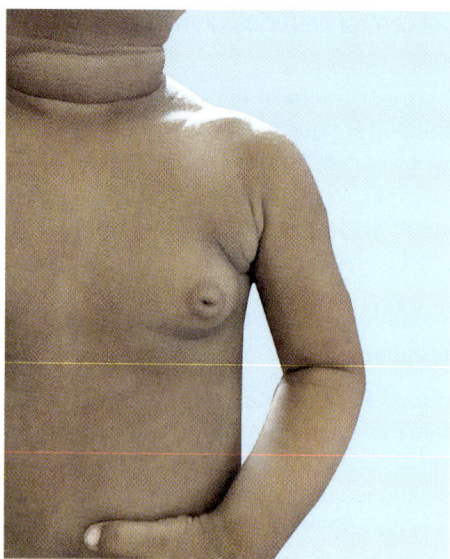

Fig. 2A: Premature thelarche in a 2 years old girl.
Courtesy: Dr Md Obaidullah Chisty

Premature Adrenarche (Pubarche)

- Isolated pubic hair development, usually less than 7–8 years old.
- Due to increase in secretion of androgens by adrenal glands earlier than normal.
- Risk factor for polycystic ovary syndrome (PCOS).
- To exclude late-onset CAH and androgen-secreting tumor.
- Androgen receptor blocker like cyproterone acetate (CA), finasteride or flutamide may be used.

Significance of Incomplete Precocious Puberty

- Normal bone age
- Normal growth rate
- Requires close monitoring up to 20% of girls with premature thelarche or adrenarche will develop central precocious puberty (CPP).

EVALUATION OF A CASE OF PRECOCIOUS PUBERTY

Q. When should be evaluated a precocious puberty?

- Children presenting with signs of secondary sexual development less than 8 years.
- Any time when pathologic cause of precocious puberty is suspected.

Q. How to approach in a case of precocious puberty?

- History
- Physical examination
- Investigations.

History

- Age of onset of pubertal changes with sequences
- Age of pubertal changes of parents, family history of any genetic disorder

- Evidence of linear growth acceleration (growth charts)
- CNS risk factors: Infections, surgery, radiation therapy, neoplasm, trauma
- Headaches, visual changes, history of seizures, laughing seizures
- History of exposure to exogenous estrogens or androgens.

Physical Examination

- Height, weight and height velocity (cm/year)
- Abnormal vital signs
- Funduscopic examination (papilledema indicates increased intracranial pressure), visual fields
- Tanner staging/genital examination
- Androgen effects: Clitoromegaly
- Skin examination:
  - McCune-Albright: *Large café-au-lait spots with irregular borders (coast of Maine)*
  - Androgen effects: Acne, hirsutism, pigmentation.

Abdominal Examination

Any lump—estrogen-producing tumor (granulosa cell, theca cell tumor) **(Fig. 3)**.

Investigations

Purpose

- To exclude the severe disease
- To determine whether pituitary inhibition is needed.

Components

- Sonography of pelvis and whole abdomen for ovary, uterus and adrenal
- X-ray left hand and wrist to determine bone age **(Figs. 4 and 5)**
- Idiopathic CPP is a diagnosis of exclusion.

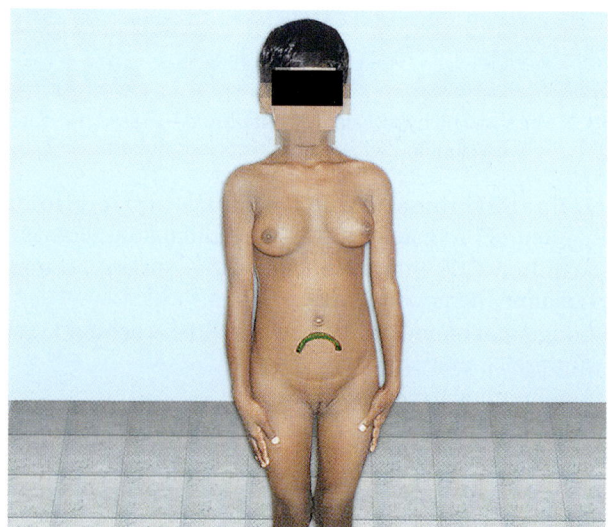

Fig. 3: Granulosa cell tumor of ovary with precocious puberty 8 years 3 months, menarche at 7 years 5 months age, breast development at 7 years age, breasts adult size, pubic hair—scanty on examination lump lower abdomen—18-week size, USG—ovarian swelling.

Further Investigations

- Brain imaging: MRI (hypothalamic hematoma, *see* **Fig. 2**)
- Serum FSH, LH, testosterone, estradiol, thyroid profile, 17-hydroxyprogesterone, DHEA, hCG
- Abdominal CT or MRI (adrenal and ovarian pathology). Initial hormones to be estimated are FSH, LH and thyroid profile.
- GnRH stimulation test to differentiate premature thelarche from true central and peripheral precocious puberty.
- Bone age (**Figs. 4 and 5**):
  - All patients with advanced pubertal changes should have a bone age done
  - If normal, unlikely to have CPP
  - If advanced, requires further evaluation
  - Determined by Galstaun's chart (**Figs. 4 and 5**).

  If bone age more than chronological age, determine the cause of precocious puberty.
- Measure basal LH level
- LH levels following administration of GnRH analog (GnRH stimulation test) (**Table 1**).

Table 1: Basal LH level and GnRH stimulation test.

	Gonadotropin-dependent precocious puberty (GDPP)	Gonadotropin-independent precocious puberty (GIPP)
Basal LH	Pubertal level	Low
GnRH stimulation test	LH↑	LH↓

Treatment

- Definitive therapy in specific causes, e.g., resection in brain tumor other than hamartoma, radiation therapy in other cases.
- Surgery in adrenal and ovarian tumor. Features of precocity regress after surgery (**Figs. 6 to 10**).

Idiopathic group—inhibition of puberty, to prevent reduction of final height.

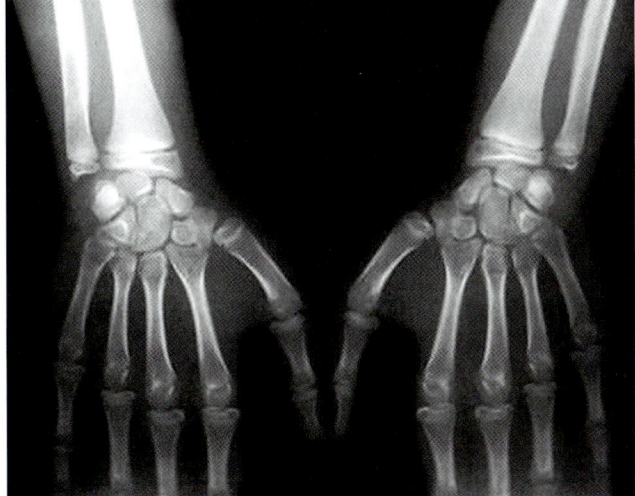

Fig. 4: Bone age determination: 10–12 years (actual age 8 years 9 months)—X-ray wrist as patient Figure 1.

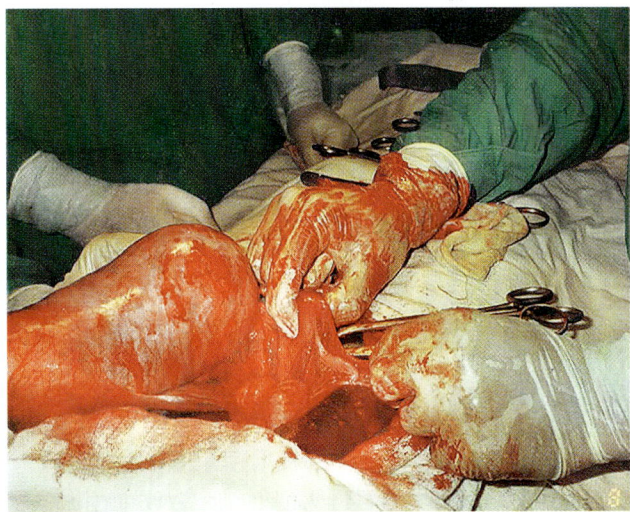

Fig. 6: Laparotomy—left-sided granulosa cell tumor of ovary as patient in Figure 3.

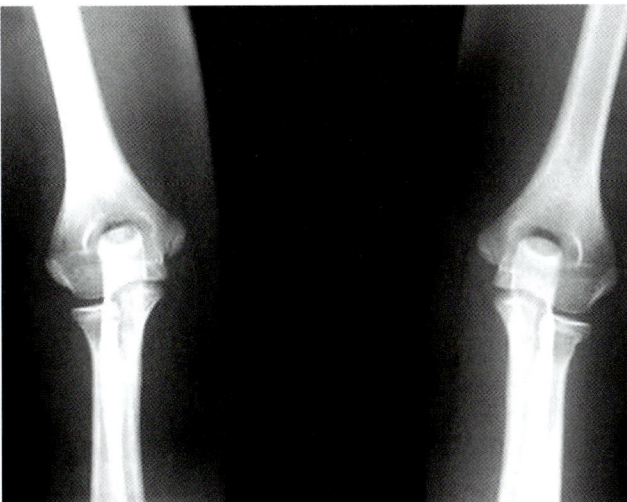

Fig. 5: Bone age determination: 10–12 years (actual age 8 years 9 months)—X-ray elbow.

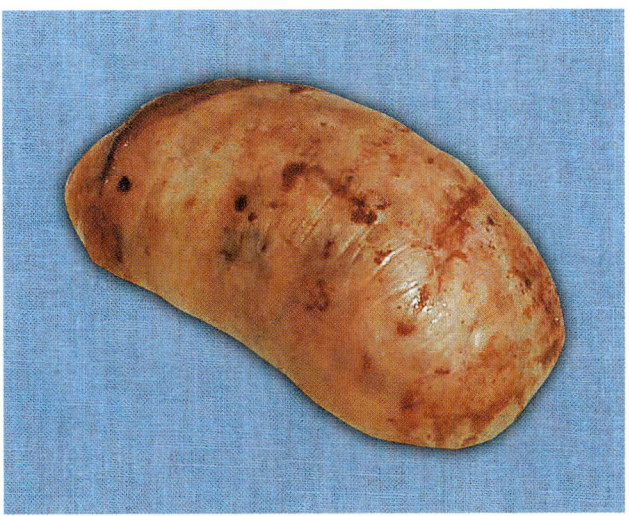

Fig. 7: Ovarian cystectomy specimen as in Figure 6.

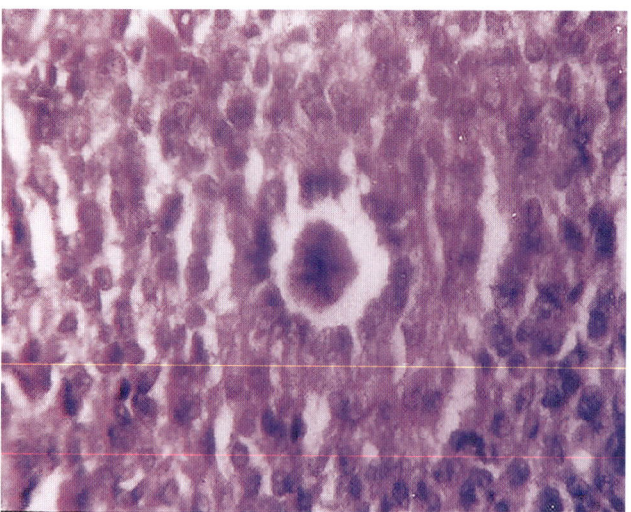

Fig. 8: HP showing granulosa cell tumor of specimen in Figure 7.

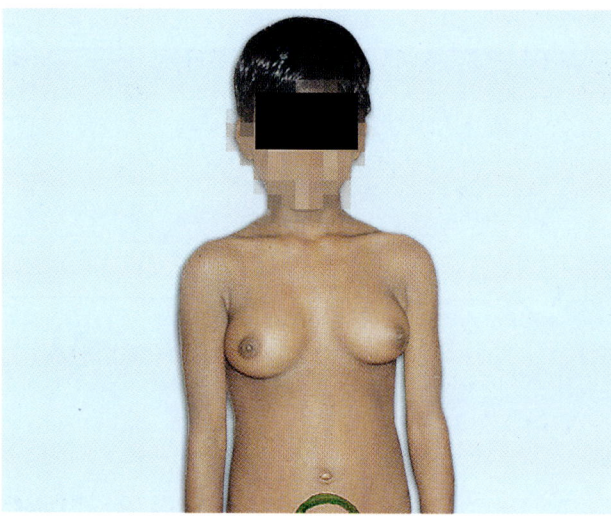

Fig. 9: Before surgery as patient in Figure 3—well-developed breasts and lower abdominal lump.

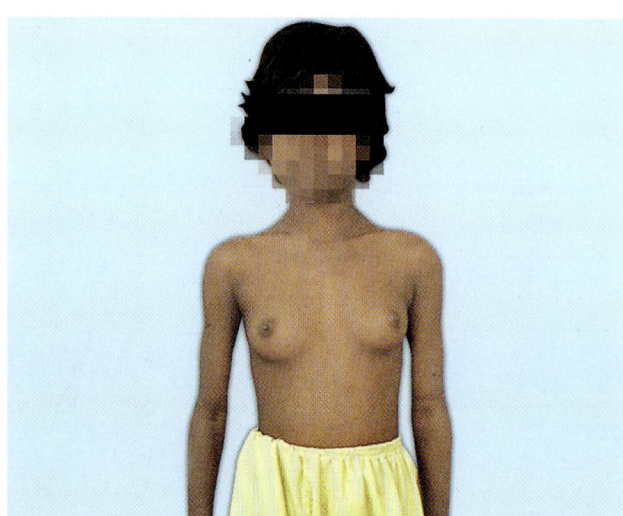

Fig. 10: Six months after surgery breasts regress, menstruation ceases in the same girl as in Figure 9.

Aims of Treatment
- Arrest of fusion of epiphysis to prevent reduction of final height
- To avoid emotional and psychological problems due to precocious development
- Reversion and prevention of further progression toward puberty.

Treatment Regimen
- Pituitary inhibition by GnRH: 1-month preparation, 3-month preparation
- Most commonly used preparation is leuprolide acetate (Lupron Depot-Ped), in a dose of 0.25–0.3 mg/kg (minimum, 7.5 mg) IM, once every 4 weeks
- Other preparations are D-Trp6-GnRH (Decapeptyl) and goserelin acetate (Zoladex).

Other route—nasal spray, subdermal histrelin implant GnRH-a (analog).

Inhibition of Pituitary by GnRH-a Therapy
- Suppress HP axis, reduces sex steroid level
- Criteria: Bone age must be 1 year difference
- Helps to gain the final height
- After the age of 8 years, beneficial effect is less. Best outcome to start below 6 years
- Duration of therapy: Usually up to 11 years of age
- Pubertal changes resume 3–12 months after stoppage of GnRH therapy.

Efficacy is assessed by:
- Clinically: 3–6 months
- Radiologically: 6–12 months
- LH and estradiol levels: 1–2 months after starting treatment or with dose adjustments.

Incomplete precocious puberty: No treatment is needed; however, close follow-up is done.

Van Wyk and Grumbach syndrome—Primary Hypothyroidism (Figs.10A and B)

Longstanding primary hypothyroidism is associated with sexual precocity. Presenting feature—is premature breast development or isolated vaginal bleeding. Galactorrhea may be present if prolactin is high. Solitary or multiple ovarian cysts may be found in USG. It is the only cause of precocious puberty that is associated with a delayed bone age. Van Wyk and Grumbach first described this syndrome, called Van Wyk and Grumbach syndrome characterized by precocious breast development, uterine bleeding and multicystic ovaries in the presence of longstanding primary hypothyroidism. Thyroxin makes normal within a few months.

ONSET OF PUBERTY

Q. How does the onset of puberty occur?
- It starts with activation of the hypothalamic-pituitary axis (between 8 years and 13.5 years of age).

CHAPTER 15: A Case of Precocious Puberty (Pediatrics and Adolescent Gynecological Problem)

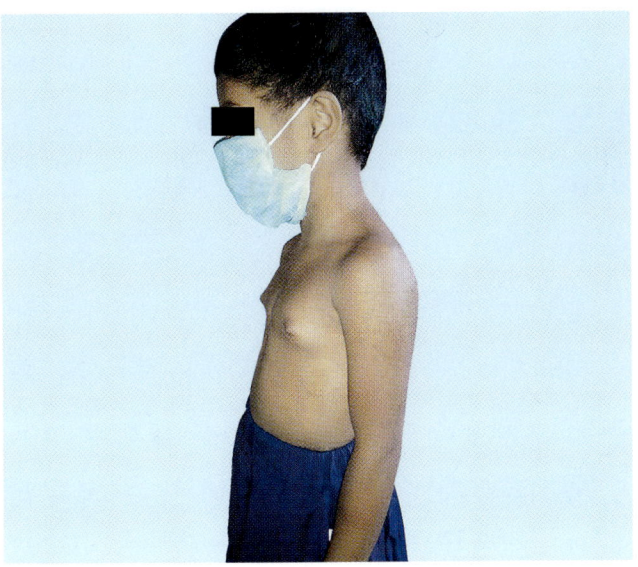

Fig. 10A: A six years girl was admitted with intermittent bleeding PV and growth of breasts for last 4–5 months. Diagnosis was made as severe primary hypothyroidism with Van Wyk and Grumbach syndrome. She was started thyroxin therapy.

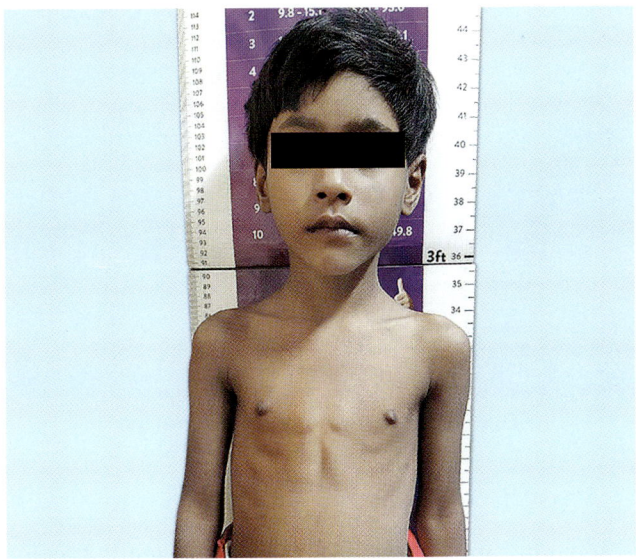

Fig. 10B: On follow up after 6 months as the girl in Figure 10A. She was found to have regression of breasts size and cessation of vaginal bleeding after treatment with thyroxin.

- The primary triggering mechanism is still hypothetical.
- Increased kisspeptin secretion from the arcuate nucleus and the anteroventral paraventricular nucleus of the hypo-thalamus triggers GnRH secretion.
- Activation of hypothalamus results sex steroids and growth hormone production, increase thyroid activity, increase adrenal activity and increase of insulin and insulin-like growth factor.

Endocrine changes during puberty can be shown in **Flowchart 1**.

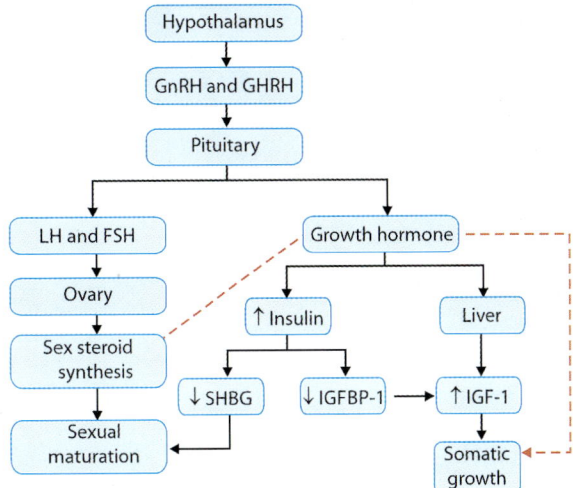

Flowchart 1: Endocrine changes during puberty.

Abbreviations: GnRH, gonadotropin-releasing hormone; GHRH, growth hormone releasing hormone; IGF-1, insulin like growth factor-1; IGFBP-1, insulin like growth factor binding protein-1

Q. Which factors determine the onset of puberty?

- Genetic
- Environment
- Socioeconomic condition/race
- Psychological state
- Nutrition
- Body weight
- Exercise
- Exposure to light.

Sequence of Pubertal Development Tanner Staging—Breasts and Tanner Staging—Pubic Hair

See Chapter 13 "Primary Amenorrhea" (**Figs. 19A and 19B**, Page 318)

PEDIATRIC AND ADOLESCENT GYNECOLOGY (PAG)

Q. Magnitude of problems—why should be addressed?

- 1.2 billion adolescents 10–19 years worldwide—18% of world population
- 88% resides developing country
- In India, it is 243 million largest, followed by China 207 million.

COMMON GYNECOLOGICAL PROBLEMS IN PEDIATRIC AND ADOLESCENT GROUP

Common gynecological problems in pediatric and adolescent group can be categorized into:

- Common gynecological problems
- Disorder of sexual development (DSD)
- Precocious puberty.

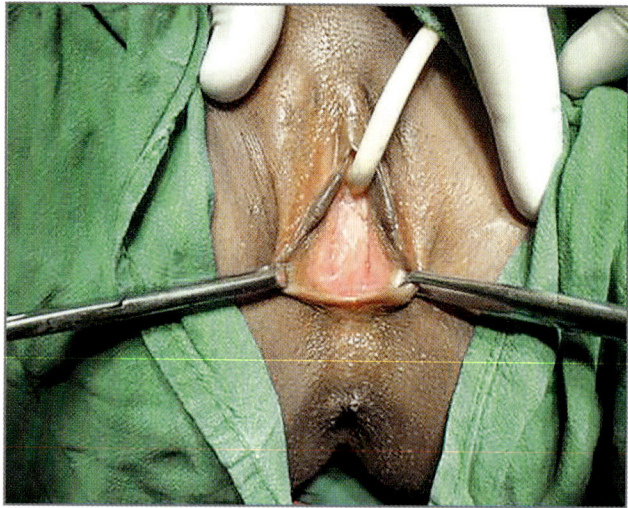

Fig. 11: Transverse vaginal septum lower third.

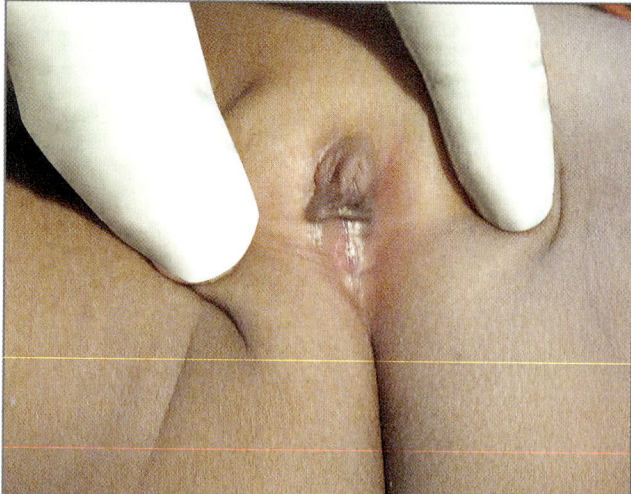

Fig. 12: Labial adhesion in 1-year child—*see* the midline raphe—fusion of labia.

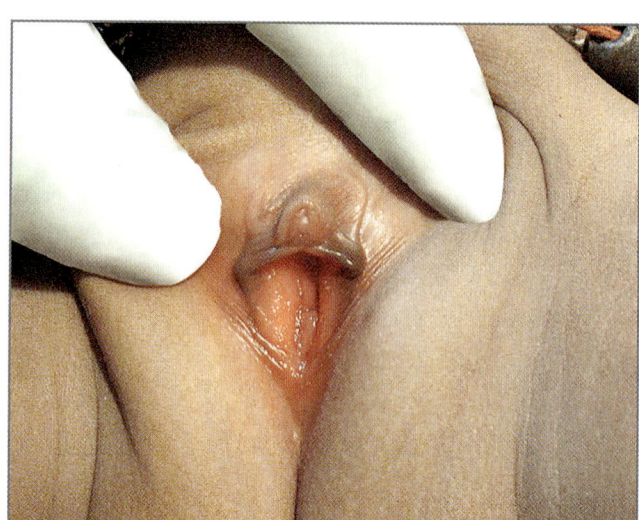

Fig. 13: After separation of adhesion in the same child as in Figure 12.

Common Problems in Pediatric Gynecology

- Vulvovaginitis
- Labial adhesion
- Vaginal bleeding
- Lichen sclerosus.

Gynecological Problems in Adolescent

- Menstrual disorders—menorrhagia, cramps, mood disturbance
- Abnormal uterine bleeding (AUB)—menorrhagia—anovular, coagulation disorder—Von Willebrand's disease
- Pelvic pain—endometriosis
- Dysmenorrhea—primary, secondary (endometriosis)
- Polycystic ovary syndrome
- Müllerian anomaly—pelvic mass, primary amenorrhea, pain, cryptomenorrhea due to imperforate hymen, transverse vaginal septum **(Fig. 11)** and cervical agenesis
- Others—ovarian neoplasm and other gynecological malignancies.

LABIAL ADHESION (FIGS. 12 AND 13)

- Labial adhesion also called labial agglutination is found 1–5% of prepubertal girls, 10% in infants in first year of life.
- Hypoestrogenism is said to be the cause. Erosion of vulva, association of lichen sclerosus, vulvar infection and trauma may be the factors.
- Diagnosis: Labia minora are fused which is identified by a midline raphe **(Fig. 12)**.
- Usually spontaneous resolution occurs at puberty with increase of estrogen level.
- Sometimes, extensive adhesion may cause pinhole meatus between labia anteriorly causing micturition problem and urinary tract infection which needs active treatment.
- Estrogen cream is applied for 2 weeks. Application of estrogen cream daily with gentle gradual traction separates the adhesion. Alternatively, gentle traction with the tip of mosquito forceps introduced anteriorly behind the fused membrane keeping the urethra in safe position separates the fused raphe **(Fig. 13)** using lignocaine ointment. Before doing that one must be sure that it is not the imperforate hymen of atresia vagina.
- Introitoplasty, midline division using electrosurgical fine tip may seldom needed in extensive adhesion cases.
- As recurrence is common routine application of ointment (vitamin A and D) or petroleum jelly to be applied nightly at least for 6 months.

VULVOVAGINITIS

Most common gynecological problem in prepubertal girl.

Symptoms

Itching, discharge, redness, bad smell.

Cause

- Nonspecific—75%; specific—25%.
- Specific: Bacterial—group a beta-hemolytic streptococcus, enteric—*Shigella*, *Yersinia*, Sex abuse—*Neisseria gonorrhoeae*, *Chlamydia*, *Trichomonas vaginalis*
- Exclude foreign bodies in vagina.
- Only vulvitis—allergic and contact dermatitis, lichen sclerosus, infective—group A β-streptococcus, pinworm (scotch tape test), candidiasis (rarely).

Diagnosis

Symptoms, physical findings, vaginoscope, detection of organism, culture.

Q. Why vulvovaginitis is more common in this age group?

- Hygiene—poorly maintained
- Proximity to anal opening
- Soiling after passage of stool
- Chemical irritants—soap, shampoo, bubble baths, bleach, etc.
- Lack of estrogen
- Lack of pad of fat and hair
- Foreign body in vagina
- Coexistent eczema
- Malnutrition, less immunity
- Abuse of sex.

Treatment of Vulvovaginitis

- Care of hygiene, topical cream, lotion, soothing ointment
- Local itching, inflammation—low dose corticosteroid
- Secondary infection—oral antibiotic—amoxicillin-clavulanic—1 week
- Anthelmintic.

VAGINAL BLEEDING IN PREPUBERTAL GIRL

Causes of Vaginal Bleeding

- Maternal estrogen withdrawal in newborn
- Bacterial vulvovaginitis
- Lichen sclerosus
- *Condyloma acuminata*
- Urethral prolapse
- Foreign body
- Trauma **(Figs. 14 and 14A)**
- Genital tumor: Pathology of upper vagina or cervix, rhabdomyosarcoma
- Precocious puberty
- Hormone intake.

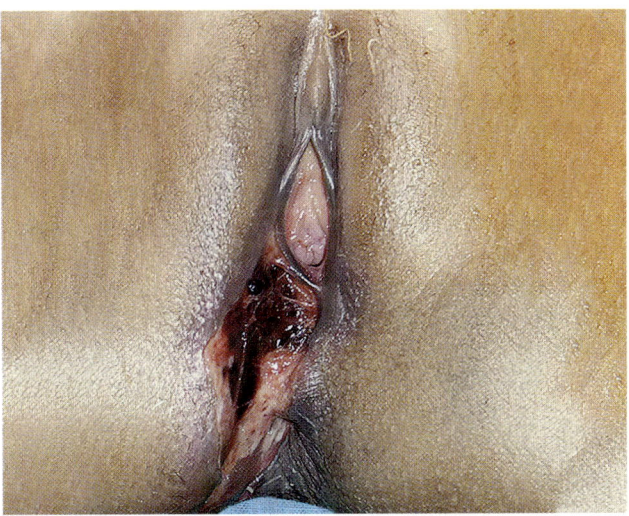

Fig. 14: Vulvar injury following fall on an object in a 7-year girl.
Courtesy: Dr Monimala Murmu, Assistant Professor

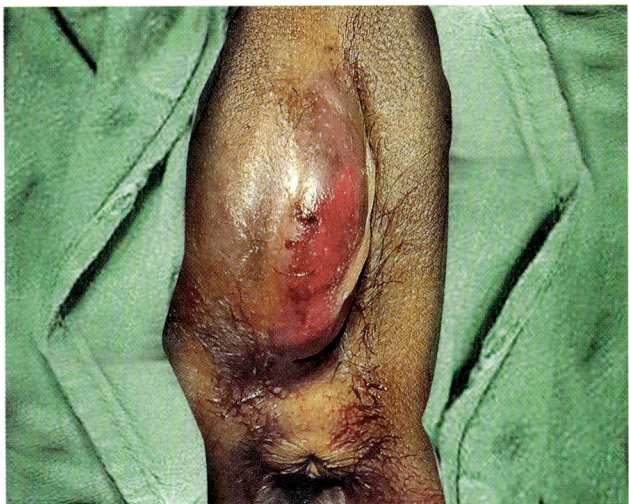

Fig. 14A: Traumatic vulvar hematoma in a 13 years girl due to fall on bed and trauma over edge of bed. Reported after 12 hours. Incision, drainage and repair done.

Diagnosis

Simple history, examination, examination under anesthesia (EUA) and saline vaginoscopy in few cases.

Treatment

According to the cause.

OVARIAN NEOPLASMS IN ADOLESCENTS AND CHILDREN (FIGS. 15 AND 16)

- Ovarian malignancy is the most common genital tract malignancy in adolescents.
- Adolescents make up only 6% of women with ovarian neoplasms.
- Ovarian tumors constitute 1–1.6% of all neoplasia in children and adolescents.

Types of Ovarian Neoplasms in Adolescents and Children

- Germ cell: (1) teratoma—benign, immature, (2) dysgerminoma, (3) endodermal sinus tumor (yolk sac tumor), (4) embryonal carcinoma, (5) choriocarcinoma, (6) gonadoblastoma, (7) mixed germ cell tumor. Germ cell tumor is common in adolescent and childhood.
- Epithelial: Serous and mucinous cystadenoma, serous and mucinous cystadenocarcinoma
- Sex-cord stromal: Granulosa-theca cell tumor, Sertoli-Leydig cell tumor, fibroma/thecoma.

Diagnostic Difficulties

- Ovarian neoplasm is not a common disease in this age group.
- Mostly asymptomatic in earlier cases.
- Vague abdominal discomfort or pain which is early symptom is frequent complaint of school going children.

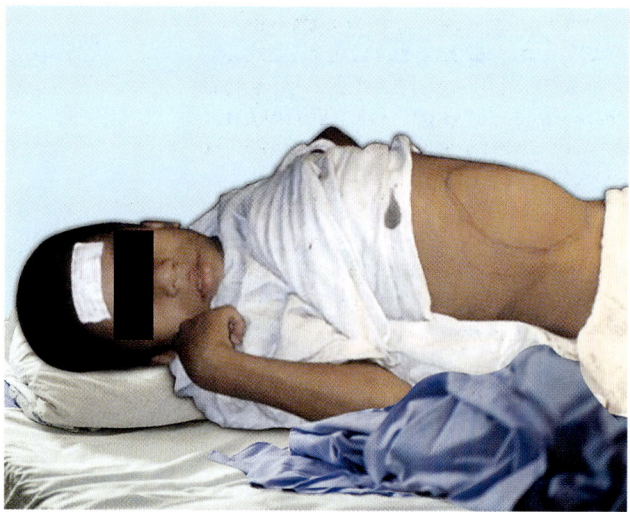

Fig. 15: A 7-year girl with swelling abdomen—mixed germ cell tumor.

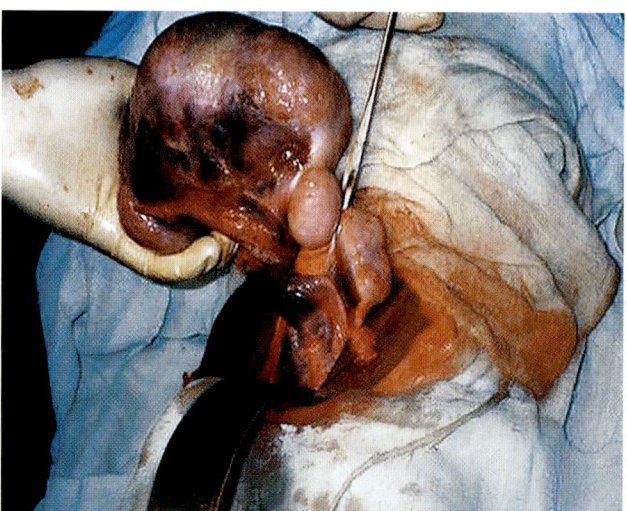

Fig. 16: Mixed germ cell tumor (bilateral) in a 7-year girl as shown in Figure 15.

Diagnosis is done in the line of approach as ovarian tumors in adult.

Management of Ovarian Tumors

Principles of Management

- During surgery conservation of reproductive structures should be a major goal of surgical therapy.
- When faced in doubt, re-exploration may be better option than to do radical approach at the initial surgery.
- Follow-up and psychological support are very important in every case.

Surgery of Ovarian Tumor in Children

- Cystectomy: Benign cysts where possible
- Unilateral oophorectomy with or without salpingectomy:
  - Benign cases with torsion and infections
  - Stage IA cases.
- Cytoreductive surgery with omentectomy in advanced cases
- Laparoscopic surgery: Cosmetic value, not practiced in malignancy.

ENDOMETRIOSIS IN ADOLESCENT

- Endometriosis is challenging to gynecology in this age group.
- Endometriosis is a possible etiology in many adolescents presenting with a complaint of chronic pelvic pain. The incidence of endometriosis among adolescents with pelvic pain is estimated to be 25–38%.
- While in adolescents with refractory to medical treatment for pelvic pain, endometriosis is found in 67% of cases at laparoscopy.
- Endometriosis has been described in premenarchal girls, and has also been documented to occur within 1 month of menarche.
- Endometriosis, when diagnosed in the adolescent versus an adult patient, is more likely to be associated with a Müllerian anomaly.

Management

- The treatment for adolescents has been adapted from adult cases of endometriosis.
- The goal of therapy is to treat the pain, cease progression of the disease and preserve fertility.
- Medical management is the initial approach in the adolescent patient.
- Surgical therapy should be reserved for the patient with persistent pain despite medical treatment.

DISORDER OF SEXUAL DIFFERENTIATION (DSD)

Presentation

At birth with ambiguous genitalia. In adolescent with atypical pubertal development.

Diagnosis

History, physical examination, karyotyping, serum testosterone, androstenedione, dihydrotestosterone (DHT).

Management of DSD

Always multidisciplinary approach.

Important issues are:
- Sex of rearing
- Disclosure
- Treatment.

Medical—steroid, hormone therapy. *Surgery*—clitorial surgery, neovagina, gonadectomy. *The details of DSD are described in Chapter 13.*

ADOLESCENT POLYCYSTIC OVARY SYNDROME

- Diagnosis is in the same line as adult PCOS.
- However as there is sometimes very difficult to differentiate the normal changes in adolescent from the diagnostic criteria of PCOS, some authorities consider all three Rotterdam criteria instead of two to diagnose PCOS.
- Careful follow-up is needed in incomplete criteria as PCOS may be diagnosed in late.

Diagnostic Difficulties

Difficulties of diagnosis of PCOS in this age group are due to:
- Normally there is irregular menses for first 2–4 years of menarche.
- Acne is a common feature in this age group.
- Instead of transvaginal route, ovarian morphology is diagnosed by transabdominally which is not accurate.
- Some authorities consider all three Rotterdan criteria instead of two to diagnose PCOS in this age group (*see* Chapter 12, Polycystic Ovarian Syndrome).

Management of Adolescent Polycystic Ovary Syndrome

Aim
- Regularization of menstrual cycle
- To reduce androgen excess
- Management of physical features of hyperandrogenism, e.g., hirsutism, acne and acanthosis.

Treatment Options
- To reduce body weight—lifestyle management, diet modification and exercises.
- Combined oral contraceptive (COC) with less androgenic progestin like norgestimate, desogestrel or drospirenone. If amenorrhea withdrawal bleeding with MPA for 10 days prior to COC.
- Insulin sensitizing agents—metformin 1,000–1,500 mg daily.
- Treatment of hirsutism—COC/ethinyl estradiol (EE) + CA, antiandrogen, androgen blocking drugs, cosmetic—temporary and permanent hair removal.

Management of Müllerian Anomaly Presenting in Adolescent

- Primary amenorrhea
- Cryptomenorrhea due to imperforate hymen, vaginal septum.

Described in Chapter of Müllerian Anomaly (Chapter 21).

PREVENTIVE GYNECOLOGY IN PEDIATRICS AND ADOLESCENT

Human papilloma virus (HPV) vaccination
- Girls aged 11 years onwards.
- Other than bivalent and quadrivalent now nonvaccine is available.

CHAPTER 16

A Case of Endometriosis Adenomyosis

CHAPTER OUTLINE

Writing a case of endometriosis and how to present the case?

- Diagnosis and Differential Diagnosis
- Etiopathogenesis
- Sites and Types of Endometriosis
- Classification
- Treatment Modalities
- Endometriosis and Infertility—Approach
- Adenomyosis—Diagnosis and Management
- Differentiation from Fibroid
- Adenomyosis—Past and Present
- Adenomyosis and Infertility
- Dysmenorrhea
- Chronic pelvic pain

PATIENT'S PARTICULARS

1. Name: Mrs XY
2. Age: 33-year-old
3. Address:
4. Occupation: Housewife
5. Married/unmarried: Married
6. History of infertility: There may be history of infertility
7. Husband's occupation:
8. Socioeconomic status: Middle-class or upper-class
9. Religion: Hindu
10. Parous/nulliparous: Parous, last child birth 7 years back

Bed No.:
Date of admission:
Date of examination:

HISTORY

- *Chief complaint/complaints*: Severe cyclical pain in lower abdomen for last 2 years mostly during menstruation admitted for laparoscopy.

- *History of present illness*: Patient states that she has been suffering from pain in lower abdomen during menstrual period for last 2 years; pain starts few days before mens and continued throughout the period. Initially pain was less and she was relieved by analgesics, later it has become more and more severe and now sometimes not relieved by analgesics completely even after hormonal treatment. Amount of bleeding during period is also heavy during last 2 years. She had also severe backache during period and deep pain during intercourse. (Elaborate if any other complaint). She has been admitted for laparoscopy.

- *Menstrual history*:
  - Last menstrual period (LMP): Write as it is
  - Duration of menstruation: 5–7 days
  - Interval in days: 28 ± 2
  - Age of menarche:
  - Regularity of cycle: Regular
  - Pain during period: Pain starts few days before period and persists throughout menses, sometimes after period
  - Amount of bleeding: More than average
  - Clot: Present
  - Intermenstrual bleeding: No

- *Obstetric history*:
  - Parity: Parous
  - Living issue (LI): 2
  - Last child birth: 7 years back

Serial no.	Year and month	Pregnancy events	Labor events	Mode of delivery	Puerperium or postabortal period	Baby

- *Past history*: Nothing significant
  - Medical:
  - Surgical:
- *Family history*: There may be history of endometriosis in family
- *Sexual history*: Deep dyspareunia
- *Functional history*:
  - Bowel: Constipation or irritable bowel syndrome. Hematuria, rectal bleeding in bladder, and rectal endometriosis very rarely.
  - Bladder
  - Sleep
  - Appetite
- *Personal history*:
  - Personal hygiene
  - Smoking or alcohol
- *Contraceptive history*: Barrier or any other
- *Drug history*:
  - History of any drug allergy
  - History of intake of corticosteroids, antiepileptic or other drugs (previous or present)
  - *Treatment history in detail*: Medical or surgical—analgesics, hormones, etc.

PHYSICAL EXAMINATION

Patient—alert, conscious, and cooperative, look anxious due to long standing pain abdomen.

- Build
- Nutrition
- Height
- Weight/body mass index (BMI)
- Edema
- Anemia: May be present due to menorrhagia
- Cyanosis
- Jaundice
- Clubbing
- Tongue, teeth, gum, and tonsil
- Neck veins
- Neck glands
- Leg veins
- Pulse:
- Respiration
- Temperature
- Blood pressure.

Systemic Examination

- *Central nervous system*
- *Cardiovascular system*:
  - Auscultation of heart
- *Respiratory system*:
  - Auscultation of chest
- *Gastrointestinal system*:
  - Liver
  - Spleen.
- *Examination of other systems*:
  - Examination of back and spines skeletal system
  - Neurological
  - Ophthalmoscopic examination
  - Urinary system.
- *Examination of breasts and nipple*:
  - Inspection
  - Palpation.

GYNECOLOGICAL EXAMINATION

- *Abdominal examination*:
  - Inspection
  - Palpation: Palpated all nine areas. There may be suprapubic tenderness and/or tenderness on both iliac fossa. Usually no lump is found.
  - Percussion
  - Auscultation.
- *Vaginal examination*:
  - Inspection and palpation of external genitalia: Nothing specific
  - Speculum examination: Rarely "blue domed cyst" in posterior fornix (*see* later)
  - Bimanual examination: Uterus—NS, retroverted (RV), mobility restricted, tenderness on examination. On right and left fornices, adnexae enlarged and tender (due to ovarian endometriosis). In pouch of Douglas (POD) (palpation through posterior fornix), there may be nodules.
  - Examination of RV septum and rectal examination: Nodules in POD, RV septum may be thickened and tender.

INVESTIGATIONS SUPPLIED OR REQUIRED

Complete hemogram, ultrasonography, cancer antigen 125 (CA 125), CT, MRI, and USG showed bilateral ovarian cyst of ____sizes Rt____, Lt____which was suggestive of endometriosis and CA 125 raised with value of _____

SUMMARY OF THE CASE (SAMPLE)

A 33-year-old married woman with two living children coming from middle-class family from rural area of Hooghly district was admitted on with chief complaint of cyclical pain in lower abdomen during menstruation for undergoing laparoscopy. She has been suffering from pain during menstruation for last 2 years, initially severity of pain was less and could be relieved by analgesics but now for last 3 months the pain is severe in nature and not relieved by analgesics completely. The pain started few days before period and persists for throughout the mens. She suffered from severe backache during period. She also complained of deep dyspareunia.

Her LMP was on____. She had dysmenorrhea as described and flow during last 2 years was heavy. She had history of infertility for 2 years following which she conceived spontaneously. She has two children, one 9-year-old girl and another 7-year-old boy both vaginal deliveries. She uses barrier method of contraception and sometimes safe period. She underwent medical treatment with analgesics and hormonal drug and relieved to some extent and following withdrawal of hormone treatment the pain recurred.

On general examination, she has mild pallor, height ____, weight ____, pulse ____, normotensive, no other abnormality on general examination.

Per abdominally there is no abnormality except suprapubic tenderness.

On per vaginal (PV) bimanual examination, uterus—NS, RV, mobility restricted, and tenderness on examination. On right and left fornices, adnexae enlarged and tender. In POD (palpation through posterior fornix), there are tender nodules. Examination of RV septum and rectal examination showed nodules in POD; RV septum is thickened.

Ultrasonography showed bilateral ovarian cyst of ____ sizes Rt ____, Lt ____ which was suggestive of endometriosis and CA 125 raised with value of____.

PROVISIONAL DIAGNOSIS

Pelvic endometriosis in a 33-year-old parous woman.

DIFFERENTIAL DIAGNOSIS

- Chronic pelvic inflammatory disease (PID)
- Adhesions postoperative or pelvic inflammation
- Ovarian cyst—torsion or hemorrhagic cyst
- Ectopic or ruptured corpus luteum—hemoperitoneum
- Large bowel disorder: Inflammatory bowel syndrome, diverticulitis, ulcerative colitis, and obstruction
- Small bowel: Crohn's disease and obstruction
- Musculoskeletal.

Q. What is your case?

Tell the summary.

Q. What is your diagnosis? Tell the provisional diagnosis.

Pelvic endometriosis in a 33-year-old parous woman.

Q. Why are you saying so?

- *Characteristic symptoms*: Progressive cyclical pain in lower abdomen (secondary dysmenorrhea), menorrhagia, backache, and deep dyspareunia.
- *Physical finding*: Bimanual examination finding—as written above
- USG report and laboratory report.

Q. How would you confirm your diagnosis?

The diagnosis would be confirmed by laparoscopy through visual examination.

Q. What treatment you want to provide to your patient after confirmation of diagnosis?

As the symptoms have recurred and progressive even after medical management with hormones patient may be tried with surgical management which can be determined by laparoscopic finding. Considering the age of the patient (33 years) conservative surgery with or without postoperative medical therapy is the treatment option for this patient.

Q. What do you mean by endometriosis?

Endometriosis is defined as the presence of endometrial-like tissue (endometrial glands and stroma) in ectopic location outside the uterine cavity.

Q. What is the incidence of endometriosis?

Endometriosis is one of the most benign gynecological conditions and second to uterine fibroid needing major gynecological surgery.

Incidence is 10% of women of reproductive age, 25–50% among women with chronic pelvic pain (CPP), and 35% of women suffering from infertility.

Q. What are the risk factors of endometriosis?

- Low BMI
- Early menopause
- Nulliparity

Q. Tell few important key points about endometriosis.

- It is one of the most common benign gynecological conditions.
- Distressing pain (in the form of dysmenorrhea) is the common symptom.
- Strongly associated with infertility.
- Deleterious sexual, reproductive and social consequences.
- The basis of medical management is estrogen–progesterone suppression which makes the cycle anovulatory which is not desirable in this group of patient of infertility.
- Recurrence is common and no permanent cure until radical surgery.
- There is no proven efficacy of medical and surgical management of minimal to mild endometriosis.

Sites of Endometriosis

Q. What are the different sites of endometriosis (Fig. 1)?

Pelvis

- Pelvis is the most common site.

CHAPTER 16: A Case of Endometriosis Adenomyosis

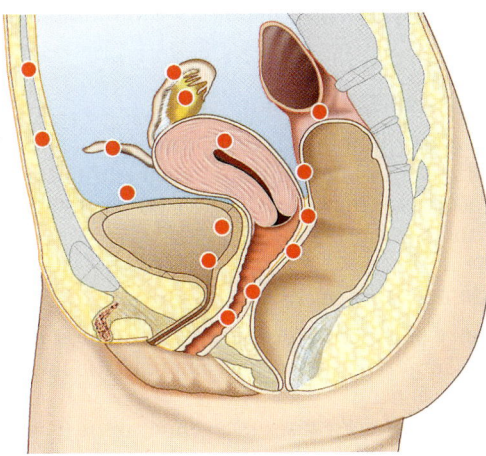

Fig. 1: Various sites of endometriosis.

walls, and the surfaces of the ovaries, tubes and uterus. For confirmation, laparoscopy is required.

Q. What are the types of ovarian endometriosis?

- Superficial: Typical lesion or subtle
- Larger ovarian cyst (endometrioma) **(Fig. 3)**: It is called chocolate cyst due to presence of thick, viscous, dark brown fluid composed of hemosiderin of old blood, resulting from the accumulation of old blood and debris inside ovary during menstruation. Three theories are implicated in pathogenesis of ovarian endometrioma, namely coelomic metaplasia, ovarian cortex implant invagination and transformation of functional cyst by ovarian surface implant.
- Rarely the wall of ovarian endometrioma becomes calcified **(Figs. 4 and 5)**.

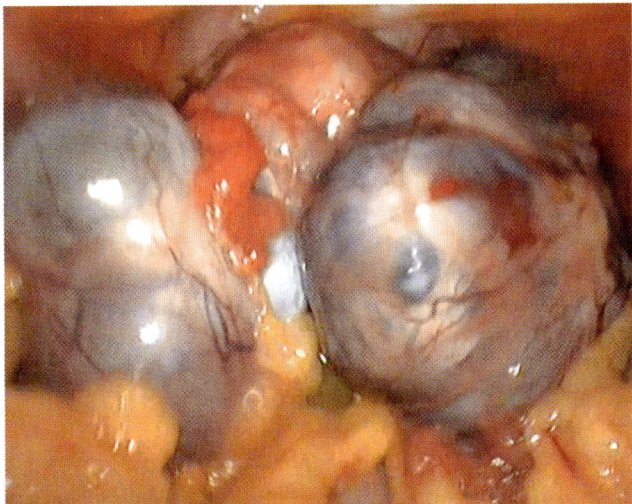

Fig. 2: Bilateral chocolate cyst (each 8 cm × 7 cm)—30 years woman presented with severe dysmenorrhea, heavy menstrual bleeding and infertility size.
Courtesy: Dr Alok De, Associate Professor

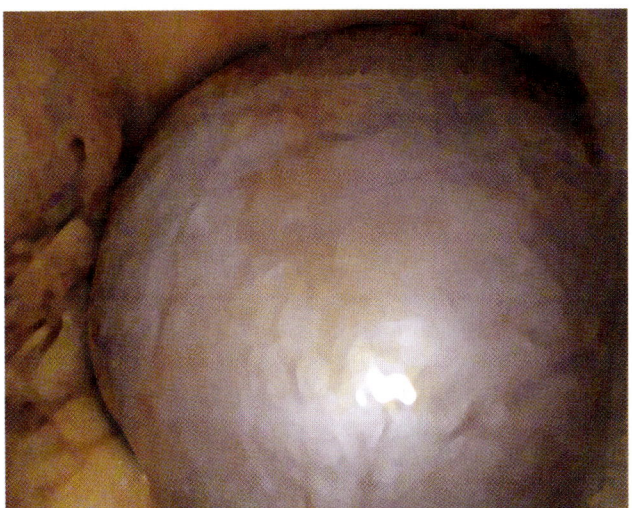

Fig. 3: Huge endometrioma size 14 cm × 12 cm.
Courtesy: Dr Alok De, Associate Professor

- The sites in pelvis are *ovaries* (most common site) **(Fig. 2)**, pouch of Douglas, uterosacral ligament, broad ligament and round ligament, RV septum, fallopian tubes, the back and front of the uterus and vagina.

Extra pelvic sites are:

- Gastrointestinal (GI) tract: Rectosigmoid, appendix, small bowel, and rectum
- Urinary tract: Bladder: ureter: kidney is 40:5:1 ratio
- Diaphragmatic or thoracic and liver.

Other Rare Sites

- Surgical scars, cutaneous nerve—commonly in sciatic nerve, brain, eyes, and umbilicus.
- The only site where extragenital endometriosis has not been reported is spleen.

Q. What do you mean by pelvic endometriosis?

Presence of endometriotic implants involving the peritoneum, anterior and posterior pouch, pelvic side

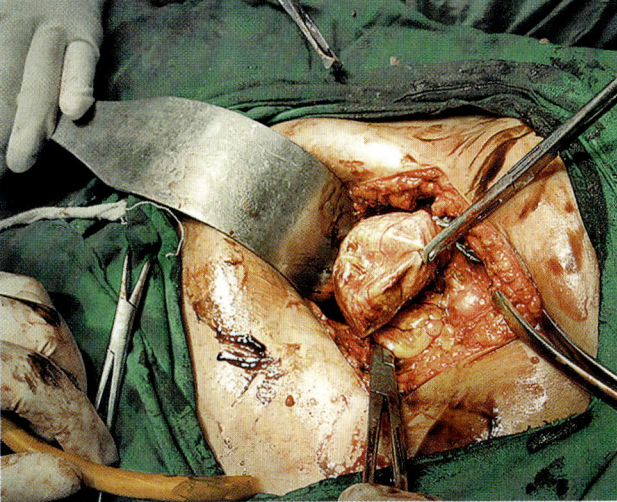

Fig. 4: Chocolate cyst—wall calcified and found radiopaque as found in Figure 10. 42 years primary infertility for 11 years with severe dysmenorrhea.

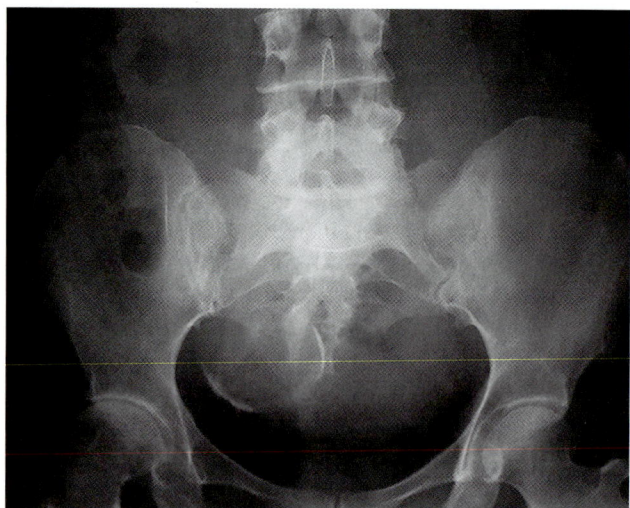

Fig. 5: Calcified chocolate cyst 42 years primary infertility for 11 years with severe dysmenorrhea in the patient as in Figure 4.
Courtesy: Dr Pradipto Sanyal, Senior Gynecologist

Lesions According to Depth

- Superficial peritoneal lesion (*see* Page 364): Types of lesion by laparoscopy.
- Cystic ovarian endometriosis (endometrioma): Chocolate cyst **(Figs. 2 and 3)**.
- Deep infiltrating endometriosis (>5 mm depth): Presence of endometriotic nodule comprising of solid mass of endometrial glands, stroma, adipose tissue, and fibromuscular tissue in between the rectum and vagina.

Deep infiltrating endometriosis (DIE) is of four types— Type I, II, III, and IV **(Fig. 6)**:

- **Type I:** Largest area exposed to peritoneal cavity—looks conical-shaped (infiltration)
- **Type II:** Entrapped nodular tissue infiltrating variety with retraction of bowel over nodule (retraction)
- **Type III:** Otherwise normal pelvis, like adenomyosis less glandular more fibromuscular tissue (adenomyosis externa)
- **Type IV:** Adenomyosis like tissue infiltrating to sigmoid colon.

Endometriosis in the Umbilicus (Fig. 7)

There may be spontaneous development of endometriosis in umbilicus and inguinal canal even without any pelvic endometriosis. The size is increased during mens and painful and appears blue.

Scar Endometriosis (Fig. 8)

Appearance of endometriosis is not uncommon in skin scar following surgery in uterus and fallopian tube without any pelvic endometriosis.

The most common cause of scar endometriosis is following hysterotomy done in midpregnancy especially for MTP. Others are cesarean delivery (more in classical), tubectomy, myomectomy, and following surgery of endometriosis.

Endometriosis in episiotomy scar is also found but rare. In scar endometriosis, the site becomes swollen, painful and appears blue during period and even there may be bleeding rarely from the site **(Fig. 9)**. In long-standing cases, it may spread widely in subcutaneous tissue, even rectus it may extend to sheath and beyond.

Cyclical pain and swelling in scar endometriosis become evident during menstruation. Sonography, CT, MRI and fine needle biopsy are useful for diagnosis and to assess depth of lesion to rectus abdominis and planning of surgery. Wide local excision may be needed **(Fig. 10)**. Occasionally, involved rectus sheath needs removal followed by repair with mesh. Recurrence is not uncommon.

Endometriosis in Vagina, Vulva, and Cervix

Endometriosis is found occasionally in vulva, vagina or over cervix, may be consequence of surgical or obstetric scar.

The most common site of vaginal endometriosis is vaginal fornix which is multiple cyst in indurated areas of vaginal vault called *"blue-domed cysts"* (*see* **Fig. 11**), if ulcerated may be confused with cancer on appearance.

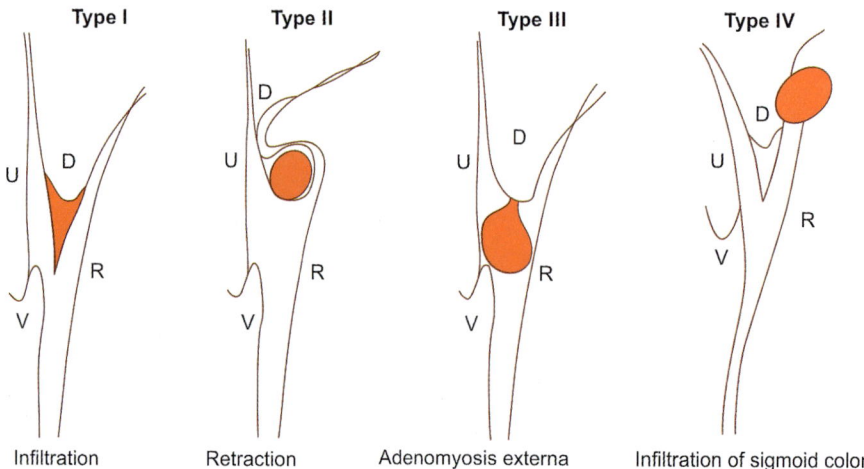

Fig. 6: Four types of deep infiltrating endometriosis—type I, II, III and IV (Koninckx PR, et al.).
Abbreviations: U, uterus; V, vagina; D, pouch of Douglas; R, rectum

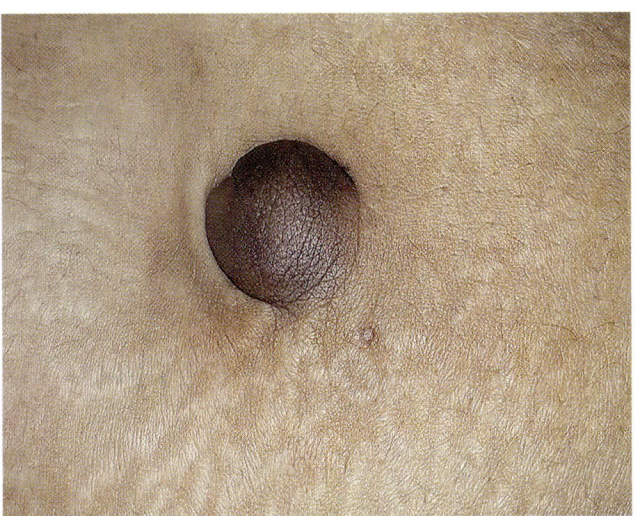

Fig. 7: Umbilical endometriosis.
Courtesy: Professor Sukanta Mishra, VIMS, Kolkata

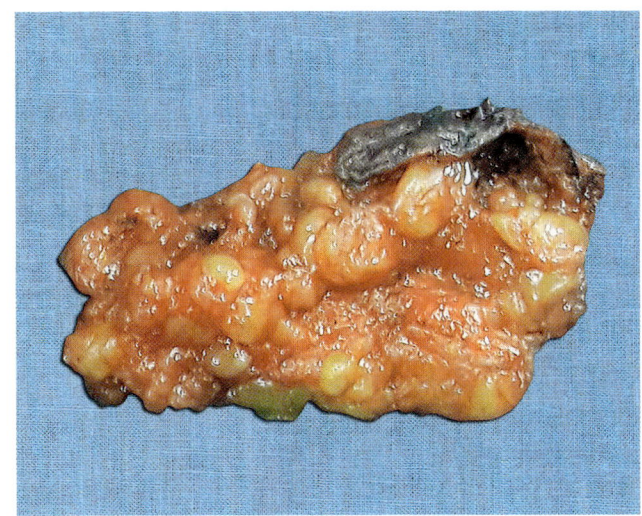

Fig. 10: Scar endometriosis after wide excision.

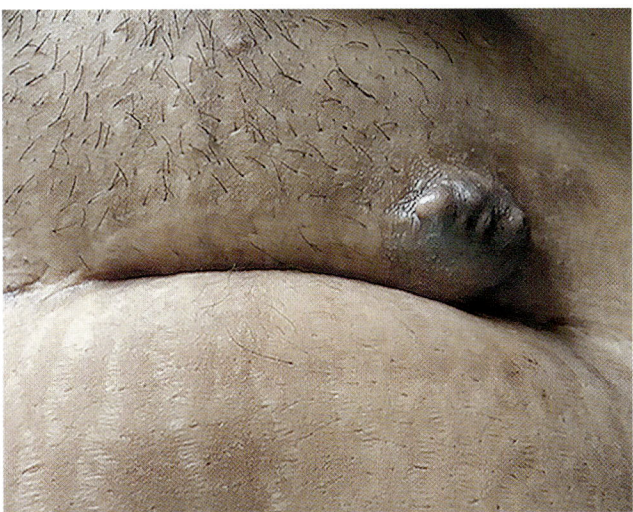

Fig. 8: Scar endometriosis following cesarean section.

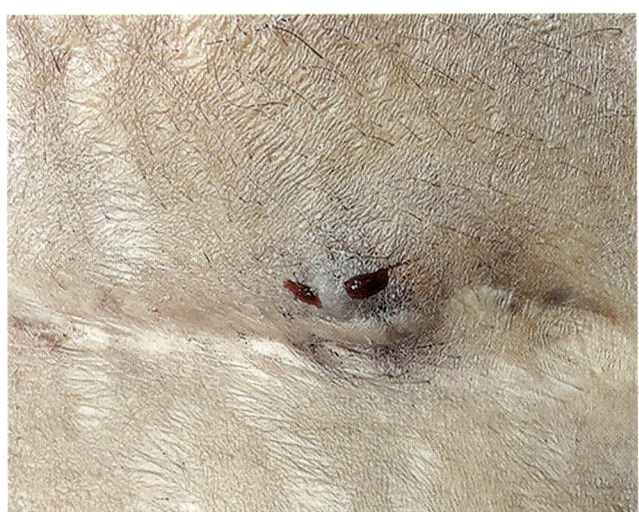

Fig. 9: Bleeding from scar endometriosis during mens.
Courtesy: Dr Anindya Das, Assistant Professor

Etiologies of Endometriosis

Q. What are the etiologies of endometriosis?

The exact etiology is not known. There have been many theories. A single theory cannot explain all endometriosis.

Theories are:

- Retrograde menstruation (Sampson's implantation theory, 1927)
- Lymphatic or vascular spread (Halban's theory, 1925)
- Coelomic metaplasia (Meyer, 1919)—rare occurrence of endometriosis in premenopausal girl is explained by metaplasia theory.
- Induction theory.
- Stem cell theory: Occurrence of endometriosis after TH BSO explains by stem cells. Both progenitor cells of the endometrium and multipotent bone marrow cells contribute to endometrial growth. Spreading of mesenchymal cells of bone marrow explain many extraperitoneal implants.

Other factors are:

- Genetic (familial clustering)—increase incidence in first degree relatives and in some races
- Immunological factors
- Anatomical defects—cervical atresia and hematometra
- Environmental toxins— 2,3,7,8-tetrachlorodibenzodioxin (TCDD)
- Hormonal dependence—intracrinology
- Iatrogenic dissemination—scar endometriosis in hysterotomy, cesarean section, hysterectomy, laparoscopic port, and episiotomy scar.

Pathology

Endometriotic lesions develop from the attachment of endometrial cells to the peritoneal surface, then invasion of these cells into the mesothelium, followed by recruitment of inflammatory cells and angiogenesis around the implant and endometrial cellular proliferation (*see* histology findings, Page 365).

Molecular mechanisms: There is aberration of molecular mechanism in endometriosis from that of eutopic endometrial growth. Formation of endometriosis is favored by estrogen dominance, estrogen dependence and progesterone resistance. Local inflammatory process and angiogenesis are involved in endometriosis. Increase aromatase activity increases estradiol production, by turn augments the production of PGE2. Cellular immunity is altered in endometriosis. Macrophages, natural killer (NK) cells, lymphocytes and numerous cytokines, especially interleukins are implicated in pathogenesis in endometriosis. Levels of vascular endothelial growth factor (VEGF), an angiogenic factor is found in higher amount in peritoneal fluid of women suffering from endometriosis.

Extraovarian production of estrogen as a cause of endometriosis (Zeitoun, et al. 1999)

- The concept is extraovarian production of estrogen from ectopic endometrium.
- Aromatase enzyme has been detected locally in endometriotic implants. An autocrine positive feedback mechanism is established which showed the continuous production of estrogen and prostaglandin E2 in the endometriotic stromal cells which do not depend on ovarian activity for estrogen production.
- This theory explains why even after total abdominal hysterectomy-bilateral salpingo-oophorectomy (TAH-BSO) endometriosis persists or recurs in some cases.
- This also justifies the use of aromatase inhibitor in treatment of endometriosis.

Classification of Endometriosis

Q. How will you classify endometriosis?

Classification system is based on laparoscopic findings.

Appearance varies from a few minimal lesions on otherwise intact pelvic organs → massive ovarian endometriotic cysts that distort tubo-ovarian anatomy → extensive adhesions involving bowel, bladder, and ureter.

American Society of Reproductive Medicine (ASRM) Classification (*see* Fig. 20, Page 370)—Stages

There have been several revisions of classification since 1979 and the current revision is on 1996. There are *four stages* with maximum rAFS (revised American Fertility Society) score of more than 40:

- Stage I (minimal): 1–5
- Stage II (mild): 6–15
- Stage III (moderate): 16–40
- Stage IV (severe): More than 40

Classified according to site, size, depth, number of endometriotic lesion, description of lesion white, red or black, and degree of adhesion of the organs involved—ovary, tube, and peritoneum (*see* Page 370, **Fig. 20**). AFS was renamed as ASRM in1995.

Limitations of ASRM Classification

It does not include retroperitoneal structures and deeply infiltrating endometriosis. Moreover, it is subjective and does not correlate well with clinical symptoms of pain or predict future fertility prospects following surgery, and it is devoid of some endometriotic locations like colon, ureter or other extra pelvic sites. To overcome these deficiencies ENZIAN staging system (2011) which focuses more on DIE and endometriosis fertility index (EFI) (2010) were developed. World Endometriosis Society (WES) agreed upon these three assessment methods (2017).

Endometriosis Fertility Index (EFI) Score

Q. What do you mean by endometriosis fertility index?

Endometriosis fertility index (EFI) score was first developed in 2010.

This index is regarded as a tool to select patient with infertility after surgical management of endometriosis whether the patient will be provided with assisted reproduction or will wait for spontaneous pregnancy.

Factors associated with history (Woman's age, duration of infertility, past pregnancy outcomes) and surgical factors (least function score with r-AFS endometriosis score and total score) are added to get the EFI score. From this EFI estimated percentage of pregnancy is calculated and advised accordingly.

(For details Adamson, et al. Endometriosis fertility index: the new, validated endometriosis staging system. Fertil Steril. 2010;94:1609-15)

Clinical Features of Endometriosis

- *Age*: Commonly in reproductive age group
- *Socioeconomic status*: More in higher socioeconomic status
- *Parity*: There may be history of infertility.

Symptoms of Endometriosis

Classical triads:
- Pain: Dysmenorrhea or menorrhagia
- Dyspareunia (deep dyspareunia)
- Infertility.

In 15% cases, there is heavy and/or irregular bleeding or premenstrual spotting. Dyspareunia is typically found in deep variety.

Others: According to site involved:
- *Urinary*: Dysuria, flank pain, back pain, abdominal pain, urgency, frequency, and hematuria. Urinary tract infection is excluded by culture and sensitivity.
- *Gastrointestinal symptoms*: Defecatory pain, constipation, diarrhea, dyschezia, tenesmus, and hematochezia. DIE of GI tract may cause pain. Sonography can diagnose rectal DIE.
- *Pulmonary*: Hemoptysis, catamenial chest pain, and pneumothorax.
- *Pain anterior abdominal wall* in scar endometriosis

It has strong adverse impact on general physical, mental and social wellbeing.

Signs of Endometriosis

- *General examination*: Looks anxious and irritable.
- *Per abdominal (PA)*: There may be suprapubic tenderness or fullness in large ovarian endometrioma.
- *Speculum examination*: Blue dome cyst **(Fig. 11)** or red powder-burn lesions may be seen over cervix or vagina.
- *Bimanual examination*: Uterus—retroverted, fixed, tender or firm, nodules in POD, enlarged cystic adnexal masses due to ovarian endometrioma.
- *RV examination*: RV septum thick and tender; POD—nodules.
- *Other sites*: Perineum, episiotomy scar, and abdominal scar.

Pain in Endometriosis

Q. What are the characteristics of pain in endometriosis?

Pain is the primary symptom.

Dysmenorrhea is of secondary onset, severe cyclical noncolicky pelvic pain during the period (70–80% cases). The pain started few days before period, worsens with onset of mens and persists for throughout the mens; pain is not normally controlled by simple analgesics or oral contraceptive (OC) pill and severe enough to cause significant in capacitation.

In approximately, 30–50% in endometriosis, there may be noncyclic chronic pelvic pain (CPP).

Endometriosis is found in 70–80% cases of women with pelvic pain. CPP seriously affects personality, working ability, social and marital life. So, pain in endometriosis may be cyclical and noncyclical.

Q. What are the causes of pain in endometriosis?

Pain is due to local peritoneal inflammation, deep infiltration with tissue damage, adhesion formation, fibrotic thickening, and collection of shed endometrial blood in endometriotic implants resulting in painful traction with the physiologic movement of tissue. Severity of pain does not always correlate with the extent of the disease.

Q. What do you mean by chronic pelvic pain (CPP)?

Chronic pelvic pain (CPP) is defined as pain, variations in cyclicity and duration, localized to the pelvis, lower abdomen, lower part of back radiating to medial side of thigh and perineum at least for six months duration not occurring solely with menstruation, intercourse and not related with pregnancy (*see* later). Endometriosis is found in 70–80% cases of women with pelvic pain.

Relation of Infertility with Endometriosis

- Incidence among subfertile women is up to 35%.
- About 30–50% endometriotic women are infertile.

Reasons of Infertility in Endometriosis

There are alterations of coital function, ovarian function, tubal function, endometrium, sperm function, and early pregnancy failure.

- *Coital function:* Less frequency and less penetration.
- *Ovarian function:* Anovulation, endocrinopathy—luteinized unruptured follicle, altered prolactin and gonadotropin midcycle surge, and oocyte maturation defect. Endometrioma reduces the quality of oocytes.
- *Tubal function:* Tubal motility disturbed due to prostaglandins and impaired oocyte pick up by fimbria.
- *Endometrium:* Interference by endometrial antibodies and luteal phase defect.
- *Sperm function:* Phagocytosis by macrophages and also inactivated by antibody.
- *Early pregnancy failure:* Increased early abortion.

It is not known whether milder form (asymptomatic) causes infertility though fecundity rate is found reduced in this group.

Diagnosis of Endometriosis

- Symptoms, signs, and examination findings
- Imaging: Transvaginal sonography (TVS), CT, and MRI
- Laboratory testing: CA 125
- Laparoscopy.

Symptoms

Symptoms have been described earlier.

Signs

Signs have been described earlier.

Examination Findings

General, PA, and PV examinations have been described earlier.

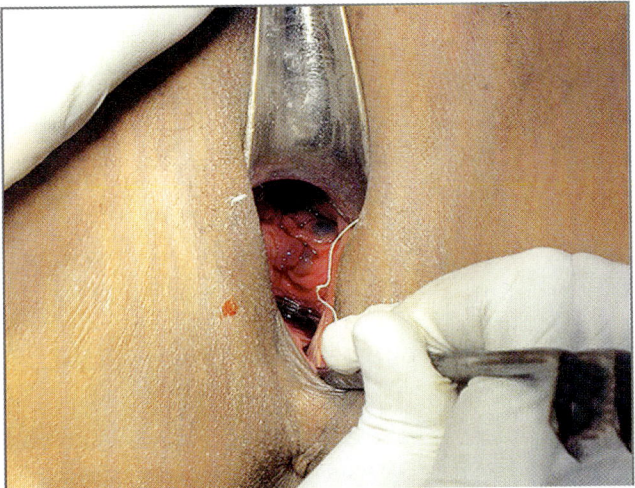

Fig. 11: Blue-domed cyst—endometriosis on the posterior fornix.

Investigations for Diagnosis of Endometriosis

* *Laboratory:* CA 125 positively correlate with severity, but sensitivity is only 28% and specificity 90%. Serum level above 35 U/mL is a cut-off point and a marker of diagnosed cases for disease recurrence after therapy. Infections and pregnancy complications are excluded by urine culture, cervical swab and serum βhCG.
* *Other biomarkers:* TSH, Vascular endothelial growth factor (VEGF) and cytokines (interleukin 6/8).
* Several MicroRNAs which are specific for modulating gene expression in endometriosis are assessed recently and may be an important noninvasive method for diagnosis in future.
* *Imaging:*
    * USG: Ovarian endometrioma and chocolate cysts **(Fig. 12)** are diagnosed by ground glass appearance and irregular wall, one to four locules and no solid part.
        * TVS is best to detect the presence of endometrioma and deeply infiltrating endometriosis of the rectum or rectovaginal septum. In smaller lesion, USG is of limited value.
        * Transrectal USG is useful in RV septum involvement cases. DIE can be diagnosed by sonography and sensitivity is about 75%. Superficial endometriosis is less accurately diagnosed by USG.
    * CT is useful in certain situation but there is no much of added advantage.
    * Role of MRI is not established. It is indicated in equivocal result in USG and where rectovaginal or bladder involvement suspected.
* *Laparoscopy:* Primary method for diagnosis of endometriosis (ACOG, 2018) **(Fig. 13)**.

Role of Laparoscopy in Endometriosis

It is gold standard in endometriosis:
* Direct visualization of the lesions: Definitive diagnosis can be done.

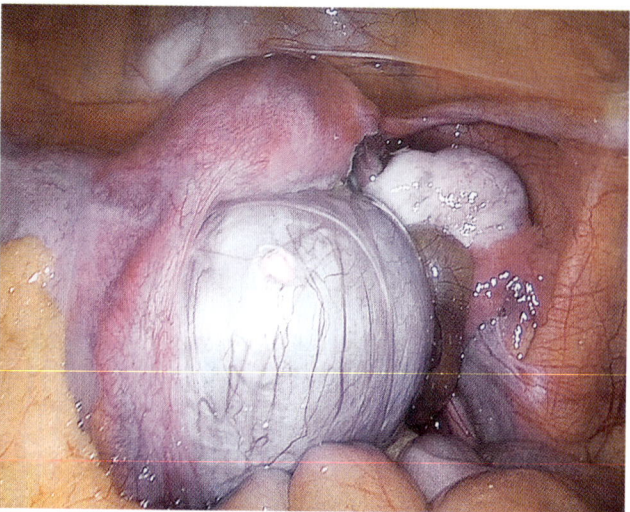

Fig. 13: Chocolate cyst left side.
Courtesy: Dr Subhas Halder, Senior Endoscopic Surgeon, Gynecology

* Stage: Type, site, adhesion, and extent of disease are determined.
* Biopsy can be taken if required.
* Ovarian endometriomas is diagnosed with laparoscopy with sensitivity and specificity of 97% and 95% respectively and no biopsy is needed to confirm.
* Concomitant surgery can be performed.
* Diagnosis is not confirmed until and unless laparoscopy is done.

Laparoscopic Findings and Types of Lesion

Other than the ovarian endometrioma and variable pelvic adhesions and scarring **(Fig. 14)**, the **followings lesions** are found laparoscopically:
* Typical black lesion: **"Powder burn" (Fig. 15)** or **"gunshot lesion"**

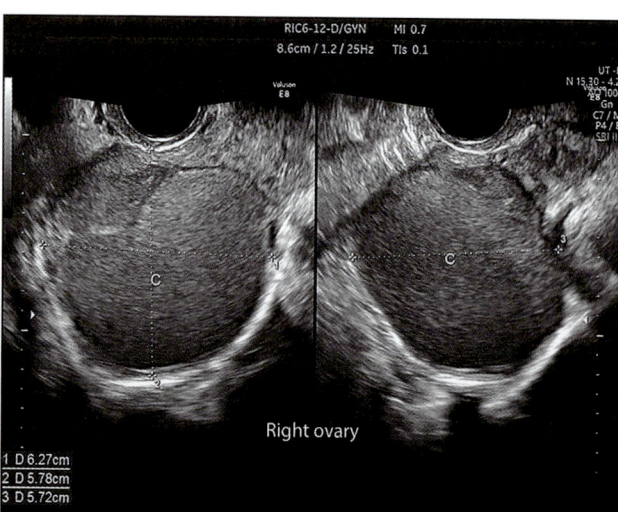

Fig. 12: Transvaginal sonography showing chocolate cyst of right ovary (6.27 cm × 5.28 cm × 5.72 cm).
Courtesy: Professor Kamal Oswal

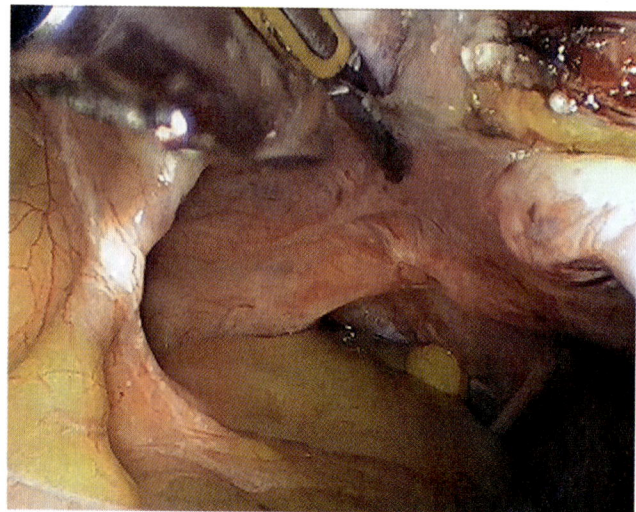

Fig. 14: Endometriotic scarring of left uterosacral ligament.
Courtesy: Dr Alok De, Associate Professor

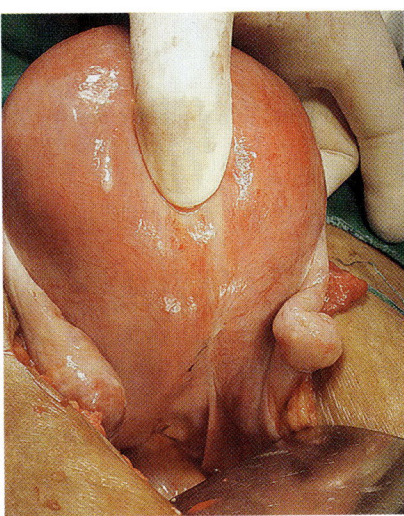

Fig. 15: Powder burn black lesion of endometriosis on posterior surface of uterus near uterosacral ligament.

- Scarring in the peritoneum and subsequently adhesion formation
- Subtle appearances: More common and active than puckered black lesion
    - Red lesions: Red flame, glandular excrescences
    - White lesion: White opacification over peritoneum
    - Yellow brown peritoneal patches (café-au-lait spots), circular peritoneal defects
    - Smooth blebs on peritoneal surface.

Q. Is biopsy needed for diagnosis?

- Biopsy confirms the diagnosis.
- However, current guideline does not suggest biopsy to avoid over diagnosis. Histopathology is needed in doubtful cases.
- Histology finding: Endometrial glands and stroma are the typical features. Hemosiderin deposition and fibromuscular metaplasia are frequently noted.

Criteria for Ovarian Endometrioma

- Diameter less than 12 cm
- Adhesion to pelvic side wall or broad ligament
- Endometriosis on surface of ovary
- Thick, tarry, chocolate color fluid content.

Other causes of chocolate cyst
Hemorrhagic corpus luteum cyst and neoplastic cyst.

Q. How will you manage endometriosis?

Goal:
- To relieve the pain
- To halt the progress of disease and reduce the disease process
- To permit satisfactory coitus
- To improve fertility where infertility is a concern.

Treatment is individualized depending on:
- *Patient's profile:*
    - Age
    - Marital status
    - Parity status and desire for children
- Presenting symptoms
- Severity of the disease
- Location of lesions
- Surgical expertise
- Patient's choice.

Prevention of Endometriosis

- Tubal patency test should be avoided immediately after curettage or around the time of mens.
- Married women with family history of endometriosis are encouraged to welcome pregnancy at the earliest.

Treatment Modalities of Endometriosis

- Expectant
- Medical
- Surgical
- Combined: Medical and surgical
- Specific treatment related to infertility like assisted-reproductive technique (ART).

Q. Is there any role of expectant management?

- Controversy exists regarding treatment of asymptomatic women diagnosed incidentally as regression occurs in significant group of patients.
- As progress occurs in many patients, treatment is justified at least to arrest progression or to eradicate for significant period. However, in mild to moderate disease in two-third of patients either regression or there is no progress and in another one third of patients' disease progression is found. Hence, follow up is important.

Q. How to relieve pain?

- Analgesics
- Induction of complete amenorrhea
- Surgical.

Medical Management

- Analgesics
- Hormones:
    - Combined oral contraceptive (COC)
    - Progestins including dienogest
    - Androgens: Danazol
    - Gonadotropin-releasing hormone (GnRH) agonist and antagonist
- Aromatase inhibitor
- Antiprogestational agent: Gestrinone
- Progesterone antagonist (mifepristone 50 mg/daily) orally for 6 months

- Selective progesterone-receptor modulators (SPRMs) and SERMs are experimental
- Angiogenic agents—cabergoline
- Others—proapoptotic agents: statin and antioxidant.

Analgesics

- Simple analgesics like paracetamol are given initially.
- In intractable cases more potent analgesics like tramadol and diclofenac are given.
- Nonsteroidal anti-inflammatory drugs (NSAIDs) are often used as first-line therapy. These are ibuprofen, naproxen, mefenamic acid and ketoprofen. These drugs inhibit both COX-1 and COX-2 enzymes nonselectively. Selective COX-2 inhibitors are used less due to the cardiovascular side effects.
- However, lowest possible dose with shortest duration should be used due to cardiovascular risk.

Mechanism of Hormonal Effects on Endometriosis

Mechanism is to induce atrophy by:

- Pseudopregnancy regime induces decidualization of endometrium—progestogens.
- Pseudomenopausal regime suppresses ovarian function—COC/GnRH.
- Anti-inflammation by anti-inflammatory drugs.

Estrogen–Progesterone Combination

- *Combined OC pill*:
  - Mainstay of treatment in pain relief.
  - Suppresses ovulation and makes decidualization of implant.
  - Can be used cyclically or continuously. Continuous (extended cycle COC) is preferable for decreased frequency of painful menses.
  - Rout: Oral, vaginal or transdermal.
  - Can be used for long-term: Initially, it is given for 6 months. If symptoms are relieved, it can be given for long-term till the planning of pregnancy. If no improvement with COC think any other diagnosis like irritable bowel syndrome.
- *Vaginal ring*: 15 μg ethinylestradiol and 120 μg of etonogestrel.
- *Transdermal patch*: 20 μg ethinylestradiol and 150 μg norelgestromin.

Progestogens

- *Oral*:
  - Dydrogesterone (20–30 mg/day).
  - Medroxyprogesterone acetate (30–40 mg/day); norethisterone (10–25 mg/day).
  - Norethindrone acetate (NETA), starting with 5 mg daily and increasing 2.5 mg daily till amenorrhea is achieved or maximum dose of 20 mg daily is reached.
  - Dienogest (2 mg/day) are used orally.
- *Injectable:* Depot medroxyprogesterone acetate 150 mg IM every 3 months. DMPA— 104 mg S/C (Syanapres) is effective in reducing pain with less impact on BMD in comparison to GnRH analogue. However, there is higher rate of irregular bleeding and slower return of ovulation after discontinuation.
- *Levonorgestrel intrauterine system* (LNG-IUS—Mirena) for 5 years
- *Implant*: Etonogestrel is used as implant (implanon). This implant is less studied in endometriosis but has comparable result with LNG-IUS in limited study. Etonogestrel is used as implant or combined vaginal ring which are primarily used as contraceptive.
- Progesterone receptor modulator, mifepristone or ulipristal acetate

Danazol

- Synthetic androgen: Isoxazole derivative of 17α-ethinyl testosterone.
- Causes hypoestrogenic and hyperandrogenic state that induces atrophy of endometrium (suppresses luteinizing hormone surge, occupies receptor sites of sex hormone-binding globulin increasing ST, binds androgen and progesterone receptor).
- 200 mg daily up to thrice daily orally for 6 months. It can be used in vaginal route with less side effect.
- Pain relief occurs in 6 months of therapy.
- The use is falling out due to androgenic side effects.
- Vaginal use of danazol in low dose is being considered as a way to preserve the benefits of the drug while reducing systemic side effects.

Dienogest

- It is a new 19-nortestosterone derivative that exhibits selective binding to progesterone receptors and with no androgenic side effects, no glucocorticoid or mineralocorticoid activity and action persists 6 months after discontinuation.
- It is an effective drug in endometriosis for relief of pain with less side effects with good compliance and well tolerated.
- It is used 2 mg daily orally, for 12–24 weeks but costly.
- It is a potential good medical option in endometriosis.

Gestrinone

Antiprogestational agent 2.5–5 mg twice weekly orally for 6–9 months. Comparable to danazol and GnRH with symptom improvement and resolution of implants. Not associated with bone loss like GnRH agonist. Important side effect is lowering of high-density lipoprotein.

GnRH

- Gonadotropin-releasing hormone agonists are currently one of the most widely used medical therapies for endometriosis.

- It induces medical menopause by down-regulating hypothalamic pituitary GnRH receptors. It decreases gonadotropin secretion, suppresses ovulation, and reduces serum estrogen levels.
- Agents: Leuprolide, buserelin, nafarelin, hitrelin, goserelin, deslorelin, and triptorelin (decapeptyl).
- It is given intramuscularly (IM), subcutaneously (SC), and intranasally. They are inactive orally. Leuprolide acetate (luprodex) 3.75 mg is given monthly or 11.25 mg, 3 monthly IM.
- Gonadotropin-releasing hormone agonists are associated with significant hypoestrogenic side effects, e.g., menopausal symptoms and reduction bone mineral density (BMD) both for spine and hip for which "add back" regimens in the form of progestin only; progestin plus bisphosphonate or progestin plus estrogen are prescribed. NETA 5 mg with or without equine estrogen 0.625 mg, or transdermal 25 µg estradiol plus 5 mg MPA combination are used as add back therapy without hampering the efficacy of pain relief by GnRH. Ideally add back therapy can be started with GnRH. Calcium 1000 mg is recommended daily with add-back therapy (ACOG, 2018).

GnRH Antagonist (Ganirelix and Cetrorelix)

GnRH antagonists are synthetic peptides used as subcutaneous injection or implantation of long-acting depots. No evidence exists on the effectiveness of GnRH antagonists for endometriosis-associated pain. Advantages are no initial flare, more rapid onset of action, quick recovery, less ovarian hyperstimulation syndrome, and less expensive.

Elagolix (Orilissa) a nonpeptide GnRH antagonist is the first and only oral tab (150/200 mg) once or twice daily used in women with moderate to severe endometriosis pain approved by FDA (2018). In United States orilissa is considered as second-line therapy next to combined E-P.

Aromatase Inhibitor

- Aromatase inhibitor like anastrozole has been successfully used in postmenopausal endometriosis or when symptoms persist following conventional treatment.
- One serious side effect is ovarian cyst formation. Use of aromatase inhibitor along with continuous COC add back therapy has been reported with significant improvement of symptoms.
- Aromatase inhibitors act by inhibiting estrogen synthesis from androgen in both ovarian and extraovarian sites.

Cabergoline

Dopamine agonist inhibits angiogenesis by reducing levels of vascular endothelial growth factor (VEGF), and thus interferes endometriotic growth and maintenance efficiently. It is used 0.5 mg twice weekly atleast for three months and can be given preoperatively, postoperatively alone or with COCs. Its advantage is it can be used alone in those patients who desire fertility, at the same time where other drugs delay conception.

Dopamine agonist decreases pain by action on nerve fibers. It does not cause hypoestrogenic and bone density changes. There is alleged risk of vulvular heart disease.

Progesteron Receptor Modulator, Mifepristone or Ulipristal

They, when used for endometriosis relieve pain and reduce extent of endometriosis. Progesterone receptor modulator-associated endometrial changes (PEACs) are common. A recent study shows that PEACs are rare in ulipristal acetate. However, serious liver toxicity of ulipristal has been reported and should never be used more than 3 months continuously.

Selective Estrogen Receptor Modulator (SERM)

Animal study and few human study shows lesion regression in endometriosis by bazedoxifene (BZA), a third generation SERM but not used clinical in endometriosia.

LNG-IUS—Mirena

- It delivers levonorgestrel to have direct effect on the endometriotic implant in the pelvic cavity through peritoneal fluid by hematogenous spread and effective for 5 years.
- Traditionally used for contraceptive. Many study though small have shown efficacy not only relief of pain but reduction of volume of the lesion as well.

Disadvantage to medical management

The most important is that recurrence rate is high after medical treatment is discontinued.

Surgical Management of Endometriosis

Endometriosis can be managed by:
- Conservative surgery
- Definitive surgery.

Conservative Surgery

Goal: Goal is to excise all visible endometriotic lesions and associated adhesions—peritoneal lesions, ovarian cysts, deep RV endometriosis, and to restore normal anatomy.

Types of surgery:
- Ablation or excision of endometrial implants
- Lysis of adhesions
- Interruption of nerve pathways:
  - Ablation of uterosacral nerves (LUNA)
  - Presacral neurectomy (PSN)
- Resection of endometriomas. Laparoscopy is preferred to laparotomy.

Combined therapy: Preoperative hormone therapy improves AFS score. There is little evidence that pain is better relieved than surgery alone. Postoperative use of OCs prevents endometrioma recurrence.

Management of Ovarian Endometrioma (Figs. 16 to 18)

* Cyst larger than 3 cm surgery (laparoscopic) by total ovarian cystectomy or by aspiration coupled with ablation of the cyst capsule is preferred.
* Cystectomy is better to drainage and coagulation of the endometrioma so far as pain relief and pregnancy outcome are concerned.
* There is chance of reduction of ovarian reserve following excision and one must be very cautious.
* Pre- and postoperative medical management by oral contraceptive pill (OCP) or GnRH agonist may be done for secondary prevention.

Definitive Surgery

* When disease is progressive or there are severe symptoms refractory to all treatment—family completed → TAH with BSO which is usually curative **(Fig. 19)**.
* Combined hormone replacement therapy may be deferred for up to 6 months following surgery particularly when active disease is found during surgery.
* Risk of surgery—technically challenging and risk of urological and colorectal complications.

Approach to Endometriosis

The **Flowchart 1** shows how a case of endometriosis is approached.

Management of Endometriosis with Infertility

The options are the followings with singly or in combination—surgery, ovulation induction, and assisted reproductive technology or intrauterine insemination (IUI).

* Medical management alone does not improve fertility.
* In minimal and mild endometriosis laparoscopic surgical ablation or excision increases fertility rate. Excision is better than ablation.

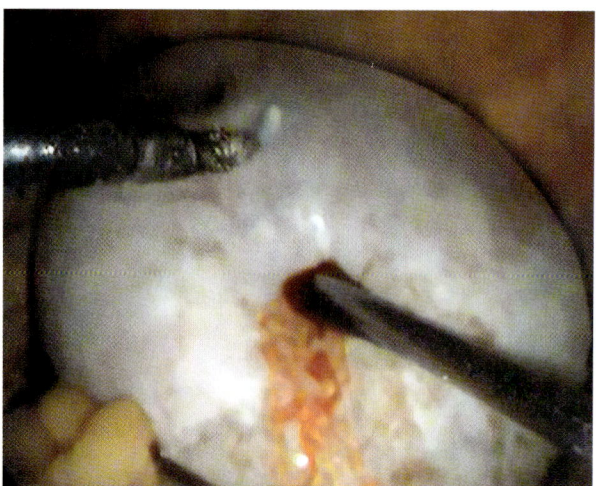

Fig. 16: Aspiration of endometrioma.
Courtesy: Dr Alok De, Associate Professor

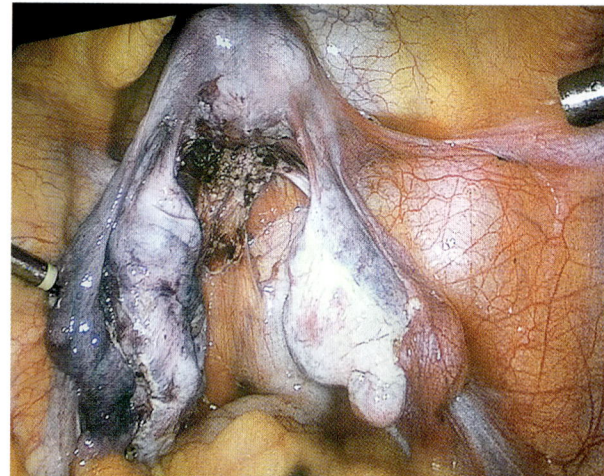

Fig. 18: Pelvic endometriosis (chocolate cyst) after surgery (cystectomy) of the patient in Figure 13.
Courtesy: Dr Subhas Halder

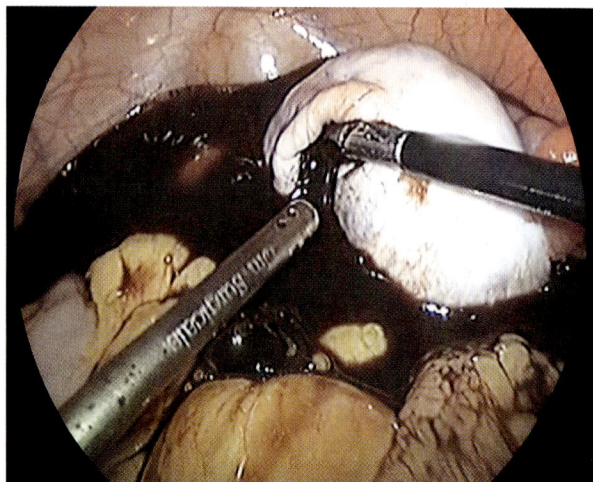

Fig. 17: Drainage of chocolate cyst before cystectomy.
Courtesy: Dr Alok De, Associate Professor

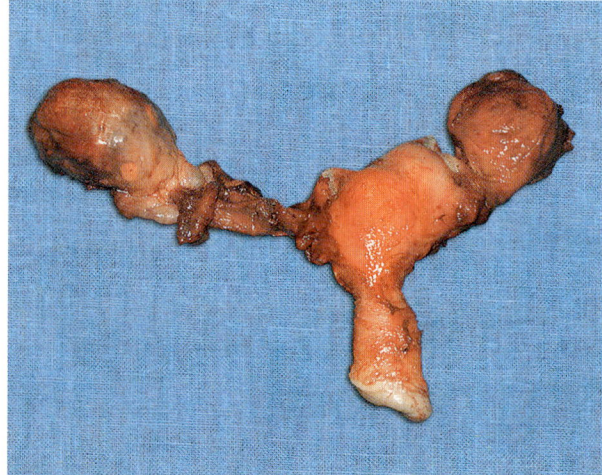

Fig. 19: Total abdominal hysterectomy with bilateral salpingo-oophorectomy in bilateral chocolate cyst in a 42-year-old woman.

CHAPTER 16: A Case of Endometriosis Adenomyosis

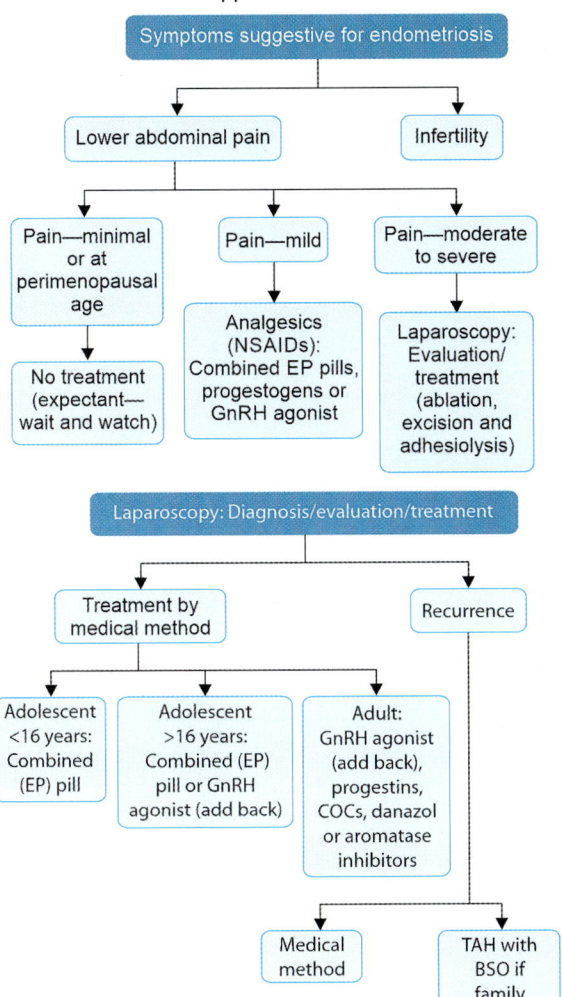

Flowchart 1: Approach to endometriosis.

Abbreviations: NSAID, nonsteroidal anti-inflammatory drug; EP, estrogen–progesterone; GnRH, gonadotropin-releasing hormone; COC, combined oral contraceptive; TAH with BSO, total abdominal hysterectomy with bilateral salpingo-oophorectomy

- Moderate and severe endometriosis may be treated surgically to restore anatomy and tubal function. In severe endometriosis, role of surgery in fertility promotion is not proved. Controlled ovarian hyperstimulation and IUI/IVF are the standard fertility treatment which may be needed in all types of endometriosis with infertility.
- Excision or cystectomy of ovarian endometrioma more than 4 cm is reasonable to do but needs meticulous technique to prevent ovarian reserve. This is also true prior to ART. Surgery in ovarian endometrioma improves both spontaneous pregnancy rate and pregnancy rate following in vitro fertilization.
- Preoperative or short course of postoperative medical therapy is suggested by many to improve fertility.

Approach to Endometriosis with Infertility

The **Flowchart 2** shows how a case of endometriosis with infertility is approached.

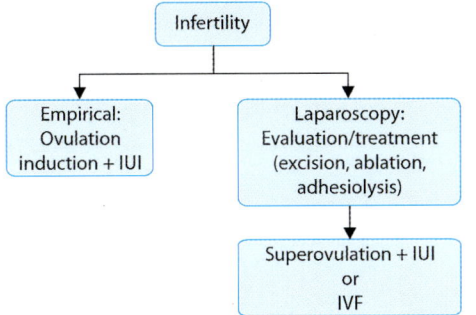

Flowchart 2: Approach to endometriosis with infertility.

Abbreviations: IUI, intrauterine insemination; IVF, in vitro fertilization

Revised American Society for Reproductive Medicine Classification of Endometriosis 1996

Revised American Society for Reproductive Medicine Classification has been shown in **Figure 20**.

ADENOMYOSIS

Q. How to define adenomyosis?

Adenomyosis is a disorder in which endometrial glands and stroma are located haphazardly deep within the myometrium with surrounding myometrial hyperplasia. It is actually benign invasion of the endometrium into the uterine musculature **(Fig. 21)**.

Q. How often does occur?

As adenomyosis is diagnosed definitely by histology. On specimen of hysterectomy of reproductive age women, it is found in 40% cases. By TVS of reproductive age women, it is reported to be as 20%.

Pathophysiology

The cause of adenomyosis is not exactly known but invagination of basal layer cells of endometrium into myometrium occurs in adenomyosis. Normal uterus lacks the submucosa, but why this deep myometrial invasion occurs is clearly not know. **Thickened junctional zone (JZ) and weakness of smooth muscle tissue of adenomyotic uterus may have role.**

Cyclical estrogen causes change in ectopic endometrium with bleeding within the myometrium resulting severe dysmenorrhea which persists throughout menses, uterine enlargement, and heavy menstrual bleeding (HMB).

As adenomyosis regresses after menopause, estrogen and progesterone have definitive role in etiopathogenesis. Aromatase level expression and high tissue estrogen levels are seen in adenomyosis which is also found in *endometrial hyperplasia, uterine fibroid, and endometriosis which are commonly associated with adenomyosis.*

Gross Pathology

Uterus becomes uniformly enlarged, usually not beyond 12 weeks pregnancy size. Surface is smooth, reddish in color and soft.

Patient's name _____ Date: _____

Stage I (Minimal) 1–5 Laparoscopy _____ Laparotomy _____ Photography _____
Stage II (Mild) 6–15 Recommended treatment _____
Stage III (Moderate) 16–40 _____
Stage IV (Severe) >40
Total _____ Prognosis _____

	Endometriosis	<1 cm	1–3 cm	>3 cm
Peritoneum	Superficial	1	2	4
	Deep	2	4	6
Ovary	Right superficial	1	2	4
	Deep	4	16	20
	Left superficial	1	2	4
	Deep	4	16	20
	Posterior cul-de-sac obliteration	Partial		Complete
		4		40
	Adhesions	<1/3 enclosure	1/3–2/3 enclosure	>2/3 enclosure
Ovary	Right filmy	1	2	4
	Dense	4	8	16
	Left filmy	1	2	4
	Dense	4	8	16
Tube	Right filmy	1	2	4
	Dense	4	8	16
	Left filmy	1	2	4
	Dense	4*	8*	16

*If the fimbriated end of the fallopian tube is completely enclosed, change the point assignment to 16.

Additional endometriosis: _____ Associated pathology: _____

To be used with normal tubes and ovaries

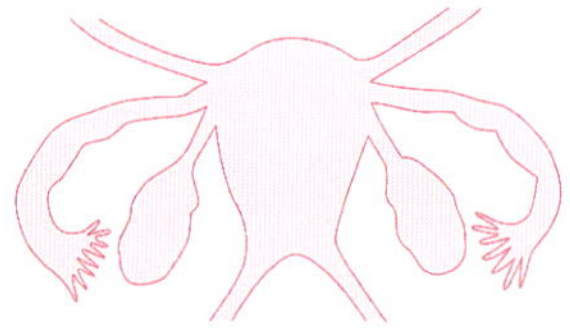

To be used with abnormal tubes and/or ovaries

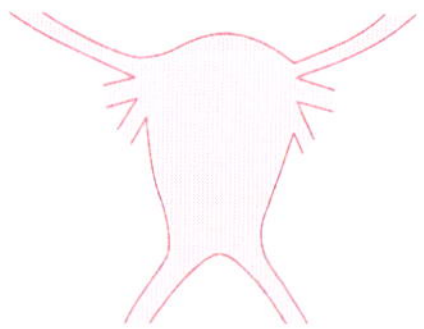

Fig. 20: Revised American Society for Reproductive Medicine Classification of Endometriosis, 1996.

Cut surface shows spongy with trabecular appearance with presence of focal areas of hemorrhage **(Figs. 21 and 22)**. Hemorrhage is minimal as the ectopic cells originate from basal layer of endometrium where proliferative and secretory changes become not so obvious like superficial layers which occur in normal menstruation.

Histopathology

Glands and stroma deep in myometrium either in scattered or in focal manner.

Types of Adenomyosis

Adenomyosis may be of two types—focal and diffuse **(Figs. 23A and B)**.

In *focal endometriosis* a focal nodular collection is seen whereas in *diffuse adenomyosis* glands and stroma are scattered in myometrium.

Junctional Zone

Q. What is junctional zone?

The area of endomyometrial junction is called junctional zone. The junctional layer consists of (from outside in):
- Myometrial layer
- Subvascular layer also called archimyometrium
- Basal endometrial layer
- Normal thickness is 7–8 mm and in adenomyosis **thickness increases to more than or equal to 12 mm.**

CHAPTER 16: A Case of Endometriosis Adenomyosis

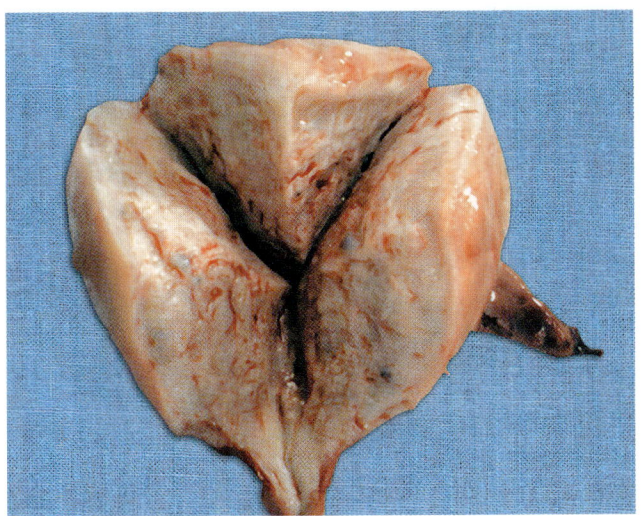

Fig. 21: Adenomyosis: Thickened myometrium, multiple endometrial glands in myometrium (same specimen after cut section as in Figure 27).

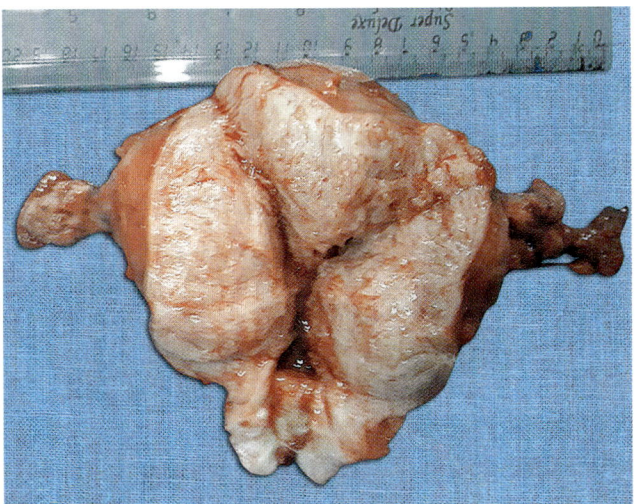

Fig. 22: Adenomyosis: Note ovaries are normal.

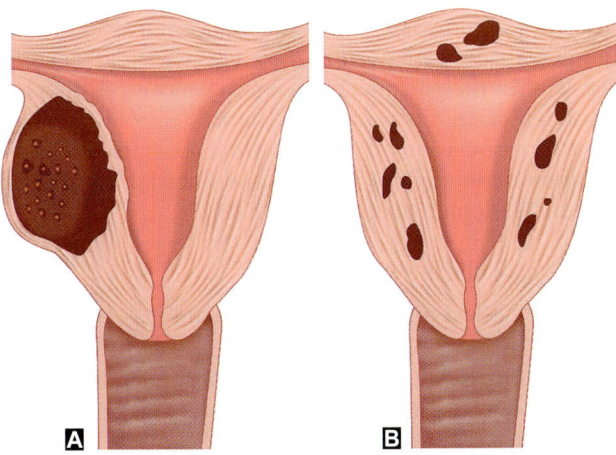

Figs. 23A and B: (A) Focal adenomyosis; (B) Diffuse adenomyosis.

Risk Factors

- *Parity and age* are important risk factors.
- About 90% occurs in *multiparous women* who are in age group of late *30 or early 40s*.
- Recently adenomyosis is diagnosed in subfertile women and second and third decades patients are not uncommon.
- Tamoxifen is a risk factor but not COC pill.

Q. How to diagnose adenomyosis?

- Adenomyosis can be diagnosed by—clinical, biopsy, TVS, 3D USG, and MRI.
- Though adenomyosis is suspected clinically, definitive diagnosis is histopathology.

Symptoms

- Heavy menstrual bleeding (HMB): 30%
- Dysmenorrhea: 30%
- Dyspareunia: 10%.

On Examination

- Uterus—bulky usually within 12 weeks can be palpated by bimanual examination, boggy, and tender.
- *CA 125*—elevated but not diagnostic.

Imaging

Transvaginal sonography is more informative and preferred to abdominal.

In diffuse adenomyosis, TVS findings are as follows **(Fig. 24)**:

- Globular enlarged uterus
- Heterogenous myometrial area
- Thicker anterior or posterior myometrial wall than the counterpart
- Small myometrial cysts representing cystic glands within ectopic endometrial foci
- Striated projection from endometrium to myometrium

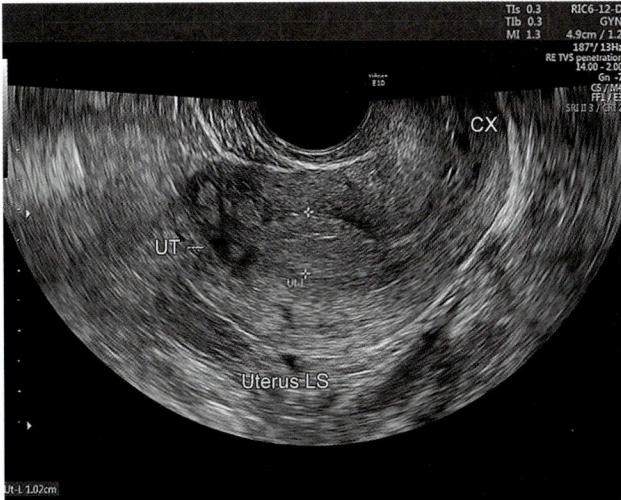

Fig. 24: Adenomyosis: Transvaginal sonography showing blurring of endomyometrial junction suggestive of adenomyosis.

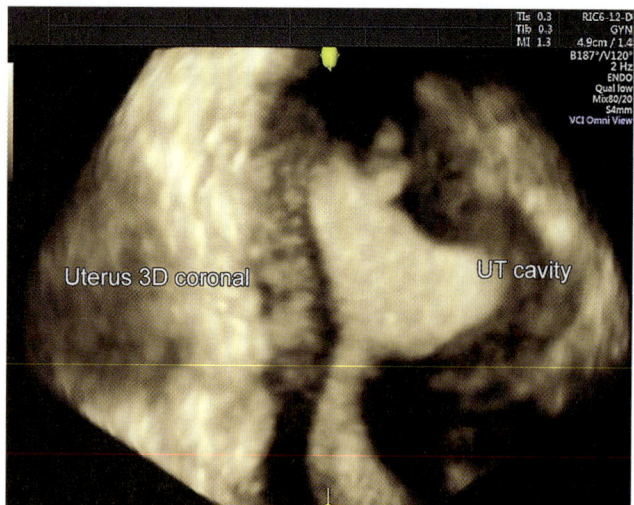 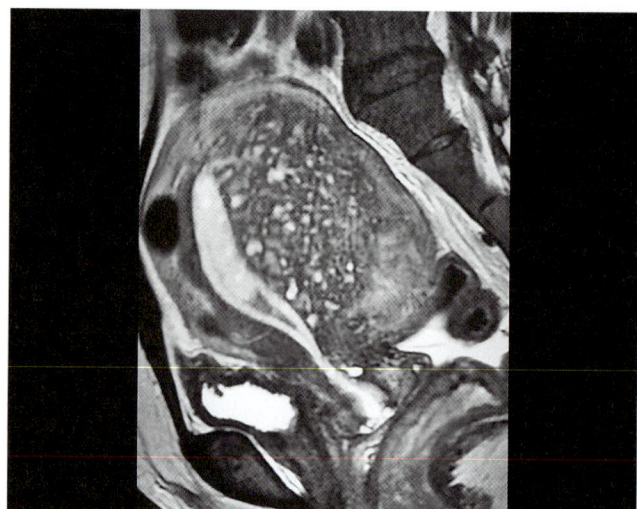

Fig. 25: 3D USG showing blurring of endomyometrial junction suggestive of adenomyosis.
Courtesy: Professor Kamal Oswal

Fig. 26: MRI showing adenomyosis—absence of well-circumscribed mass which is found in fibroid. Presence of multiple glands inside adenomyosis.
Courtesy: Professor M Karmakar, IPGMER

- Ill-defined endometrial echo
- Poor differentiation of endometrial and myometrial junction.

In focal adenomyosis difference between adenomyosis and leiomyoma are essential which can be done on the following points by TVS:
- Shape is elliptical rather than spherical
- Discrete hypoechoic nodule or nodules with poorly defined margins (in contrast to fibroid where margin is clear)
- Presence of anechoic cysts of different diameters
- Pressure effect on surrounding tissue is less
- By 3D ultrasound JZ looks blurred in adenomyosis **(Fig. 25)**.

Role of MRI in Adenomyosis (Fig. 26)
- An MRI provides very good images of endometrium, myometrium, and ectopic endometrium in adenomyosis.
- Large globular irregular mass without fibroid.
- Myometrial foci are of high intensity.
- It can differentiate leiomyoma and adenomyosis better than TVS by delineating the junctional zone. JZ is at least 12 mm and/or ill-defined low signal intensity myometrial area whereas there is a well-circumscribed mass related to leiomyoma.

Q. Which imaging would you prefer in adenomyosis?
- Sonography and MRI both are useful.
- Transvaginal sonography is less expensive and available clinically. Operators experience has influence on diagnostic accuracy.
- An MRI is little superior to TVS. In inconclusive diagnosis, MRI is helpful.

Biopsy
Biopsy is not ideal as TVS and MRI are equally informative. It can be done through laparoscopy and hysteroscopy guidance from posterior wall near posterior JZ full thickness with 14-gauze needle.

Laparoscopy and hysteroscopy may be suggestive but cannot do the exact diagnosis.

Laparoscopy
Large and boggy uterus

Hysteroscope
"White ridges and black opening" in the endometrium.

Q. Relation between endometriosis and adenomyosis—is it a variety of endometriosis?

Though common association, epidemiologically and mechanism are separate.

In the past, it was thought that the diseases were separate entities. Adenomyosis was called endometriosis interna but many recent studies show they have strong association **(Fig. 27)**. In the past, the association was only 8–15% but recent data states it is as high as 50–90%.

Other associations with adenomyosis— fibroid (7%), endometrial polyp (3%), atypical endometrial hyperplasia (4%), and endometrial carcinoma (1.5%).

Adenomyosis and Infertility
- Subfertility is common in younger age group, late marriage is a factor.
- Subfertility is caused by defective sperm migration, bad quality oocyte, defective implantation, and miscarriage due to macrophages.

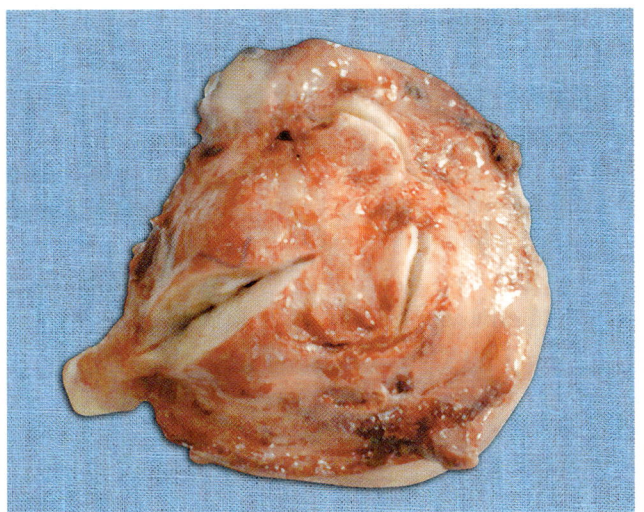

Fig. 27: A 42-year-old nulliparous woman married or 18 years with history of infertility presented with heavy menstrual bleeding with severe dysmenorrhea, right ovary chocolate cyst with pelvic adhesion— association of adenomyosis and endometriosis.

Adenomyosis—Past and Present

There are some noticeable changes regarding adenomyosis. These are:
- Previously, it was thought the disease is of entirely of parous women and is found in late 30 and 40s; now it is found more in infertile women and relatively in younger group of second and third decade age.
- Association with endometriosis was 8–15% and considered as two separate disease entities, now both are found in more frequent association in 50–90% range.
- Main symptoms were dysmenorrhea, menorrhagia, and dyspareunia; now subfertility is a major issue.
- In the past, treatment trend was radical—hysterectomy; now more attitude is toward conservative and fertility preservation.

Management

Medical

Relief of pain and bleeding and improvement of fertility where it is the issue:
- NSAIDs
- *Hormones*: Aim is to induce amenorrhea and to make the ectopic endometrium quiescent and to relieve dysmenorrhea and HMB by altering prostaglandins:
  - COCs
  - Only progestogen—LNG-IUS and depo-provera.
    - Expulsion rate of LNG-IUS is higher in adenomyosis.
  - Danazol—less preferred due to androgenic effect.
  - GnRH agonist: It is particularly useful in adenomyosis with infertility.
- Symptoms return with ceasing treatment in most of the patients.

Adenomyosis with Infertility
- Conservative treatment of different modalities, mostly GnRH agonist with or without ART.
- Adenomyosis has negative impact on ART result.

Hysterectomy

It is the definitive treatment especially in parous women.

In diffuse adenomyosis of uterus more than 10 cm (>12 weeks size—palpable abdominally) with intractable HMB and dysmenorrhea is beyond conservative treatment. In infertile women, hysterectomy with preservation of ovary for future surrogacy is considered.

Other Options
- Endometrial ablation—attempted but less successful to eradicate deeper lesion.
- Uterine artery embolization and MRI-guided focused ultrasound (MRgFUS) have been found to be effective in small series.
- Laparoscopic partial resection of uterus with uterine artery occlusion.

Obstetric Outcome

Abortion, preterm labor, uterine rupture, ectopic, and postpartum hemorrhage (PPH) are more common.

DYSMENORRHEA

Q. What do you mean by dysmenorrhea?

Cyclical pain during period incapacitating to the woman from normal activity is called dysmenorrhea though any painful menstruation is commonly regarded as dysmenorrhea.

Q. What are the types?

Two types:
- Primary dysmenorrhea
- Secondary dysmenorrhea

In **primary dysmenorrhea** no identifiable cause is detected and is not associated with any identifiable pathology and associated in ovulatory cycles. It begins shortly after onset of menarche and most intense just before and during period. Usually, it improves following childbirth and decreases with increasing age.

Secondary dysmenorrhea develops over time, and starts few days before menstruation and ceases after menstruation. It is due to some pathology.

Q. What are the causes of secondary dysmenorrhea?
- Endometriosis and adenomyosis
- PID
- Outlet obstruction, e.g., cervical stenosis
- Endometrial polyp and submucus leiomyoma

Q. What do you mean by spasmodic dysmenorrhea and congestive dysmenorrhea?

In **spasmodic dysmenorrhea** pain is crampic in nature and perceived on 1st or 2nd day of period and found in primary dysmenorrhea.

In **congestive type** pain starts before the onset of menstruation and relieved after its onset and nature is pelvic discomfort which is felt in secondary dysmenorrhea.

Q. What do you mean by membranous dysmenorrhea?

Here, menstruaion is associated with expulsion of big pieces of endometrial cast, nature of pain is cramping and it is one rare variety of primary amenorrhea. It may have family history. Drugs reducing blood flow is effective.

Q. What are the causes of pain in primary dysmenorrhea?

- Prostaglandin-prostaglandins secreted by endometrial cells increase myometrial contraction, increase active pressure and also ischemia causing pain. Higher levels of prostaglandins is found in menstrual blood of women with severe dysmenorrhea.
- Neurogenic factors
- Increase vasopressin and endothelin
- Anatomical abnormality like rudimentary horn, bicornuate uterus
- Psychosomatic in adolescent girl

Q. How will you differentiate primary and secondary dysmenorrhea?

Parameters	Primary	Secondary
Nature of pain	Spasmodic pain in lower abdomen	Pelvic discomfort colicky, congestive
Cause of pain	Prostaglandins	Pathology like endometriosis adenomyosis, etc., prostaglandin is one factor
Age of onset	Begins shortly after onset of menarche. Usually, it improves following childbirth and decreases with increasing age	Develops over time in reproductive years
Relation with menstruation	Most intense just before and during period	Starts few days before menstruation and ceases after menstruation
Other symptoms	Flushing, nausea, vomiting related to prostaglandin	AUB, dyspareunia and infertility, abnormal discharge in PID
Physical findings	Almost normal	There may be adnexal swelling, tenderness, restricted mobility of uterus, enlarged uterus in fibroid and adenomyosis and other finding as per cause
Investigations	Within normal limit	USG and laparoscopy may help to diagnose the pathology

Abbreviations: AUB, abnormal uterine bleeding; PID, pelvic inflammatory disease; USG, ultrasonography

Q. How to approach a case of dysmenorrheal to reach diagnosis?

History

Age of onset, relationship with menstruation, nature of pain, associated symptoms, severity of pain which can be ascertained by whether she has to take analgesics or need to take leave from work or school due to pain. These will determine the type.

Physical Examination

Abdominal examination—lump in fibroid, large endometrioma

Pelvic examination (not done in adolescent)—adnexal mass in endometrioma, tenderness in PID and endometriosis, fixed uterus in endometriosis and pelvic adhesion, enlarged uterus in fibroid, nodules in POD (endometriosis) and abnormal cervix.

Investigations

- Total blood count, CA125
- Vaginal and endocervical swab for pelvic infection
- TVUS, CT, MRI
- Laparoscopy in case of clinical suspicion of pelvic pathology e.g., endometriosis, adenomyosis or to rule out any pathology

Treatment of Primary Dysmenorrhea

- NSAIDs: Ibuprofen, naproxen and mefenamic acid
- Hormones:
  - COC
  - Progesterones: Oral, desogestrel, Parenteral- Inj DMPA, LNG-IUS, subdermal implant
  - GnRH: Side effects precludes its use and not a first line treatment
- Heat—old method but beneficial
- Lifestyle: Diet-low fat vegetarian diet, vitamin E, vitamin B_1, few herbal products
- Others: Acupuncture, transcutaneous nerve stimulation (TENS)
- Surgery: Cervical dilatation under GA—it damages sensory nerve endings in the cervix, laparoscopic uterine nerve ablation (LUNA), presacral neurectomy (Cotte's operation).

Treatment of Secondary Dysmenorrhea

- NSAIDs
- Treatment of pathology:
  - Endometriosis
  - Pelvic adhesions
  - Submucous polyp
- Hysterectomy

CHRONIC PELVIC PAIN

Q. How to define chronic pelvic pain (CPP)?

Chronic pelvic pain (CPP) is defined as pain, variations in cyclicity and duration, localized to the pelvis, lower abdomen, lower part of back radiating to medial side of thigh and perineum at least for six months duration not occurring solely with menstruation, intercourse and not related with pregnancy. However, definition of chronic pelvic pain is not without controversy.

Incidence: Prevalence is 15% worldwide.

Causes of CPP and Pathology

Pathophysiology and etiology remain unclear in many cases, in more than half of the cases more than single factor is present and strongly associated with neuropathic pain.

The causes of CPP can be gynecological and nongynecological like gastrointestinal, urological, musculoskeletal, neuropathic and psychosocial as given in the **Table 1**.

Table 1: Causes of CPP.

Gynecological	Endometriosis, adenomyosis, uterine fibroid, PID, adhesions, ovarian cyst and vulvodynia
Gastrointestinal cause	Irritable bowel syndrome
Urological	Interstitial cystitis/painful bladder syndrome
Musculoskeletal	Pelvic floor myalgia, pain from pelvic joints, postural muscle strain, damages of muscle of abdomen and pelvis
Neurological	Neuropathic pain—central and peripheral, nerve entrapment by scar tissue, fascia and in narrow foramen and postsurgical
Psychosocial	Sexual and physical abuse

Evaluation and Diagnosis

History, examination, investigations.

Clinical history taking and examination can give clue to the diagnosis.

History

- Pain—localization of pain (mapping of pain) may indicate the site of origin. Nature of pain may give clue to probable cause **(Table 2)**. "Pain log" is useful for realizing the pattern of pain and impact on quality of life. Dates of episode of pain, location, severity, relation with mens, urination, coitus, physical activity, posture and use of analgesics will help to reach at diagnosis. Characteristics of pelvic pain of different origin is expressed by mnemonic SOCRATES (*see* Page 5, **Table 2**). Predesigned questionnaire in relation to pain and use of various pain scales (visual analogue scale, numerical rating scale and verbal rating scale) are useful to assess different aspects of pain.
- Previous surgery or history of infection: Adhesions
- History of abuse, trauma
- Unexplained weight loss—malignancy. Systemic disease
- Postcoital bleeding may indicate cervical cancer
- Postmenopausal bleeding: There may be endometrial cancer.

Table 2: Nature of pain and probable cause of CPP.

Nature of pain	Probable cause
Pain related with menstrual cycle	Adenomyosis, endometriosis
Pain—no relation with menstrual cycle	Interstitial cystitis, irritable bowel syndrome, adhesions musculoskeletal etiologies
Pain with urinary urge	Interstitial cystitis, urethral syndrome
Cramp-like pain	Inflammatory bowel disease, irritable bowel syndrome
Burning, or electric shock-like pain	Nerve entrapment
Onset of pain in postmenopausal period	Malignancy

Examination

Abdominal and Pelvic Examination

- Pain on palpation on back, sacroiliac joint, symphysis pubis may indicate musculoskeletal origin.
- Superficial pain on parities: Source of pain on abdominal or pelvic wall.
- Carnett test positive indicates abdominal wall or myofascial source of infection.

Carnett test: The patient with chronic pelvic pain is asked to raise both legs or the head off the table while in supine position. One finger by the examiner is placed on the painful abdominal site when rectus muscles are contracted. In case of myofascial pain such as trigger points, entrapped nerve, hernia, or myositis pain is increased whereas pain becomes less if it is of intra-abdominal visceral origin.

Bimanual Examination

- Uterus—enlarged, tender, mobility restricted-adenomyosis, endometriosis, endometritis, pelvic adhesions.
- Adnexal swelling—ovarian tumor, hydrosalpinx.
- Uterosacral involvement—endometriosis, malignancy
- Vulva/vagina—suburethral swelling, tenderness—urethral caruncle, vulvovaginal pain may indicate vulvodynia.
- Any point tenderness over vulva, vagina and bladder is looked for.

Investigations

- Urinary pregnancy test, complete blood count, urine examination for infection and hematuria.
- Genital tract swab to detect STIs like Chlamydia to rule out PID.

- TVS—adnexal masses, TO abscess, ovarian cyst, endometrioma, uterine adenomyosis, fibroid, hydrosalpinx
- MRI—suspected deep infiltrating endometriosis, for assessment of pelvic mass
- Laparoscopy—when pain is severe and cause is unclear, to confirm adnexal mass, endometriosis, adhesions and to treat concurrently if needed.

Management

Aim is to maximize quality of life. There is limited evidence on treatment of CPP and are mostly based on symptomatic treatment.

Therapy consists of:
- General health improvement (diet, hydration, exercise and sexual health).
- Medical—analgesics, hormonal, tricyclic antidepressant (amitriptyline, nortriptyline, gabapentin, pregabalin) or selective serotonin reuptake inhibitor
- Local steroid injection in nerve involvement
- In resistant case—referred to pain clinic
- Surgical management: Conservative laparoscopic surgery in endometriosis, pelvic adhesions. Neurolysis consists of nerve transection or injection of neurotoxic chemical. Presacral neurectomy (PSN), laparoscopic uterine nerve ablation (LUNA) are two procedures attempted for pain reduction. Hysterectomy is done as last resort but not always effective to reduce pain completely.
- Others: Pelvic floor physical therapy, local steroid injection in nerve involvement, nerve blocks or neuromodulation by surgical implanted device, behavioral interventions (hybrid of cognitive psychotherapy and physiotherapy), ear acupuncture and Chinese herbal medicine.
  Chronic pelvic pain should be considered a regional pain syndrome or functional somatic syndrome in absence of known etiology and a biopsychosocial approach should be considered.

Monitoring: A numeric pain scale is useful to quantify and measure any change in pain.

Treatment Protocol

- If cause is explored treatment is done according to the disease, e.g., endometriosis, adenomyosis, PID, adhesions. Irritable bowel syndrome, interstitial cystitis, painful bladder syndrome—refer to respective discipline, etc.
- When cause is not known the options in order of sequence are:
  - Simple analgesic: NSAIDs, paracetamol, opiates
  - Hormonal treatment as therapeutic trial—COC pill, LNG-IUS, GnRH-analogues.
  - Tricyclic antidepressant (amitriptyline, nortriptyline, gabapentin, pregabalin) or selective serotonin reuptake inhibitor in suspected neuropathic pain and underlying mood disorder.

OVARIAN REMNANT SYNDROME AND OVARIAN RETENTION SYNDROME

Q. What is ovarian remnant syndrome and what is ovarian retention syndrome?

Symptoms created by remnants of excised ovary is called ovarian remnant syndrome whereas symptoms arising from of an ovary intentionally left during previous gynecological surgery is known as ovarian retention syndrome or residual ovary syndrome.

In both cases evaluation is necessary by history taking, careful pelvic examination and investigations by sonography and/or CT, MRI. Surgical treatment is often needed by laparoscopy or laparotomy.

Pelvic Congestion Syndrome

Q. What is pelvic congestion syndrome?

Pelvic congestion syndrome is due to tortuous and congested ovary due to retrograde flow of blood through incompetent valves. Dilatation of pelvic veins in late pregnancy, ovarian hormonal imbalance and estrogen are thought to be involved in pathophysiology of pelvic congestion syndrome

Patient complains of heaviness and chronic pelvic pain and worsens premenstrually. Bimanual examination reveals tenderness at the junction of outer and middle third of a line drawn in between anterior superior iliac spine and symphysis pubis. There may be varicosities in vagina, perineum and thigh.

Diagnosis is done by pelvic venography or by sonography, CT, MRI and laparoscopy to visualize varicosity.

Treatment options: Medical—progestogen (MPA) or GnRH agonists. Embolization or ligation of ovarian vein, and hysterectomy.

CHAPTER 17

A Case of Vesicovaginal Fistula and Urinary Incontinence

CHAPTER OUTLINE

Writing a case of vesicovaginal fistula (VVF) and how to present the case?

- Diagnosis of VVF—Sim's Triad
- Types of VVF
- Management of VVF
- Repair of VVF—Steps of Surgery
- Anatomy of Ureter
- Ureteric Injury—Management

Stress Incontinence:
- Types
- Pathophysiology
- Diagnosis—Evaluation
- Management—Kelly-Burch Colposuspension
- TVT and TOT—Detailed Surgical Steps

HISTORY TAKING

Patient's Particulars
Patient of obstetric fistula usually comes from low socioeconomic status or neglected medical background.

History
- *Chief complaint/complaints*: Patient usually complains:
  - Continuous leakage of urine per vagina
  - Cannot pass urine herself through via naturalis
  - Emission of offensive uriniferous odor
  - Itching around the vulva (pruritus).
- *History of present illness*: Detailed history is taken when she first noticed this leakage of urine. Following an obstructed and prolonged labor fistula usually develops 4–7 days after delivery due to sloughing after ischemic necrosis. Following an operative delivery or hysterectomy she complains of leakage of urine from the very first day of the procedure (operative fistula). Sometimes, ureteric fistula presents little late after surgery. Whether there is any history of trauma over the genitalia like fall on a sharp object. History of tuberculosis and cervical malignancy are important to diagnose infective or malignant fistula, respectively.
- *Menstrual history*: Routine history is taken. Sometime, there may be secondary amenorrhea.
- *Obstetric history:*
  - Parity-obstetric fistula is more common in primipara
  - Living issue:
  - Last child birth:

  It is taken in tabular form in usual manner.

Serial no.	Year and month	Pregnancy events	Labor events	Mode of delivery	Puerperium or postabortal period	Baby

History of prolonged labor, obstructed labor, any vaginal instrumental delivery, and cesarean section are noted. Home delivery or instrumental delivery is also noted. The day of appearance of urinary leakage is enquired.

- *Past history*:
  - Medical: Tuberculosis, malignancy, and history of radiotherapy.
  - Surgical: History of any type of previous surgery is taken. Whether the complaint is following abdominal

or vaginal hysterectomy or there is any other vaginal operation.
- *Family history*:
- *Social history*: Socially isolated due to offensive odor from her body. Looks irritable.
- *Functional history*: Patient cannot pass urine herself; there is continuous leakage of urine. Any incontinence of stool may be due to complete perineal tear (CPT) or low rectal fistula.
- *Personal history*: Insomnia.
- *Contraceptive history*:
- *Drug history*:

PHYSICAL EXAMINATION

- Detailed general survey is recorded
- Usually patient had poor nutritional status
- Short stature in obstetric fistula suggests contracted pelvis.

Systemic Examination
Routinely cardiovascular system, respiratory system, gastrointestinal systems, and urinary systems are examined.

Examination of Breasts
Routinely done.

GYNECOLOGICAL EXAMINATION

Abdominal Examination
Routine inspection, palpation, and percussion (if required) are done. There may be scar of cesarean section or other abdominal surgery.

Vaginal Examination
Woman is examined in *dorsal supine position*, in thigh flexed and knee flexed condition.

Bad uriniferous smell is obtained from long distance. Patient usually lies on a rubber cloth on bed. (For undergraduate examination, only inspection is allowed).

- *Inspection*:
  - Vulva and labial skin is excoriated, redness, wet and sometimes with ulceration and scratch marks.
  - Continuous leakage of urine through the introitus may be visible.
  - Uriniferous smell is emitted from the body.
- *Speculum examination*: It is done in:
  - Dorsal lithotomy position
  - Knee chest position or
  - Sims' position (*see* below).

With the help of Sims' speculum perineum is retracted and anterior vaginal wall is seen.
Site of fistula, number of fistula, size, and fistulous margins are noted. A large fistula is identified by protrusion of mucosa through the fistulous opening.

A catheter (metal or rubber) introduced through the external urethra can be seen through fistulous opening. Condition of cervix and vagina is noted.
On the posterior wall, presence of any rectal fistula and CPT is searched for.

- *Palpation*: Fistula is palpated; its size, margin, and fixity are assessed. Inspectory findings are confirmed. Bimanual examination is also done. Condition of cervix, rectum, and uterus is noted.

Rectal examination and rectovaginal examination are also done to detect any CPT and rectal fistula.

SUMMARY OF THE CASE (SAMPLE SUMMARY)

Mrs XY, a 24-year-old woman, para 1+0 with no living issue coming from a low socioeconomic status was admitted on.... with history of continuous leakage of urine per vagina since last 6 months following a difficult vaginal delivery after prolong labor giving a birth of a stillborn baby. Patient first observed urinary leakage 7 days after the childbirth.

On general examination, her general condition is poor, short stature (4 ft 6 inches) weight is, pallor-mild, pulse/min, and normotensive.

Per abdominal examination revealed nothing and on vaginal examination was done; there was gush of urine coming out of vagina with redness, wetend excoriated labial and vulvar skin (no need of further examination in UG examination).

On speculum examination, fistula was found (describe accordingly as your finding) and palpatory findings are noted as described later.

INVESTIGATIONS SUPPLIED OR REQUIRED

Investigations supplied are Hb%, routine blood count (TC, DC, ESR), urine analysis, ABO, Rh factor, urine examination, blood sugar, urea, creatinine, X-ray chest, ECG, and any urodynamic study report.

PROVISIONAL DIAGNOSIS

A case of genitourinary (GU) fistula (describe type, site, noumber, etc., if vaginal examination is done).

DIFFERENTIAL DIAGNOSIS

Differential diagnosis includes stress or urge incontinence, ureterovaginal fistula, vesicovaginal fistula, and urethrovaginal fistula.

Q. Why are you saying it is genitourinary fistula?

- By symptoms—chief complaints, history of present illness, and obstetric history
- Signs—inspectory and palpatory findings (as written in case taking)
- A metal catheter when introduced through the external urethra can be seen through fistulous opening (in case of big fistula).

Diagnosis of Genitourinary Fistula

Patient's profile:
- Patient usually comes from low socioeconomic status or neglected medical background
- Young primipara.

Symptoms

Patient usually complains:
- Continuous leakage of urine per vagina
- Cannot pass urine herself through via naturalis
- Emission of offensive uriniferous odor
- Itching around the vulva (pruritus).

Timing of first leakage of urine—following an obstructed and prolonged labor fistula usually develops 4–7 days after delivery due to sloughing after ischemic necrosis. Following an operative delivery or hysterectomy she complains of leakage of urine from the very first day of the procedure (operative fistula). Sometimes, ureteric fistula presents little late after surgery.

There may be history of trauma over the genitalia like fall on a sharp object. History of tuberculosis and cervical malignancy is important to diagnose infective or malignant fistula, respectively.

- *Menstrual history:* It is usually normal. Occasionally, there may be secondary amenorrhea— exact cause is not known, probably central in origin.
- *Obstetric history*: Obstetric fistula is more common in primipara. There may be history of prolonged labor, obstructed labor, followed by instrumental delivery or cesarean delivery.
- Socially isolated due to offensive odor from her body, irritable. History of insomnia.
- History of malignancy and tuberculosis.
- History of surgery—abdominal or vaginal hysterectomy or there is any other vaginal operation in case of operative fistula.

Signs

- General survey
- Usually patient had poor nutritional status
- Short stature in obstetric fistula
- Looks irritable.

Local Examination

- *Inspection*:
    - Vulva and labial skin is excoriated, redness, wet and sometimes with ulceration and scratch marks
    - Continuous leakage of urine through the introitus may be visible
    - Uriniferous smell is emitted from the body.
- *Speculum examination*: With the help of Sims' speculum perineum is retracted and anterior vaginal wall is seen **(Figs. 1 and 2)**. Site of fistula, number of fistula, and fistulous margins are noted. A large fistula is identified by protrusion of mucosa through the fistulous opening. A catheter (metal or rubber) introduced through the external urethra can be seen through fistulous opening **(Fig. 3)**. Condition of cervix and vagina is noted. On the posterior wall, there may be rectal fistula and CPT.

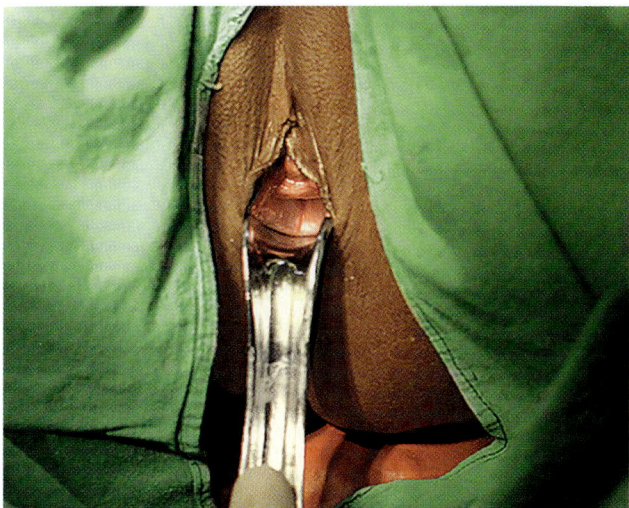

Fig. 1: Examination in dorsal position by retracting the posterior vaginal wall with Sims' speculum.

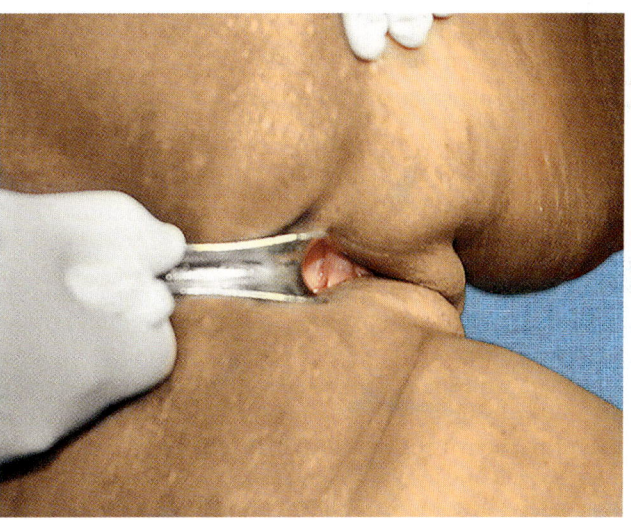

Fig. 2: Examination in Sims' position with the help of Sims' speculum. Note the anterior wall is visible well.

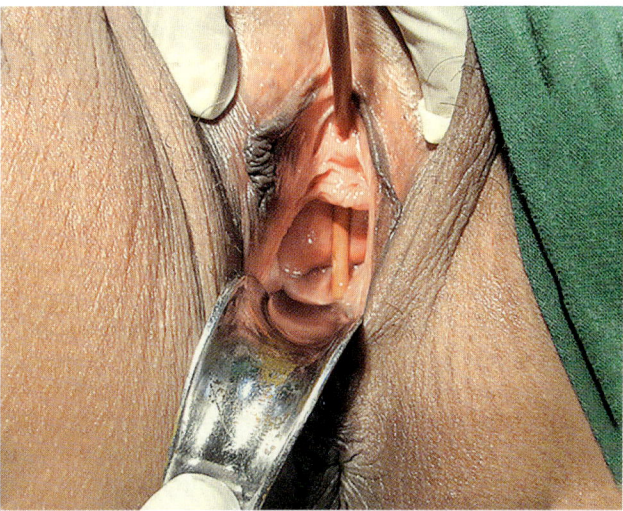

Fig. 3: Catheter introduced through urethra is visible inside vagina indicating presence of fistula.

- *Palpation*: Fistula is palpated; its size may be small to large, margin and fixity are assessed. There may be multiple in number. Inspectory findings are confirmed.
  Bimanual examination is also done. Condition of cervix, rectum, and uterus is noted.
  Rectal examination and rectovaginal examination are also done to detect any CPT and rectal fistula.

Q. Sometimes vaginal discharge may be confused with excessive vaginal discharge. How would you differentiate?

By creatinine level of the fluid. Creatinine level of urine is usually greater than 17 mg/100 mL, may be higher value with a mean of 113.5 mg/100 mL.

Q. You are not sure of fistula, how will you confirm?

By dye test using methylene blue or indigo carmine.

Q. How would you perform the dye test?

A diluted solution containing methylene blue or indigo carmine is instilled into the bladder through the urethra by a catheter and anterior wall is inspected. Dye is seen coming through the fistula and site is also determined. Sterile milk can also be used. Usually, 200 mL solution is sufficient. In ureterovaginal fistula, dye is not visible.

Q. What is three swab test? Why it is done? How it is done?

Three swab test is done to detect small fistula and to determine the location. This test is also called "tampon test".

Procedure

Three pieces of cotton wool swab or gauze are placed into the vagina, one in the upper part of vagina, one in middle part, and last one in lower part of vagina near introitus and the bladder is instilled with 300 mL of diluted solution of methylene blue or indigo carmine through a catheter. The patient is asked to do normal activity or walk for 15–30 minutes and the swabs are removed one by one and inspected.

Inference

If the lower one is soaked with dye, it is likely due to urethral incontinence. Cotton swab of middle part of urethra stained with dye indicates midvaginal vesicovaginal fistula. The swab of uppermost part of vagina is stained with dye in case of upper vesicovaginal or vesico-cervico-vaginal fistula. The uppermost swab not stained with dye but soaked with urine is indicative of ureterovaginal fistula.

Q. What is pyridium and three swab combined test (combined dye test)?

This is done to detect the ureteral involvement.

Phenazopyridine hydrochloride (pyridium) when given orally acts as bladder analgesia and the color of urine becomes orange. A few hours before three swab test to be done patient is given oral 200 mg pyridium tablet and then three swab test is done.

If uppermost swab is stained orange ureteric fistula is likely and if both uppermost swab becomes orange stained and middle swab becomes blue both ureter and bladder involvement is suspected.

Q. What are the other tests used for diagnosis of GU fistula?
- Cystoscopy or cystourethroscopy
- Intravenous urography or retrograde pyelography or voiding cystourethrography.

Q. Which one is very important diagnostic method for GU fistula?

Cystoscopy, better to say cystourethroscopy.

Q. How does cystourethroscopy help?
- It helps to locate the site of the fistula
- To diagnose total number of fistulae
- Relation of fistula with orifice, the knowledge of which is very important for management
- Evaluation of marginal mucosa of fistulous opening.

Q. How would you do the cystoscopy if there is large fistula?

Fistula opening is temporarily blocked by introducing Foley catheter and then cystoscopy is done.

Q. What is the role of intravenous pyelography?

Condition of kidney and ureter is assessed by intravenous pyelography (IVP). Retrograde pyelography and IV urography can be done. Voiding cystourethrography is also helpful to diagnose the number and position of fistulas.

SUMMARY OF DIAGNOSIS

- Symptoms
- Signs
- Introduction of metal catheter
- Dye test
- Three swab test
- Combined dye test
- Cystourethroscopy
- IVP.

Genital Fistula

Q. What do you mean by genital fistula?

Genital fistula means where there is abnormal communication between the genital tract (vagina, cervix, and uterus) and the urinary (ureter, bladder, and urethra) or alimentary tract singly or in combination.

Q. How would you classify genital fistula?
- Genitourinary
- Genitofecal
- Vaginoperineal.

Q. How would you classify genitourinary fistula?
- Based on anatomy
- Based on complex or simple nature of fistula
- New classification (Goh, 2004).

Classification of GU fistula based on anatomy: All types of communication may occur except urethra-uterine **(Fig. 4)**:

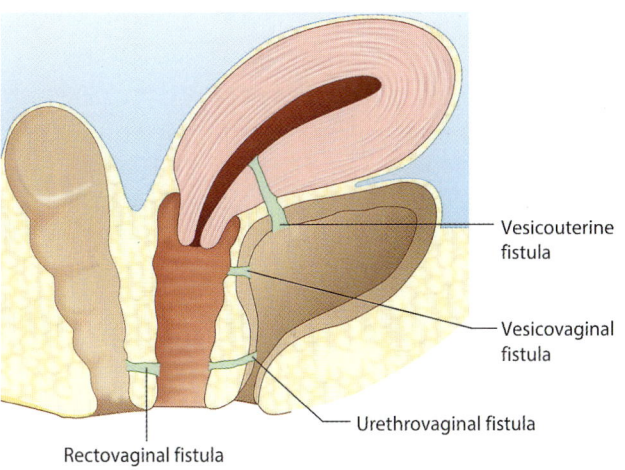

Fig. 4: Varieties of fistula—vesicouterine, vesicovaginal, urethrovaginal and rectovaginal fistula.

- *Vesical fistula*: Vesicovaginal fistula (VVF), vesicocervical, and vesicouterine
- *Ureteric fistula*: Ureterovaginal, ureterocervical, and ureterouterine
- *Urethral fistula*: Urethrovaginal and urethrocervical.

Classification of VVF based on complexity:
- *Simple*: Less than 2–3 cm measurement, located near the cuff (supratrigonal), normal vaginal length, and no history of radiation or malignancy.
- *Complicated*: More than 3 cm measurement, located away from cuff (trigonal), small vaginal length history of radiation, and malignancy present.

New classifications (Goh, 2004) of GU fistula:
This classification is based on the distance from the external urinary meatus (EUM), size, extent of fibrosis and vaginal length, or special considerations.
Based on the distance from the external urinary meatus:
- Type 1—distal margin of fistula more than 3.5 cm from EUM
- Type 2—distal margin of fistula more than 2.5–3.5 cm from EUM
- Type 3—distal margin of fistula more than 1.5–2.5 cm from EUM
- Type 4—distal margin of fistula less than 1.5 cm from EUM.

Based on size:
- Size less than 1.5 cm in the largest diameter
- Size 1.5–3 cm in the largest diameter
- Size more than 3 cm in the largest diameter.

Based on extent of fibrosis:
- None or only mild fibrosis (around fistula and/or vagina) and/or vaginal length more than 6 cm, normal capacity
- Moderate or severe fibrosis (around fistula and/or vagina) and/or reduced vaginal length and/or capacity

- Special consideration, e.g., postradiation, ureteric involvement, circumferential fistula, or previous repair.

Types of vesicovaginal fistula:
- High vaginal—in upper part of vagina like posthysterectomy VVF
- Mid vaginal—in central position of vagina
- Low vaginal—low in vagina.

Q. Write the different etiological causes of VVF.

Mostly acquired, rarely congenital.
- *Obstetric causes*: In developing countries, 90% of GU fistulas are from obstetric trauma, specifically obstructed labor.
    - Obstetric trauma: Obstructed labor—ischemic necrosis—infection—sloughing-fistula formation after first week of delivery, female circumcision, or female genital mutilation are important cause of introital injury.
    - Obstetric operations: Instrumental-destructive operation, forceps and abdominal-rupture uterus, and cesarean section.
- *Gynecological or pelvic surgery:* In developed countries, 90% VVF are following pelvic surgery, 80–90% by obstetrician-gynecologists, and rest by urologists or general surgeons.
- *Other causes:*
    - Malignancy—advanced cancer cervix, vagina or bladder
    - Radiation—develops after 1–2 years
    - Trauma or foreign body—fall on a pointed object, sexual assault, fracture of pelvic bone, forgotten pessary, bladder calculi, mesh used in tension in sling operation.
    - Infective—tuberculosis, lymphogranuloma venereum, actinomycosis, and autoimmune disease, etc.

Q. Which is the most common pelvic surgery causing VVF?

Hysterectomy is responsible for 75% cases.

Incidence

The **overall incidence** of VVF following hysterectomy is 0.8/1,000 cases; highest following laparoscopic hysterectomy is 2/1,000, abdominal is 1/1,000 and following vaginal hysterectomy, it is 0.2/1,000 procedures.

Milestones of Genital Fistula

- Documentation of genital fistulae dates back to 2050 BC when a CPT was discovered in Egyptian mummy.
- Roonhuyse from Amsterdam is the first to report in 1676 the surgical correction of genital fistula.
- J Marian Sims (1813–1883) of the United States of America was the first to repair VVF successfully in 1852 and is called the pioneer of VVF surgery. The first speculum used by Sims was a bent spoon.
- Mahfouz of Egypt is called the greatest fistula expert in the world because of personal experience of more than 1,000 fistulae cases.

Q. Who was Marion Sims?

See above.

Q. What is Sims' triad?
- Sims' position
- Sims' speculum and
- Silver wire suture originally used by JM Sims.

Q. Describe Sims' position (Figs. 5 and 6).
- Patient in left lateral position with left arm behind.
- Both legs are flexed. Right leg is more flexed than left. (*see also* **Fig. 33**, Chapter 1)

Q. How would you manage a case of vesicovaginal fistula?
Surgical local repair is the treatment. However, occasionally small VVF may spontaneously heal following continuous bladder drainage.

Q. What is the role of conservative management?
When the diameter of fistula opening is small (up to 2 cm) immediate continuous bladder drainage for 2–8 weeks the fistula may heal. Many studies agree to provide conservative management in fistulous size of 1 cm or less. It is said that if it does not heal within 4 weeks unlikely that it will heal.

Effectivity of fibrin sealant monotherapy is not proved yet.

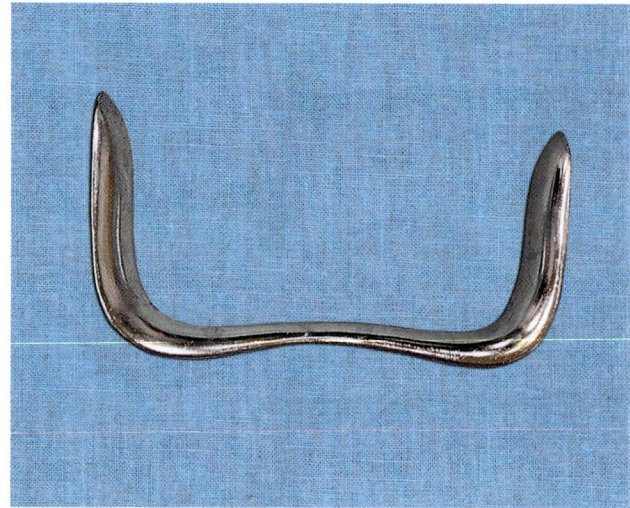

Fig. 6: Sims' speculum.

Q. Which is the best time to repair?
- If it is detected within 24 hours immediate repair is done
- As most of the fistula becomes evident in second week, continuous bladder drainage is done for 6–8 weeks expecting spontaneous healing. If it persists, it is repaired after 3 months.

Optimal time of repair is 3–6 months **(Figs. 7 and 8)**. Recently, earlier repair is advocated with similar success.

Q. What are the different approaches of surgical treatment of VVF and which one is preferred?
- Vaginal
- Abdominal.

It depends on the type of fistula and surgeon's choice.
In general, gynecologists prefer vaginal approach and urologist through abdominal approach.
Obstetric fistulas are better dealt through vaginal route and high up fistula especially after hysterectomy is done through abdominal route.

Advantages of vaginal approach:
- Direct and satisfactory
- Inflicts minimum injury to patient
- Strong vaginal wall is used
- Shorter operative times, shorter hospital stay
- Less blood loss
- It allows use of ureteric stents if needed.

Indications of abdominal approach:
- Fistula is at very high up not is accessible well from below
- Previous unsuccessful repair
- Vagina is stenosed
- Vaginal tissue is fibrosed and mobilization is difficult
- Associated with suspected ureteric involvement
- Need for abdominal graft, either omental or peritoneal
- Very near to ureteric opening
- Fistula is big and complex in nature.

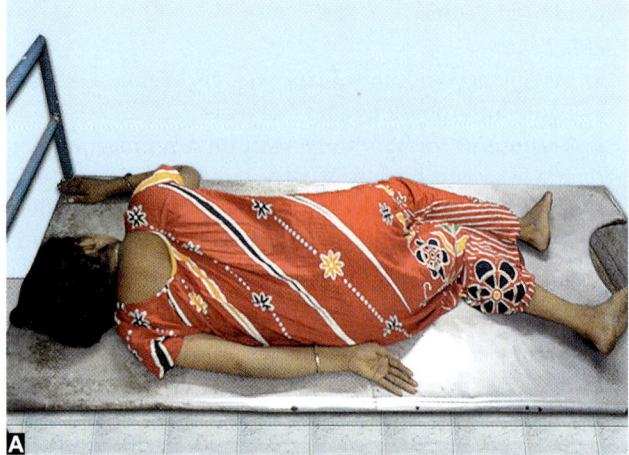

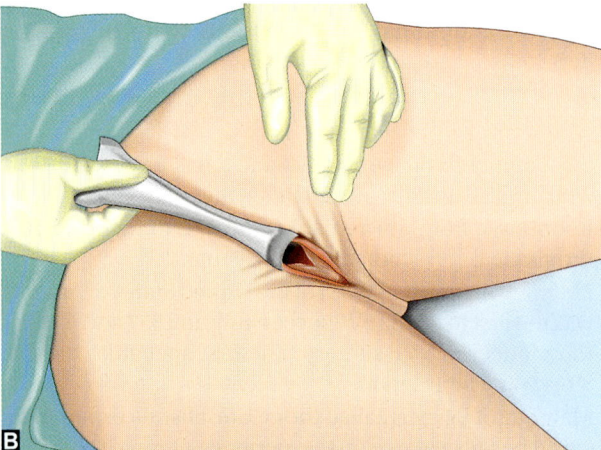

Figs. 5A and B: (A) Sims' position. Patient in left lateral position with left arm behind, both legs are flexed. Right leg is more flexed than left; (B) Sims' speculum to retract posterior vaginal wall.

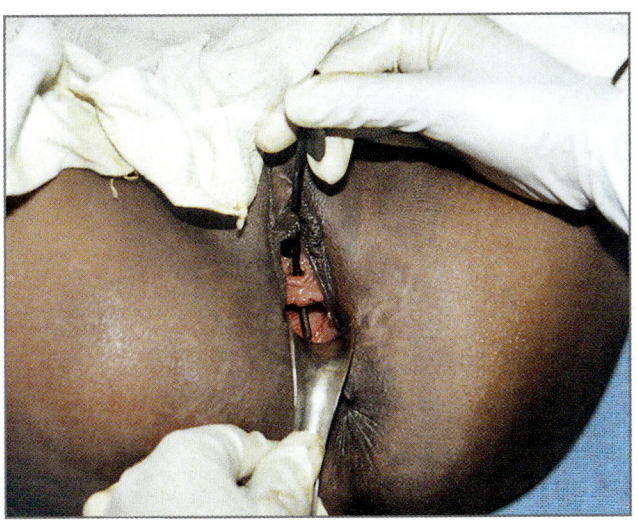

Fig. 7: Vesicovaginal fistula (VVF).

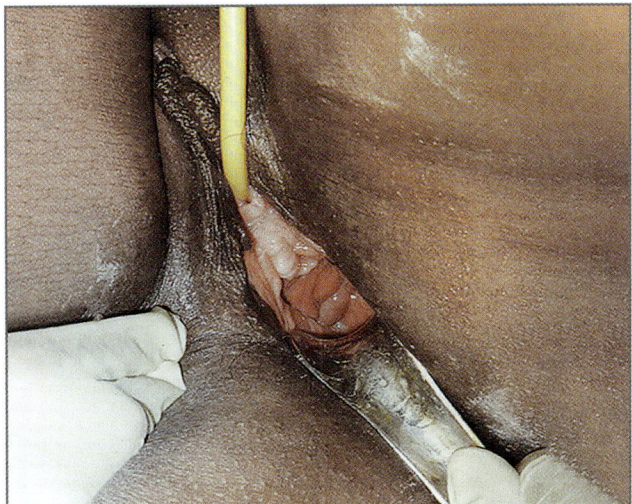

Fig. 8: Healed VVF after repair as in Figure 7.

Figs. 7 and 8: Vesicovaginal fistula (VVF) following obstructed labor. A 20-year-old primipara 4 feet 10 inch height attended with gaping of episiotomy and incontinence of urine with history of forceps delivery of a stillborn baby following a prolonged labor in eclampsia 1 month back. She noticed leakage of urine at home 8 days after delivery. VVF was of 1.5 cm diameter and urethra was patulous. VVF was repaired through vaginal approach 5 months after delivery in 3 layers. First layer with 3-0 Vicryl, second layer with 3-0 Vicryl, and vaginal mucosa with 2-0 Vicryl stitches. She was discharged after 3 weeks with complete cure.

The woman came with pregnancy of 12 weeks after one and half years (Fig. 8; Healed VVF). She was antenatally cared and elective cesarean section was done at term delivering a healthy female baby weighing 2.9 kg. The age of that girl at present is 12 years. Mother is well and did not take further issue.

Principles of Repair

- Maintenance of adequate asepsis
- Good exposure
- Complete removal of scar tissue making availability of viable tissue in surrounding
- Good mobilization
- Suturing without tension
- Repair in multilayer
- Use of appropriate suture material
- Proper hemostasis
- Postoperative bladder drainage for prolong period.

Q. What are the various types of vaginal surgery?

- Vaginal flap splitting technique
- Sims' saucerization (edge-pairing technique)
- Latzko vaginal repair.

Difficult vaginal surgery using graft:
- Using bulbospongiosus (Martius graft)
- Using gracilis muscle transplantation (Ingelman-Sundberg).

Preoperative care and investigations before surgery:
- Confirmation of diagnosis—as above
- Physical examination
- Routine preoperative investigations
- *Urine for culture sensitivity*: Urine is collected by sterile Sims' speculum or by transurethral catheterization after blocking the fistula by a Foley catheter.

Vaginal Approach—Flap Splitting Method (Figs. 9 to 12)

- Position of the patient—high lithotomy or Sims' position (**Fig. 13**)
- Anesthesia—general anesthesia or regional
- Incision—a circular incision 1–2 cm surrounding the fistulas opening (**Fig. 9**)
- A vertical or horizontal incision is made extending the encircling incision on two sides
- Flaps of vaginal wall are dissected from bladder wall on two sides and mobilized (**Fig. 9**)
- Fistula margin scar tissue is excised (**Fig. 9**)
- Repair in three layers (**Figs. 10 to 12**):
    1. Bladder wall with 3-0 delayed absorbable interrupted avoiding bladder mucosa
    2. Second layer over bladder inverting the first layer with interrupted 3-0 sutures
    3. Third layer is the approximation of vaginal flaps with 3-0 delayed absorbable interrupted stitches.

  All sutures will be tension free. Following second layer bladder is filled with 100 mL of fluid to test water tightness.
- Cystoscopy is done finally to check repaired site and ureteral patency to exclude its involvement.

Postoperative Care

- Continuous bladder drainage with Foley catheter for at least 10 days. Catheter is changed every 5 days. In some centers, catheter is kept for 3 weeks.
- Following repair of large fistula bladder drainage through suprapubic cystostomy is suggested.

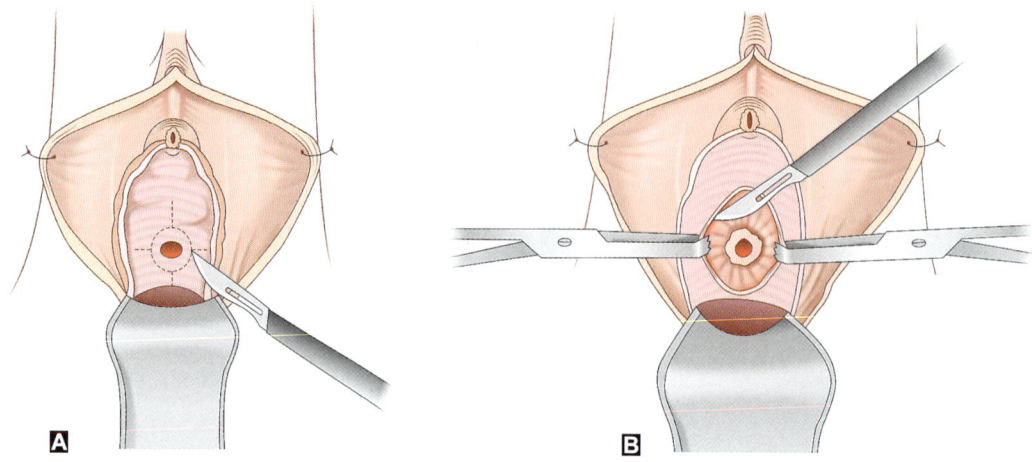

Figs. 9A and B: (A) Flap splitting method of vesicovaginal fistula repair. A circular incision is given surrounding the fistula; (B) Vaginal wall dissected, mobilized, and scar tissue removed.

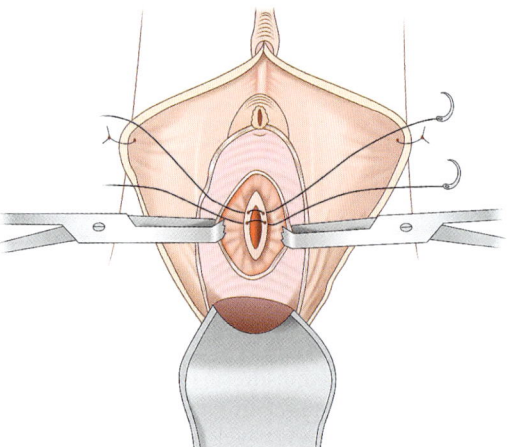

Fig. 10: Flap splitting method of vesicovaginal fistula repair. Bladder wall repaired with 3-0 delayed absorbable avoiding bladder mucosa.

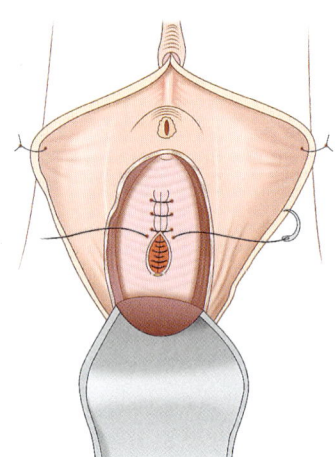

Fig. 12: Flap splitting method of vesicovaginal fistula repair. Third layer is the approximation of vaginal flaps with 3-0 delayed absorbable interrupted stitches.

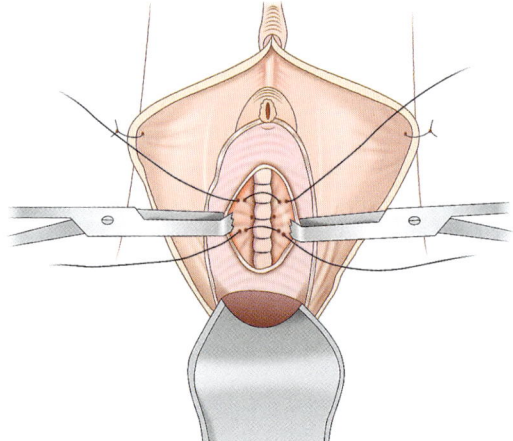

Fig. 11: Flap splitting method of vesicovaginal fistula repair. Second layer over bladder inverting the first layer with interrupted 3-0 sutures.

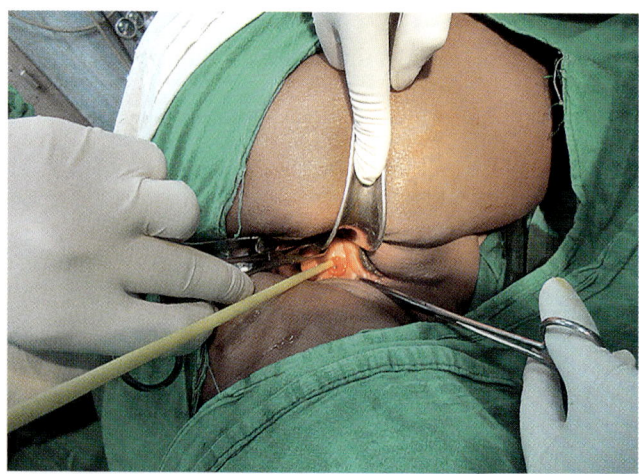

Fig. 13: Repair of vesicovaginal fistula in Sims' position. A Foley (small) catheter is introduced, inflated and traction is done to make the fistula's margin prominent.
Courtesy: Professor RP Ganguly and Dr Sanjoy Mukherji

- Plenty of fluid by mouth
- Antibiotics
- Discharged after third week.

Advice Following Repair

- Abdominal delivery in next pregnancy
- Avoidance of coitus for 3 months
- Better to avoid pregnancy for 3 years
- If fails repair after 3 months.

Favorable Prognosis Following Repair

- Easily accessible fistula
- Site—midvaginal or juxtacervical, away from ureteric opening and urethral meatus
- Size—not big
- Margins are healthy, pliable
- First time repair
- Experienced surgeon
- Good postoperative care.

Sims' saucerization (edge-pairing technique)

- This is the classical method done when the fistulas opening is very small.
- After denuding the scar margin the fistula is repaired in single layer avoiding the bladder mucosa. No bladder mobilization is done.
- This method is not popular at present.

Latzko vaginal repair

- In this technique, part of the upper vagina (2–3 cm) is obliterated (partial colpocleisis). This method is preferred in posthysterectomy apical fistula (*see* Chapter 10, Pelvic Organ Prolapse Le Fort's operation).
- To bring the fistula in operative field either a pediatric catheter is introduced and after inflation of balloon the catheter is drawn or four stay sutures are given surrounding the fistula to draw the fistula and a mediolateral episiotomy may be needed for good exposure.
- A vaginal incision of 1–2 cm surrounding the tract is given, mobilized, and excised with scissors.
- Tract of the fistula may or may not be removed. If tract is excised bladder mucosa is approximated with 3-0 delayed absorbable suture.
- Then, anterior and posterior vaginal fibromuscular wall is apposed with interrupted 3-0 delayed absorbable sutures. A second layer and if needed a third line of sutures are given over the first fibromuscular layer.
- Bladder is tested for water tightness with 100 mL of fluid. If there is no water tightness further sutures are given.
- As there is shortening of vagina in this method, prior counseling especially for dyspareunia is mandatory.

Types of Abdominal Approach

- Transvesical
- Transperitoneal.

Abdominal Method of Repair

- A midline or Pfannenstiel incision is made to open the peritoneal cavity.
- Space of Retzius is opened and bladder is opened by extraperitoneal vertical incision on its dome (intentional cystotomy).
- Ureteral orifices and fistula are identified.
- Placement of ureteric tents is needed if the fistula is near to ureter. The incision is extended up to the fistula tract which is then excised.
- Vagina is dissected from the bladder by sharp dissection.
- Vagina is repaired with 2-0 delayed absorbable suture in two layers and the bladder is repaired with 3-0 delayed absorbable sutures in two layers covering the first layer by the second.
- Omentum may be mobilized and sutured with the anterior wall of vagina which will cover the incision line and also interpose between bladder and vagina.
- This will help better healing by increasing blood flow. Cystoscopy is helpful to detect ureteric inclusion and to see the repaired area.
- Postoperatively, both suprapubic and urethral drainage is given. Urethral drainage is removed first followed by suprapubic. For obstetric fistula, drainage is kept for 3 weeks, for surgical fistula 2 weeks and for radiation fistula it may need up to 6 weeks.

Principal Steps of Repair in Abdominal Route

It can be done by transvesical approach and transperitoneal approach.

- *Transvesical approach*: In this method, bladder is approached through suprapubic route and repaired by flap splitting technique.
- *Transperitoneal approach*: Following laparotomy, bladder and vaginal walls are separated and repaired separately.

Management of Irreparable VVF

- *Urinary diversion*:
  - Ureterocolic anastomosis
  - Ileal loop bladder.
- *Management of VVF with CPT*: Repair of VVF first followed by repair of CPT or rectovaginal fistula in the same sitting.

URETEROVAGINAL FISTULA

Q. What is the incidence of ureterovaginal fistula?

The incidence is 2% of all urinary fistula.

Ureter

Course, Anatomy, and Blood Supply of Pelvic Part of Ureter (Figs. 14 and 15)

Course (Figs. 14B and 15): Ureter enters into the pelvis by crossing over the bifurcation of common iliac artery (**Fig. 15B**) or the proximal part of external iliac artery and lying

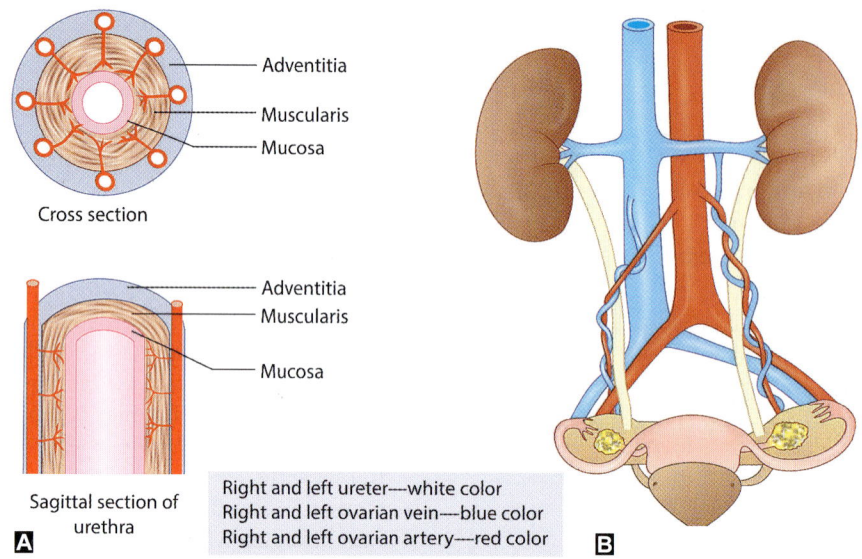

Figs. 14A and B: (A) Vasculature of ureter showing both in longitudinal and transverse section; (B) Course of ureter.

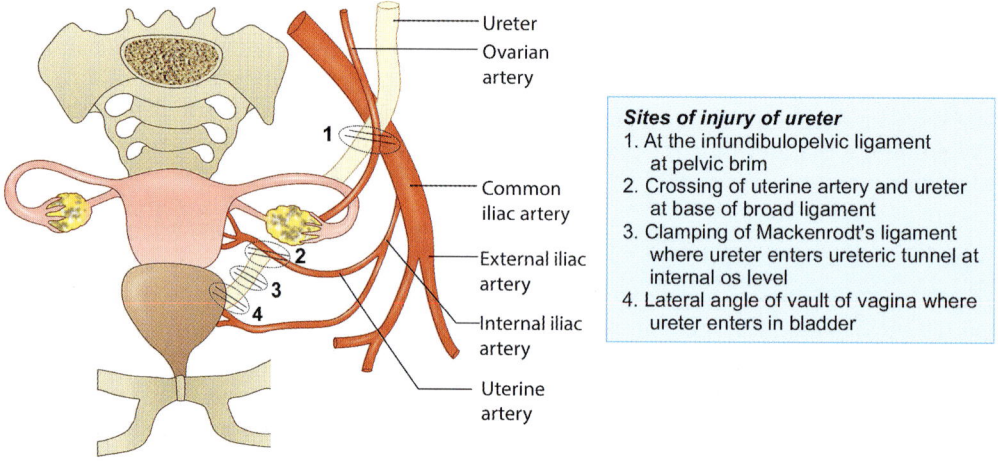

Fig. 15A: Course of ureter: Four danger points where injury of ureter may occur during hysterectomy.

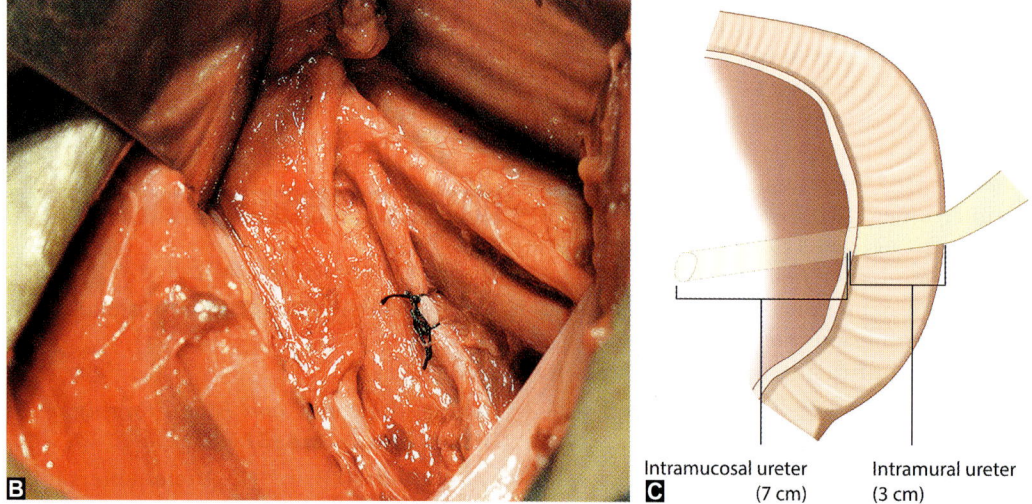

Figs. 15B and C: (B) Ureter crossing the common iliac artery above its bifurcation. Here, internal iliac is tied (left side); (C) Course of ureter inside the bladder.

medial to ovarian vessels and is retroperitoneal throughout its entire course.

It follows the course of internal iliac artery for a short distance slightly in front and medial to it until it passes near the ischial spine where it changes it direction. It courses anteriorly along the anterolateral aspect of uterosacral ligament, passes into the base of broad ligament to enter into the cardinal ligament *tunnel of Wertheim* 1–2 cm lateral to cervix.

Near the isthmus it courses under the uterine artery (water below the bridge) and passes lateral to anterior vaginal fornix, and passes anteromedially toward the bladder base and runs close to upper one-third of anterior vaginal wall. It finally enters the bladder and travels obliquely for 1–1.5 cm to open in ureteral orifice **(Fig. 15C)**.

Anatomy: Length of pelvic part of ureter is about 13 cm, total length 25–30 cm. It is a tubular structure. Diameter at the pelvic brim is 1 cm and at the bladder 0.5 cm. The wall is composed of fibromuscular tissue, inner and outer longitudinal and middle circular muscle layer and the mucous layer is lined by transitional epithelium.

Blood supply and surgical importance (Fig. 14A): Ureter is supplied by common iliac, external iliac, internal iliac, uterine artery, and superior vesicle arteries. Most of the blood supply *comes from lateral sides* as pelvic part of ureter lies medial to vessels in contrast to abdominal part which gets supply from medial side. This is very important during dissection of pelvic part of ureter so that lateral dissection should be less to prevent avascular damage which may cause ureteric fistula. Attempts should be made to keep the ureter as much as attached to adjacent peritoneum as possible. The anastomosis in ureteral adventitia is extensive and forms a longitudinal network.

Causes of Ureterovaginal Fistula

- Congenital—very rare
- Acquired—mostly following pelvic surgery e.g. difficult hysterectomy like endometriosis, pelvic inflammatory disease, cervical fibroid, broad ligament fibroid, radical hysterectomy in cancer cervix. In vaginal hysterectomy, there is also chance but less.

Types of Injury of Ureter

- Division by through and through cutting
- Partial occlusion by kinking or by crushing due to accidental clamping
- Ligature or clamping
- Devascularization resulting ischemic necrosis.

Q. How would you manage ureteric injury?

It should always be managed by consultation with urologist or a gynecologist trained in urogynecology training.

Management depends on whether it is identified during operation or diagnosed in postoperative period.

Ureteric Injury Diagnosed During Operation

Crush injury by ligature or clamp—the ligature or clamp is released and a ureteric tent is introduced.

Following ligation:
- End-to-end anastomosis
- Ureteroureteric anastomosis **(Fig. 14)** with opposite ureter or
- Reimplantation of the ureter into the bladder.

Q. How would you diagnose ureterovaginal fistula postoperatively?

- Escape of urine per vagina few days following a history of surgery, from drain or from surgical incision.
- Stormy postoperative period—abdominal distension and pain, rigor, fever due to urinoma formation.
- In unilateral injury, there may not be severe symptoms and kidney on that side becomes atrophy and nonfunctioning.
- Patient can pass urine per urethra as bilateral involvement is unlikely.
- Three swab test.
- Combined pyridium and three swab test.
- Ultrasonography may detect hydronephrosis or urinoma.
- A CT scan with/without contrast.
- Intravenous urography
- Cystoscopy—no urine is seen to come from damaged ureteric side.
- Serum creatinine.

Q. When does the fistula appear following an injury of ureter?

It depends on the type of injury sustained on ureter:
- In case of division or partial occlusion it occurs in *first week*
- Ligation and subsequent sloughing results fistula formation in *second week*
- Ischemic necrosis causes fistula formation in *third week onward*.

Danger Points of Injury of Ureter (see Fig. 15A)

Q. What are the danger points where injury may occur during hysterectomy (see Fig. 15A)?

- At the infundibulopelvic ligament at pelvic brim—during infundibulum ligament clamping.
- Crossing of uterine artery and ureter at the base of broad ligament during ligation of uterine artery.
- Clamping of Mackenrodt's ligament where ureter enters ureteric tunnel at internal os level.
- Lateral angle of vault of vagina where ureter enters the bladder during clamping or suturing of vaginal vault.

Q. How would you prevent ureteric injury?

- Surgeon must be ureteric conscious during pelvic surgery.
- Four danger points—1, 2, 3, 4—must be remembered and surgeon will be very careful during dealing with those areas; as above (*see* **Fig. 15A**).

- To separate the vesicouterine space adequately before clamping the uterine stump.
- The dictum is to cut nothing until ureter is identified and isolated in its entire extent.
- If in doubt always trace the ureter from pelvic brim by opening medial leaf of peritoneum.
- Too much skeletonization of ureter is prohibited in radical hysterectomy.
- During laparoscopy cautery at uterosacral region in endometriosis will be used very cautiously. Harmonic scalpel is better instrument for this.
- Preoperative IVP in pelvic pathologies altering ureteric course.
- Preoperative stenting.

Management of Ureteric Fistula

Detection during operation—placing of stent, anastomosis or implantation.

Postoperative detection:
- Transureteric anastomosis—ureter is anastomosed with opposite ureter **(Fig. 16)**
- End-to-end anastomosis—done over a ureteric catheter **(Figs. 17A and B)**
- Ureterovesical anastomosis **(Figs. 18A to E)** with/without bladder mobilization
- Using bladder flap (Boari's technique) **(Fig. 19)**
- Nephrostomy immediately followed by definite surgery in later date
- Nephrectomy.

Ureterovesical anastomosis (Figs. 18A to E):

Indication: Injury at the base of broad ligament or near the bladder so that it can be implanted in bladder.

Procedure of ureterovesical anastomosis (Figs. 18A to E)

The distal end of the proximal part of cut end of ureter is split longitudinally for 0.5 cm and fine suture is passed through

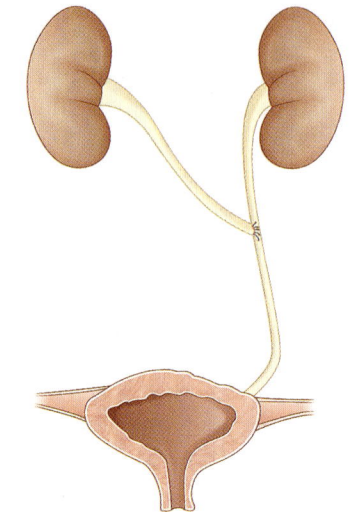

Fig. 16: Transureteric ureteroureteric anastomosis.

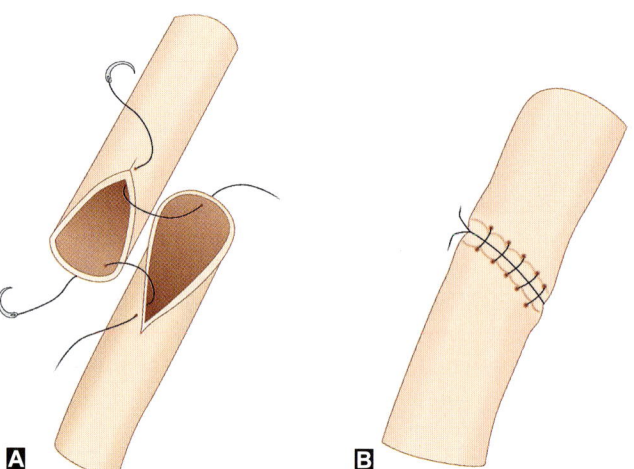

Figs. 17A and B: Ureteroureteric anastomosis.

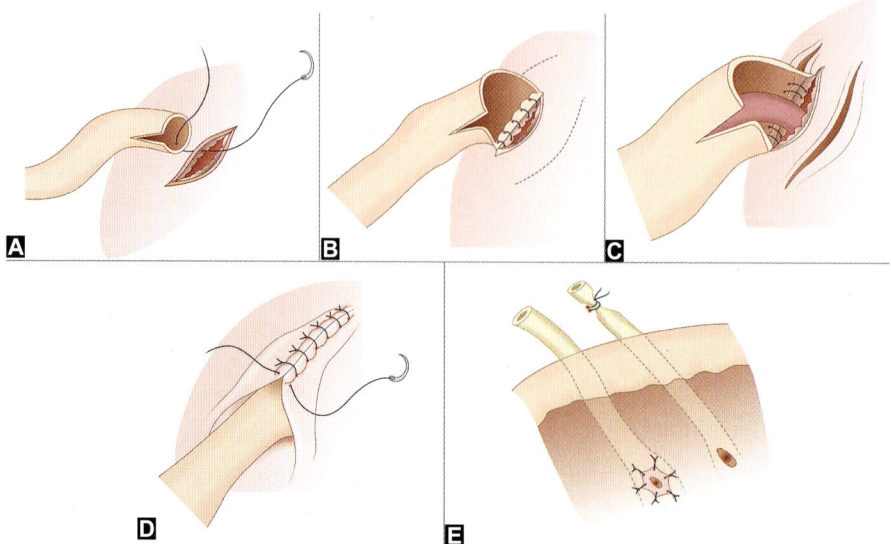

Figs. 18A to E: Ureterovesical anastomosis with ureteric catheter.

the flaps. A ureteric catheter is passed through the ureter and fixed.

The end of distal part of the ureter is tied. Cavity of the bladder is opened by 4 cm incision at the fundus. An artificial ureteric tunnel is made by putting an artery forceps inside the cavity near original orifice and pierced through the wall with small incision. The ureteric catheter and the threads are drawn inside the bladder by the forceps and ureteric wall is fixed to the bladder wall. The end of catheter is passed through the urethra to bring it through external urinary meatus (EUM). Bladder is closed in layers. To prevent the stenosis tunnel is made in such a way that the ureter traverses through the wall obliquely to some extent not directly through and through.

Ureterovesical anastomosis with bladder flap (Boari's flap method) **(Fig. 19)**:

In case, fistula is high up a tongue of bladder wall is separated from the bladder wall and made ureteric like tube and anastomosis is done without tension **(Fig. 19)**.

Rectovaginal Fistula

This is due to abnormal communication between rectum and vagina with epithelial lined tracts. This results because of involuntary escape of flatus and feces into the vagina. The details are described in the Chapter 18, Complete Perineal Tear.

URINARY INCONTINENCE

Q. What do you mean by urinary incontinence?

Urinary incontinence is defined as involuntary leakage of urine.

Types

- *Urethral*:
  - Stress incontinence
  - Urge incontinence
  - Mixed incontinence (stress and urge)
  - Others (overflow, neurogenic, etc.).
- *Extraurethral*:
  - Vesicovaginal fistula
  - Ureterovaginal fistula
  - Other congenital defect of lower urinary tract (ectopia vesicae and ectopic ureter).

Sometimes, a term is used known as *"true incontinence"* which is continuous leakage of urine. The conditions are any genitourinary fistula, development anomaly, and urethral dilatation and stretching.

Stress incontinence is involuntary leakage of urine during coughing or sneezing, laughing or due to increase of intra-abdominal pressure. It is the most common type of incontinence.

Urge incontinence is the involuntary leakage of urine with awareness accompanied or preceded by voiding urge.

Overflow incontinence is an old term used in an entity when woman cannot empty her bladder resulting retention of urine and incontinence occurs in urgency and recently, it is considered as one variant of urge incontinence.

Overactive bladder: It is a condition of urinary urgency with/without incontinence and usually associated with daytime frequency and nocturia.

Q. What is urodynamic stress incontinence and genuine stress incontinence?

When symptom or sign of stress urinary incontinence (SUI) is confirmed by objective urodynamic study in absence of detrusor muscle contraction it is called urodynamic stress incontinence and previously it was known as genuine stress incontinence.

Detrusor Overactivity or Detrusor Instability

When urge incontinence is confirmed by urodynamic study, it is called detrusor overactivity (DO) and previously, it was known as detrusor instability (DI).

Bladder Filling and Emptying: Mechanism of Micturition

Bladder is filled and becomes emptied by voiding in a cycle, called micturition cycle. Detrusor muscle due to its three smooth muscles layers arrangement in plexiform fashion has huge capacity to expand during filling of bladder.

When the capacity of bladder is reached, stretch receptors send sensory signals. The sphincter becomes closed by inhibition from cortex through the spinal voiding reflex till a convenient place of voiding is available in case of adult woman.

As soon as the voluntary inhibition is withdrawn bladder starts to be emptied by relaxation of pelvic floor and urethral sphincters and contraction of detrusor in a synchronization fashion.

Parasympathetic cholinergic nerves supply the detrusor for contraction and urethral sphincter is supplied by both sympathetic and somatic nerves (pudendal nerves).

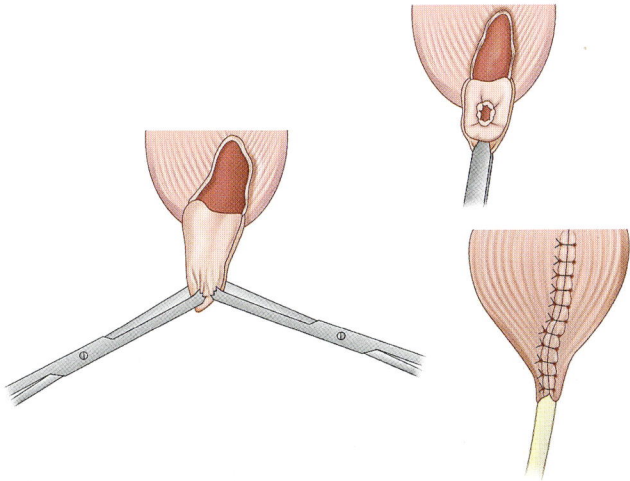

Fig. 19: Ureterovesical anastomosis with bladder flap (Boari's flap method).

Q. **How continence is maintained?**

Continence is maintained by anatomical support and sphincter support.

* *Anatomical support (Figs. 20A and B):* Neck of bladder and urethra are supported by pubourethral ligament, arcus tendineus fascia, vagina, and its fascia and levator ani muscles.

  In normal continent woman, increase of abdominal pressure is transmitted equally to bladder, base of the bladder, and neck **(Fig. 20A)**.

  When support is lost, there is hypermobility of urethra and urethra is not retained in position. There is loss of pressure transmission to the urethra; urethra and bladder neck become unable to close resulting reduced urethral closing pressure which in turn makes the loss of continence **(Fig. 20B)**. This is most common variety. The basis of colposuspension operation like Burch and MMK procedures is to restore this anatomical support.

* *Sphincter support*: Continence is maintained by urethral mucosa, urethral vasculature, urethral epithelium, and surrounding urethral musculature.

  Three muscles form the sphincteric complex namely, *sphincter urethrae, urethrovaginal sphincter, and compressor urethrae*.

  Urethral epithelium is highly vascular in premenopausal women and is a contributory factor for continence.

The inner to outer layers in urethra are:

1. Mucosa
2. Submucosa (lamina propria) with vascular plexus
3. Longitudinal smooth muscle layer
4. Circular smooth muscle layer, and
5. Striated urogenital sphincter muscles.

Intrinsic sphincteric defect:

Urinary incontinence may occur in defect of these components by preventing urethral closure and is called *intrinsic sphincteric defect (ISD)* and urethra behaves like "lead pipe".

Diabetic neuropathy, degenerative neuropathy, pelvic surgery, hypoestrogenemia, pelvic radiation, and childbirth diminish the urethral integrity. Vascular changes in the urethra due to atrophy of lower genital tract results poor coaptation and greater chance of incontinence. This loss of integrity can be treated by pelvic floor exercise, injection of urethral bulking agents, and urethral sling procedures [tension-free vaginal tape (TVT) and transobturator tape (TOT)].

Q. **What is coaptation of urethral mucosa?**

Connective tissue layer supports the epithelium of urethra and is made into deep folds. Coaptation is the urethral mucosal approximation caused by the vascular capillary network which runs in the subepithelial layer and serves as *inflatable cushion*. Coaptation is the most important factor of maintaining continence. This vasculature is reduced due to hypoestrogenemia especially in menopause leading to urinary incontinence.

Pathophysiology of Stress Incontinence

Continence is lost by loss of anatomical support and sphincteric support (internal sphincteric defect) as described above.

Causes of urge incontinence or overactive bladder (OAB) are mostly neurological and idiopathic.

Q. **What are the risk factors of stress incontinence?**

* Age
* Multiparity
* Vaginal births: Due to injury to pelvic muscle and connective tissue, damage of pudendal nerve
* Forceps delivery
* Vaginal birth of macrosomic baby (>4 kg)
* Prolonged labor
* Obesity: High body mass index increases intra-abdominal pressure which in turn exceeds urethral closing pressure. Decrease weight loss reduces urinary incontinence.
* Menopause: Hypoestrogenemia causes urethral mucosal atrophy and bladder irritation causes urge and stress incontinence. Systemic estrogen therapy worsens incontinence but local estrogen improves the condition.
* Family history: Incontinence is common among sisters
* Cognitive impairment
* Smoking
* Connective tissue disease
* Chronic obstructive pulmonary disease
* Chronic increased abdominal pressure: Chronic cough, long-standing weight lifting work and constipation.

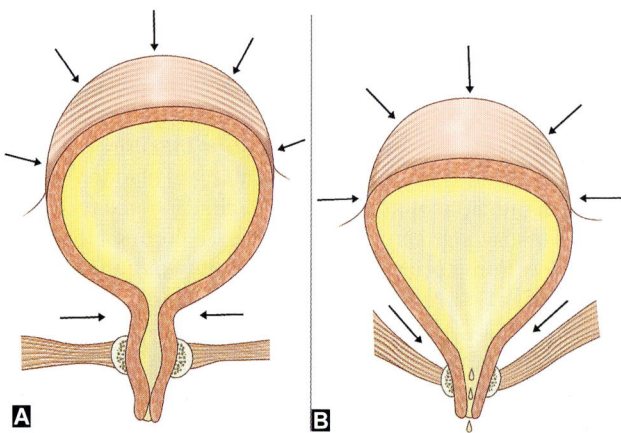

Figs. 20A and B: (A) In normal continent woman, increase of abdominal pressure is transmitted equally bladder, base of the bladder, and neck; (B) Continence is lost. There is loss of pressure transmission to the urethra; urethra and bladder neck become unable to close resulting reduced urethral closing pressure.

Q. **What are the drugs which may contribute to incontinence?**

Anticholinergics, thiazolidinediones, α-adrenergic agonists, and blockers, angiotensin- converting-enzyme inhibitors, calcium channel blockers, diuretics, alcohol, and narcotics all contribute to incontinence.

Diagnosis of Stress Incontinence

History is taken in details. Enquiry is made regarding:
- The type of incontinence—only stress, only OAB or mixed
- Number of voids per day, urgency, and leakage, if any continence pad is taken, if so type and number of pads, if the underclothes are changed.
- Whether leakage occurs due to physical activity or any urgency to void or leaking without urgency, whether any symptom of prolapse.
- A voiding bladder diary can be maintained where intake of fluid and voided urine amount is recorded.
- Constipation or stool impaction
- Any medical history—diabetes, past surgery or any medication are taken.

General Physical Examination

General examination:
- Anxious look
- Obesity.

Gynecological Examination

- *Per abdominal examination*: Any lump, e.g., fibroid or ovarian cyst that may be responsible for urinary frequency, whether there is any abdominal scar.
- *Pelvic examination*: Presence of prolapse, pelvic mass, presence of stress incontinence, and occult stress incontinence during coughing or Valsalva maneuver as demonstrated in Chapter 10, Pelvic Organ Prolapse.

Q. How will you demonstrate stress incontinence? What is occult or "hidden" stress incontinence?

Presence of stress incontinence (spurting of urine through urethra) is noted on coughing. For this examination, patient is asked not to evacuate of bladder before examination.

"Occult" or "hidden" stress incontinence is a condition which is revealed after the prolapse is reduced and supported by pessary *(Pessary test)* or large cotton swab or ring forceps or speculum. In these cases, due to direct compressive effect or urethral kinking there is no demonstrable stress incontinence normally. Urethra should not be overly straightened (showing false positive test) or obstructed (showing false-negative test) or tension is not placed over puborectalis muscles by excessive posterior retraction during elicitation. If this test is not done preoperatively, occult incontinence may remain undetected, hence not corrected and patient may present with stress incontinence postoperatively (*see also* Page 222, Chapter 10).

Q. What is Bonney's test and Marshall's test?

These two tests are done to detect whether surgical repair will be successful or not in incontinence. In positive test, repair is expected to be successful.

Bonney's Test

At the urethrovesical junction two fingers are kept on two sides of urethra and neck is elevated and patient is asked to cough. Test is said to be positive if there is no leakage after coughing, i.e. it is a stress incontinence case.

Marshall's Test

Here instead of fingers Allis tissue forceps are used to elevate bladder neck after local anesthetic agent infiltration.

Tone of pelvic floor muscle and sacral reflexes (bulbocavernosus) are elicited. Pelvic organ prolapse assessment is done if any as in Chapter 10.

Pad Test

Patient uses a preweighted sanitary pad while doing work or climbing stairs, hand washing, etc. The weight of the pad is taken after a variable period may be up to 24 hours. Deducting the two weight urine voided is measured which is then converted to mL.

Q-Tip Test

A small piece of *swab* applied with 1% lignocaine jelly is placed into the urethra and a Valsalva maneuver is performed. At rest and during Valsalva maneuver the swab-excursion angle is measured. A resting angle or an angle change more than 30° to the horizon is suggestive of *urethral hypermobility*.

Complete bimanual and rectovaginal examination is done.

Investigations

- *Urine examination*: A fresh midstream urine is collected for detection of infection or culture sensitivity.
- *Post-void residual urine (PVR)*: It is measured either by catheterization or with sonography after voiding.

Causes of large PVR are recurrent infection, neurologic defect, and pelvic mass.

- *Urodynamic studies*: *Cystometry, urethrocystometry, and uroflowmetry.*

Indications of Urodynamic Studies

- When conservative treatment is unsuccessful and surgical treatment is planned
- Recurrent symptoms
- A complex history with incongruous physical findings
- To know which treatment is necessary for individual case—if there is mixed incontinence both urge and stress urodynamic study can make it clear that urge component is responsible for symptom. Conservative management with physical and or pharmacotherapy is sufficient avoiding unnecessary surgical therapy.

Cystometry

Cystometry helps to diagnose type of incontinence by reproducing micturition cycle by measuring bladder pressure and abdominal pressure.

Procedure: Two type of cystometrics—simple cystometrics and multichannel cystometrics.

Simple cystometrics has some limitations as it cannot assess ISD. Multichannel cystometrics can assess for ISD.

Procedure of multichannel cystometrics: In this method, two catheters are used, one for bladder and another for rectum or vagina. Vagina is preferred to rectum if the former is not obscured by prolapse as stool in the rectum may obstruct the catheter.

The bladder pressure is the combination of detrusor pressure and pressure in the abdominal cavity and rectal or vaginal pressure is the pressure in the abdominal cavity.

Hence, detrusor pressure = bladder pressure – rectal or vaginal pressure.

Bladder is filled with warm saline during which the pressure measurement is taken and woman usually lies in standing position, upright position or sits on a commode where leakage is recorded.

In every 50 mL, the patient is asked to cough and external urethral meatus is observed for leakage of urine.

The woman is asked to tell the onset of sensation of bladder filling and at which amount (usual amount 150 mL) it is recorded.

The volume at which strong desire to void is noted (usually at 350 mL) and also noted the amount at the onset of urgency (usually up to 500 mL).

The patient is asked to cough every 50 mL and leakage of urine is observed through external urethral meatus.

Urodynamic stress incontinence is diagnosed when there is leakage with increase abdominal pressure in absence of detrusor activity.

Diagnosis of detrusor overactivity: Diagnosis is made when the woman has involuntary detrusor contraction during urodynamic test with/without leakage.

Usefulness of urodynamic study—it can diagnose:
- Detrusor overactivity with/without sensation during filling
- Detrusor overactivity with incontinence
- Urodynamic stress incontinence
- Mixed incontinence.

Urethrocystometry and uroflowmetry: Other than intravesical pressure urethral pressure is also measured. Normal urethral pressure is approximately 40 cm of water. Less than 20 cm may result incontinence.

Resting bladder pressure is 2–8 cm of water with 150 mL urine. At filling, it rises to 15 cm of water. Voiding function is assessed by uroflowmetry.

Micturition cystourethrography: Posterior urethrovesical angle is measured by micturition cystourethrography. Normal angle is 100°.

Corrective surgery by sling or colposuspension is effective in loss of urethrovesical angle.

Videocystourethrography is very informative procedure for urodynamic study.

Imaging:
- *Ultrasonography*: It is useful to detect total urine volume, residual volume, and thickness of urinary bladder. In detrusor instability, thickness may be more than 6 mm.
- *Magnetic resonance imaging (MRI)*: For detection of pelvic floor musculature and fascial defect MRI is a useful tool.

Management of Urinary Incontinence

- Conservative: Diet, fluid balance, loss of weight, bladder retraining, and pelvic floor exercise
- Drugs: Mostly anticholinergic and also local estrogen
- Surgery
- Others: Devices, electric stimulation-sacral neuromodulation and percutaneous tibial nerve stimulation (PTNS) and magnetic stimulation.

Q. Which treatment where?

- Conservative method—for all types of incontinence
- Drugs—overactive bladder (OAB)
- Surgery—in stress urinary incontinence not improved by conservative management
- Others—specific situation.

Conservative

Diet: To avoid food that may have high acidity and caffeine as they cause urgency and frequency. Artificially sweetened or carbonated drinks are avoided as they are associated with urgency and incontinence symptoms. Diet containing calcium glycerophosphate decreases urgency and frequency.

Fluid balance: Not too much and not too less water as more fluid increases frequency and less fluid (concentrated urine) increases the sense of urgency. Average between 1.5–2.5 L.

Loss of weight: Weight loss in obese woman improves both stress incontinence and OAB.

Bladder retraining: Bladder drill or retraining is to train the woman to increase voiding interval in stepwise fashion to achieve normal frequency. Combining with pelvic floor exercise it works very well to reduce frequency and urgency. Schedule voiding may also beneficial in reducing stress urinary incontinence.

Pelvic floor strengthening: Active pelvic floor muscle training improves mild-to-moderate symptoms of urinary incontinence. It is also called Kegel's exercise which involves voluntary contraction of levator ani muscle. Individualized exercise program is offered for each patient with increasing number of contraction and also duration of each contraction for 4–6 months. In both bladder training and pelvic floor strengthening motivation of the patient is important.

Electric and magnetic stimulation for nerve damage: Electric stimulation is effective if incontinence is due to denervation. Magnetic stimulation has been tried with success in pelvic floor muscle weakness in very elderly.

Vaginal devices: These are ring pessary, silastic vaginal cone, and other pessaries. Some pessaries called "incontinence pessaries" have been developed to treat incontinence as well as pelvic organ prolapse. They act by giving bladder neck support. Success is inconsistent.

Q. Role of medical management in incontinence.

The main role of medical management is to treat *OAB symptoms and OAB*. Medical agent has minimum role in the treatment of stress urinary incontinence.

Drugs Used in Urge Urinary Incontinence and Overactive Bladder

The drugs used are mostly anticholinergic drugs by reducing the detrusor contractility **(Table 1)**.

Mechanism of action: The contraction of the detrusor muscle is under control of parasympathetic nerves. The anticholinergic drugs act by competitively inhibiting the acetylcholine at muscarine receptors. Recently, it is known that acetylcholine is also neurotransmitter in afferent sensory pathway thus has direct effect on reducing sensation of bladder filling.

Drugs, dose and mechanism of action are given in **Table 1**.

Local agents: Topical vaginal estrogen cream improves in bladder sensation and urgency especially in postmenopausal woman and there is no role of oral estrogen.

Side effects of the drugs: As the muscarine receptors are present on the sites other than the bladder side effects are significant. Side effects are:

- Dry mouth—gingival and buccal ulceration
- Vision problems—photophobia and blurred vision
- Decrease sweating—hyperthermia
- Diminished detrusor function—urinary retention
- Constipation.

Surgery

Surgery is a highly effective option for stress urinary incontinence.

Q. What is the aim of surgery?

- To restore the urethrovesical angle
- To restore urethral sphincter mechanism
- To elevate the proximal urethra
- To restore urethral conduit.

Q. When to do surgery?

All conservative managements fail.

Proper diagnosis of type of incontinence (stress) is done. Detrusor instability must be excluded before surgery otherwise symptoms may aggravate.

Pessary test, Bonney's test, and Marshal test help to speculate the result of surgery.

Q. What are the surgical options in stress incontinence?

- Kelly's operation—plication of pubocervical fascia
- Colposuspension—classical—Burch colposuspension/Marshall-Marchetti (MMK) colposuspension and laparoscopic colposuspension
- Midurethral sling using tape:
    - TVT
    - TOT
- Pubovaginal sling
- Needle suspension
- Repair of paravaginal defect
- Artificial urinary sphincters.

Table 1: Drugs, dose, and mechanism of action.

Drugs	Dose	Mechanism of action	Comments
Oxybutynin	2.5–5 mg up to thrice daily Release preparation 5 mg once daily can be increased by 5 mg weekly up to 20 mg daily	Antimuscarine	• First choice as recommended by NICE • More effective than tolterodine • Transdermal patch/gel is available to decrease side effects
Tolterodine	2 mg twice daily Release preparation 4 mg once daily	Antimuscarine	Less side effects
Fesoterodine	4 mg once daily, maximum dose 8 mg once daily	Antimuscarine	Better than tolterodine
Trospium	20 mg twice daily	Antimuscarine quaternary amine	Increased urgency warning time with decreased muscarine side effects
Solifenacin	5–10 mg once daily	M3-selective antimuscarine	do
Darifenacin	7.7–15 mg daily	M3-selective antimuscarine	do
Imipramine hydrochloride	10–25 mg 1–4 times daily	Tricyclic antidepressant, anticholinergic, α-adrenergic	Dose required is less in comparison to as antidepressant. Used in mixed urgency
Mirabegron	25–50 mg daily	β_3 adrenergic agonist	Recent drug, acting more on storage function than anticholinergic and can be used simultaneously with anticholinergic

Abbreviation: NICE, National Institute for Health and Care Excellence.

Kelly's Operation

Kelly's operation (1914) is like anterior colporrhaphy (see Page 226, Chapter 10) with adding reefing mattress sutures in the urethrovesical fascia at the level of bladder neck. Pacey (1949) made further lateral dissection and apposed the medial fibers of puborectalis in the midline beneath the buttressed urethra and the bladder neck.

Burch Colposuspension (Fig. 21)

It is an old operation and performed widely before the development of new techniques using tapes. It is indicated in SUI.

A suprapubic Pfannenstiel incision is given to open the retropubic space. After retracting the bladder medially two or three nonabsorbable or delayed absorbable sutures on each side of bladder neck are placed through iliopectineal ligament (Cooper ligament) of pubic symphysis to tie with the paravaginal fascia to support neck of the bladder.

In Marshall-Marchetti colposuspension procedure, the tissues are fixed to periosteum of symphysis pubis. Osteitis pubis is added risk of MMK. Its success rate is 80–85%.

Complications: Operative complications—hemorrhage, injury of bladder and urethra, osteitis, and long-term posterior vaginal wall prolapse.

Midurethral Sling (Figs. 22A and B)

It can be done by retropubically called:
❖ *Tension-free vaginal tape (TVT)(Fig. 22A)* or
❖ *Transobturator procedure (TOT) (Fig. 22B).*

Tension-free vaginal tape (TVT) is indicated in both SUI and ISD. Transobturator procedure (TOT) is indicated in SUI.

One cm wide nonabsorbable mesh of polypropylene made into tape is passed via the vaginal incision under the midurethra to be placed behind the symphysis pubis (TVT) through the small suprapubic incision or behind the inferior pubic rami via obturator foramen (TOT) through small incision on groin on each side.

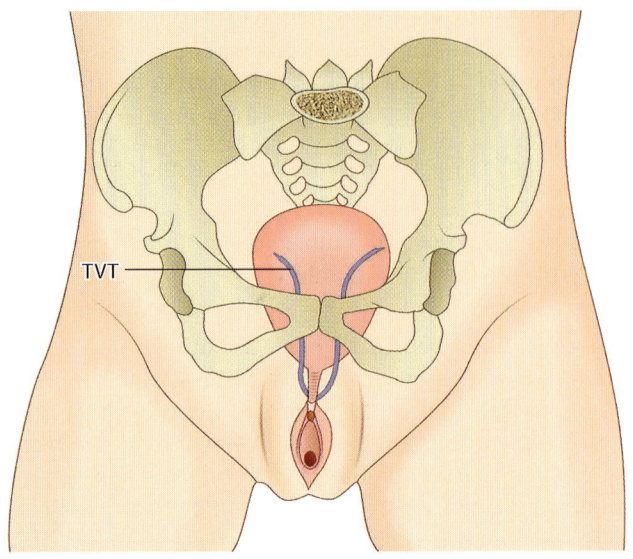

Fig. 22A: Midurethral sling: Tension-free vaginal tape (TVT).

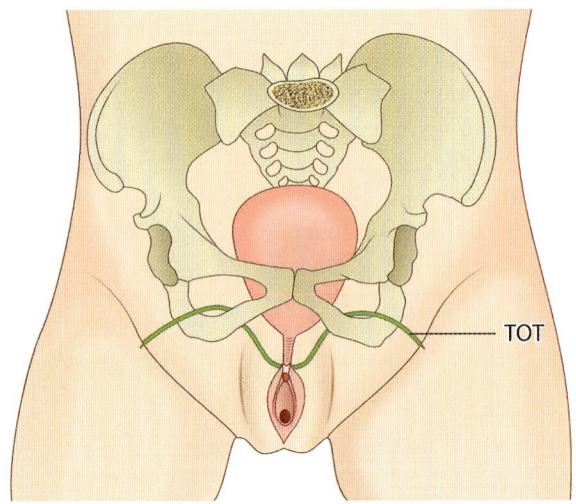

Fig. 22B: Midurethral sling: Transobturator (TOT) procedure.

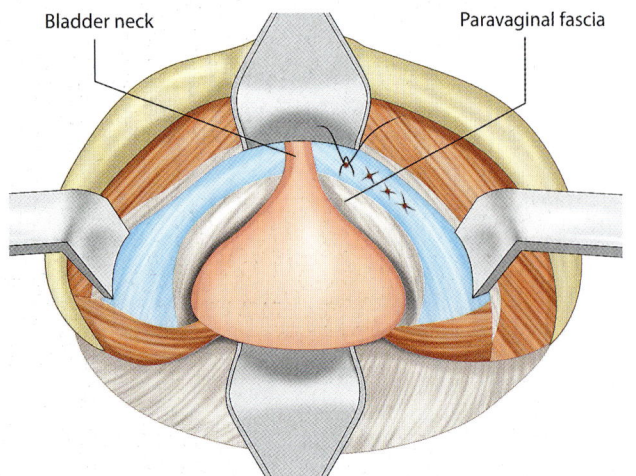

Fig. 21: Burch colposuspension.

The surgical procedures of TVT (see Page 395, **Figs. 23 to 28**) and TOT are (see Pages 396-398, **Figs. 29 to 37**) described later.

Periurethral Injection of Bulking Agent

In this method under local anesthesia synthetic polymer materials either as microscopic beads or viscous liquid that bulk up the bladder neck is injected into urethral submucosa to prevent leakage. This indicated when patient is physically unfit or there is still leakage after midurethral sling or colposuspension operation.

Success rate is 70% and longer-term cure rate is less.

Pubovaginal Sling

Bladder neck is supported by fascia of rectus sheath by vaginoabdominal approach. It is indicated in ISD and failed SUI procedure.

Needle Suspension

Proximal urethra is suspended to anterior abdominal wall. It is indicated in SUI but no longer done nowadays.

Artificial Urinary Sphincters

This device is comprised of an inflatable cuff, a balloon to control pressure and a pump. It is indicated in other treatment and previous surgical failure. It is expensive. Its complications are infection and erosion.

Surgery for Detrusor Overactivity

Botulinum toxin A, a neurotoxin, is injected in various sites across the dome of the bladder through cystoscopic approach. This will inhibit detrusor contraction by flaccid paralysis of detrusor which is responsible for symptoms. This is the second-line treatment of DO next to medical.

Surgical Procedure of Tension-free Vaginal Tape (Figs. 22 to 28)

Patient is in lithotomy position. Anesthesia—regional or general anesthesia.

After proper dressing and draping, the bladder was catheterized by Foleys catheter. Anterior lip of cervix is held by multiple teeth vulsellum and pulled downward and outward.

Anterior vaginal wall is grasped by two Allis tissue forceps one at 1cm and the other at 4 cm posterior to the external urethral meatus in midline. A vertical incision of 2.5 cm is made in the midline between two forceps. The lateral flaps are dissected through the vesicovaginal space.

The TVT needle (Fig. 23) is passed initially through a 5 mm skin incision (the site of incision is at the midpoint of a line joining one labiocrural fold to the midline just above the symphysis pubis) in the suprapubic region beneath the pubic symphysis and the descending pubic ramus to appear through the vaginal incision.

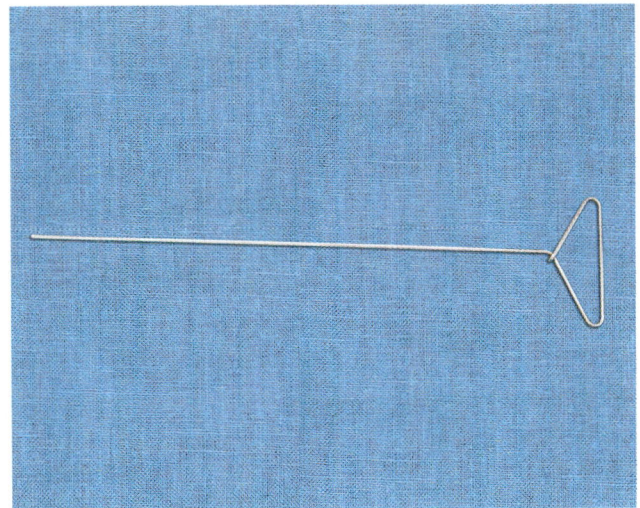

Fig. 24: Tension-free vaginal tape guidewire for Foley catheter.

During insertion of the needle a guidewire fitted with a Foley catheter (best 18 size) **(Fig. 24)** is passed through the urethra about 5 cm to move the urethra away from the needle insertion site in order to prevent injury of the bladder and urethra. For this, handle of the guidewire is moved toward the side to which the needle is inserted and by this way bladder neck will go away from the needle.

After keeping the needle in that position other needle is inserted on opposite side moving the guidewire opposite way.

Now, cystoscopy **(Fig. 25)** is done to see whether there is any injury to the bladder or urethra. After being sure that there is no injury, one end of the tape **(Fig. 26)** tied with the needle and the needle was then withdrawn so that the lateral end of the tape taken out through the tract made by the needle. Same procedure is done on the opposite side so that the other end of tape was taken out through the tract on the opposite side.

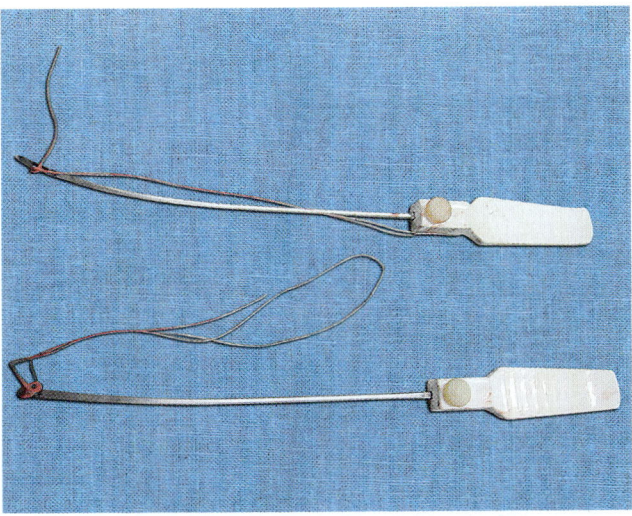

Fig. 23: Tension-free vaginal tape needle.

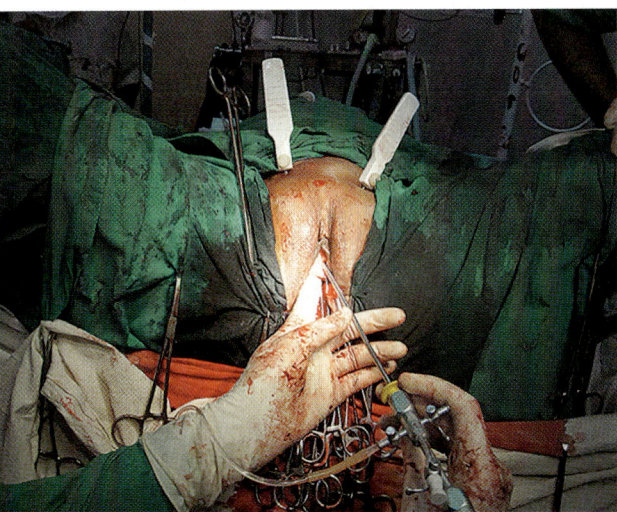

Fig. 25: Cystoscopy to see whether there is any bladder injury.

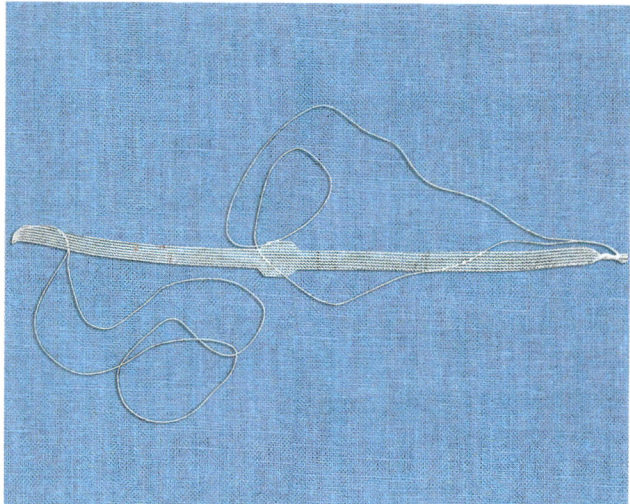

Fig. 26: Tension-free vaginal tape.

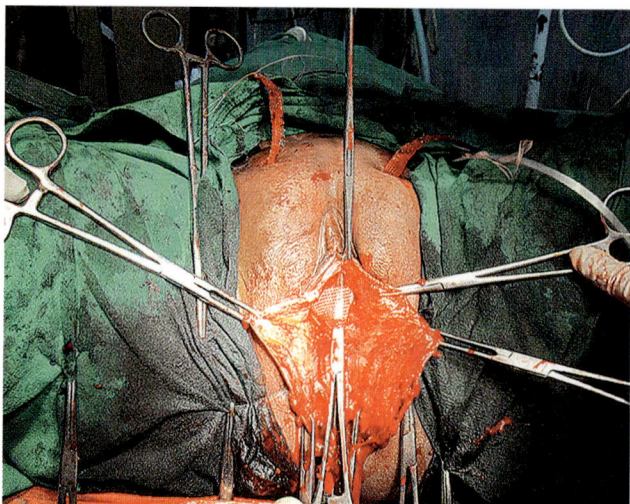

Fig. 28: Tension-free vaginal tape after placing the tape. A artery forceps has been kept to prevent excess tightness.

Both ends of the tape were pulled simultaneously so that the broader part of the tape is placed in the midurethral region.

It was taken care that the tape in the midurethral part was not too tight which was ascertained by placing an artery forceps between the tape and the urethra **(Figs. 27 and 28)**.

The excess part of the mesh is cut flushed with the skin.

Anterior vaginal wall is closed by continuous interlocking vicryl sutures, while doing so it was taken care that the mesh could not be taken in the bite of vaginal wall.

In the presence of cystocele, initially incision for anterior colporrhaphy is done and then proceeded. In that case before final pulling of tape cystocele is repaired with two or three interrupted stiches following which final pulling of mesh is done, after which vaginal wall is repaired.

Cystoscopy is done following the procedure to check the injury of bladder and urethra.

Surgical Procedure of Transobturator Tape (Outside in Technique) (Figs. 22 and 29 to 37)

Patient is in lithotomy position. Anesthesia—regional or general anesthesia.

After proper dressing and draping, the bladder is catheterized by Foleys catheter. Anterior lip of cervix is held by multiple teeth vulsellum and pulled downward and outward.

Anterior vaginal wall is held by two Allis tissue forceps 1 cm and 4 cm posterior to the external urethral meatus in the midline.

A vertical incision of 2.5 cm made in the midline between two forceps **(Fig. 29)**. The lateral flaps dissected through the vesicovaginal space using scissor and blunt finger dissection.

A 0.5 cm to 1 cm incision is made in the genitourinary fold (thigh crese) 4–6 cm lateral to the clitoris on both sides (at the insertion of adductor longus by palpation) on both sides.

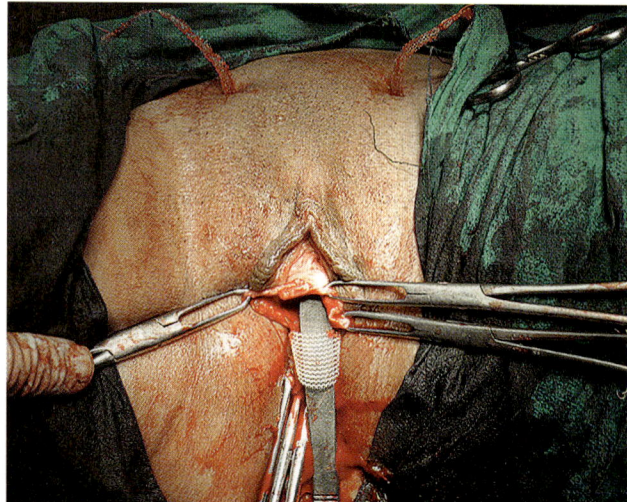

Fig. 27: Tension-free vaginal tape after placing the tape before final stretching.

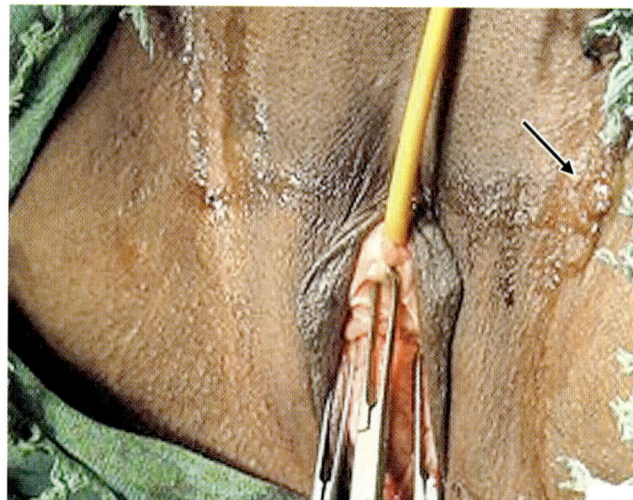

Fig. 29: Transobturator tape. Anterior vaginal wall is held by Allis tissue forceps before incision (arrow indicates the site of groin incision).

Courtesy: Professor Subhash Chandra Biswas, IPGMER, Kolkata

Left index finger is inserted in the vesicovaginal space to assess the ischiopubic rami and the obturator foramen of left side to make submucosal tunnel beneath the vaginal epithelium which extends up to and behind the ischiopubic rami.

The TOT needle is then inserted perpendicularly through groin fold incision on left side and guided by the finger until it penetrates the obturator foramen in its upper and medial part **(Figs. 30 to 32)** which is understood by "popping" sensation.

The needle is then passed under the pubic ramus and taken out through the vaginal incision **(Fig. 33)**.

One end of the tape is tied with the needle and the needle is then withdrawn so that the lateral end of the tape is taken out through the tract made by the needle **(Fig. 34)**.

Same thing is done on the opposite side so that the other end of tape is taken out through the tract on the opposite side.

Both ends of the tape were pulled simultaneously so that the broader part of the tape is placed in the midurethral region **(Fig. 35)**. It is taken care that the tape in the midurethral part was not too tight which was ascertained by placing an artery forceps between the tape and the urethra **(Fig. 36)**.

The excess part of the mesh is cut flushed with the skin.

Anterior vaginal wall is closed by continuous interlocking vicryl sutures, while doing so it was taken care that the mesh could not be taken in the bite of vaginal wall.

Cystoscopy is not necessary in TOT as injury of bladder is unlikely in this procedure.

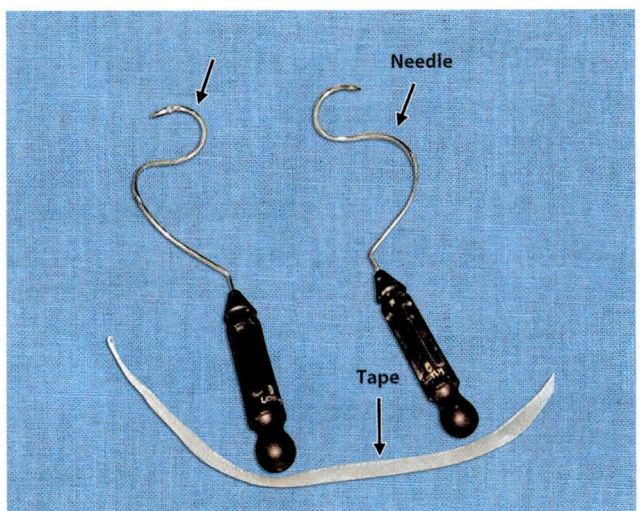

Fig. 30: Transobturator needle and tape.
Courtesy: Professor Subhash Chandra Biswas, IPGMER, Kolkata

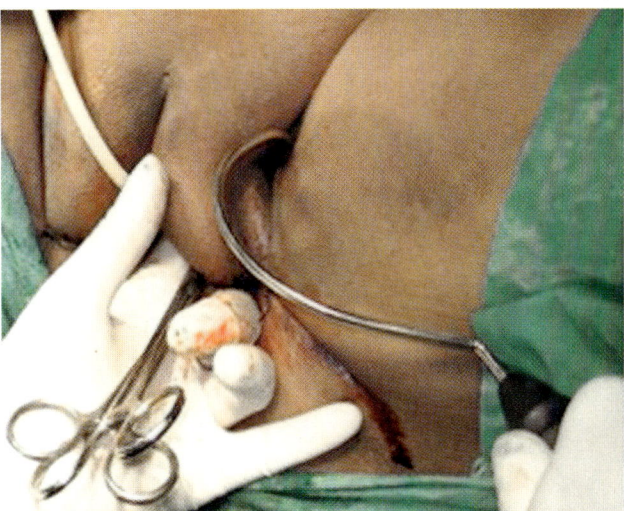

Fig. 32: Transobturator tape (TOT). Left index finger is introduced in left vesicovaginal space and TOT needle is inserted through groin fold incision perpendicularly.
Courtesy: Professor Subhash Chandra Biswas, IPGMER, Kolkata

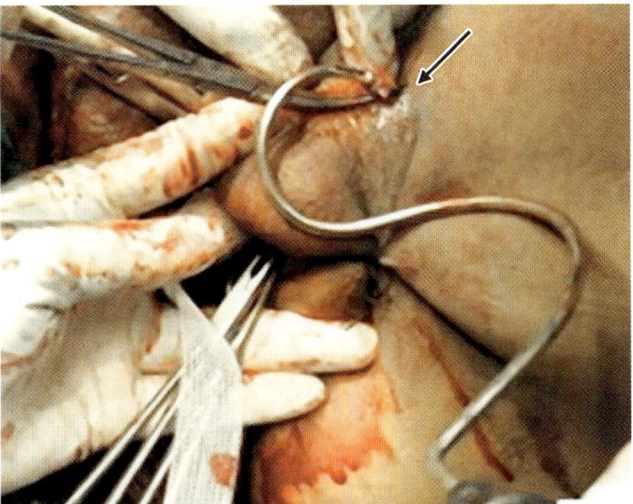

Fig. 31: Transobturator tape needle is inserted through groin fold incision perpendicularly (outside in).
Courtesy: Professor Subhash Chandra Biswas, IPGMER, Kolkata

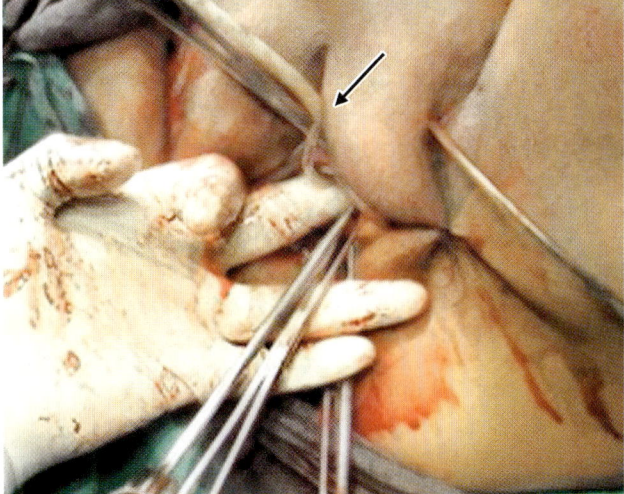

Fig. 33: Transobturator tape—TOT needle is inserted to get through vagina.
Courtesy: Professor Subhash Chandra Biswas, IPGMER, Kolkata

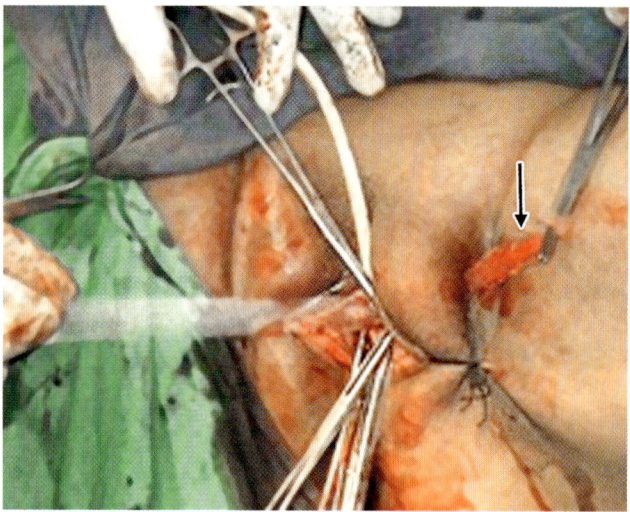

Fig. 34: Transobturator tape—tape is withdrawn on left side. Arrow indicates the end of tape outside.
Courtesy: Professor Subhash Chandra Biswas, IPGMER, Kolkata

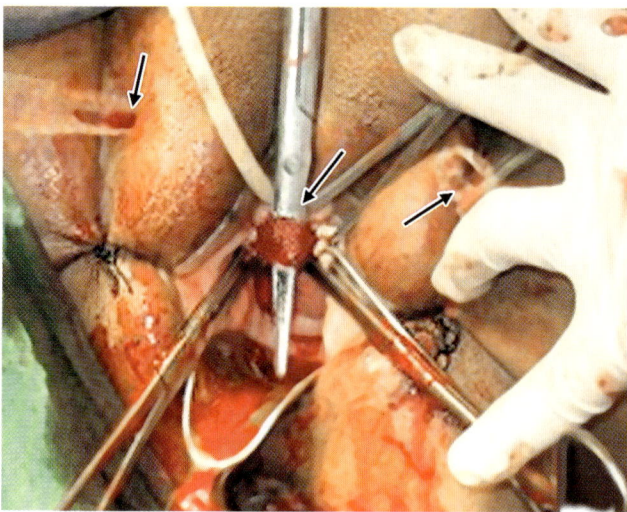

Fig. 36: Transobturator tape. An artery forceps is placed between the tape and urethra to prevent too tight tightness.
Courtesy: Professor Subhash Chandra Biswas, IPGMER, Kolkata

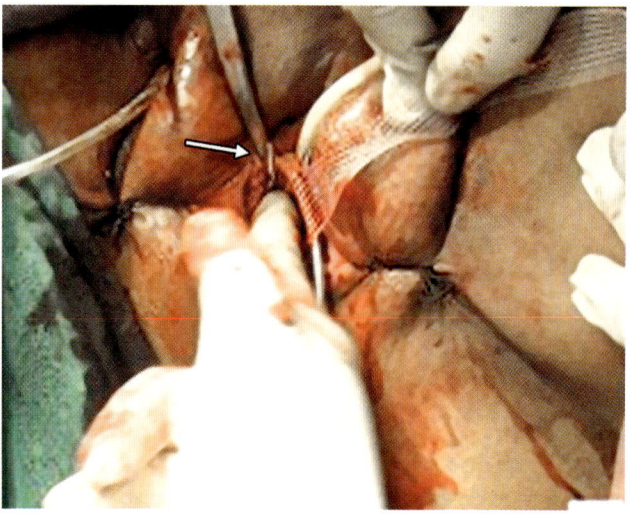

Fig. 35: Transobturator tape—same thing is done on opposite side.
Courtesy: Professor Subhash Chandra Biswas, IPGMER, Kolkata

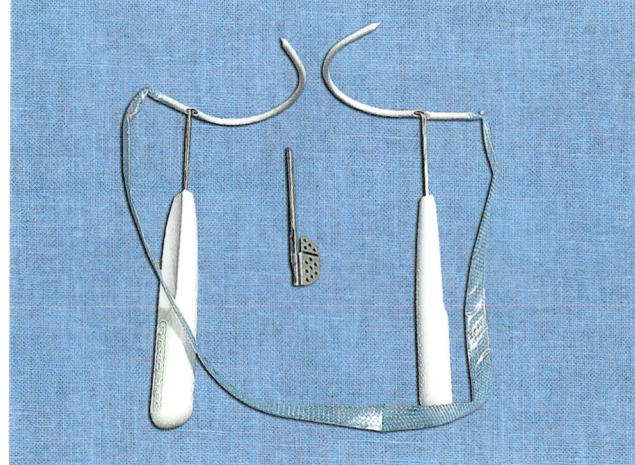

Fig. 37: Composite set of obturator device, helical passers and atraumatic winged guide.
Courtesy: Professor Subhash Chandra Biswas, IPGMER, Kolkata

Transobturator Tape (TOT) by Inside out Technique (Figs. 37 to 40)

For this method, a composite device is available which contains obturator device, helical pressers, and atraumatic winged guide. Following incision on vagina in the same manner as the previous method after creating a vesicovaginal space needle along with the tape is introduced *from inside out* through obturator foramen with the help of atraumatic winged guide **(Figs. 37 to 40)**.

Advantages of TVT and TOT

Recovery time is very short and success is good.

Complications

Complication is due to mesh, peroperative bladder injury, and retropubic vessel injury. This complication is less in TOT. The complications are:

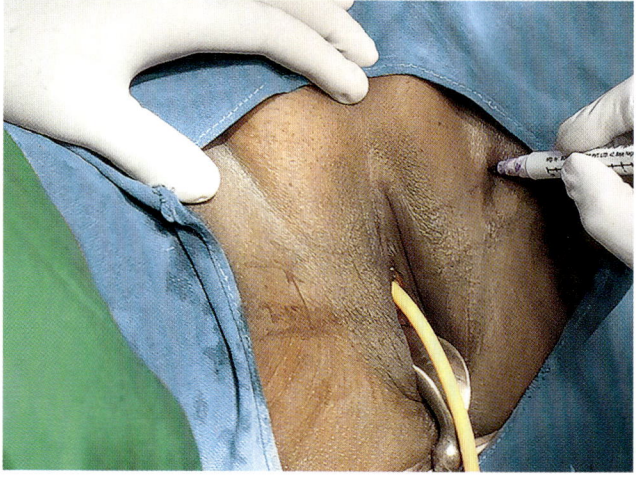

Fig. 38: Marking at the groin fold.
Courtesy: Professor Subhash Chandra Biswas, IPGMER, Kolkata

CHAPTER 17: A Case of Vesicovaginal Fistula and Urinary Incontinence

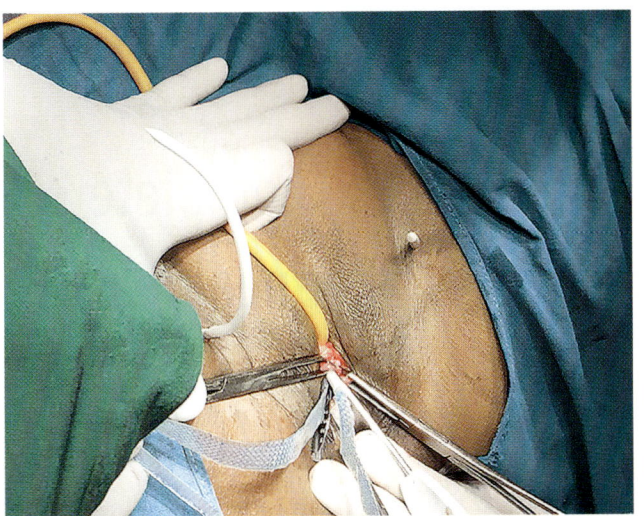

Fig. 39: Needle is introduced inside out technique.
Courtesy: Professor Subhash Chandra Biswas, IPGMER, Kolkata

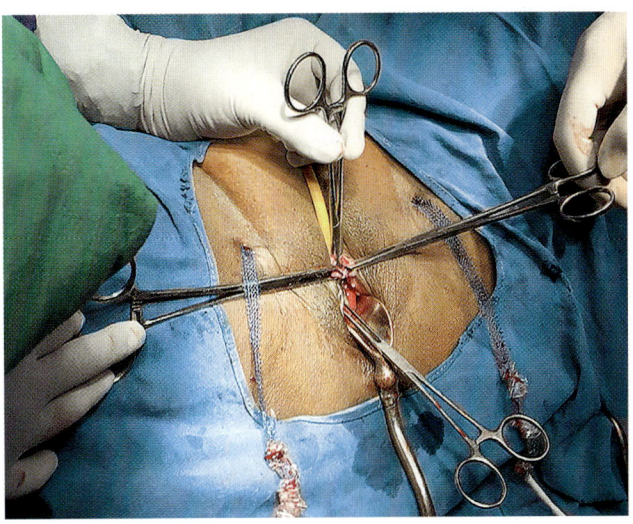

Fig. 40: Tape is placed properly.
Courtesy: Professor Subhash Chandra Biswas, IPGMER, Kolkata

- Difficulty in voiding and appearance of OAB symptoms
- Failure.

TVT versus TOT
- The TVT is technically difficult in comparison to TOT
- Complication is more in TVT
- Cystoscopy is mandatory in TVT
- The TVT is more effective in both SUI and ISD whereas TOT is effective only in SUI.

CHAPTER 18

A Case of Old Complete Perineal Tear

Chapter Outline

Writing a case of old complete perineal tear (CPT) and how to present the case?

Complete Perineal Tear:
- Definition and Etiology
- Types and Diagnosis
- Prevention
- Management—Steps of Layer Method

Rectovaginal Fistula (RVF):
- Etiology
- Diagnosis
- Management

PATIENT'S PARTICULARS

1. Name: Mrs PM
2. Age: 23 years
3. Address: Remote village of North 24 PGs
4. Occupation: Housewife
5. Married/unmarried: Married
6. History of infertility: Nil
7. Husband's occupation: Farmer
8. Socioeconomic status: Low
9. Religion: Hindu
10. Parous/nulliparous: Primipara

Bed No.:
Date of admission: 24.3.2017
Date of examination: 29.3.2017

HISTORY

- *Chief complaint/complaints*: Inability to hold the stool and flatus.
- *History of present illness*—describe in detail: Patient complains of inability to hold the flatus and feces for last 9 months since her childbirth. The passage of stool and flatus becomes more during increase of intra-abdominal pressure like coughing.

- *Menstrual history*:
  - Last menstrual period: Amenorrhea, lactation—if mens write down all points
  - Duration of menstruation:
  - Interval in days:
  - Age of menarche:
  - Regularity of cycle:
  - Pain during period/if pain is related with menstruation:
  - Amount of bleeding:
  - Clot:
  - Intermenstrual bleeding:

- *Obstetric history*:
  - Parity: Primipara
  - Living issue: 1
  - Last childbirth: 9 months back, home delivery.

Q. Describe the labor in detail which is usually difficult, if hospital delivery whether there was forceps or ventouse application?

Serial no.	Year and month	Pregnancy events	Labor events	Mode of delivery	Puerperium or postabortal period	Baby

- *Past history*: Nothing significant
  - Medical
  - Surgical
- *Family history*:
- *Sexual history*: Sexually active (usually difficulty in sex)
- *Functional history*:
  - Bowel: Inner garment is soiled with stool
  - Bladder
  - Sleep
  - Appetite
- *Personal history*:
  - Personal hygiene poor
  - Smoking/alcohol
- *Contraceptive history*:
- *Drug history*: Nil
  - History of any drug allergy
  - History of intake of corticosteroids, antiepileptic or other drugs (previous or present).

PHYSICAL EXAMINATION

- Patient: Alert, conscious, and cooperative
- Write down all the points according to Chapter 1
- Look: Irritable

Systemic Examination
Write as usual as Chapter 1.

Examination of Breasts and Nipple
- Inspection
- Palpation.

GYNECOLOGICAL EXAMINATION

Abdominal Examination
- Inspection
- Palpation
- Percussion
- Auscultation.

Vaginal Examination (Figs. 1 and 2)
- *Inspection of external genitalia*:
  - Vagina and anal canal open into almost together, complete absence of gynecological perineum, protrusion of pinkish anal mucosa through the opening (or sometimes rectal prolapse) **(Fig. 2)**.
  - Vagina and anal canal is separated by a septum formed by posterior vaginal mucosa and anterior wall of anal mucosa with a lower transverse margin, absence of anal rugae on two anterolateral aspects of anal canal, present only posteriorly.
  - Two dimples-like points on two anterolateral aspects of anal canal (3 and 9 o'clock position) indicating torn ends of anal sphincter. Dimples become prominent on

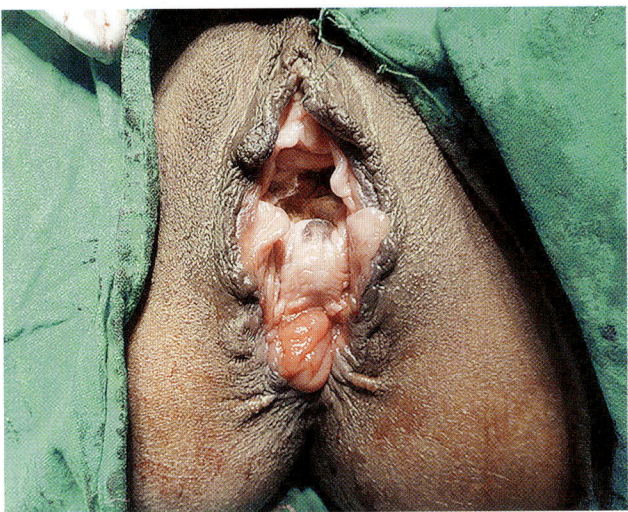

Fig. 1: Old complete perineal tear (in a young woman of 23 years old).

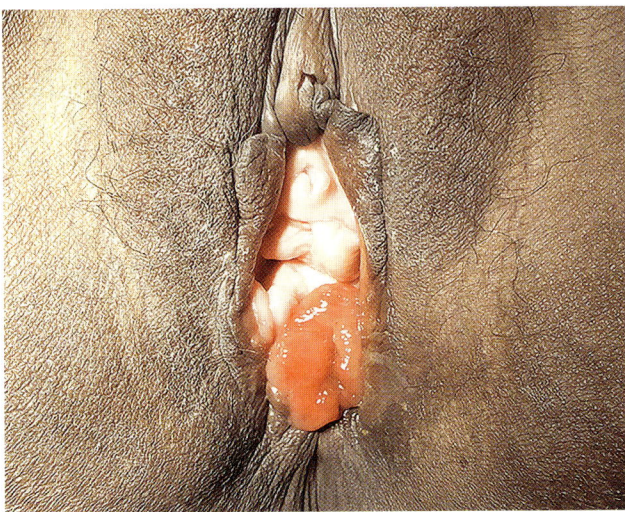

Fig. 2: Old complete perineal tear (in a postmenopausal woman of 56 years old).

  asking the patient to hold the stool like action (*see* **Figs. 3A and B**, Page 404).
- *Palpation of external genitalia*: There is absence of sphincteric grip. Vagina and anal canal are separated by a septum formed by vaginal wall and anal wall with a fibrosed lower concave margin.
- *Speculum examination*: Describe the cervix.
- *Bimanual examination*: As usual write the findings—uterus, adnexa, and fornices.

SUMMARY OF THE CASE (SAMPLE)

A 23-year-old P1+0 has been admitted on with complain of incontinence of stool and feces since her last childbirth. She is primipara and delivered at home by untrained dai. There was difficulty during delivery. Her perineum was not repaired (or if repaired not healed) following which incontinence of stool started.

On examination, patient looks irritable, she is normotensive, no abnormality detected on general physical and abdominal examination.

On local examination vagina and anal canal are found to open into almost together in the perineum, complete absence of gynecological perineum, protrusion of pinkish anal mucosa through the opening (or sometimes rectal prolapse), absence of anal rugae on two anterolateral aspects of anal canal, rugae was present only posteriorly, two dimple-like points (at 3 and 9 o'clock position) on two anterolateral aspects of anal canal indicating torn ends of anal sphincter.

Investigations Supplied
To be written as supplied.

Provisional Diagnosis
A case of old complete perineal tear.

Differential Diagnosis
Differential diagnosis is rectovaginal fistula (RVF).

COMPLETE PERINEAL TEAR

Q. What do you mean by complete perineal tear? When would you call it old?

Complete perineal tear (CPT) means tear of the perineum involving the external anal sphincter with or without the involvement of anal wall (anal mucosa and internal sphincter).

It is called "old" after 3 months of delivery.

Q. What are different types of perineal tear (lacerations)?

Perineal tear or laceration is categorized into four degrees (RCOG, 2015).
1. *First degree*: When injury occurs involving perineal skin, fourchette, and/or vaginal mucosa only.
2. *Second degree*: Tear extends to the fascia, muscles of the perineal body, and but not the anal sphincter.
3. *Third degree*: Injury to the perineum extending involving anal sphincter complex (external and internal anal sphincter)*:
   - 3a: Less than 50% of external sphincter complex (EAS)
   - 3b: More than 50% thickness involved
   - 3c: Both EAS and internal sphincter (IAS) torn.
4. *Fourth-degree tear*: Perineal injury involving anal sphincter complex (EAS and IAS) and anorectal mucosa to expose the lumen of rectum.

The term anorectal mucosa is used instead of anal mucosa as proximal part of anus is lined by rectal mucosa (columnar) whereas distal 1–1.5 cm is lined by modified squamous epithelium.

Q. What do you mean by OASIS?

It means obstetric anal sphincter injuries including both third- and fourth-degree perineal tears.

---
*As per other view, third degree laceration means involving the external anal sphincter.

Q. What do you mean by rectal buttonhole tear?

When tear involves rectal mucosa but sphincter complex becomes intact. It is not under the fourth degree. If unrecognized during repair, it may lead to a RVF.

ANATOMY OF ANAL CANAL AND ANAL SPHINCTER

The length of anal canal is 4–5 cm and it starts as continuation of rectum at the level of levator ani attachment. From inside outwards it has mucosa, internal anal sphincter, intersphincteric space outside which lies the external anal sphincter in lower part and puborectalis in upper part. Internal anal sphincter is the continuation of smooth circular muscle fiber of rectum. Intersphincteric space contains the extension of the rectal longitudinal smooth muscle layer. The mucosa contains the columnar epithelium in cephalad and simple stratified squamous epithelium caudally, in between lies the dentate or pectinate line. Anal cushions are the three submucus arteriovenous plexuses which are highly vascular and helps for complete closure and continence of the anal canal to some extent.

Hemorrhoids are the venous engorgement in the cushion and may result from pregnancy, excess straining and hard stool as a result of degeneration and loss of support by connective tissue. External hemorrhoids which lie below the pectinate line may be painful and may be seen as mass. Above the pectinate line there may be internal hemorrhoids which may bleed or prolapse but unlikely painful.

Anus has two sphincters, namely internal anal sphincters (IAS) and external anal sphincters (EAS). IAS and EAS along with puborectalis muscle form the anal sphincter complex.

Outside IAS lies the external anal sphincter in its lower part and puborectalis in upper portion. The length of IAS is 3–4 cm and at its distal part there is overlapping with EAS.

IAS maintains the anal canal resting pressure and responsible for fecal incontinence significantly. It becomes relaxed before defecation.

EAS is a circular muscle ring throughout the circumference of IAS on its lower part. It is attached anteriorly with perineal body and posteriorly with coccyx by anococcygeal ligament. It has three parts namely subcutaneous, superficial and deep. For anal continence it has great role. In addition to keep the resting continence it prevents incontinence in urgency by squeezing pressure.

Puborectalis which is one of the three muscles of levator ani (the other two are pubococcygeus and iliococcygeus) lies medially and extends from pubic bone on either side and comes behind the anorectal junction acting as a sling maintaining the continence.

Hence, the continence of anal canal is maintained by EAS (major role), IAS, puborectalis and anal cushion.

As the sphincters are close to the vagina, it is likely that they are torn during vaginal delivery. IAS is injured in fourth degree tear and advanced third degree laceration (3c) resulting anal incontinence.

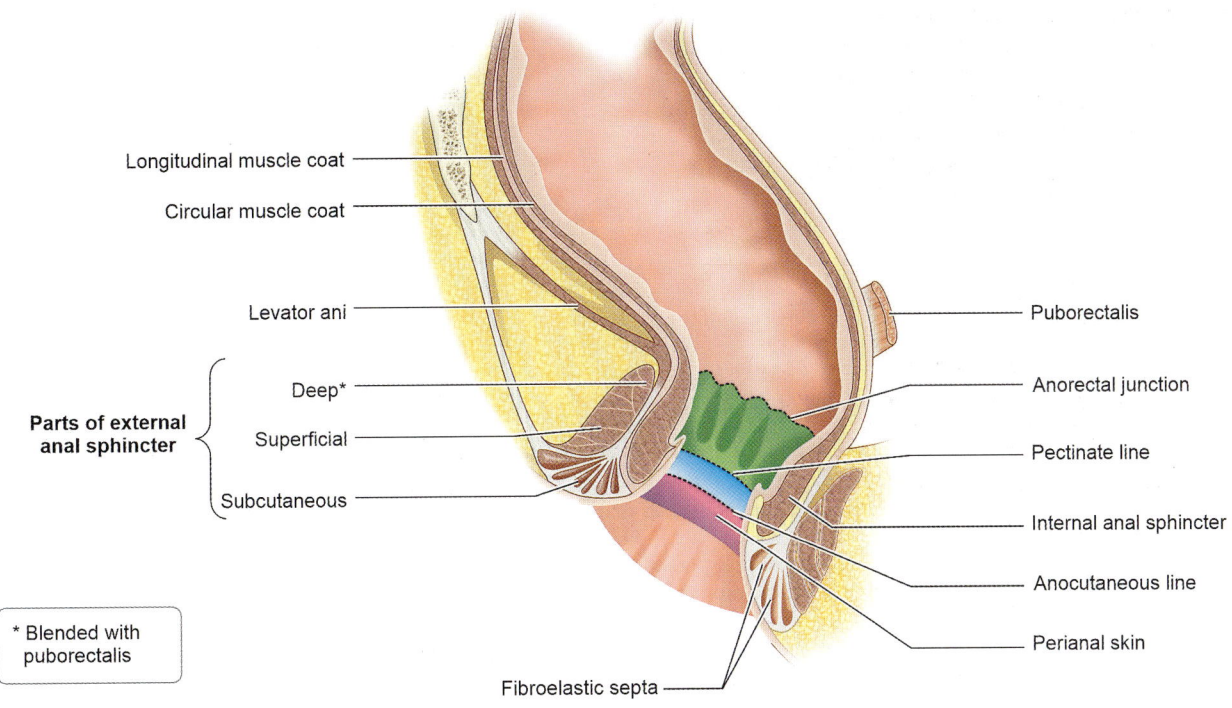

Fig. 2A: Anatomy of anal canal and anal sphincter.

Q. What do you mean by anal incontinence?

Anal incontinence is defined as the complaint of involuntary loss of flatus and/or feces affecting quality of life.

ANAL INCONTINENCE

Q. How does continence of flatus and/or feces occur and how disrupted (pathophysiology of anal incontinence)? Discuss the anatomy.

- The perineal body lies between the vagina and the rectum. It is mostly formed by the bulbocavernosus and transverse perineal muscles and other muscles are puborectalis and the external anal sphincter. The anal sphincter complex (EAS and IAS) lies below the perineal body and extends for a distance of 3–4 cm.
- The external anal sphincter is composed of skeletal muscle. The internal anal sphincter, which overlaps and lies above the external anal sphincter, is composed of smooth muscle which is continuous with the smooth muscle of the colon.
- In urgency, external anal sphincter and puborectalis maintain the continence. Puborectalis muscle provides continence of hard stool whereas external and internal sphincters are responsible for maintenance of flatus and liquid stool.
- The internal anal sphincter provides most of the resting tone of anus and is essential for maintenance of continence.
- Laceration of this sphincter is associated with anal incontinence.

DIAGNOSIS OF OLD COMPLETE PERINEAL TEAR

Q. How would you diagnose complete perineal tear?

Symptoms

- Inability to hold the flatus and feces since her childbirth.
- The involuntary passage of stool and flatus occurs more during increase of intra-abdominal pressure like coughing.
- She is usually young primipara with history of home delivery or difficult labor.

Signs

Local Inspection (Figs. 3A and B)

- Vagina and anal canal open into almost together, complete absence of gynecological perineum.
- Protrusion of pinkish anal mucosa through the opening (or sometimes rectal prolapse).
- Vagina and anal canal are separated by a septum formed by posterior vaginal mucosa and anterior wall of anal mucosa with a lower transverse margin.
- Absence of anal rugae on two anterolateral aspects of anal canal, present only posteriorly.
- Two dimple-like points on two anterolateral aspects of anal canal (at 3 and 9 o'clock position) indicating torn ends of anal sphincter. Dimples become prominent on asking the patient to hold the stool-like action.

Palpation of External Genitalia

- There is absence of sphincteric grip

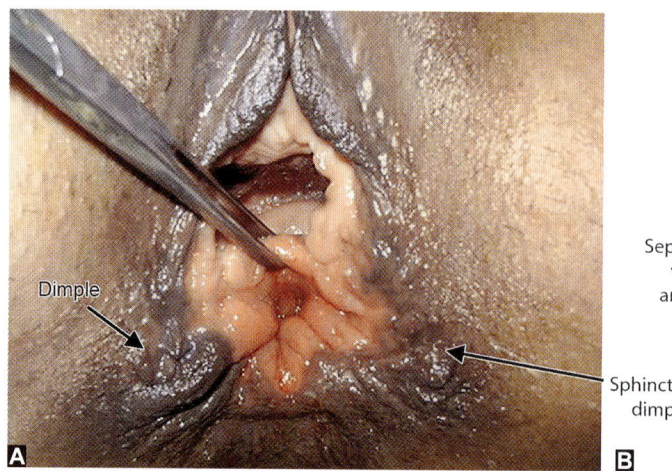
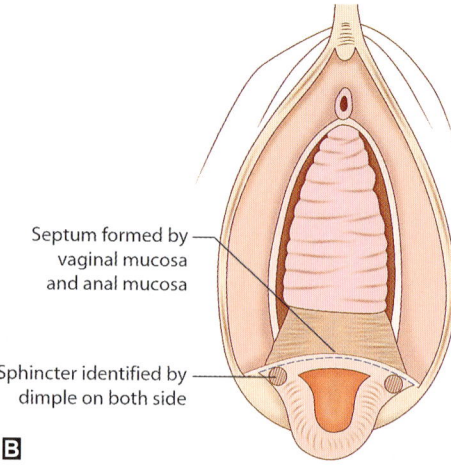

Figs. 3A and B: Complete perineal tear. Vagina and anal canal open into almost together, complete absence of gynecological perineum, protrusion of pinkish anal mucosa through the opening, vagina and anal canal are separated by a septum formed by posterior vaginal mucosa and anterior wall of anal mucosa with a lower transverse margin (held by Allis tissue forceps), absence of anal rugae on two anterolateral aspects of anal canal, present only posteriorly, two dimple-like points on two anterolateral aspects of anal canal (3 and 9 o'clock position) indicating torn ends of anal sphincter. Dimples become prominent on asking the patient to hold the stool-like action.

- Vagina and anal canal are separated by a septum formed by vaginal wall and anal wall with a fibrosed lower concave margin.

Q. What is the significance of incontinence of hard stool and liquid stool?

Puborectalis muscle provides continence of hard stool whereas external and internal sphincters are responsible for maintenance of continence of flatus and liquid stool.

Q. What are the different causes of incontinence of stool?

- *Congenital*: Weakness of sphincter or development defect of perineum
- *Traumatic*: Complete perineal tear, RVF
- *Malignancy*: Rectum, vagina, postradiotherapy
- *Neurological*
- *Infective*: Abscess, Koch's disease (tuberculosis).

Q. What constitutes perineum? Structure of perineum.

Structures from superficial to deep in the perineum:
- Skin
- Fascia of Colles
- Contents of superficial perineal pouch: Superficial transverse perinei, external anal sphincter
- Inferior layer of urogenital diaphragm
- Contents of deep perineal pouch: Transverse perinei profundus, sphincter vaginae
- Superior layer of urogenital diaphragm
- Levator ani
- Pelvic cellular tissue.

Causes of Complete Perineal Tear

Q. What are the causes of complete perineal tear?

Obstetric causes:
- Mismanaged second stage
- Instrumental delivery—more on forceps than ventouse
- Malpresentation—occipitoposterior, after-coming head of breech
- Precipitate labor
- Delivery of large baby
- Shoulder dystocia
- Extension of median episiotomy wound.

Traumatic causes:

Fall on sharp object, trauma by animals, force sodomy, operations for hemorrhoid, and following repair of RVF.

Risk Factors of Complete Perineal Tear

- Nulliparity
- Prolong second stage
- Median episiotomy
- Prolonged second stage
- Precipitate labor
- Persistent occipitoposterior
- Operative delivery
- Large baby
- Asian race.

Prevention of Perineal Tear During Delivery

Q. How would you prevent perineal tear during delivery?

- Proper management of second stage of labor—timely episiotomy, to maintain flexion before extension, to deliver in between contraction, and perineal protection at crowning.
- Mediolateral episiotomy is preferred; angle should be 60° away from the midline when the perineum is distended.
- Episiotomy should be given in instrumental deliveries and of mediolateral type.

Q. During delivery, how would you detect CPT?

Diagnosis at birth—after vaginal birth careful inspection and/or palpation of the local area is done to detect the extent of perineal injury.

Both vaginal and anorectal palpation is extremely important to detect the sphincter injury.

Endoanal ultrasound—**occult OASIS** is better diagnosed by ultrasonography. Intrapartum endoanal ultrasound during labor is used to diagnose clinically occult tear but is not routinely recommended by ACOG (2020).

Treatment of Complete Perineal Tear (OASIS)

Q. What is the treatment of complete perineal tear?

Surgical management is the treatment of complete perineal tear—layer method of perineorrhaphy and sphincteroplasty.

Q. If any CPT occurs during delivery when would you like to repair it and what are the reasons?

Immediately it should be repaired. The advantages are identification of structures is easy, the area is highly vascular with chance of healing and alignment is good and infection is less.

Q. If it is missed to repair in the initial period what is your advice?

If it is not repaired within 24 hours patient is asked to come after 3 months for repair as old CPT. The reasons are during this period involution will be good and the area would be free of infection. In recent days, the concept of early repair has come that will correct sexual and bowel function early. This is also true for dehiscence following episiotomy/OASIS repair.

Q. What preoperative preparation would you like to take in repair of CPT?

- Assessment of the patient clinically
- Routine preoperative investigations, e.g., complete hemogram, VDRL test, blood sugar, urine examination, stool for ova, parasite and cyst, and other investigations as needed for anesthetic fitness.
- Patient should be admitted at least 3 days before surgery.
- Bowel preparation: Low residual diet like milk and fluid with less vegetable, few days before surgery. Bowel should be emptied by aperients and enema. Intake of phthalylsulfathiazole or neomycin oral (350 mg thrice daily) 3 days prior to surgery helps control bacterial flora.
- Vaginal disinfection by douching and insertion of gauze pack soaked with Savlon or betadine in preoperative consecutive few days.
- Consent and preoperative counseling regarding success, recurrence, and complications of surgery.

Q. State the principles of surgery.

- Dissection of the anatomical structures as far as possible.
- Removal of scar tissues, proper apposition without tension with complete hemostasis.
- Prevention of infection as far as possible
- Proper postoperative care.

STEPS OF SURGERY FOR REPAIR OF CPT

Q. Describe the basic steps of surgery for repair of CPT.

It is commonly done by **layer method**, the basic steps of which are:
- Incision for separation of vaginal and anorectal mucosa
- Dissection for exposure of perineal muscles and external sphincters
- Debridement of scar tissue especially of anorectal mucosa
- Repair is done sequentially:
  - Anorectal mucosa
  - Repair of prerectal fascia (internal sphincter)
  - Apposition and repair of external sphincters in midline
  - Repair of musculofascial structures of pelvic floor (perineal body including levator ani)
  - Repair of vaginal mucosa
  - Superficial muscle and subcutaneous tissue
  - Finally skin.

Q. Describe the details of steps of layer method of perineorrhaphy and sphincteroplasty (Figs. 4 to 9).

- Regional saddle block, epidural or general anesthesia
- Patient in lithotomy position, antiseptic dressing, draping and catheterization and final vaginal examination done.

Incision (Figs. 4A and B)

Two lateral ends of rectovaginal septum near the lower edges of labia minora on either side are held by two Allis tissue forceps and stretched from two sides. Other two Allis tissue forceps are applied on either side posterolaterally over the dimple representing the torn end of external anal sphincter. An elliptical incision is made along the junction of posterior vaginal wall and the rectal mucosa. This incision is extended on either side posterolaterally over the dimple (almost H-shaped incision) **(Figs. 4A and B)**.

One tissue forceps is applied over posterior vaginal mucosa corresponding to midpoint of rectovaginal septum about 5 cm away from the margin of rectovaginal septum. A vertical incision of about 2 cm along the midpoint of the septum is made over posterior vaginal wall.

Dissection (Fig. 5): The two flaps of posterior vaginal wall are separated from the anterior wall of rectal mucosa by sharp dissection so that the rectum is separated from the vagina and laterally the perineal muscles are reached and a good rectovaginal space is exposed. The incisions over the dimples are deepened to expose the torn end of sphincter ani externus.

The sphincter is identified by pulling the torn end with Allis tissue forceps and feeling tightness of sphincter as a cord behind the anus.

Lower scarred part of vaginal mucosa near margin is excised. Any scar tissue along the lower margin of torn rectum and anus is excised. And this will freshen the cut edges.

SECTION 2: Clinical Cases

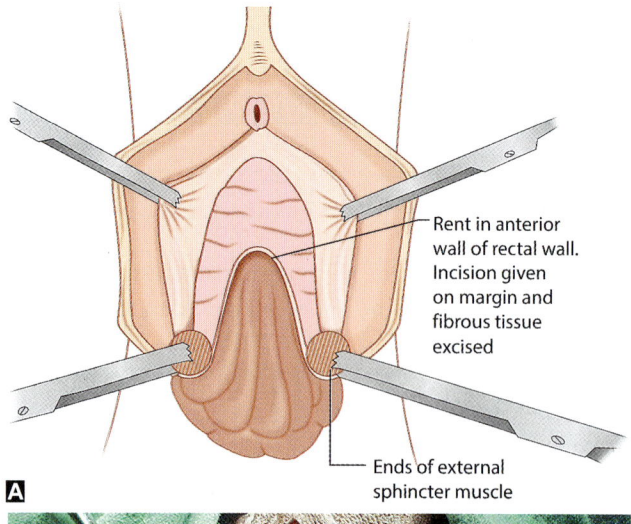

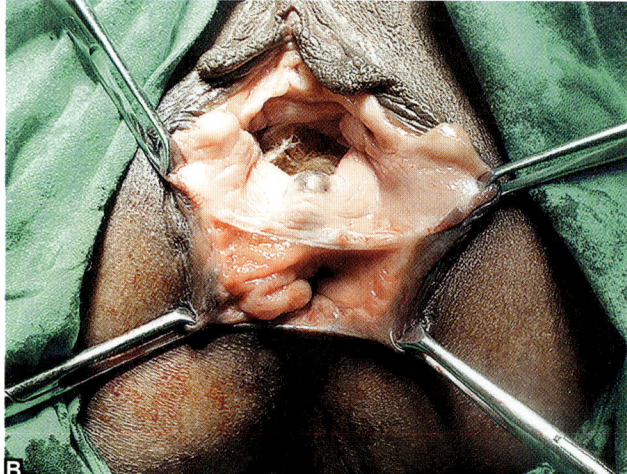

Figs. 4A and B: Holding with four Allis tissue forceps. Two lateral ends of rectovaginal septum near the lower edges of labia minora on either side are held by two Allis tissue forceps and stretched from two sides. Other two Allis tissue forceps are applied on either side posterolaterally over the dimple representing the torn end of external anal sphincter (almost H-shaped).

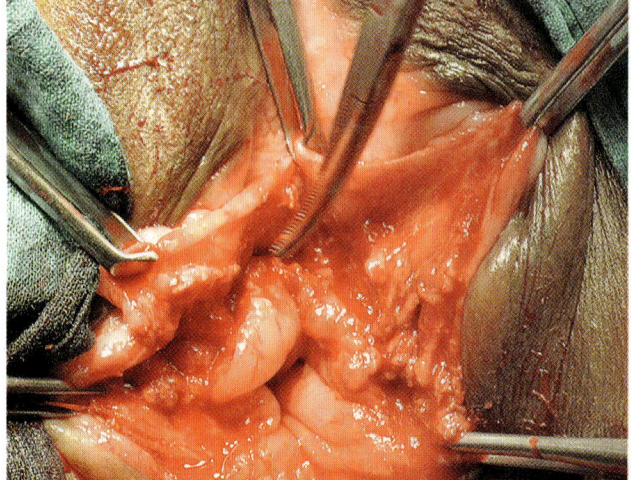

Fig. 5: Dissection of rectovaginal space. Torn ends of external sphincters are held by two Allis tissue forceps.

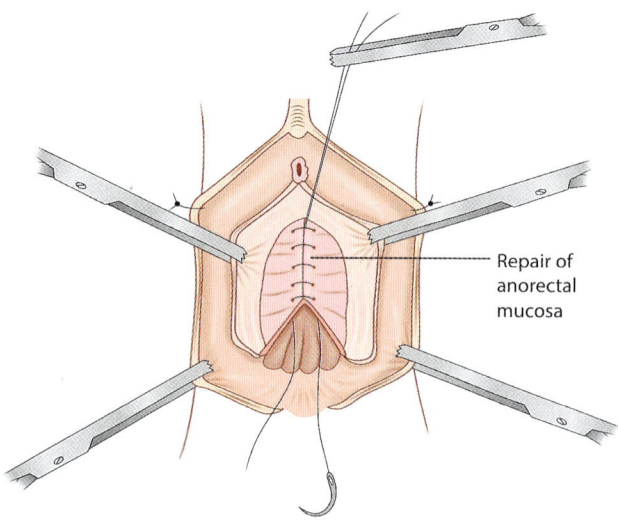

Fig. 6: Anorectal mucosa is repaired with 3-0 continuous or interrupted delayed absorbable suture.

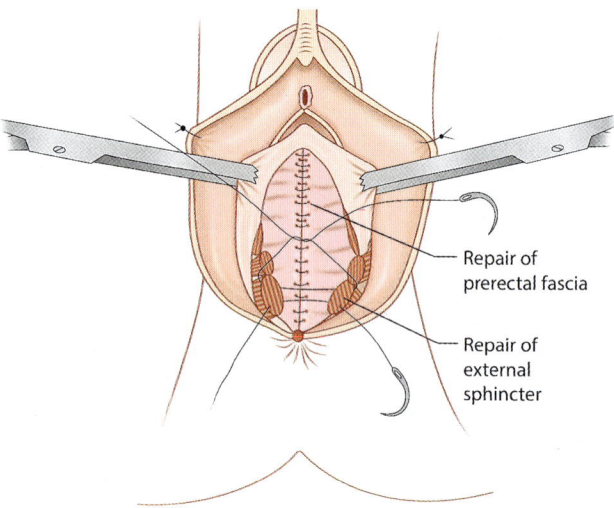

Fig. 7: Repair of prerectal fascia.

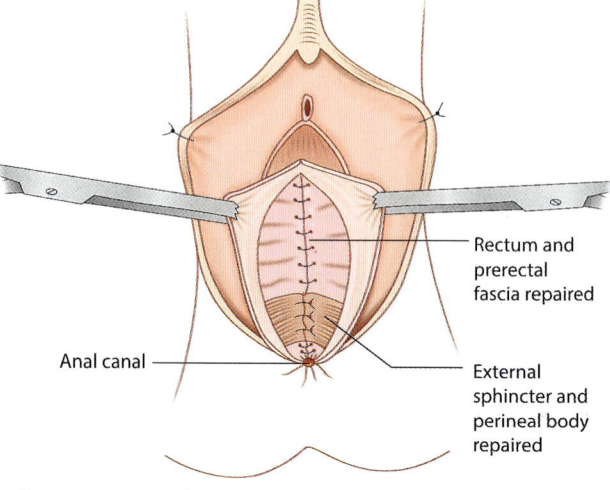

Fig. 8: Rectum and prerectal fascia, perineal body and external sphincter repaired.

CHAPTER 18: A Case of Old Complete Perineal Tear

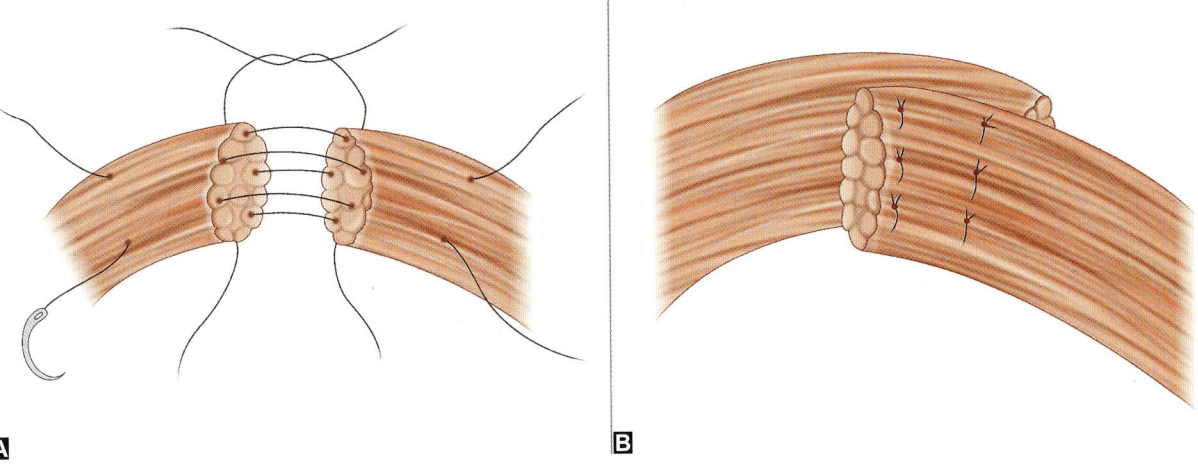

Figs. 9A and B: (A) Repair of external ani sphincter—end to end; (B) Repair of external ani sphincter— overlapping.

Removal of scar tissue and mobilization of rectum are important steps so far as success of the operation is concerned.

Repair is done in following sequences:

Anorectal mucosa: Upper edge of her torn rectum is held by Allis forceps, and the anorectal mucosa is repaired with 3-0 continuous or interrupted delayed absorbable suture to reach the mucocutaneous margin of the anal opening, so as to make a normal anus. These sutures take the entire thickness of lumen of anorectum **(Fig. 6)**.

Prerectal fascia (internal sphincter): First layer of sutures is reinforced and buried with a second layer which is the prerectal fascia, recently regarded as internal anal sphincter. This suture should be of Lambert type. This layer is given either interrupted or continuous 3-0 delayed absorbable sutures **(Figs. 7 and 8)**.

Repair of external sphincter: The freshened torn ends of both sides are brought to midline and sutured end to end **(Fig. 9A)** or overlapping technique **(Fig. 9B)** with 2-3 interrupted figure of eight or interrupted sutures.

Repair of the perineal body: The two levator ani muscles are drawn together in between posterior vaginal wall and the anterior wall of rectum and anal canal and sutured by interrupted stitches **(Fig. 8)**.

Repair of posterior vaginal margins: These are repaired by continuous 2-0 or 1-0 delayed absorbable sutures from apex to near perineal skin **(Fig. 10)**.

Repair of subcutaneous tissue and skin: These are repaired with interrupted 1-0 delayed absorbable sutures. Following these stitches the formation of anus is completed, so that rugae radiate from it like the spokes of a wheel **(Figs. 10 and 11)**.

Postoperative Management after Repair of CPT

- Care of the wound daily with antiseptic solution and after micturition. Wound should be kept dry.
- Continuous catheterization is done as reflex retention is common after this operation.

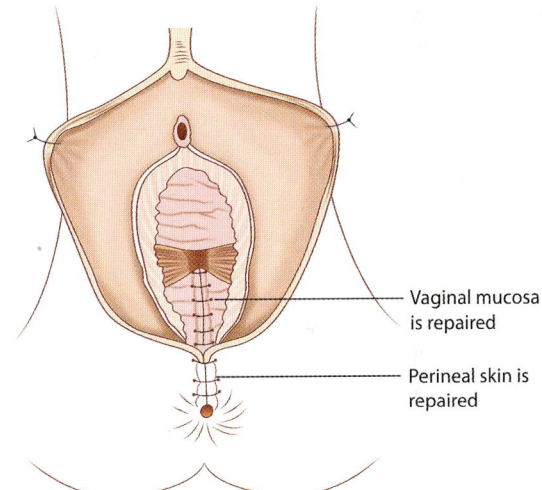

Fig. 10: Vaginal mucosa and perineal stitches completed. The formation of anus is completed, and rugae radiate from it like the spokes of a wheel.

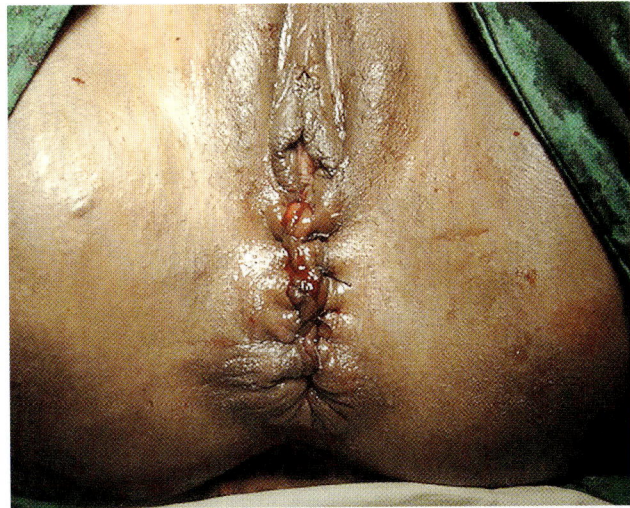

Fig. 11: Vaginal mucosa and perineal stitches completed. The formation of anus is completed, and rugae radiate from it like the spokes of a wheel.

- Patient is kept for intravenous fluid for first 24 hours.
- Bowel should be confined for 5 days—nutrition and laxative are adjusted accordingly.
- Diet—low roughage diet is given for 4 postoperative days. Tea, soup, fruit juice, milk, and gradually boiled egg and biscuits are given. Vegetables are avoided. After clear of bowel normal diet is allowed which is usually after 5 days.
- Good analgesia.
- Broad-spectrum antibiotics.
- Patient is asked to lie on lateral position or in a posture so that thighs are adducted.
- Laxative—from first postoperative day lactulose is prescribed, the dose of which is gradually increased. Laxative is given from fourth postoperative day. Bulk laxative is avoided.
- Patient is discharged on third week.

Advice During Discharge

- To come on follow-up after 4 weeks or earlier if necessary and regular follow-up for 6 months.
- Avoid constipation.
- Physiotherapy
- To avoid pregnancy for 1 year.
- To avoid sexual intercourse for 8 weeks.
- In next pregnancy and delivery always under specialized hospital care.

Postoperative Complications

- Wound disruption and failure—sometimes only in wait and watch policy it may heal and for this secondary repair should not be attempted before 3 months.
- Infection
- Secondary hemorrhage
- Hematoma
- Functional failure in spite of anatomical apposition
- Dyspareunia
- Rectal and anal canal stenosis.

Prognosis

About 60–80% of women become asymptomatic after 12 months after delivery in repair of recent CPT.

Preoperative Counseling and Consent

- The complications are described
- Success rate of surgery is 80%.

Management of Pregnancy and Labor in Case of Post CPT Repair

Pregnancy should be cared in a specialized hospital.

There is no clear recommendation for routine cesarean section after repair though many advise for routine cesarean section in post-repair pregnancy.

In patients with persisting fecal incontinence, reduced sphincter function or suspected fetal macrosomia an elective cesarean section is suggested.

Q. What are the other lesions may be associated with CPT?

As this is a case of mismanaged labor the other lesions like vesicovaginal fistula (VVF) and RVF are looked for.

Q. Is there genital prolapse a common association with CPT? Why not?

In spite of tear of decussating fibers of the levator ani muscles the incidence of prolapse in CPT is uncommon. As the patient draws together the levator ani continuously in an effort to close the bowel the levator ani on both sides acquire good tone thus preventing genital prolapse. This can be evident on palpation of levator during clinical examination.

Q. If there is amenorrhea what do you exclude?

When there is amenorrhea, exclude the pregnancy.

Q. If CPT is detected in antenatal period when would you repair?

Not during pregnancy and not immediately after delivery.

RECTOVAGINAL FISTULA (RVF)

Q. What do you mean by RVF?

Rectovaginal fistula is a communication between the rectum and anal canal with the vagina resulting passages of feces and flatus through the vagina **(Figs. 12 to 15)**.

Q. What are the causes of RVF?

- *Congenital*: It is rare.

In vestibular anus, anal canal opens into the vagina instead of its normal position.

- *Acquired*:
    - Traumatic:
        - Obstetric trauma: (1) Faulty repair of obstetric CPT or nonhealing of repaired CPT **(Figs. 13A and B)** or (2) Obstructed labor; (3) Instrumental delivery, and (4) Inclusion of rectal mucosa during episiotomy repair.

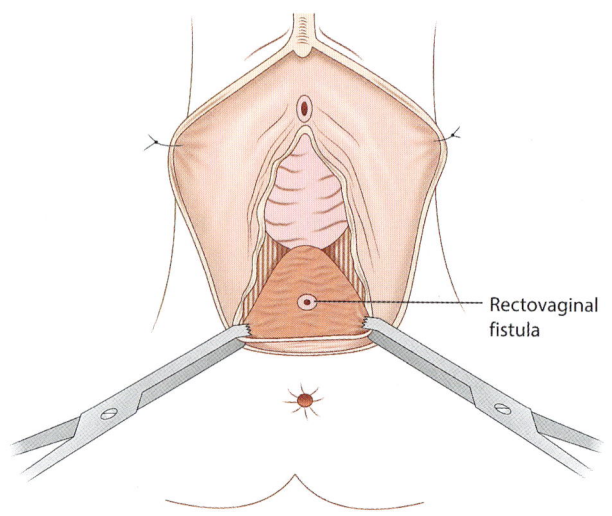

Fig. 12: Rectovaginal fistula.

CHAPTER 18: A Case of Old Complete Perineal Tear

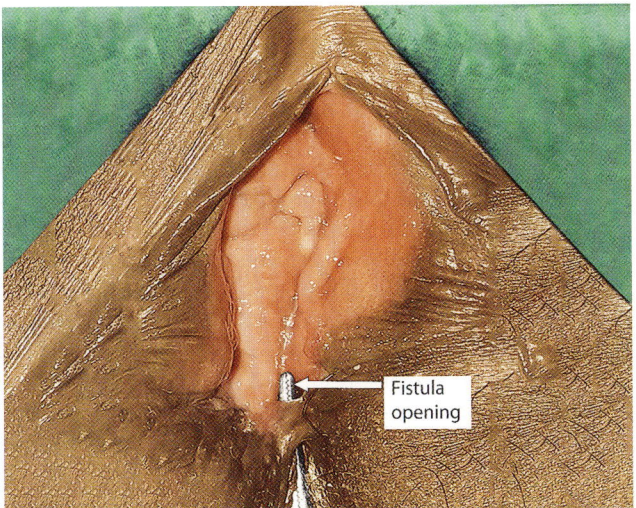

Fig. 13A: Rectovaginal fistula—a small mosquito forceps introduced through RVF following an episiotomy.

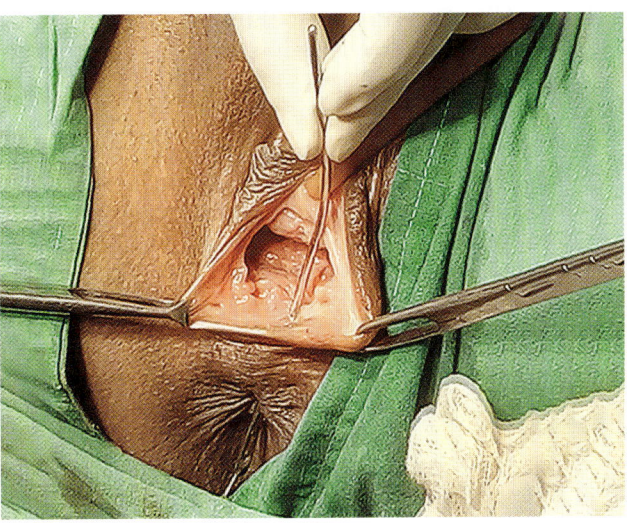

Fig. 13B: Rectovaginal fistula showing by a probe.
Courtesy: Professor Sukanta Mishra, HOD, VIMS, Kolkata

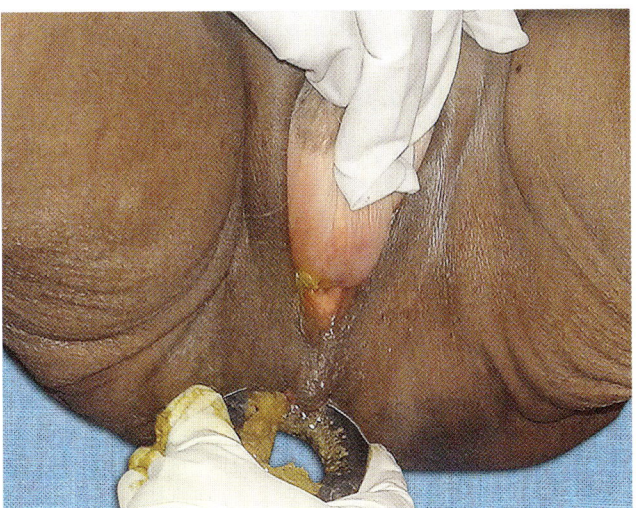

Fig. 14: The ring pessary was removed from the rectum.

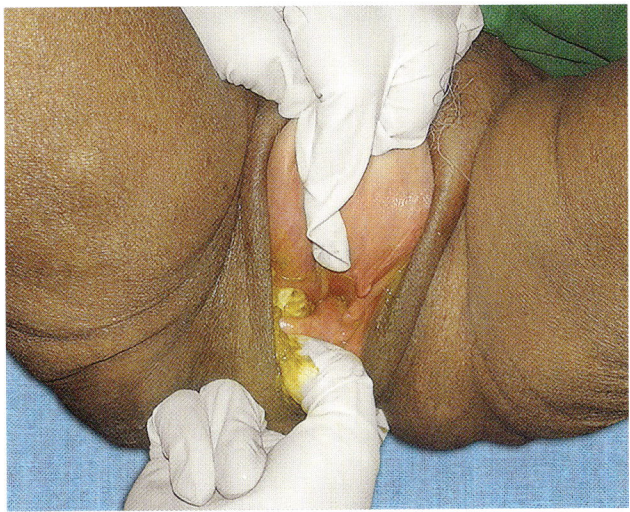

Fig. 15: Tip of the finger is seen in vagina through the rectovaginal fistula on rectal examination.

Figs. 14 and 15: Rectovaginal fistula (RVF) due to ring pessary.

A 75-year-old woman attended outpatient department with complain of mild pain, constipation and difficulty in defecation. On per vaginal examination she had 2nd degree uterine prolapse with fecal contamination of vagina due to a rectovaginal fistula of 3 × 3 cm size situated at upper part of posterior wall of vagina. On rectal examination a rubber ring pessary was found in rectum which was removed digitally. On interrogation patient gave history of introduction of such device more than 15 years back but she had forgotten.
Courtesy: Professor Ramprasad Dey, Obstetrics and Gynecology, Chittaranjan Seva Sadan

- Operative trauma: During hysterectomy both abdominal or vaginal, radical hysterectomy, perineorrhaphy, repair of enterocele and colpotomy
- Penetrating injury: Fall on a sharp object.
- Infective: Pararectal abscess and pelvic abscess
- Malignant: Cancer of cervix, vagina, and rectum
- Radiation fistula: Radiotherapy in cervical cervix
- Forgotten pessary **(Figs. 14 and 15)**.

Causes of high fistula are during difficult hysterectomy and radiation.

Location of RVF

- Low
- Middle
- High

Q. How would you diagnose RVF?

From symptoms and signs.

Symptoms of RVF

Passage of flatus and stool into the vagina (most common). In small fistula, only flatus comes out. Incontinence of stool through a large fistula is very destressing. Symptoms may appear immediately after delivery, sometimes after a week.

Signs of RVF

In big fistula it is easily diagnosed by pelvic examination, speculum examination, and rectovaginal examination. The sites and sizes are noted. In opening there may be pinkish rectal mucosa or stool is visible. There may be scarring even vaginal stenosis. In small fistula, examination under anesthesia may be needed. Following repair of CPT fistula becomes evident usually after 7–10 days. Small fistula may heal spontaneously.

Probe Test

In case of small fistula a probe is passed through the vagina and the tip can be seen and felt through rectal examination (*see* **Fig. 13B**).

Prevention of RVF

To take care during conduct of delivery and to repair the CPT by experienced surgeon.

Management of RVF

Q. What is the treatment of RVF?

Surgical repair after 8–12 weeks. Sometime small fistula heals spontaneously.

For low or middle fistula, vaginal approach is sufficient. In upper fistula, abdominal method may be needed.

- *Fistula situated in lower third of vagina*: It is converted into complete perineal tear and repaired as CPT.
- *Fistula situated at middle or upper part*: Repair is done by flap splitting method. A circular incision is given around the fistula. Vagina is separated from the rectum with sharp dissection circumferentially and entire fistula tract is excised.

  It is repaired in three layers: (1) This includes rectal muscularis mucosa and submucosa extramucosally with interrupted or continuous 3-0 absorbable sutures. (2) The second layer of bowel is given to invert the first layer and this includes internal sphincter. (3) Third layer is the approximation of vaginal wall by 3-0 delayed absorbable suture.

  No suture is preferably entered the lumen. In between second and third layer puborectalis and the external anal sphincter reconstruction may be needed if the fistula is very low down.
- Fistula situated near vault is difficult to repair from below and abdominal approach may be needed.
- Preoperative bowel preparation is mandatory.
- **For difficult RVF or postradiation fistula** *temporary colostomy* is done first followed by repair of fistula after 10 days and closure of colostomy done after 6 weeks.
- **In vestibular anus,** Rizzoli's operation is performed by following steps:
  - Anus is dissected free
  - Incision over perineum
  - Anal margins are sutured to the skin of perineum, and finally
  - Suturing of perineal wound. Congenital fistula is better to repair after puberty after full development of vagina.

Section 3

Reproductive Physiology

Section Outline

19. Physiology of Ovulation, Menstruation, Spermatogenesis and Implantation
20. Menopause and its Management
21. Development of Genital Organs and Müllerian Anomaly

CHAPTER 19

Physiology of Ovulation, Menstruation, Spermatogenesis and Implantation

Chapter Outline

- Oogenesis
- Development of Ovarian Follicles—Ovarian Cycles
- Cyclical Hormonal Changes
- Endometrial Cycles
- Spermatogenesis
- Structure of Spermatozoa
- Fertilization
- Transport of Fertilized Ova
- Implantation
- Premenstrual Syndrome (PMS) or Premenstrual Tension (PMT)

INTRODUCTION

Menstruation occurs in a cyclical fashion due to the effect hormonal changes in ovarian cycle.

Ovarian cycle consists of:
- Follicular phase
- Ovulation phase
- Luteal phase.

Endometrial cycle consists of:
- Menstruation
- Proliferative phase
- Secretory phase.

Follicular phase corresponds to proliferative phase and luteal phase corresponds to secretory phase.

PHYSIOLOGY OF OVULATION

Process of Oogenesis (Fig. 1)

Development of Primordial Follicles

At the early embryonic life the germ cells differentiate (mitosis) into oogonia and enter into the first meiotic division as *primary oocytes,* when development is arrested until puberty. Arrest occurs in prophase phase (diplotene stage) of meiosis I (Meiosis has four phases, namely prophase, metaphase, anaphase, and telophase. Prophase has five stages: leptotene, zygotene, pachytene, diplotene, and diakinesis).

The number of oocytes reaches maximum in the fetus to *6-7 million by 20 weeks of gestation* and parallely atresia of oogonia occurs rapidly followed by follicular atresia. No new oocyte is formed during rest of life. At the diplotene stage, the oocyte is surrounded by single layer of 8-10 granulosa cells and will form *primordial follicle* which will be used up for follicular development at menarche till menopause.

In each month of reproductive years several primordial follicles mature into primary follicles. Only few of the primary follicles will develop into *secondary follicles.*

One or two of the secondary follicles will progress to *tertiary or Graafian follicle,* at the stage of which meiosis I is completed to produce *secondary oocyte (haploid) and first polar body.*

The secondary oocyte halts meiosis at its second metaphase. *One secondary oocyte is released at ovulation.*

Completion of second meiotic division and *release of second polar body occur only after fertilization.*

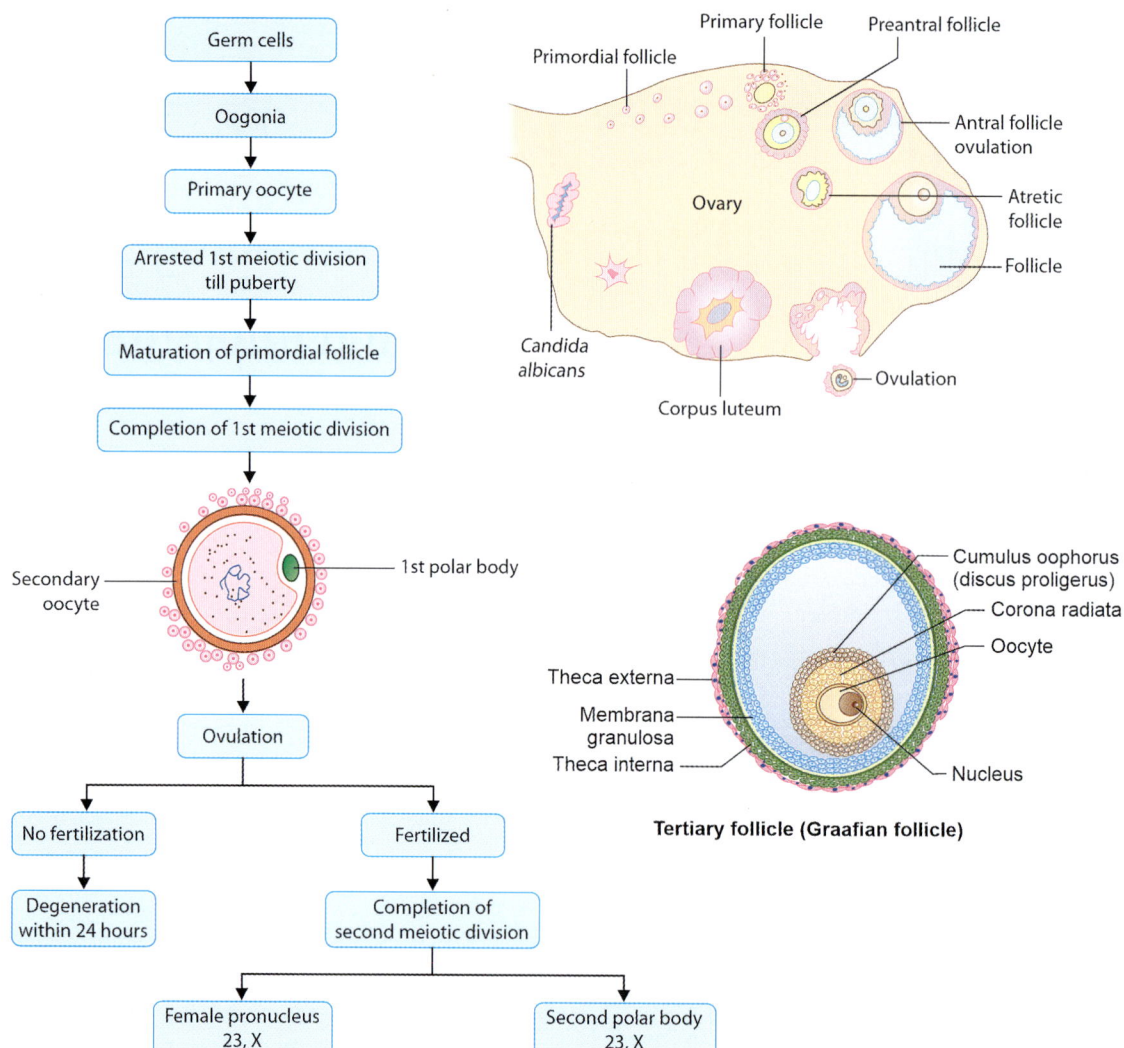

Fig. 1: Oogenesis is from germ cell—look secondary oocyte contains one polar body and the ovulated oocyte is secondary oocyte containing only one polar body. Second polar body is only formed after fertilization (see Fig. 15).

The Sequence of Phases is as Follows (see Fig. 1)

Primordial follicles → Primary follicles → Secondary follicles (preantral follicles) → Tertiary or antral follicles → Preovulatory or Graafian follicles → Ovulated as secondary oocyte.

The oogonia devoid of granulosa cells will undergo atresia. To survive, i.e. to be rescued from atresia, oogonia must enter into meiotic prophase.

At birth only *300,000 oocytes* remain for ovulation, others undergo atresia and of these 300,000 only 400–500 will be ovulated throughout reproductive life. Oogonia begin to enter meiotic prophase I at about 8 weeks of gestation and called **primary oocyte.**

Hence, the *primordial follicle* is nongrowing and consists of primary oocyte, arrested at in diplotene stage of meiotic prophase, surrounded by single layer spindle-shaped granulosa cells and will remain so until the time of ovulation when the process of meiosis will resume.

Oocyte maturation inhibitor (OMI) produced by granulosa cells is said to be responsible for this stasis at meiosis I. OMI acts by getting access to oocytes via gap junctions at surrounding cumulus of granulosa.

Just before ovulation with the midcycle luteinizing hormone (LH) surge gap junctions between granulosa and oocyte are disrupted and OMI cannot act and meiosis I is resumed.

Further Developments of Ovarian Follicles

With the onset of puberty *primordial follicles* will be activated and grow in a cyclical fashion through stages of *preantral follicle, antral follicle, preovulatory follicle* finally causing ovulation, *corpus luteum* formation, and subsequent menstruation in the event of nonfertilization.

Hence with each normal menstrual cycle ovary will pass through three phases **(Fig. 2)**:

1. Follicular phase

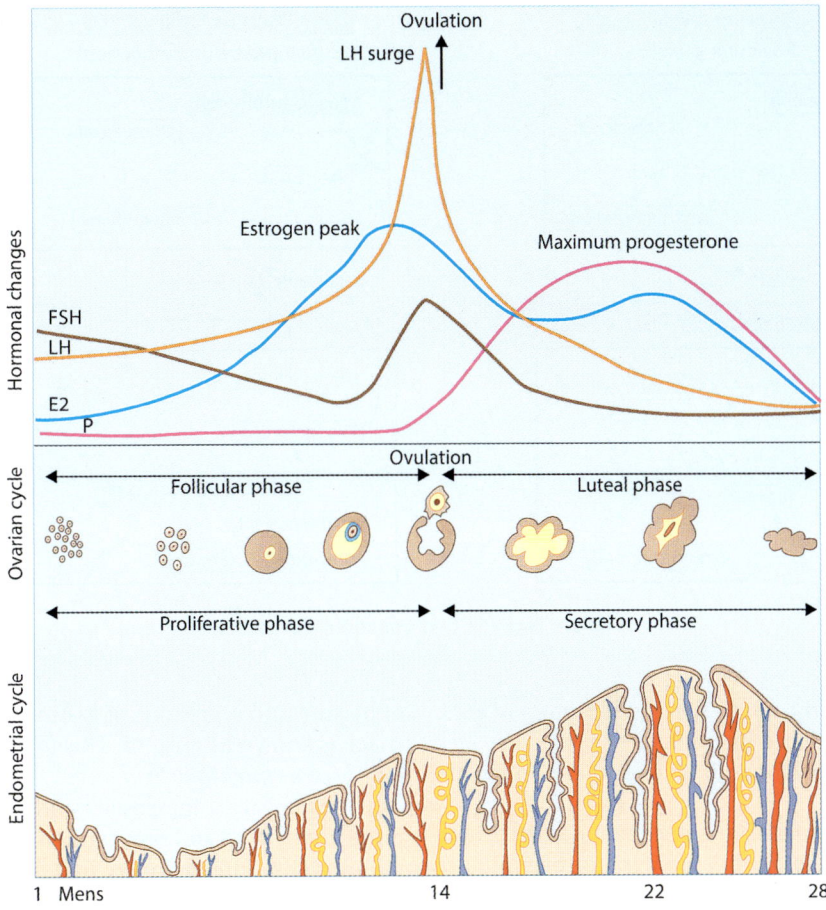

Fig. 2: Endometrial cycle, ovarian cycle, and cyclical changes of pituitary and ovarian hormones.

2. Ovulation phase
3. Luteal phase.

Follicular phase

For single ovulation from a dominant follicle in each cycle a cohort of follicles are recruited over the time span of several menstrual cycles, but the ovulatory follicle is one of a cohort recruited at the time of the *luteal follicular transition* at the preceding month. The mechanism of determining which follicles and how many follicles will be recruited is unknown. Total duration of time taken to reach preovulatory status is about 85 days. Recruitment and initial growth of the cohort of primordial follicles is gonadotropin independent.

Soon after initial recruitment cohort of follicles is assumed to go under control of follicle- stimulating hormone (FSH) for further growth (gonadotropin-independent to gonadotropin-dependent growth). In late luteal phase of previous cycle when there is decline in estrogen, progesterone and inhibin A FSH starts to increase which stimulates follicular growth. The first changes seen are increase in the size of oocyte and transformation of single layer of granulosa cells to multilayer of cuboidal cells.

Formation of secondary or preantral follicle: As the oocyte is enlarged it is surrounded by a membrane, zona pellucida which is formed by glycoprotein-rich substance secreted by oocyte to form preantral follicle. Simultaneously, there is mitotic proliferation of granulosa cells surrounding oocyte and theca cells in the stroma bordering granulosa cells and stroma is differentiated into theca interna and theca externa. At this point, one follicle of the cohort will be selected for dominance which becomes evident at about fifth day of cycle and others undergo atresia.

The *theca cells will produce androgen and granulosa cells will produce estrogens* under influence of pituitary LH and FSH, respectively. This is called *two-cell, two-gonadotropin theory.*

TWO-CELL, TWO-GONADOTROPIN THEORY (FIG. 2A)

According to this theory, there is subdivision and compartmentalization of steroid hormone synthesis property in the developing follicles.

Androgens (mostly androstenedione) are synthesized from cholesterol by the theca cells in response to stimulation by LH as theca cells at this stage are abundant of LH receptors.

These androgens are transferred to granulosa cells where androgens are aromatized to produce estrogens under the influence of FSH and aromatase activity is mostly found

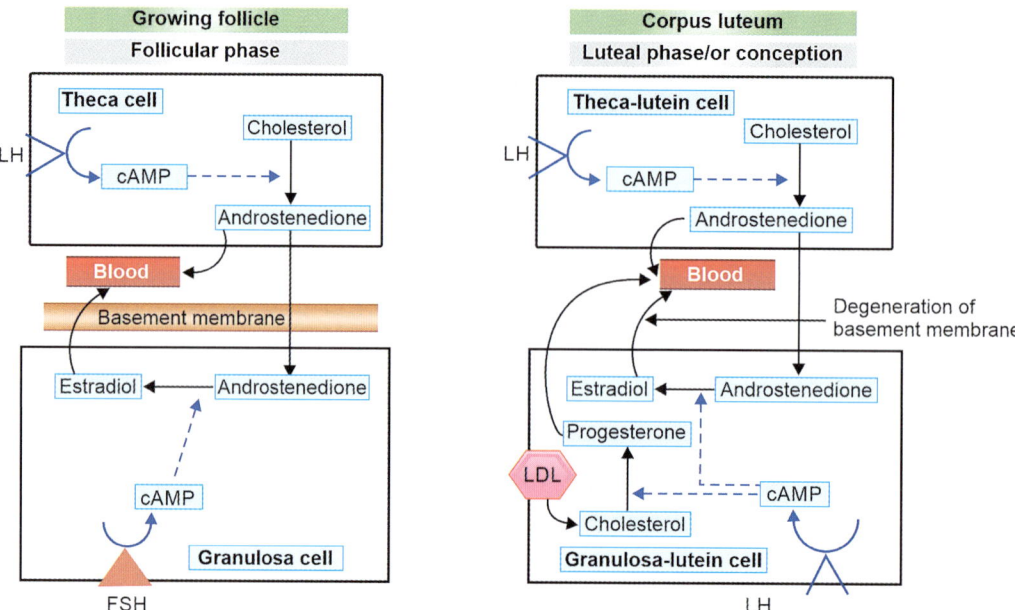

Fig. 2A: Two-cell, two-gonadotropin theory.
Abbreviations: LH, luteinizing hormone; FSH, follicle-stimulating hormone; cAMP, cyclic adenosine monophosphate

in granulosa cells which contain specific receptors of FSH. Androgens are not produced in granulosa cells as they lack several enzymes essential for androgen synthesis which are present in theca cells.

Estrogen has a great role in creating a microenvironment and along with FSH it helps further proliferation of granulosa cells, estrogen production, and FSH receptor synthesis.

Androgens promote granulosa cell proliferation, aromatase activity and will inhibit granulosa cell death. However, chronic elevation of androgens suppresses H-P secretion of FSH and is detrimental to any follicular growth as found in polycystic ovary syndrome (PCOS).

Q. How dominant follicle is selected?

With follicular development peripheral estrogen and inhibin B increase, which in turn give negative feedback to pituitary and hypothalamus to decrease FSH levels. This falling FSH level results a threat to continue follicular growth and helps in selection of a single "dominant follicle".

The follicle which has the *greatest number of FSH receptors* with a richly estrogen microenvironment will escape from atresia and will be *"dominant follicle"* and the others will cease to grow. This dominant follicle will produce more estrogen which will further decrease FSH by negative feedback and with this decline of FSH other follicles of initial cohort except dominant one will suffer atresia. In exogenous gonadotropin administration this natural synchronization is lost and multiple follicles will grow as found in ovulation induction.

Rise of estrogen level in spite of decrease of FSH at this stage is *explained* by the fact the dominant follicle acquires maximum number of receptors for FSH.

Formation of antral or tertiary follicle and preovulatory or Graafian follicle: With further development of dominant follicle there is accumulation of fluid which is composed of plasma and secretions of granulosa cells. The fluid-filled space is known as antrum. This follicle is now called *antral follicle or tertiary follicle.*

Follicular size is increased rapidly due to accumulation of more antral fluid and now termed preovulatory or Graafian follicle. Thus preovulatory follicle is composed of fluid-filled antrum (*antrum folliculi*) and granulosa cells are differentiated into heterogeneous population.

The wall of the antrum is formed by a few layers of cuboidal granulosa cells called *membrana granulosa*. The oocyte is surrounded by granulosa cells and in one side it is connected with follicle by specialized granulosa cells which is called *cumulus oophorus or discus proligerus.*

The granulosa cells immediately surrounding the oocyte are arranged in radial fashion and called *corona radiata.* The granulosa cell mass is avascular and gets nutrition from vascular ovarian stroma.

The ovarian stroma is differentiated into inner highly vascular layer, *theca interna* and outer fibrous stromal cell layer called *theca externa.*

Just before ovulation unequal division occurs with formation of secondary oocyte and first polar body (*see* **Fig. 1**). The diameter of mature or secondary oocyte is 100 µ.

Second polar body and mature oocyte are formed only after fertilization by second meiotic division. The mature follicle diameter is about 18 mm. It occupies outer layer of cortex and lies near the surface prior to ovulation.

Primary oocyte contains 46 chromosomes, secondary oocyte 23 chromosomes, and mature oocyte also 23 chromosomes.

Ovarian and pituitary hormones in follicular development: Circulating *estrogens* has biphasic pattern of effect on pituitary LH secretion. Lower estrogen concentration inhibits LH and higher concentration gives positive feedback to LH release.

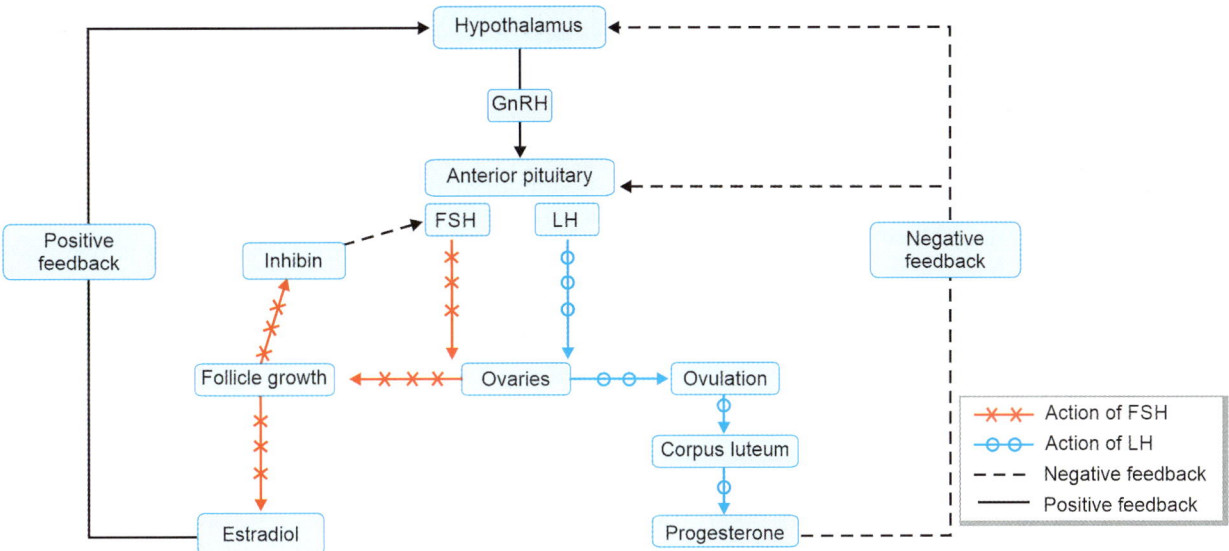

Fig. 2B: Regulators of gonadotropins.
Abbreviations: GnRH, gonadotropin-releasing hormone; LH, luteinizing hormone; FSH, follicle-stimulating hormone

When the estrogen level is sustained at a higher level of 200 pg/mL for more than 48 hours LH surge occurs by positive feedback to both hypothalamus and anterior pituitary gland. At the same time estrogen-FSH interaction induces the formation of LH receptors on the granulosa cells of dominant follicle.

Luteinizing hormone surge results luteinization of granulosa cells and production of progesterone which further gives positive feedback for LH secretion and also small preovulatory rise in FSH. From the theca cells androgens secretion also rises around the time of ovulation and this androgen is thought to increase libido to ensure sexual activity at the highest time of fertility.

The LH surge also stimulates the resumption of meiosis of oocyte prior to ovulation and triggers ovulation. Mean duration of LH surge is 48 hours and *ovulation occurs about 34–36 hours after the onset of LH surge.*

The basal level of serum FSH and LH ranges 5–10 IU/L and in midcycle levels peaks to 2 times in FSH and 3 times in LH than basal level in normal ovulatory woman.

OVULATION PHASE (*SEE* FIG. 2)

Under the influence of LH, FSH and progesterone local concentration of prostaglandins and proteolytic enzymes are increased in follicular wall which becomes weakened and an opening is formed through which *slow extrusion of secondary oocyte occurs, called ovulation* (Fig. 3).

Ovulation is not an explosive rupture rather a slow extrusion of oocyte. Ovulation occurs 10–12 hours of LH peak or 34–36 hours after the onset of midcycle LH rise.

Regulators of Gonadotropins (Fig. 2B)

Steroid hormones are the main regulator. Other than steroid hormones there are autocrine and paracrine mediators. The two peptides are *inhibin* and *activin* produced by granulosa cells. Inhibin has two forms A and B.

Inhibin B is produced in follicular phase and *inhibin A* is produced in luteal phase. Both inhibins inhibit (negative feedback) FSH synthesis and release. *Activin* is structurally similar to inhibin but has opposite action. It stimulates FSH release from the pituitary and potentiates its action on ovary.

There are several *paracrine regulators* found in the ovary. These are insulin-like growth factor (IGF-I and IGF-II), epidermal growth factor (EGF), transforming growth factor-alpha (TGFα, β1), interleukin-1, tissue necrosis factor-b, etc. They in several ways promote the normal ovulatory process.

Luteal Phase—Formation of Corpus Luteum

After release of ovary the remaining follicular shell containing granulosa and theca cells is transformed into corpus luteum.

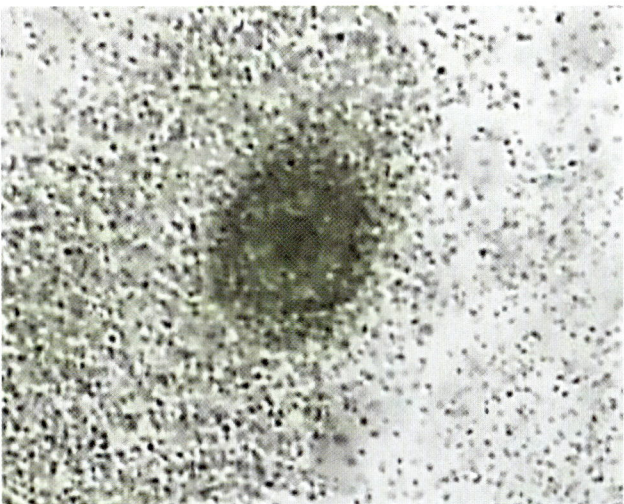

Fig. 3: Mature oocyte surrounded by cumulus cells.
Courtesy: IRM, Kolkata

Membranous granulosa cells take up yellow lutein pigment and lipids. In the corpus luteum basement membrane degenerates (**Fig. 2A**) and undergoes extensive vascularization in order to rich blood supply to granulosa cells for continued steroidogenesis and supply to systemic circulation. This is helped by secretion of angiogenic factors, such as vascular endothelial growth factor (VEGF).

Corpus luteum passes through *three stages,* namely:
- *Stage of proliferation*
- *Stage of vascularization, stage of maturity and*
- *Stage of involution.*

Pituitary LH secretion and granulosa cell activity produce progesterone which prepares the endometrial bed for implantation. Corpus luteum also produces estradiol and inhibin A.

Progesterone and estradiol will give negative feedback to decrease FSH and LH secretion. Inhibin also potentiates FSH withdrawal.

Decline of FSH and LH will go in such a level that further recruitment and development of ovarian follicles will not occur.

Ovarian apoplexy: Sometimes though rarely, corpus luteum cyst is formed following ovulation due to hemorrhage in the corpus luteum which usually regresses spontaneously. There may be pain due to excessive bleeding inside the cyst. Rarely, rupture occurs resulting profuse intraperitoneal hemorrhage which needs immediate surgical intervention (ovarian apoplexy) which usually occurs within 21–25 days of the cycle. Picture is like ectopic pregnancy. For detail *see* Chapter 3: A Case of Lump Abdomen (Ovarian Tumor).

Q. What is luteal-placental shift?

If conception does occur human chorionic gonadotropin (hCG) will be secreted by placental trophoblasts and will stimulate corpus luteum to secret progesterone and luteal function is essential at least *up to 5 weeks* of gestation following which placenta itself will produce required progesterone and will take the charge to maintain pregnancy (*luteal-placental shift*).

Luteolysis and corpus albicans formation

In absence of implantation and lack of hCG production corpus luteum will invariably regress after 12–16 days of ovulation which is known as *luteolysis* and will form *corpus albicans*. The exact mechanism of luteolysis is not known, probably a local paracrine regulation plays a role.

Due to the regression of corpus luteum progesterone production stops and shedding of endometrium occurs resulting menstruation.

Waning of estrogen, progesterone, and inhibin A will withdraw the central negative feedback to gonadotropin and will allow FSH and LH levels to rise and new preantral follicles start to be stimulated and a new cycle begins.

Progesterone level reaches maximum in midluteal phase (40 mg/day). *Progesterone level more than 3 ng/mL on day 21 indicates ovulation*. Level of more than *10–15 ng/mL indicates luteal phase adequacy* and no progesterone supplementation is needed.

PHYSIOLOGY OF MENSTRUATION (*SEE* FIG. 2)

Endometrium

Endometrium consists of three layers, namely:
- Stratum compactum (superficial compact zone)
- Stratum spongiosum (intermediate zone)
- Stratum basalis (deepest zone).

The superficial two zones comprising of two-thirds is called *decidua functionalis* and shed with each cycle in absence of pregnancy.

The deep stratum basalis also called *decidua basalis* is not shed and from this the zone superficial zones regenerate. Stratum compactum contains gland necks and dense stroma, stratum spongiosum contains glands, loose stroma, and interstitial tissue.

Blood Vessels in Uterus

Uterus gets blood supply from *uterine* and *ovarian arteries* from where *arcuate arteries* arise to supply myometrium.

Radial arteries arise from arcuate artery at right angle to extend toward endometrium.

Radial artery bifurcates at myoendometrial junction to divide into *basal arteries* and *spiral arteries*. Basal arteries supply the basal layer and spiral arteries to functional layer to form subepithelial plexus. Basal arteries are relatively unresponsive to hormones whereas spiral arteries respond to hormonal changes with more coiling and spasm resulting bloodshed in mens.

Endometrium is under the influence of sex steroids, estrogen, and progesterone secreted by ovary and due to the cyclical hormonal changes the histological character of endometrium alters in different phases of menstrual cycle. Endometrium passes through *three phases* in the menstrual cycle (*see* **Fig. 2**).

1. *Proliferative phase*—corresponds to follicular phase of ovary
2. *Secretory phase*—corresponds to luteal phase of ovary
3. *Menstrual or bleeding phase* following which proliferation starts.

Menstrual cycle starts with the onset of menstruation and traditionally first day of menstruation is called day 1 of menstrual cycle.

Proliferative Phase (Figs. 4 and 5)

Endometrium enters in the proliferative phase after the completion of repair of endometrium which is manifested by cessation of menstrual bleeding within 5–7 days.

During the proliferative phase *glandular* and *stromal* growth occurs to prepare the endometrium for implantation of embryo due to the effect of estrogen secreted by developing follicles.

Thickness of endometrium increases from 0.5 mm at mens to 3.5–5 mm at the end of proliferative stage.

The straight, narrow, and small *endometrial glands* become long and tortuous. Lining of endometrial gland changes from single columnar to pseudostratified epithelium with increase mitotic activity before ovulation.

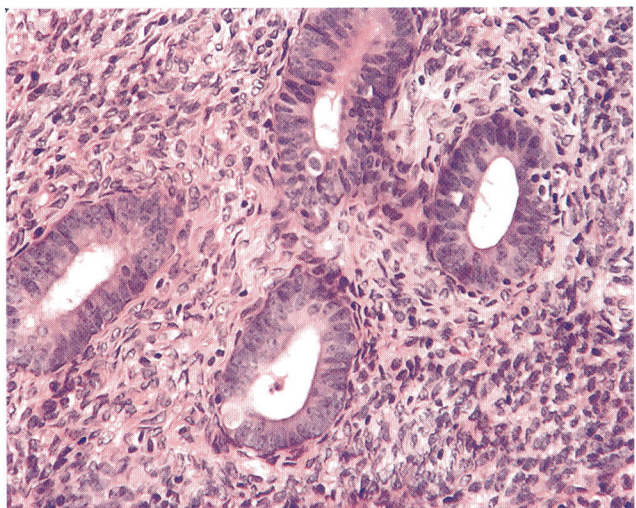

Fig. 4: Proliferative endometrium.
Courtesy: Dr Anup Boler, Associate Professor

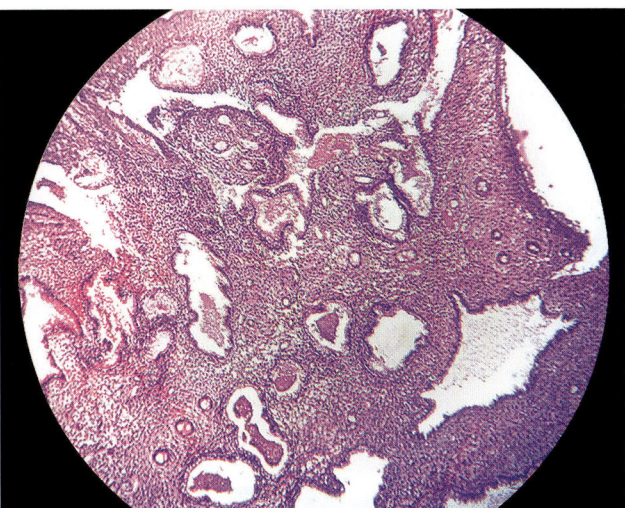

Fig. 6: Secretory endometrium.
Courtesy: Dr Anup Boler, Associate Professor

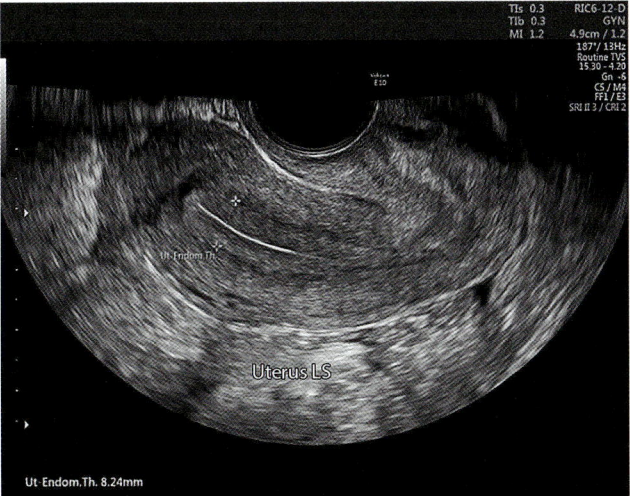

Fig. 5: Transvaginal sonography showing proliferative endometrium (preovulatory).
Courtesy: Professor Kamal Oswal

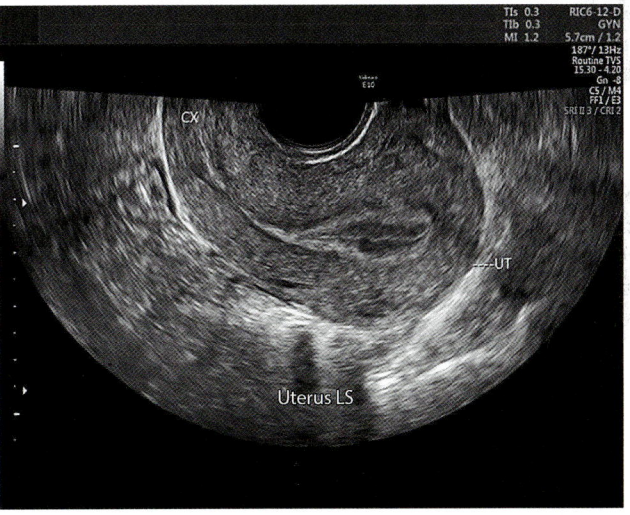

Fig. 7: Transvaginal sonography showing early secretory endometrium.
Courtesy: Professor Kamal Oswal

The *stroma* remains dense but infiltrated with cells derived from bone marrow and *vessels are infrequent*.

Secretory Phase (Figs. 6 and 7)

Following ovulation which usually occurs in day 14 of 28 days cycle histological appearance of endometrium goes to secretory phase due to the effect of progesterone and lasts from 14 to 28th day of cycle.

Progesterone reduces the estrogen receptors in the endometrial cells and antagonizes the estrogenic action.

Glandular lumen becomes filled with protein rich secretions. Initially glycogen containing vacuoles are seen subnuclear which first appears on day 16 of menstrual cycle, the nucleus pushed toward the lumen, later nucleus is pushed basal and looks saw-toothed appearance and secretion in gland lumen is seen from day 20 onward.

Glands become more tortuous and cork screw shaped.

Spiral arteries grow and become coiled.

Stroma becomes vascular and edematous. Secretory activity becomes maximum generally on day 6 or 7 postovulatory. Edematous stroma is termed *"pseudodecidua"* due to its similarity on staining appearance with that of pregnancy.

Around 2 days before menstruation, there is dramatic increase of lymphocytes which indicates the onset of menstrual flow. The spiral arteries increase their number and coiling.

In spite of continued availability of estrogen the endometrial height remains roughly at preovulatory extent—*5–6 mm* as proliferation of epithelium ceases 3 days after ovulation, believed to be due to inhibition by progesterone.

Menstruation—Bleeding Phase

Shedding of functional layers of endometrium due to ischemic necrosis as a result of withdrawal of estrogen and progesterone is termed *menstruation.*

In absence of implantation sex steroids are withdrawn, *spiral arterioles are highly coiled and vascular spasm* of spiral artery results endometrial ischemia.

Prostaglandins are produced maximum throughout mens. Prostaglandin F2 alpha (PGF2α) causes vasoconstriction which is also responsible for vasospasm. Myometrial contraction due to the effect of PGF2α removes sloughed out endometrial tissue.

Breakdown of lysosomes and release of proteolytic enzymes promote local tissue destruction. The entire functional layer is exfoliated leaving behind the basalis layer from which endometrium regenerates. Re-epithelialization starts within 2–3 days after the onset of menstruation and completed within 48 hours.

Platelet aggregation and thrombi control blood loss initially following which vasoconstriction of endometrial arteries occur.

The regulation of steroid receptors in the endometrium controls steroids effects on endometrial development and function.

Peak estrogen receptor concentration is found in proliferative phase and estrogen receptor expression is decreased in luteal phase due to rising progesterone level. Progesterone receptors peak at midcycle in response to rising estrogen levels.

Normal duration of menstrual cycle ranges from *21 days to 35 days*, lasts for *2–6 days* and in each cycle blood loss is *20–60 mL*.

Summary of Endocrinal Changes in Ovarian and Endometrial Cycles (see Fig. 2)

Menstruation is the end result of coordinated activity of hypothalamo-pituitary-ovarian-uterine axis.

Arcuate nucleus of the hypothalamus secretes gonadotropin-releasing hormone (GnRH) in pulsatile fashion into portal circulation traveling to anterior pituitary and controls the gonadotropin (FSH and LH) secretion.

Interplay among the gonadotropins and ovarian steroids aided by ovarian autocrine and paracrine regulation results ovarian phases namely follicular phase, ovulation and luteal phase, and endometrial phases, e.g., menstruation, proliferative phase, and secretory phase.

The sequences are as follows (*see* **Fig. 2**):

- Due to *fall of estrogen and progesterone* at the last part of luteal phase in absence of implantation onset of *menstruation occurs*. FSH level starts to rise resulting activation of cohorts of ovarian follicles.
- Growing follicles under the influence of *FSH will secret estrogen*. Estrogen has two functions: proliferation of endometrium and negative feedback to FSH secretion by pituitary. Inhibin B secreted by granulosa cells also gives negative feedback to FSH. Consequently, level of FSH falls.
- Falling level of FSH results threat to the growing follicles. Only one follicle which contains the maximum FSH receptors will be escaped and will grow and called *"dominant follicle"* which will produce more estrogens. Rise of estrogen level in spite of decrease of FSH is explained by the fact the dominant follicle acquires maximum number of receptor for FSH at this stage. Increase estrogen further decreases FSH causing regressing of other follicles except the dominant one.
- Very high estrogen level at late follicular phase gives positive feedback to LH secretion. In early follicular phase low estrogen level has negative feedback to LH and high estrogen at late follicular phase causes dramatic increase of LH secretion (biphasic response). There is secondary rise of FSH with LH peak. Normal level of estradiol—in follicular phase 30–200 pg/mL. In ovulation phase it becomes 200–600 pg/mL.
- At the preovulatory period there is formation of LH receptors on granulosa cells and progesterone starts to be produced before ovulation with the stimulatory effect of LH.
- *With the sustained high level of estrogen LH peak occurs which triggers the ovulation*. Ovulation occurs after 24–36 hours of LH surge. Preovulatory progesterone secretion is essential for rupture of ovarian follicle. Basal levels of FSH and LH are 5–10 IU/L both and in midcycle FSH level becomes 2 times and LH 3 times.
- Following ovulation corpus luteum is formed from follicular cells and *secretes progesterone*, essential for secretary changes of endometrium to form implantation bed. *Maximum progesterone secretion occurs (>10–15 ng/mL) on midluteal phase (day 22 of menstrual cycle)*.
- After ovulation level of estrogen drops in early luteal phase which gradually shows secondary peak following complete formation of corpus luteum along with progesterone peak. Rising estrogen increases progesterone receptor whereas rising progesterone decreases estrogen expression in luteal phase.
- *Progesterone:* Basal level of progesterone is 0.6 ng/mL or little more in proliferative stage. It starts to rise just before ovulation and becomes peak at midluteal phase.
- Estrogen, progesterone, and inhibin A together give negative feedback to gonadotropin secretion which shows low level till the later part of luteal phase which prevents further recruitment of ovarian follicle.
- *In absence of implantation luteolysis* occurs resulting fall of estrogen and progesterone level.
- Absence of negative back enhances the pituitary gonadotropin secretion with activation of cohort of follicles for the next cycle.
- *Fall of estrogen and progesterone level causes shedding* of endometrium resulting menstruation as described above.

NORMAL COMPOSITION OF SEMEN (FIG. 8)

It was *Anthony van Leeuwenhoek* who first described spermatozoa in 1685.

Human semen is a gray-yellow opalescent fluid which is made up of a suspension of spermatozoa in seminal plasma (**Fig. 8**).

pH is alkaline: 7.2–7.8. Normal volume is 2.0 mL or more per ejaculate.

Composition of Semen

- More than 90% of the seminal plasma is contributed by secretion of accessory glands of male genital tract of which major part (46–80%) is formed by alkaline seminal *vesicular secretion* which is the source of fructose, prostaglandins, and coagulating proteins. Fructose is the energy source of sperm.
- *Prostatic secretion:* About 13–30% of seminal plasma comes from *prostatic secretions* which contain proteolytic enzymes (which liquefies the semen within 20–30 minutes), citric acid, acid phosphatase, zinc, etc., and acidic.
- *Testicular secretion* contributes only 5% of ejaculate which is composed of testosterone, inhibin, transferrin, etc.
- *Epididymis* add little which is more important biochemically (carnitine, inositol, glycerophosphorylcholine, lipids, cholesterol) than volumetric contribution.
- *Bulbourethral and urethral glands* contribute 1–2 mL of ejaculate containing immunoglobulin G (IgG) and mucoprotein which is responsible for lubrication.

The normal parameter of semen (WHO criteria) is described in Chapter 11: A Case of Infertility.

Functions of Seminal Plasma

Seminal plasma provides a *support medium* for transporting male gametes out of the body and for buffering the pH of the vagina. In natural insemination (coitus) ejaculated spermatozoa have to traverse the cervix and uterus where role of seminal plasma is crucial.

Besides, seminal plasma contains *both reactive oxygen species (ROS) and antioxidants* normally in a balance manner. Minimal ROS is essential for normal function of sperm whereas excess is detrimental for sperm function. In healthy men, a delicate balance exists between physiological ROS and antioxidants in the male reproductive tract.

Structure of Spermatozoa (Figs. 9 and 10)

Spermatozoa consist of:
- Head
- Neck or connecting piece
- Tail.

Sperm is the smallest cell in the body with the length of sperm head 4–5 µm.

Head

- Major area (65%) of sperm head is occupied with nucleus with scanty space left for cytoplasm.
- Anterior aspect of sperm head (two-thirds) is covered by the acrosomal cap.
- Acrosomal cap has two layers—outer acrosomal and inner acrosomal layer. Acrosomal cap contains various types of enzymes of which two are significant namely, acrosin and hyaluronidase.
- Covering the outer acrosomal layer is the plasma membrane, which is the outermost layer of the sperm head. The posterior part of the sperm is postacrosomal region.
- Immediately behind the acrosome lies the equatorial region which is very important because this part attaches to and fuses with the egg. The shape of human spermatozoa is highly pleomorphic (**Fig. 11**).

Neck

- Neck or connecting piece measures 0.3 µm and contains proximal and remnants of the distal centriole.
- Sperm centriole has an important function during fertilization. Following entry of sperm head into the oocyte sperm centriole triggers up formation of female pronucleus inside the ooplasm.

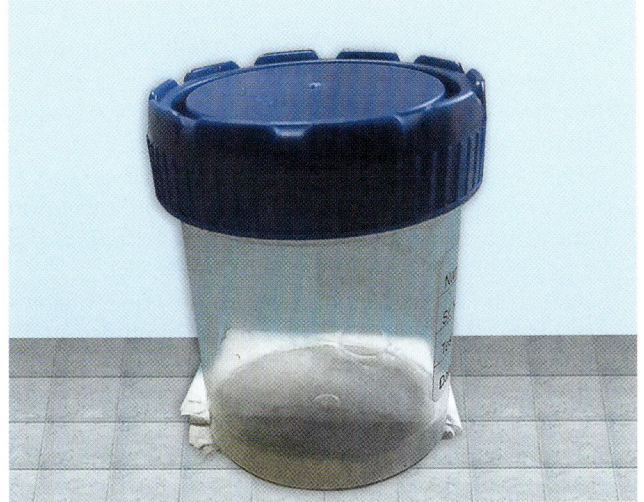

Fig. 8: Ejaculated semen in wide mouth clean container for examination. Normal semen is a gray-yellow opalescent fluid.

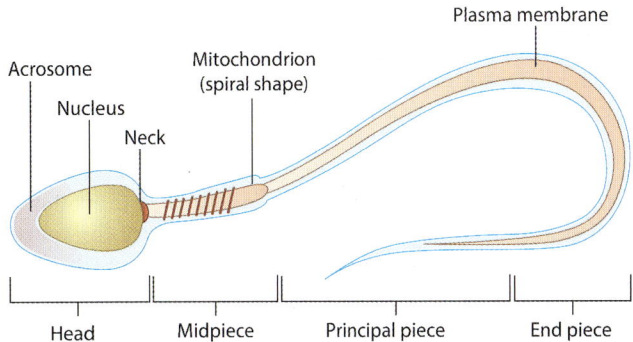

Fig. 9: Mature spermatozoa: It consists of head, neck, and tail. Tail has three parts—midpiece, principal piece, and end piece.

SECTION 3: Reproductive Physiology

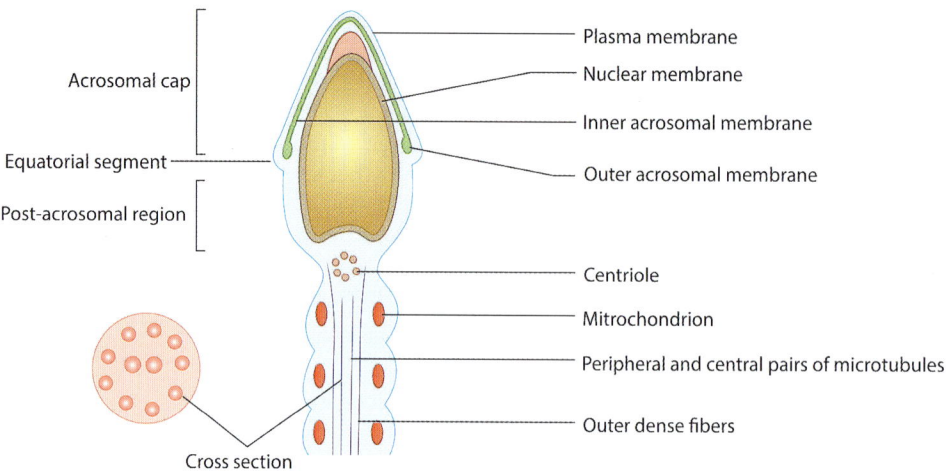

Fig. 10: Structure of sperm head, midpiece, and cross section of midpiece.

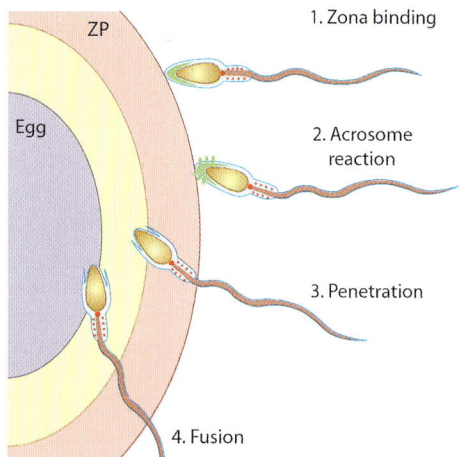

Fig. 11: Fertilization: Zona binding, acrosome reaction, zona penetration, and sperm-oocyte fusion. Due to zona reaction immediately after entry of one sperm zona becomes hardened preventing entry of other sperm thus avoiding polyspermia.

- This area (centriole) has been termed as *"black box"* (preserving all informations of fertilization) of the spermatozoa.

Tail
Tail or flagellum is further divided into *midpiece* (7 μm), *principal piece* (main piece) (40 μm), and *terminal or end piece* (5–7 μm).
- **Midpiece** contains a cytoplasmic portion and lipid-rich mitochondrial sheath. In the central region **(Fig. 10)**, there are 11 central axis fibrils surrounded by outer ring of 9 coarse fibrils surrounding which mitochondria lie in spiral fashion. Mitochondria are involved in oxidative mechanism and also offer energy necessary for sperm motility (called *"power house"*). Coarse nine fibrils of outer ring diminish in thickness and terminate in end piece.
- **Principal piece** is the longest part of the tail and provides most of the propellant machinery (*motor apparatus*).
- **Endpiece** is the last narrow part.
- Presence of *dynein* bands (a type of protein) in the tail is the source of energy and offers propellant force for the spermatozoa. Absence of dynein or deformity of tail is the factor responsible for sperm immotility. This dynein protein is also present in respiratory tract. In immotile cilia syndrome (*Kartagener syndrome*) patient suffers from bronchiectasis and having immotile sperms and infertility.

PHYSIOLOGY OF SPERMATOGENESIS (FIGS. 12 AND 13)

- Testes has two distinct components, the seminiferous tubules and the Leydig cells. Leydig cells lie in the connective tissue outside seminiferous tubules. After migration of germ cells to genital ridges.
- During embryogenesis there is 300,000 spermatogonia in each gonad after migration of germ cells to genetic ridge. By puberty the number becomes 600 million by mitosis. There is production of 100–200 million sperms each day and more than 1 trillion in reproductive span.
- Spermatozoa are produced from the primary germ cells (stem cells) situated in the wall of seminiferous tubule through multiple steps.
- Stem cells form spermatogonia A and B by mitosis. Spermatogonia A are similar to mother cell.
- Spermatogonia undergo next step of spermatogenesis to form *primary spermatocyte* (diploid cells-46) by mitosis from which two *secondary spermatocytes (haploid)* is formed by phase I meiosis division (*see* **Fig. 12**).
- Each secondary spermatocyte, in turn by final meiosis, produces two haploid *spermatid* containing *23 chromosomes*.
- Large spermatid is matured into compact spermatozoa, the process called *spermiogenesis* by which condensation of nucleus, formation of flagellum and development of acrosome occur.
- New cohort of spermatogonia goes into the maturation process every 16 days.

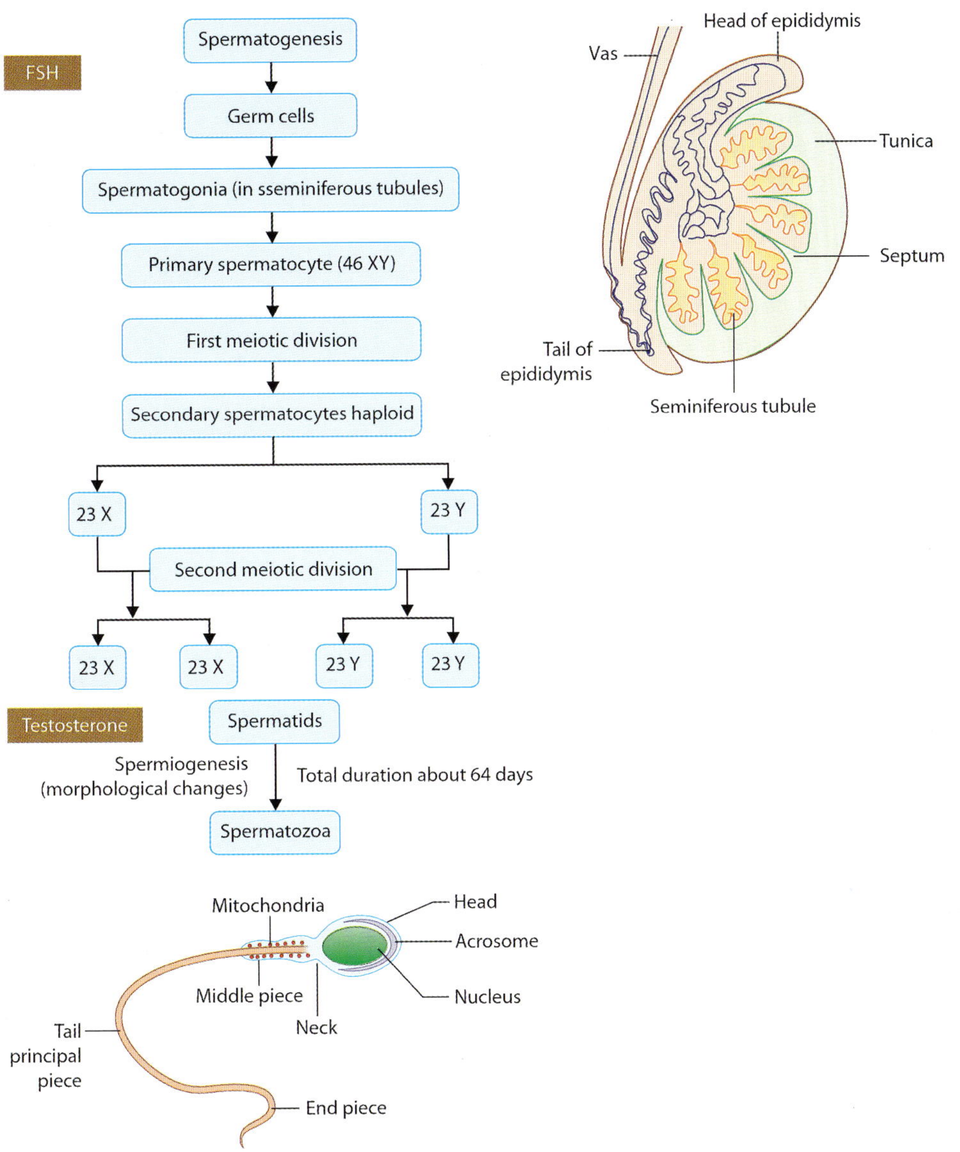

CHAPTER 19: Physiology of Ovulation, Menstruation, Spermatogenesis and Implantation

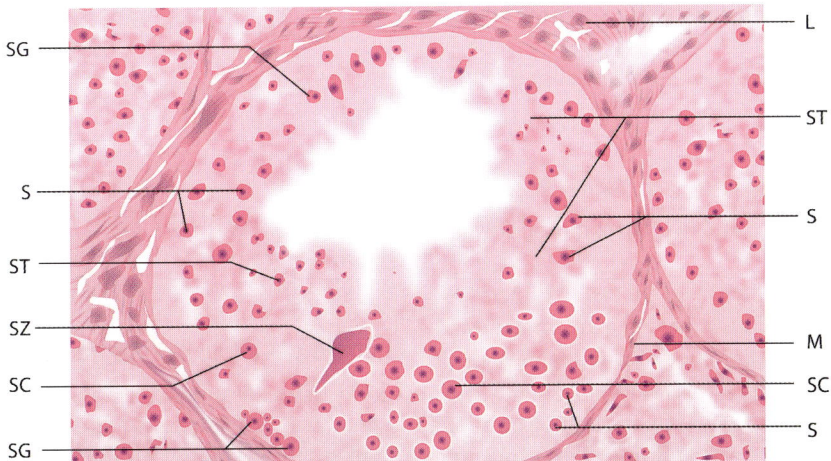

Fig. 12: Spermatogenesis from spermatogonia in sequence of primary spermatocyte, secondary spermatocyte, spermatid, and mature spermatozoa.

Fig. 13: Microscopic view of cross section of seminiferous tubule.
Abbreviations: SG, spermatozoa; S, Sertoli cells; ST, spermatids; SZ, spermatozoa; SC, primary spermatocytes; L, Leydig cell; M, myoid cells

- Process of *spermatogenesis*, i.e., from spermatogonia to mature spermatozoa *takes about 64 days*.
- *Spermiation* is a process through which mature sperms are released into lumen of seminiferous tubule.
- After releasing into lumen sperms enter into epididymis where more maturation takes place and acquire progressive motility during 3–5 days traversing through tortuous structure for reaching to vas.

Hormonal Control of Spermatogenesis (Flowchart 1)

Endocrinal control of spermatogenesis is not so clear like that of oogenesis and it is evident from the fact that medical induction of ovulation is a successful therapeutic option where the medical induction of spermatogenesis is not. Though gonadotropin is essential for spermatogenesis probably local paracrine regulation has strong impact on production of good fertilizable spermatozoa the knowledge about which is limited.

- GnRH acts on anterior pituitary to synthesize FSH and LH.
- LH acts on Leydig cells to synthesize testosterone (5–10 mg/day approx.).
- Inhibin and androgen binding globulin (ABG) are produced by Sertoli cells which are under control of FSH. FSH indirectly supports the action of LH by formation of LH receptors on Leydig cells.
- Testosterone goes both into circulation and seminiferous tubules. The concentration of testosterone in testes is 50–100 times higher than in blood.
- Testosterone binds with ABG to be carried to luminal wall for spermatogenesis.
- Leydig cells lie outside the tubules. So, testosterone to be carried from Leydig cell to inside the lumen at the site of spermatogenesis is dependent on ABG production by Sertoli cell which is under control of FSH secretion.
- Follicle-stimulating hormone is crucial for the initiation and maintenance of spermatogenesis and testosterone is essential for major part of spermatogenesis and maturation (last part) of sperms, even in epididymis.
- Inhibin gives negative feedback for FSH secretion and testosterone for LH secretion through hypothalamo-pituitary axis.
- Hence, both FSH and LH are essential for spermatogenesis.

The Flowchart 1 shows the hormonal control of spermatogenesis.

Use of Gonadotropin and Testosterone in Clinical Practice

Gonadotropin has been tried extensively in seminopathy but the result is not satisfactory.
In clinical practice, testosterone is used in two regimes:
1. Low-oral dose of testosterone is used in an expectation to increase libido and also to enhance spermatogenesis.
2. High injectable-dose of testosterone is used in an expectation that it will give negative feedback to hypothalamo-pituitary axis and sudden stoppage of drug may increase endogenous testosterone and enhances spermatogenesis. Both regimens are not found to be so effective in practice. In testosterone-related seminopathy, it is thought that it is not the absolute deficiency of testosterone, it is the defect of utilization of testosterone locally (defective paracrine regulation) which is responsible for impaired spermatogenesis.

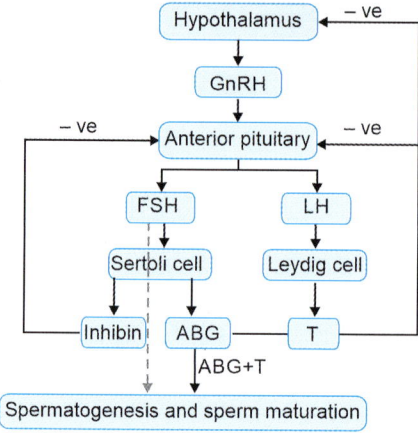

Flowchart 1: Hormonal control of spermatogenesis.

Abbreviations: GnRH, gonadotropin-releasing hormone; FSH, follicle stimulating hormone; LH, luteinizing hormone; ABG, androgen binding globulin

Sperm Transport and Fertilization (Fig. 14)

After ejaculation sperms are released through vas and mixed with fluid from accessory glands prostate, seminal vesicles, and bulbourethral glands. The secretion of accessory glands constitutes more than 90% of ejaculate mostly contributed by seminal vesicles. Near the prostate from the common ejaculatory duct seminal fluid containing sperms after mixing with prostatic secretions passes through the urethra and also mixed with secretions of bulbourethral glands (as described above) is emitted through external urethral meatus.

Important Events Related to Sperm Following Deposition in Female Genital Tract (*see* Page 267, Fig. 32)

- Transport
- Capacitation
- Cumulus separation
- Zona recognition
- Acrosome reaction
- Zona penetration
- Sperm oocyte fusion.
- Following sperm-oocyte fusion, cytoplasmic syngamy and nuclear syngamy occur to form the zygote finally.

From Ejaculation to Fertilization

- The released semen is a gray-yellow opalescent gelatinous mixture (coagulum) of sperms and seminal plasma. It takes 20–30 minutes for liquefaction.
- During coitus, semen is deposited in the upper vagina and external cervical surface. Vaginal pH is strongly acidic

CHAPTER 19: Physiology of Ovulation, Menstruation, Spermatogenesis and Implantation

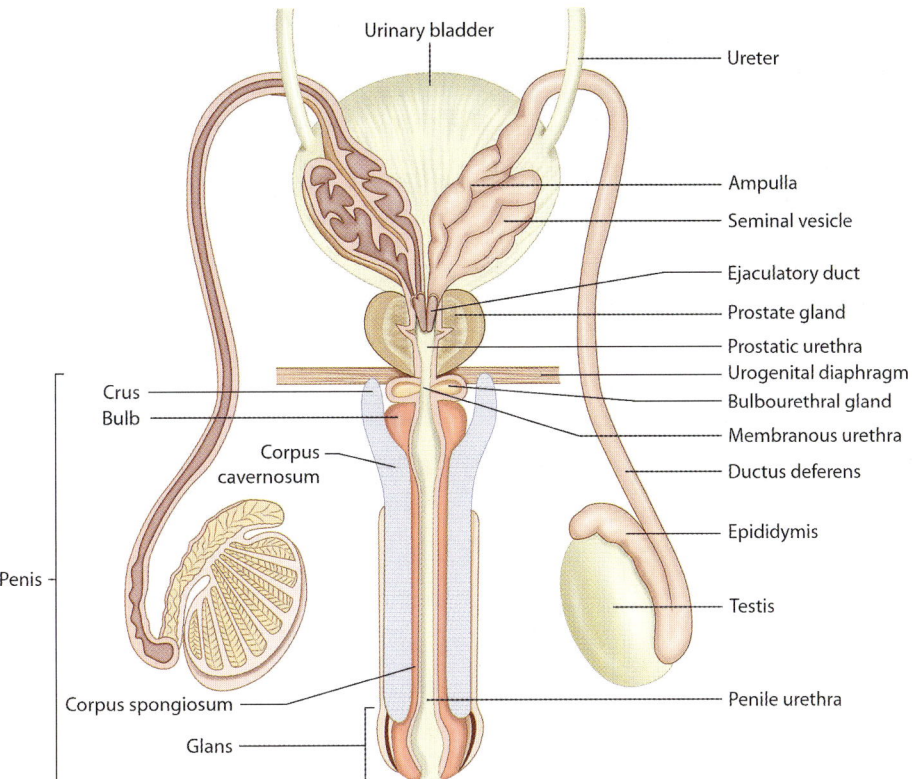

Fig. 14: Male reproductive tract—sperms produced in seminiferous tubules of testes, stored in epididymis. During ejaculation sperms traverse through vas, mixed with secretion of accessory glands—seminal vesicles, prostate and bulbourethral glands. Semen containing sperms is emitted through the external urethral meatus.

- and detrimental to sperms and that of cervix is neutral or near alkaline where sperms can survive. To escape from vaginal pH good motile sperms quickly move to cervix.
- Ninety-nine percent of sperms are lost by leakage from the vagina in spite of coagulum formation (only <0.1% ejaculated semen reaches the fallopian tube).
- Of the remaining a small minority gain access to cervical crypts and undergo *capacitation* to become competent to fertilize the oocyte.
- Sperm has to cross the *three barriers,* namely cervix, uterus, and uterotubal junction to reach the middle third of the fallopian tube, the site of fertilization.
- Cervical canal is the first selective filtering barrier. At each barrier the sperm population is reduced so that eventually near about *only 200 or so* of the most active spermatozoa have the opportunity to reach the ovum and have a scope to fertilize.
- In follicular phase, sperms from posterior fornix to fallopian tube may reach within 2 minutes as in highly estrogenized cervical mucus glycoprotein forms parallel micelle to facilitate sperm transport with an average time to reach uterine cavity within 90 minutes. Maximum number of sperms may lie in cervix for 24 hours.
- Although many of these spermatozoa help digest the path of extracellular matrix (composed of glycosaminoglycan and hyaluronan) covering the cumulus cells only one (the luckiest one) will be able to penetrate the zona.

- Zona pellucida is the acellular covering of the oocyte. Zona pellucida contains ligands of sperm which are relatively species specific. Initial contact of sperm and oocyte is receptor mediated where glycoproteins secreted by zona (ZP1, ZP2, ZP3) take a vital role.
- Acrosome reaction helps the spermatozoa to penetrate the zona pellucida. The proteases and glycosidases released as a result of acrosome reaction, in addition to hyperactivated motility, enable sperm to penetrate the zona pellucida.
- Following *zona penetration*, the equatorial head region of the spermatozoa binds the oocyte plasma membrane in the perivitelline space after which *sperm-oocyte fusion* occurs.
- Fusion of sperm-oocyte membranes trigger cortical reaction which leads to enzyme induced *zona reaction*, the hardening of zona which *prevents polyspermia* by providing obstacle to the entry of other sperms.
- Sperm-oocyte fusion results *cytoplasmic syngamy* followed by *nuclear syngamy* and finally *zygote* is formed.

Transport of Egg, Fertilization, and Blastocyst Formation

Transport of Egg after Ovulation

- Oocyte pick-up in the fallopian tube is caused by the adhesive character of the cilia present (which are abundant there) in the fimbriae and the presence of follicular cumulus cells surrounding the egg has great role on this adhesive process. In the tube egg transport is dependent on smooth muscle contractions and ciliary-induced flow of secretory fluid.

- *Fertilizable lifespan of oocyte is approximately 12–24 hours and that of sperm is 48–72 hours.*
- Fertilization occurs in midportion of tube (ampulla) where the fertilized egg lies maximum (90%) time.
- Fallopian tube has an important holding action till the endometrium becomes prepared and competent for implantation of blastocyst. And this time may be up to 80 hours.

Cleavage, Formation of Morula and Development of Blastocyst Competent for Implantation (Figs. 15 to 18)

Formation of Compact Morula

- Following fertilization, and formation of zygote cell division is continued with morphological refashioning and genetic reprogramming.
- The eight-cell stage embryo (3–4 days postovulation) undergoes compaction during transit from fallopian tube to uterine cavity to form a 8–16 cell compact morula (Fig. 15).
- Cell number in this stage is not accompanied by appreciable increase in embryonic size inside the zona.

Blastocyst Formation

- Shortly after entering into the uterine cavity the 32–64 cell stage blastocyst is formed (4–6 days postovulation).
- It is characterized by the presence of a cavity and the presence of two cell types: an outer cell mass, called *trophectoderm (TE) and inner cell mass (ICM).*
- Formation of blastocyst is identified by the appearance of inner cavity within the cells.
- Several genes have been identified which are crucial for segregation of the TE and ICM lineages at the morula-to-blastocyst transition.

IMPLANTATION

Q. What is implantation?

- Implantation means embedding of the blastocyst in the endometrial stroma and in placentation blood flow interchange occurs between mother and fetus.
- Successful implantation depends on two important factors—blastocyst competency and endometrial receptivity.

Preparation of Endometrium (Embryonic Bed)

- Endometrium undergoes a complex series of organized proliferative and secretory changes in menstrual cycle as

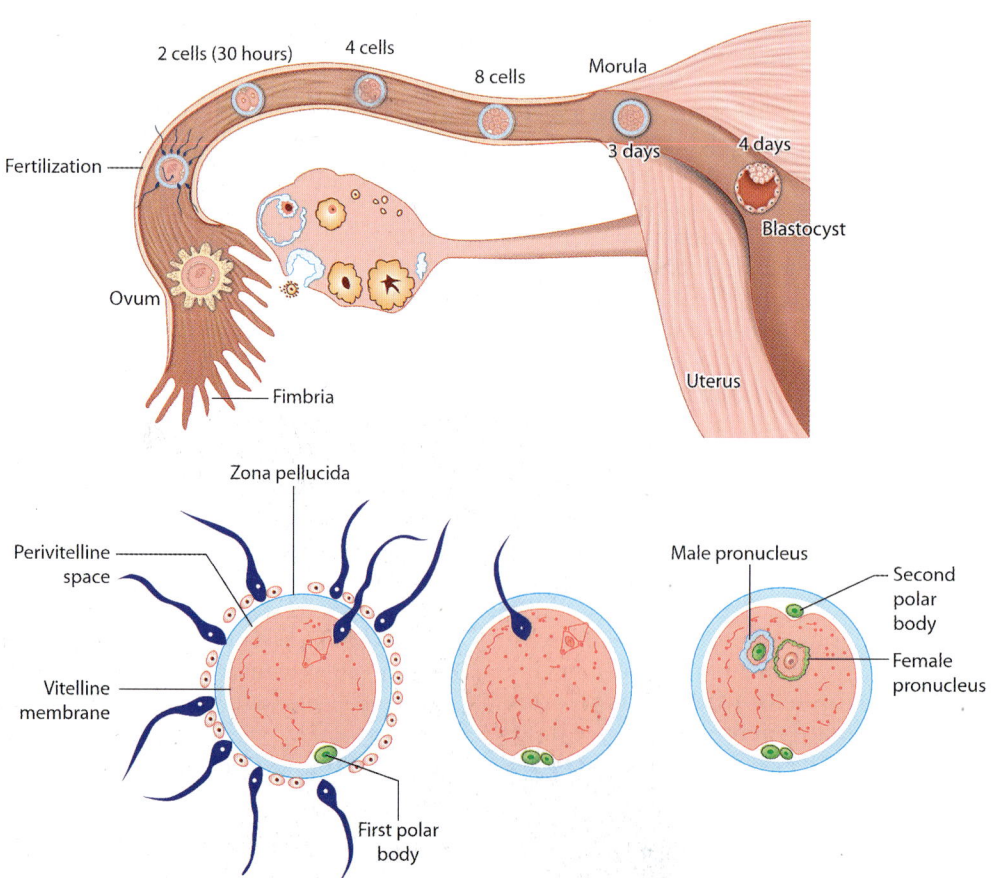

Fig. 15: Fertilization, formation of pronuclei, and successive stages of cleavage of embryo, formation of morula and blastocyst with their transport in female reproductive tract to enter into uterine cavity.

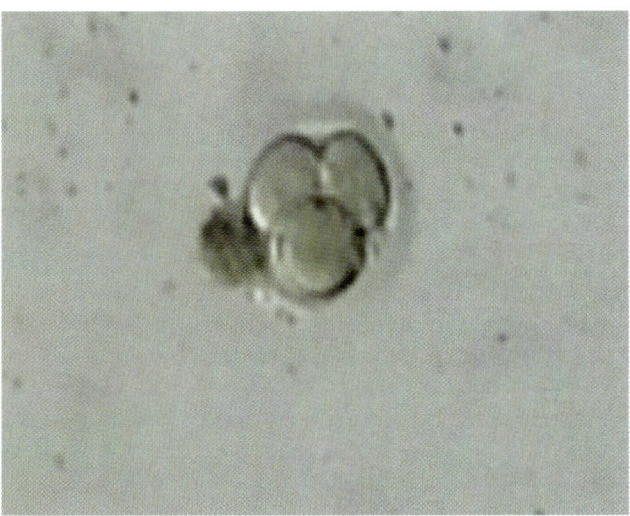

Fig. 16: Second day cleaved embryo (2–4 cell stage).
Courtesy: IRM, Kolkata

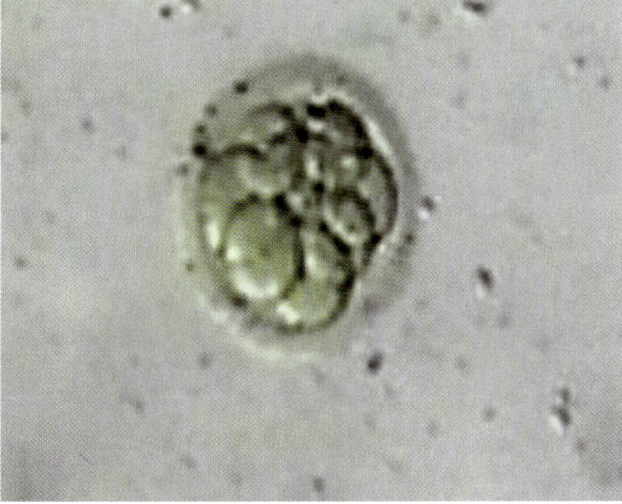

Fig. 17: Third day cleaved embryo (8-cell stage).
Courtesy: IRM, Kolkata

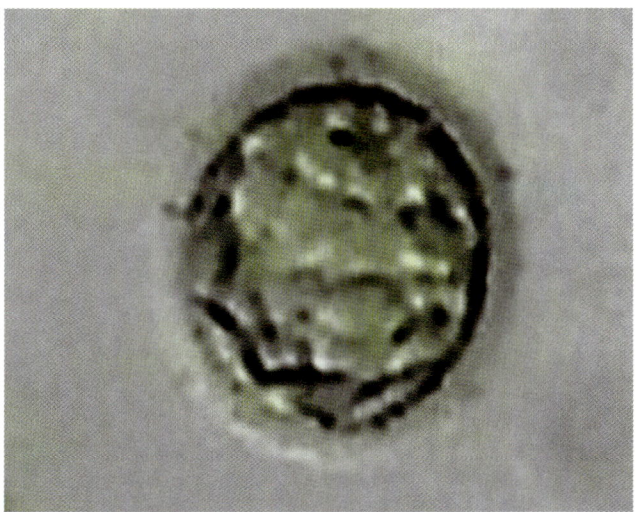

Fig. 18: Blastocyst (4–5 days after fertilization).
Courtesy: IRM, Kolkata

described above. Enormous histological, molecular, and biochemical changes occur in the endometrium from proliferative to secretory stage to make it receptive.

❖ Between days 22 and 25 predecidual transformation of the upper two-thirds of the functionalis layer occur and the glands exhibit extensive coiling and secretions found in lumen.

❖ Changes within the endometrium also can mark the so-called *implantation window* and is seen on days 20–24.

❖ Epithelial surface cells show decreased microvilli and cilia but appearance of bleb like luminal protrusions on the apical cell surface, called *pinopodes* which are important for blastocyst implantation.

❖ At the same time changes in the surface glycocalyx occur which allow acceptance of a blastocyst.

❖ The endometrium is *10–14 mm thick* in the midluteal phase at the time of implantation.

At this time, there is maximum secretory activity with abundant glycogen and lipids in the endometrial cells.

Spiral artery development reflects a marked induction of angiogenesis. Angiogenesis is the key feature of the endometrial cycle and implantation. This process of the growth of blood vessels from pre-existing vessels is regulated by the sex steroids and directly by growth factors like vascular endothelial growth factor (VEGF).

Decidualization

Q. What is decidualization?

Transformation of secretory endometrium to decidua is called *decidualization* and dependent on estrogen and progesterone and factors secreted by the implanting blastocyst. The decidua is a specialized, highly modified endometrium of pregnancy and is essential for hemochorial placentation.

Endometrial Receptivity

❖ Endometrial receptivity can be defined as the ability of the uterine mucosa to facilitate successful embryonic implantation.

❖ The receptive phase has now been firmly established, around 5–9 days after ovulation, corresponding to days 20–24 of an idealized 28-day menstrual cycle.

❖ The principal regulators of endometrial receptivity are ovarian steroids, estrogen, and progesterone through nuclear estrogen receptors (ERα and ERβ) and progesterone receptors (PRα and PRβ).

❖ Estrogen stimulates epithelial and stromal proliferation and induces progesterone receptor expression.

❖ On the other hand progesterone is responsible for promotion of stromal transformation or decidualization, glandular secretion, and vascular remodeling.

❖ *Pinopodes* are preferred sites of embryoendometrial adhesions and serve as morphological markers of uterine receptivity and under the influence of progesterone.

Embryoendometrial Synchronization

- Embryoendometrial synchronization is essential for successful implantation.
- During natural conception, 2–3 days postfertilized embryo (cleavage stage) crosses the fallopian tube and nourished in tubal environment, while blastocyst-stage embryo (4–6 days postfertilized) synchronizes with the endometrium (*see* **Fig. 15**).
- In IVF program, better implantation rates accrue after transferring blastocyst stage embryos into uterine cavity instead of cleavage-stage embryo.

Morphological Steps of Implantation (Fig. 19)

The most difficult part of implantation is for the floating blastocyst to become attached to endometrium. Like entering to dock a tanker coming into port, the blastocyst is first drawn by large molecules that extend from the endometrium, followed by a cascade of molecules that bring the trophoblasts into closer contact with the endometrium.

Once intimate contact is made, the trophoblasts begin to be attached with the endometrium. The site of implantation is usually upper posterior wall of uterus in midsagittal plane.

The process of implantation is classified into three continuous phases:
1. Apposition
2. Attachment (adhesion)
3. Penetration (invasion).

Apposition

- *Apposition* is the unstable adhesion of blastocyst to the endometrial surface which usually occurs 2–4 days after the morula enters the uterine cavity.
- A prerequisite for this contact is a *loss of the zona pellucida (zona hatching)* by proteolytic digestion.

Attachment

- *Attachment* is a *stable adhesion*.
- Local paracrine interaction between the embryo and endometrium is believed to occur to trigger a stronger attachment.
- Shortly after attachment, "primary decidualization reaction" occurs in the endometrium followed by secondary decidualization after 2–3 days with stronger attachment.

Penetration (Invasion)

- *Penetration (invasion)* process starts within a few hours of attachment which involves invasion of the embryo through the luminal epithelium and its basal lamina into the stroma, to establish a vascular relationship between the embryo and the mother.
- In humans, implantation is "interstitial" as the embryo invades the stroma deeply enough for the luminal epithelium to be reconstituted over it.
- Trophoblastic cells are differentiated into *syncytiotrophoblast* and *cytotrophoblast*. The former

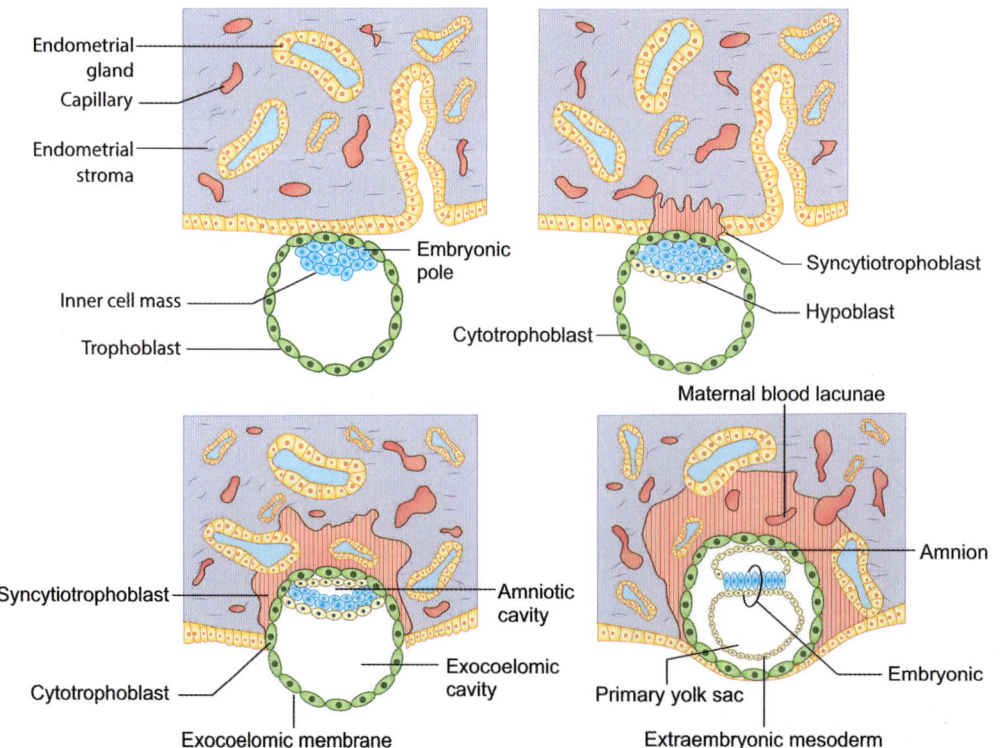

Fig. 19: Process of implantation—apposition, attachment, penetration, and placentation.

is formed by fusion of trophoblastic cells and the latter retain their cellularity.
- *Human chorionic gonadotropin secreted by the embryo is detectable in maternal serum within 8–10 days of ovulation in most of the pregnancies.*

Concept of Early Pregnancy Factor

After hatching from the zona pellucida even before blastocyst adheres with the surface epithelium, a dialogue between the mother and the early embryo starts. Early pregnancy factor (EPF) can be detected in the maternal circulation within 1–2 days after fertilization. EPF is initially produced by the ovary in response to a signal from the embryo. And after implantation, EPF is derived from embryo. EPF has immunosuppressive properties and has a role in cell proliferation and growth. There is reason to believe that endometrial receptivity for implantation requires appropriate signals from the embryo.

Molecular Cross Talk

- A reciprocal interaction between the embryo and endometrium takes place during implantation and it is thought that embryo is not a passive component rather directs many activity of implantation process.
- Theses interactions take place through various molecular factors better called biochemical tools like cell adhesion molecules (CAMs), cytokines, growth factors, matrix metalloproteinase (MMP), and prostaglandins.

Cell adhesion molecule: Various members of CAM family like selectins, integrins, and cadherins are important for cell adhesions process of implantation.

Cytokines: Endometrium produces at least three cytokines which are involved in implantation. Interleukin has a pivot role in implantation.

Growth factors: Growth factors and their receptors are another group of proimplantation mediators and include members of the EGF family, TGFβ, fibroblast growth factors, IGF, and platelet-derived growth factors.

Matrix metalloproteinases: Matrix metalloproteinases (MMP-9) and tissue inhibitors of MMP (TIMP-1) are thought to be principal mediators for matrix degradation during implantation and decidualization.

Prostaglandins: Prostaglandins are important for change of vascular events which are necessary for implementation process. These are produced from the phospholipids of membrane under the sequential action of phospholipase A_2 (PLA_2), cyclooxygenase (COX), and prostaglandin synthase enzymes.

Immune Acceptance in Pregnancy

- Immune tolerance is the unique feature in normal pregnancy in spite of the fact that half of its gene of embryo is paternal in origin.
- To prevent the maternal immune system rejecting the embryonic transplant some kinds of immunomodulation occur about the nature of which little is known.
- The factors like trophoblastic human leukocyte antigen expression and an increase in decidual regulatory T cells are said to be associated with maternal tolerance of immune system. The role of natural killer cells in pregnancy loss is not clear.

Placentation (see Fig. 19)

- Chorionic villi (from the embryo) on the embryonic pole grow, forming chorionic frondosum and becomes attached tightly with the decidua basalis (also called decidual plate) and forms the actual placenta.
- Villi on the opposite side degenerate and form the chorionic laevae and lie beneath the decidua capsularis.
- The placenta is formed in the second week of after ovulation.
- Invasion of the trophoblast should be optimal as too much deep invasion is associated with *placenta accrete* and *placenta percreta* and shallow placentation is said to be the etiopathogenic factor for *preeclampsia* and *fetal growth restriction*.

PREMENSTRUAL SYNDROME (PMS) OR PREMENSTRUAL TENSION (PMT)

Q. How to define premenstrual syndrome (PMS) or premenstrual tension (PMT)?

PMS or PMT is defined as the cyclic physical and behavioral symptoms during late luteal phase of the menstrual cycle which interfere with the work and lifestyle followed by symptom free interval.

PMS is very common and reported by 75% of women but mostly mild and self-limiting, but in approximately 15% cases it is moderate to severe variety.

Premenstrual dysphoric disorder (PMDD) is a severe form of PMS characterized by severe irritability, tension, anger, dysphoria and mood swing. Sometimes it is considered as a distinct clinical entity.

Etiologies of PMS

- Not exactly known
- Effects of estradiol and progesterone due to cyclical ovarian activity are the major factor.
- Central neurotransmitters: Gamma aminobutyric acid (GABA), serotonin and noradrenaline influenced by E and P play a role.
- Alteration of electrolyte and fluid balance by renin-angiotensin-aldosterone system (RAAS) influenced by sex steroids which result bloating and weight gain.

Diagnosis of PMS

Symptoms and signs—typically occurs in late luteal phase and cyclical in nature
- Bloating, weight gain, mastalgia, headache
- Abdominal cramps

- ❖ Tiredness, fatigability, lethargic
- ❖ Psychological depression, mood swing
- ❖ Anxious, tense
- ❖ Loss of interest in working place or in school
- ❖ Sleepy and increase appetite (overeating)

ACOG Criteria (2000) for Diagnosis of PMS

- ❖ Invariably starts 5 days or one week before onset of period.
- ❖ Should be cyclical.

Diagnosis of PMS and PMDD requires a maintenance of prospective symptoms diary and evidence of socioeconomic dysfunction.

Differential Diagnosis

Primary psychiatric symptom, anemia, hypothroidism, endometriosis, fibromyalgia, fibrocystic breast disease and irritable bowel syndrome, etc.

Management

Principle of management:
- ❖ Symptomatic treatment
- ❖ Modification of hormonal disturbance
- ❖ Referral to psychiatrist in severe PMS

Treatment modalities:
- ❖ Lifestyle management, nutrition and exercise: Food and beverages containing high sugar and caffeine are avoided. Less fat, salt and alcohol, frequent starchy foods with high fiber are taken. Isoflavones and primrose oil may be helpful to treat PMS.
- ❖ Stress management: Regular exercise and meditation alleviate symptoms.
- ❖ Vitamins and minerals: Vitamin B_6 (pyridoxine—50 mg/day), Calcium (1 g/day), Vitamin D (10 μg/day) Magnesium (250 mg/day) and Vitamin E
- ❖ Selective serotonin-reuptake inhibitors (SSRIs): Efficacy and tolerance have been proved by several well controlled trials. Fluoxetine (20–40 mg/day), Citalopram (10–20 mg/day), Escitalopram (10–20 mg/day) are used continuously or only in luteal phase.
- ❖ Alprazolam, a benzodiazepine is useful in treatment of PMA and PMDD by relieving depression.
- ❖ Diuretic like spironolactone is used widely in treatment of PMS.
- ❖ Hormonal treatments:
  - Combined estrogen and progesterone (COCs) acts by cycle suppression with variable result. Continuous two or three cycle without break is more effective. COC containing spironolactone derivative like drospirenone is beneficial.
  - Transdermal patch of estrogen.
  - Only progestogen and progestogen blocking drugs- Utrogestan 200 mg (D17-D28), Danazol or Mirena.
  - GnRH analogues (3.6 mg SC/month) is indicated in severe form and resistance cases. HRT is used as add back therapy to prevent osteoporosis.

CHAPTER 20: Menopause and its Management

Chapter Outline

- Menopause—Definition
- Menopausal Transition—STRAW Classification
- Physiology of Menopause
- Effects of Menopause—Immediate, Intermediate and Long-term
- Evaluation of Menopause
- Management
- Scope and Indications of Hormone Therapy—Current Recommendation

MENOPAUSE

Q. Define menopause.

Menopause is the point in time of permanent cessation of menstruation due to loss of ovarian activity (WHO). **Menopause is declared at a point in time after 1 year of cessation of menstruation.** Average age is 51.5 years and Indian average is about 47 years. Premature ovarian failure is called when menopause occurs before the age of 40 years.

Factors Influencing the Age of Onset of Menopause

- Environmental
- Genetic
- Surgical—oophorectomy and hysterectomy
- Chemotherapy
- Radiation
- Smoking.

Q. What do you mean by menopausal transition?

Menopausal transition is not a point but over a span of 4–7 years before permanent cessation during which endocrine and biological changes occur with appearance of symptoms. Average age of onset of transition is 47 years.

Postmenopausal is years following the point of permanent cessation of menstruation.

Perimenopausal or Climacteric

The time period in the late 40s to early 50s around the menopause and starts with menstrual cycle irregularity and extends up to 1 year after permanent cessation. The term climacteric is derived from the word "*Klimax*" in Greek, which means ladder climb to the menopause.

All these terms are now replaced by menopausal transition.

Q. What is STRAW?

Full form of it is *Stages of Reproductive Ageing Workshop* (STRAW), where standard classification guideline for female reproductive aging was proposed in 2001 and the term menopausal transition was introduced.

Q. How female reproductive and postreproductive life is divided in STRAW original classification?

- The phases of reproductive aging are broadly classified into reproductive, menopausal transition (MT), and postmenopausal.
- The main anchor for the staging system is final menstrual period (FMP).

Table 1: Stages of Reproductive Aging Workshop (STRAW) staging system.

Stages	−5	−4	−3	−2	−1	+1		+2
Terminology	Reproductive			Menopausal transition		Postmenopause		
	Early	Peak	Late	Early	Late*	Early*		Late
				Perimenopause				
Duration of stage	Variable			Variable		(a) 1 year	(b) 4 years	Until demise
Menstrual cycles	Variable to regular	Regular		Variable cycle length (>7 days different from normal)	≥2 skipped cycles and an interval of amenorrhea (≥60 days)	Amenorrhea x 12 months	None	
Endocrine	Normal		↑FSH	↑FSH		↑FSH		

Abbreviations: FMP, final menstrual period; FSH, follicle-stimulating hormone; ↑,elevated; *Stages most likely to be characterized by vasomotor symptoms

- There are **five stages before FMP** and **two stages after FMP**
- *Stage-5*—early reproductive period, *stage-4*—reproductive peak, *stage-3*—late reproductive period, *stage-2*—early MT, *stage-1*—late MT.
- *Stage+1a*—1st year after FMP, *stage+1b*—2-5 years postmenopausal, and *stage+2*—later postmenopausal years till demise.

Table 1 shows the STRAW staging system.

Characteristics of MT Stages

- In early MT (*stage-2*) menstrual cycles are still regular, but cycles typically shorter (7 or more days different), follicle-stimulating hormone (FSH) increased, estrogen unchanged, or slightly elevated in follicular phase probably due to high FSH. Ovulatory cycle becomes anovulatory. Pregnancy may occur accidentally.
- Late MT (*stage-1*) is characterized by 2 or more missed menses or one interval of amenorrhea longer than 60 days. Anovulation occurs more frequently. This stage is mostly to have menopausal symptoms.
- In the established menopause (*stage+1b*), FSH and luteinizing hormone (LH) rise fourfold higher than in reproductive year. Levels of FSH more than 40 IU/L and LH more than 20 IU/mL are considered to be in postmenopausal range.

STRAW classification is subject to modification and modified in 2010 and again in 2015.

PHYSIOLOGY OF MENOPAUSE

Endocrine Changes

Reproductive Life

Mechanism of regular normal ovulatory menstrual cycle (see also Chapter 19):

- Gonadotropin-releasing hormone (GnRH) released from the arcuate nucleus of basal hypothalamus binds with GnRH receptors of gonadotropes present in anterior pituitary and stimulate to release of gonadotropins—FSH and LH cyclically.
- FSH and LH, in turn, acting on ovary produce estrogen, progesterone (steroid hormones) and inhibin (peptide).
- Estrogen and progesterone giving the positive and negative feedback to pituitary and hypothalamus regulate the amplitude and frequency of GnRH release and gonadotropin production from pituitary.
- Inhibin produced from ovarian granulosa cells gives negative feedback to pituitary over FSH secretion.

Late Reproductive to Menopausal Transition to Menopause

- In late reproductive stage and early menopausal transition near the age of late 40s, level of FSH increases slightly due to decrease production of inhibin and in turn increases estrogen level.
- Thus, inhibin is the first hormone, which is decreased first not the estrogen.
- Rather estrogen initially increased and in fluctuates in perimenopausal women. However, in spite of regular cycle progesterone levels become lower in early MT than in peak reproductive years. In one period, there may be unopposed estrogen action on endometrium.
- Estrogen starts to decrease in late MT. In menopausal transition, testosterone level remains almost unchanged.
- In late menopausal transition, follicular depletion occurs more rapidly and along with increase FSH and decrease inhibin, level of AMH (anti-Mullerian hormone) decreases progressively. AMH is a glycoprotein produced by the secondary and preantral follicle and regarded as a marker of ovarian reserve.

In Postmenopause

- In postmenopause, estrogen and progesterone production cease with increase of gonadotropins fourfold by negative feedback.

- *Adrenal steroids*—dehydroepiandrosterone sulfate (DHEA-SO$_4$) and androstenedione are reduced. Androgen (from both ovary and adrenal) is converted to less potent estrone, which is characteristic of aging process.
- *Sex hormone-binding globulin (SHBG)*: Following menopause production of SHBG by liver declines resulting free estrogen and testosterone.

Summary of Sequence of Hormone Changes in Menopause Transition and Menopause

- Depletion of ovarian follicles (low antral follicular count) → decrease of inhibin B → increase of FSH, and increase and fluctuation of estrogen, low progesterone, normal testosterone (early MT) → increase of FSH, decreased inhibin B, decrease AMH (late MT) → in post-menopause estrogen and progesterone production stopped by ovary, FSH and LH level increased fourfold but testosterone and androstenedione are produced by ovary but in less amount. Androstenedione is converted peripherally to estrone (E1).

- Estradiol (E2) is the main estrogen in premenopause and varies from 40 pg/mL to 400 pg/mL. In postmenopause, predominant estrogen is estrone (E1), which is derived from conversion from androgen produced by both ovary and adrenal gland.

Endometrium in Menopause Transition

- In late MT, anovulation is frequent and endometrium exhibits estrogenic effect unopposed by progesterone resulting proliferative or disordered endometrium (hyperplasia and endometrial cancer).
- *Abnormal bleeding*: Abnormal bleeding occurs more than 50% cases at the stage of MT; however, etiology should be carefully determined depending not solely on MT irregularity. Abnormal bleeding should be evaluated by sonography, hysteroscopy, and endometrial biopsy. Anovulation is the most common cause of abnormal bleeding in menopause transition but endometrial hyperplasia, carcinoma, endometrial polyp, fibroid, and pregnancy-related bleeding should be kept in mind and excluded.

Oocyte Depletion

In the different life cycle, oocyte depletion occurs continuously with highest at 20 weeks of intrauterine period:
- 20 weeks intrauterine period—7 million
- At birth—2 million
- At puberty—20,000
- Only 400 exhaust in reproductive life
- In late 30s and early 40s, rapid depletion of follicles occurs.
- In menopause, complete depletion of follicles occurs.

Consequences (Effects) of Menopause

- In menopause, there is depletion of ovarian follicles and cessation of production of steroid hormones (estrogen and progesterone).

Table 2: Effects of menopause.

Effects of menopause	Symptoms
Immediate effect	• Vasomotor symptoms—hot flashes, sweating, sleep disturbance, and palpitation • Psychological and mood disturbances • Sexual dysfunction • Urinary symptoms—frequency, dysuria, and recurrent UTI • Somatic symptoms—headache, dizziness, mastalgia, joint aches, and back pain
Intermediate effect	• Urogenital atrophy and urinary incontinence • Skin changes • Urogenital problems • Pelvic organ prolapse
Long-term effect	• Bone changes • Cardiovascular changes • Dementia and cognitive decline

Abbreviation: UTI, urinary tract infection

- Several effects occur on the health of the woman in menopausal transition and following menopause. These health hazards are solely due to estrogen deprivation or combined with aging process that is not clearly understood.

These effects can be categorized into *three groups* according to their time of appearance, namely:
1. Immediate
2. Intermediate
3. Long-term (Table 2).

Vasomotor Symptoms

- Explained by central thermoregulatory dysfunction due to estrogen withdrawal and neurotransmitters concentration.
- Interestingly, these changes are *contemporary to LH pulses*.
- Occurs in late MT and early postmenopausal phase in 75% cases and severe in 10% cases. Disappears within 1–5 years. May extend up to 70 years, duration is 2–3 minutes and 1–2 times even more per day.
- The *symptom* is characterized by sudden feeling of heat (*hot flash*) over trunk and faces quickly spreading to rest of the body, which is followed by shivering, sweating, palpitation, and anxiety. Women suffering from hot flashes frequently complain of sleep disturbance, which hampers day-to-day work, impairs cognitive function, and makes her irritable, lethargic, and depressive.
- Symptoms are more common and severe in surgical menopause. Smoking and high-body mass index (BMI) are important risk factors for vasomotor symptoms.

Psychological and Mood Disturbances

- Psychological and mood disturbances are in the form of mood swings, anxiety, irritability, poor memory, loss of concentration and depression, and attributed to deficiency of neurotransmitter caused by estrogen

deficiency, the administration of which may reduce the symptoms.
- Previous psychological problems and present stress appear to increase the risk.

Urinary Problems

- These are urinary frequency, dysuria, and recurrent lower urinary tract infection (UTI). Incontinence, both urge and stress incontinence, is common (45–50%) in postmenopausal women.
- Predisposing factor for incontinence (both urge and stress) is estrogen deficiency-induced thinning of urethral mucosa, which favors urine leak, ascending infections, and colonization of yeast and bacteria, which becomes recurrent.
- Urogenital atrophy is found in 25% of women even after estrogen therapy. Vaginal epithelium becomes thinner, increased rugosity, easily abrased, and petechial hemorrhage occurs more frequently.

Sexual Dysfunction

- These are decreased libido, vaginal dryness, and painful intercourse.
- Loss of elasticity and atrophy are accompanied by decreased blood flow to vagina, vulva, decreased lubrication due to vaginal dryness resulting pain and difficult intercourse.
- Reduction in libido and arousal are linked to estrogen withdrawal and also androgen deficit.
- Woman may stay sexually active until their 8th or 9th decades of life. Sexual problems are common with one in two women.
- With age, interest in sex declines in both sexes, more in female. Low desire—43%, difficulty in lubrication problem—39%, and inability to climax—34%.

Dementia and Cognitive Decline

- Dementia means impairment of cognitive function including loss of memory, language, thought process, and judgment, which impart tremendous impact in day-to-day life in family, society, and in working place losing confidence.
- Alzheimer's disease is the most common cause of dementia in elderly.

Skin Changes

Skin changes are characterized by thinning and wrinkling due to loss of collagen; there may be pigmentation and more prone to be bruised by trauma.

Pelvic Organ Prolapse

- Pelvic ligaments and fasciae become relaxed due to deficiency of estrogen resulting POP.

Osteoporosis

- Osteoporosis is a skeletal disorder characterized by low-bone mass and architectural deterioration of bone tissue predisposing to increase risk of fracture.
- Bone loss in postmenopausal women is largely attributed to estrogen deficiency. Postmenopausal bone loss occurs more in trabecular bone (spine, pelvis, and proximal femur) than cortical bone (bone of peripheral skeleton).
- In estrogen deficiency, bone resorption increases with increase chance of fracture hip, vertebrae, and distal radius (*Colles' rogen deficiency*).
- Kyphosis with back pain is the frequent clinical manifestation. Osteoporosis is a major global problem affecting 52 million out of which 35 million are women.
- Other than estrogen deficiency, some risk factors modifiable and nonmodifiable factors increase the chance of osteoporosis.
- Modifiable factors are sedentary lifestyle, less calcium, and vitamin D intake.
- Nonmodifiable factors are age, race (Asian or Caucasian), family history, early menopause, P/H of fracture and surgical menopause, and other medical conditions like hyperthyroidism, hyperparathyroidism, prolong use of steroid, and chronic renal disease.

Bone Mineral Density

- Bone mineral density (BMD) is measured to diagnose osteoporosis and to determine fracture risk.
- *Dual energy X-ray absorptiometry (DEXA)* is the primary technique for BMD measurement.
- *Bone marrow density* is expressed as T score, which is the number of standard deviation by which the targeted bone differs from the young normal mean.
- *T score above –1 is considered normal, a score between –1 and –2.5 denotes low bone mass (osteopenia), and T score below –2.5 indicates osteoporosis.*
- *FRAX (an online fracture risk assessment tool) has been developed by the WHO to evaluate fracture risk. BMD by DEXA is recommended for all women aged 65 years or older irrespective of risk factor and for younger postmenopausal women with one or more risk factors.*

Cardiovascular Disease

- Women have a much lesser risk before menopause in comparison to men with same age.
- Estrogen is a cardioprotective in several ways by decreasing low-density lipoprotein (LDL) and total cholesterol, increasing high-density lipoprotein (HDL), reducing atheroma formation directly acting on vascular wall.
- After menopause with decrease of estrogen protection from CVD diminishes with similar incidence with men at age of 70. Cardiovascular disease is the leading cause of death in postmenopausal women.

- Modifiable risk factors are sedentary lifestyle, obesity, smoking, diabetes, hypertension (HT), and hyperlipidemia.
- Nonmodifiable are family history and age.

Cardiovascular Disease and Hormone Therapy

- Though observational studies initially showed that postmenopausal hormone therapy is beneficial for preventing heart disease, but *large Women's Health Initiative (WHI) randomized controlled trial showed that hormone therapy did not prevent heart disease in healthy women,* instead there was *increased risk of CVD in older women.*
- Increased risk of CHD occurred principally on older women, and no increase risk in women of ages 50–59 or within 10 years of menopause.
- This analysis does not support the hormone therapy for prevention of heart disease, but indicates that there is no contraindication of HT to treat the hot flashes and night sweats in otherwise healthy women for short period.

Q. How to evaluate menopausal women or women in menopausal transition?

Goal is to optimize menopausal women or women in menopausal transition:
- History taking
- Physical examination
- Laboratory studies.

History

It should be taken to know the problems of the woman, risk factors for menopausal consequences, any other disease other than menopause and need of specific treatment. It includes:
- Age
- Duration of menopause
- History of vaginal discharge
- History of lifestyle, diet, and type of food taken
- Pattern of bleeding, if still no menopause
- Family history bleeding, if still no menopause woman, fracture
- Past history: (i) medical—diabetes, HT, hyperlipidemia, and thyroid disorder; (ii) surgical— surgical menopause.
- Drug history—prolong steroid therapy, history of smoking.

Physical Examination

- *Height*: History of height loss may be due to osteoporosis, spinal compression (annual height measurement)
- Weight
- BMI, obesity—waist circumference
- Blood pressure (BP)
- Skin changes
- Breast examination including nipple
- Vulva, vagina—shrinkage of labia majora, labia minora may disappear, narrowing of introitus.
- Per vaginal examination—atrophy of vagina is characterized by loss of rugae of vagina, which is thin, pale, and dry and vaginal pH is high 5, there may be bacterial infection. Presence of cystocele, rectocele, and uterine descent looked for strength of pelvic musculature and fascia is examined by palpation.

Laboratory Study

- *Hormones:* FSH, LH, estradiol, and inhibin. FSH level more than 10 mIU/mL on day 3 of period is considered as bad outcome in vitro fertilization (IVF); more than 40 mIU/mL is documented as established menopause. Estradiol may be normal, elevated, or low depending upon the stage of menopausal transition as described previously. At menopause, E2 level is extremely low or undetectable.
- *Maturation index* of vaginal mucosal exfoliated cells indicates the hormonal status. Parabasal/intermediate/superficial cells are in the range of 0/40/60 in estrogenic phase (out of total 100 cells counted). Shifting to left means increase of intermediate or parabasal cells denoting low estrogen.

Markers of Bone Mass

- *BMD-DEXA* as described previously
- *Urinary and serum markers of bone resorption and formation*—there are several bone formation markers synthesized by osteoblast and bone degradation products produced by osteoclasts, which can be measured in blood or urine and may be valuable in bone remodeling rate. Till now, they are not estimated in routine clinical management but in future will become a useful adjunct.

MANAGEMENT OF MENOPAUSE

- *Counseling*—common sense education
- Lifestyle management
- Exercise
- Diet
- Vitamin D_3 and calcium
- Hormone therapy
- Other nonhormone therapy.

Q. What is called hormone therapy?

In menopause, as there is deficiency of hormone due to loss or decrease of estrogen, hormone is administered in anticipation to regain the function of hormone and to restore the problems associated with hormone deprivation.

Hormone therapy is called *hormone replacement therapy (HRT), hormone therapy (HT), menopausal hormone therapy (MHT), and estrogen therapy (ET).* The term HRT is now less favored.

HT encompasses both estrogen- progesterone therapy (EPT) and only estrogen therapy (ET). HT therapy has been extensively studied for a long period and the evidence-based recommendations are yet to be evolved.

Treatment of Vasomotor Symptoms

Lifestyle Interventions

Keeping the room temperature low, wearing light garments, and losing weight by exercise and diet modification, meditation and smoking cessation improve vasomotor symptoms.

Estrogen Therapy

Most effective treatment is systemic estrogen therapy.

Route

Estrogen can be given by oral, parenteral, topical, vaginal, or transdermal route with similar efficacy.

Preparation and Dose

- In *presence of intact uterus intermittent progesterone is added.* Short-term therapy with lowest effective dose needed to treat is the approach at present.
- In menopausal transition, combined pill may be given. Low-dose oral conjugated estrogen (0.3 mg/day), estradiol (0.5 mg/day or transdermal estradiol) can be given with minimal side effects.
- In "*menopausal transition*", estrogen and progesterone combination is given continuously without any pill-free interval thus women will be complete amenorrheic.
- In *cyclic therapy*, estrogen is given for 25 days and in last 10 days progesterone is added and no drug is given for 5 days resulting withdrawal bleeding. Or, estrogen is given continuously and progesterone is added first 10 days.
- Continuous therapy is usually given following menopause and cyclic therapy in menopausal transition.
- In contraindication to estrogen [history of venous thromboembolism (VTE) or breast cancer] *only progesterone* (20 mg daily) is used.

Tibolone

- Tibolone is a synthetic steroid compound and used as selective tissue estrogenic activity regulator (STEAR). It has estrogenic, progestogenic, and mild androgenic activity.
- It reduces hot flush, prevents bone loss, prevents vaginal dryness, and improves libido.
- It is given 1.25 mg or 2.5 mg daily without any progestogen.
- Its use is restricted to postmenopausal woman only.

Nonhormonal Drug

- Nonhormonal drug is *clonidine*.
- Others are selective serotonin reuptake inhibitor like *paroxetine* and *aminobutyric acid gabapentin*, which significantly reduce hot flashes.
- Other agents like *phytoestrogens, soy products, phytoprogestogens, vitamin E*, etc., have been used with variable results.

Treatment of Sexual Dysfunction

- Important cause of dyspareunia is vaginal atrophy and dryness due to deficiency of estrogen.
- *Estrogen* orally or vaginally improves dyspareunia.
- Vaginal products like estrogen creams (CEE), tablet (17E-estradiol), and rings (estradiol- releasing vaginal ring) had greater patient acceptance. Each unit of ring contains 2 mg of estradiol and is worn for 3 months.
- Use of water-soluble *vaginal lubricants* like K-Y jelly and Astroglide is very effective before intercourse. Estrogen has also strong positive effect on mood and libido other than improvement of local vaginal symptomatology.

Treatment and Prevention of Osteoporosis

- *Calcium* (1,000–1,500 mg) and vitamin D (400 IU) should be taken daily to prevent and to treat osteoporosis.
- *Hormone therapy with estrogen* prevents and treats osteoporosis with good efficacy. Chance of fractures is reduced to 50%, if hormone therapy is given soon after menopause and continued for long-term.
- The largest trial, WHI trial, has proved the high efficacy of hormone therapy with conjugated estrogen (0.625 mg/day) or low-dose estrogen (0.3 mg) with calcium and vitamin D in prevention of fracture.

Nonhormonal Antiresorptive Agents

- For treatment of osteoporosis, the common pharmacological agents recently used are nonhormonal antiresorptive agents.
- *Bisphosphonates* like alendronate (daily 35 or 70 mg oral), risedronate (35 mg weekly or 150 mg monthly oral) or zoledronic (5 mg intravenously) are very effective for prevention and treatment of osteoporosis. Major side effects of oral route are gastrointestinal (GI) problems.
- *Raloxifene*, a selective estrogen receptor modulator (SERM), provides with an estrogenic action on bone and lipid profile without stimulating breast or endometrium and in a dose 60 mg orally daily prevents vertebral fracture with low bone mass. This is the only SERMs approved for osteoporosis. *Bazedoxifene* is another SERM and its combination with conjugated estrogen, known as tissue-selective estrogen complex (TSEC) is approved by FDA. Benefits of estrogen and to offset estrogen stimulation of the endometrium and breasts by the SERM are obtained on use of TSEC. Hence, TSEC is a good choice as systemic HT for women with intact uterus without using progesterone.
- *Calcitonin* (200 IU/day) nasal spray and parathyroid hormone (20 µg/day SC) are the other agents used to treat osteoporosis.

Treatment of Depression

- Antidepressant drugs along with psychotherapy and counseling are effective treatment to alleviate depression.

- As menopausal symptoms are considered as the principal cause of depression, mood symptoms are improved by hormone therapy due to concurrent resolution of hot flush and disturbed sleep.

Prevention of Cardiovascular Disease

Current evidence shows that *there is no role of hormone therapy in prevention of cardiovascular disease.* Treating the HT, diabetes, and hyperlipidemia along with addressing the modifiable factors are the effective measure to reduce the risk.

Risks and Benefits of Hormone Therapy (Summary)

Risks

- There is increased risk of coronary heart disease in older women with hormone therapy. Risk of stroke, thromboembolism, and cholecystitis increases.
- Long-term uses increase breast cancer and ovarian cancer.

Benefits

- BMD increases fracture and colorectal cancer decreases with long-term hormone therapy.
- Menopausal syndrome improved with HT.
- Overall mortality rate decreases in women less than 60 years of age.

Contraindication of Estrogen Therapy (ET)

Recent liver disease, history of thromboembolism, breast cancer, estrogen-dependent tumor, undiagnosed uterine bleeding and suspected pregnancy are all contraindications of estrogen therapy. ET should be used with caution in many conditions like in gallbladder disease, hypothyroidism, severe hypocalcemia, elevated breast cancer risk and prior endometriosis, etc.

Current Recommendation of Hormone Therapy in Menopausal Transition and Menopause

- *Indication*: Only for treatment of vasomotor symptoms, vaginal atrophy, prevention and treatment of osteoporosis, in surgical menopause and in premature ovarian insufficiency
- Type, dose, route and duration are guided by the treatment objective and increase of safety
- In general, it should be given in *lowest effective* dose for *shortest period* of time
- Every 6–12 months interval, *re-evaluation* is done whether to continue or not, only with shared decision making.
- *Duration:* No time limit of duration of therapy is specified in well-informed symptomatic women and can be used till the benefit outweighs the risk. However, women must be informed that risks increase with the age and duration of treatment.
- *Low-dose local vaginal estrogen* given for extended period is safe.
- *Bone-specific agent* is appropriate for long-term use for prevention and treatment of osteoporosis.
- Progesterone is added with estrogen in presence of uterus to prevent endometrial carcinoma.
- In "*presence of uterus*", estrogen and progesterone combination is given continuously without any pill-free interval, thus women will be completed amenorrheic.
- In *cyclic therapy*, estrogen is given for 25 days and in last 10 days progesterone is added and no drug is given for 5 days resulting withdrawal bleeding. Or, estrogen is given continuously and progesterone is added first 10 days.
- Continuous therapy is usually given following menopause and cyclic therapy in menopausal transition.

Q. What are the important trials in relation to hormone therapy in menopause?

The important trials are:
1. Postmenopausal Estrogen/Progestin Interventions (PEPI) trial
2. Heart and Estrogen/Progestin Replacement Study (HERS) trial
3. Women's Health initiative (WHI) trial
4. ELITE trial

CHAPTER 21

Development of Genital Organs and Müllerian Anomaly

Chapter Outline

- Development of Male Genital System
- Development of Female Genital System
- Classification of Müllerian Anomaly—Old and New
- Diagnosis of Müllerian Anomaly
- Gynecological and Obstetric Outcome of Effects of Müllerian Anomaly
- Description of Individual Anomaly—Diagnosis, Reproductive Outcome and Management
- MRKH Syndrome—Vaginoplasty
- Surgical Methods of Müllerian Anomaly—Strassman, McIndoe and Williams' Operation

Q. Describe the development of genital organs.

- Primordial gonads appear during 6th week of development.
- Associated undifferentiated ducts (Müllerian and Wolffian) also begin to develop at this stage.

DEVELOPMENT OF MALE GENITAL SYSTEM

- Presence of *SRY* gene and other testes determining factor (TDF) on *short arm of Y chromosome* will determine the development of testes and the undifferentiated gonad will be differentiated into testicular tissue.
- Testosterone produced by the Leydig cells influences the formation of epididymis, vas deferens and seminal vesicles from Wolffian structure. Anti-Müllerian hormone (AMH) secreted by Sertoli cells will regress the Müllerian structures.

DEVELOPMENT OF FEMALE GENITAL SYSTEM (FLOWCHART 1 AND TABLE 1)

In XX gonad ovarian structures are developed passively due to absence of *SRY* gene and other TDFs and facilitated by the antitesticular action of the genes *DAX1*, *RSPO1* and *WNT4*.

Development of Uterus, Cervix and Vagina

- In absence of AMH, Müllerian ducts (paramesonephric ducts) continue to develop caudally and medially to develop fallopian tubes, uterus, cervix, and upper vagina after midline fusion. Fusion takes place at 7th week.
- The cranial ends of fusion are the site of the future *fundus of uterus* and unfused paramesonephric ducts form the *fallopian tubes*.
- *Uterine corpus and cervix:* The caudal ends of fused paramesonephric ducts form the uterine corpus and cervix.

Flowchart 1: Normal development of female reproductive tract.

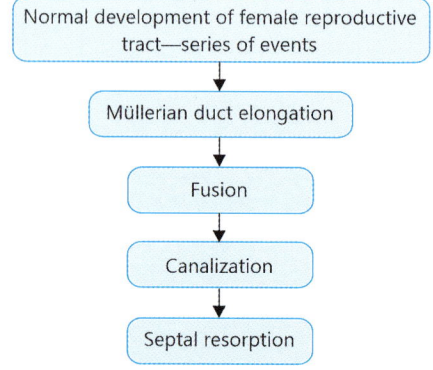

CHAPTER 21: Development of Genital Organs and Müllerian Anomaly

Table 1: Timeline of developments and results of defective developments.

Period of embryonic life	Developments	Defects of developments
6–9 weeks	• Appearance of Müllerian ducts • Caudal midline fusion • Connection with urogenital sinus	Failure of development of Müllerian ducts—uterine aplasia
10–13 weeks	Upward midline fusion of the caudal parts	Failure of fusion—uterine didelphys, bicornuate uterus
14–18 weeks	Resorption of medial septum to form uterovaginal channel— uterine cavity and upper two-thirds of vagina	Failure of resorption—septate uterus

Cervix

Cervix develops from elongation of caudal aspects of fused Müllerian ducts and differentiation (canalization) takes place at 20th week as a result of condensation of stromal cells at a specific site of fused Müllerian ducts. Hence, cervix is of Müllerian origin.

Vagina

- Further caudal development brings this structure into contact with urogenital sinus. At the point of contact, there is proliferation and elongation of fused Müllerian ducts to form vaginal cord (Müllerian origin).
- The vaginal cord invaginates into elongated sinovaginal bulb (urogenital sinus origin) which arises from the posterior aspect of the urogenital sinus to form vaginal plate.
- Vagina develops from vaginal plate. Canalization of vaginal cord occurs both from below and above and is not completed until 21 weeks.
- Epithelialization of vagina including ectocervix occurs by the cells derived mostly from urogenital sinus. Hence, vagina is developed from both Müllerian duct (upper 3rd) and urogenital sinus.

Hymen

Hymen is embryologic septum between the sinovaginal bulb above and the urogenital sinus below. Hymen is lined by an internal layer of epithelium and an external layer of epithelium derived from the urogenital sinus, with mesoderm between the two. It is not derived from the Müllerian ducts. It usually becomes perforated before or shortly after birth.

External Genitalia

- External genitalia consists of genital tubercle, urogenital sinus, urethral, and labioscrotal folds.
  - *Clitoris:* Genital tubercle becomes the clitoris.
  - *Labia minora:* Urethral folds become labia minora.
  - *Labia majora:* Labioscrotal folds develop into labia majora in female.
- The external genitalia of fetal gender is identifiable by sonography by the end of first trimester.
- In males, scrotum and penis are developed by the action of androgens.

MÜLLERIAN ANOMALY CLASSIFICATION

There many classification systems. Three classification systems are given here.

(1) The American Fertility Society (AFS), (2) 1988, ESHRE/ESGE Classification System (2013) and (3) ASRM Müllerian Anomaly Classification (MAC), 2021.

The American Fertility Society (AFS), 1988 (Fig. 1)

1. Segmental Müllerian hypoplasia or agenesis:
   - Vaginal
   - Cervical
   - Uterine fundus
   - Tubal
   - Combined anomalies
2. Unicornuate uterus:
   - Communicating rudimentary horn
   - Noncommunicating horn
   - No endometrial cavity
   - No rudimentary horn
3. Uterine didelphys
4. Bicornuate uterus:
   - Complete (septum to internal os)
   - Partial
5. Septate uterus:
   - Complete (septum to internal os)
   - Partial
6. Arcuate
7. Diethylstilbestrol (DES) related.

Specific Defects in Development and the Resultant Structures

The specific defects in development and the resultant structures have been given in **Table 2**.

Genital tract anomalies are often associated with urinary tract anomalies (Wolffian duct origin) (30–50% cases) due to close embryologic interaction.

Classification System for Müllerian Anomaly (2013 ESHRE/ESGE) (Fig. 2)

The European Society of Human Reproduction and Embryology (ESHRE) and the European Society for

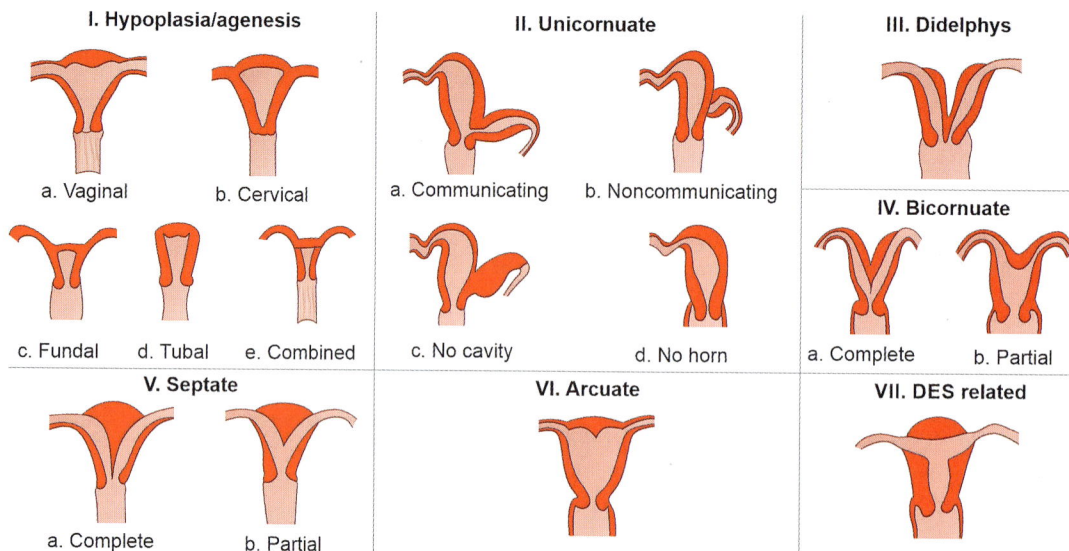

Fig. 1: Müllerian anomaly classification (The American Fertility Society, 1988).

Table 2: Specific defects in development and the resultant structures.

Defects in development	Result
Incomplete development of Müllerian duct	Unicornuate uterus (II): (a) with communicating horn; (b) with noncommunicating horn; (c) horn with no cavity; (d) no horn
Complete failure of fusion	Didelphic uterus (III)
Incomplete lateral fusion	Arcuate or bicornuate uterus (IV). Bicornuate may be: (a) complete or (b) partial
Failure of reabsorption of septum between two Müllerian ducts	Septate uterus (V): (a) complete; (b) partial
Failure in development of Müllerian ducts and their fusion with urogenital sinus	Mayer-Rokitansky-Küster-Hauser (MRKH) syndrome (complete agenesis of uterus and vagina)
Sinovaginal bulbs will fail to proliferate from the urogenital sinus	
Failure of elongation of caudal end of fused Müllerian ducts may lead to failure of canalization of entire vagina	Cervical atresia and complete vaginal agenesis
Failure of both elongation and canalization of the vaginal cord from the caudal end of the fused Müllerian ducts	Cervical atresia and agenesis of upper 3rd of vagina
Failure of contact between the caudal end of fused Müllerian ducts and the cranial end of sinovaginal bulb or failure of resorption of tissues at that area of contacts	Transverse vaginal septum
Segmental failure of differentiation of the normally elongated fused Müllerian ducts	Isolated cervical atresia

Table 3: Main classification of uterine anomaly according to new classification system.

U0	U1	U2	U3	U4	U5	U6
Normal uterus	Dysmorphic uterus	Septate uterus	Bicorporeal uterus	Hemiuterus	Aplastic	Unclassified

Gynaecological Endoscopy (ESGE) have developed a new classification system for Müllerian anomaly in 2013 though old classification AFS 1988 is still widely used.

Anatomy is the basis for the systematic categorization of anomalies in new classification. For the sake of simplicity, an extremely detailed subclassification is avoided.

Table 3 shows seven main classification of uterine anomaly. New classification is shown in **Figure 2**. Subclassification of cervical/vaginal anomaly is shown in **Table 4**.

Subclassification of cervical/vaginal anomaly is given in **Table 4**.

Table 4: Subclassification of cervical/vaginal anomaly.

Cervix		Vagina	
C0	Normal cervix	V0	Normal vagina
C1	Septate cervix	V1	Longitudinal non-obstructing vaginal septum
C2	Double 'normal' cervix	V2	Longitudinal obstructive vaginal septum
C3	Unilateral cervical aplasia	V3	Transverse vaginal septum and/or imperforate hymen
C3	Cervical aplasia	V4	Vaginal aplasia

CHAPTER 21: Development of Genital Organs and Müllerian Anomaly

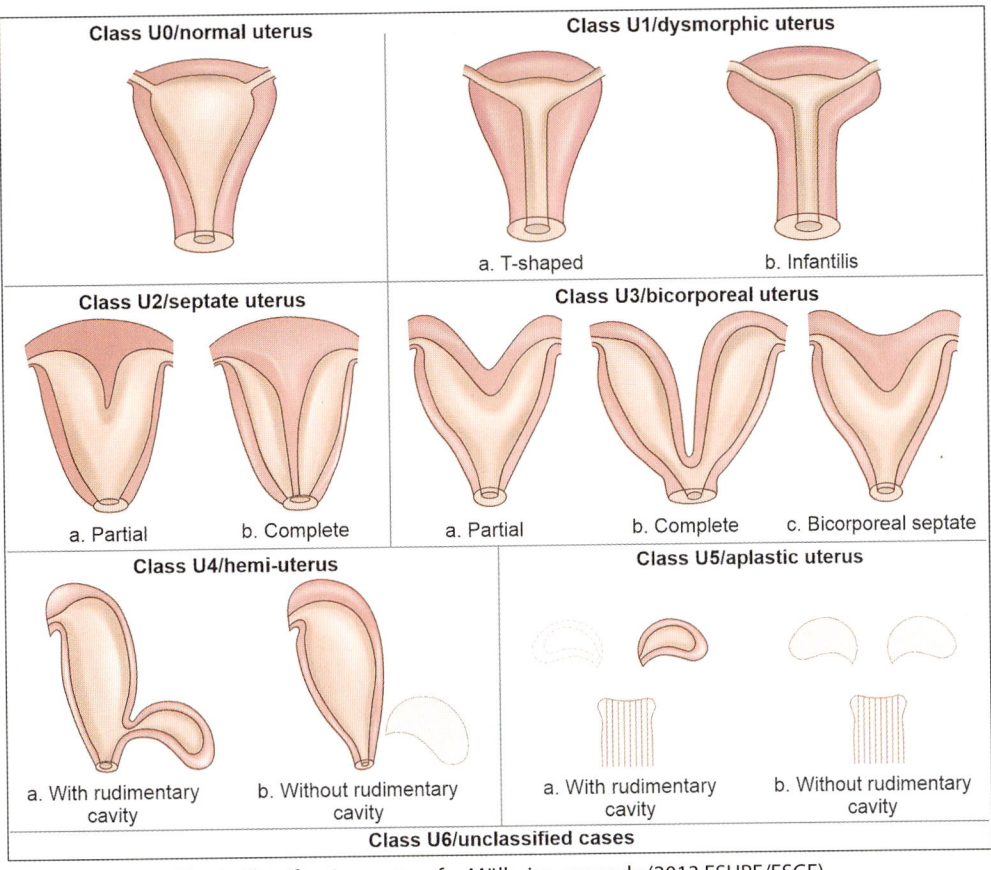

Fig. 2: Classification system for Müllerian anomaly (2013 ESHRE/ESGE).

Class U0: Normal uterus; Class U1: Dysmorphic uterus; Class U2: internal indentation more than 50% of the uterine wall thickness and external contour straight or with indentation less than 50%; Class U3: external indentation more than 50% of the uterine wall thickness, Class U3b: width of the fundal indentation at the midline more than 150% of the uterine wall thickness

ASRM MÜLLERIAN ANOMALY CLASSIFICATION 2021 (MAC, 2021)

Among many classification systems of Mullerian anomalies AFS classification 1988 is most accepted and useful classifications till now, but not without criticism due to many lacunae. To overcome those lacunae as much as possible ASRM Müllerian Anomaly Classification (MAC), 2021 has been created. The new MAC, 2021 system has classified Mullerian anomalies into nine systems based on similar elements in presentation, appearance, and treatment. In this system some anomalies may appear in more than one category as anomalies represent a continuum of development and combine elements and some anomalies may appear in more than one category: (1) Müllerian anomalies, (2) cervical agenesis, (3) Unicornuate uterus, (4) uterus didelphys, (5) bicornuate uterus, (6) septate uterus, (7) longitudinal vaginal septum, (8) transverse vaginal septum and (9) Complex anomalies.

ASRM Müllerian Anomaly Classification (MAC), 2021 is given in **Figure 2A**.

Prevalence of Müllerian Anomalies

- 0.5–6% of women.
- Most cases are diagnosed during pregnancy or gynecological examination.
- In absence of symptoms, many remain undiagnosed.
- In women with recurrent pregnancy loss (RPL), prevalence is 13.3%.
- In women with infertility, it is 24.5%.

Effects of Müllerian Anomalies

- Gynecological problems.
- Adverse pregnancy outcome.
- Associated anomalies—*associated renal anomalies: 30–50% cases and other systems like skeletal system.*

Gynecological Problems

- Abnormalities of menstrual cycle especially primary amenorrhea with or without cyclical pain abdomen.
- Pelvic pain.
- Dyspareunia/apareunia.
- Infertility
- Endometriosis.

Adverse Pregnancy Outcome

- Spontaneous abortion—RPL.
- Ectopic pregnancy in rudimentary horn of unicornuate uterus.
- Preterm labor (PTL).
- Fetal growth restriction (FGR).

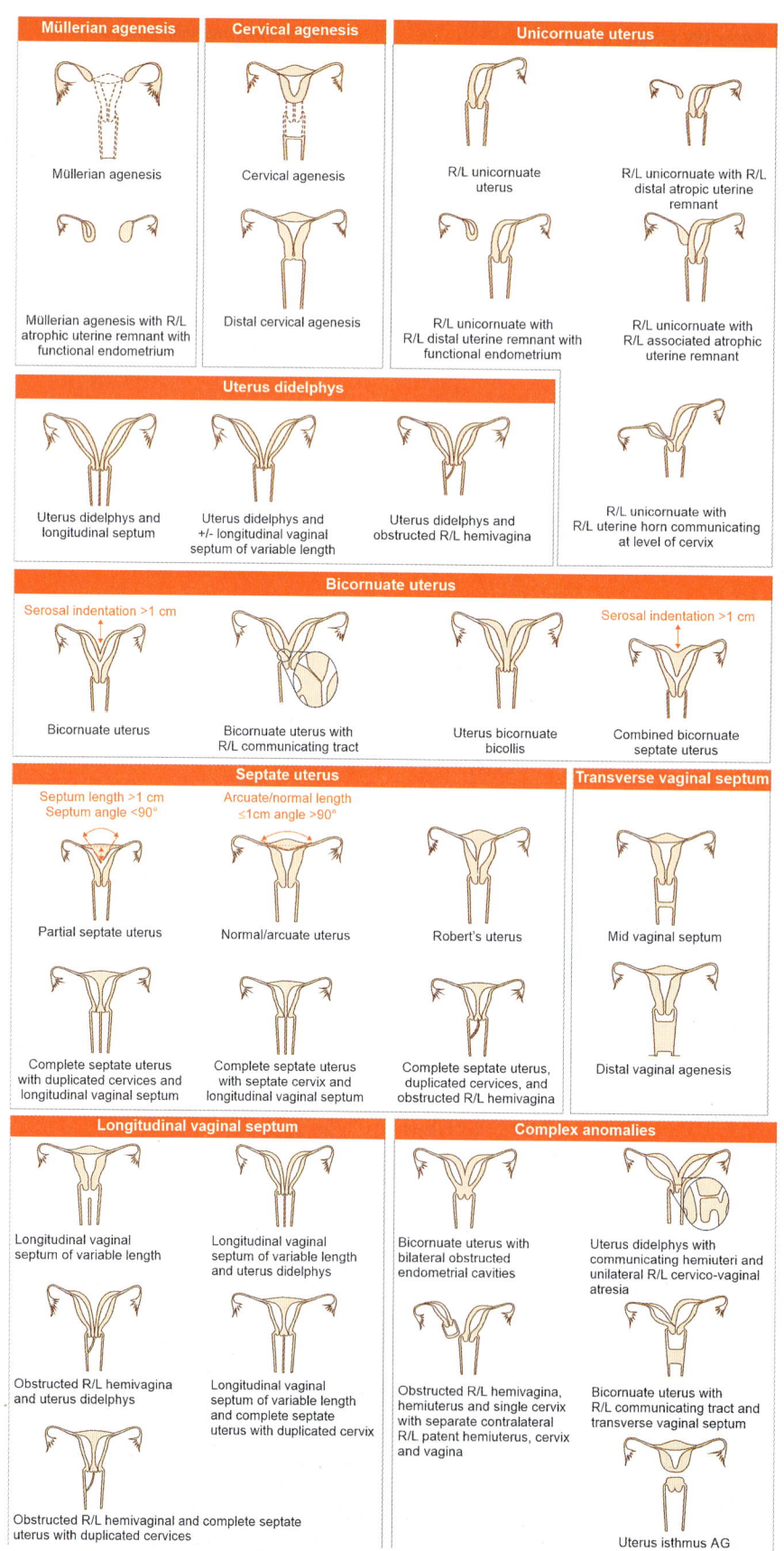

Fig. 2A: ASRM Müllerian Anomaly Classification (MAC) 2021.

- Malpresentation: Transverse is more common in arcuate and subseptate uterus and breech is in bicornuate, unicornuate and complete septate uterus.
- Preterm premature rupture of membranes (PPROM).
- Prolonged labor—incoordinate uterine action.
- Obstructed labor—by nongravid horn of bicornuate or rudimentary horn.
- Retained placenta and postpartum hemorrhage (PPH)—due to implantation of placenta over septum.
- Increase cesarean rate—increase perinatal mortality.

Diagnosis of Müllerian Anomaly

- Clinical symptoms and physical examination.
- Many are asymptomatic—diagnosis during pregnancy, during infertility workup and workup of miscarriage.
- Hysterosalpingography (HSG).
- Sonography-2D USG and 3D USG.
- Computed tomography (CT) scan.
- Magnetic resonance imaging (MRI).
- Laparoscope.
- Hysteroscope.

Role of 3D USG and MRI: It is very difficult to differentiate between bicornuate uterus and septate uterus by imaging. Initially, by HSG and 2D TVS anomaly is diagnosed. This differentiation is very important as septate uterus can be managed by hysteroscopic resection. To differentiate the two types 3-D TVS or MRI are performed (*see* later).

UNICORNUATE UTERUS (FIGS. 3 AND 4)

- Incidence—14%.
- Four types according to the AFS classification—most common is noncommunicating rudimentary (IIb) (*see* **Fig. 1**).
- Unilateral complete agenesis—type IId—true unicornuate uterus.
- Incomplete unilateral agenesis—type IIa, IIb, IIc—also called pseudounicornuate uterus— much more frequent (65%)—30% contain endometrial tissue and onehalf communicating.

Diagnosis

- Clinical—uterus is markedly deviated to one side.
- HSG **(Fig. 5)**, ultrasonography (USG) and MRI.
- HSG—a deviated banana-shaped cavity with single fallopian tube.

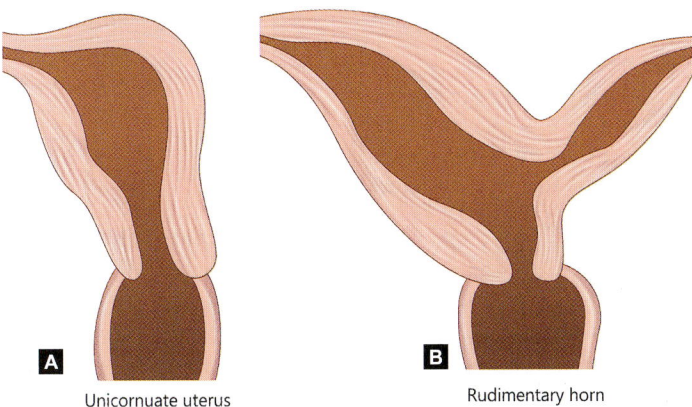

Figs. 3A and B: (A) Unicornuate uterus; (B) Unicornuate uterus with communicating horn.

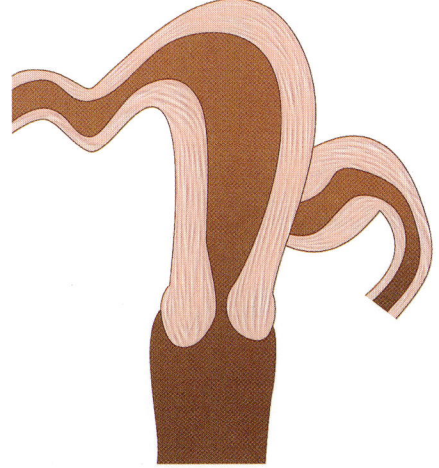

Fig. 4: Unicornuate uterus with noncommunicating rudimentary horn.

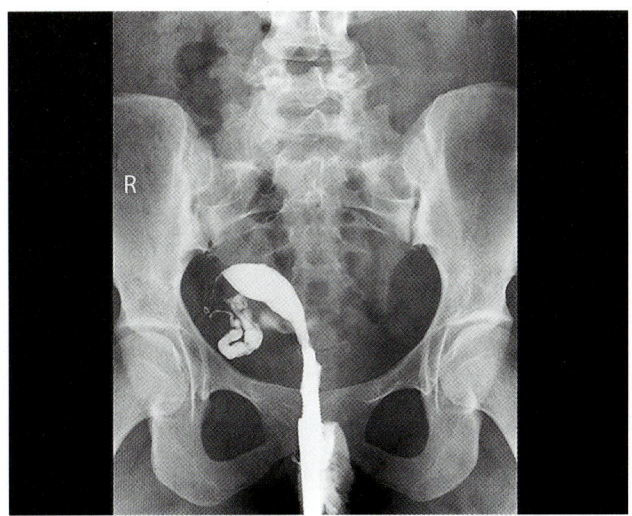

Fig. 5: HSG suggestive of unicornuate uterus.

- USG by two-dimensional (2D) rudimentary horn tissue is diagnosed situated between hemicavity and contralateral ovary.
- Three-dimensional (3D) **(Fig. 6)** or MRI is more precise to diagnose. Solid horn may mimic pedunculated subserous myoma. Transvaginal sonography (TVS) and MRI may be helpful to diagnose. Sometimes laparoscopy may be needed.

Adverse Impacts of Unicornuate Uterus

- *Gynecological problems:* Pelvic pain—if a noncommunicating horn contains functional endometrium, the girl presents with abdominal pain with or without mass. Increase incidence of infertility, endometriosis and dysmenorrhea.
- *Adverse pregnancy outcome:* Impaired uterine blood flow, diminished uterine cavity and less muscle mass of hemiuterus and cervical incompetence are considered to be adverse obstetrics outcome.
- Preterm labor—16%.
- Miscarriage—36%.
- Fetal growth restriction.
- Fetal demise.
- Live birth rate—54%.
- Malpresentation commonly breech presentation **(Fig. 7)**.
- Dysfunctional labor and high cesarean rate.

Ectopic pregnancy and uterine rupture: Pregnancy in rudimentary horn is a potential site for ectopic pregnancy and when it occurs in noncommunicating horn—risk of uterine rupture is high. Sperm comes from contralateral fallopian tube.

Management

- A noncommunicating horn containing functional endometrium should be resected and can be done laparoscopically. If there is no functional endometrium or it is solid removal is not indicated. Prophylactic excision of a horn having a cavity is recommended by many.

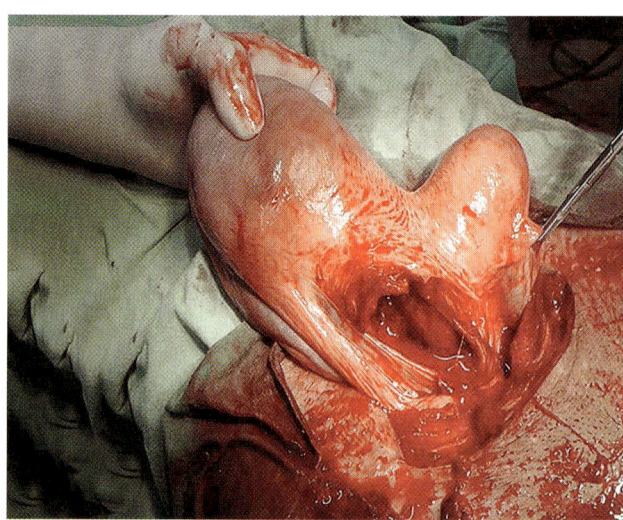

Fig. 7: Pregnancy in right horn (unicornuate, left horn—rudimentary)—breech presentation.
Courtesy: Professor S Laha and Dr Rupali Modak, Assistant Professor

- Pregnancy in rudimentary horn is excised **(Fig. 8)** with or without laparoscopy or medically (methotrexate) treated as soon as diagnosed. Rudimentary uterine rupture occurs mostly before 20 weeks of pregnancy.
- *Pregnancy in unicornuate uterus:* No specific treatment—hence monitoring and management accordingly keeping in mind the chance of PTL and malpresentation. Prophylactic cerclage is advocated but role is not established.

Differentiation of Bicornuate, Septate and Arcuate Uterus

Figure 8A shows diagrammatic representation of 3-D TVS of Bicornuate, Septate and arcuate uterus in coronal plane. Fundal indent is more than 1 cm, in bicornuate uterus, in ASRM classification. In septate uterus partition depth is more than 1.5 cm and partition angle is less than 90° and in arcuate uterus partition depth is less than 1 cm and partition angle is

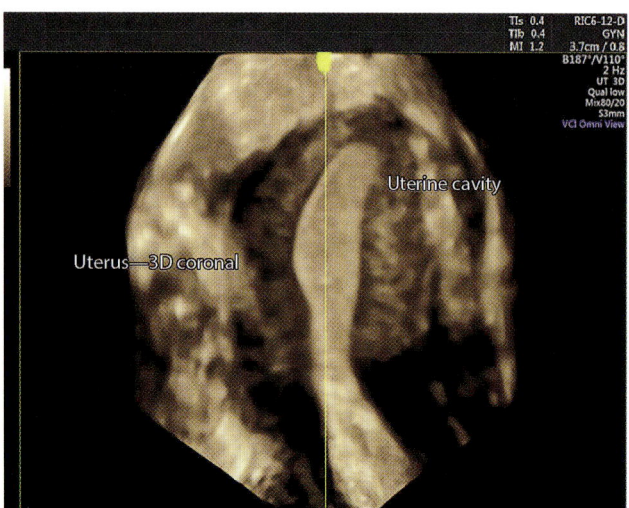

Fig. 6: 3D USG suggestive of unicornuate uterus.
Courtesy: Professor Kamal Oswal, HOD, Radiology, VIMS, Kolkata

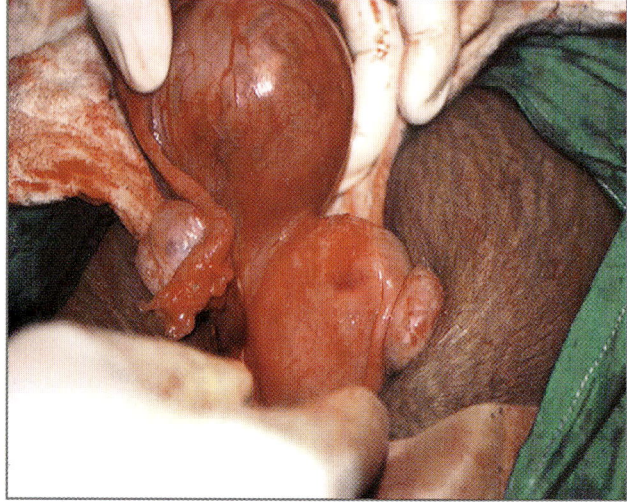

Fig. 8: Pregnancy in rudimentary horn—excision is treatment.

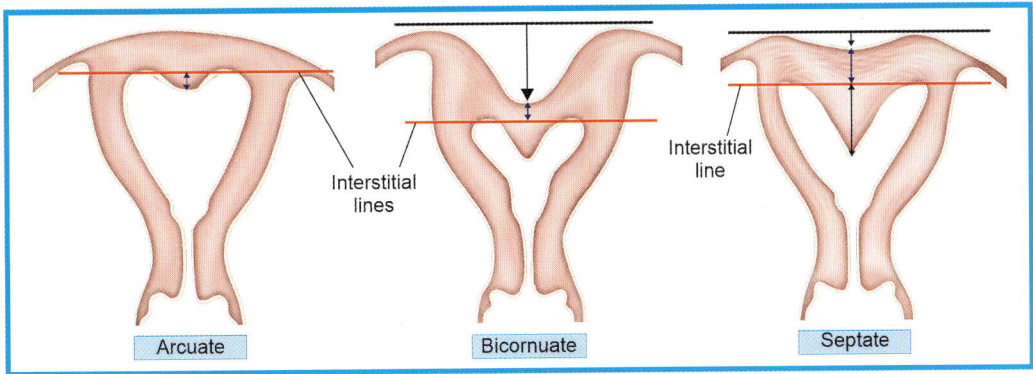

Fig. 8A: Diagrammatic representation of 3-D TVS of bicornuate, septate and arcuate uterus in coronal plane.

more than 90° (American Society for Reproductive Medicine, 2016). ESHRE/ESGE also made different differentiating features in the same way.

UTERINE DIDELPHYS (FIGS. 9 TO 14)

- Failure of fusion of Müllerian ducts results uterine didelphys (two cervices).
- Presence of two noncommunicating endometrial cavities *each with a cervix* and a fallopian tube may be associated with a longitudinal vaginal septum.
- Obstruction may occur by septum at one-half of vagina [obstructed hemivagina and ipsilateral renal anomaly (OHVIRA) syndrome] **(Fig. 15)**.
- It constitutes 10% of uterine anomalies.
- *Diagnosis:* Uterine didelphys is suspected if a longitudinal vaginal septum or two separate cervices are found. Confirmation is done by HSG by which two completely separate canals are seen.

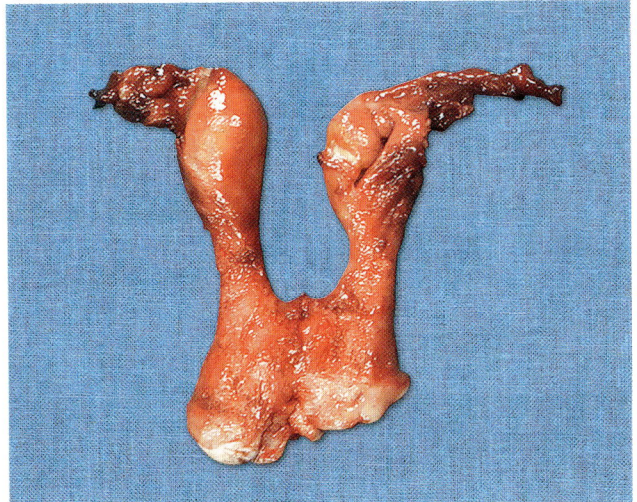

Fig. 10: Uterine didelphys. Abdominal hysterectomy with sacrocolpopexy done in a 41-year parous woman with genital prolapse.
Courtesy: Professor SL Seal and Dr Sanjay Bhattacharyya, Assistant Professor

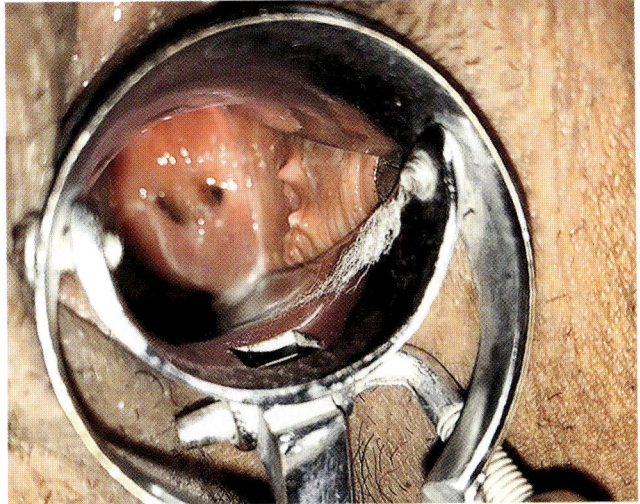

Fig. 9: Double cervical os in didelphys uterus.
Courtesy: Dr Sunita Sharma, IRM, Kolkata.

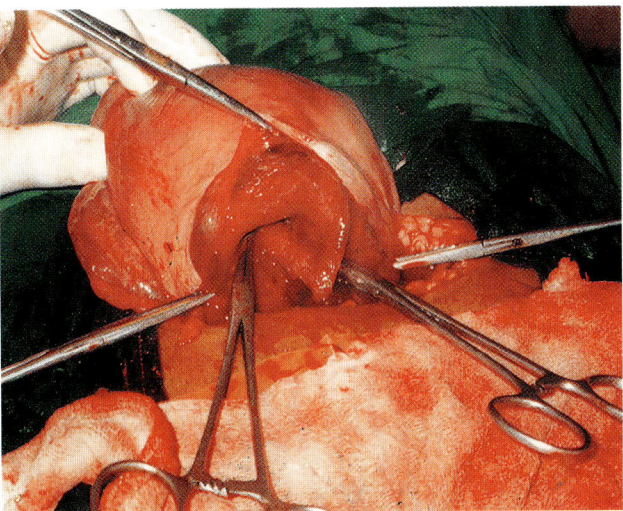

Fig. 11: Double uterus, double cervix, double vagina (during cesarean section).

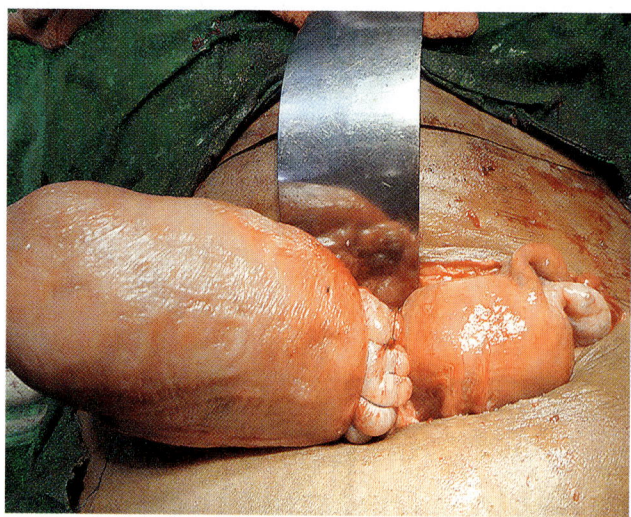

Fig. 12: Cesarean section done in uterus didelphys (pregnancy in left hemiuterus) with bicolis with septate vagina.

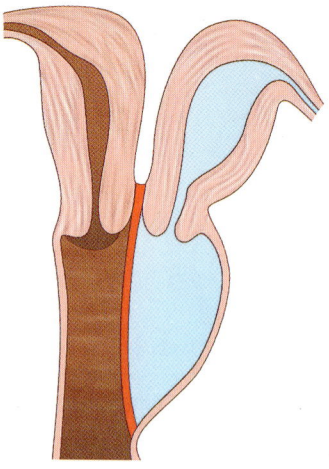

Fig. 15: OHVIRA (obstructed hemivagina and ipsilateral renal anomaly) syndrome.

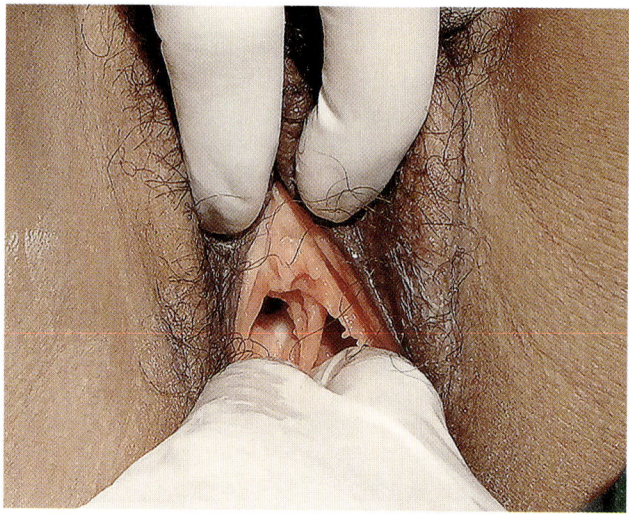

Fig. 13: Vaginal longitudinal septum in uterine didelphys.
Courtesy: Dr Keka Mandal

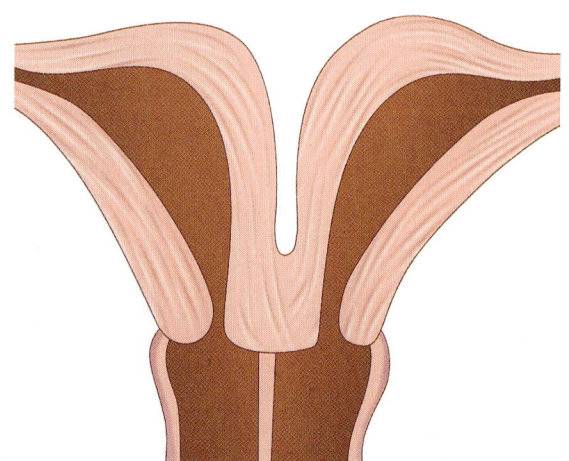

Fig. 14: Didelphic uterus with vaginal septum.

- Two-dimensional not always can differentiate from bicornuate and 3D and MRI are helpful to differentiate didelphic, bicornuate and septate uterus.

Reproductive outcome in uterine didelphys:
- Better in compared to unicornuate uterus possibly due to improved blood supply from contralateral side in contrast to unicornuate uterus.
- Pregnancy occurs more in right horn (76%). Fetal survival is 75%.
- There is significant risk of PTL (RR 3.58, p <0.001) and malpresentation (RR 3.70, p <0.001) when compared with normal uteri. There is increased risk of miscarriage but not statistically significant.

Treatment
Surgery is rarely indicated to improve reproductive outcome only in selected patients with repeated late trimester pregnancy loss.

BICORNUATE UTERUS (FIGS. 16 TO 20)

- Accounts for 25% of uterine anomalies.
- One cervix with two divergent horns.
- Two separate but communicating endometrial cavities. Myometrium is present surrounding each cavity.
- The upper surface of fundus is "heart-shaped" **(Fig. 16)**.
- The difference between bicornuate and septate uterus is made visually (in septate—normal looking fundus and in bicornuate—midline indentation), 3D USG, MRI or by laparoscopy where heart-shaped uterus is differentiated from normal-shaped septate uterus.
- HSG is initial diagnostic step-marked divergence (wide angle >105) **(Fig. 17)**. Intercornual angle more than 105° suggests bicornuate uterus, whereas less than 75° indicates a septate uterus.

CHAPTER 21: Development of Genital Organs and Müllerian Anomaly

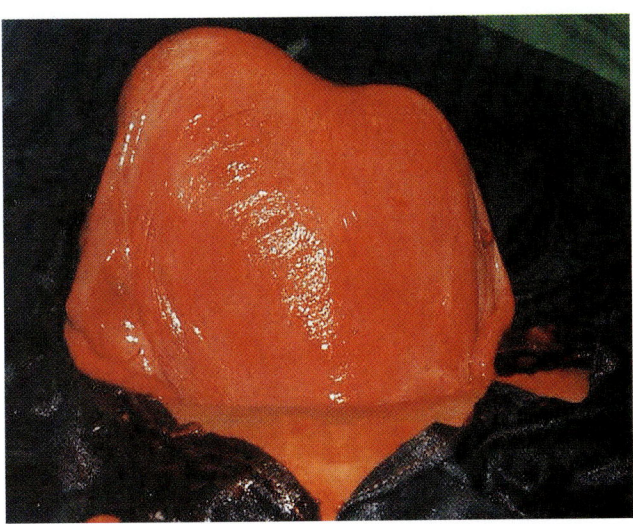

Fig. 16: Bicornuate uterus—look the fundal appearance.

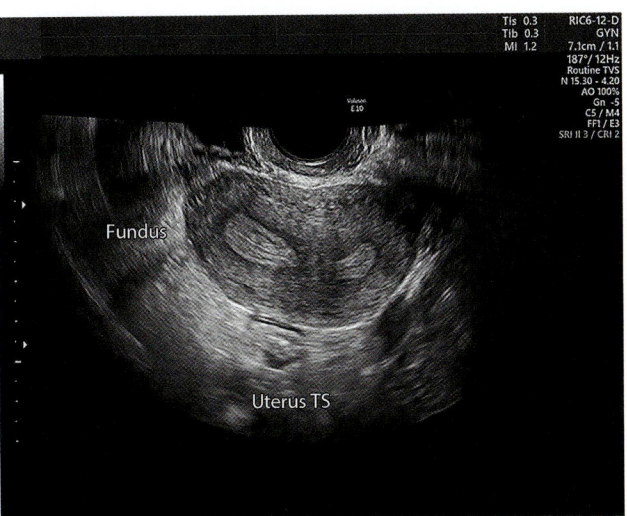

Fig. 18: TVS suggestive of bicornuate uterus.

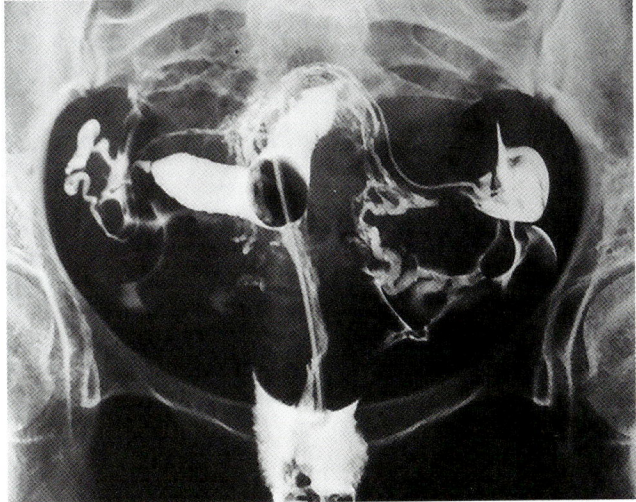

Fig. 17: HSG showing bicornuate uterus. Hysterosonosalpingography catheter has been used instead of HSG cannula.
Courtesy: Dr Subir Roy

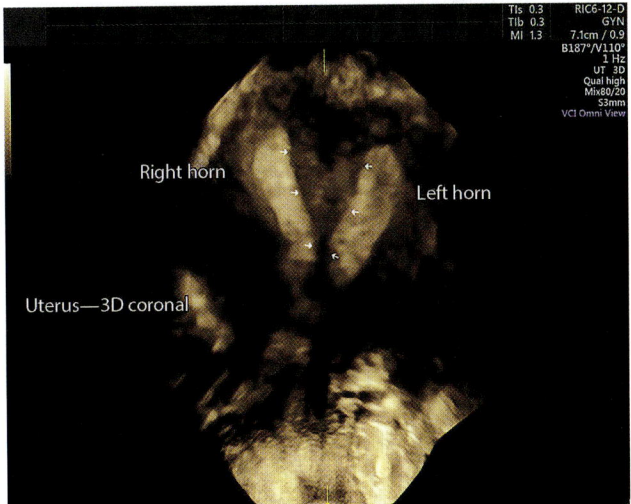

Fig. 19: 3D USG suggestive of bicornuate uterus.
Courtesy: Professor Kamal Oswal

- USG—uterine duplication with invagination of fundus. "V" sign is the spacing between the horns and urinary bladder.
- Fundal invagination more than 1 cm by 3D and MRI **(Fig. 8A-coronal plane)** and distinct vascularization in color Doppler testify bicornuate uterus (<1 cm septate uterus). 2D can differentiate a bicornuate from septate but not from didelphic. 3D **(Fig. 19)** and MRI are more helpful.
- *Diagnosis* is confirmed by laparoscope when hysteroscopic resection of septum is attempted.

Reproductive Outcome in Bicornuate Uterus

- Success of delivering live baby is 60%.
- Premature onset of labor occurs around 22–32 weeks as pregnancy grows in half a uterus.

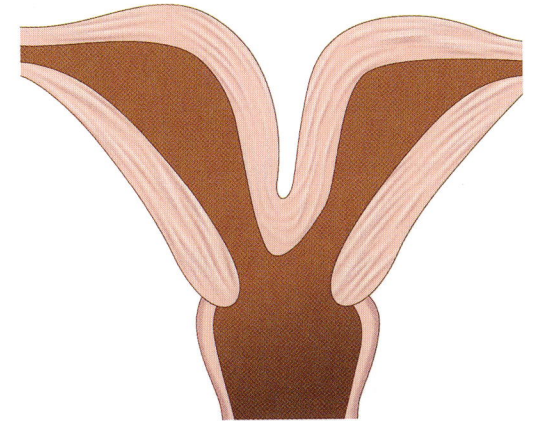

Fig. 20: Bicornuate uterus.

- Chance of preterm delivery more than 60%. Increased risk of miscarriage (RR 3.40, $p < 0.05$), preterm birth (RR 2.55, $p < 0.001$) and malpresentation (RR 5.38, $p < 0.001$).

- Reproductive outcome is better in comparison to septate uterus, hence surgical interference is needed less.
- Other than monitoring of pregnancy, no specific treatment is advocated.

Indications of Surgery in Bicornuate Uterus

- Unification operation (*Strassman technique*) is indicated with good outcome in women with multiple spontaneous abortions with bicornuate uterus in absence of other cause. More than 85% end in live birth following surgery (*see* Page 453, **Figs. 34A to C**).
- Cesarean section is indicated following metroplasty.

Different Surgical Techniques of Uterine Unification due to Lateral Fusion Defect

- Transcervical lysis of uterine septum.
- Modified Jones metroplasty (*see* below).
- Jones metroplasty.
- Tompkins procedure.
- Strassman metroplasty (*see* below). See **Figs. 34A to C**, Page 453.

SEPTATE UTERUS (FIGS. 21 TO 24)

- Results from failure of resorption of medial part of fused Müllerian ducts.
- Most common (35%) of all Müllerian anomalies.
- This anomaly is not usually with renal anomalies.
- External contour of uterus is normal. On coronal section, fundal serosa is rectilinear or less than 1 cm invagination.
- Cavity is divided by fibrous hypovascularized myometrium. It may be *partial*, *complete* and sometimes *asymmetric septate uterus* (this variety is given in Musset's classification, not in AFS). Rarely, a complete vaginocervicouterine septum is found.

Diagnosis

- Septate uterus is diagnosed during investigations of infertility or RPL or may be incidental finding without adverse obstetric outcome.
- HSG (**Fig. 21**), sonography and MRI.
- In HSG, finding is almost similar with bicornuate uterus but acute angle in septate uterus is less (<75°).
- USG—two endometrial cavities separated by hypoechoic myometrium and fundal contour slightly concave or flat. 3D (**Figs. 22 and 23**) USG and MRI precisely depict size and extend of septum. By 3D partition depth is more than 1.5 cm and partition angle is less than 900 than in coronal plane (**Fig. 8A**).

Reproductive Outcome in Septate Uterus

- Septate uterus is associated with subfertility, miscarriage, and malpresentation. Preterm delivery is not increased.
- Spontaneous abortion (8–12 weeks) rate is 42%. There may be fetal malformation infrequently.

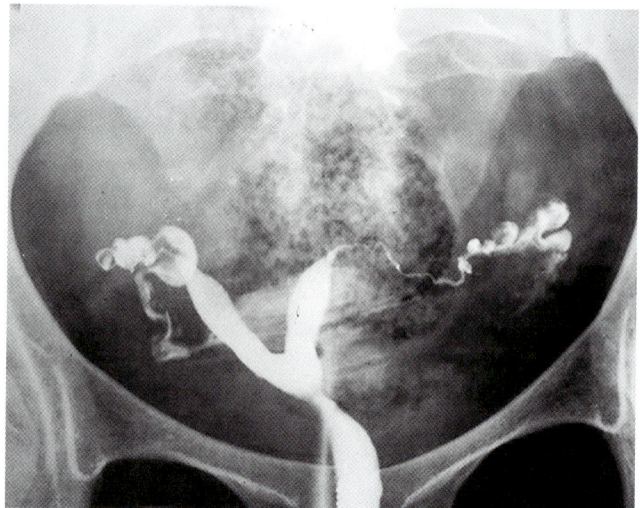

Fig. 21: Septate uterus.

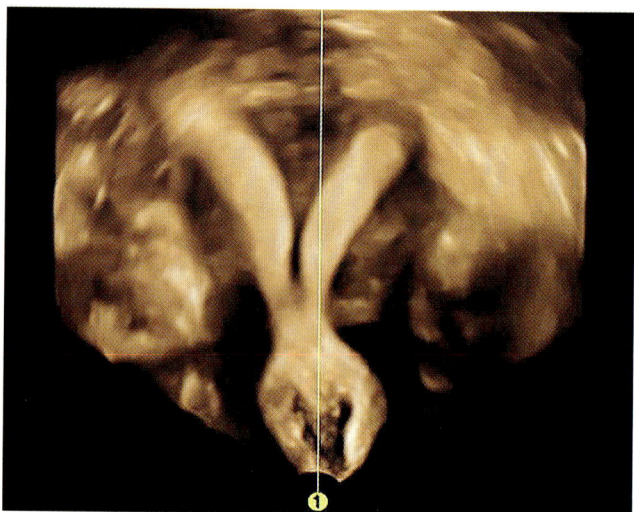

Fig. 22: 3D USG suggestive of complete septate uterus.

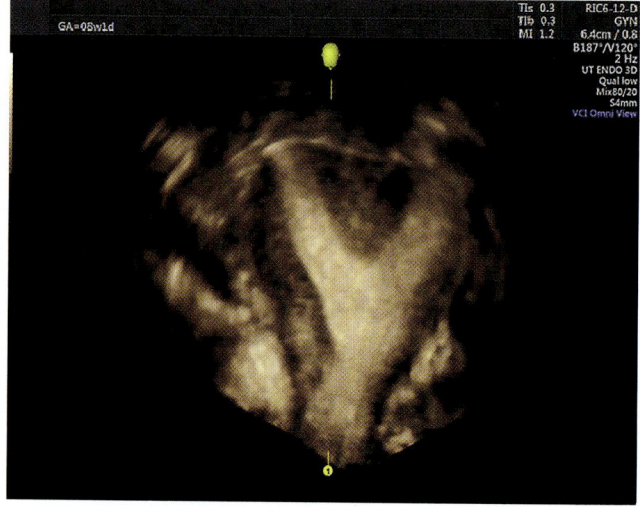

Fig. 23: 3D USG suggestive of subseptate uterus.

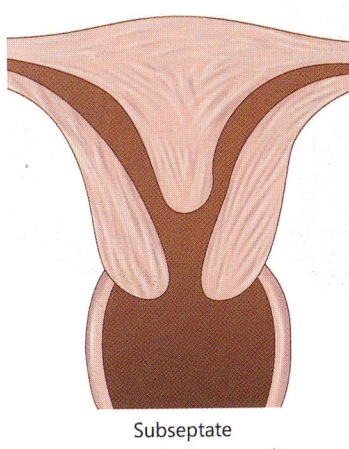

Fig. 24: Subseptate uterus.

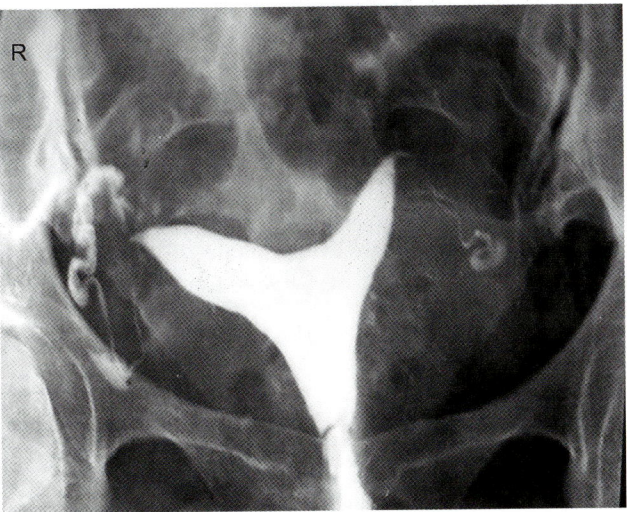

Fig. 26: HSG showing arcuate uterus.

- The cause of first trimester abortion is diminished blood supply, implantation on avascular septum, distorted uterine cavity and cervical and endometrial abnormalities.
- Reproductive outcome is poor in comparison to bicornuate uterus, hence surgical interference is needed more.

Treatment

- Surgical resection via hysteroscopic metroplasty (Fig. 25) is considered when associated with infertility or RPL.
- Hysteroscopic procedure is easy, safe and effective procedure showing improved reproductive outcome; however, there is no randomized controlled trial (RCT) comparing hysteroscopic resection and non-intervention. Adjunctive laparoscopy is preferred to be vigilant for uterine perforation. 60% pregnancy rate and 45% live birth are reported following hysteroscopic resection.
- Open surgical method is discarded due to adhesion, rupture uterus, infertility and increase cesarean section rate.

ARCUATE UTERUS (FIG. 26)

- There is slight indentation in the fundus. Ratio of height to fundal indentation to intercornual distance is less than 10%.
- HSG and USG can diagnose. To differentiate from bicornuate and septate uterus 3D TVS (Fig. 8A) is helpful where partition depth is found less than 1cm and partition angle is more than 900.
- Most women have no adverse reproductive consequences and no treatment needed.
- Only few series show second trimester loss and PTL.
- Surgery is indicated in excessive pregnancy losses when other reasons are not found.

Q. What is the role of cerclage in uterine anomaly?

- Cerclage—transvaginal and transabdominal method may be useful for many women with uterine anomalies and repetitive pregnancy losses.
- Indication is determined by the criteria used for women without such defects.

TRANSVERSE VAGINAL SEPTUM (FIG. 27)

- Results from failure of canalization of vaginal plate at the point where the urogenital sinus meets the Müllerian duct.
- Incidence—rare: 1:2,100–1:72,000.
- May be perforation, vary in thickness and location in vagina.
- In complete septum—amenorrhea, hematocolpos, hematometra.
- In presence of perforation—normal menses but dyspareunia.

Types

Low—less than 3 cm from introitus (Fig. 28); mid—3–6 cm; high—more than 6 cm.

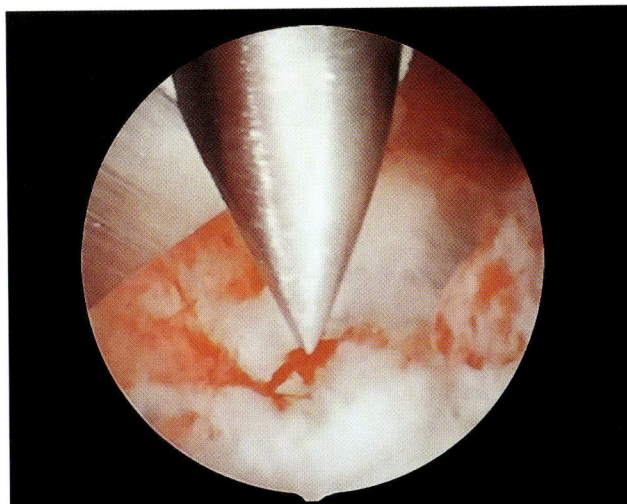

Fig. 25: Hysteroscopic septal resection.
Courtesy: Dr Bani Mitra

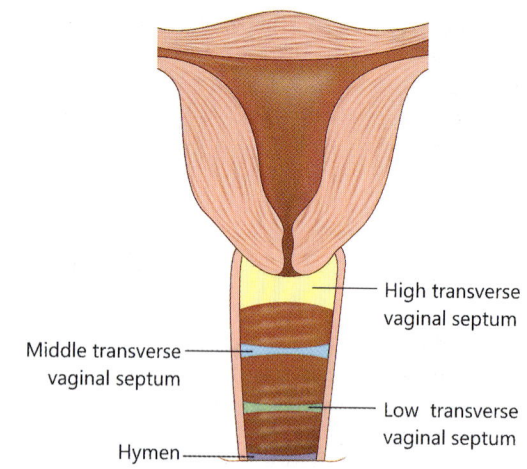

Fig. 27: Transverse vaginal septum at various levels of vagina.

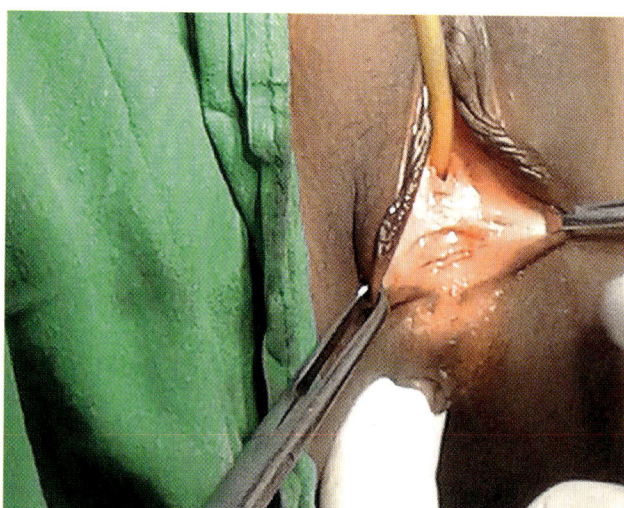

Fig. 28: Low transverse vaginal septum.

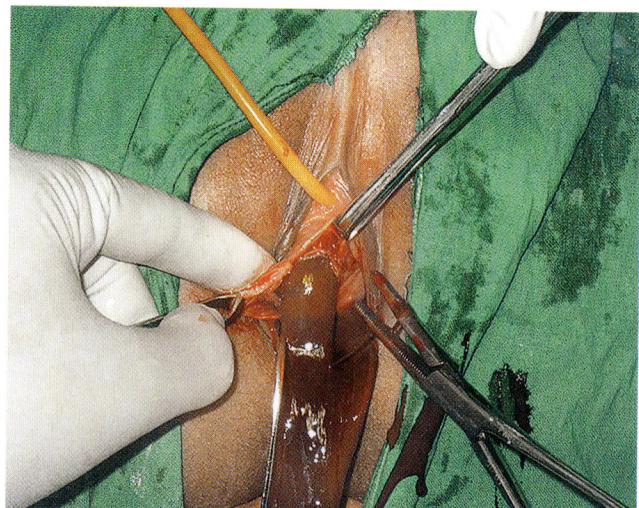

Fig. 29: Transverse vaginal septum— drainage of cryptomenorrhea.

- USG
- MRI—it is especially useful to confirm diagnosis and to determine the site and thickness of the septum and also to detect the presence of cervix whether it is only vaginal septum or with cervical atresia (see **Figs. 17 and 18**, Page 316).

Management (Table 5)

- Surgical resection with anastomosis of proximal with distal vagina after drainage of blood **(Fig. 29)**.
- Occasionally skin grafts or buccal mucosal grafts are used. Diagnostic needle aspiration is helpful to determine the direction of dissection in suspected hematocolpos.
- In high type abdominovaginal approach using laparoscopy is suggested recently.
- Stenosis with dyspareunia is a real problem. All cases of laparoscopic and abdominoperineal cases, vaginal dilatation is recommended.
- In less than 2 cm thick septum, prognosis is good. In thick septum (>2 cm), scarring, stenosis and fistulae formation are common.

LONGITUDINAL VAGINAL SEPTUM (SEE FIG. 14)

- Due to failure of canalization of vaginal plate.
- Variety:
  - Complete—from cervix to introitus (see **Fig. 13**).
  - Partial **(Fig. 30)**.
- About 90% cases are associated with uterine anomaly, commonly didelphys or complete uterine septum.
- *Diagnosis*: It may be asymptomatic. Dyspareunia or difficulty inserting tampons or may be diagnosed in labor. Clinically diagnosed.
- *Treatment*: Surgical resection of entire septum and hemostasis.
- OHVIRA is special variety (see **Fig. 15**).

Table 5: Management of transverse vaginal septum.

Types/position	Management	Result
Thin	Vaginal resection Perineal skin flap may be needed occasionally	Good
Mid or high <2 cm thick with good lower vaginal length	Laparoscopic resection	Good
>2 cm imperforate	Abdominoperineal approach All cases of laparoscopic and abdominoperineal cases, vaginal dilatation is recommended	Scarring, stenosis and fistulae formation common

Diagnosis

- Clinical—similar to imperforate hymen— amenorrhea, cyclical pain abdomen, abdominal or pelvic mass, short vagina and nonvisibility of cervix.

CHAPTER 21: Development of Genital Organs and Müllerian Anomaly

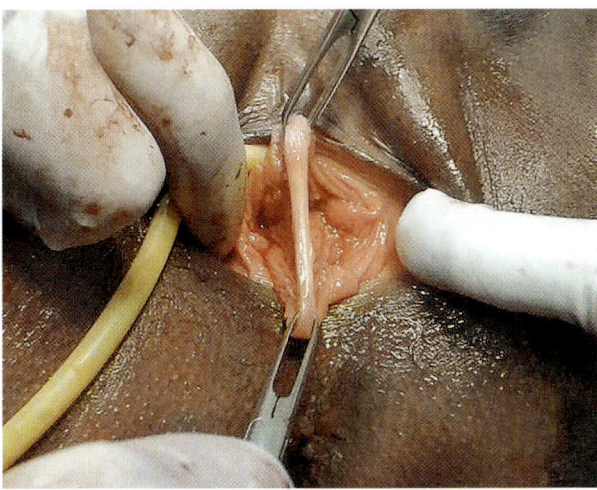

Fig. 30: Longitudinal septum of vagina.

- Gonadotropin-releasing hormone (GnRH) or combined oral contraceptive (OC) is used to suppress the menstruation as a temporary method to prevent endometriosis till a definite treatment plan is arranged.
- Recently various conservative surgeries are recommended in selected cases.

Various conservative surgeries in atretic cervix are:
- Simple canalization of uterus (uterovaginal fistula) with vagina through atretic cervix.
- Anastomosis or implantation of uterus with vagina with or without resection of atretic cervical tissue (Deffarges et al., and by Acien P).
- Creation of neocervix from atretic cervical tissue and fix it to the vagina by pulling (Chakravarty).
- Canalization of cervix using graft or flaps—amniotic membrane and pudendal graft for cervical reconstruction.
- Laparoscopically-assisted uterovestibular anastomosis. (Creighton, et al. and by Fedele, et al.) or uterovaginal anastomosis (Kriplani, et al.).

Pregnancy by zygote intrafallopian tube transfer (ZIFT) and transmyometrial transfer of embryo by in vitro fertilization (IVF) have been reported.

VAGINAL AGENESIS (FIG. 32)

Sometimes isolated vaginal agenesis may occur with normal cervix and uterus. Prognosis is better than cervical agenesis.

MAYER-ROKITANSKY-KÜSTER-HAUSER SYNDROME (*SEE* ALSO CHAPTER 13)

- Uterus, cervix and upper part of vagina are absent resulting from complete Müllerian agenesis and only a small vaginal pouch measuring 1–2 inches deep is present.
- Distal parts of fallopian tubes are present and ovaries are normal.
- A transverse Müllerian ridge (knob) (**Fig. 33A**) is present in between urinary bladder and sigmoid colon. The fallopian

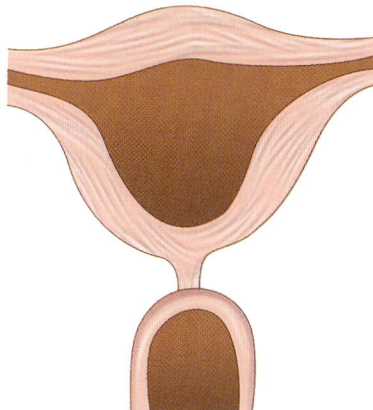

Cervical atresia

Fig. 31: Cervical agenesis.

CERVICAL AGENESIS (FIG. 31)

- Incidence—very rare: 1:80,000–100,000.
- Presentation—primary amenorrhea, worsening lower abdominal pain with or without a mass secondary to hematometra.
- Associated with vaginal aplasia in almost 40% of cases.
- In presence of functional endometrium, uterus is distended and endometriosis develops secondary to retrograde menstrual flow.

Diagnosis
- Clinical
- Radiographic study.
- Sonography and MRI.

Treatment
- Surgical canalization in cervical atresia with functional uterus.
- Previously conservative surgery was not encouraged due to serious complications including death and hysterectomy was recommended.

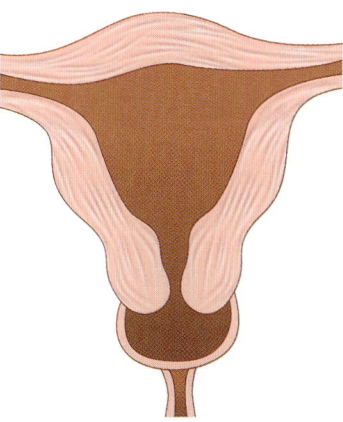

Vaginal atresia

Fig. 32: Vaginal agenesis.

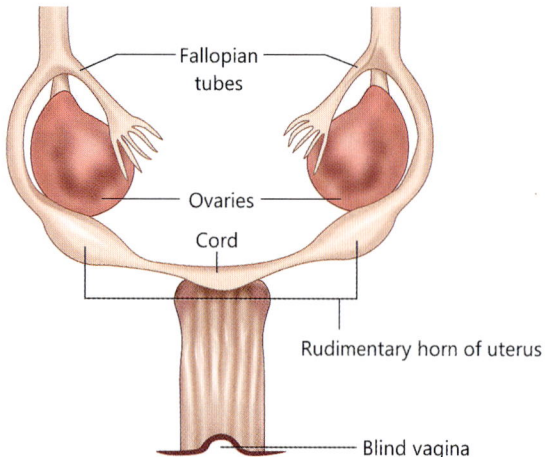

Fig. 33A: Schematic diagram of RKH syndrome— complete absence of uterus, cervix and vagina. Uterus may be rudimentary.

tubes and ovaries are normal. Mostly, Müllerian knob is devoid of any active endometrium. Rarely (2–7%) active endometrium may be present resulting accumulation of menstrual blood and causing cyclical lower abdominal pain. In these cases, excision of rudimentary knob is needed.

- *Associated abnormalities*: *Renal* (15–40%) and *skeletal abnormalities* (12%) may be present in this syndrome. Renal abnormalities may be in the form of absent, pelvic kidney, horseshoe-shaped kidney or double urinary collective system. Scoliosis, spina bifida, sacralization of lumbar vertebra, lumbarization of sacral vertebra and cervical vertebra malformation are the skeletal abnormalities. MURCS syndrome includes Müllerian duct aplasia, renal aplasia and cervicothoracic somatic dysplasia.
- Karyotype is typical female 46 XX with normal secondary sexual character.
- Clinical presentation—primary amenorrhea with developed secondary sexual character.
- On examination—looking like female. All secondary sexual characters are present with well-developed breasts. Labia well-developed and vagina is blind and only lower part of vagina is present.

Incidence of MRKH Syndrome

It is 1 in 5,000 newborn girls second to gonadal dysgenesis as a cause of primary amenorrhea.

Investigations

- USG—uterus absent. Renal abnormalities may be detected.
- Karyotype—46 XX.
- Laparoscopy—tubes present, ovaries normal and a transverse ridge with Müllerian knob present.
- Intravenous pyelogram (IVP) is done to exclude urinary tract abnormalities.
- X-ray may be needed for skeletal abnormality.

Treatment Plan

- Restoration of genital tract function—coital function, reproductive function and menstrual function:
  (1) Vaginoplasty for coitus; (2) reproduction by surrogacy and adoption; and (3) resumption of menstruation is not possible.
- Uterine transplantation is an exciting hope (*see* later in detail).
  - A Swedish team (Brannstrom M, et al. 2014) has reported a series of nine cases of first human uterine transplant—eight MRKH and one cervical cancer.
  - Seven cases have viable uteri with regular menses on 6 months follow-up and two cases resulted graft rejection. There was one live birth in that series.
- Usually, no need of general health management except to take care of any renal and skeletal abnormality.

Vaginoplasty: Methods of Creating Vagina (Fig. 33B)

- Goal is to create a functional vagina.
- It may be achieved by surgery or conservative.
- Postoperative dilatation is important after vaginoplasty either regular intercourse or manual dilatation.
- Nonsurgical methods (gradual dilatation—**Fig. 33B**) are preferred to surgical methods recently.

Q. What are the different methods of vaginoplasty?

- Progressive vaginal dilatation is first choice.
- **Frank** (1938): Conservative method by using graduated hard dilators, plastic or glass dilators.
- **Ingram** (1981): Frank method was modified by Ingram affixing the dilators over bicycle—half- to two-hour per day.
- **McIndoe-Reed operation**—using skin graft over a solid mold.
- **Williams' vulvovaginoplasty.**
- **Vaginoplasty** using amnion (Chakravarty), peritoneal graft (Davydov, et al.), bladder mucosa or sigmoid colon (Freudndt, et al.)

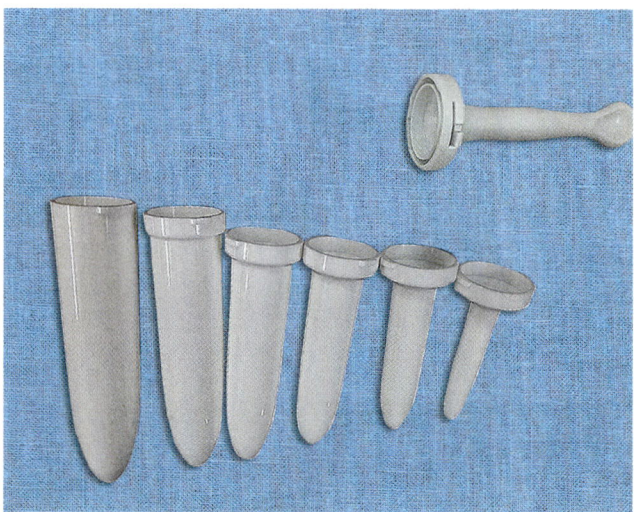

Fig. 33B: Vaginal dilators.

- *Vecchietti's technique:* Sphere connected to two metal wires and guided through potential vaginal space using laparoscope to anterior abdominal wall where they are attached to traction device which is tightened daily. This causes progressive dilatation to create vagina.
- **Laparoscopic vaginoplasty** with peritoneum (Davydov, et al.).
- **Use of engineered autologous** tissue for creation of vagina is a novel technique reported by Mexico group (2014).

SURGICAL METHODS IN MÜLLERIAN ANOMALY

Transcervical Resection of the Septum (see Fig. 25)

- Done by: (1) hysteroscopic scissors; (2) resectoscope; (3) electrocautery, or by (4) laser removal.
- Should be done with laparoscopic guidance to prevent uterine perforation.
- In complete septum with double cervix, a Foley catheter is placed in other cavity and resection is done till catheter is visible.
- Foley tamponade is given sometimes to control postoperative bleeding. Pretreatment GnRH is helpful.
- Postoperative estrogen can be given for better healing.
- Patient may try for pregnancy after 2 months.

Modified Jones Metroplasty in Uterine Septum

- It is a type of wedge resection, containing myometrium and septum.
- Tip of wedge should be in middle of fundus to avoid transection of interstitial portion of tubes.
- After wedge resection uterus is repaired in three layers.

Tompkins Procedure in Uterine Septum

- One vertical incision through the middle of the fundus up to endometrium reached.
- Divide the septum in the septum in two halves.
- Then both of them are incised up to 1 cm of tube.
- Advantage—most anatomical. There is no or minimal loss of endometrial and myometrial tissue.

Strassman Metroplasty (Figs. 34A to C) [Ferdinand Strassman (1866–1938)]

- Ideal for bicornuate uterus, where hysteroscopic resection is not possible due to chance of adhesion.
- Vertical incision is given for both the cornua so as to reset their median portion to open both cavities, then sutured in layers.
- If chances of cervical incompetence to extend procedure till cervix to unify it, cervix may be left doubled.

Different Methods of Vaginoplasty—Creation of New Vagina

Frank (1938) Method of Dilatation

Passive dilatation of vaginal dimple using gradual dilators—a set of dilators of increasing length and width is available.

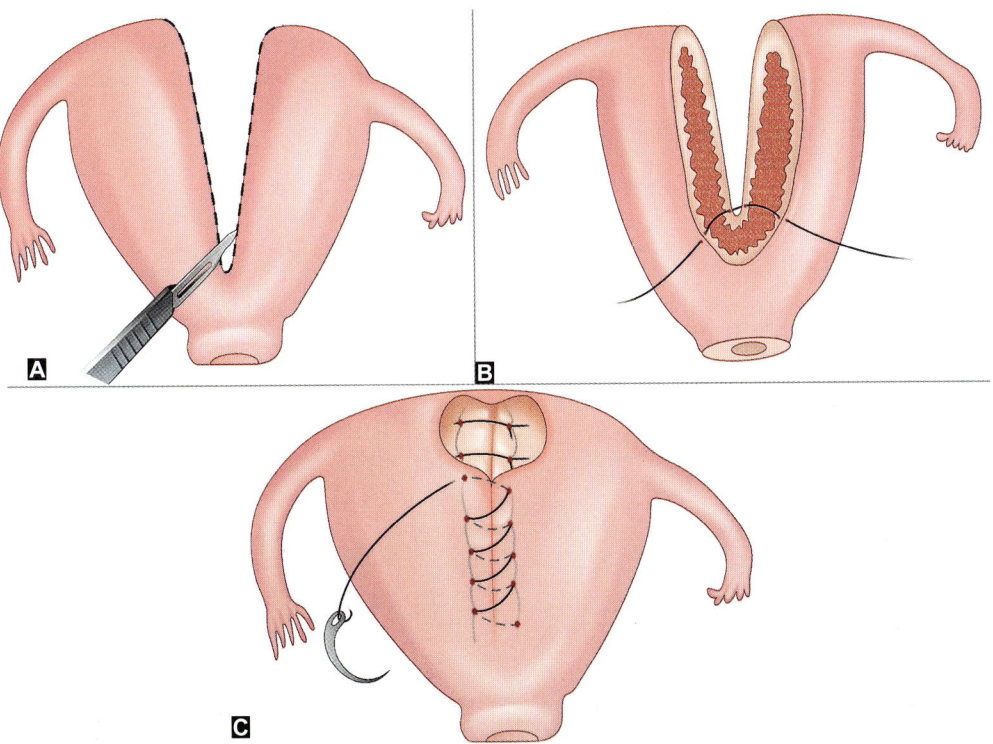

Figs. 34A to C: Strassman metroplasty: (A) Incision; (B) Removal of septum; (C) Repair of the wound.

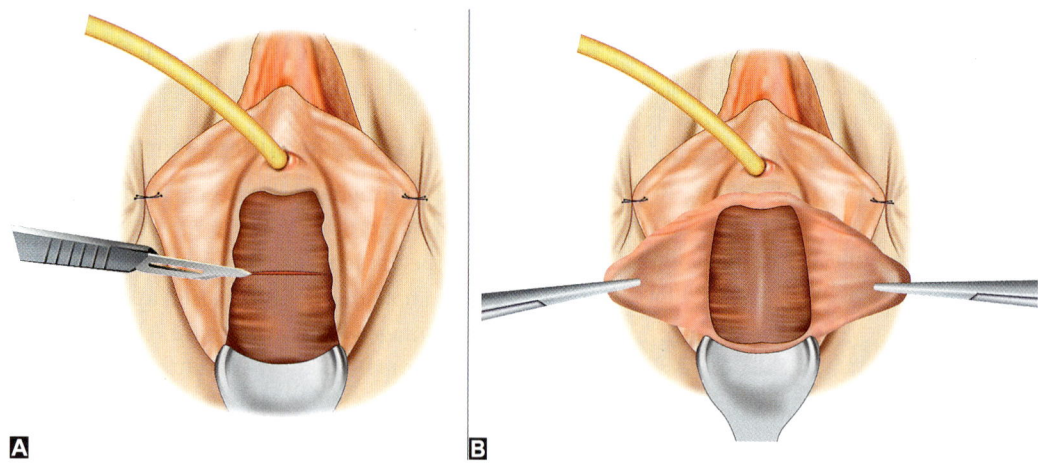

Figs. 35A and B: (A) Transverse incision is given over blind vaginal mucosa; (B) Space is created by blunt and sharp dissection.

Ingram (1981)—Dilators Fixed with Bicycle

Dilators built on a bicycle seat and tool with height of 24 inches at least 2 hours/day for 1 month the swifting to next size. Attempt to sexual intercourse after using largest dilator for 1–2 months, therefore continued dilatation is recommended if intercourse is infrequent.

Abbe-Wharton-McIndoe Operation

- Operation of choice in absent vagina.
- 80–100% success rate.

Timing: Previously, it was done just before marriage, but due to chances of nonhealing and postoperative complication marriage becomes delayed. Now it is advised to do in between 17 years and 20 years of age with good intellectual development to followup postoperative period regularly.

Principles of Procedure

- Dissection is done to make adequate space between rectum and bladder **(Figs. 35 and 36)**.
- *Inlay split-thickness skin grafting:* In Counsellor-Flor modification of *McIndoe technique*, vaginal form (mold) is made from foam rubber block covered by condom over which skin graft is sutured to insert into vaginal space **(Figs. 37A and B).**
- Continuous and prolonged dilatation during contractile phase of healing.

Contraindications

- In case of solitary kidney low in pelvis (does not provide room for adequate dissection). choice is William's operation.
- Should not be done in poor follow-up patient.

Complications

- Enterocele formation—when vaginal mucosa brought in close proximity to pelvic peritoneum.
- Genitourinary fistula (4%)—urethrovaginal, vesicovaginal and rectovaginal.
- Postoperative infection.
- Graft rejection.

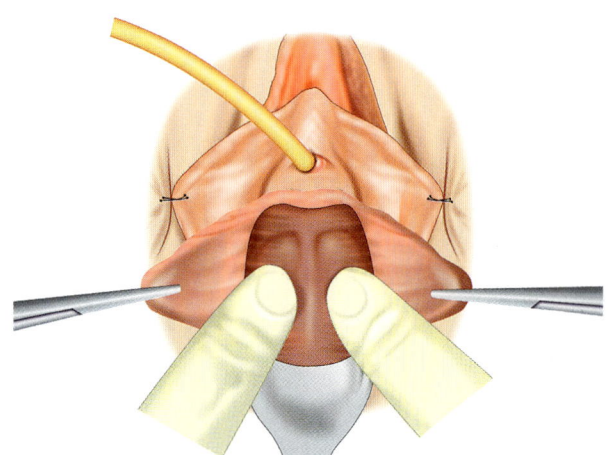

Fig. 36: Creation of vaginal space in between urethra in front and rectum behind—by blunt and sharp dissection, median raphe is seen for which sharp dissection may be necessary.

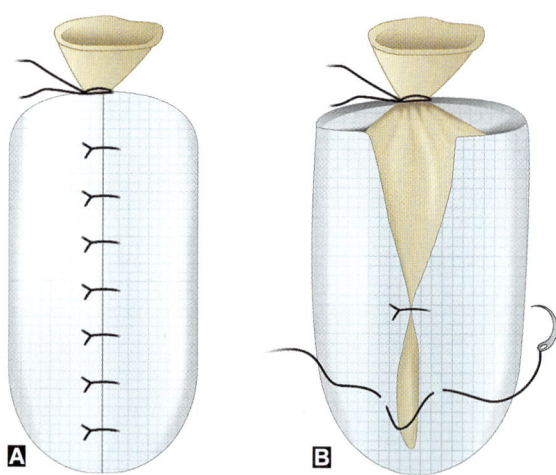

Figs. 37A and B: McIndoe vaginoplasty— vaginal mold (form).
(*see* text—Inlay split-thickness skin grafting)

CHAPTER 21: Development of Genital Organs and Müllerian Anomaly

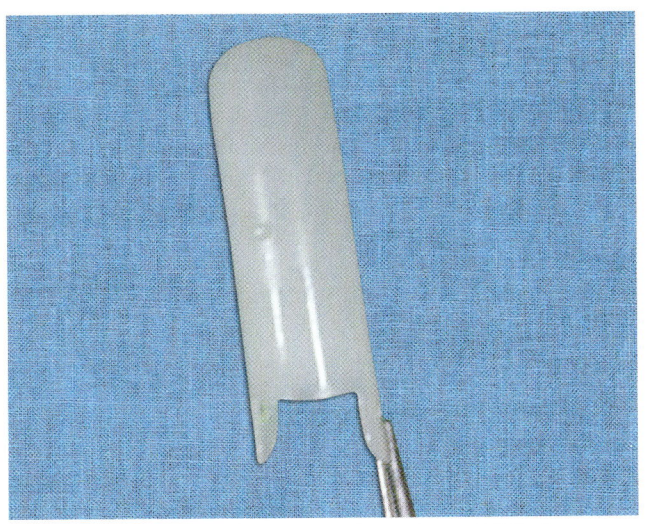

Fig. 38: Plastic vaginal mold—used by Professor BN Chakravarty.

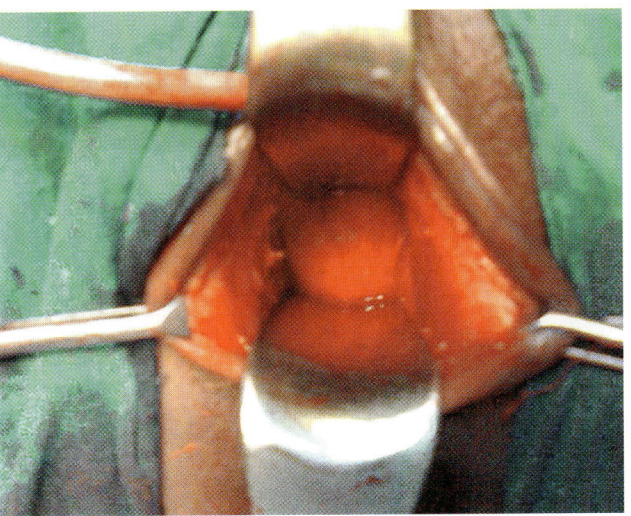

Fig. 39: Vaginoplasty—vagina is created—peritoneum at vault is visible.

Chakravarty BN designed a special plastic mold (**Fig. 38**) for this purpose and used to insert into the space (**Fig. 39**) created in between urethra in front and rectum behind using amniotic graft over it.

Regular dilatation with artificial dilator or regular intercourse is needed to prevent the stenosis and obliteration of vagina.

Williams' Vulvovaginoplasty (Figs. 40A to C)

- **Horseshoe-shaped incision** is given over vulva extending medially through inner side of labia majora up to the level of urethral meatus.
- Then **perineal pouch is created** by suturing inner margin of vulvar skin, then reinforce neovagina by suturing labial fat and perineal muscle. Lastly outer margin of skin of both sides is approximated by interrupted stitches.
- Postoperatively rest is given and intercourse is avoided for 6 weeks.
- Disadvantage—normal anatomy is not restored which makes an awkward angle for intercourse.
- Not popular. Indicated when other methods fail.

UTERINE TRANSPLANTATION

A Swedish team (Brannstrom, M et al. 2014) has reported first a series of nine cases of first human uterine transplant—eight MRKH and one cervical cancer. Dr Shailesh Puntambekar from India reported uterine transplantation in 2017 and first bay was delivered in October 2018.

Indications of **uterine transplantation** are absolute uterine factor. Absent of uterus due to complete mullerian agenesis, prior hysterectomy, obliterating intrauterine adhesions and distorting leiomyomas.

There are various issues in relation to uterine transplantation like ethical issue, donor issue, recipient issue and graft rejection issue one major. The various concerns of recipient is need of major surgery, long term immunosuppression therapy, chance of rejection, for pregnancy to achieve IVF and ET is essential. Uterus should be removed after 1–2 child to avoid continuation of immune suppression. Donor needs surgery. Criteria for recipients are absolute uterine factor infertility, no medical contraindications, there is personal or legal

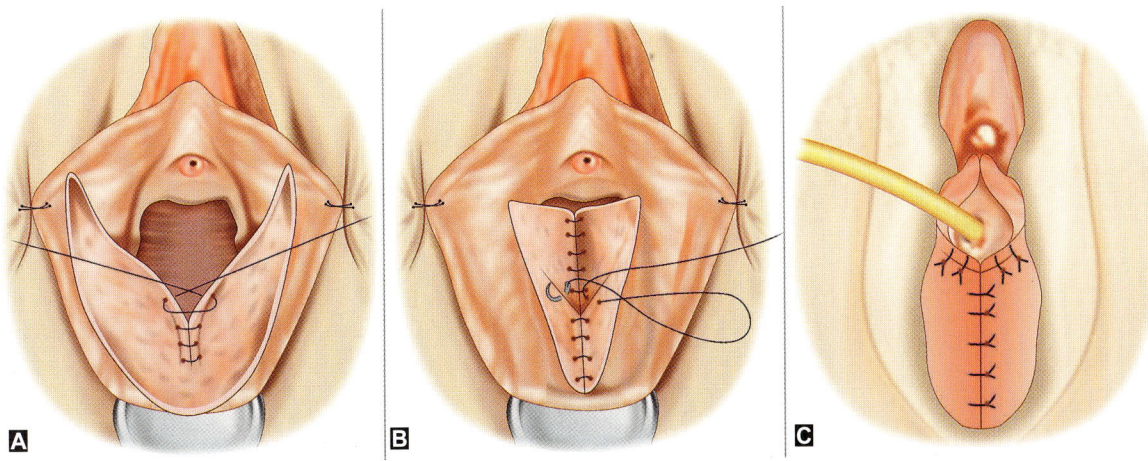

Figs. 40A to C: Williams' vaginoplasty (*see* text for description).

contraindications to alternative like adoption and surrogacy. She must be compliant to all advice and follow-up. She should have informed consent of all risks and benefit. Donor should be fulfilled some criteria regarding age, completion of child bearing and informed consent of the procedure.

Uterine transplantation is not a live shaving procedure like other transplantation, e.g., kidney and liver, etc. There are significant risks of recipient and there is alternate method like gestational surrogacy. Experienced surgeons with cardiothoracic expert in vascular surgery are mandatory. Uterine transplantation is a debatable issue. It is always under institution review and under purview of state law. THOTA rules (Transplantation of Human Organs and Tissue rules, 2014) under Ministry of Health and Family Welfare should be strictly followed.

Section 4

Birth Control and Population Demography

Section Outline

22. Family Planning and Contraception
23. Demography and Family Planning Programs in India—Present Scenario

CHAPTER 22

Family Planning and Contraception

Chapter Outline

- Combined Oral Contraceptives
- Progesterone Only—Oral Pill, Injectable, Subdermal Implants, Vaginal Ring
- Centchroman
- Transdermal Combined Patch
- Transvaginal Combined Ring
- Emergency Contraceptives
- Intrauterine Contraceptive Devices
- Postpartum Intrauterine Contraceptive Device
- Barrier Contraceptives—Male, and Female
- Fertility Awareness-based Methods
- Permanent Sterilization: Female—Tubal Ligation, Laparoscopic Ligation, Essure; Male—Vasectomy—Surgical Steps
- Male Contraceptives
- Birth Control Vaccine

COMMON VIVA QUESTIONS ON CONTRACEPTIVES

Questions on Combined Pill (Fig. 1)

For answers see Page 466 and onwards

- What is this?
  Combined oral contraceptive (COC) pill.
- What is the composition?
  Estrogen and progestogen.
- Which one is estrogen and which one is progestogen?
  Ethinyl estradiol is estrogen and other is progestogen (*see* the strip. It is written on strip).
- What are respective doses? How many tablets? Why different color?
- What is the mechanism of actions?
- When to start?
- What are noncontraceptive benefits?
- What are the noncontraceptive uses?
- What are the side effects?
- What is failure rate? How it is expressed? What is pearl formula?
  0.3/HWY (100 woman-years) in perfect users and 8/HWY in typical users.
- What are contraindications?
- What will be your advice in missing pill?

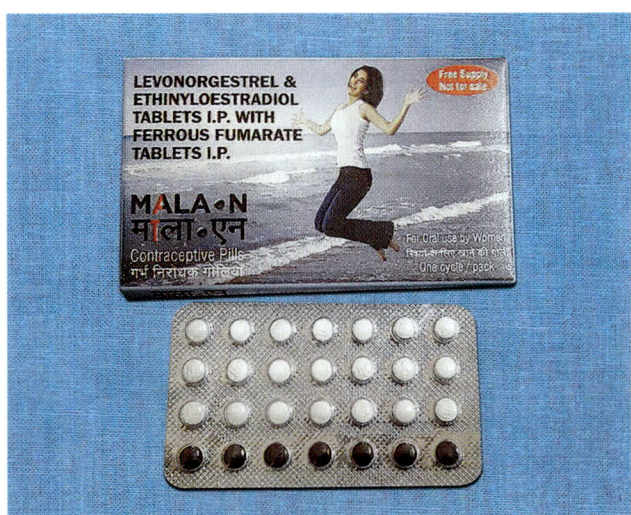

Fig. 1: Combined oral contraceptives.

Question on Intrauterine Contraceptive Device (IUCD) (Figs. 2 to 4)

For answers see Page 478 and onwards

❖ What is it?
Look whether CuT 380A or Multiload 375. If it is Multiload do not say Cu-T which is a common mistake.
❖ What is 380/375? What does A in 380A stand for?
❖ What is the mechanism of action?
❖ How many years it is used?
CuT 380A—10 years; Multiload 375—5 years, and Mirena 5 years.
❖ What are the advantages?
❖ What is failure rate?
Cu-intrauterine device (IUD) in perfect use—0.6 and in typical use 0.8/HWY and in levonorgestrel-intrauterine system (LNG-IUS) both are 0.2/HWY.
❖ Noncontraceptive uses of IUCD.
❖ How will you insert?
CuT 380A, Multiload 350 and Mirena.

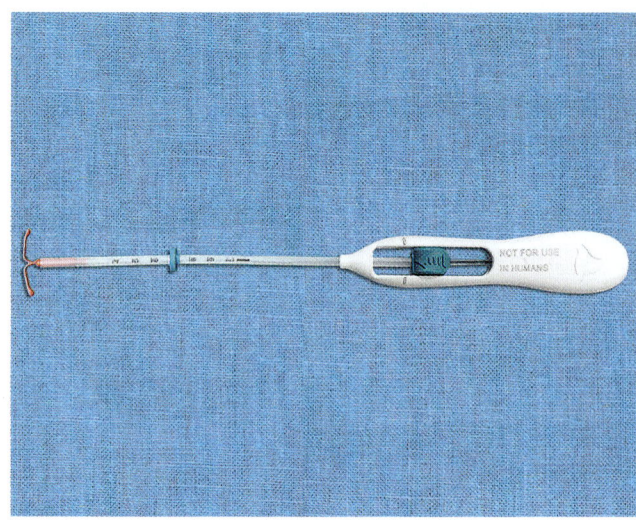

Fig. 4: Mirena with applicator.

❖ What are the complications and side effects?
❖ What are the causes of missing thread and what will you do?
❖ What will you do in perforation?
❖ What is your approach in pregnancy with IUCD in situ?
❖ What is the relation between IUD and ectopic pregnancy?
❖ What do you mean by postpartum intrauterine contraceptive device (PPIUCD)?

Question on Condom—Nirodh (Fig. 5)

For answers see Page 491 and onwards

❖ What is it? What type of contraceptive it is?
❖ Noncontraceptive benefits.
❖ What is the most important reason for promoting this method of contraception?
❖ What are the advantages?
❖ What are the disadvantages?
Failure rate in perfect use 2/HWY and in typical use it is 18/HWY.
❖ What are the noncontraceptive uses?

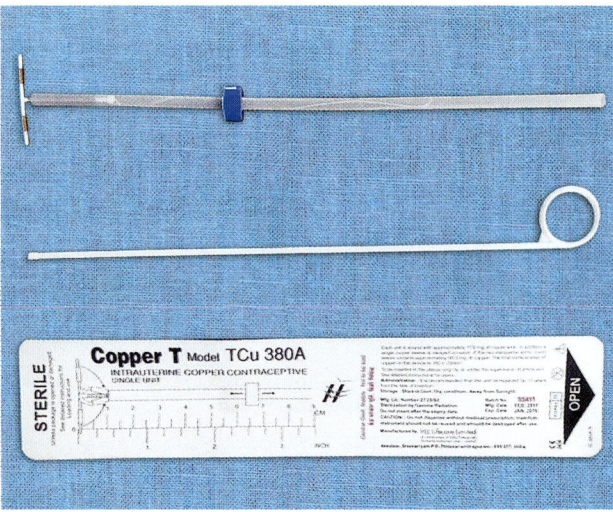

Fig. 2: CuT 380A with plunger and inserter tube.

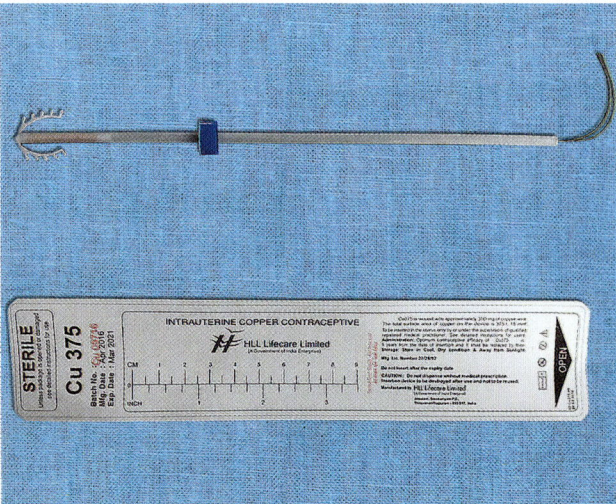

Fig. 3: Multiload 375 with inserter tube.

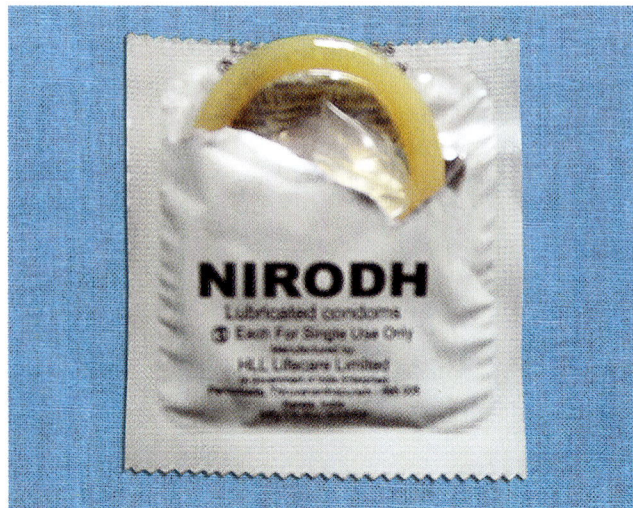

Fig. 5: Male condom.

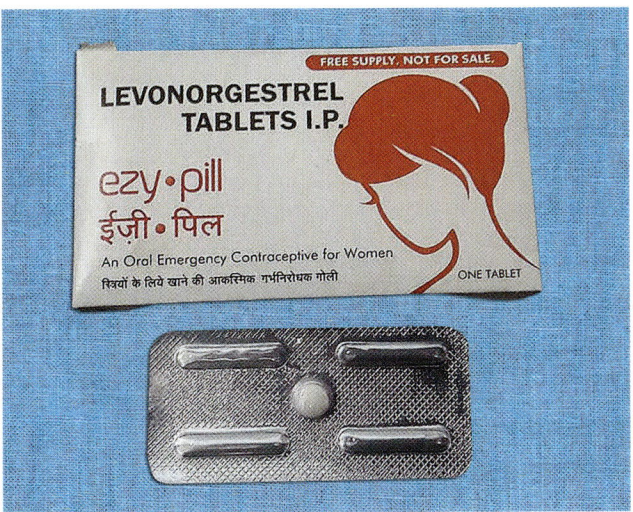

Fig. 6: Emergency contraceptive pill.

Question on Emergency Pill (Fig. 6)

For answers see Page 477 and onwards

- When you will advise to take?
- What is the composition?
- What are the other agents used as emergency contraceptive?
- Can you advise to use on regular basis?
- What are the side effects?

Question on Progestogen-only Pill (POP) (Fig. 7)

For answers see Page 471 and onwards

- What is the composition?
- In which case it is most suitable?
  Best for breastfeeding woman particularly for first 6 months when combined pill cannot be given.
- When will you start?
- How does it act (mechanism of action)?
- Situations where POP is indicated superior to COC?
- What are the other contraceptive methods that can be used in postpartum period and during lactation?

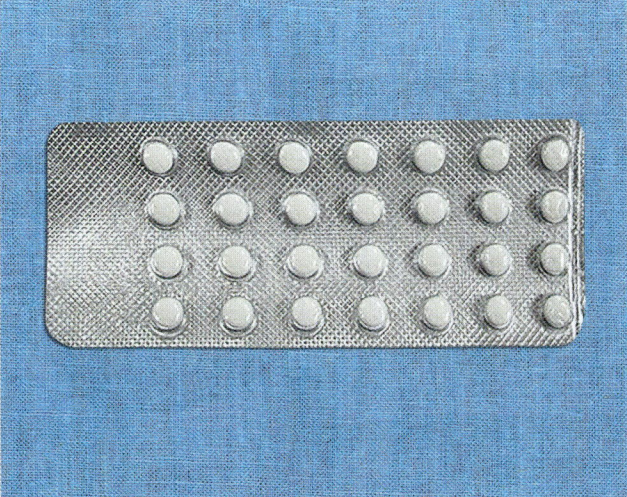

Fig. 7: Progesterone-only pill.

- What is failure rate?
  1–3/HWY
- Side effects.
- Contraindications.
- How will you advise in missing POP pill?

Q. What do you mean by contraception?

Contraception is a procedure to prevent conception as a consequence of intercourse. By contraception fertilization is prevented.

Q. What do you mean by birth control and family planning?

Birth control or family planning means limitation of pregnancy and family size by which population is controlled. Birth control or family planning involves not only contraception but also interception such as emergency contraception and induced abortion.

Emergency contraception prevents the implantation and is used after the act of coitus. Induced abortion [medical termination of pregnancy (MTP)] is a method in which continuation of pregnancy is prevented by removal of product of conception after implantation.

Q. What do you mean by fertility control?

Fertility control was used originally to mean fertility prevention, but now the term is broadly used which also includes fertility promotion.

HISTORY OF BIRTH CONTROL

History of fertility control dates back to 4000 years ago when a prescription was discovered written on an ancient Egyptian papyrus for local use of a paste containing ground acacia as contraception.

Using sheath to cover the penis during intercourse as barrier contraceptive is the oldest method of contraception. Condom is the most popular contraceptive used in the world. A physician Dr Condum is given credit for its invention and he recommended it to Charles II (1660–85) for prevention of illegal offspring. The term "Condom" was first appeared in printed form in 1717 and is also thought to be derived from the Latin word "condus" which means a receptacle.

The idea of intrauterine device came from the practice of using pebbles insertion inside the uteri of camels by Arabs and Turks while journeys through deserts for long distance to prevent pregnancy. Avicenna, an Islamic scientist is reported to use contraceptive intrauterine pessary first in humans in the 11th century.

It was Margarate Sanger, a nurse by profession who first dreamt about a "Magic Pill" in 1912 and started birth control movement in New York for which she was imprisoned but continued her movement. Dr Marie Stopes is another pioneer in the movement on contraception from England and published first book on contraception named "Married Love" in 1918.

Discovery of progestogens from the plant mexicans wild yam (diosgenin) by Russel Marker in 1941 is the important cornerstone in the history of hormonal birth control. Carl Djessary in 1951 first prepared the synthetic progesterone pill. Gregory Pincus in 1951 confirmed that progestogens worked as antiovulatory. First successful human trials were given by Pincus and John Rocks in 1954 among 50 patients. Rock, Gracia, and Pincus in 1956 first published that fertility control can be achieved by using norethynodrel (a progestational agent) by suppressing ovulation. Combining mestranol, an estrogenic agent with it was shown to improve efficacy and lessening breakthrough bleeding. *"Enovid" containing 10 mg noretynodrel and 0.15 mg mestranol is the first combined oral contraceptive (COC) pill and it was approved officially in USA in 1959.*

Estrogen was isolated first by Doisy in 1929 and ethinyl estradiol was synthesized in 1938. Progestin-only pill was released first in 1971.

CRITERIA OF AN IDEAL CONTRACEPTIVE

Q. What should be the criteria of an ideal contraceptive?

It should be:
- 100% effective
- Reversible
- No side effect or risk
- Cheap
- Easily available
- Highly acceptable
- Does not interfere sexual pleasure
- Intercourse independent and no regular action is needed by the user
- Should have noncontraceptive benefits.

In fact, in practice there is no ideal contraceptive. The goal is to make available a contraceptive which achieves the above criteria as near as possible.

CLASSIFICATION OF BIRTH CONTROL METHODS

Q. How will you classify birth control methods? Birth control methods are described in Table 1.

- Temporary (birth spacing methods)
- Permanent (birth limiting).

WHO TIER METHOD (GROUPS) CLASSIFICATION

Q. How contraceptive methods are grouped now? Tier system.

Now (by *WHO*), contraceptives are grouped according to the effectiveness and their failure rate [pregnancy per 100 woman-years (HWY)] are as follows from most effective (<1/HWY) to least effective (30/HWY) from first (top) tier to fourth tier.

Table 1: Birth control methods.

Broad categories of contraception	Methods of contraception
Temporary:	

• Natural methods (behavioral)	• Breastfeeding (lactational amenorrhea method)
	• Fertility awareness methods: Identification of fertile period and abstinence or using barrier method during fertile phase by:
	  – Calendar-based method
	  – Symptoms-based method
	  – Combined
	• Withdrawal method (coitus interruptus)

• Hormonal methods—regular contraceptives	• Estrogen progesterone combination • Only progesterone • Progesterone containing intrauterine device (IUD)
• Barrier methods or spermicidal gels	• Male condom • Female condom • Diaphragm and cervical cap • Spermicides: Creams, jellies, suppositories, aerosol foams, and vaginal contraceptive films • Contraceptive sponge—today
• Intrauterine contraceptive device	• Inert: Lippes loop (not used now in India) • Copper containing IUD • Progesterone containing IUD
• Emergency contraceptives	• Combined oral contraceptive pills • Progesterone only pill (0.75 mg levonorgestrel, 1.5 mg levonorgestrel) • Copper containing IUD • Antiprogestin: Mifepristone (RU486)
• Nonsteroidal oral contraceptive	• Selective progesterone receptor modulator (Ulipristal acetate) • Ormeloxifene (Centchroman)
Permanent • Female sterilization • Male sterilization	• Tubal ligation and essure • Vasectomy

- **Top tier** or **first tier** methods **(most effective)**—<2:
  - Implants
  - Intrauterine device (IUD)
  - Female sterilization
  - Male sterilization.
- **Second tier** methods **(very effective)**—3-9:
  - Injectables
  - Lactational amenorrhea methods (LAMs)
  - Pills
  - Patch
  - Vaginal ring.
- **Third tier** methods **(effective)**—10-20:
  - Male condoms
  - Diaphragm
  - Female condom
  - Fertility awareness methods.
- **Fourth tier** methods **(least effective)**—21-30:
  - Withdrawal
  - Spermicides.

EXPRESSION OF FAILURE RATE

Q. How would you express failure rate?

Pearl Rate or Index (1932)

- Rate of failure in terms of pregnancy per HWY of exposure.
- Failure rate = Number of accidental pregnancies ×1200/ total months of exposure.
- Failure rate is expressed as per HWY. A failure rate of 3/HWY means that if the couple uses that particular method of contraception for 1 year 3 women will become pregnant.
- Drawback of this method is that there can be resultant high failure rate in short-term user as there is no standard for duration of use. This is overcome by the life-table method.

Life Table Method (1962)

In this method, cumulative rates per 100 users to the end of n months used are derived (n = multiple of 12 corresponding to successive years of use). In this method, the continuation rate, number of users, rate of pregnancy, and side effects are expressed per 100 women users.

Failure rates of individual method in *perfect use* and typical use per HWY in first year of use have been shown in **Table 2**.

Q. What do you mean by GATHER?

It is a method of counseling which is known as "GATHER Approach" for Family Planning Counseling.

Counseling often has six elements, or steps. Each letter in the word *GATHER* stands for, as follows: G: Greet; A: Ask; T: Tell; H: Help; E: Explain; R: Return.

GATHER is a useful memory aid to help counselors or service providers to remember the basic steps in the counseling process and to add structure to a complex activity and to avoid leaving out important steps.

Table 2: Failure rates of individual method.

	With perfect use	With typical use
Combined oral contraceptive pill	0.3	8
Progesterone-only pill breastfeeding Non-breastfeeding	1–3 0.3 0.9	1 3–10
Centchroman	1–2	Not documented
Emergency pill	Only progestin—1/100 women EP—2/100 women Efficacy increases as soon earliest taken after coitus	
Depot medroxyprogesterone acetate	0.2	6
Implanon	0.05	0.05
Copper intrauterine device	0.6	0.8
Levonorgestrel-intrauterine system	0.2	0.2
Combined hormonal patch	0.3	9
Combined vaginal ring	0.3	9
Male condom	2	18
Female condom	5	21
Diaphragm	6	12
Female sterilization	0.5	
Vasectomy	0.1	
Fertility awareness method	0.4–5	25
Withdrawal	4	25

Hormonal Methods of Contraception

- *According to composition:*
  - Estrogen–progesterone combination
  - Only progesterone.
- *According to route of administration:*
  - Oral:
    - Hormonal: Combined oral contraceptives (COCs), progesterone-only pill, emergency contraceptive
    - Nonhormonal: Centchroman (ormeloxifene).
  - Injectable
  - Dermal implant
  - Transdermal patch
  - Transvaginal
  - Intrauterine.

Types of Combined Preparations (Estrogen and Progesterone)

- *Combined oral contraceptives:*
  - Monophasic
  - Biphasic
  - Triphasic
  - Quadriphasic
  - Extended pill
  - Shorter pill-free interval
- *Emergency contraceptive*
- *Monthly-combined injectable preparation*
- *Vaginal ring (Nuvaring)*
- *Transdermal patch.*

Types of Progesterone-only Preparation

- *Oral preparations:*
  - Progesterone-only pill
  - Emergency contraceptive.
- *Injectable:* Injection depot medroxyprogesterone acetate (DMPA) and norethisterone enanthate (NET-EN)
- *Implants:* Norplant, implanon, and nexplanon
- *Intrauterine device:* LNG-IUS
- *Vaginal rings—progering:* Used 3 monthly for lactating woman.

CLASSIFICATION OF STEROIDAL CONTRACEPTIVES

Q. Steroidal contraceptives—how will you classify?

Steroidal contraceptives can be categorized according to the **Flowchart 1**.

COMBINED ORAL CONTRACEPTIVES PILLS

Q. What are the other names?

Combined oral contraceptive pills are also named as COCs, oral contraceptives (OC), oral contraceptive pills (OCPs), and pill.

Q. What is the composition of COCs?

Its composition is estrogen and progestin.

Estrogen

- Ethinyl estradiol is used mostly
- Mestranol which is 3-methyl ether (not available in India) and
- Estradiol valerate—recently approved by Food and Drug Administration (FDA) (2010).

Progestin

Varieties of progestin are used—first generation, second generation, third generation, and also other newer progestogens.

[Progesterone is a natural substance produced by corpus luteum. Progestogens, progestins, gestagens, gestogens or progestational agents are synonyms whose actions are like natural progesterone, but they differ structurally. Progestogens used in clinical practice are broadly classified into two groups:

1. Progesterone and its derivatives in which the natural progesterone, dydrogesterone (stereoisomer of progesterone), and ester derivatives, etc. lie and mostly used for noncontraceptive purposes. Injectable contraceptive like DMPA only lies in this group.
2. Testosterone or 19-nortestosterone derivatives. Most of the contraceptives including NET-EN lie in this group. Replacement of methyl group by hydrogen atom in 19 position in testosterone yields nortestosterone. 19-nortestosterone derivatives exhibit primarily progestational activity rather than androgenic.]

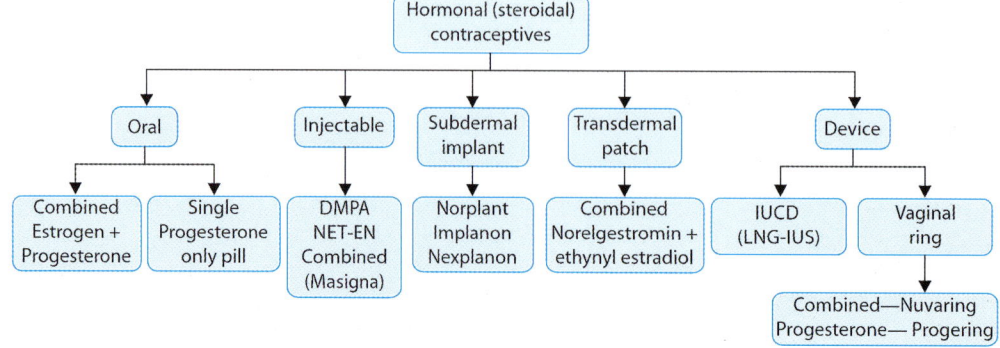

Flowchart 1: Steroidal contraceptives.

Q. What are the first generation progestins?

These are norethynodrel, norethindrone acetate, ethynodiol diacetate, and lynestrenol.

Q. What are the second generation progestins?

These are levonorgestrel and dl-norgestrel.

Q. What are the third and fourth generation progestins?

Third generation progestins are desogestrel, gestodene and norgestimate—more effective, lipid friendly, and less androgenic.

Fourth generation progestins are drospirenone, dienogest, nestorone, nomegestral acetate and trimegestone.

Other Newer Progestin

- *Drospirenone:* It is a spironolactone derivative, antimineralocorticoid, and antiandrogenic. Drospirenone is described as *fourth generation progestin*. And it is used in women with moderate acne vulgaris and premenstrual syndrome (premenstrual dystrophic disorder) requesting contraceptive. As theoretically, it is associated with potassium retention it should not be given in renal or adrenal insufficient patients and monitoring is needed.
- *Dienogest*—2 mg
- *Cyproterone acetate (CA):* The combined pill containing cyproterone acetate is primarily used for acne and hirsutism due to the antiandrogenic effect of CA.
- *Nomegestrol and nestorone* are pregnane group of progestogens.

Goal to Achieve a Best Hormonal Contraceptive—Changing Path

- Combining estrogen with progestin
- Changing types of estrogen and progestin:
    - Estrogen—ethinyl estradiol, mestranol, and estradiol valerate
    - Progestin—first, second, third, and newer generation.
- Minimizing the dose to reduce side effect but retaining the efficacy:
    - Estrogen: 50 µg → 35 µg → 30 µg → 20 µg → 15 µg (Minesse) → 10 µg
    - Progestins: Levonorgestrel 0.15 mg → 0.10 mg (Loette).
- Increasing the days of COCs at a stretch—to increase the duration from 20 days → 21 days → 24 days → 84 days (extended pill) to increase efficacy and to decrease the chance of dysphoria and dysmenorrhea due to delayed menstruation in long extended pill
- Administering the dose in phasic manner—monophasic → biphasic → triphasic → quadriphasic. Cochrane review does not see any benefit over monophasic
- Altering the rout of administration—nonoral delivery system by topical patch and vaginal ring which started the year 2000 onward.

Q. Concept of combined formulation of estrogen and progesterone—how and why?

Rock, Gracia, and Pincus in 1956 first published that fertility control can be achieved by using *norethynodrel (a progestational agent)* by suppressing ovulation. The initial progestin products were contaminated with 1% mestranol, an estrogenic agent. To get more pure progestin by lowering estrogen more break-through bleeding was observed. Combining mestranol with progestin was shown to lower break-through bleeding and to improve efficacy of contraception.

Every progestogen has estrogenic, antiestrogenic, and androgenic effects. The type of progesterone is such selected that they have more selective action of ovulation inhibition and lesser side effects. In fact the dose of progestin in COC is such low that none of the side effects are significantly manifested.

The daily dose of ethinyl estradiol in COC available now varies from 50–20 µg, majority 30 µg. The lowest acceptable dose is guided by ability to prevent break-through bleeding.

The lowest dose of EE *approved is* 10 µg *(FDA 2011).*

Reasons of lowering dose of estrogen: Thrombosis is more serious effect and dose related. Water retention, bloating, weight gain, breast engorgement, nausea and decreased libido become less with lowering of dose.

Types of Combined Pills

Various types of combined pills **(Table 3)** are as follows:

- *Monophasic pills:* These are commonly used. The dose of estrogen and progestin is constant throughout the cycle. They are packed either 21 days or for 28 days. In 28 days pack seven pills are either placebo or iron containing tablets making separate from hormone containing tablet. Most of the pills are monophasic.
- *Multiphasic pill: Biphasic and triphasic* pills are developed to lower the total amount of progesterone in the cycle to reduce side effects and the dose of progestin varies from one phase to other marked by different color, low dose in the beginning, and increasing the dose later to make more physiological. Triquilar is a triphasic pill available in India but not popular. *Quadriphasic pill containing estradiol valerate and dienogest (NATAZIA) is now approved in Europe.* The disadvantages of multiphasic pills are increase break-through bleeding and difficulty in intake due to different tablets in different days.
- *Estrophasic approach-(estrostep):* Combination of low dose progestin and gradually increasing the dose of estrogen. In early period there is less nausea and with increasing SHBG by increasing dose of oestrogen gradually there will be less free androgen and less acne.
- *Extended cycle oral preparation* (yet to be available in India): In every 3 months, 7 days are pill free. Out of 91 days, 84 days contain hormones (EE 30 µg and levonorgestrel 0.15 mg or EE 20 µg and levonorgestrel 0.10 mg) and 7 days placebo. Extended cycle formulation is becoming popular for high contraceptive efficacy and reduced incidence of menstrual related dysphoria and dysmenorrhea. Example is Seasonale. Seasonique

SECTION 4: Birth Control and Population Demography

Table 3: Types of combined pills.

According to changes of dose in different phases of cycle	Number of days at a stretch before pill free	According to change of types of progestin	According to type of estrogen	According to decreasing of dose of estrogen
Monophasic Biphasic Triphasic Quadriphasic	Commonly 21 days in a cycle with 7 hormone-free days	Levonorgestrel Desogestrel Gestodene Drosperidone	Ethinylestradiol is used in all pills now Mestranol and estradiol valerate are approved but pill containing the last two not available in India	Common dose of EE is 30 μg Low dose pill—ethinyl-estradiol-20 μg Currently 10 μg of EE is approved
	Shorter pill-free interval—24 days with 4 days hormone-free days			
	Extended cycle pill-continuous 84 days with 7 days hormone free			
	Even continuous 365 days without break is proposed			

contains 84 tablet of EE 30 μg and levonorgestrel 0.15 mg (*see* later).

* *Shorter pill-free gap:* Here 24 days hormone containing pill (example 20 μg EE and 3 mg drospirenone) with 4 days placebo instead of 7 days. The aim of 24/4 regimen is to increase the efficacy of very low-dose pills. Minesse and Yaz are two examples both available in India.

Questions on COC Pills

Q. What is this?

This is combined oral contraceptive pill.

Q. What is the composition?

Its composition is estrogen and progestogen.

Q. Which one is estrogen and which one is progestogen?

Ethinyl estradiol is estrogen and other is progestogen (written in strip).

Q. What are respective doses?

Mala N: Ethinyloestradiol 30 μg levonorgestrel 0.15 mg.

Available Formulations

See **Table 3**.

Q. Which phasic pill is commonly used?

Monophasic Pill

* 28 days pill pack—21 sequential color code tablet followed by 7 days inert tablet or iron containing tablets are commonly used (Mala N) **(Fig. 8)**, Or
* 21 days pill pack—to be taken 21 days continuously followed by 7 pill-free days (Ovral-L, Novelon and Femilan).

Mechanism of Actions

* *Central action:* It prevents *ovulation* by inhibiting gonadotropin-releasing factor which inhibits follicle-stimulating hormone (FSH) and luteinizing hormone

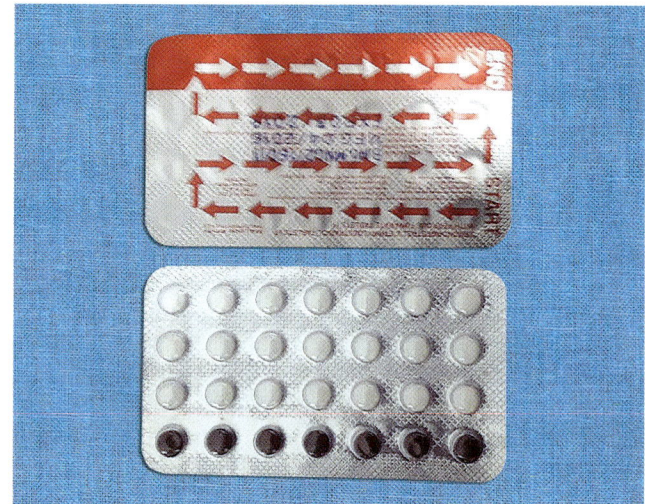

Fig. 8: Mala N—combined estrogen progesterone pill.

(LH) secretion. Both estrogen and progestogen inhibit FSH and LH.
* *Peripheral action:* Endometrium-progestogen prevents *implantation* by making endometrium atrophic and hostile.
* *Cervical mucus becomes hostile* for sperm penetration due to effect of progestogen.
* Tubal motility is reduced by the effect of progestogens thus hampering transfer of fertilized ova.

Q. When to start the pill in first cycle?

* *In normal nonpuerperal or non-postabortal women:*
  * It should be started ideally on first day of menstrual period and no additional protection is needed. This is commonly done.
  * It can be started any day within 5 days, no back up protection is needed.
  * Sunday start—started first Sunday after onset of menstruation.
  * Quick start—started immediately after getting prescription, at any day of period, pregnancy is excluded.

If on Sunday or quick start method, it is more than 5 days additional method or abstinence is needed for 1 week to prevent pregnancy.

- *In puerperal or postabortal women:*
  - **After delivery**: In breastfeeding mother, COC is started after 6 months of childbirth as it will affect lactation if started earlier. Progesterone—only pill or injection can be started earlier. In nonlactating women, COC should be started after 3 weeks of delivery. To avoid risk of thromboembolism, it is not started within 3 weeks.
  - **After MTP or abortion**: It is started within 7 days after evacuation.

Q. How to take?

- *In 28 days strip (Mala N commonly used/Government supply):* The color tablet (hormone containing) is started on first day of period and continued for 21 days followed by 7 days nonhormonal tablet. From next day another pack is started so that there is no tablet-free day. Patient is getting 21 days hormone containing tablet and 7 days placebo or iron containing tablet. Women will experience mens in any of the days of hormone-free period.
- *In 21 days pack (Ovral-L, Novelon/Femilon):* It is started on first day of mens and continued for 21 days. There will be tablet-free days for 7 days during which mens (with bleeding) occurs and next strip started after 7 days irrespective of day of menstruation.

Key instruction: One pill each day till pack is finished. To take same time each day—it will help to remember and also reduces side effect. Linking pill intake time with any regular activity like teeth cleaning, etc.

NONCONTRACEPTIVE BENEFITS OF COMBINED ORAL PILLS

Q. What are the noncontraceptive benefits of combined oral pills?

- Menstrual bleeding becomes less and anemia is improved
- Menstrual cycle becomes regular
- Premenstrual symptoms become less
- Reduces dysmenorrhea—both primary and secondary
- Reduces pelvic inflammatory disease (PID)—by preventing spread of bacteria from cervix, reduces intensity of acute salpingitis
- Reduces ectopic pregnancy
- Hirsutism and acne improved
- Using in premenopausal age vasomotor symptoms decreased
- Rheumatoid arthritis progress less
- Bone mineral density (BMD) is increased
- Reduces benign breast disease
- Reduces development of new ovarian cyst, neoplasia
- Reduces endometrial carcinoma to half—one-tenth, reduces ovarian carcinoma and colorectal cancer.

NONCONTRACEPTIVE USES OF COCs

Q. What are the noncontraceptive uses of COCs?

- Dysfunctional uterine bleeding
- Endometriosis
- Dysmenorrhea
- Polycystic ovary syndrome
- Hirsutism and acne
- Hypothalamic amenorrhea
- Hormone replacement therapy in primary hypogonadism.

Benefits of COCs in Comparison to Other Contraceptives

- Failure rate is low: 0.3/HWY in perfect users and 8/HWY in typical users
- No privacy is needed
- No hindrance in sexual pleasure
- Free of cost by Government or reasonable cost
- There are several noncontraceptive benefits
- Can be used for noncontraceptive purposes.

Q. What are the side effects of COC pill?

Major adverse effects are less, mainly minor side effects.

Minor Side Effects—Common

- *Gastrointestinal system:* Nausea and vomiting
- *Genital system:* Excessive white discharge, vulvovaginitis, cervical mucorrhea and eversion of cervix
- *Bleeding abnormalities:* Break-through bleeding, spotting, scanty period, and amenorrhea
- *General:* Increase weight gain—fluid retention, facial pigmentation (chloasma)
- *Breast changes:* Mastalgia, enlarged breasts
- *Central nervous system:* Headache or dizziness, mood swings, depression, and loss of libido.

Major Side Effects—Less

- Thromboembolism: 3–5 times due to estrogen
- Myocardial infarction: Especially who smoke and hypertensive
- Stroke
- Hypertension: 1% among COC users
- Gallbladder disease.

Neoplastic Disease

Reports of neoplastic changes and COC use are conflicting.

- Breast cancer in current users—not significant. Age more than 40 with family history—chance is higher. However relation of COCs and breast tumorogenesis is inconclusive.
- Cervical dysplasia and cancer rates are increased and related with duration. However, this is more speculative. More frequent human papilloma virus (HPV) exposure due to less use of barrier contraceptive may be the reasons.

Postpill Amenorrhoea

See Chapter of secondary amenorrhoea.

MEDICAL ELIGIBILITY CRITERIA (MEC) WHEEL FOR CONTRACEPTIVE USE

Q. What are the contraindications of oral contraceptives?

Government of India has published *medical eligibility criteria (MEC) wheel for contraceptive use 2015 based on WHO criteria*; the details of MEC are given in **Table 4**.

Some Important Contraindications

Absolute Contraindications of Combined Oral Pills (Category 4)

- Active liver disease and recent history of jaundice
- Liver cirrhosis, adenoma or carcinoma
- History of current thrombophlebitis or thrombotic, embolic disorder, myocardial infraction, stroke–thromboembolic disorder is increased 3–5 fold in COCs.
- Uncontrolled hypertension
- Diabetes with vascular complications
- Migraine aura (with focal neurological deficit)
- Woman aged above 35 years who smokes
- Carcinoma breast (known or suspected)
- Endometrial cancer
- Undiagnosed vaginal bleeding
- Complicated valvular disease
- Breastfeeding within 6 months
- Postoperative prolonged immobilization

Table 4: Category of WHO Medical Eligibility Criteria (MEC) of any contraceptive.

Category	Criteria	Use clinical judgment	Limited clinical judgment
1	No restriction for use	Can be used in any circumstances	Yes
2	Advantages outweigh the theoretical or proven risks	Generally the method can be used	Yes
3	Theoretical or proven risks out weight the advantages	Not usually recommended unless more appropriate methods are available or not acceptable	No
4	Unacceptable health risk	Methods not be used	No

The examples of MEC for combined oral contraceptives are Category 1—uterine fibroid, benign breast disease; Category 2—high body mass index; Category 3—within 6 months of breastfeeding women; at drugs intake; Category 4—history of thromboembolic phenomenon, severe hypertension.

Relative Contraindications (Category 2/3)

- Allergy
- Controlled hypertension (within 140/90 mm Hg)
- Asymptomatic gallbladder disease
- Jaundice with pill use
- Diabetes
- Women taking AT (antitubercular) drugs like rifampicin and anticonvulsive drug
- Body mass index (BMI) above 30 kg/m^2
- Most of the contraindications are related to effect of sex steroid over cardiovascular and hepatobiliary systems
- Before planning of pelvic or leg surgery COC should be stopped 2 months prior surgery
- Age (no age is contraindicated including adolescent and above 40 years, irrespective of marital status and irrespective of parity OCP can be used).

Q. What preliminaries you will do before prescribing a pill?

Nearly all women can use COCs safely and effectively except where there is contraindication (as above).

What is done only to fulfil *the medical eligibility criteria* to find the contraindications.

These can be done mostly by questionnaire (history taking) and minimal examination (baseline blood pressure measurement-not mandatory) and no laboratory investigations.

Breasts examination, pelvic examination, routine blood or other routine tests, and cervical cancer screening can be done but not mandatory (WHO 2011). However, pregnancy is always excluded.

Questionnaire (history taking) before COCs advice:
Pregnancy status, breastfeeding, smoking, liver disease, hypertension, diabetes, gallbladder disease, breast cancer, seizure disorder, migraine, abnormal uterine, history of stroke, personal and family history of thromboembolism, planning for any surgery, and risk factors for heart disease.

Drug Interaction

The COCs may interfere with the action of some drugs and on the contrary some drugs reduce the efficacy of COCs.

Barbiturates, carbamazepine, phenytoin, primidone, topiramate, rifampicin and anticonvulsants increase oral contraceptive metabolism and efficacy of COC decreased and higher doses containing 50 µg may be needed. Some broad-spectrum antibiotics hamper intestinal absorption, hence additional protection is needed.

MISSING PILL

Q. What will you do in missing pill?

Management depends how many pill missed and in which period of cycle it is missed **(Table 5)**.

CHAPTER 22: Family Planning and Contraception

Table 5: Management of missing pill.	
Missing pills	Advice
Missed 1 or 2 pills	• One pill to be taken as soon as possible or two pills at schedule time • Little or no risk of pregnancy
Started new pack 1 or 2 days late	• Advice same as above
Missed 3 pills or more in first week or second week or started new pack 3 or more days late	• One hormonal pill is taken as soon as possible and continue the schedule pill • Use backup method or abstinence for next 7 days • If she had sex in past 72 hours consider to take also emergency pill
Missed 3 or more pills in the third week	• One hormonal pill is taken as soon as possible and all hormonal pills in the pack are finished as scheduled. 7 nonhormonal pills in a 28 day pill pack are to be discarded • A new pack is started next day • Use backup method or abstinence for next 7 days • If she had sex in past 72 hours consider to take also emergency pill
Any nonhormonal pill missing (last 7 days of 28 days pack)	Missed nonhormonal pill or pills discarded. Continue to take tablet as usual and new pack is started on schedule day
Severe vomiting or diarrhea	When there is vomiting within 2 hours after taking pill another pill to be taken as soon as possible and rest of the schedule pills are continued as usual

Q. How many years COCs can be continued?

❖ The OCPs can be continued up to established menopause or up to 51 years which one is later if no indication for withdrawal develops.
❖ For birth spacing 3–5 years.

Q. How to follow-up in a case of COC pill user?

First follow-up after 3 months, then after 6 months, and then yearly. If the women is above 35 years of age followedup more frequently. To report at any time if there is any problem.

Components of each follow-up visit: Any adverse complaints, weight change, BP examination, breasts examination, and pelvic examination and Pap smear.

Q. What are the indications of stoppage of pill?

Majority of women can tolerate the COC pill well, but only a few cannot tolerate well for which it should be stopped. Or patient desires pregnancy planning or going for surgery.

The indications of stoppage of pill are:

❖ Desires pregnancy planning
❖ Going for surgery (before 2 months)
❖ Sudden chest pain
❖ Calf pain or recurrent cramps
❖ Severe migraine and loss of vision
❖ Sudden respiratory distress
❖ Excessive weight gain
❖ Fainting attack or repeated vertigo
❖ Uncontrolled BP more than 160/100 mm Hg
❖ Severe depression
❖ Unexplained convulsion
❖ Liver disease—jaundice and hepatitis
❖ Prolong immobilization for any disease or orthopedic problem or surgery.

Q. What is your opinion regarding selection of pills?

❖ Combined oral contraceptive containing 30 µg ethinylestradiol and levonorgestrel or norethisterone is still the pill of choice universally.
❖ For efficacy 20 µg ethinyl estradiol and desogestrel/gestodene is best but break-through bleeding is slightly more in 20 µg EE than 30 µg EE and venous thromboembolism (VTE) is more in desogestrel or gestodene than levonorgestrel or norethisterone.
❖ In presence of acne vulgaris and premenstrual syndrome drospirenone containing pill is the choice but as it causes potassium retention monitoring is needed and in drospirenone there is slightly higher risk of VTE than second generation.
❖ There is no extra-benefit of biphasic and triphasic pill over monophasic (Cochrane review).

Q. Which one is the lowest estrogen-containing pill available now in India?

Minesse—contains ethinyl estradiol 15 µg and gestodene 0.060 mg of 24 tablets + 4 days placebo.

Q. Which one is the lowest progesterone-containing pill available now in India?

Loette: Ethinyl estradiol 20 µg and levonorgestrel 10 mg, estrogen also less—21 days duration.

Q. Name the 24 days containing pill (with 4 days placebo) which are available in India.

❖ *Yaz:* containing ethinyl estradiol 20 µg and drospirenone 3 mg for 24 days 4 days placebo
❖ *Minesse:* Ethinyl estradiol 15 µg and gestodene 0.060 mg of 24 tablets + 4 days placebo.

Q. Name the pill containing gestodene.

Minesse, Femovan

SECTION 4: Birth Control and Population Demography

Q. Name the pill containing drosperinone.

Yasmin, Doris, Yaz

Q. Name the extended pill.

Seasonale containing ethinyl estradiol 30 μg levonorgestrel 0.15 mg 84 days + 7 days placebo (91 days pack).

Extended pill is still not available in India **(Fig. 9)**.

Seasonique 7 pills 10 μg of ethinyl estradiol after 84 days active pills like seasonale.

Q. Advantages of extended regimen.

Extended regimen (a) reduces break through bleeding, (b) reduces the total length of withdrawal bleeding, (c) reduces ovarian activity, thus less failure of contraception and due to long period and amenorrhea dysmenorrhea, headache and bloating become less.

Q. Name the pill which contains natural estrogen.

1. Zoely: It is comprised of nomegestrol acetate (pregnane group of progestogen—2.5 mg) and estradiol valerate (natural estrogen 1.5 mg) with a strip of 28 tablets containing 24 white tablets and 4 yellow placebo tablets.

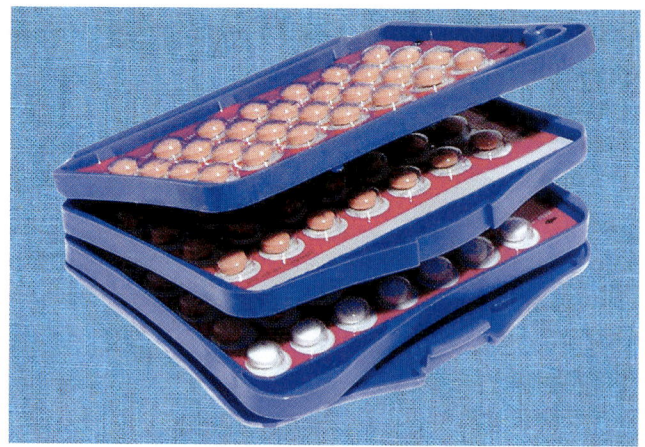

Fig. 9: Extended pill 84 + 7.

2. Natazia: Estradiol valerate + dienogest —28 pills—multiphasic.

Various Types of Oral Pill or Steroid Contraceptives.

Various types of oral pill or steroid contraceptives have been listed in **Table 6**.

Route	Market name	No. of tablets	Estrogen	Progestogens
Oral monophasic	Mala N (Government supply)	21 + 7 iron tablets	Ethinyl estradiol 30 μg	Levonorgestrel 0.15 mg
	Ovral-28	21 + 7 iron tablets	Ethinyl estradiol 30 μg	Levonorgestrel 0.15 mg
	Mala-D	21 + 7 iron tablets	Ethinyl estradiol 30 μg	Levonorgestrel 0.15 mg
	Ovral-L*	21 tablets + 7 days gap	Ethinyl estradiol 30 μg	Levonorgestrel 0.15 mg
	Novelan/ Ovuloc	21 tablets	Ethinyl estradiol 30 μg	Desogestrel 0.15 mg
	Femilon/ Ovuloc LD	21 tablets	Ethinyl estradiol 20 μg	Desogestrel 0.15 mg
	Femovan	21 tablets	Ethinyl estradiol 30 μg	Gestodene 0.075 mg
	Minesse	24 tablets + 4 days placebo	Ethinyl estradiol 15 μg	Gestodene 0.060 mg
	Yasmin	21 tablets	Ethinyl estradiol 30 μg	Drospirenone 3 mg
	Doris	21 tablets	Ethinyl estradiol 30 μg	Drospirenone 3 mg
	Yaz	24 tablets + 4 days placebo	Ethinyl estradiol 20 μg	Drospirenone 3 mg
	Freedase	21 tablets	Ethinyl estradiol 30 μg	Dienogest 2 mg
	30 Loette	21 tablets	Ethinyl estradiol 20 μg	Levonorgestrel 10 mg
Oral triphasic	Triquilar	21 tablets	Ethinyl estradiol 30 μg Ethinyl estradiol 40 μg Ethinyl estradiol 30 μg	Levonorgestrel 50 μg (1–6 days) Levonorgestrel 75 μg (7–11 days) Levonorgestrel 125 μg (12–21 days)
Progesterone only pill	Cerazette	28 tablets	No estrogen	Desogestrel 75 μg
Emergency pill	Ezy pill (Government of India)	1 tablet	No estrogen	Levonorgestrel 1.5 mg
Injectable	Antara (Government supply) Safe-3	1 mill vial deep intramuscularly every 3 monthly	No estrogen	Medroxyprogesterone acetate 150 mg/mL
Intrauterine system	Mirena Emily (HLL)	5 years	No estrogen	52 mg levonorgestrel
Vaginal ring	Nuvaring	21 days single use	Etonogestrel (11.7 mg)	Ethinyl estradiol (2.7 mg)

*Ovral G which contains ethinyl estradiol 50 μg and norgestrel 500 μg is available in 20 tablets strip and is not used as contraceptive but used in conditions like abnormal uterine bleeding.

Contraceptives Available at Present through Government of India

- Combined pill: *Mala N*
- Emergency pill: *ezy-pill* containing levonorgestrel 1.5 mg
- Intrauterine device: Cu-T 380A for 10 years and Multiload Cu-375 for 5 years
- Injectable: Injection DMPA intramuscular—*Antara*
- Male condom: *Nirodh*
- Nonhormonal nonsteroidal oral contraceptives centchroman (ormeloxifene) in the name of *Chhaya*.

Mala N, ezy-pill, Nirodh and Chhaya each distributed in two different packs—one type of pack is distributed directly from Government facility which is free of cost and other type of pack distributed by Asha with a nominal cost.

PROGESTERONE-ONLY PILL

It is also called "mini pill".

Composition

Progesterone-only pill contains very low dose of synthetic progestin either levonorgestrel or desogestrel and no estrogen. POP was first released in 1971.

The available preparation is *cerazette* which contains desogestrel—each tablet is of 75 µg. Each pack contains 28 tablets of same color.

The other preparations are: Norethisterone 350 µg (Micronor, Noriday), Levonorgestrel 30 µg (Norgeston, Microval), Lynestrenol 500 (Mini-kare).

Mechanism of Action

- The POP makes the cervical mucus thick and prevents entry of sperm and prevents implantation by changing endometrium.
- It also inhibits ovulation, but antiovulatory effect is not reliable like estrogen–progesterone combination. Desogestrel inhibits ovulation 95% cases and levonorgestrel only in 50–60% cases. The higher dose progestogen only methods act centrally and inhibit ovulation well to make highly effective.

Situations where POP is Indicated Superior to COC

- *Best for breastfeeding woman particularly for first 6 months* as it does not affect milk production when COCs should not be given. Breastfeeding and POP combinedly 100% effective for up to 6 months.
- In old age, it is safe.
- The POPs do not cause or increase hypertension and ideal for women who have cardiovascular disease risk factors like hypertension, diabetes, history of thrombosis, migraine aura, and women above 35 years who smoke.
- Cerebrovascular disease.
- Systemic lupus erythematosus with nephritis and vascular disease.
- Ideal where estrogen is contraindicated.

Advantages of POP

- In many situations, estrogen cannot be given
- Fertility returns immediately after stoppage of pill.

Q. How to take and when to start?

One pill to be taken every day at the same time and to be taken continuously. As the mucous changes do not persist for more than 24 hours, pill should be taken at the same time of the day. Even if a pill is taken 4 hours late additional protection is needed for next 48 hours.

Can start POP at any time if pregnancy is excluded. Depending on situation starting is depicted in **Table 7**.

Table 7: Timing for starting progesterone-only pill.

Lactating mother	
Within 6 months after giving birth	Can be started at any time if menstruation has not returned. No backup method is needed
More than 6 months after giving birth	If menstruation is not returned it can also be given at any time provided pregnancy is excluded and a backup method like condom or abstinence is needed for first 2 days of taking pill
Nonlactating puerperal mother women	
Within 4 weeks of delivery	Can be started any time, no backup method is needed
After 4 weeks of birth	If menstruation is not returned it can also be given at any time provided pregnancy is excluded and a backup method like condom is needed for first 2 days of taking pill
If menstruation is resumed, progesterone-only pills (POPs) can be started as menstruating women written below
Women with normal menstrual cycles (nonpuerperal)	
Couple not using any method	Starting within 5 days of menstrual cycle no additional protection is needed provided pregnancy is excluded. A backup method like condom or abstinence is needed for first 2 days of taking pill if started after 5 days
If pregnancy is not ascertained POPs should be started during next menstruation and to use condoms till that period
Immediately, if switching from an intrauterine contraceptive device
If switching from other method	POP should be started immediately if the other method was taken correctly and there is no pregnancy. Backup is not needed
Following abortion or miscarriage	Immediately, no backup if started within 7 days
After 7 days can be started on any day after exclusion of pregnancy, backup with condom for 2 days

Q. Missing progesterone-only pill—how you will advise?

Advice for missed progesterone-only pill is described in **Table 8**.

Table 8: Management of missed progesterone-only pill.	
3 or >3 hours delay in taking pill or missed one pill (12 or more hours late taking a POP containing desogestrel 75 µg) or	A pill is taken at earliest and continue as usual Two pills may be taken on next day same time
In menstruating woman	A backup method is used for next 2 days Consider emergency contraceptive pills if she has intercourse last 72 hours
In severe vomiting or diarrhea	If within 2 hours another pill is taken as soon as possible and continue as usual

Side Effects

- Nausea
- Bleeding irregularities
- Headaches
- Dizziness
- Mood swing
- Breast tenderness.

Disadvantages

- Irregular vaginal bleeding—amenorrhea (25% cases), irregular bleeding, frequent bleeding, and prolonged heavy menstrual bleeding is more
- Functional ovarian cyst develops more.

Failure Rate

- More failure rate than COCs—1 to 3/HWY. If taken every day at the same time failure rate is less –0.3/HWY
- Compliance of on time taken is very important to avoid failure
- In case of failure chance of ectopic is more
- No protection against sexually transmitted diseases.

Contraindication

Contraindications include breast cancer, unexplained vaginal bleeding, liver tumor, and active severe liver disease.

CENTCHROMAN (FIG. 10)

Centchroman (ormeloxifene) is a nonsteroidal and nonhormonal once a week OCP. It contains ormeloxifene which is developed by Central Drug Research Institute, Lucknow, India. It was known as "Saheli". It is supplied by Government of India in a pack of OCP containing 8 tablets in the name of "*Chhaya*" recently. Centchroman can also be used as an emergency contraceptive.

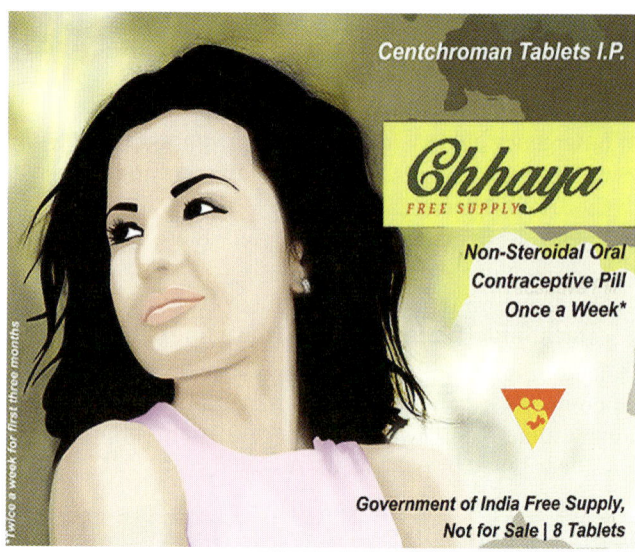

Fig. 10: Chhaya.
Centchroman nonsteroidal–nonhormonal tablet, 8 tablets, each tablet 30 mg

Composition and Schedule of Intake

One tablet contains 30 mg ormeloxifene. One pill is taken orally twice a week for first 3 months, followed by once weekly thereafter. First pill is started from first day of period and second pill after 3 days.

Mechanism of Action

It works by preventing implantation. It has no antiovulatory effect. It acts as selective estrogen receptor modulator. In some body tissues like bones it has weak estrogenic action and in some tissues like breasts and uterus it has strong antiestrogenic action.

Side Effects

- It is relatively safe
- Delayed period in few women
- No significant side effect.

Contraindication

Contraindicated in liver disease and renal disorder.

Pregnancy Failure

It is an effective contraceptive. With perfect use 1–2/HWY.

INJECTABLE CONTRACEPTIVES (FIG. 11)

Q. What are the different types of injectable contraceptives?

- **Two types:** (1) Only progesterone, and (2) combined—estrogen and progesterone
- Combined injectable contraceptives are not available in India (written later, *see* Page 474).

CHAPTER 22: Family Planning and Contraception

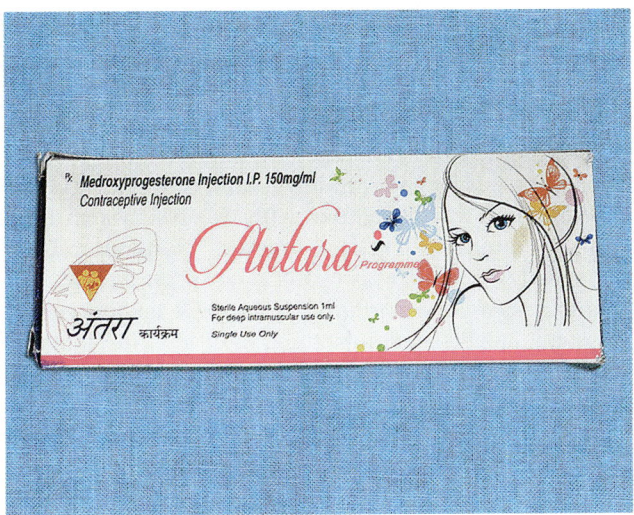

Fig. 11: Antara.
Injection DMPA 150 mg for intramuscular (India Government supply)

Progesterone-only Injectable Contraceptive

Types and Formulation

Progesterone only injectable—three depot preparations are used worldwide.
1. **Depo-provera:** Injection DMPA containing 150 mg in 1 mL vial for intramuscular injection every 3 months (Antara **Fig. 11**).
2. **Depo-subQ provera** which is a derivative of DMPA containing 104 mg dose (equivalent to 150 mg DMPA intramuscular) for subcutaneous use for every 3 months. **Sayana-press,** medroxy progesterone acetate 104 mg for subcutaneous injection every three months is available in India **(Fig. 11A)**.
3. Injection norethindrone enanthate 200 mg marketed as Norgest/Noristerat for 2 monthly intramuscular injection. It is commonly called norethisterone enanthate *(NET-EN)*. Among the three only DMPA is available in India. Recently, Government of India has made available injection

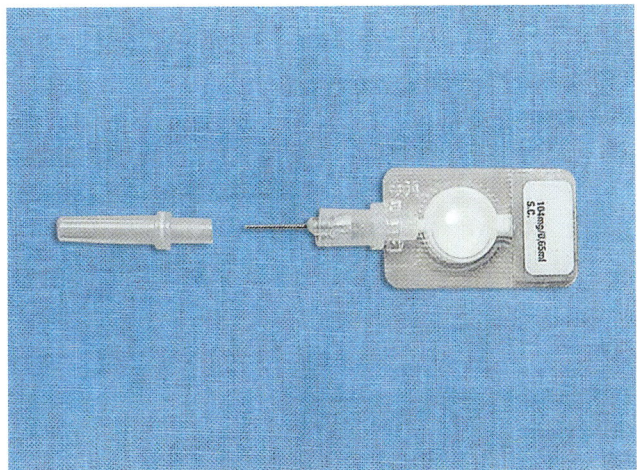

Fig. 11A: Sayana-press.

DMPA in the National Family Planning Programme in the name of *"Antara"* for intramuscular use **(Fig. 11)**.

Mode and Site of Injection (Antara)

Site is upper arm (deltoid muscle), buttocks (gluteal muscle, upper outer portion) or thigh (outer anterior) and is given deep intramuscular. The site should not be massaged after administration.

Mechanism of Action of DMPA

Like progesterone-only pill by: (A) changes of cervical mucosa, (B) ovulation inhibition, and (C) making endometrium unreceptive.

Efficacy or Failure Rate

Equivalent to or better than COCs. Failure rate is 0.2% in perfect use and 6% in typical use.

Q. When and how to start?

Contraindications are ascertained on questionnaire. Routine examination and laboratory investigations are not needed.
* In lactating mother (fully or near fully)—to start after 6 weeks of birth.
* In nonlactating puerpera—to start after 3 weeks or can be started immediately.
* In menstruating woman—within 7 days of menstrual cycle, no additional protection is needed. If started after 7 days a backup method or abstinence is needed for 7 days.

Q. How to follow-up?

Patient is asked to come at the time of next injection. She is asked for any complaints and blood pressure is checked. Next dose is given as per schedule —DMPA, after 3 months; NET EN, after 2 months. Next dose if delayed up to 4 weeks there is no need for additional contraceptive.

Advantages

* Estrogenic side effects are avoided
* Does not suppress lactation
* Anemia is improved as less blood loss
* As only progesterone, it is relatively less effect on lipid metabolism, blood sugar level, hemostatic function, thyroid function, liver function, and blood pressure
* Chance of thromboembolism, cerebrovascular disease, and stroke are less as there is no estrogen
* Endometrial and ovarian cancer risk diminished.

Q. Who are suitable for progesterone only injectives?

All women can use except who have contraindications and also the women who forget to take daily pill. Counseling regarding bleeding pattern and delayed fertility return increase the acceptance.

Disadvantages and Side Effects

* Irregular bleeding—irregular and continuous bleeding occurs for first 3 months. Later woman becomes amenorrheic and irregular infrequent bleeding—she

should be counseled about this. In irregular bleeding mefenamic acid has good help.
- Return of fertility after withdrawal takes a long time even up to 1 year.
- Bone mineral density is decreased due to hypoestrogenemia; it should be used cautiously for adolescent and perimenopausal women. However bone density recovers after stoppage. Hence on this ground-its use is not limited (American College of Obstetricians and Gynecologists 2014).
- Carcinoma in situ increased but no cancer cervix or liver neoplasm.
- Others side effects—weight gain 2–3 kg in first year, breast tenderness, and mood changes.

Hence, most important side effects are irregular bleeding, amenorrhea, and delayed return of fertility.

Q. What are the noncontraceptive benefits of DMPA?
- Improves anemia
- Improvement of endometriosis and its symptoms—pain and bleeding
- Prevents PID
- Dysmenorrhea becomes less
- Protects endometrial cancer.

Cancer and Progesterone-only Contraceptives
- Carcinoma in situ increased but no increase of cancer cervix or liver neoplasm.
- Endometrial and ovarian cancer risk diminished.

Contraindications of Injectable Contraceptives
- Unexplained vaginal bleeding
- Pregnancy
- Breast cancer
- History of active thromboembolism
- Significant liver disease
- Cerebrovascular disease—stroke
- Severe hypertension
- Ischemic heart disease
- Diabetic vasculopathy or >20 years.

Combined Injectable Preparations
1. Medroxyprogesterone acetate (25 mg) and estradiol cypionate (5 mg) marketed as **Cyclofem** and
2. Norethisterone enanthate (50 mg) and estradiol valerate (5 mg) marketed as **Masigna**. They are given 28 days interval intramuscularly.
   These are not available in India.

SUBDERMAL IMPLANTS (FIGS. 12 TO 17)

Q. What is implant?

It is a progestin containing device inserted subdermally into the upper arm under local anesthesia and it releases hormone for many years.

Till now implant is not available in India for general use.

Device and Varieties Generated

The system is coated with a polymer to prevent fibrosis. The varieties of implants are as follows:

- *Norplant system:* In *Norplant I,* there were *six* silastic rods **(Fig. 12)** which release levonorgestrel and effective for 5 years. Now it is withdrawn from USA market. Later *Norplant II* was developed with two-rod system **(Fig. 13)** containing 75 mg levonorgestrel. Norplant rod was inserted subcutaneously by trocar and cannula **(Fig. 14)**.
- *Jadelle and Sino-implant II: Two-rod* levonorgestrel system. Jadelle is manufactured in China. Norplant and Jadelle are radiopaque. Jadelle and Sino-implant are licensed for 5 and 4 years, respectively.
- *Implanon (Fig. 15):* Single-rod subdermal implant containing etonogestrel and releases 25–70 µg etonogestrel daily which decreases with time. This is metabolized to desogestrel and becomes effective for 3 years. It can be easily removed and another device can be implanted. Implanon is not radiopaque and in difficult removal help of ultrasound is needed.

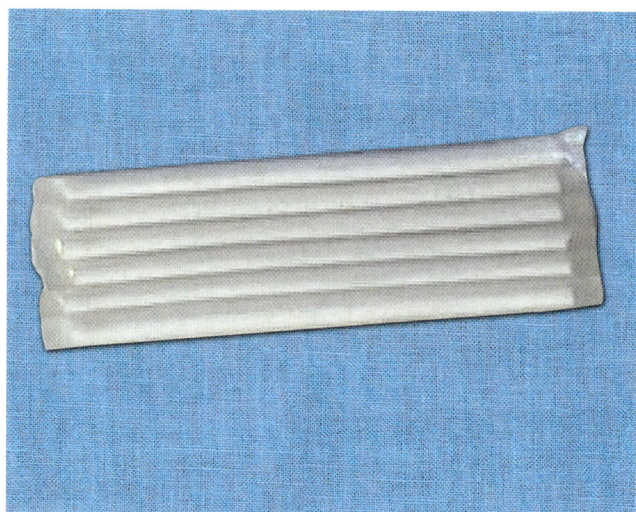

Fig. 12: Norplant 6 rods.

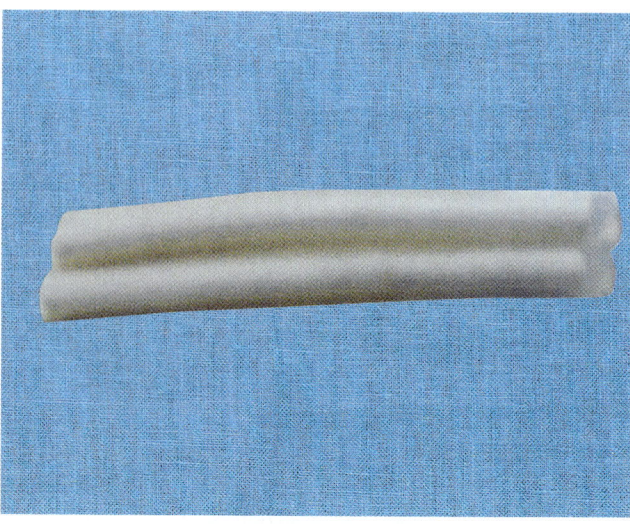

Fig. 13: Norplant 2 rods.

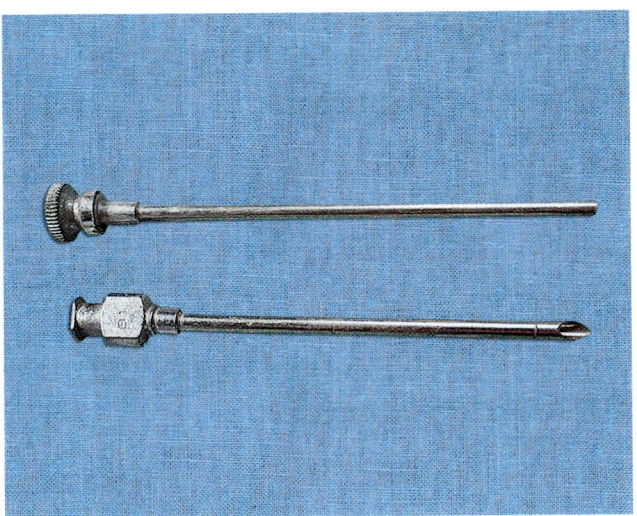

Fig. 14: Trocar cannula for insertion of Norplant rod.

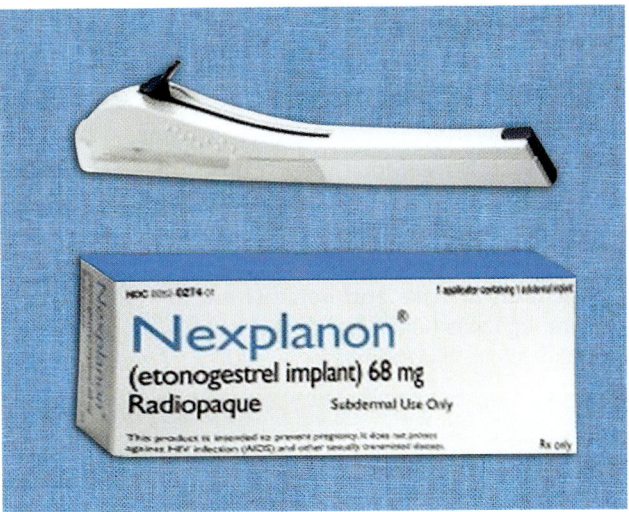

Fig. 16: Nexplanon with applicator.

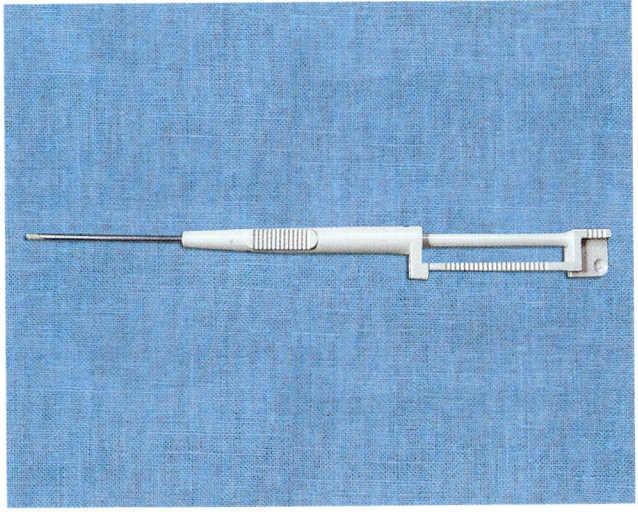

Fig. 15: Implanon—applicator containing 1 implant 68 mg etonogestrel.

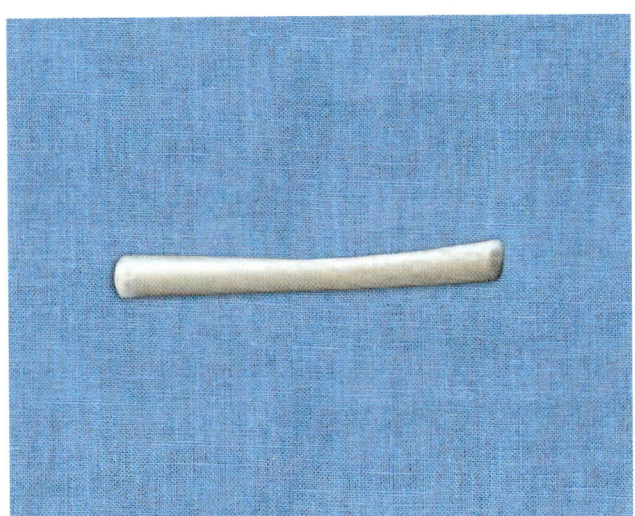

Fig. 17: Nexplanon rod with 68 mg etonogestrel.

❖ *Nexplanon (Fig. 16):* It has replaced the implanon. It is a single-rod **(Fig. 17)** bioequivalent implant containing 68 mg of etonogestrel which is covered by ethylene vinyl acetate copolymer. Initially releases 60–70 μg daily, gradually reduces to 25–30 μg daily after 3 years. It is also effective for 3 years.

Method of insertion of Nexplanon: The rod-shaped single implant is available preloaded in a needle with disposable applicator **(Fig. 16)**. It is inserted subdermally along the bicep groove of the inner arm 6–8 cm from the elbow and the device can be palpable beneath the skin. As it is superficial its removal is easy with a small hemostatic forceps after small incision after which another device is placed within same incision site. It is radiopaque.

Q. When to insert?

It is inserted:
- In lactating woman 6 weeks after childbirth.
- Within 3 weeks in nonlactating puerpera.
- Menstruating woman within 5 days of period.

Mechanism of Action

- Like progesterone-only pill by (A) changes of cervical mucosa, (B) ovulation inhibition, and (C) making endometrium unreceptive.
- *Efficacy:* Highly effective—0.05/HWY.

Advantages

- A long-acting reversible contraceptive (LARC)
- Only progesterone, no side effect of estrogen
- Return of fertility occurs immediately after withdrawal in contrast to injectable
- Insertion and removal easy with Nexplanon.

Disadvantages and Side Effects

- Irregular bleeding which is very common for which woman needs counseling before insertion. It is important cause of early discontinuation.
- Others are weight gain, mastalgia, and mood changes.

COMBINED HORMONAL TRANSDERMAL PATCHES (FIG. 18)

- A square-shaped flexible thin plastic patch containing releasing norelgestromin 203 µg (progestin) and ethinyl estradiol 33.9 µg (estrogen) in every 24 hours.
- One patch is used for 1 week. Consecutive 3 weeks are used with one patch-free week.
- It is applied over dry skin of body usually outer arm, abdomen, back or thighs.
- Mechanism, risks and benefits are like other COCs. Compliance is better. Accidental removal without notice make failure. It is expensive.

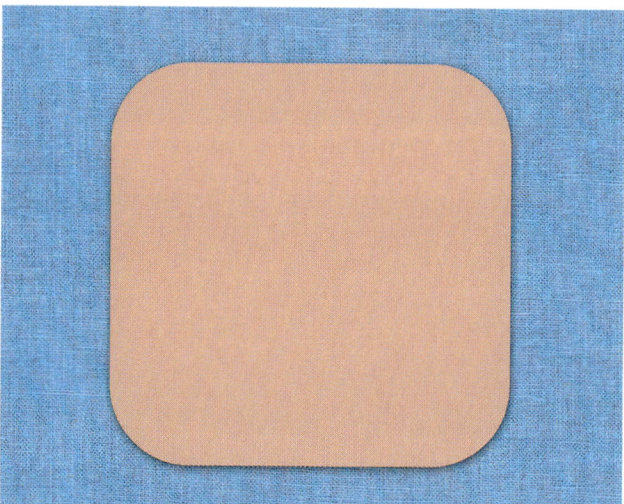

Fig. 18: Transdermal combined hormonal patch.

TRANSVAGINAL COMBINED HORMONAL RING (FIG. 19)

- *Nuvaring:* It is a flexible ring made of polymer containing etonogestrel (11.7 mg) and ethinyl estradiol (2.7 mg). Daily release of etonogestrel and ethinyl estradiol is 120 µg and 15 µg, respectively. Outer diameter of the ring is 54 mm and inner diameter is 50 mm. It is marketed as Nuvaring.

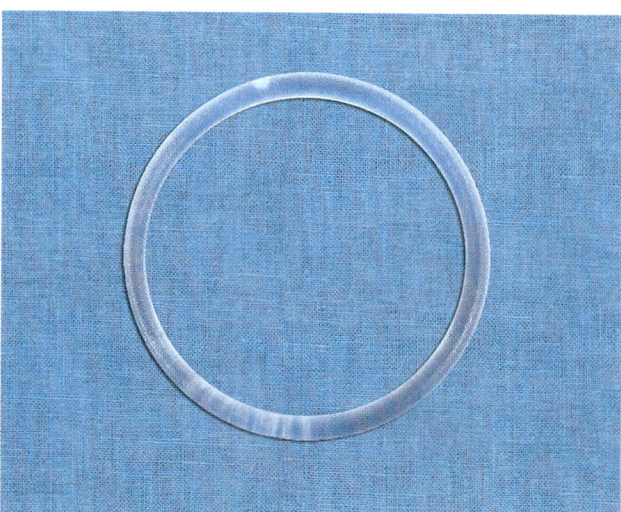

Fig. 19: Nuvaring combined hormonal ring.

- It is worn within 5 days of period and kept for 21 days with 7 days gap during which withdrawal bleeding may occur. A fresh ring is used for each cycle. There is no need to insert it in any special site in vagina and insertion and removal is easy.
- Cycle control is excellent and works mainly by anovulation with good efficacy and failure rate is 0.65/HWY. Sometimes both or any partner may feel the ring during intercourse. In case of displeasure, it can be removed during intercourse but to be worn within 3 hours.
- *Annovera:* A new vaginal ring containing new progestin segesterone acetate and ethinyl estradiol. It is also used for 21 days. However, Annovera can be used for up to one year. It is FDA approved.

PROGESTERONE VAGINAL RING (FIG. 20)

Progesterone vaginal ring (PVR) in the name of *Progering* is available in some south and central American countries. One vaginal ring is used for 3 months. The vaginal ring is made of silastic elastomer containing 1 g total progesterone with releasing rate of progesterone 10 mg/day for lactating women. Failure rate is 1.5/100 women.

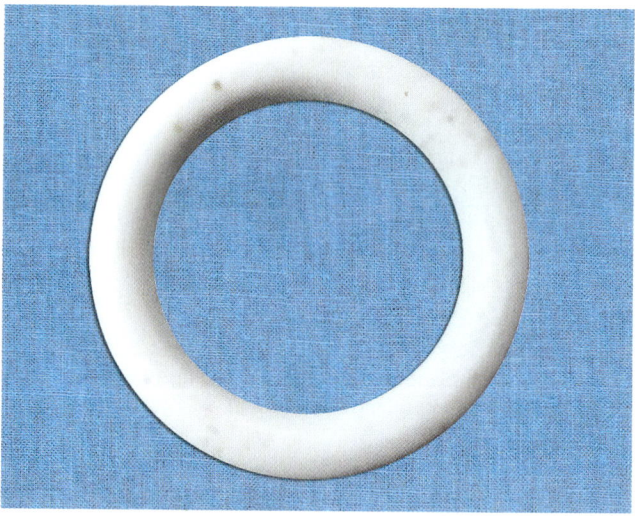

Fig. 20: Progesterone vaginal ring.

EMERGENCY CONTRACEPTIVES (FIG. 21) (SYNONYMS: MORNING AFTER PILL, POSTCOITAL CONTRACEPTION)

Definition

Emergency contraception is a method using drug or any device to prevent the pregnancy after unprotected or inadequately protected act of coitus.

The indications are: (1) Unprotected coitus without contraception, (2) Sexual assault without effective contraception, and (3) Incorrect use of contraception/concern about contraceptive failure, e.g. condom breakage, slippage, missed pill, too much delayed injectable contraceptives, improper use of diaphragm, cervical cap and expulsion of IUCD and implant, etc.

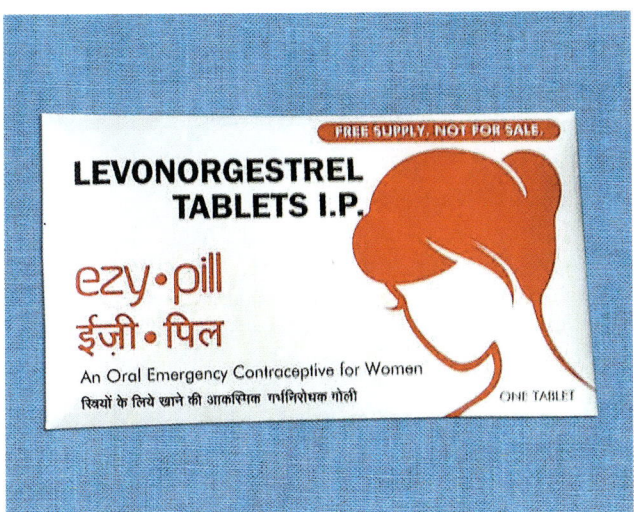

Fig. 21: Emergency contraceptive pill—single tablet levonorgestrel 1.5 mg.

The method was first gained popularity in 1970s as "*morning after pill*". And it also may be called "*postcoital contraception*".

First concept of postcoital contraceptives with sex steroids to prevent pregnancy began in 1960 using high-dose estrogen for 5 days. Later, it was replaced by COCs and more recently progestogen-only pill.

Q. Which is the most common EC pill used?

The most common EC used is progesterone-only pill containing levonorgestrel. In the National Family Program EC pill containing levonorgestrel 1.5 mg per tablet is available. It should be taken immediately after accidental or unprotected coitus or as soon as possible within 72 hours. The name of the tablet is *ezy-pill* which is available in free of cost in all family planning center.

Q. What are the different varieties of ECs available?

Various types are (A) Hormonal pill—progesterone-only pill and combined pill; (B) Nonhormonal tablet—ulipristal acetate (Ella—30 mg single tablet), a selective receptor modulator, mifepristone, and centchroman; and (C) Mechanical—IUCD.

The agents and their dosage schedule are given in **Table 9**.

Q. Mechanism—how do the ECs work?

It depends on which day of menstrual cycle intercourse occurs. The probable mechanisms are:
- Inhibition or delay ovulation
- Endometrial changes thus preventing implantation
- Interfering sperm transport
- Hampering corpus luteal function. IUCD prevents implantation and has gametotoxic and embryotoxic effect.

Q. Does EC cause abortion?

No. It differs from medical abortion that later is used to terminate an existing pregnancy, whereas EC is effective only before a pregnancy is established.

Q. Which IUD is used?

Any Cu containing like Cu-T 380 A. Mirena is not suitable as EC.

Q. When to remove IUD if it is used as EC?

It is removed after onset of next mens or can be kept in situ for ongoing contraception.

Q. What to do if another accidental unprotected coitus occurs in the same cycle?

The previous EC will not prevent pregnancy except IUD and further administration is needed. Barrier method is best to use after first EC intake until next menses if they have intend to act of coitus.

Q. What are the side effects of hormonal EC?

Side effects include nausea, vomiting, and sometimes irregular bleeding after few days of administration and also alteration of onset of menstruation. To avoid vomiting it is taken 1 hour prior to intake of high dose combined EC.

Table 9: Agents and their dosage schedule of emergency contraceptives.

Methods	Content	Content-1 tablet	Schedule of intake
Hormonal	Progestogen-only pill	Levonorgestrel 0.75 mg	One tablet as soon as possible after coitus, second dose after 12 hours within 72 hours
		Levonorgestrel 1.5 mg	Single dose 1 tablet as soon as possible after coitus within 72 hours
	Combined estrogen progestogen pill (Yuzpe method, 1974)	High dose COC—EE 50 µg + levonorgestrel 250 µg	Two tablets as soon as possible after coitus, 2 tablet after 12 hours within 72 hours
		Low dose combined oral contraceptive—EE 30 µg + levonorgestrel 0.15 mg	Four tablets as soon as possible after coitus, 4 tablet after 12 hours within 72 hours (Vomiting is the main problem. Antiemetic should be taken before 1 hour)
Antiprogesterone	Ulipristal Mifepristone	30 mg 25–50 mg single dose	Both can be used up to 120 hours of unprotected coitus
Mechanical device	Intrauterine contraceptives	Cu-T 380A	Can be used up to 120 hours within unprotected coitus

Q. Is EC can be used as a regular contraception?

No, as there is chance of more failure and on regular use there will be irregular bleeding and irregular mens.

Q. Fact about EC methods.

IUD is most effective EC, and can be continued as a regular method, but needs office visit for insertion. Ulipristol is the most effective oral regimen. Progesterone—only contraception is most commonly used and more effective and lesser side effects than COC which is less used now.

Efficacy of EC

It depends on the type of EC used and time of interval from intercourse. Earlier from intercourse it is used better is the efficacy. So far as efficacy, convenience and tolerability are concerned levonorgestrel—only is the ideal choice.

Shifting to Regular Contraceptive

Immediately following use of EC regular contraceptive is started. IUD is continued. If Ulipristol is used COC or progesterone only is taken on 6th day, not within 5 days.

Failure Rates

- Progesterone only—1/100 women
- Combined—2/100 women
- Mifepristone—0.6/100 women
- IUD—0.5/100 women.

Q. If failure occurs after administration of EC, does teratogenicity occurs?

No, no such effect.

INTRAUTERINE CONTRACEPTIVE DEVICES (IUDs OR IUCDs)

Q. What do you mean by IUCDs?

The IUDs or IUCDs are the devices made of plastic or metal or combination of these with/without hormonal agent used for insertion in uterine cavity for purpose of contraception. IUCDs are safe, effective, convenient long-acting reversible method of contraceptive. It is the *second most commonly used method* next to female sterilization worldwide.

Q. What are the types of IUDs?

According to content:
- *Inert:* Lippes loop (**Fig. 22**, not used nowadays in India), Ota ring, Saf T coil, and Mahua ring.
- *Copper-containing IUD:* Copper 7, Copper T200, *Copper T380A*, Copper T380Ag, Multiload Copper 250, and *Multiload Copper 375*.
- *Hormone releasing IUD:* Progesterone IUD (Progestasert) and *Levonorgestrel IUD* (*Mirena*, LNG 20).

Copper and hormone releasing IUDs are called *medicated* IUDs and inner IUDs are called *nonmedicated*.

Skyla and Liletta are newer LNG releasing IUDs and can be kept for 3 years.

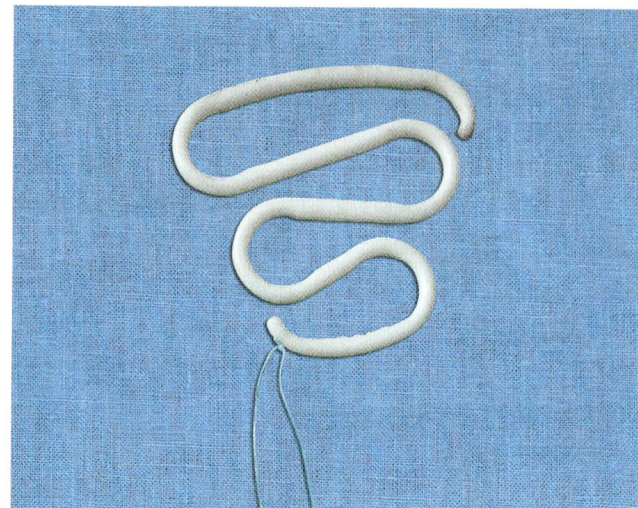

Fig. 22: Lippes loop.

According to design:
- *Open:* Lippes loop (**Fig. 22**), Cu-T 200, 380A, Multiload copper 250, 375, Mirena are examples. If perforation occurs chance of strangulation cannot occur due to absence of aperture.
- *Closed:* Grafenberg ring [made of silver wire devised by E Grafenberg (Germany, 1920)] and Brinberg bow are not used due to the chance of strangulation of gut if perforation occurs.
- *Frameless IUD: GyneFix* is a frameless copper-containing IUD and *Fibroplant* is a frameless levonorgestrel IUD (*see* later in detail) (*see* **Fig. 55**).

Of these *Lippes loop* (**Fig. 22**), an inert oldest IUD made of polythene made radiopaque by impregnating with barium sulfate is commonly used in Pakistan, Indonesia, and China. Once popular it is not used in India from 80s and is gradually being replaced by medicated IUD throughout the world.

Copper T380A (model name *TCu 380A*) and *Multiload copper 375* (model name Cu375) are supplied by Government of India free of cost. *Remember Cu375 is Multiload not T-shaped and hence not called copper T.*

Q. Describe each device-CuT-380A (Figs. 23 and 25) and Multiload Cu375 (Figs. 24 and 26)

Difference between Cu 380A and Multiload Cu375		
Types	Cu 380A (Fig. 23)	Multiload Cu375 (Fig. 24)
Shape and morphology	T shaped 'A' stands for arm—means Cu is present also on arm Length—36 mm, more wider transversely	Horizontal arm is replaced by inverted U shaped flexible plastic serrated fins with 5 stubs on each side. The fins keep the device in uterine cavity without stretching Length —36 mm, less wider transversely

Contd...

Contd...

Types	Cu 380A (Fig. 23)	Multiload Cu375 (Fig. 24)
Duration of use	Recommended for use for 10 years	Recommended for 5 years
Plunger	Plunger (solid white rod) present Available in a sterilized sealed packet along with plunger (Fig. 25)	Provided with a preloaded inserter tube without plunger (Fig. 26) in a sterilized pack. Insertion is easier
Amount of copper surface area and weight	Total copper surface area 380 mm^2 [stem wrapped with 314 mm^2 of fine copper wire (approximately 175 mg) and each arm has a 33 mm^2 copper sleeve (66.5 mg of Cu each arm)]	Total copper surface area 375 mm^2 350 mg weight which is present only on vertical limb
Location of Cu	Cu present on both vertical and horizontal limb	Cu present only on vertical limb
Cu type wire/solid	Wire on vertical limb. Solid bracelet on horizontal limb	Wire on vertical limb
Made of	Polyethylene impregnated with barium sulfate	Polyethylene impregnated with barium sulfate
Color of strings/threads and length	Polyethylene double strings-white in color Shorter (11.5 cm)	Monofilament nylon double threads- Fluorescent Green- longer (19.5 cm) in size which is useful for postpartum insertion
Base	Base is round shaped with 3 mm ball which will prevent perforation through cervix	Base is wide and split. Standard length is 36 mm

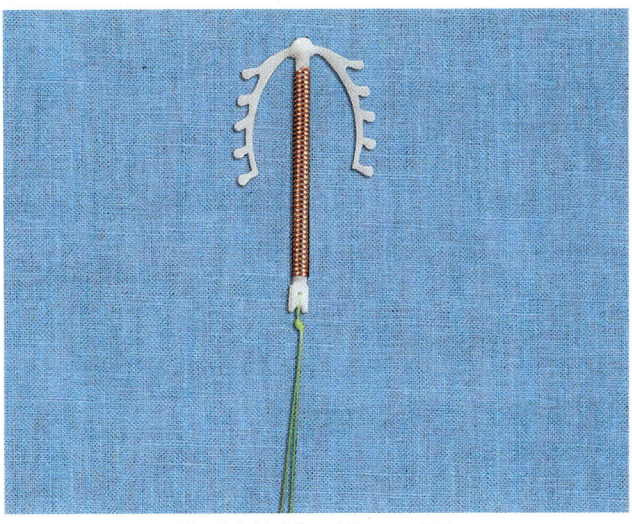

Fig. 24: Multiload Copper 375.

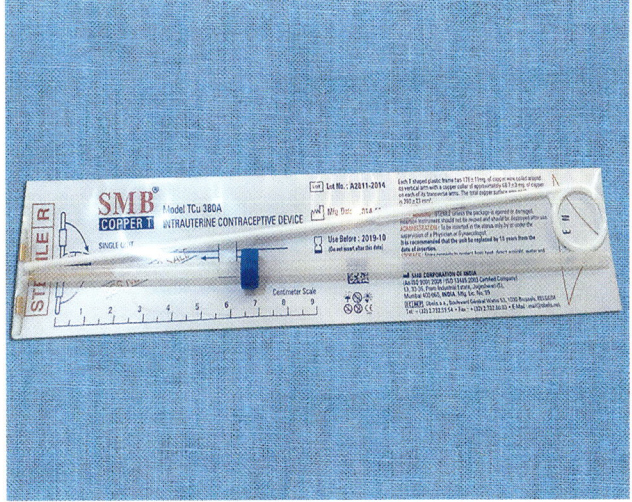

Fig. 25: CuT 380A.

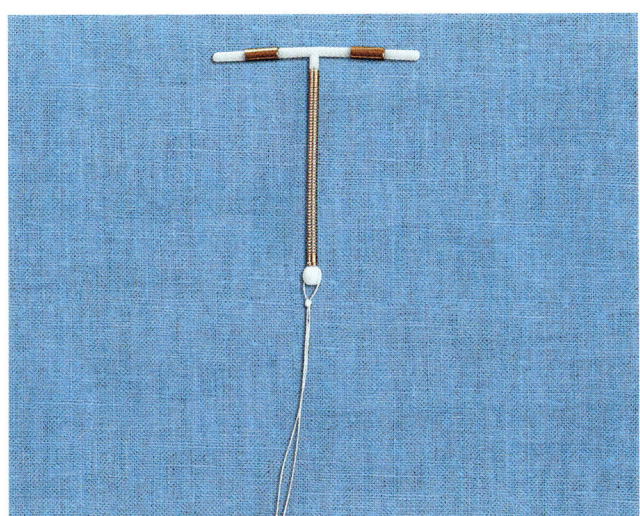

Fig. 23: CuT 380A.

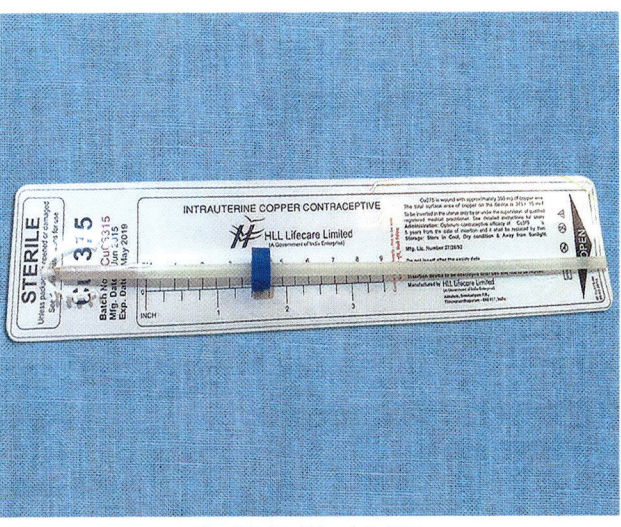

Fig. 26: Multiload Cu375.

Q. What does A stand for in Cu-T 380A?

"A" in CuT-380A stands for arms which signifies that there is additional copper in the arm other than vertical arm. In Cu-T 200 copper is present only in vertical arm with surface area of 200 mm².

LNG-IUS (Mirena) (Figs. 27 to 29)

Levonorgestrel-intrauterine system (Mirena) is a T-shaped plastic device covered with a membrane of polydimethylsiloxane containing levonorgestrel of 52 mg. Daily release rate of LNG is 20 µg in the uterine cavity. A blue-colored monofilament thread is attached to the loop of the device. It is radiopaque. *LNG-IUS is recommended for 5 years*. Other than contraception it has noncontraceptive benefits and use.

The LNG-IUS with lower dose and smaller frame (Skyla-13 mg LNG with release of 6 µg daily) for 3 years has been designed. Frameless LNG-IUS Fibroplant14 is used for 3 years.

LNG-IUS (Emily) Figs. 29A and B: Progesterone containing IUD is also available in a shape looking like multiload Cu375 with inverted U shaped flexible plastic serrated fins and a vertical limb containing levonorgestrel of 52 mg with daily release of 20 µg (same as Mirena) with preloaded inserter. It is simpler to insert and available in India.

Noncontraceptive uses of LNG-IUS are dysfunctional uterine bleeding (DUB), endometriosis, adenomyosis, simple endometrial hyperplasia, etc. It is not recommended for emergency contraceptive.

Mechanism of Action of Copper-containing Devices

- Gametotoxic, both for sperm and egg thus prevent fertilization due to local inflammation by Cu-containing device leading to lysosomal activation and other inflammatory action—this is the most important mechanism.
- Toxic to blastocyst.
- Endometrial hostility leading to failure of implantation.

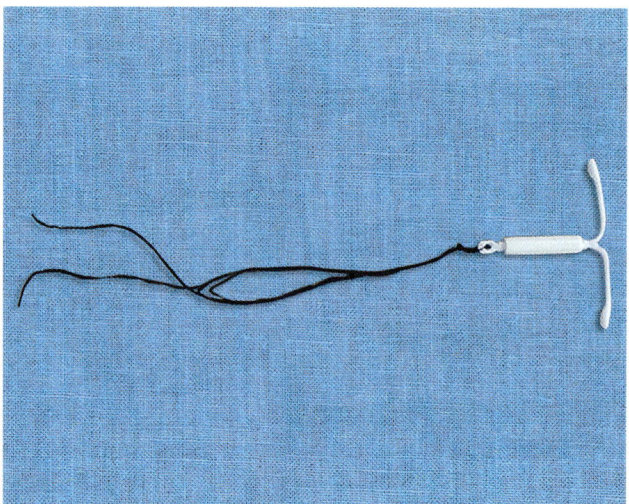

Fig. 27: Mirena (LNG 20).

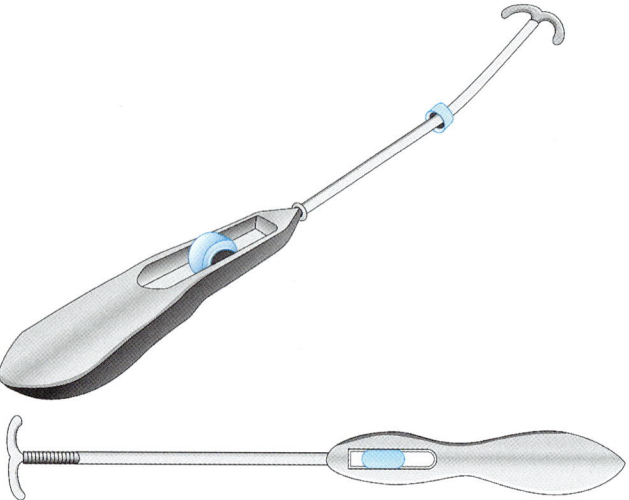

Fig. 29: Levonorgestrel-intrauterine system Mirena (LNG–IUS).

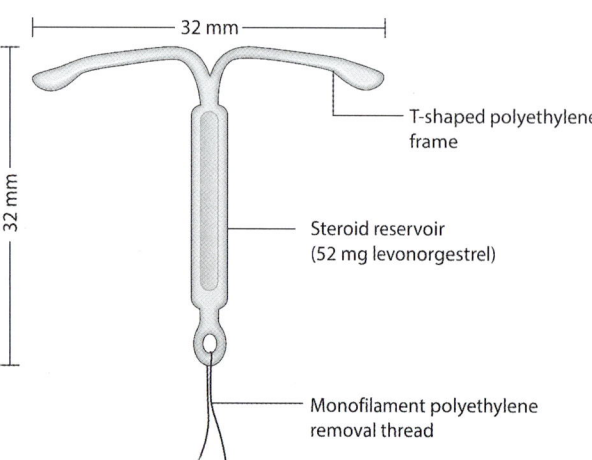

Fig. 28: Schematic diagram of levonorgestrel-intrauterine system (Mirena).

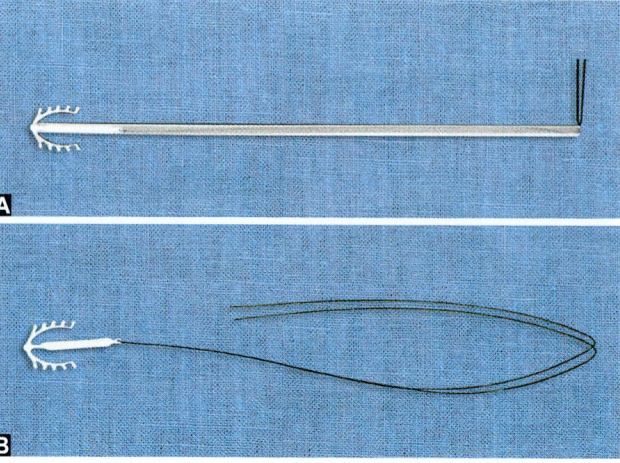

Figs. 29A and B: Levonorgestrel-intrauterine system Emily.

- The LNG-IUS prevents pregnancy by progesterone-mediated mechanism—makes cervical mucus hostile thus preventing sperm penetration, decrease tubal motility thus preventing fertilization, makes the endometrium atrophy, and makes anovulation which is however not consistent.

Q. How many years you can keep IUD?

- The device CuT-380A is recommended to use for 10 years, though it is shown to prevent pregnancy for up to 20 years.
- Multiload Cu375 is recommended for 5 years.
- The LNG-IUS is recommended for 5 years.

CONTRAINDICATIONS OF COPPER-CONTAINING IUDs

Q. What are the contraindications of copper-containing IUDs? [As per medical eligibility criteria (MEC) WHO 2015]

Absolute contraindications (Category 4—a condition which represents an unacceptable health risk if the contraceptive method is used):

- Pregnancy
- Puerperal sepsis
- Immediate post-septic abortion
- Unexplained vaginal bleeding
- Persistently elevated beta human chorionic gonadotropin (hCG) or malignant disease following gestational trophoblastic disease
- Carcinoma cervix
- Endometrial cancer
- Fibroid uterus with distortion of uterine cavity
- Current PID
- Anatomical uterine anomaly with distortion of uterine cavity
- Pelvic tuberculosis
- Current purulent cervicitis or chlamydial infection or gonorrhea
- Current breast cancer *(only for LNG-IUS)*.

Relative contraindications (Category 3—a condition where the theoretical or proven risks usually outweigh the advantages of using the method):

- Postpartum more than or equal to 48 hours to less than 4 weeks
- Severe or advanced HIV clinical disease (who stage 3 or 4)
- Severe thrombocytopenia
- Ovarian cancer
- Increase risk of sexually transmitted disease (STD).

Q. What are the contraindications of LNG-IUS? [As per medical eligibility criteria (MEC) WHO 2015]

Absolute contraindications (Category 4) of LNG-IUS:

- Pregnancy
- Undiagnosed vaginal bleeding pre-evaluation
- Presence of puerperal or immediate postabortal sepsis
- Gestational trophoblastic disease—persistently elevated β-hCG levels or malignant disease
- Cervical cancer and endometrial cancer
- Breast cancer—past and no evidence of current disease for 5 years
- Uterine fibroid with distortion of cavity
- PID
- Current purulent cervicitis or chlamydial infection or gonorrhea
- Pelvic tuberculosis.

Relative contraindications (Category 3) of LNG-IUS:

- Postpartum more than or equal 48 hours to less than 4 weeks
- Acute deep vein thrombosis/pulmonary embolism (DVT/PE)
- Positive (or unknown) antiphospholipid antibodies
- Migraine with aura at any age
- Breast cancer past and no evidence of current disease for 5 years
- Ovarian cancer
- Increase risk of STI.

Advantages of IUD as Contraceptive

- One time motivation
- Good efficacy, failure rate low—Cu IUD 0.6/HWY and in typical use less than 0.8/HWY. LNG-IUS in both perfect use and typical use failure rate is 0.2/HWY
- Safe, complication less
- LARC
- No further costs after insertion
- Does not require the user anything to do after insertion
- No interference in sex
- No systemic side effect and life risk is minimum
- No effect on breastfeeding
- Health benefits—protects against risk of pregnancy and protects against endometrial cancer
- After withdrawn she can conceive immediately.

Disadvantages of IUD

- A health worker or medical personnel is essential for screening and introduction
- They have some complications like pain, bleeding, infection and perforation
- Insertion is painful
- Expulsion occurs spontaneously without knowledge
- Does not prevent STDs including AIDS/HIV infection.

Q. What is efficacy?

- Copper-containing IUD: With perfect use failure rate is 0.6/HWY and in typical use failure rate is less than 0.8/HWY.
- LNG-IUS: With perfect use failure rate is 0.2/HWY and in typical use failure rate is less than 0.2/HWY.

Q. What are the noncontraceptive uses of IUDs?

- CuT 380A and Multiload Cu375—in Asherman syndrome (uterine synechiae)

- LNG-IUS—in DUB, endometriosis, adenomyosis, simple endometrial hyperplasia, and selected cases of uterine fibroids, etc.

Q. For whom you can prescribe copper containing IUDs (i.e. Who can use IUD)?

It can be given to woman who has no contraindication.

As per WHO, woman can begin using IUDs without STI testing, without an HIV test, without any blood tests or routine laboratory tests, without breast examination, and without cervical cancer screening.

Q. When to insert IUDs?

- *Interval:* Patient has had regular menstrual cycle. Best time is to insert 2–3 days after period is over (as cervix becomes softer and dilated to make the procedure easy), however any time can be given. If it is inserted 12 days within onset of period no back up is needed. During lactational amenorrhea (fully or nearly fully) breastfeeding it can be offered any time within 6 months. After 6 months if no period IUD can also be inserted provided reasonably sure she is nonpregnant.
- *Postabortal* (miscarriage or after): Immediately following abortion or within 12 days no back up is needed. Infection is to be ruled out.
- Postpartum intrauterine contraceptive device: The postpartum intrauterine contraceptive device (PPIUCD) can be placed immediately (within 10 minutes) following delivery of the placenta, during cesarean section or within 48 hours following childbirth.
- *Emergency contraceptive:* Within 5 days of unprotected coitus.

Q. Who can insert and where it is done?

A especially *trained* healthcare provider can insert IUD into the uterus through the vagina in an approved center as an *outpatient procedure*.

Selection of the Patient

Selection can be done by history taking and examination including pelvic (P/V) examination to exclude any *contraindication* according to MEC (medical eligibility criteria).

Woman is *explained* the procedure and informed about the problems those may arise associated with it, follow-up protocol, to report in case of any problem and written *consent* is taken.

Steps of Insertion of IUCD

Woman may be given a nonsteroidal anti-inflammatory drug such as ibuprofen (200–400 mg) half an hour before the procedure.

Infection prevention: The instruments used should be high level *disinfected* (boiling, steaming or soaking in disinfectant chemicals) and for insertion "*no touch*" method is employed.

Q. What is no touch technique?

No touch technique involves: (1) The device (CuT 380A) is loaded inside the inserter tube before taking out the device and partially opening the pack (this procedure is not needed in multiload). The solid rod is introduced into the insertion tube from the bottom alongside the threads until it touches the bottom of T380A; (2) Pack is opened only (see the pack—open is written in which end) on opposite end of the site of the device, not on the side where the CuT is; (3) The device is taken out by holding the proximal end and not to touch the distal end where the device has been made fixed; and (4) During insertion, care should be taken so that the uterine sound and the loaded end do not touch the vaginal wall anywhere.

The procedure of fitting the CuT in inserter tube and introduction of solid white bar inside the tube can be done after taking out the unit outside with gloves finger but no touch technique method by keeping the device inside the pack is the ideal for infection prevention and on doing practice it becomes easier and should always be practiced.

Always presterilized closed pack is used.

Proper Procedure of Insertion of CuT 380A (Figs. 30A to G)

Woman is asked to evacuate blabber normally.

She is put in lithotomy position and a gentle per vaginal bimanual examination is done to note the position, size of the uterus, and adnexae. If any contraindication (pathological discharge, abnormality in uterus and adnexae) is detected procedure is not done.

- *Fitting of the device before application:* This involves the fitting the arms of CuT inside the inserter tube by bending and introduction of solid white bar inside the tube from the opposite end of tube preferably by no touch technique. CuT 380A should not be loaded **(Figs. 30A and B)** into the inserter tube *not more than 5 minutes before* insertion because the malleable arms may remain bent inward even after releasing it.
- A *posterior vaginal speculum* is inserted, anterior of cervix is held by Allis tissue forceps. An uterine sound is introduced to note the position and length of the uterocervical canal. By moving the blue plastic flange (guard) the length of the inserter tube is adjusted according to the length of uterocervical canal.
- The inserter tube loaded with IUD and the solid white rod is introduced into the endometrial **(Fig. 30C)** cavity till the blue guard touches the cervix **(Fig. 30D)**. It is kept in notice that the IUD arm should lie in the same plane as the plane (transverse plane) of blue guard so that after releasing the arms will lie transversely.
- Now, to release the IUD arms, the inserter tube is withdrawn (no more than 1 cm) while the solid white rod is held steady *(withdrawal technique)* **(Fig. 30E)**.
- Inserter tube is gently moved upward to feel slight resistance. Now the solid white rod is withdrawn and then followed by withdrawn of inserter tube one after another **(Fig. 30F)**.

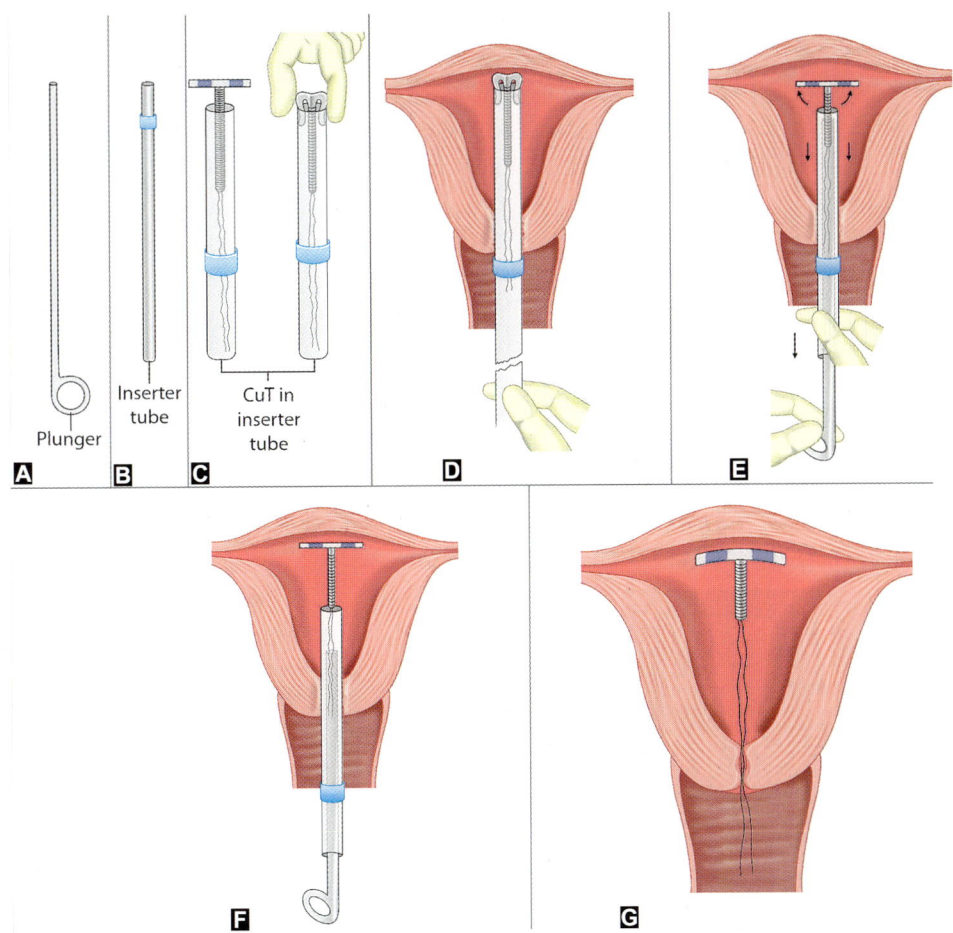

Figs. 30A to G: (A) Plunger; (B) Inserter tube; (C) CuT in inserter tube and horizontal arms are bent to introduce into inserter tube; (D) CuT with inserter tube and plunger is introduced into uterine cavity. Before that length of uterine cavity is measured by uterine sound and guard is adjusted to make the length of the system according to cavity length; (E) Inserter tube is withdrawal fixing the plunger by other hand so that the CuT is released; (F) Inserter tube with plunger is brought out to leave the CuT in place; and (G) CuT is in place, the thread is trimmed to keep the length outside external os 2–3 cm.

- The threads which are visible protruding through the cervix are trimmed so that 2–3 cm remains **(Fig. 30G)**.
- Speculum and the Allis forceps are removed.

Procedure of Insertion of Multiload Cu375

- The principle is same.
- The inserter tube with the device is taken out from the pack in no touch technique.
- Here there is no white solid rod needed.
- As there is a bent fin mild dilatation of cervix may be needed.
- The inserter tube with the device is introduced up to the fundus.
- The inserter tube is withdrawn.
- The thread is trimmed keeping 2–3 cm outside the external os **(Figs. 31A to C)**.

Method of Insertion of Mirena (Figs. 32 to 38)

- Patient is put in lithotomy position, P/V examination done. Posterior vaginal wall retracted posteriorly and anterior lip is held by Allis tissue forceps and length of uterine cavity is measured by uterine sound.
- Packet is opened completely on sterile technique.
- The slider is pushed forward to load Mirena in insertion tube **(Fig. 33)**.
- Upper edge of flange (guard) is set corresponding with the length of uterine cavity as measured by uterine sound **(Fig. 34)**.
- Inserter is introduced through the cervix to the extend so that flange (guard) lies 1.5–2 cm outside external os **(Figs. 35 and 36)**.
- Now keeping the inserter steady slider is pulled up to the mark to open the horizontal arms of Mirena **(Fig. 37)**.
- The inserter is advanced so that flange touches the cervix.
- Holding the inserter in place the slider is pulled all the way down. This will release the Mirena.
- Now inserter is removed by pulling it out **(Fig. 38)**.
- Thread is cut leaving 2–3 cm outside the cervix.

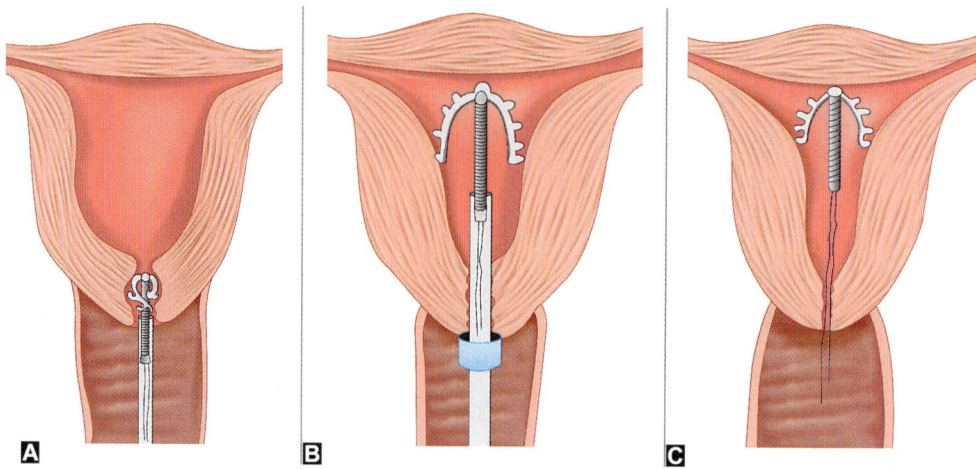

Figs. 31A to C: (A) Technique of insertion of Multiload Cu375. The inserter tube with the device Multiload Cu350 is introduced, here there is no plunger; (B) The device is introduced up to the fundus; (C) The introducer has been withdrawn keeping the Multiload in situ. The thread is trimmed keeping 2–3 cm outside external os.

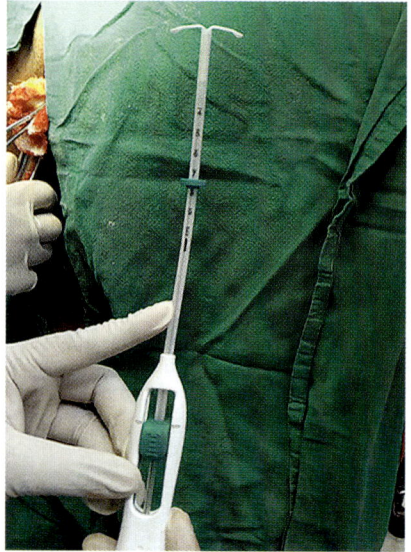

Fig. 32: Mirena insertion-made ready.
Courtesy: Dr Sudipto Jana

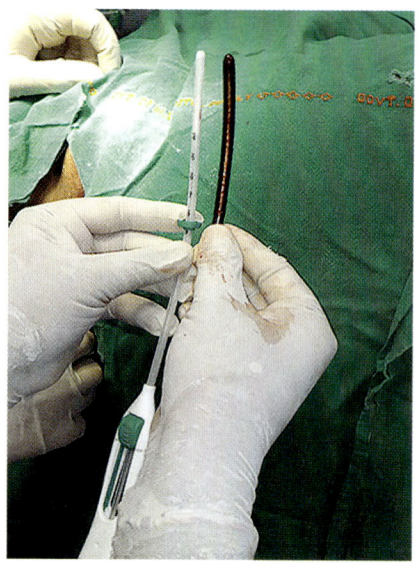

Fig. 34: Length is adjusted by moving guard.

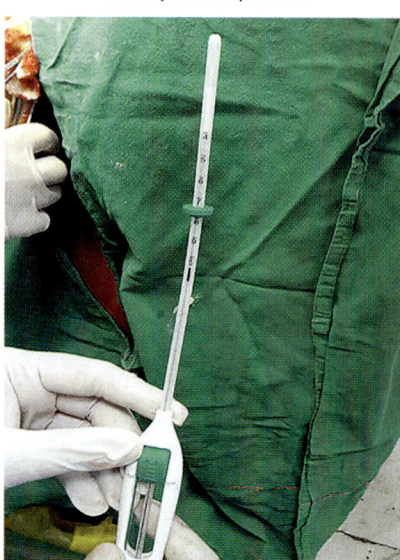

Fig. 33: Mirena is loaded.

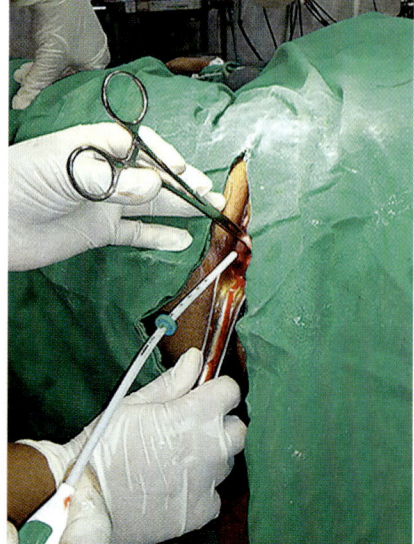

Fig. 35: Mirena is inserted in uterine cavity.

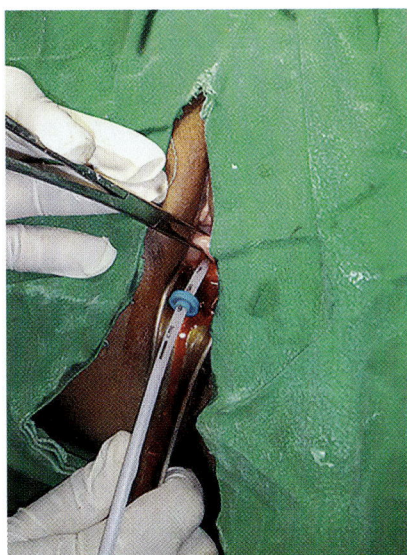

Fig. 36: Mirena insertion—flange (guard) lies 1.5–2 cm outside external os.

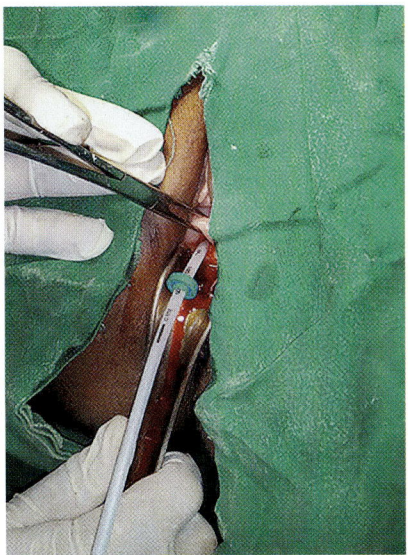

Fig. 38: Mirena introducer withdrawn gently.

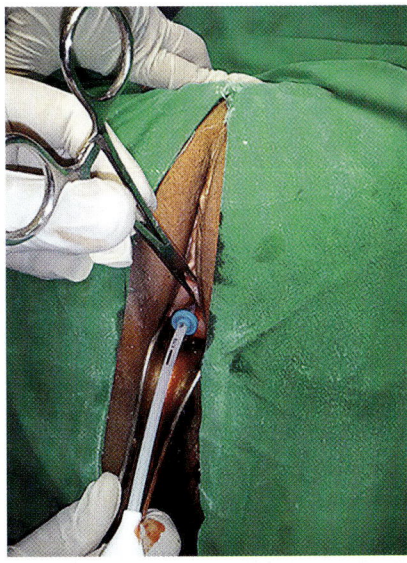

Fig. 37: Mirena insertion—Mirena is released inside uterine cavity.

Q. How you will follow-up?

- Patient is counseled that initially, there may be pelvic cramp and increase vaginal bleeding.
- Patient is usually asked to come for follow-up after next period or 3–6 weeks after insertion. In the visit, she is asked for any side effects and presence of IUD is confirmed by presence of string.
- Woman is asked to feel the thread after next period and time-to-time for first few months, and then annually.
- If any excessive symptoms or amenorrhea she is advised to come.
- She should be advised after how many years she will come for changing the device or for alternate contraceptive or for further issue.

Complications of IUCD

Immediate

- Cramping uterine pain—lasts for few hours and if not relieved analgesic or antispasmodic is given.
- Vasovagal attack rarely occurs immediately after insertion.

Late

Menorrhagia (5–10%) and anemia—NSAIDs like ibuprofen, diclofenac for first few days of period reduces heavy bleeding. Few women may need iron tablet for anemia.

- Dysmenorrhea (5%)
- Expulsion: up to 5%
- Perforation: Incidence is 0.1%
- Infection
- Failure—pregnancy rate given above—for Cu IUD in perfect use 0.6/HWY and in typical use 0.8/HWY and in LNG-IUS both are 0.2/HWY
- PID: 2–5%
- Ectopic pregnancy—not increased (see Page 487).

Q. Perforation—what is the cause, how will you diagnose, and how will you manage? (Figs. 39 to 46)

- Uterine perforation is rare (0.1%) but happens. Increase risk of perforation is due to inexperience of provider, breastfeeding, and less than 6 months following childbirth.
- It may occur during insertion when more pain occurs or may occur spontaneously later.
- It may occur partial or completely and migrated commonly to omentum, adhered to adnexa or to the parieties. Bowel perforation or fistula is also reported.
- Extrauterine copper—bearing device induces local inflammatory reaction and adhesion formation.
- Patient usually presents with missing thread. X-ray shows device but in USG no device is seen in the uterine cavity.

SECTION 4: Birth Control and Population Demography

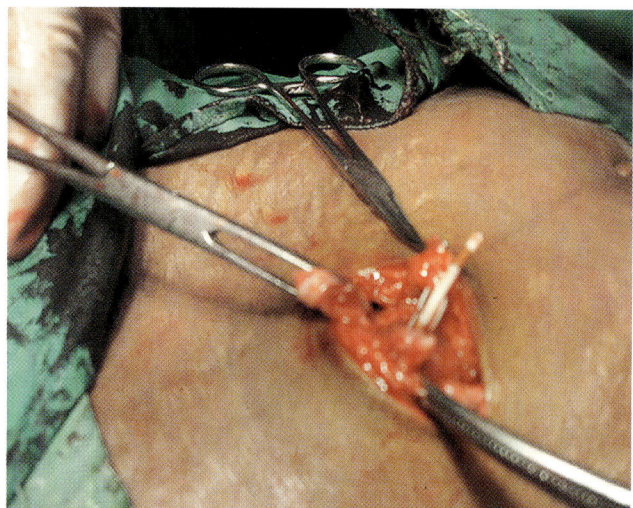

Fig. 39: Perforation of CuT removed from anterior abdominal wall which was introduced 2 years back. Woman came with missing thread.

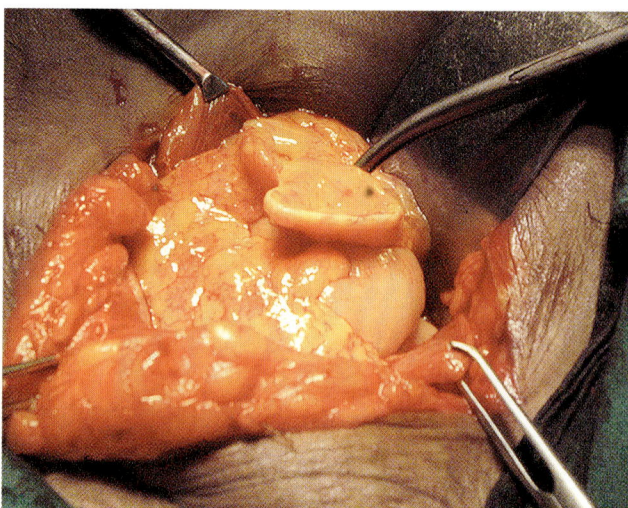

Fig. 42: Lippes loop after perforation removed after 27 years of insertion (this was removed in 2006).

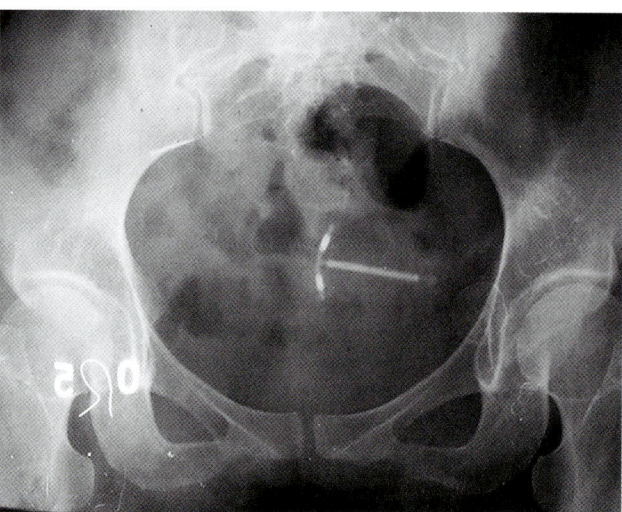

Fig. 40: X-ray abdomen of the same patient as Figure 39.

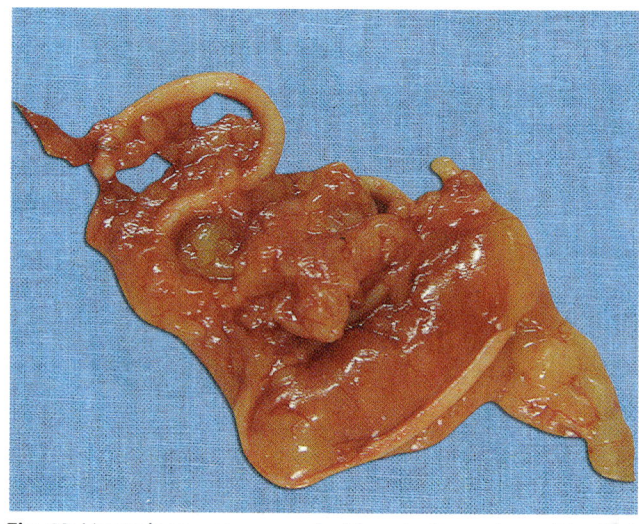

Fig. 43: Lippes loop was removed with part of omentum with which it was adhered as shown in Figure 42.

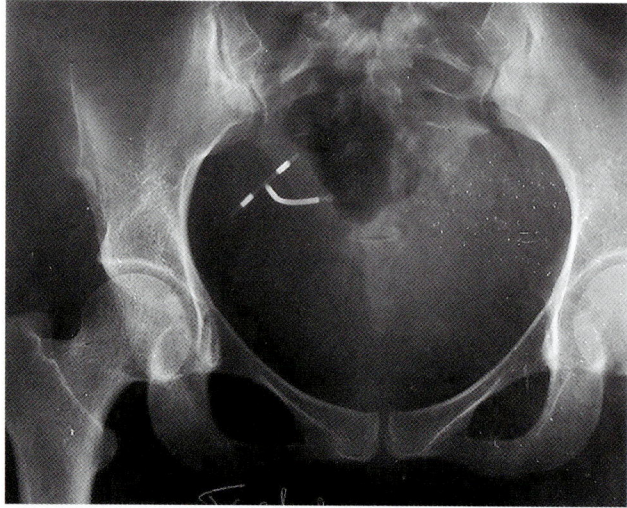

Fig. 41: X-ray showing CuT in pelvis. Laparotomy showed CuT adhered with right adnexa.

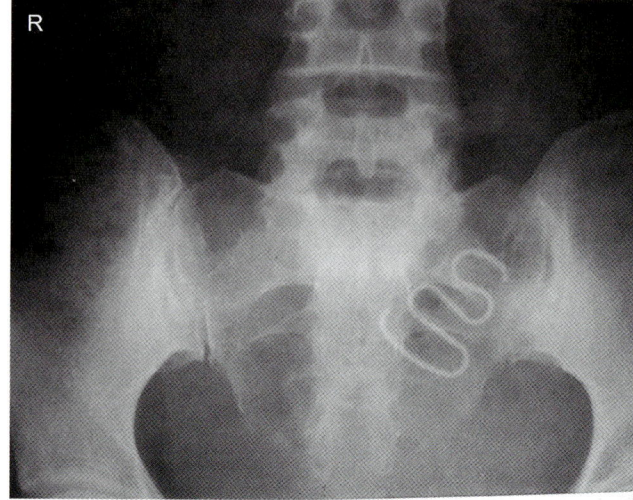

Fig. 44: Straight X-ray of the patient as Figures 42 and 43.

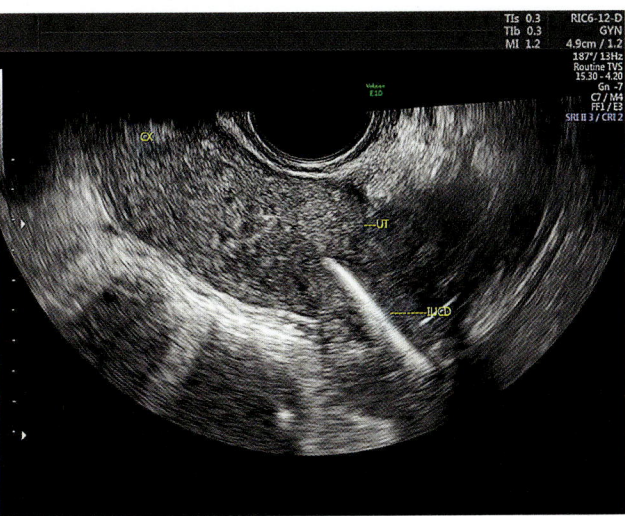

Fig. 45: Transvaginal sonography showing misplaced intrauterine contraceptive device.

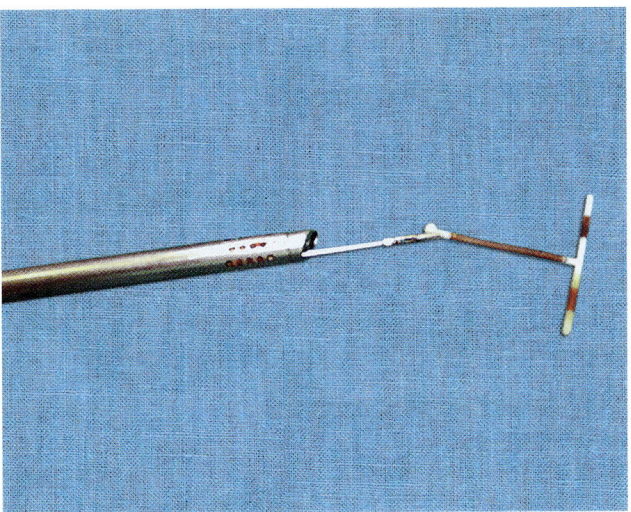

Fig. 47: Hysteroscopic removal of CuT in missing thread due to torn thread (look thread is absent).
Courtesy: Dr A Rakshit, Associate Professor, Obstetrics and Gynecology

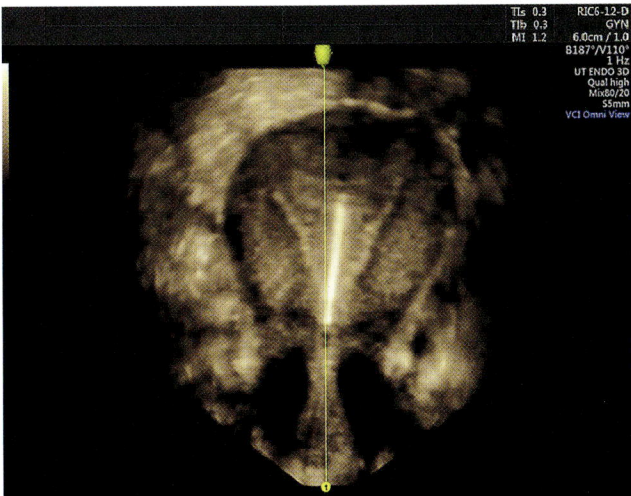

Fig. 46: 3D USG showing normal position of intrauterine contraceptive device inside uterine cavity.
Courtesy: Professor Kamal Oswal, VIMS, Kolkata

- Once diagnosed removal is mandatory.
- Laparoscopical removal is possible in most of the cases. Rarely laparotomy is needed.

Expulsion

The incidence is 5% in first year and commonly occurs during first month and more common (10%) in postpartum cases. The woman is asked to palpate the string periodically through vagina by advancing her middle finger toward cervix either in squatting or in sitting position on the edge of chair. On first follow-up, the string is checked.

Infection

Commonly occurs in first 3 weeks and thereafter chance becomes less. Common organism is actinomyces-like organisms (ALOs). If symptomatic it is removed and penicillin-based antibiotic is administered. In suspected case before insertion antibiotic to cover Chlamydia is given and procedure is deferred.

Q. Missing thread—what are the causes of missing thread and how would you manage?

- The causes are torn of the thread, expulsion of device, twisting of the thread inside, perforation, or pregnancy.
- X-ray of pelvis can detect whether it has been expelled.
- It is detected by ultrasonography whether it is intrauterine or extrauterine.
- If it is intrauterine, it is removed by a hook or best managed by hysteroscopic removal **(Fig. 47)**.
- If it is outside uterus, it is removed laparoscopically or sometimes laparotomy may be needed. Sometimes, the device may penetrate the uterine wall in varying degrees. Hysteroscopically or laparoscopically removal depends on how much it is uterine and how much it has perforated.

Q. Pregnancy with IUD in situ—what to do?

Woman usually comes with amenorrhea. On examination, the string is visible up to 14 weeks, thereafter it goes inside. As it is contraceptive failure counseling is needed whether she wants termination or continuation. MTP is done if she wants. If she wants continuation woman is counseled that there is increase chance of abortion, infection, and preterm birth if the device lies in situ. If the thread is visible it is removed with slight increase chance of abortion. If continuation is done with device in situ chance of birth defect is usually not increased.

Q. Relation of ectopic pregnancy and IUCD—does IUD cause ectopic pregnancy?

Intrauterine device is effective in preventing all pregnancies. IUD reduces the absolute number of ectopic pregnancy by half compared with rate in women who do not use contraceptive. However IUD mechanism reduces the intrauterine pregnancy more than in other places. When pregnancy occurs, IUD in situ ectopic pregnancy must be excluded though *absolute number of ectopic is reduced by IUD.*

Q. When you will remove IUD?

If the patient cannot tolerate due to side effects the problem is addressed with sympathy and if still persists it should be removed. Best time of removal is during monthly period when cervix becomes soft. If removed in mid-cycle abstinence or back-up procedure is needed.

In failure, it is removed.

In suspected perforation, she is referred to higher center for diagnosis and removal.

After stipulated period of use, it is changed or alternate method is advised or woman is allowed to conceive if she desires.

POSTPARTUM IUCD

Q. What do you mean by postpartum IUCD?

Provision of IUCD in the immediate postpartum period is called PPIUCD and it offers an effective and safe method for spacing and limiting births.

Considering the huge potentiality and abundant scope in India, especially after increase of institutional delivery Government of India has given special emphasis in PPIUCD started the training on immediate postpartum insertion of IUCD from 2010 and it is one of the important components of family planning program of India.

Q. Why to stress on PPIUCD?

- In India a significant percentage of population in the first year postpartum have an unmet need for family planning.
- Maximum chance of unplanned pregnancy due to unreliability of LAM, unpredictable ovulation time, and lack of awareness regarding need of contraception.

Advantages of PPIUCD

- Counseling during antenatal period and in early labor is very successful and woman and family become highly motivated to accept it as a reliable birth spacing method.
- It is safe to use as it is certain that the woman is not pregnant at the time of insertion.
- There is minimal risk of uterine perforation because of the thick wall of the uterus.
- There is reduced perception of initial side effects (bleeding and cramping) and reduced chance of heavy bleeding, especially among LAM users, since they experience amenorrhea.
- There is no effect on amount or quality of breast milk.
- It saves time as performed on the same delivery table for postplacental or intracesarean insertions. Additional evaluations and separate clinical procedure are not required.
- It needs minimal additional instruments, supplies, and equipment.
- The woman has an effective method for contraception before discharge from hospital.
- The increased institutional deliveries are the opportunity to provide women easy access to immediate PPIUCD services.
- *It is effective long-active reversible contraceptive method.*

Effectiveness

Failure rate is low: 0.6 to 0.8 pregnancies per 100 women in first year of use. The CuT-380A is effective for 10 years for continuous use. Multiload Cu375 is effective for 5 years.

Disadvantages

- Provider needs specific training in postpartum insertion.
- Expulsion rates appear to be higher. In general, expulsion rates for PPIUCD range between 10% and 14% where in interval, it is 5%. Good technique can reduce expulsion to 4–5%.
- Nonvisibility of string per vagina may occur in spite of in situ position.
- The other limitations of the immediate PPIUCD are the same as the interval IUCD.

Timing of PPIUCD Insertion

The PPIUCD can be placed immediately following delivery of the placenta, during cesarean section or within 48 hours following childbirth:

- *Postplacental:* Insertion within 10 minutes after expulsion of the placenta following a vaginal delivery on the same delivery table.
- *Intracesarean:* Insertion that takes place during a cesarean delivery, after removal of the placenta, and before closure of the uterine incision.
- *Immediate postpartum*—within 48 hours after delivery: Insertion within 48 hours of delivery and prior to discharge from the postpartum ward.
- Insertion any time after 6 weeks postpartum is called *extended postpartum or interval PPIUCD.*
- The IUCD should not be inserted from 48 hours to 6 weeks following delivery because there is an increased risk of infection and expulsion.

Procedure of IUCD Insertion—Technical Aspects (Figs. 48 to 54)

Fundal placement of IUCD is the most important.

In *postplacental insertion* long placental forceps *(Kelly's forceps)* is needed to insert. Negotiation of the "bend" where the uterine body flops over the lower uterine segment is a common challenge during insertion. *For insertion technique, see the Figures 49 to 54 with description in legends.*

For intracesarean insertion, it is best done manually with the fingers. Alternatively, regular ring forceps can be used. After

CHAPTER 22: Family Planning and Contraception

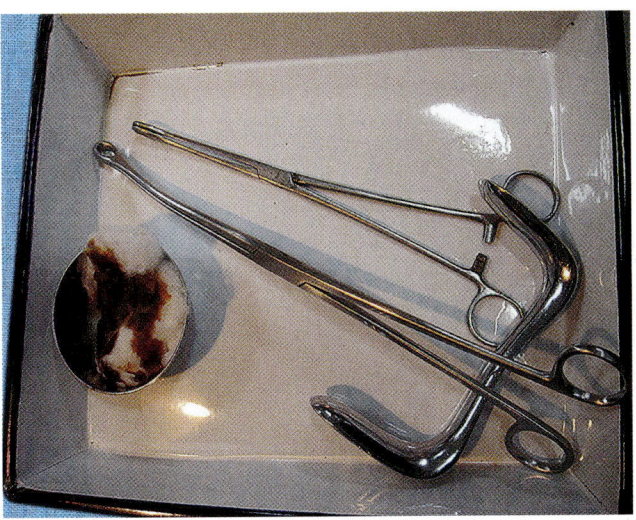

Fig. 48: Instruments necessary for postpartum intrauterine contraceptive device including Kelly's forceps.

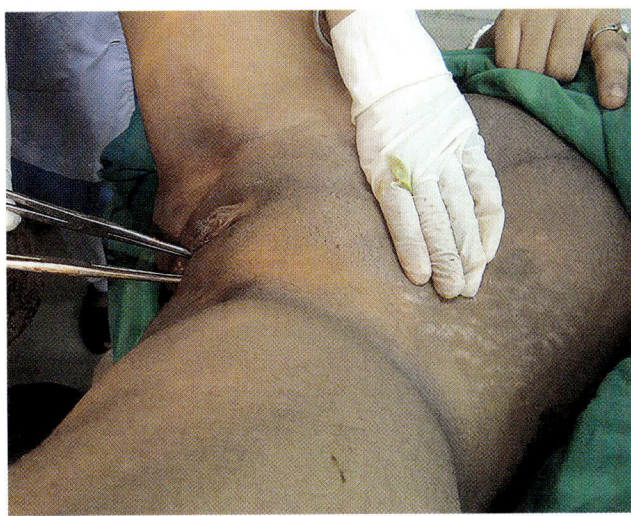

Fig. 51: During insertion left hand kept over uterus to make uterus straighten.

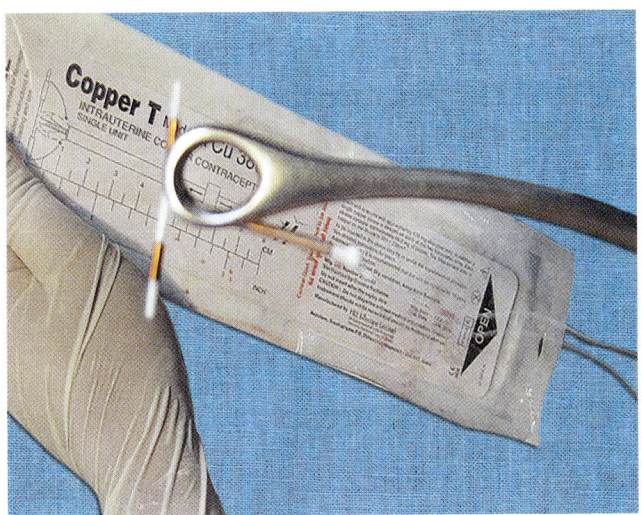

Fig. 49: CuT removed in nontouch technique.

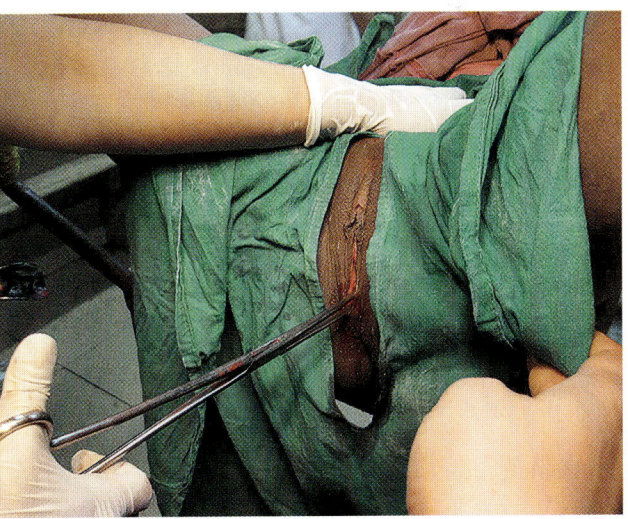

Fig. 52: Before withdrawal of Kelly's forceps, it is opened and shifted to left side away from the device and then withdrawn.

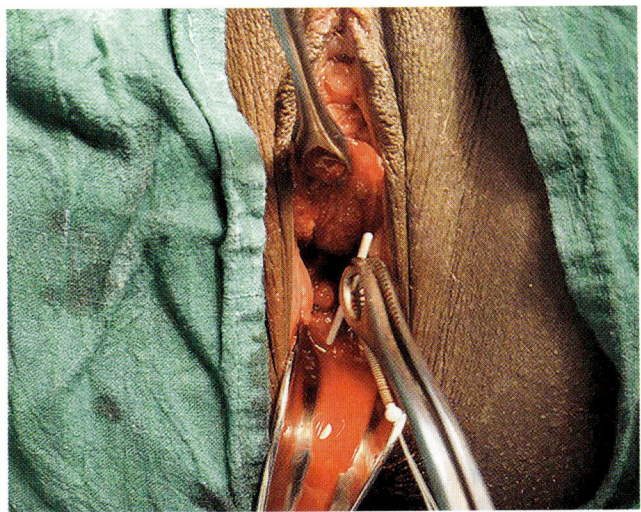

Fig. 50: Intrauterine device with the help of Kelly's forceps is introduced.

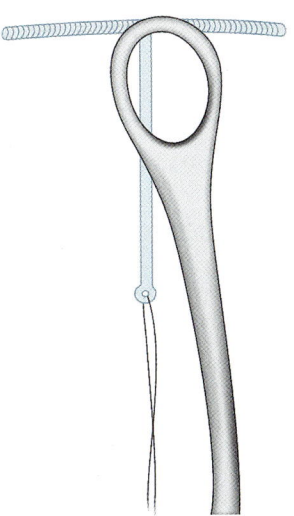

Fig. 53: Method of holding the intrauterine contraceptive device with the Kelly's forceps.

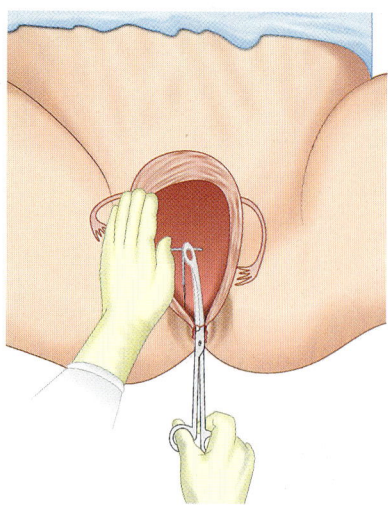

Fig. 54: During insertion left hand kept over uterus to make uterus straighten.

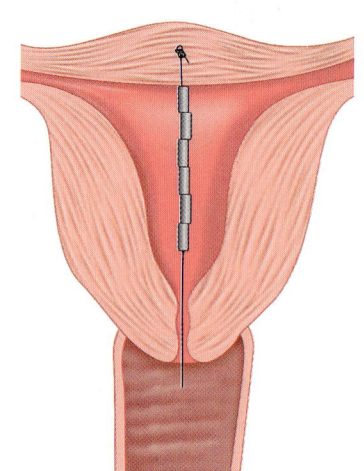

Fig. 55: Frameless intrauterine contraceptive device containing six copper sleeves (GyneFix 330 IUD).

the placenta is removed, the provider inserts the IUCD, and then closes the uterine incision. It is important not to attempt to pass the strings of the IUCD through the cervical os before closure of the uterus as this will displace the IUCD and leave it lower down in the uterine cavity. There is no need to fix the IUCD with a ligature.

In immediate postpartum (within 48 hours after delivery) insertion regular ring forceps is sufficient for insertion.

The provider must insert the IUCD by following all recommended clinical and infection prevention measures for successful insertion.

Patient should be selected according to WHO Medical Eligibility Criteria.

Contraindications

Medical eligibility criteria—Category 3 (relative contraindications):
- Chorioamnionitis
- Prolonged rupture of membranes (>18 hours)
- 48 hours to 6 weeks within delivery.

Medical eligibility criteria—Category 4 (absolute contraindications):
- Postpartum hemorrhage (unresolved)
- Puerperal sepsis
- Extensive genital trauma.

Follow-up

- Woman is advised to return to the clinic for postpartum care at 6th week routinely or earlier if she has serious problems.
- Routine immediate PPIUCD follow-up care should be integrated with standard postpartum services.
- A pelvic examination is done to examine the visibility of the strings and to cut them if the woman finds them uncomfortable.

- At 6 weeks postpartum, the IUCD strings can be felt by some women and majority within 6 months. It is not necessary for her to check the strings. In suspected expulsion or misplaced IUCD sonography is advised.

Frameless IUCD (GyneFix and Fibroplant) (Fig. 55)

Frameless IUCD, *GyneFix 330 IUD* contains 6 copper sleeves **(Fig. 67)** and *GyneFix 200 IUD* contains four copper sleeves are under trial. Copper beads are tied together on a monofilament polypropylene thread. Polypropylene thread is provided with a single knot on the top of thread which is inserted in the myometrium of uterine fundus of 1 cm depth. The minimum effective life of GyneFix 200IUD is 5 years.

Failure rate is 2.5/HWY.

Fibroplant 14 (also 20): A frameless LNG-IUS releasing 14 μm or 20 μg LNG daily and is anchored in the endometrium. Fibroplant 14 is used for 3 years. Frameless IUDs are of smaller size. Pain, bleeding, expulsion, and incidence of ectopic pregnancy are claimed to be less.

LONG-ACTING REVERSIBLE CONTRACEPTIVE (LARC)

Q. What do you mean by LARC?

LARC is long-acting reversible contraceptive. The type of contraception which needs use of once in more than 1 month is called LARC.

LARC includes:
- Injectable progestogens
- Subdermal implant and
- IUCD.

Two injectable progestogens are commonly used namely *DMPA* (150 mg IM every 12 weeks) and *NET-EN* (200 mg IM every 8 weeks) and used as contraceptives from 1960s. Recently, India Government has made available DMPA in the name of "Antara".

Norplant system containing six silastic rods was launched in 1991, later two-rod system *Norplant II* was developed. Subsequently, *Jadelle and Sino-implant II* with *two-rod* followed by development of single-rod implant *Implanon* and latest is *Nexplanon*, a single-rod implant which is effective for 3 years.

Intrauterine device was first described in 1909 containing silkworm gut. Later, Grafenberg made it popularized with silver, later replaced by alloy of copper and zinc. Now, levonorgestrel IUS is available with more advantages and designed by a Finnish doctor, Jouri Valter Tapani Luukkainen. LNG-IUS Mirena, a highly effective contraceptive with a release of constant dose of 20 µg is widely used for using in heavy menstrual bleeding. Very recently, lower dose system with 13.5 mg levonorgestrel for 3 years has been approved. At present in family planning program of Government of India, Cu-T 380A and Multiload 375 are available. LNG-IUS is not provided in family planning program.

Advantages of LARC

- It can be used in all ages.
- LARC is very safe, irrespective of parity, breastfeeding, obese, and diabetes.
- Unplanned pregnancy is less in LARC in comparison to other methods.
- Efficacy very high comparable to sterilization.
- Reversible
- Does not need user's daily attention and high continuation rate. It is not user dependent method.
- Client becomes satisfied.
- No effect on sex.
- Though initial cost is high but cost-effective, less than OCP in 1 year use.
- There are several noncontraceptive benefits.

Contraindications

There are some contraindications of the respective LARC described in respective place.

BARRIER METHODS OF CONTRACEPTIVE

Q. What are the different types of barrier methods?

- Male condom
- Female condom
- Occlusive caps—diaphragm and cervical cap
- Spermicides—creams, jellies, suppositories, aerosol foams, and vaginal contraceptive films
- Contraceptive sponge—today
- Combined.

History and Development of Condom

As written before (*see* Page 461).

Male Condom (Figs. 5, 56 and 57)

Q. What material it is made of and what are the types?

Condoms are mostly made from latex rubber, less commonly lamb cecum, or polyurethane. They are available in various colors and shapes. Length is 15–20 cm, cylindrical, diameter 3–3.5 cm, thickness 0.03–0.07 mm, one end is closed and other end with inbuilt rim.

These may be dry, semidry prelubricated, and may be provided with spermicidal jelly with nonoxynol-9 in outer and inner surface. Individual condom is packed rolled and sealed in aluminum or plastic foil packs.

The male condom is supplied by Government of India free of cost in the name Nirodh and now supplied in new pack (*see* **Fig. 5**).

Efficacy and Failure Rate

Condom is an effective contraceptive method with failure rate in perfect use 2/HWY in first year of use and failure in typical use is 18/HWY.

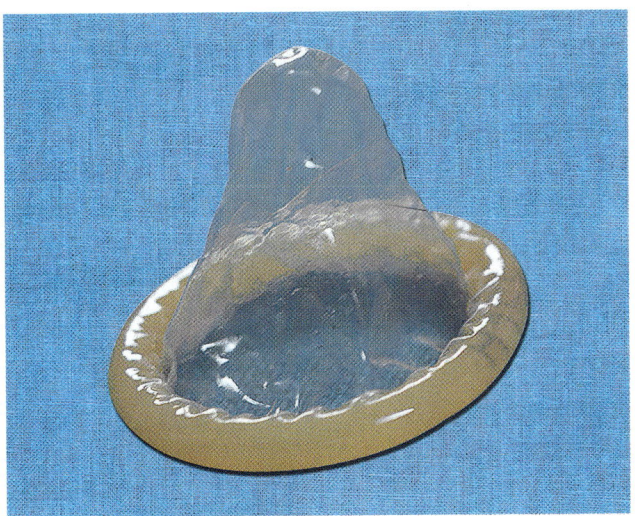

Fig. 56: Male condom.

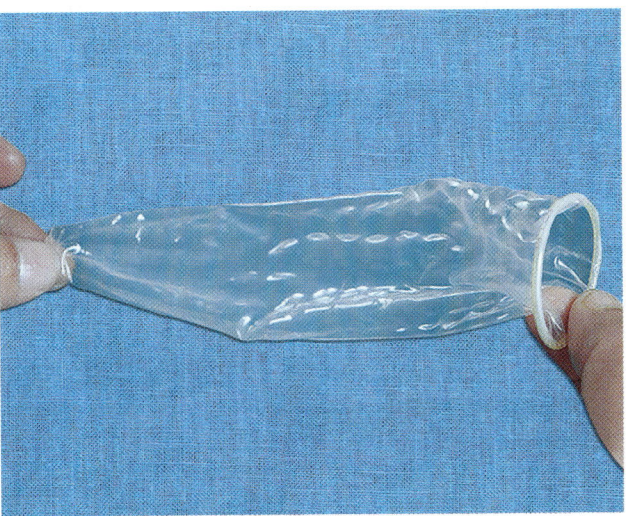

Fig. 57: Male condom—to show the full length.

Q. How efficacy can be improved?

- It will be worn before contact of penis and vagina.
- Penis is withdrawn in erect condition with holding its base.
- Using with spermicide.

Advantages

- Safe, effective, and less costly.
- No medical help or prescription is needed.
- Ideal for couples or partners with infrequent intercourse, e.g., in old age, teen age, and premarital.
- During lactation.
- In case of intolerance to oral contraceptive and IUD.
- Highly protective against STIs, HIV, syphilis, gonorrhea, trichomonas, monilia, non-gonococcal urethritis, and Chlamydia.
- Prevents transmission of herpes virus and HPV.
- Reduces the chance of severe cervical dysplasia and cervical cancer in prolong use in comparison to oral pill or no use of contraceptive.

Q. What is the most important benefit of condom?

Prevention of HIV transmission—80–95% in comparison with nonuser.

Disadvantages

- Interference with sexual pleasure—usually adjusted with practice
- Breakage of condom
- Hypersensitization rarely
- Failure is more than COCs and IUDs
- Problem of disposal for rural village people.

Q. Other than contraceptive what are the other purposes it can be used (noncontraceptive use)?

- For male catheterization
- Prevention of STIs
- Condom tamponade in postpartum hemorrhage
- In transvaginal probe for sonography
- In premature ejaculation.

Q. How to use?

- Condom is unrolled over the erected penis after retracting the foreskin.
- During unrolling over penis, the tip of condom is squeezed to make it air free.
- Prelubricated condom has advantages.
- Immediately after ejaculation penis should be withdrawn in erect condition and holding its base against his body.
- In case of breakage and slippage a spermicidal agent should be inserted into the vagina and she will use emergency contraceptive earliest within 72 hours.

Contraindication

Severe allergy to condom material.

Female Condom (Fig. 58)

Q. What material it is made of and what are the types?

Female condom is made of polyurethane, looks like cylindrical sheath with two rings on two ends, closed and open. The open ring lies outside the vagina and closed ring is placed behind the symphysis pubis beneath the cervix. It is 17 cm long and 7 cm in diameter (larger diameter than male condom). It is prelubricated with dimethicone. It is available in the name of *Femidom*, *Reality*, *Velvet*, etc.

Female and male condoms should not be used together, as there may be slip, displacement, and breakage more.

Efficacy and Failure

Failure rate in typical use is 21/HWY and in perfect use is 5/HWY. Failure is higher than male condom.

Advantages

- It prevents pregnancy by preventing sperms not in contact with female genital tract.
- It prevents STIs including HIV, CMV, and hepatitis B virus.
- It is a method under Woman's control.

Disadvantages

- It is expensive.
- Woman needs motivation and she should acquire the technique of use.
- Slippage is more (1 in 10), sometimes penis may go outside the condom into vagina.
- Chance of breakage is less (0.6%) than male condom.

Vaginal Diaphragm and Spermicide (Fig. 59)

Diaphragm is nearly hemispherical dome of various diameters with a circumferential flexible metal springs. It is made of rubber or latex materials. The common size varies from 60 mm to 80 mm. The required size is determined by the vaginal examination by service provider. In India, it is available as Ortho diaphragm.

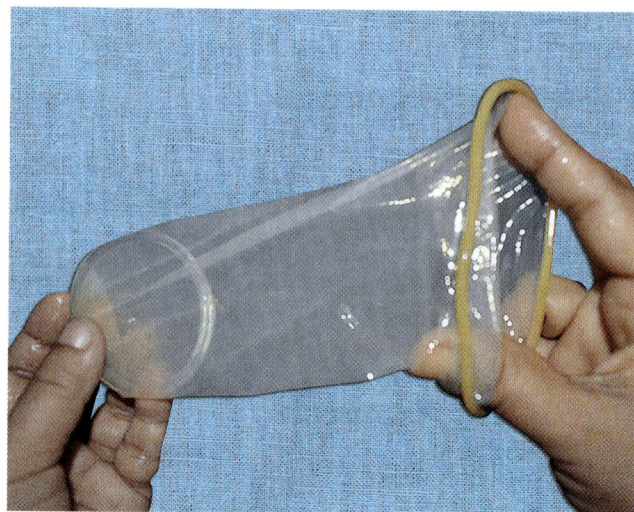

Fig. 58: Female condom.

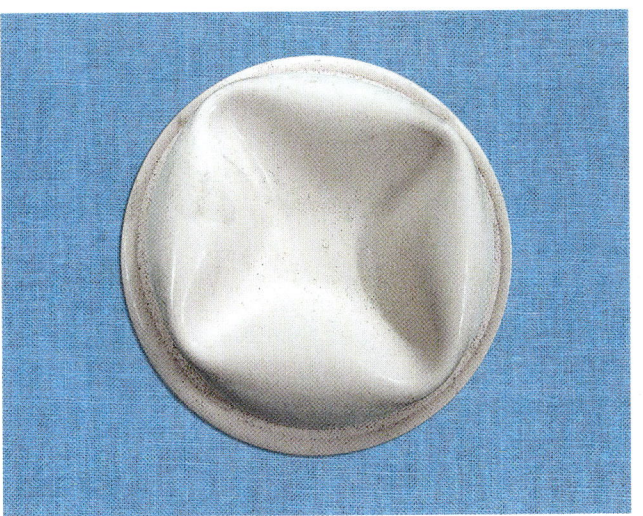

Fig. 59: Vaginal diaphragm.

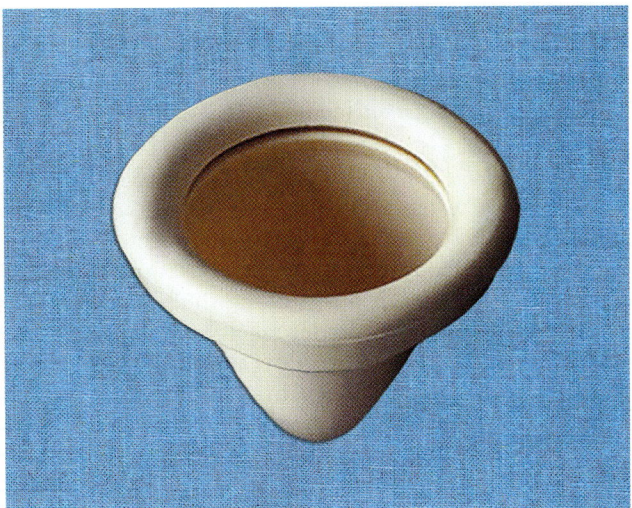

Fig. 60: Cervical cap.

It is used combinely with spermicidal jelly or cream and efficacy becomes very good.

Spermicide is applied over the cervical surface and placed in the vagina to cover the cervix; the rim is placed in the posterior fornix and anteriorly to the inner surface of symphysis pubis. It acts by preventing sperms into the cervical pool and damaging sperms.

Diaphragm is introduced 2 hours before intercourse and kept at least up to 6 hours after intercourse but should not be kept for more than 24 hours for fear of toxic shock syndrome.

Advantage

It prevents pregnancy with good efficacy if properly used. Failure rate in compliant user is 1.9–2.4/HWY.

Disadvantage

It needs high degree of motivation. Irritation to vagina and penis are other factors. In women with prolapse, it cannot be given. Urinary tract infection and vaginal infection may occur.

Cervical Cap or Check Pessary (Fig. 60)

Dome-shaped or thimble like reusable appliance made of silicone or rubber especially designed to fit with the cervix and remain in position by suction. Act by preventing sperm entry into cervix and spermicide are also combined to increase the efficacy. The different diameter available is 22 mm, 26 mm, and 30 mm. It can be introduced any time before intercourse but must be kept at least for 8 hours after intercourse. It is not suitable when cervix is lacerated and irregular. Ortho cervical cap is one commercially available cap.

Spermicides

Spermicides are contraceptive chemical agents capable of destroying sperms. They are available as jellies, creams, foams, suppositories, and film.

The chemical agent is *nonoxynol-9 or otoxynol-9*. They act by physical barrier to sperm penetration and chemical sperm killing action.

They should be given shortly before intercourse as their period of action is maximum 1 hour. Douching should not be done within 6 hours of intercourse. Failure rate is 5–12 pregnancies/ HWY in correct user.

Only spermicidal agents have no protective effects on Chlamydia, HIV, and gonorrhea. Use with male condom has the best result and protecting STIs. The combined spermicide-microbicide agents are under trial and have effect on protecting STIs including HIVs.

The disadvantages are irritation on vagina and penis, and vaginal discharge.

Contraceptive Sponge

Contraceptive sponge *Today* is available in polyurethane disk impregnated with noloxonol-9. It can be inserted up to 24 hours before coitus and to be kept at least for 6 hours after intercourse but not longer than 30 hours. It is more convenient than condom or diaphragm but less effective than those methods. Contraceptive sponge is available in India.

Fertility Awareness-based Methods

Q. What do you mean by fertility awareness-based methods?

Fertility awareness-based methods are defined as identification of fertile days of the menstrual cycle. In the fertile days, the couple either become abstinent or use alternate contraceptive like barrier or spermicidal agents. This is sometimes called *periodic abstinence or natural family planning*.

Broadly, there are two types of fertility awareness-based methods and their combination.

- *Calendar-based method* (standard days method with or without memory aids like CycleBeads or calendar rhythm method by calculating from last 6 months).

- *Symptoms-based method* [two-day method, basal body temperature (BBT) method, ovulation method (also known as Billing's method or cervical mucus method)]
- *Symptothermal method* (combined).

Calendar-based Method

Standard days method: Safe period is from 1st day to 10th day and 18th day to 28th day avoiding unprotected coital act from 11th to 17th day in a 28 day cycle. WHO recommends day 8th to 19th as fertile days during which couple avoids sex or will use any method as described. For memory couple may use CycleBeads (In India, It is available as *Ritumala*) **(Fig. 61)**, a color-coated string of beads indicating fertile and nonfertile days. Where there is variation of cycle days, it is considered that luteal phase is almost constant (14 days).

Calendar rhythm method: As there is variation of days in a cycle of different months woman is asked to record menstrual calendar for last 6 months. About 18 is subtracted from the shortest recorded cycle and this is considered as first day of fertile time. About 11 is subtracted from longest recorded cycle and this estimated day is the last day of her fertile time and risk days are calculated. Couple is advised to avoid unprotected coitus in the risk days.

Symptoms-based Method

This is based on observing signs of fertility. Methods may be two-day method, BBT method, and ovulation method (also known as Billing's method or cervical mucus method). In *two-day method*, the woman is asked to check for cervical secretions at every afternoon and/or evening on fingers, underwear, tissue paper or around the vagina. As soon as she notices any secretion of any type that day and the following day is considered as fertile period. Couple will avoid unprotected sex on those days and following two dry days (without secretion). Drawback is that in vaginal infection or in another condition two-day method is difficult to use.

Billing's method or cervical mucus method: The woman checks the cervical mucus by fingers. Intercourse is safe immediately after period during the dry days till the mucus is detected. Then the couple will avoid sex or use barrier method till the fourth day of peak day and then have unprotected sex till man starts. Peak day is the last day of clear, slippery, stretchy, and wet.

Basal body temperature method: The couple avoids intercourse or uses condom or any other barrier contraceptive from day 1 of menstrual cycle till 3 days after the rise of temperature and then can go for unprotected coitus. This method is hardly used.

Symptothermal method: The combination of BBT method and cervical mucus method is more effective.

Advantages of Fertility Awareness Methods

No side effects and health risk, and no cost.

Disadvantages

Failure rate is high, requires partner's cooperation and motivation, must track of days and be aware of body changes according to method and cannot prevent HIV and AIDS.

Failure Rate of Fertility Awareness Methods

It is very high, pregnancy rate is 25 per/HWY using periodic abstinence. But with consistent and correct use and abstinence in fertile days failure rate is low 0.4–5/HWY.

Withdrawal Method (Coitus Interruptus)

In this procedure, penis is withdrawal from the vagina before ejaculation and ejaculation is done away from vagina. This method is practiced commonly.

Advantage

No cost and no device and always available in every situation.

Disadvantage

Unreliable, pre-ejaculatory prostatic fluid may contain sperms, high failure rate, cause strain to male partner and woman may not be fully satisfied. Male involvement and motivation are most important.

Failure Rate

It is 25/HWY in typical use but in perfect use, it is 4/HWY.

Lactational Amenorrhea Method (LAM)

It is a temporary family planning method based on fertility effect of breastfeeding. LAM inhibits ovulation and causes amenorrhea and prevents pregnancy.

This method requires three conditions, namely:
1. Mother's menstrual period has not returned
2. Baby is fully breastfeeding or nearly fully breastfed and fed often, day and night
3. Baby is less than 6 month old.

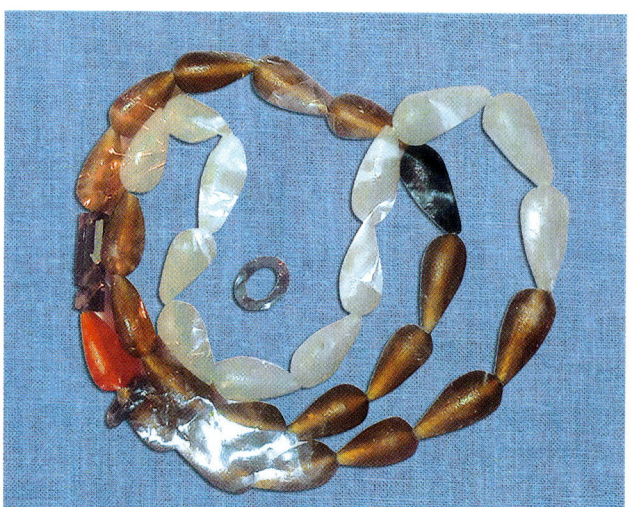

Fig. 61: Ritu mala CycleBead—indicating fertile and nonfertile days.

"Fully breastfeeding" includes both *exclusive breastfeeding* (the infant receives no other fluid, not even water, in addition to breast milk) and *almost-exclusive breastfeeding* (the infant receives vitamins, water, juice, or other nutrients once in a while in addition to breast milk).

"Nearly fully breastfeeding" means that infant receives some liquid or food in addition to breast milk, but the majority of feedings (more than three-fourth of all feeds are breast milk).

Failure Rate

It is 2 pregnancies/100 women using LAM in the first 6 months after childbirth.

Advantage

It is a natural family planning method, provides optimal breastfeeding giving health benefit to both baby and mother and it has no direct cost or no device is needed.

Disadvantages

- "Fully breastfeeding" or "near fully breastfeeding" is not assured.
- Breastfeeding may not be possible always and there is contraindications in certain medications.
- Some newborn cannot breastfeed, e.g., small for date, premature needing intensive care, cleft lift, cleft palate, etc.

Persona

Persona is a combination of mini laboratory and microcomputer. Based on the measurements of the first significant rise in the levels of estrone-3-glucuronide and luteinizing hormone in *urine*, it displays the "safe" (green) and "unsafe" (red) days of woman's cycle. The failure rate is high, 6/HWY, in perfect use.

PERMANENT CONTRACEPTION

Contraception is by:
- Female sterilization
- Male sterilization.

Female Sterilization

Female sterilization is a surgical method by which female losses her ability to conceive permanently.

Occlusion of the fallopian tube in some form is the underlying principle of female sterilization. It is done by: (1) ligation of fallopian tube with—without resection or by (2) blocking both the tubes by any means so that sperm and oocyte cannot come together.

Female sterilization can also be done by nonsurgical method. Hysterectomy causes permanent sterilization but not done for sterilization solely.

Tubal occlusion can be done by:
- Tubal ligation
- Chemical agent in transcervical approach
- Mechanical method—*Essure* by hysteroscopic method.

Tubal Ligation

Tubal ligation is an operation where resection of both the fallopian tube is done to achieve permanent sterilization.

Q. Who introduced the tubal ligation?

In 1823, it was Dr J Blundell from London who first performed tubal ligation. Initially, it was done only for therapeutic purpose. In late 1950s and 1960s, it was accepted as permanent contraceptive technique by many countries and from 1970, it has become very popular globally and at present in many countries including India, it is the most common method of contraception.

Q. How would you categorize tubal ligation according to timing of the surgical procedure?

- *Interval ligation or sterilization:* It is done within 7 days of the beginning of menstrual period (in the follicular phase of the menstrual cycle) or anytime during the cycle if the woman and the provider are reasonably sure that she is not pregnant.
- *Postpartum ligation or sterilization:* It should be done within 7 days of delivery. Usually, first 24 hours are avoided as this period is very vital for the neonate.
- *Postabortal ligation:* Ligation following spontaneous abortion can be performed concurrently or within 7 days of abortion, after excluding infection.
- *Medical termination of pregnancy ligation:* Ligation following MTP can be performed immediately after the procedure if the provider has ensured that the abortion is complete and there is no infection.
- *Medical abortion:* In the next menstrual cycle, if client had undergone medical abortion.
- *Cesarean ligation:* Concurrent with lower segment cesarean section. Sometimes, it can be done with other surgery, e.g., ovarian cystectomy.

Q. What are the various approaches of tubal ligation?

Approach may be:
- Abdominal
  - Conventional
  - Minilaparotomy
  - Laparoscopic
- Vaginal.

Abdominal method (Figs. 62 to 68):

Procedures: Woman is brought to the table after emptying of bladder herself or catheterized and position is dorsal supine.

Anesthesia: General, spinal or local anesthesia is administered. In case of local anesthesia, good sedatives are given.

After dressing and draping a skin incision of 3–4 cm length is given either transverse, midline vertical or paramedian. In interval ligation abdominal incision is given (1 finger

SECTION 4: Birth Control and Population Demography

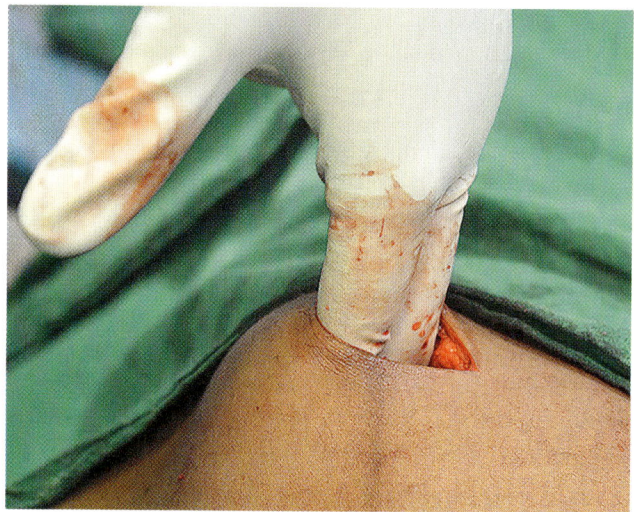

Fig. 62: Tubal ligation—tube is brought out by index and middle finger.

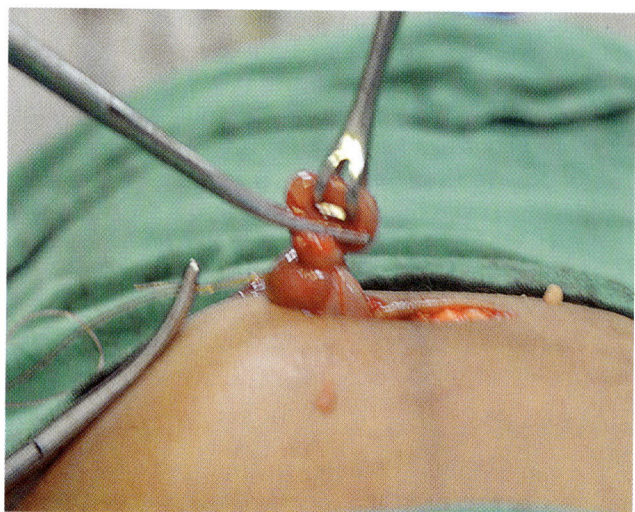

Fig. 65: Pomeroy technique.

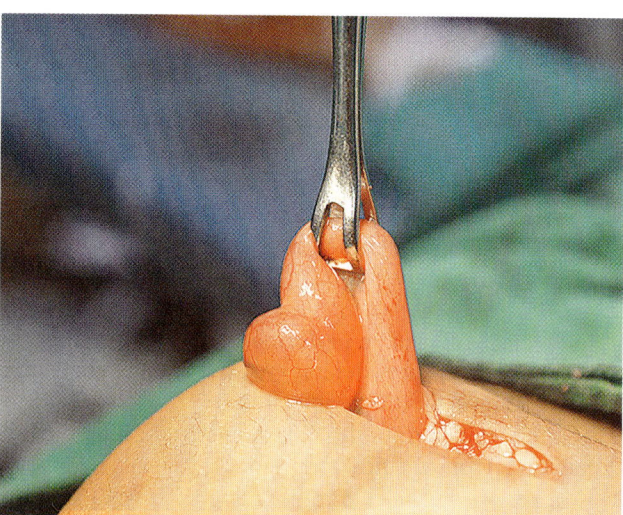

Fig. 63: Tubal ligation—loop of tube is held.

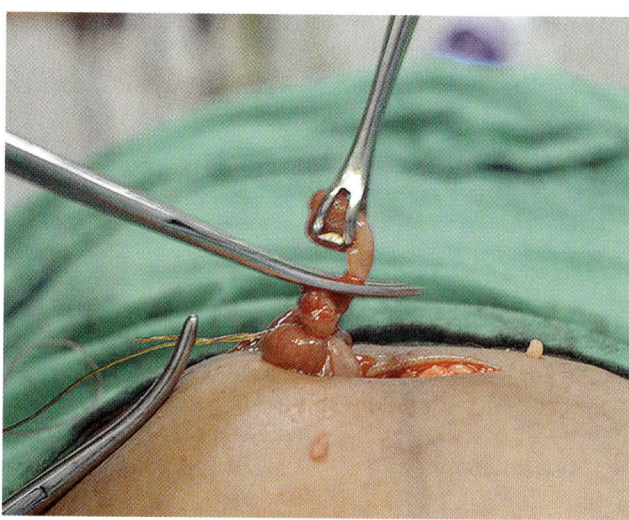

Fig. 66: Pomeroy technique—loop of tube excised.

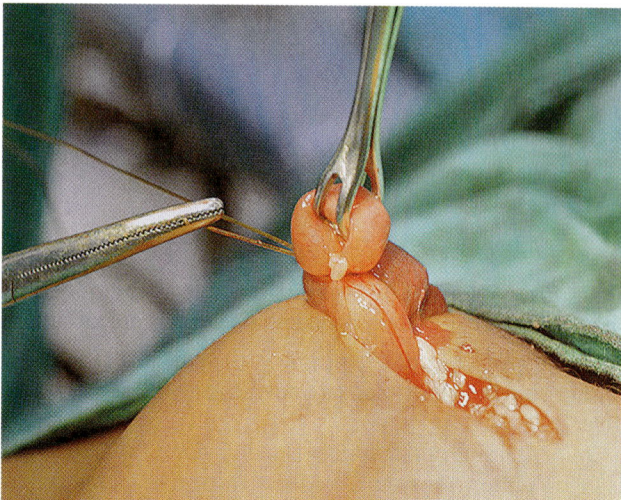

Fig. 64: Ligation by Pomeroy technique.

breadth) 2.5 cm above the symphysis pubis, but in puerperal ligation an incision of 3–4 cm (2 finger breadth) is given 2 cm below the highest point of fundus.

The index finger is passed behind the uterus then laterally behind broad ligament and the tube is hooked **(Fig. 62)**. Fallopian tube is identified by seeing the fimbria. Pomeroy's procedure should be followed for excision and ligation of tube, using a square knot with 1-0 chromic catgut.

POMEROY TECHNIQUE (FIGS. 63 TO 68)

After bringing out the tube through the incision a clamp is placed about 4 cm lateral to the fundus and tube is pulled up so as to form a loop by Allis tissue forceps or Babcock forceps.

- Avoiding the blood vessels by observation against light a round bodied needle is passed through the mesosalpinx.
- The base of the loop is tied with 1-0 catgut stitches keeping about 2 cm of the loop above. The loop is cut and about 1.5

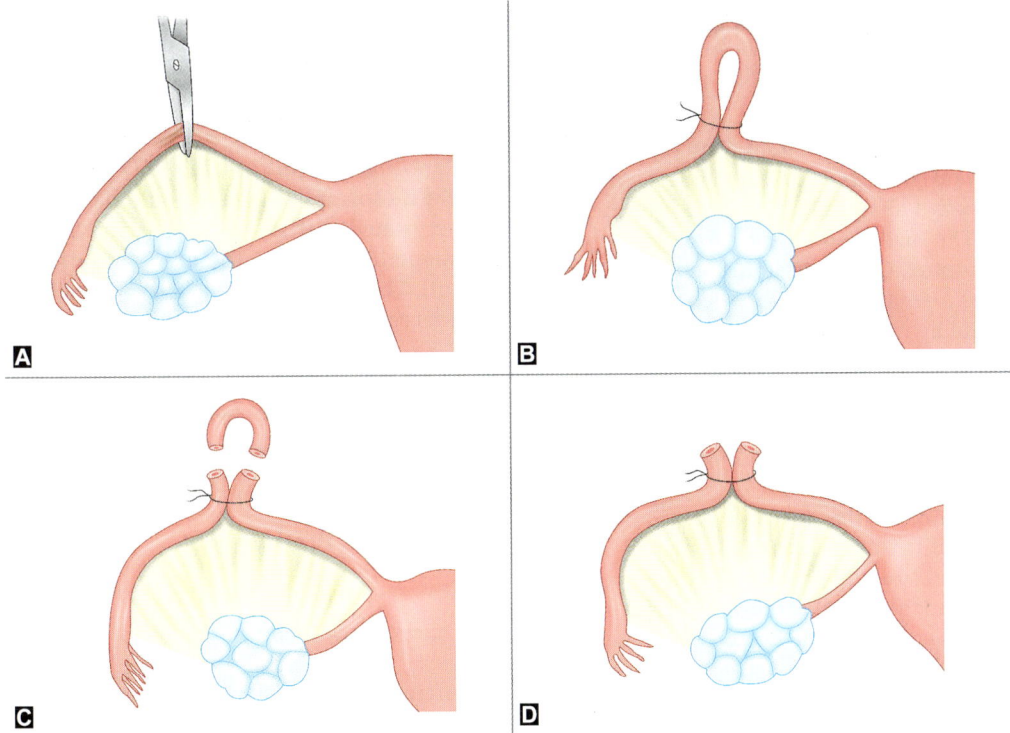

Figs. 67A to D: Pomeroy method of tubal ligation: (A) Tube is pulled up by clamp or forceps (Allis or Babcock) to make a loop; (B) The base of the loop is tied with catgut stitches; (C) Loop is excised; (D) Stump after excision.

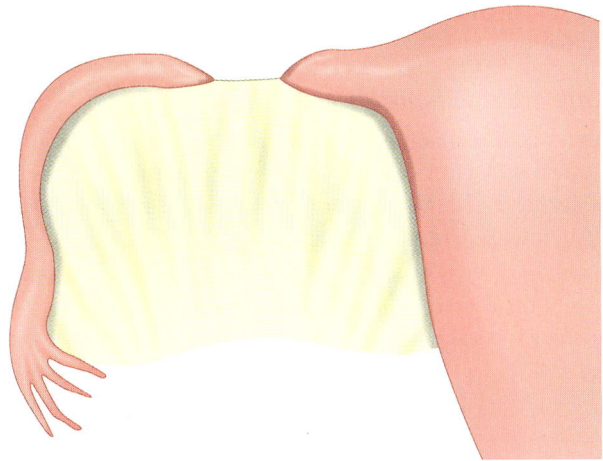

Fig. 68: Look of the cut ends of the tube are separated away after healing.

cm of the loop is removed taking care that the cut margins are not very near to the tie. Care must be taken to avoid damage to the blood vessels, ovaries, and surrounding tissues.

- The stumps are inspected carefully to make sure that the tube is cut completely and to ascertain that there is no bleeding from the stump. Tubal mucosa is seen in resected tubal end. The excised segment of the tube is also examined to be sure that tubal segment is removed and sent for histopathological examination. Both sides are done one after other.
- The skin incision is to be closed with an absorbable or nonabsorbable suture, and a small dressing or bandage applied.

(If the possibility of sterilization reversal is kept in mind the following precautions are taken. The site of the occlusion should be 2–3 cm from the uterine cornu in the isthmal region. Excision of 1 cm of the tube should be done. Use of cautery and crushing of the tube should be avoided.)

Q. Conventional and minilaparotomy—what is the basic difference?

The term minilaparotomy was first described by Osathanondh (1974). The method is suitable as outpatient procedure in health center and camp. It is done with local infiltration of lignocaine under injection pethidine (100 mg), Phenergan (25 mg) intramuscular sedation half an hour before the operation. The operation is done in *semilithotomy or Trendelenburg position*. The abdominal *incision is relatively small*, 2–3 cm in length. *A especially designed uterine elevator* introduced transvaginally is used to push the uterus to one side to bring the tube closed to incisional area. Ligation is done by Pomeroy technique. The method is very suitable for interval ligation. Patient is kept for 4 hours before discharge or if required for overnight. Analgesic is given for 3 days and antibiotics for 5 days. *Time taken, postoperative discomfort, and hospital stay are less* with equal success in minilaparotomy in comparison to conventional technique. Minilaparotomy is safe, convenient, and suitable for mass sterilization.

OTHER TECHNIQUES OF TUBAL STERILIZATION

Q. What are the other techniques of tubal sterilization other than Pomeroy? Describe each in short.

The different techniques for tubal ligation are described next.

- *Irving technique (Figs. 69 and 70):* The tube is ligated twice with chromic catgut about 2.5 cm from the uterine cornu and then cut. The medial end is mobilized by dissecting it from mesosalpinx. On the posterior surface of uterus near the cornu a small tunnel is made in an avascular area. One of the ligatures attached to the medial stump which was kept long is threaded in a needle. The needle is passed through the tunnel to bring about 1.5 cm through the uterine wall. The medial end of tubal is buried and tied in the tunnel. The distal tubal stump is buried in the mesosalpinx which is then closed.
- *Uchida technique:* In the mesosalpinx saline with epinephrine is infiltrated. The muscle layer of the tube is made separated from the serosa. The mesosalpinx is incised to open and the denuded tube is pulled out to form a loop. Tube is cut after putting two clamps. The medial end of the tube is made free from the mesosalpinx and 5 cm of the tube is removed. The medial end of the tube is buried inside the mesosalpinx which is then repaired. The lateral stump is kept outside the mesosalpinx after ligation.
- *Parkland technique (Fig. 71):* An avascular area in the mesosalpinx is selected adjacent to the tube and perforated with a small artery forceps and the jaws are opened to separate the tube from the mesosalpinx (2.5 cm). The freed tube is ligated proximally and distally and intervening segment of the tube of about 2 cm is excised.
- *Kroener's fimbriectomy technique (Fig. 72):* The fimbrial end is ligated twice with silk and then excised.
- *Madlener technique:* In the middle part of the tube, a loop of tube is crushed at the base and ligated with silk suture material.

Failure Rate of Tubal Ligation

Q. What is the failure rate of tubal ligation?

The overall failure rate in tubal ligation is less than 1%; lowest in Irving and Uchida and *highest* in Kroener's fimbriectomy (Pomeroy technique 0.3%, Irving technique 0.1%, Kroener's fimbriectomy 2–3%, Madlener technique 0.3-2%, and Parkland technique 0.25%).

The reasons for failure are surgical error (30–50%), spontaneous recanalization, or the woman was already pregnant at the time of pregnancy—a so called luteal phase pregnancy.

Transcervical Sterilization

Tubal occlusion achieved by transcervical approach either by mechanical device or chemical compounds:
- Mechanical device: Essure (microcoil) and Adiana
- Chemicals: Quinacrine pellets.

Essure (Fig. 73) by hysteroscopic approach: Essure permanent birth control system consists of a spring-like device. This coil device is called microinsert and is enclosed in polyester

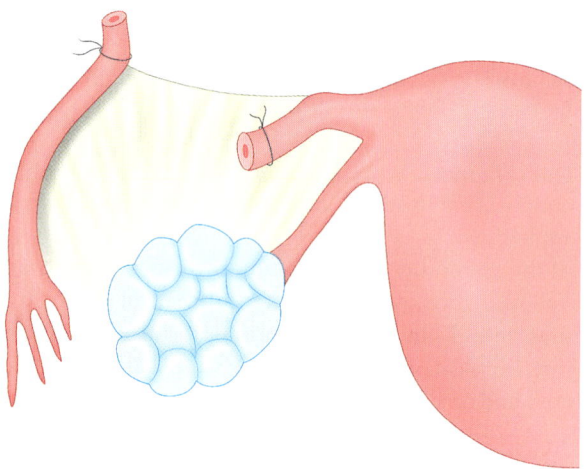

Fig. 69: Irving technique—tube is ligated first (will be placed and numbered first before 5).

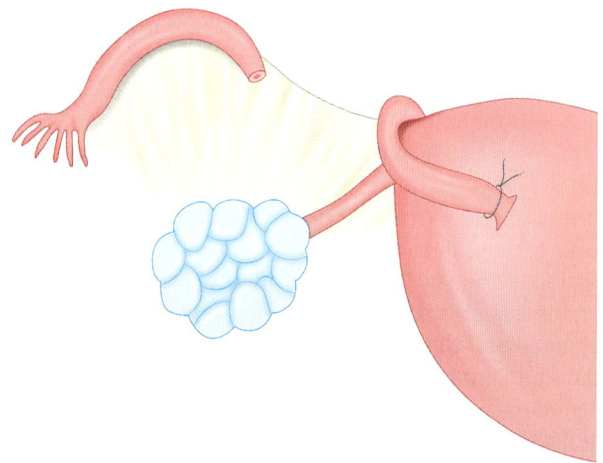

Fig. 70: Irving technique—medial tubal end is buried into a tunnel behind the uterus.

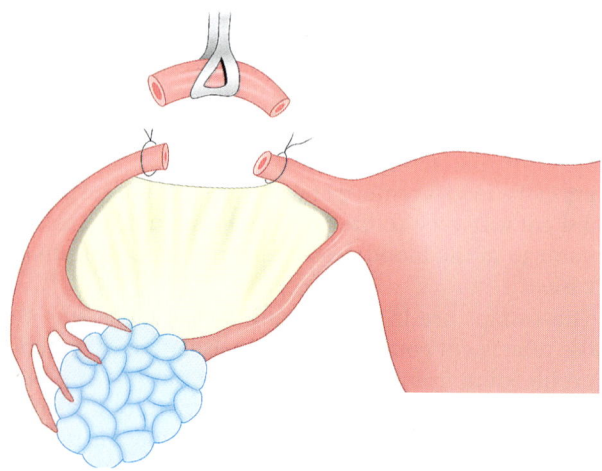

Fig. 71: Parkland technique—intervening segment of tube is excised.

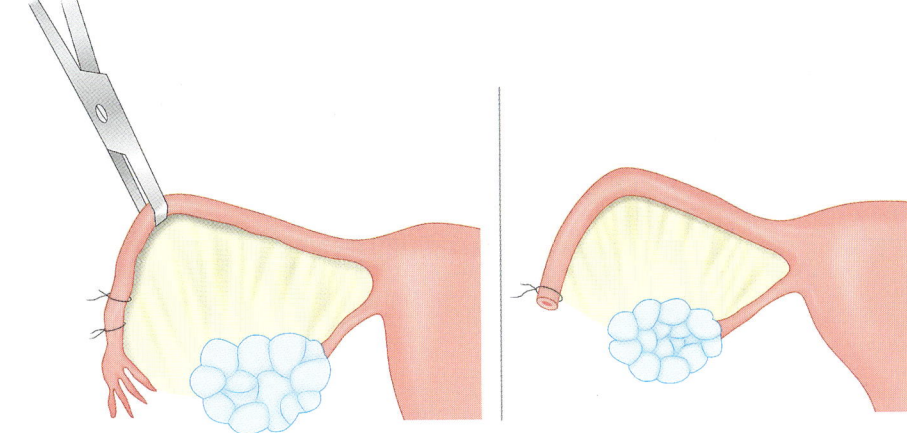

Fig. 72: Kroener's fimbriectomy.

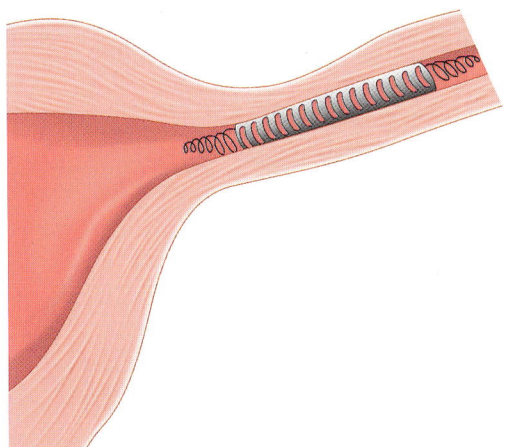

Fig. 73: Essure—a spring-like device is placed in fallopian tube by hysteroscopic approach.

fibers. An expandable outer coil made of nitinol (alloy of nickel and titanium) surrounds these fibers.

Microinsert is introduced through the vagina into the uterus through a **hysteroscope** into the fallopian tube under intravenous sedation or paracervical block. In 3 months' time scar tissue grows into the device and plugs the fallopian tube. The placement of Essure should always be confirmed by hysterosalpingography (after 3 months) or transvaginal sonography, until then the woman must have protected intercourse. Essure is FDA approved. It is done as office procedure and takes less than 20 minutes.

Failure rate is 1–5% after 1 year. Essure placement is considered as permanent sterilization. Contraindications are recent pelvic infection, pregnancy or pregnancy within prior 6 weeks and allergy to its composition.

Adiana—permanent contraception is withdrawn from market since 2013.

Quinacrine pellets: Quinacrine pellet is placed into the uterine fundus near ostia by an IUD-type inserter. It incites an inflammatory response to cause tubal occlusion. It is an effective method and used in resource poor countries. WHO does not recommend its use due to concern of its carcinogenesis.

LAPAROSCOPIC STERILIZATION (FIG. 74)

Female sterilization with laparoscopy has become more popular because its safety, efficacy and simplicity, and with small incisions. But there is need of special instrument and expertise training.

It is done either by single puncture or double puncture technique. In built operating system for applying clips either straight type or angled type is also available for laparoscopic ligation. The instruments needed are fiberoptic lighting system, gas insufflations apparatus for pneumoperitoneum, Verses needle, trocars, and uterine manipulator.

Tubal occlusion methods: Tubes may be occluded by:
- Falope ring (silastic band made of rubber with barium sulfate) **(Figs. 75A to C)**
- Filshie clip (made of titanium) **(Fig. 76)**
- Hulka–Clemens Spring clip **(Fig. 77)**

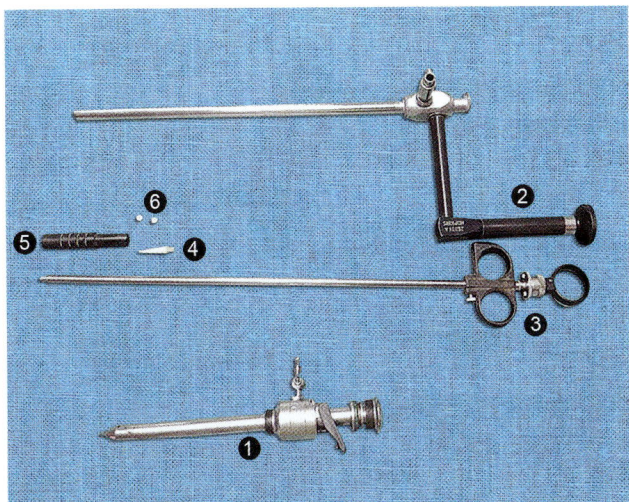

Fig. 74: Instruments for laparoscopic ligation: (1) Trocar cannula, (2) Scope, (3) Tong, (4) Loader, (5) Pusher, and (6) Falope ring.

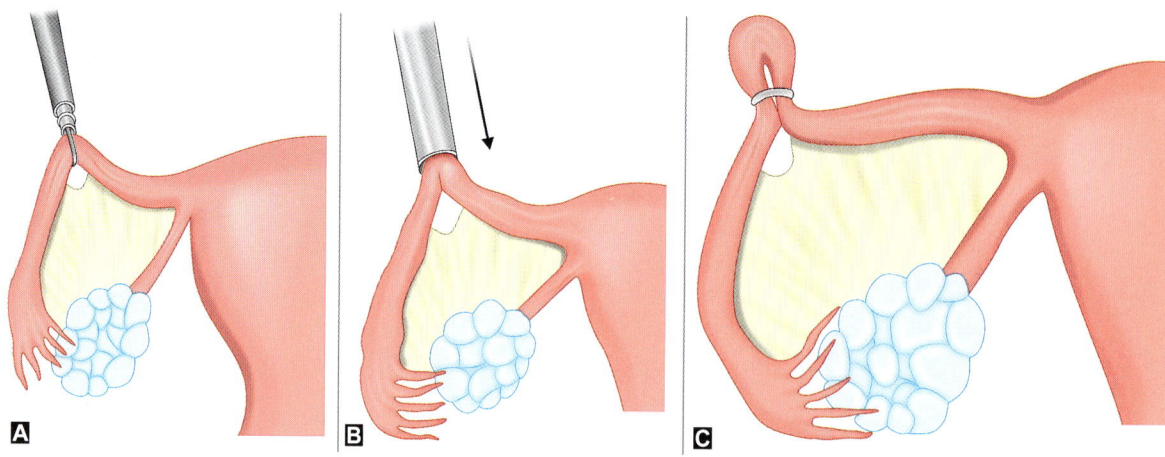

Figs. 75A to C: Laparoscopic tubal ligation by Falope ring (silastic ring).

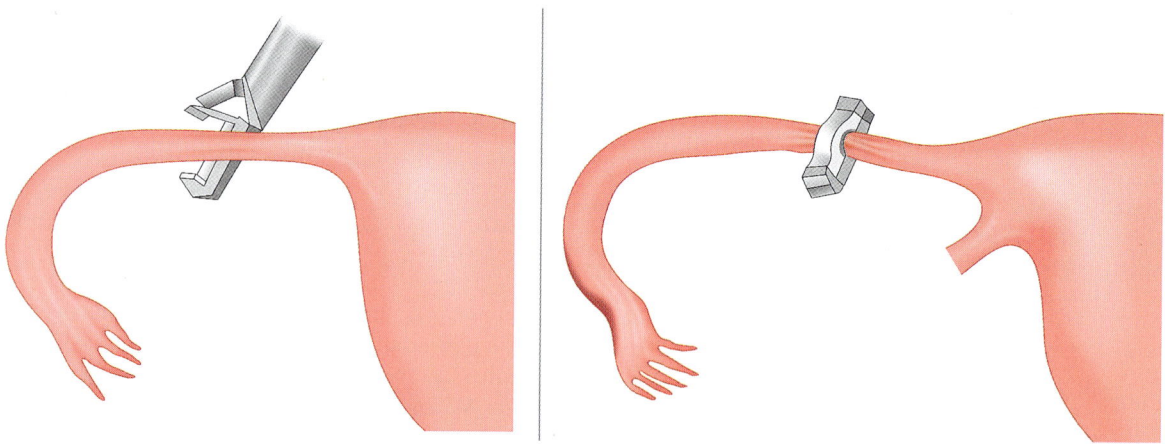

Fig. 76: Laparoscopic ligation by Filshie clip.

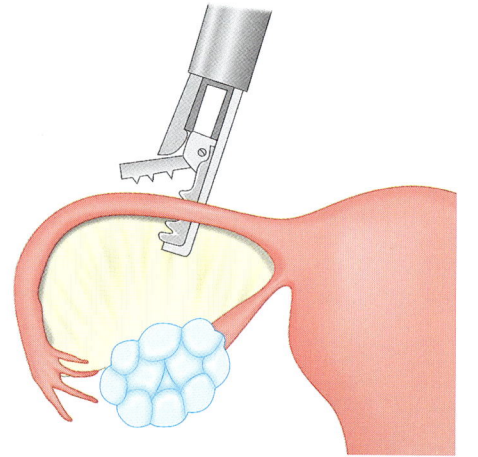

Fig. 77: Laparoscopic ligation by Hulka-Clemens spring clip.

- Tubular coagulation with unipolar or bipolar diathermy (**Fig. 78A**).

Falope ring is popular in India and commonly employed in mass sterilization. Diathermy has a higher failure rate and electrosurgical system is needed.

Procedures of Laparoscopic Tubal Ligation by Falope Ring (Figs. 75A to C and 78B)

Anesthesia: Sedation with pethidine, phenergan and local anesthesia is satisfactory though many surgeons prefer general anesthesia even in outpatient procedure. Position—modified lithotomy position with thigh at 45° angle to the body.

Antiseptic dressing, draping and catheterization is done. Uterine manipulation is done after P/V examination.

After local infiltration with 10 cc of 1% lignocaine Veress needle is introduced at 45° after a small infraumbilical skin incision. The abdomen is inflated with 2 L of CO_2, N_2O, oxygen or air depending upon type of sterilization and availability. In electrocoagulation air or oxygen is not used.

Trocar and cannula is introduced after elevating the abdomen with left hand. After removing the trocar the laparoscope with the ring applicator (tong) preloaded with two silastic ring (Falope) is introduced through the cannula (in single puncture technique). Two Falope rings are loaded in the applicator before insertion with the help of loader and pusher.

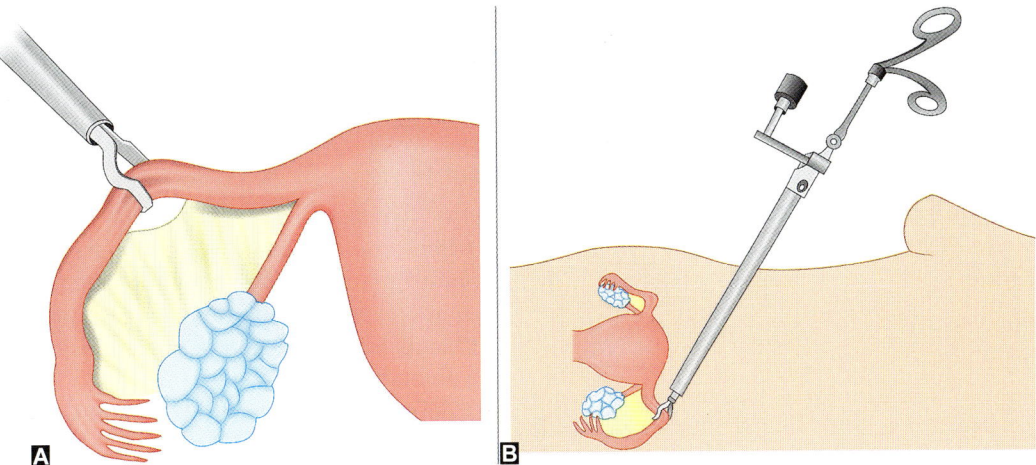

Figs. 78A and B: (A) Laparoscopic ligation by electrocoagulation; (B) Laparoscopy.

The loaded applicator is brought to any one tube first and grasped at the junction of proximal and middle third of tube making a loop and the silastic ring is slipped into the base of the loop and the tube is released from the grasping tong (*see* **Figs. 75A to C**). The same procedure is repeated on other side. When the rings are applied the loops become white due to avascularity.

After final checking of abdominal cavity deflation done and laparoscope is removed. Wound is stitched with catgut stitches.

Advantages of laparoscopic sterilization:
- Very effective like minilaparotomy, can be done as outpatient procedure.
- Safe and complication rate low.
- Can be done under local anesthesia.
- Incision is very small, postoperative pain is less.
- Incidental diagnosis of pelvic pathology.
- Success rate of sterilization reversal is good except in electrocoagulation where there is increased risk of ectopic pregnancy.

Disadvantages of laparoscopic sterilization:
- Though rare serious and life-threatening complication may occur. Embolism, cardiorespiratory distress, and cardiac arrest occur rarely.
- Expensive instrument is needed.
- Surgeon should be properly trained and should be gynecologist.
- It is not suitable for puerperium and large gravid uterus where MTP is done in second trimester.
- Contraindicated in heart disease, respiratory dysfunction, abdominal tumor, and hernias.

Vaginal tubal ligation:
Tubal ligation is done through colpotomy.

Patient is in lithotomy position. After applying the posterior vaginal speculum posterior lip of cervix is held by Allis tissue forceps. Pouch of Douglas is opened by transverse incision and inserting fingers fallopian tube is grasped and brought down by Babcock or curved atraumatic forceps. Tube is ligated with Pomeroy or fimbriectomy method. Colpotomy wound is closed by single layer of catgut stitches.

Advantage: There is no abdominal scar, minimal postoperative pain, can be done as outpatient procedure, and no special instrument is needed.

Contraindications of vaginal ligation: Endometriosis, pelvic infection, and vaginal infection. Trauma and injury of tube, ovaries and gut and severe hemorrhage may occur. Needs expertization in this procedure. Occasionally, failure may occur even by experienced surgeon. General or regional anesthesia is mostly needed. To tackle complication laparotomy may be needed.

Q. What are the complications of tubal sterilization?

Complications of ligation depend on:
- Method of sterilization
- Method of anesthesia
- Route of ligation
- Patient profile
- Technical capability of surgeon.

Minor complications may amount to 14% and major complications may reach a maximum of 1–2%. Complications are more in vaginal than abdominal. It is more following cesarean and MTP than in interval ligation.

Operative complications include:
- Anesthetic hazards
- Cardiorespiratory arrest
- Respiratory depression
- Bowel injury
- Bladder injury
- Injury to tube and ovary
- Broad ligament hematoma
- Bleeding from mesosalpinx
- Convulsion and toxic reaction to anesthetic drugs.

Postoperative complications include:
- Wound infection

- ❖ Wound hematoma
- ❖ Wound dehiscence
- ❖ Pelvic infection
- ❖ Peritonitis
- ❖ Intestinal obstruction
- ❖ UTI
- ❖ Intraperitoneal hemorrhage
- ❖ Bladder or bowel fistula
- ❖ Incisional hernia.

Long-term effects include:

- ❖ Failure—0.4 to 15%.
- ❖ *Ectopic pregnancy:* Incidence of ectopic pregnancy is not increased, however following failure ectopic pregnancy may occur and must be excluded. If pregnancy does occur, 15–20% of such pregnancies are likely to be ectopic. Of all ectopic pregnancies poststerilization ectopic contributes 12%. The probable explanation for ectopic gestations after tubal ligation is recanalization or formation of a tuboperitoneal fistula.
- ❖ *Post-tubal sterilization syndrome:* Gynecologic and psychologic problems following ligation called "post-tubal sterilization syndrome".
- ❖ Psychological problem.

Mortality Following Female Sterilization

1.5/100,000 procedure in USA, in India, it is high 10–70/100,000 procedure. The three major causes of death are anesthetic hazard, sepsis, and hemorrhage.

Efficacy and Failure (WHO) of Female Sterilization

Less than 1 pregnancy per 100 women over the first year after operation (5 per 1,000).

Health Benefits (WHO) of Female Sterilization

- ❖ Protect against risk of pregnancy and PID.
- ❖ *Ovarian cancer prevention*: Bilateral salpingectomy during sterilization may reduce ovarian cancer and the idea has come from the theory of origin of ovarian cancer from epithelium of fallopian tube (*opportunistic salpingectomy*).

Q. How would you select the patients and what are the formal procedures before tubal ligation?

- ❖ Informed choice, informed consent, and preoperative counseling is mandatory.
- ❖ Cases should be selected on the basis of medical eligibility criteria laid by WHO.

Informed Choice and Informed Consent

The purpose of *informed choice* is to ensure that all clients choose the best option/s for their healthcare needs after getting full information about all available options.

Informed consent means that a client understands the surgical procedure and other options and then decides to receive the care.

Q. Who will give consent for permanent sterilization?

Woman herself will give consent. *The consent of the partner (spouse) is not required for sterilization.* However, the partner should be encouraged to come for counseling.

Counseling

Steps before signing the consent form:

- ❖ Clients must be informed of all the available methods of family planning and should be made aware that for all practical purposes this operation is a permanent one.
- ❖ Clients must make an informed decision for sterilization voluntarily.
- ❖ Clients must be counseled whenever required in the language that they understand.
- ❖ Clients should be made to understand what will happen before, during, and after the surgery, its side effects, and potential complications.

The following features of the sterilization procedure should be explained to the client:

- ❖ It is a permanent procedure for preventing future pregnancies.
- ❖ It is a surgical procedure that has a possibility of complications, including failure, requiring further management.
- ❖ It does not affect sexual pleasure, ability or performance.
- ❖ It will not affect the client's strength or ability to perform normal day-to-day functions.
- ❖ Sterilization does not protect against reproductive tract infections, STIs, and HIV/AIDS.
- ❖ A reversal of the surgery is possible, but the reversal involves major surgery and the success of which cannot be guaranteed.
- ❖ In the unlikely event of any complication or failure or death, there is a redressal mechanism available in the form of an indemnity coverage.

Eligibility Criteria for Clients Undergoing Female Sterilization

Self-declaration by the client will be the basis for compiling this information. No eligible client should be denied female sterilization service.

- ❖ Clients should be ever-married.
- ❖ *Female clients should be above the age of 22 years and below the age of 49 years.*
- ❖ *The couple should have at least one child, whose age is above one year, unless the sterilization is medically indicated.*
- ❖ Clients or their spouses/partners must not have undergone sterilization in the past (not applicable in cases of failure of previous sterilization).
- ❖ Clients must be in a sound state of mind, so as to understand the full implications of sterilization.
- ❖ Mentally ill clients must be certified by a psychiatrist and a statement should be given by the legal guardian

or spouse regarding the soundness of the client's state of mind.
- A relevant medical history, physical examination, and laboratory investigations need to be completed to ascertain eligibility for surgery (*see* below—accept, caution, delay, and special).

Q. How will you assess and screen the client?

Assessment and screening of woman are done according to MEC (as detailed below) by the following ways:
- *Patient's particular:* Age, marital status, occupation, religion, educational status, number of living children, and age of the youngest child.
- *Medical history:* History of illness to screen for the diseases mentioned under the medical eligibility criteria immunization status of women for tetanus, current medications, contraceptive used.
- *Menstrual history:* LMP.
- *Obstetric history:* Interval from last pregnancy.
- *Physical examination:* Pulse, BP, respiratory rate, temperature, body weight, general condition and pallor, auscultation of heart, and lungs.

Examination of Abdomen, Pelvic Examination, and Other Examinations as Indicated by the Client's Medical History or General Physical Examination

Laboratory investigations: Routine investigations like hemoglobin (hemoglobin should be ≥7 g/dL) and urine examination for albumin and sugar are necessary. Other investigations may be conducted, if indicated:

Assessment for Eligibility to Undergo Female Sterilization

Client assessment for eligibility to undergo female sterilization is important in minimizing risk of complications.

No medical conditions prevent a woman from undergoing female sterilization (no absolute contraindication) but may limit when, where or how the female sterilization procedure should be performed on the basis of *A, C, D and S* as guided by WHO eligibility criteria.

A = accept: There is no medical reason to deny sterilization to a person with this condition.

C = caution: The procedure is normally conducted in a routine setting, but with extra preparation and precautions.

D = delay: The procedure is delayed until the condition is evaluated and/or corrected. Alternative temporary methods of contraception should be provided.

S = special: The procedure should be undertaken in a setting with an experienced surgeon and staff, equipment needed to provide general anesthesia, and other back-up medical support. Alternative temporary methods of contraception should be provided if referral is required or there is otherwise any delay.

The following are the conditions included in caution, delay, and special categories:

Caution: Previous abdominal or pelvic surgery, obesity, controlled BP (140-159/90-99), uncomplicated heart disease, history of ischemic heart disease, stroke, history of cerebrovascular accident, history of DVT or pulmonary embolism, epilepsy, depressive disorders, current breast cancer, uterine fibroids, PID without subsequent pregnancy, uncomplicated diabetes, hypothyroidism, mild cirrhosis, liver tumors, kidney disease, thalassemia and sickle cell disease, and HIV.

Delay: Severe iron deficiency anemia (hemoglobin <7 g/dL), current pregnancy, 8-42 days postpartum, pregnancy with severe pre-eclampsia or eclampsia, postpartum or postabortion complications (infection, hemorrhage, and trauma), current DVT/PE, major surgery with prolonged immobilization, abdominal skin infections, current ischemic heart disease, lung disease like pneumonia, systemic infection, unexplained vaginal bleeding, large collection of blood in uterus, malignant trophoblastic disease, cancers of the genital tract, current PID, current purulent cervicitis, chlamydia, gonorrhea, current gallbladder disease, and uncontrolled diabetes.

Special: Conditions that increase chances of heart disease or stroke, i.e., older age, smoking, high BP or diabetes; blood pressure above 160/100 mm Hg, complicated heart disease, coagulation disorders, chronic lung diseases (asthma or emphysema), endometriosis, pelvic tuberculosis, fixed uterus due to previous surgery or infection, abdominal wall or umbilical hernia, postpartum or postabortion uterine rupture or perforation, diabetes of 20 years standing with organ damage, hyperthyroidism, severe cirrhosis of liver, and AIDS.

Offer the client another contraceptive method till the procedure can be performed.

Q. Who can do tubectomy?
- For minilap any MBBS doctor with training can do the procedure.
- For laparoscopic ligation: Person with recognized postgraduate degree, Diploma in Obstetrics and Gynecology, and also by MS surgery degree holder trained in laparoscopic sterilization.

Certificate of Sterilization

A certificate of sterilization is given by the medical officer of the facility after 1 month of sterilization or after first menstrual period.

Male Sterilization

Permanent sterilization of men is *bilateral vas ligation and also called vasectomy* which is accepted universally (**Figs. 79 and 80**).
- Vasectomy is one of the safest and very effective contraceptive methods with very low complication and failure rates.
- Vasectomy is a very simple minor surgical procedure that takes about 10-15 minutes to perform, with minimal

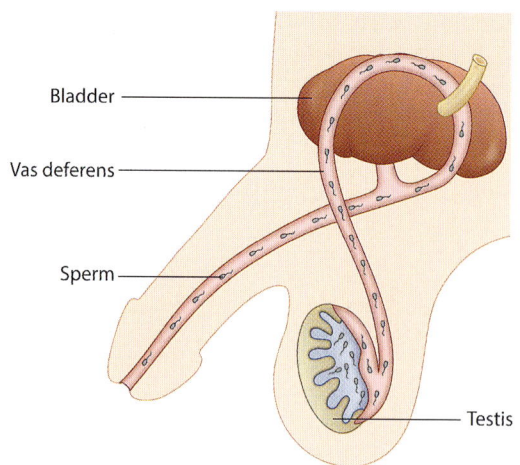

Fig. 79: Normal anatomy of male genital tract.

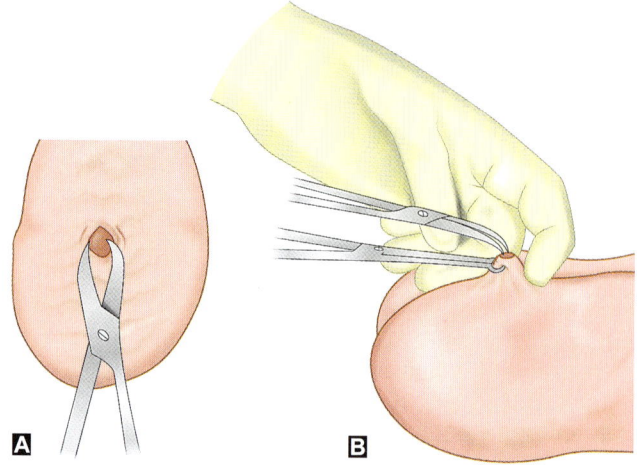

Figs. 81A and B: (A) Vas is grasped extracutaneously by the ringed clamp; (B) Puncture is made with dissecting forceps and puncture site is enlarged.

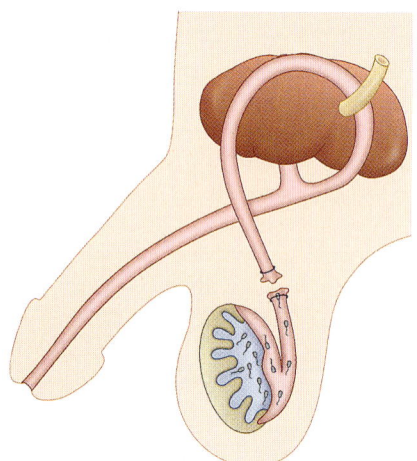

Fig. 80: Schematic diagram of vas ligation (vasectomy).

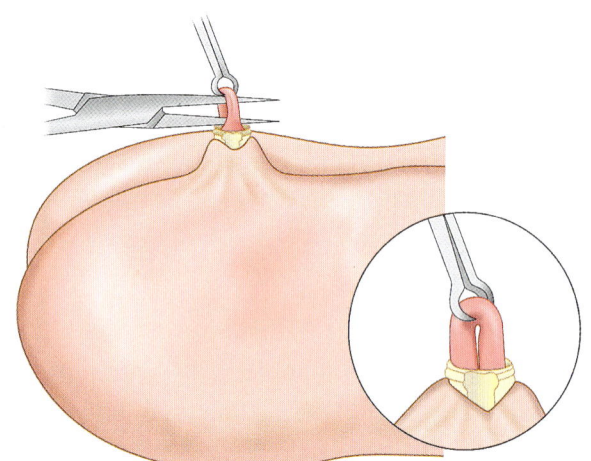

Fig. 82: A loop of vas is brought out.

bleeding during the procedure. The man can walk back home within 30 minutes after the procedure.
- Vasectomy involves identification of vas at the top of the scrotum after small skin incision or puncture, transection of both vas and ligation of both sides done under local anesthesia as an outpatient procedure.
- Sperm cannot pass to the distal part of vas and the seminal ejaculate does not contain any sperm and pregnancy does not occur.

Types

Types include conventional and nonscalpel vasectomy.

Nonscalpel vasectomy (Figs. 81 to 89): Nonscalpel vasectomy is now popular with many advantages over conventional as scalpel is not used instead only single puncture is done, hence no stitch is needed and in contrast to conventional method multiple punctures is not needed for anesthesia and single needle prick is sufficient and less time is needed, postoperative pain and complications are less.

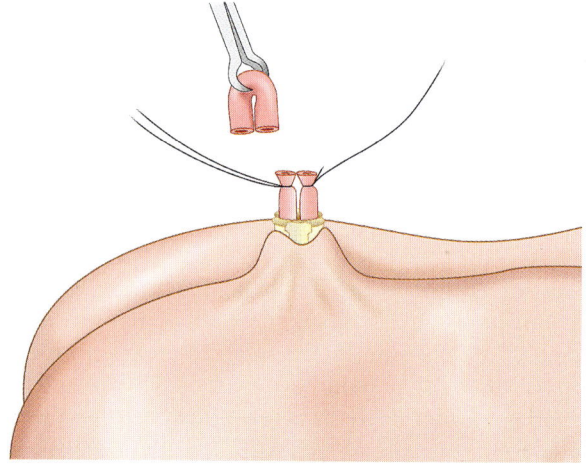

Fig. 83: 1–2 cm vas is excised after silk suture tying of each end separately.

CHAPTER 22: Family Planning and Contraception

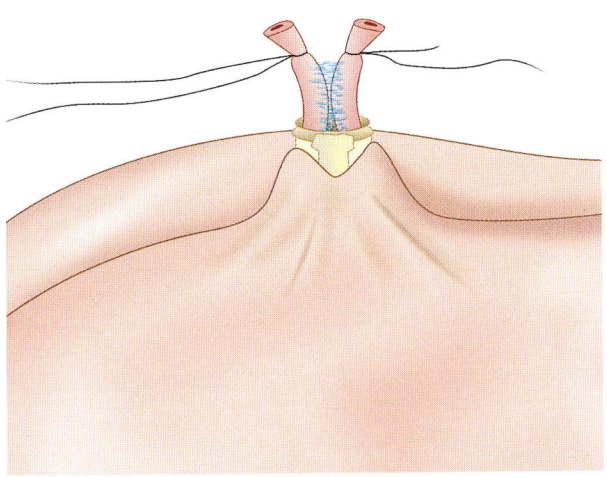

Fig. 84: Tied cut ends of vas.

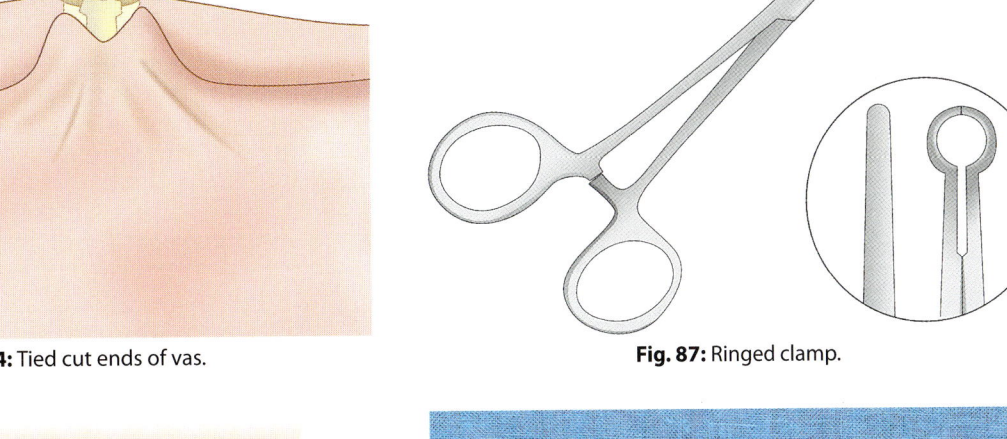

Fig. 87: Ringed clamp.

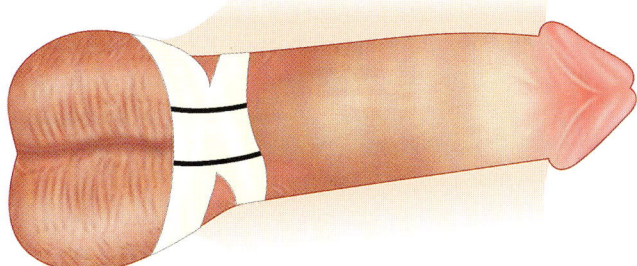

Fig. 85: Dressing of puncture site without stitch.

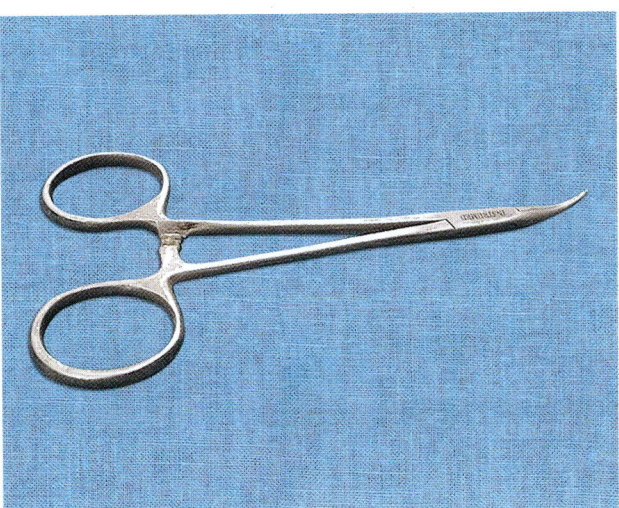

Fig. 88: Dissecting forceps for nonscalpel vasectomy.

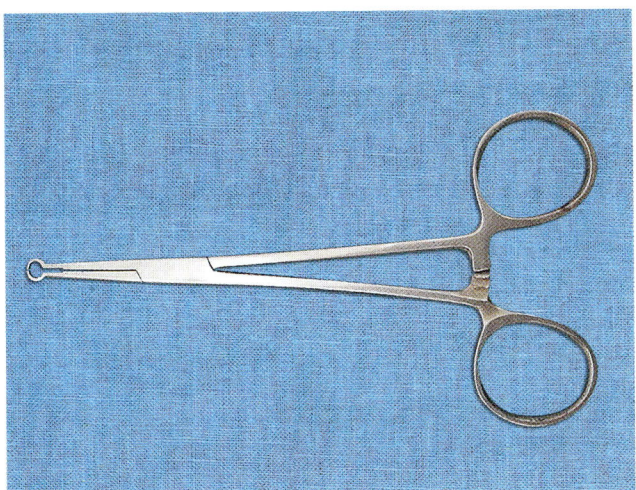

Fig. 86: Ringed clamp for nonscalpel vasectomy.

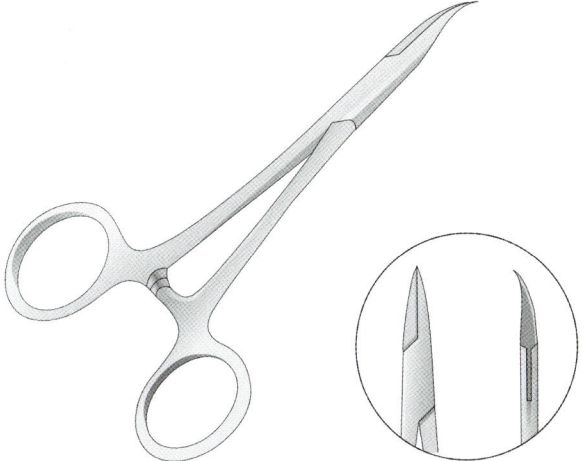

Fig. 89: Sharp pointed tip dissecting forceps.

Nonscalpel vasectomy was introduced by Dr Li Shunqiang in 1974 from China.

Instrument needed: Two special instruments are needed:
- Extracutaneous ringed clamp—a special variety of clamp when closed a ring is formed of 3–4 mm which is used to hold the vas extracutaneously without injuring it **(Figs. 86 and 87)**.
- Dissecting forceps looking like mosquito forceps with sharply pointed tip **(Figs. 88 and 89)**.

Procedure: Genital area is washed with soap and water and the man is brought to the table with surgical gown. Following antiseptic dressing and draping and retracting the penis away from the area 10 mL of 1% lignocaine is injected into the

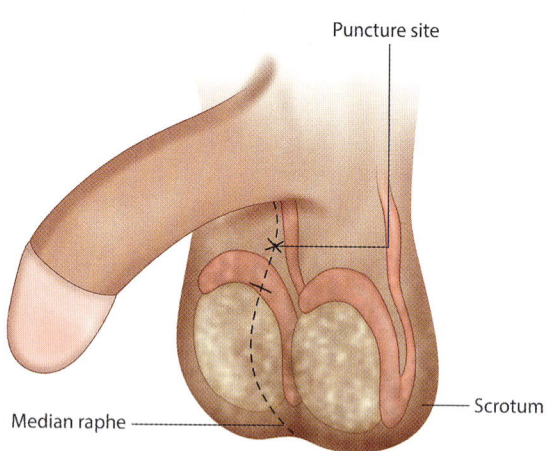

Fig. 90: Nonscalpel vasectomy—puncture site.

scrotal skin in the midline (median raphe) and then along the vas usually on the right within the external spermatic fascia toward inguinal ring. The other side is anesthetized with the same puncture site **(Fig. 90)**.

After fixing by the three-finger technique, the vas is grasped extracutaneously by the ringed clamp (*see* **Fig. 81A**) and elevated.

A puncture is made on scrotal skin directly over the vas using one blade of the dissecting forceps and pushed. It is withdrawn and both blades are introduced in closed condition and spread to enlarge the puncture hole including the perivascial sheath (*see* **Fig. 81B**).

A loop of vas is brought out by dissecting forceps after removing the ringed clamp (*see* **Fig. 82**). The vas is then ligated, 1–2 cm of vas is excised and cut ends of vas are tied with nonabsorbable 2-0 silk stitches (*see* **Figs. 83 and 84**). The other vas is dealt in similar manner.

Then puncture site is pinched for a minute to arrest any oozing and dressing is done with sterile gauze and adhesive tape (*see* **Fig. 85**).

After taking rest for half an hour man can stand and can leave after 1 hour.

Postoperative advice: The scrotum is supported by tight underwear or suspensory bandage for 24 hours. Man will take rest for 24–48 hours in supine position. He can join his work after 1 week, even after 3 days if he feels comfortable and can have sex after 3 days.

Any hemorrhage, swelling or severe pain should be reported. Antibiotic and mild analgesics are given. For first 3 months, additional contraceptive is advised. It needs 20 ejaculations to clear all stored sperms.

Semen analysis is done after 4 months. After 4 months if two samples are found without sperm on two occasions the procedure is declared as successful.

Complications:
- Immediate: Infection, hematoma formation, and pain
- Delayed: (1) Postvasectomy syndrome (chronic local pain); (2) Sperm granuloma; (3) Failure; and (4) Impotency following vasectomy is a myth.

Failure rate: It is 0.15/HWY.

Myth about vasectomy:
- Does it make the man impotent? No
- Does it decrease sex drive? No
- In this procedure is testes removed? No
- Following vasectomy does the man become weak? No
- Does vasectomy cause any other disease? No

Sterilization does not protect against STIs, including HIV. If there is a risk of STI/HIV, the correct and consistent use of condoms is recommended.

ELIGIBILITY OF MALE STERILIZATION

Self-declaration by the client will be on the basis of compiling this information:
- Clients should be *at least 22 years old and should be below the age of 60 years.*
- Clients should be *ever-married.*
- The couple *should have at least one child, whose age is above 1 year* unless the sterilization is medically indicated.
- Clients or their spouses must not have undergone sterilization in the past (not applicable in the cases of failure of previous sterilization).
- Clients must be in a sound state of mind, so as to understand the full implications of sterilization.
- Mentally, ill clients must be certified by a psychiatrist, and a statement should be given by the legal guardian or spouse regarding the soundness of the client's state of mind.

Eligibility of providers: Any trained and empanelled MBBS doctor can provide vasectomy services in government institutions and accredited private/NGO facilities.

The state maintains a district-wise list of doctors empanelled for performing sterilization operations in government institutions and accredited private/NGO facilities.

Medical Eligibility Criteria for Male Sterilization

No medical conditions prevent a man from using vasectomy. All men can have vasectomy. There are some medical conditions that may limit when, where, or how the vasectomy should be performed.

The criteria is categorized like female sterilization—*A = accept; C = caution; D = delay, and S = special.*

The following are the conditions included in caution, delay, and special categories in male sterilization:
- *Caution:*
  - Young age
  - Depressive disorders
  - Diabetes
  - Previous scrotal injury
  - Large varicocele
  - Large hydrocele.

- *Delay:*
  - Local skin infection: (1) Scrotal skin infection; (2) Active STI; (3) Balanitis (4) Epididymitis or orchitis
  - Systemic infection or gastroenteritis
  - Filariasis and elephantiasis
  - Intrascrotal mass.
- *Special:*
  - Coagulation disorders
  - Cryptorchidism
  - Inguinal hernia

Consent

Consent of wife is not necessary.

OTHER MALE CONTRACEPTIVES

Q. What is the present scenario of male contraception?

Presently male method of contraception accounts for only 30% of worldwide use. Up till now, the male contraceptive methods are restricted to condom, natural method (withdrawal method, abstinence) and vasectomy and there is no method approved clinically for pharmacological regulation of male fertility at present.

Recent renewed interest has been focused on male fertility regulation partly due to arousal of women's rights even in developing countries and partly for searching newer methods of contraception to combat population explosion.

Q. How male fertility regulation can be achieved?

The male fertility regulation can be achieved by:
- Preventing the deposition of sperm in the female genital tract.
- By vas occlusion (blocking) thus preventing the emission of sperm with seminal fluid.
- Inhibiting spermatogenesis or its maturation or destroying fertilizing capacity or by killing or by hormonal or nonhormonal methods.

Prevention of Deposition of Sperm in the Female Genital Tract

It can be achieved by: (1) Barrier method, e.g., condom or by (2) Natural family planning method, e.g., withdrawal method and rhythm method (abstinence).

Q. How vas occlusion can be done?

This may be done by:
- Vasectomy
- Injection of sclerosing agents into the vas lumen
- Intravasal introduction of nylon thread as intravasal contraceptive device (IVCD)
- By using clips or by vas valves.

Vasectomy: Vasectomy is very safe, simple, effective, and is widely used. A technique of "NO SCALPEL VASECTOMY (NSV)" developed by Dr Li Shunqiang in China in 1974 is used in many countries since 1986 and is very popular.

The *sclerosing agents* like liquid polyurethane after injection into the vas lumen hardens and blocks the passage of sperm. The disadvantages are: (1) the procedure is technically difficult to perform and (2) disappearance rate of sperm from the ejaculate may be slower than in conventional vasectomy.

Solid silicone plugs: Two for each vas are inserted surgically inside the vas lumen to block the passage of sperm. Each plug is fixed with nylon thread. One such device is called "SHUG".

The *IVCD* has been attempted with thick nylon but is not popular due to high failure rate.

Application of *metallic clip* through a tiny puncture hole has been tested in dogs but has not been attempted on humans.

Attempts have been made to prepare *vas valves* so that the passage of sperm can be controlled but none is found to be promising till now.

Inhibiting spermatogenesis or its maturation or destroying fertilizing capacity or by killing:
- Hormonal method and
- Nonhormonal method.

Hormonal Method of Male Contraception

Various drugs have been tried for male contraception; ideally, a male version of the female oral contraceptive should be available.

Because spermatogenesis is dependent on gonadotropins, an obvious contraceptive approach is suppression with exogenous steroids.

Resultant suppression of testicular steroidogenesis due to suppression of gonadotropin requires coadministration of androgen to prevent the symptoms and consequences of hypogonadism. On this physiological basis, steroid hormones have been attempted to suppress spermatogenesis and studies have been carried out.
- Androgen alone
- Androgen-progestogen combination:
  - Medroxyprogesterone acetate
  - Cyproterone acetate
  - LNG
  - Desogestrel and etonogestrel
  - Norethisterone.
- Estrogens
- Testosterone with gonadotropin-releasing hormone (GnRH) analogs: GnRH agonists and GnRH antagonists.

Testosterone alone: Different preparations of testosterone in various routes have been studied. Various preparations are: (1) Testosterone propionate; (2) Testosterone enanthate; (3) Testosterone undecanoate; (4) Testosterone buciclate. It can be used in subdermal, implant, pellete, and intramuscular route.

Due to long-term side effects, it is unlikely that testosterone alone will be developed as a male contraceptive.

Androgen-progestogen combination: Progesterone-androgen combination should be the ideal male pill where progesterone component suppresses pituitary gonadotropin release and androgen component maintains libido and male secondary sexual character. Norplant, DMPA, NET-EN, desogestrel, and etonogestrel are used along with testosterone.

Nonhormonal Agents and Plant Products

Nonhormonal agents and plant products inhibiting spermatogenesis and sperm maturation: Gossypol, *Tripterygium wilfordii,* and 6-chloro-6-deoxy sugars and α-chlorohydrin.

- *Gossypol,* a polyphenolic yellow pigment found in the seed, stem, and roots of the cotton plant, whose antifertility effects were first identified in the 1950s. Due to high incidence of irreversibility and potential serious hazards, use of gossypol as contraceptive has not been very popular.
- *T. wilfordii* is a multiglycoside extract of the plant *T. wilfordii*, long used in China for the treatment of psoriasis and has been attempted as a reversible male fertility control agent
- *6-chloro-6-deoxy sugars and α-chlorohydrin* acts on epididymal spermatozoa by inhibition of glycolytic activity. Unfortunately, the neurotoxic effects of these compounds prohibit their use in male fertility regulation.
- *Reversible inhibition of sperm under guidance (RISUG)* is a nonhormonal male method and has been studied in India (Guha SK, et al. 1997). It contains styrene maleic anhydride which when injected into the vas inhibits the sperm transport by changing the pH incompatible for sperm. *Vasagel* with different combination with similar approach has been studied in United states.

Summary of Male Contraceptive

- ❖ Other than condom, rhythm method, coitus interruptus, and vasectomy no clinically approved pharmacological methods or agents are still available as male contraceptive.
- ❖ At present, the study on using a long-acting injectable testosterone and depot progestin is well advanced and may be available for clinical use in near future.

ANTIFERTILITY VACCINE

Development of contraceptive vaccines for both male and female has been tried. Theoretically, a vaccine against any component of regulatory pathway of reproduction is possible.

Phase I trial for contraceptive vaccine shows promising hope and phase II trial is on the way in different centers in India. Passive or active immunization against FSH has been tried but its use been discarded for fear of creating autoimmune reactions. Work on anti-GnRH vaccines for fertility control has shown bad effects on sex hormone production and sex organs of both males and females and inconsistent effect on spermatogenesis. Anti-hCG vaccine shows a great promise but far way to bring in clinical practice. In practice, it will take many more years before a vaccine is successfully developed for contraception. Vaccine production in male is at present concentrated for treatment of prostate cancer rather than fertility control.

23 CHAPTER

Demography and Family Planning Programs in India—Present Scenario

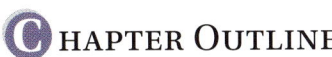HAPTER OUTLINE

- Magnitude of Problems
- Fertility Indicators
- Modern Contraceptive Uses in India
- Unmet Need
- Milestones of Family Planning in India
- RMNCH+A
- Contraceptives—India Government Supply

MAGNITUDE OF THE PROBLEM

India is the second most populous country of the world next to China. It harbors 17.5% of the world's population in only 2.4% of the global land mass. India contributes about 20% of births worldwide. In the last census 2011, total population of India had reached to 121 crores. Total absolute increase in population during the last decade was 18.15 crores. Population growth during that decade is 17.64% which was though lower in comparison to 21.15% of 2001 census still it is higher considering the need of arresting population growth. The combined population of Uttar Pradesh and Maharashtra is bigger than that of the United States.

At present, world's population is estimated to be almost **7.98 billion** (2022). China is the most populous nation. At present (2022), **India's** population is **1.41 billion** contributing **17.7%** and that of **China** is **1.45 billion** contributing **18.47%** of World's population (**Fig. 1**). It was estimated from the last census that India is on course to overtake China by 2030, recent trend shows that will happen much before 2030 though growth rate of India is also falling. Very soon, India will be the most populous country in the World and China will be second.

FERTILITY INDICATORS

Crude Birth Rate

Crude birth rate (CBR) is the number of live births during a year per 1,000 population at mid-year.

India's CBR is 21.6 as per Sample Registration System (SRS) 2012. The CBR is showing a consistent decline each year recording total decline of 16% from the year 2000 to 2012. India is in latter half of the third stage of demographic transition whereby the death rate has declined substantially and the birth rate is also declining.

Total Fertility Rate

Total fertility rate (TFR) is average number of children a woman would have throughout her child-bearing years. The TFR has declined from 2.2 to 2.0 at the national level between National Family Health Survey (NFHS-4) and 5. There are only five states in India which are above replacement level of fertility of 2.1. These states are Bihar, Meghalaya, Uttar Pradesh, Jharkhand and Manipur.

Women age 20–24 years married before age 18 years (%) is 23.3% according to NFHS-5.

SECTION 4: Birth Control and Population Demography

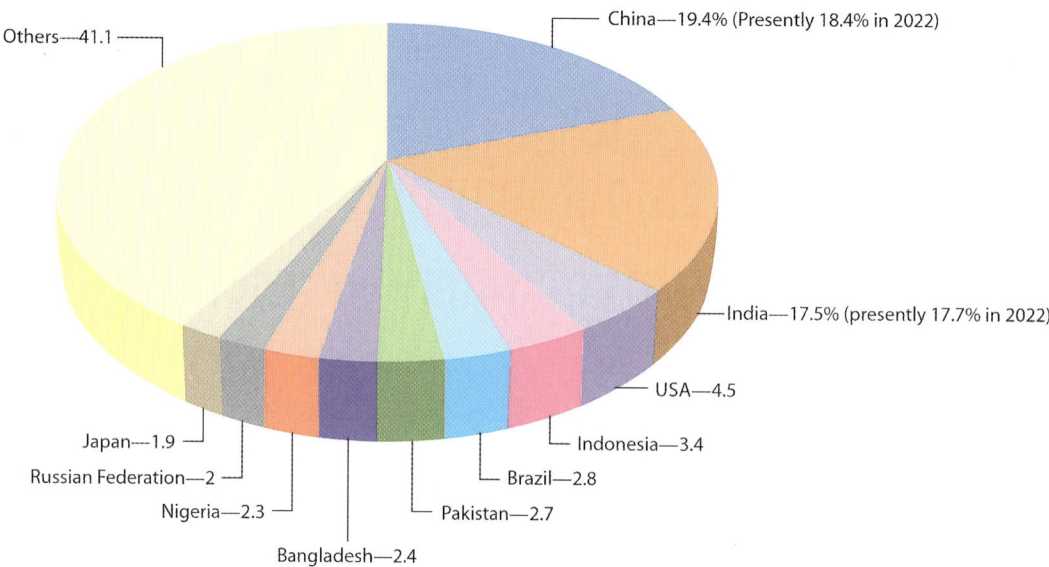

Fig. 1: Percentage of population of major countries of the world.
Source: Adapted from FP Vision 2020.
Presently (2022) India contributes 17.7% and China 18.4% (*see* the text)

CURRENT USE OF FAMILY PLANNING METHODS (CURRENTLY MARRIED WOMEN AGE 15–49 YEARS) AS PER NFHS-5 (2019-21) DATA

The National Family Health Survey 2019-21 (NFHS-5), the fifth in the NFHS series, provides information on contraceptive use of different methods.

Contraceptive prevalence rate is defined as percentage of eligible couples using any modern method of contraception.

Overall Contraceptive Prevalence Rate (CPR) has increased in the country in NHFS 5. Use of modern methods of contraceptives has also increased in almost all States/Union territories (UTs).

Any modern method used by currently married women age 15–49 years in India is 56.5 (%). The most popular modern contraceptive in India is female sterilization. Female sterilization accounts for 37.9%, male sterilization: 0.3%, intrauterine device (IUD)/postpartum intrauterine device (PPIUD): 2.1%, pill: 5.1%, condom: 9.5% and injectables: 0.6%.

UNMET NEED IN INDIA

Total unmet need for family planning (currently married women age 15–49 years) is 9.4% and unmet need for spacing is 4.0%.

Government has now stressed on all types of spacing method. Postpartum intrauterine contraceptive device program is now becoming more popular in various states of India. Recently, injection depot medroxyprogesterone acetate (DMPA) been made available from government sector in free of cost in the name of "Antara".

MILESTONES OF FAMILY PLANNING PROGRAM IN INDIA

India is the first country in the world to have launched a National Family Planning Program way back in 1952.

In 1952, National Family Program launched → 1976, First National Population Policy → 1983, First National Health Policy → 1994, India signed the plan of action at International Conference on Population and Development Cairo 2002 → 1996, Target Free Approach → 1997, Reproductive and Child Health Program launched → 2000, Second National Population Policy → 2002, Second National Health Policy → 2005, National Rural Health Mission and Reproductive and Child Health Program II launched → 2012, National Rural Health Mission extended to 2017 → 2012, London summit on Family Planning (FP) to fulfill India's "Vision FP 2020".

RMNCH+A

Q. What is RMNCH+A?

RMNCH+A is abbreviation of "Reproductive, maternal, newborn, child and adolescent health".

The RMNCH+A strategic approach has been developed to provide an understanding of "continuum of care" to ensure equal focus on various stages of life **(Fig. 2)**. It is based on the evidence that maternal and child health cannot be improved in isolation as adolescent health and family planning have an important impact on outcome.

RMNCH+A program has been launched in India in 2013 and is at the heart of flagship program National Health Mission (NHM). India's Vision FP 2020 builds on integrated RMNCH+A approach.

CHAPTER 23: Demography and Family Planning Programs in India—Present Scenario

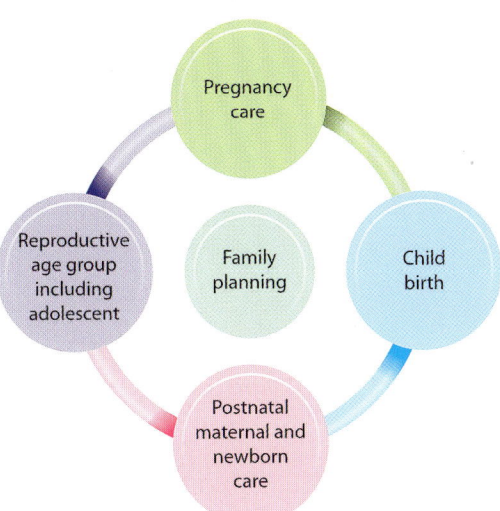

Fig. 2: RMNCH+A strategy with equal focus on various stages of life.

CONTRACEPTIVES AVAILABLE AT PRESENT THROUGH GOVERNMENT OF INDIA

- Combined pill: *Mala N*
- Emergency pill: *Ezy-pill* containing levonorgestrel 1.5 mg
- Intrauterine device: Cu-T 380A for 10 years, Multiload Cu-375 for 5 years
- Injectable: Injection DMPA intramuscular—*Antara*
- Male condom: *Nirodh*
- Nonhormonal nonsteroidal oral contraceptives centchroman (ormeloxifene) in the name of *Chhaya*.

Mala-N, ezy-pill, and Nirodh and Chhaya each is distributed in two different packs—one type of pack is distributed directly from government facility in free of cost and other type of pack distributed by accredited social health activist (ASHA) with a nominal cost.

Besides these methods, permanent sterilization (male and female) is one of the important programs of Government of India.

Section 5

Instruments and Operation

Section Outline

24. Identify the Instruments—Know Your Instruments
25. Operative Gynecology
26. Endoscopic Surgery: Laparoscopic/Hysteroscopic/Robotic Surgery
27. Routine Postoperative Management in a Gynecological Surgery

CHAPTER 24

Identify the Instruments—Know Your Instruments

CHAPTER OUTLINE

- **Instruments at a Glance—Identify All**
- **Questions on common instruments asked in viva:**
  Sponge Holding Forceps, Ovum Forceps, Female Metallic Catheter, Foley Catheter, Sims' Speculum, Cusco's Speculum, Anterior Vaginal Wall Retractor, Allis Tissue Forceps, Multiple Teeth and Single Tooth Vulsellum, Uterine Sound, Cervical Dilator, Uterine Curette (All Types), Uterine Dressing Forceps, Lane's Tissue Forceps, Hysterectomy Clamp, Babcock's Tissue Forceps, Myoma Screw, Bonney's Myomectomy Clamp, Landon's Bladder Retractor, Aneurism Needle, Hodge-Smith Pessary and Ring Pessary

INSTRUMENTS AT A GLANCE

All the instruments have been shown in **Figures 1 to 68**.

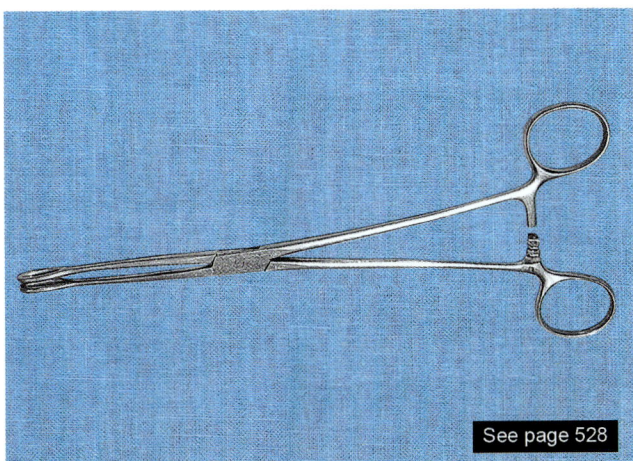

Fig. 1: Sponge holding forceps.

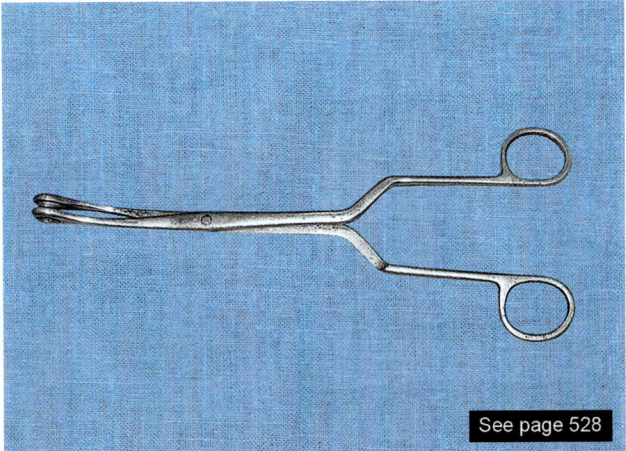

Fig. 2: Ovum forceps.

SECTION 5: Instruments and Operation

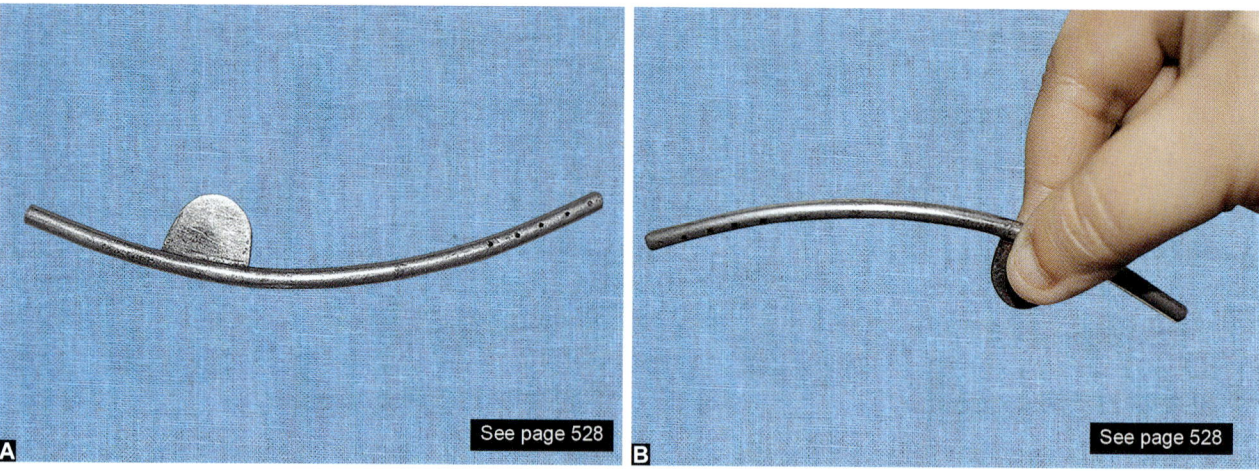

Figs 3A and B: (A) Female metallic catheter; (B) Procedure of holding metal catheter during evacuation.

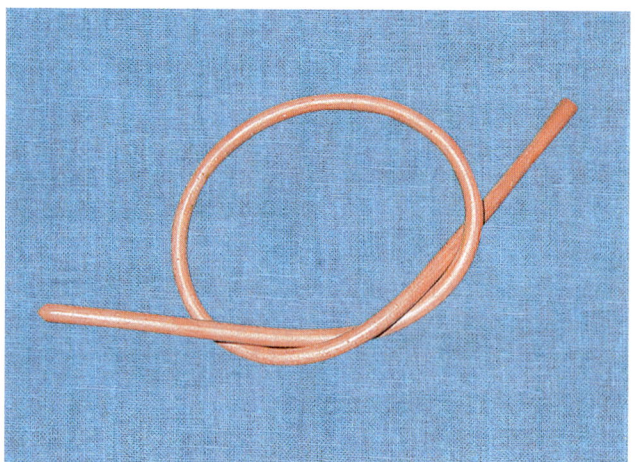

Fig. 4: Simple rubber catheter.

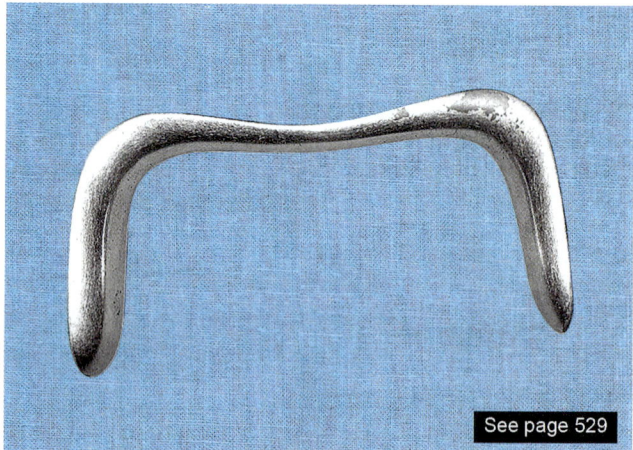

Fig. 6: Sims' posterior vaginal speculum (double-bladed).

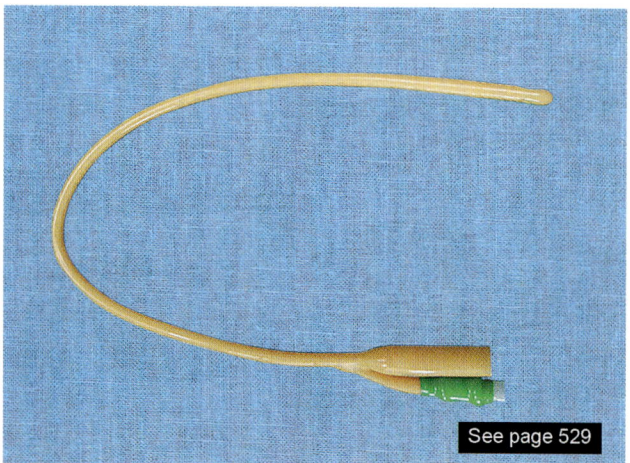

Fig. 5: Foley catheter.

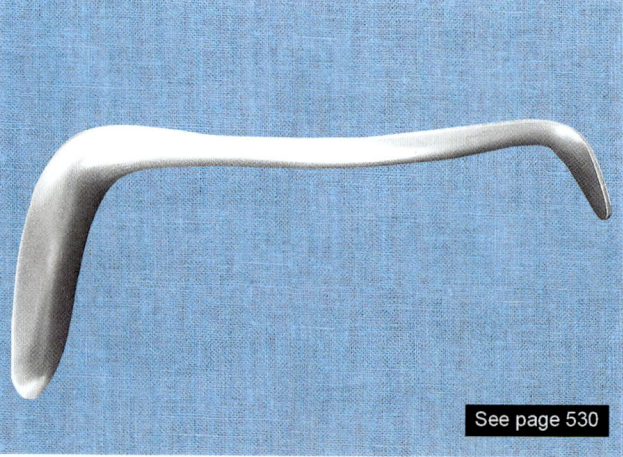

Fig. 7: Single-bladed posterior vaginal speculum.

CHAPTER 24: Identify the Instruments—Know Your Instruments

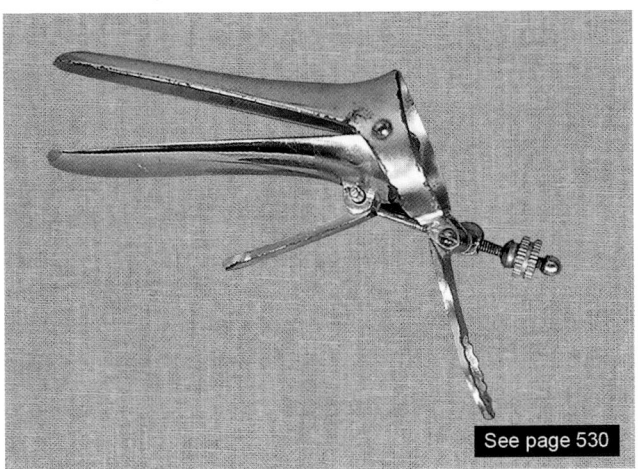

Fig. 8: Cusco's speculum.

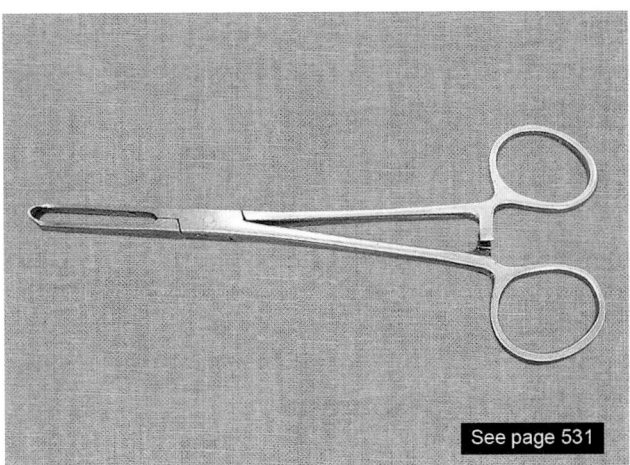

Fig. 11: Allis tissue forceps.

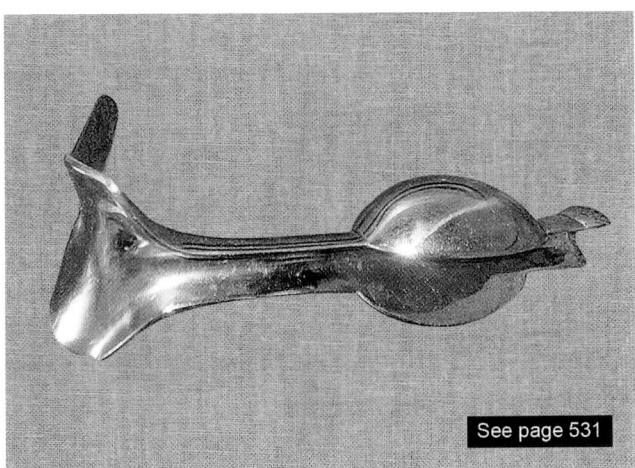

Fig. 9: Auvard's self-retaining speculum.

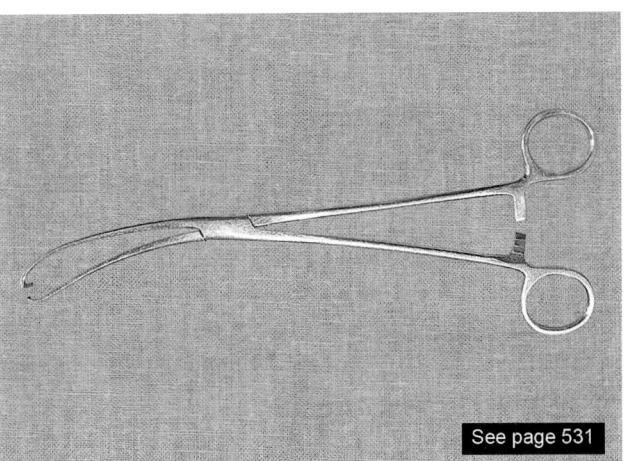

Fig. 12: Multiple teeth vulsellum.

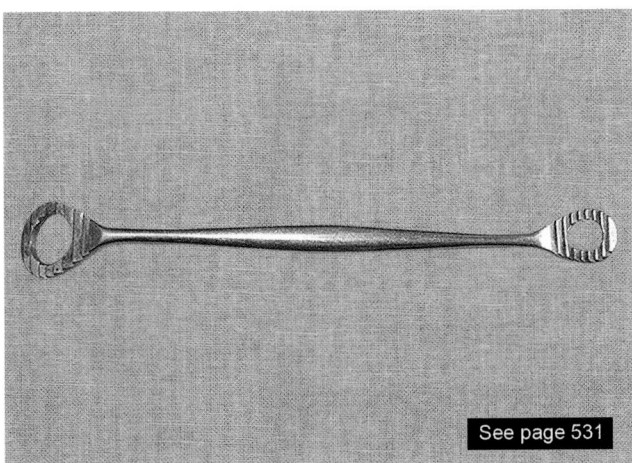

Fig. 10: Anterior vaginal wall retractor.

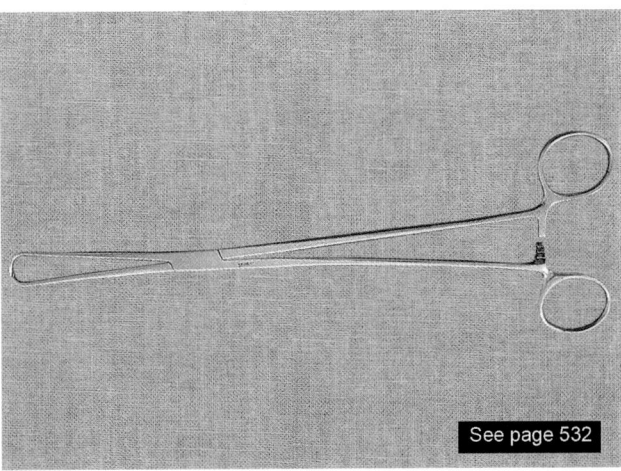

Fig. 13: Single tooth vulsellum.

SECTION 5: Instruments and Operation

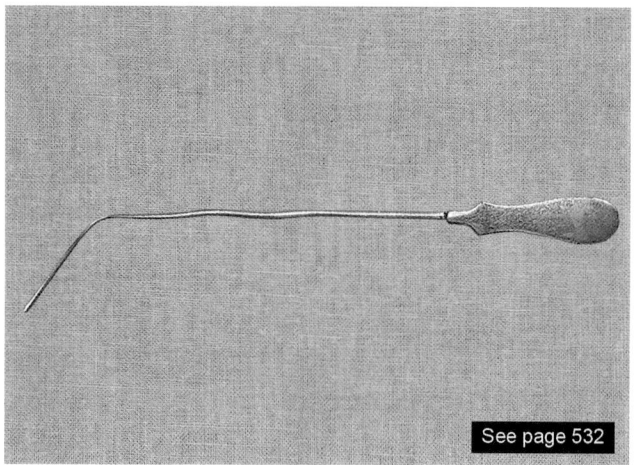

Fig. 14: Olive pointed graduated metallic malleable uterine sound.

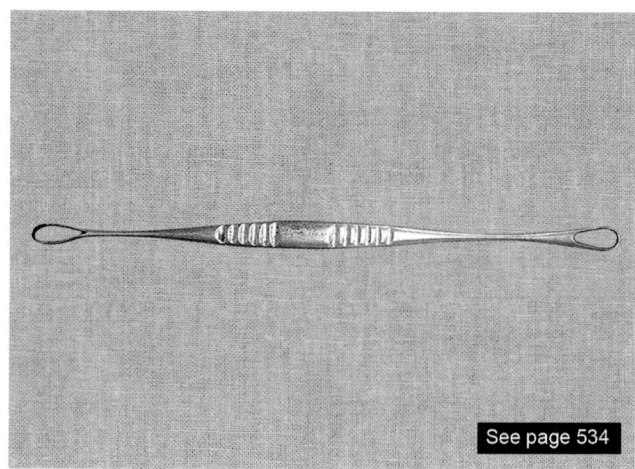

Fig. 17: Uterine curette (blunt and sharp).

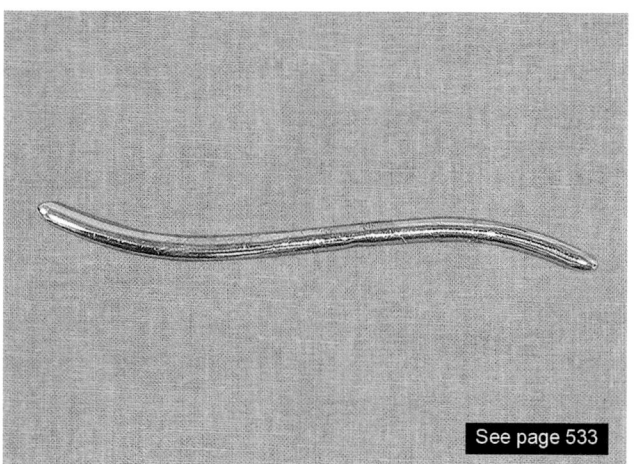

Fig. 15: Hegar's cervical dilator.

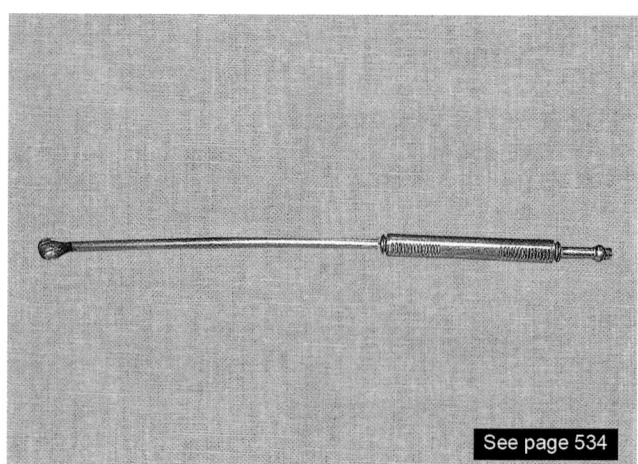

Fig. 18: Flushing curette.

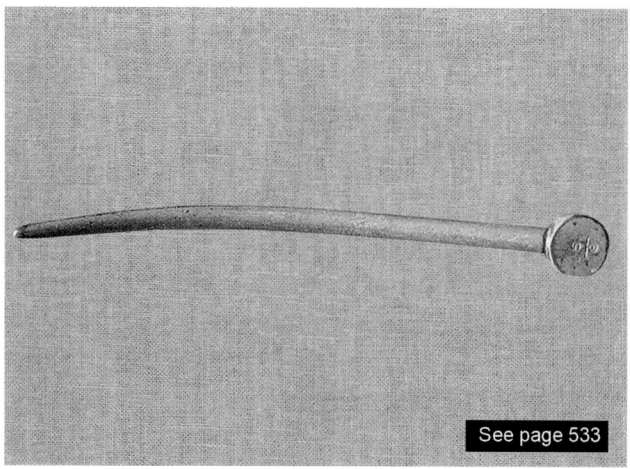

Fig. 16: Hawkin–Ambler's cervical dilator.

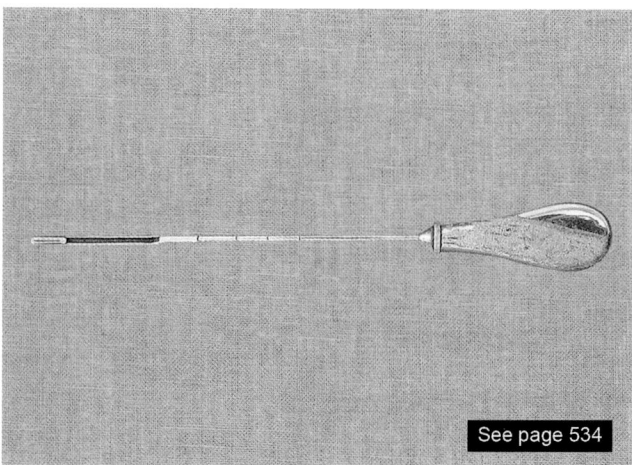

Fig. 19: Sharman's curette.

CHAPTER 24: Identify the Instruments—Know Your Instruments

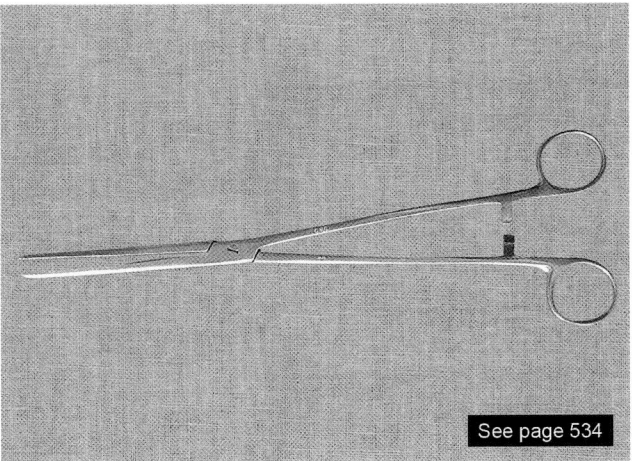

Fig. 20: Uterine dressing forceps.

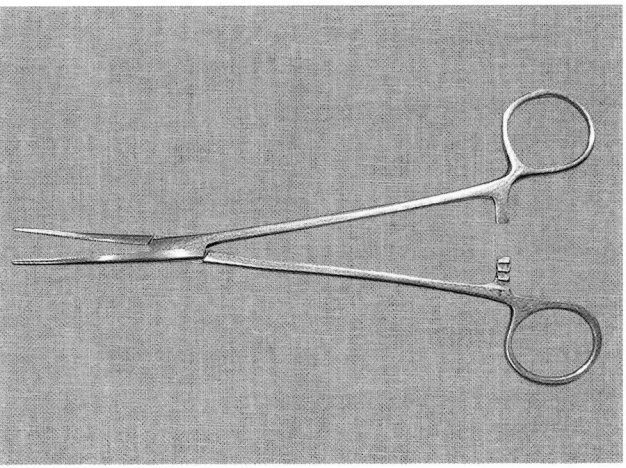

Fig. 22B: Long (hemostatic) forceps—Spencer Wells variety—curve.

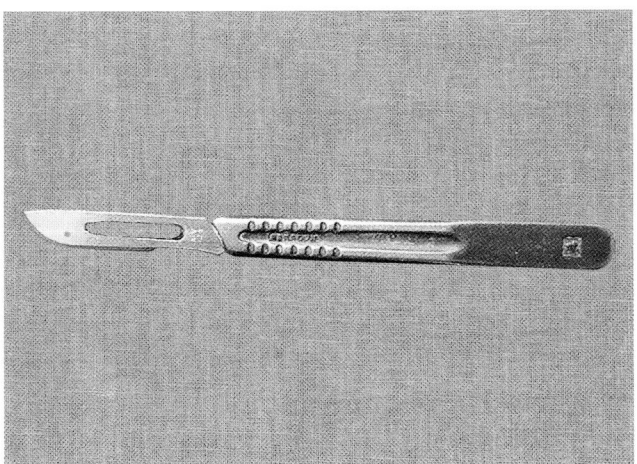

Fig. 21: Scalpel blade fitted with handle.

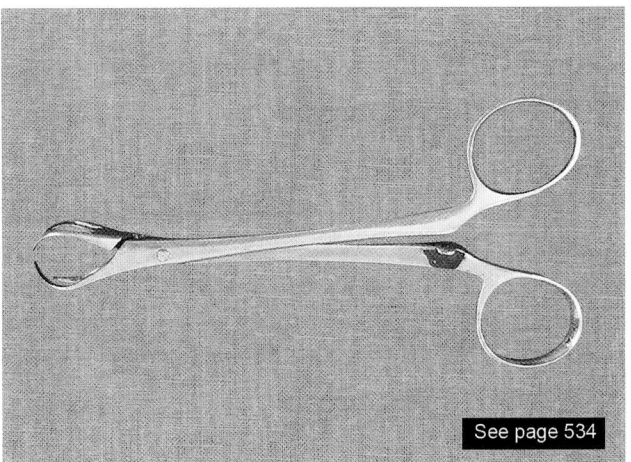

Fig. 23: Lane's tissue forceps.

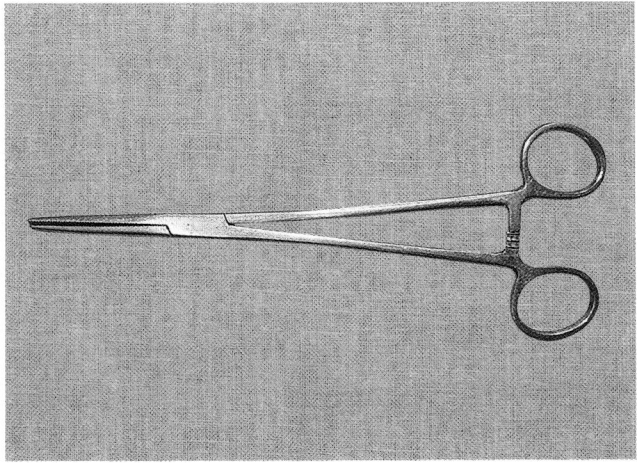

Fig. 22A: Long (hemostatic) forceps—Spencer Wells variety—straight.

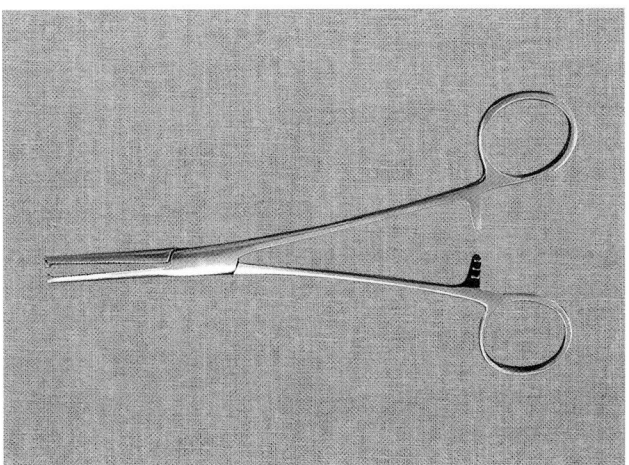

Fig. 24: Kocher's artery forceps.

SECTION 5: Instruments and Operation

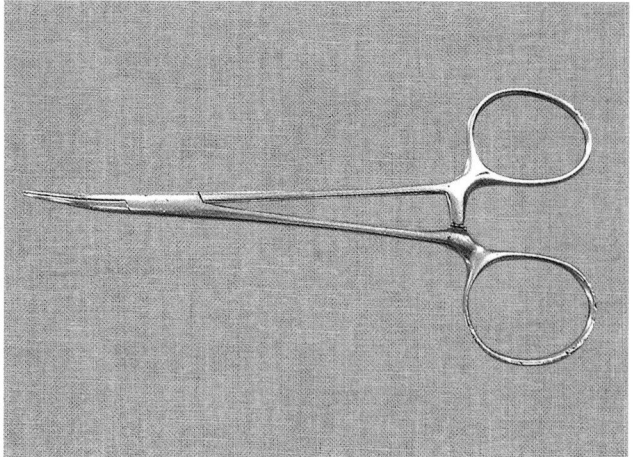

Fig. 25: Mosquito forceps.

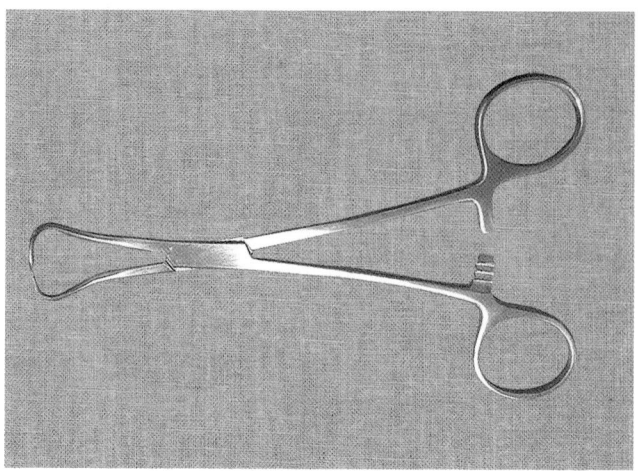

Fig. 28: Towel clip.

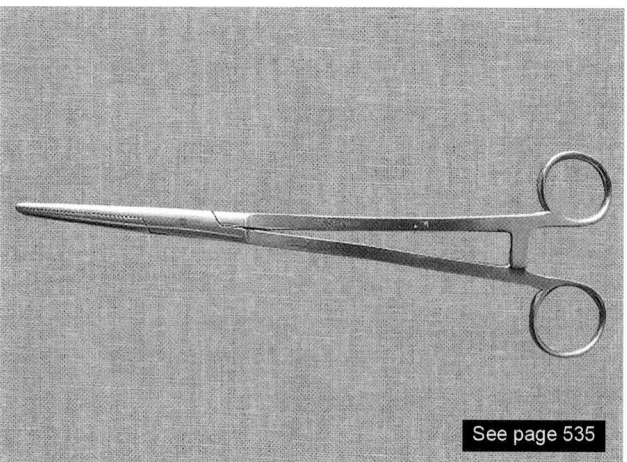

Fig. 26: Hysterectomy clamp (straight) (Spencer Well's).

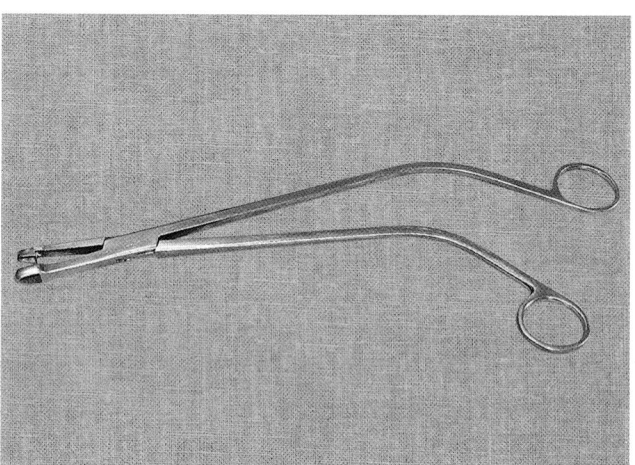

Fig. 29: Punch biopsy forceps for biopsy from cervix.

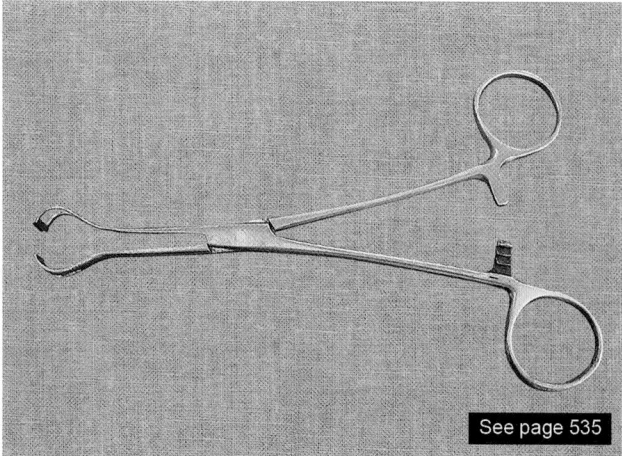

Fig. 27: Babcock's tissue forceps.

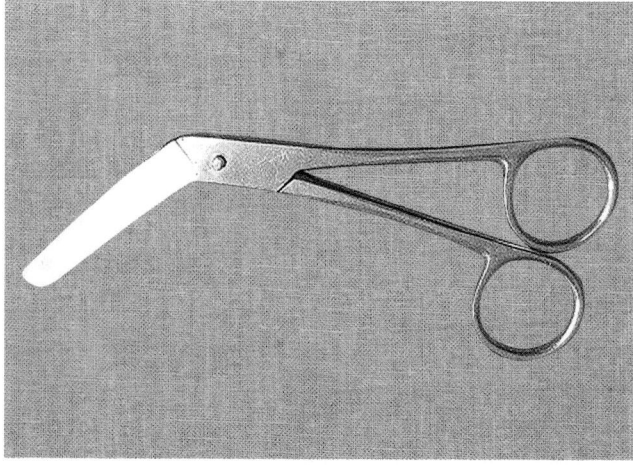

Fig. 30: Curved scissor (perineorrhaphy, episiotomy scissor).

CHAPTER 24: Identify the Instruments—Know Your Instruments

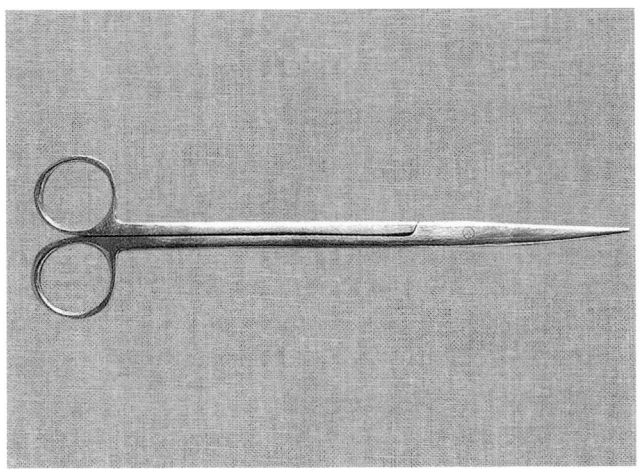

Fig. 31A: Fine scissor (Metzenbaum scissor).

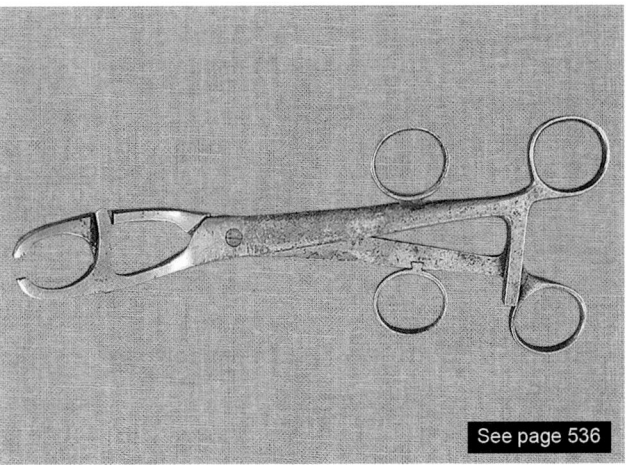

Fig. 33: Bonney's myomectomy clamp.

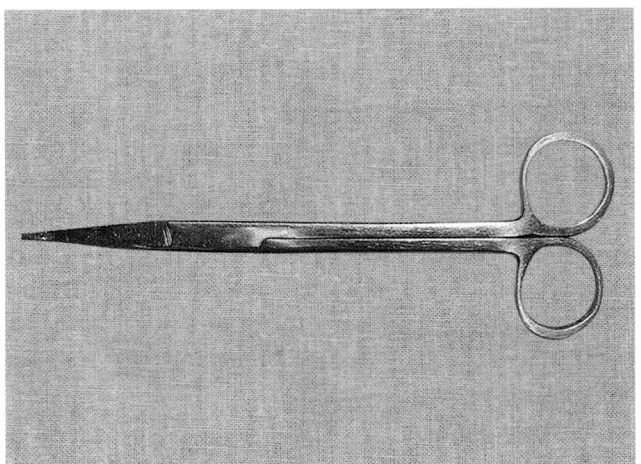

Fig. 31B: Straight scissor (Mayo's scissor).

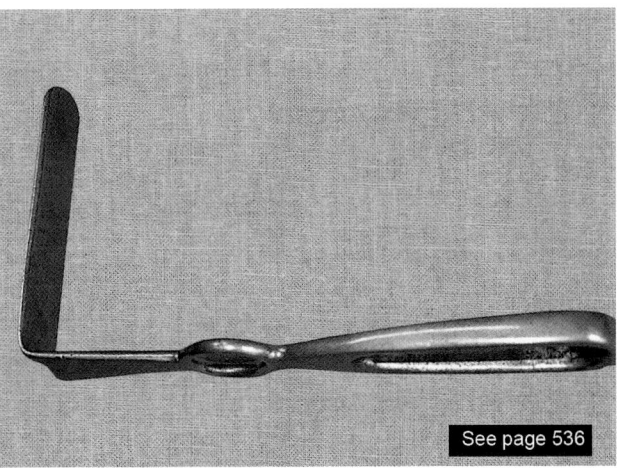

Fig. 34: Landon's bladder retractor.

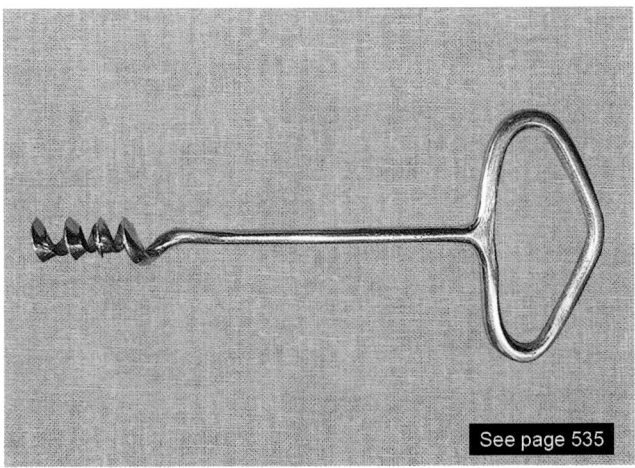

Fig. 32: Myoma screw.

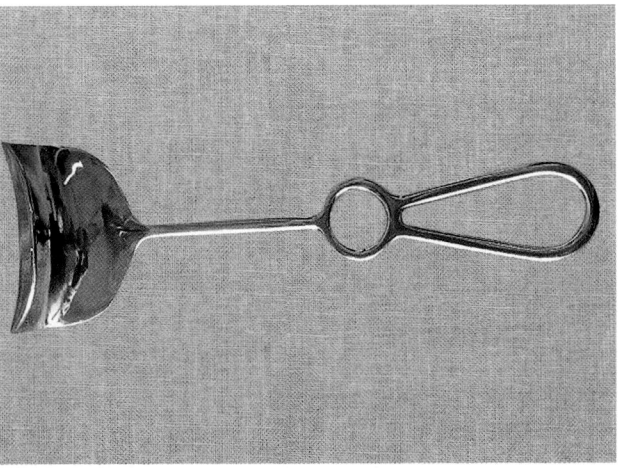

Fig. 35: Doyen's retractor.

SECTION 5: Instruments and Operation

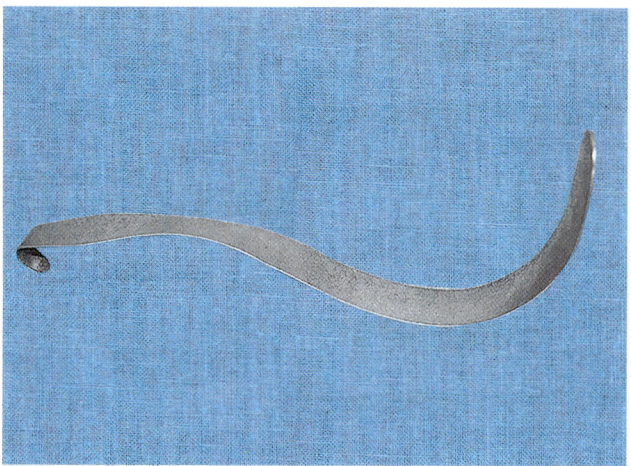

Fig. 36: Deaver's retractor.

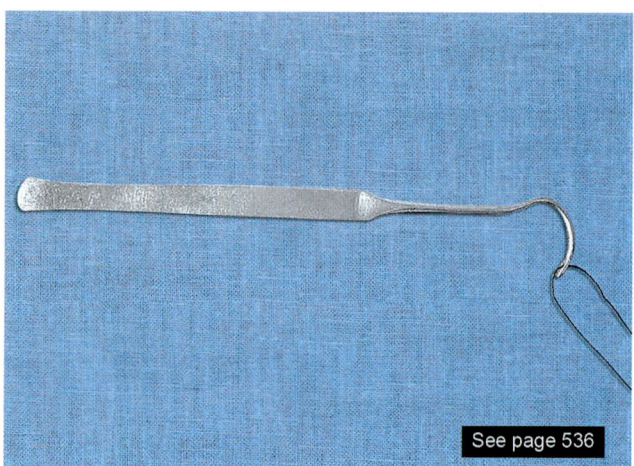

Fig. 39: Aneurysm needle.

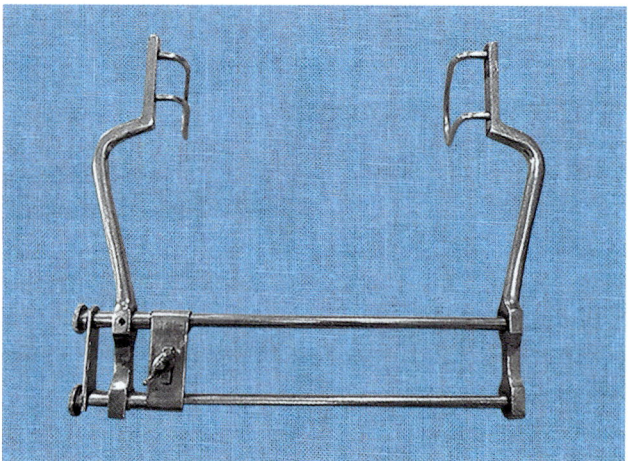

Fig. 37: Balfour abdominal self-retaining retractor.

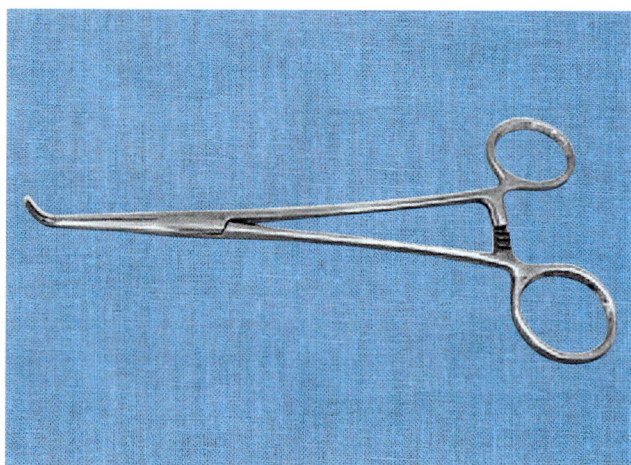

Fig. 39A: Right angled forceps (Meigs-Navratil forceps) for ligation of internal iliac artery or deep vessel.

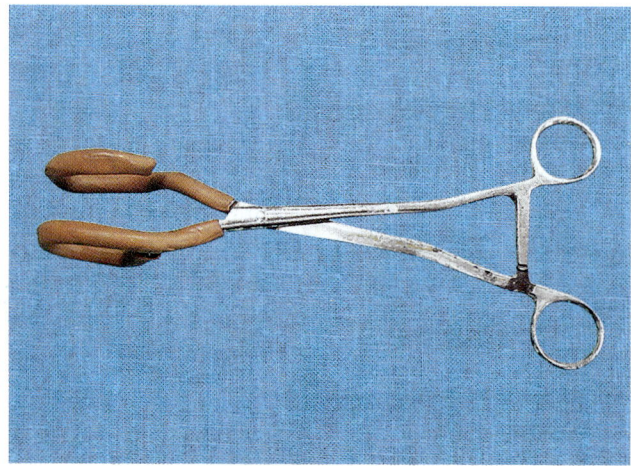

Fig. 38: Uterus holding forceps—uterus held in tubal surgery.

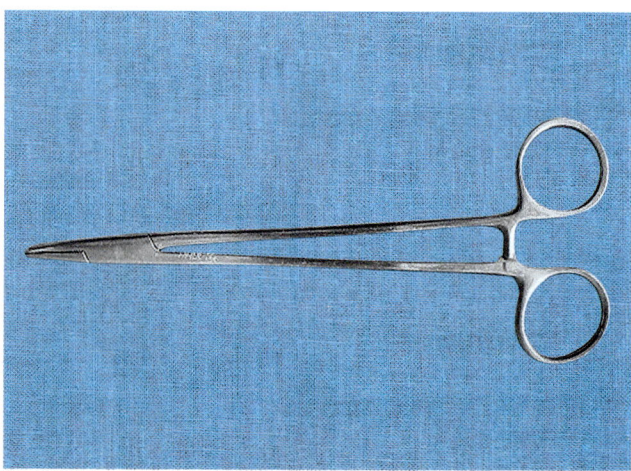

Fig. 40: Needle holder.

CHAPTER 24: Identify the Instruments—Know Your Instruments

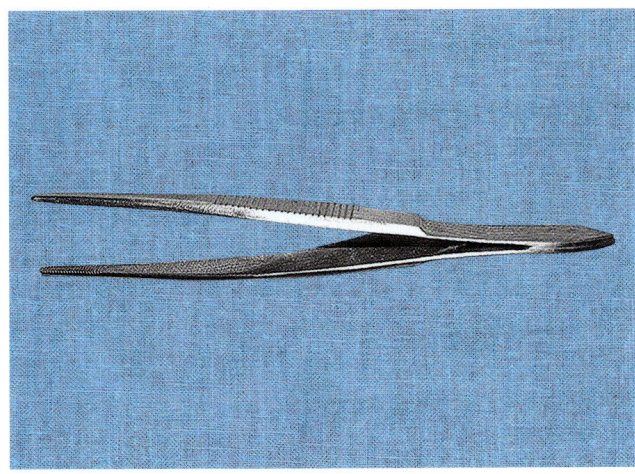

Fig. 41: Dissecting forceps—nontoothed.

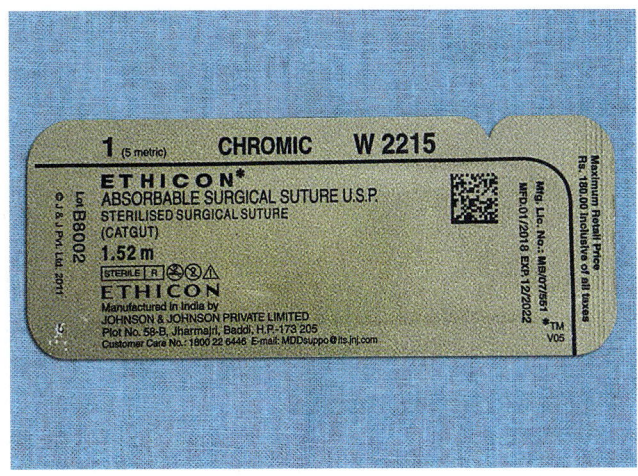

Fig. 44: Pack of catgut.

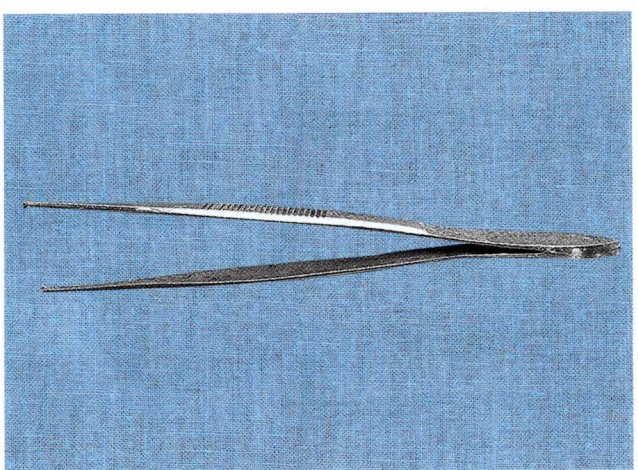

Fig. 42: Dissecting forceps—toothed.

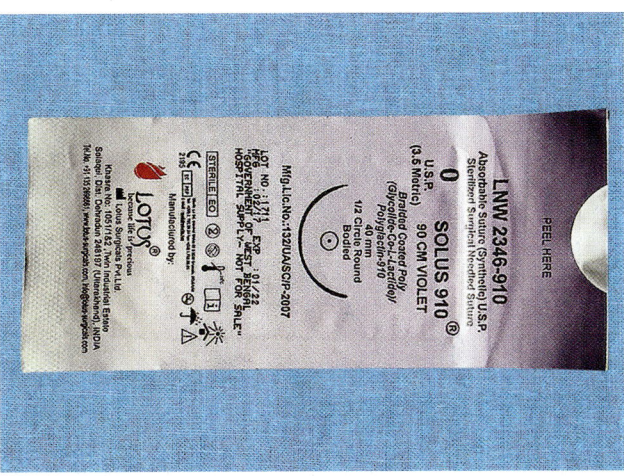

Fig. 45: Pack of vicryl delayed absorbable suture.

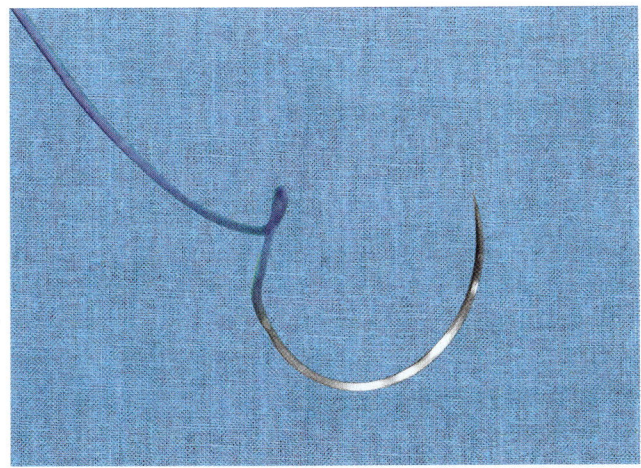

Fig. 43: Curved round body needle atraumatic with vicryl.

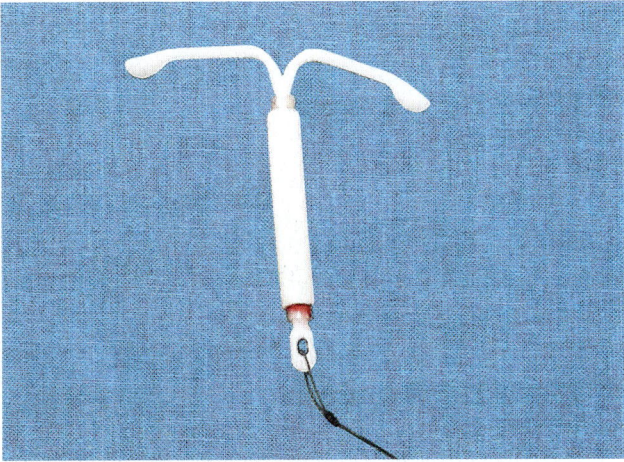

Fig. 46: LNG-IUS Mirena used for contraceptive, AUB, endometriosis, fibroid (*see* Chapter 22).

SECTION 5: Instruments and Operation

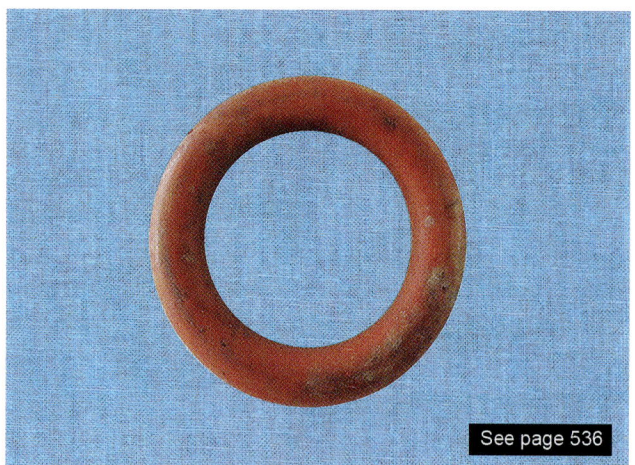

Fig. 47: Ring pessary used for pelvic organ prolapse.

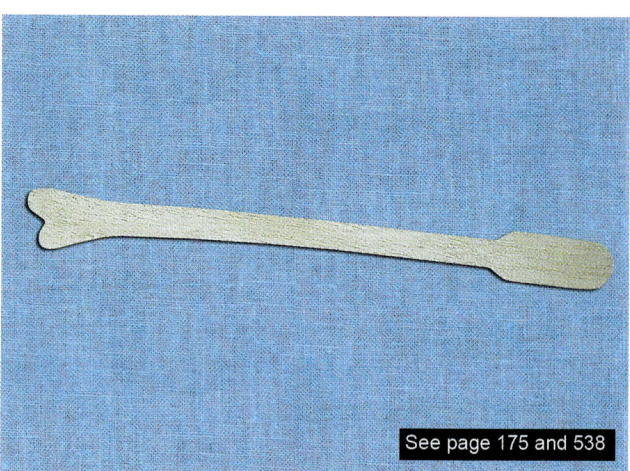

Fig. 50: Ayre's spatula (wooden).

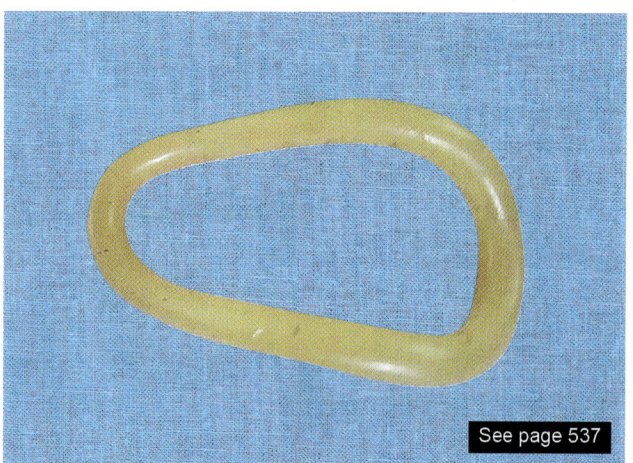

Fig. 48: Hodge–Smith pessary for correction of mobile retroversion.

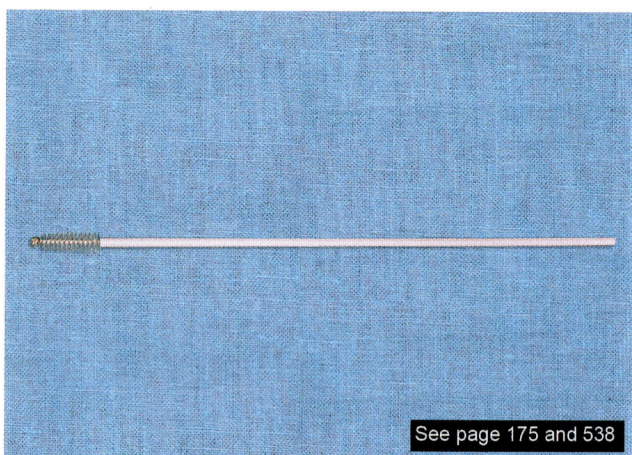

Fig. 51: Cytobrush.

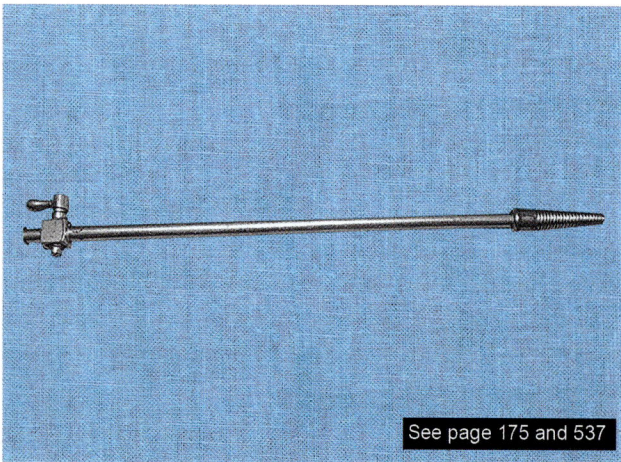

Fig. 49: Hysterosalpingography (Leech Wilkinson HSG cannula).

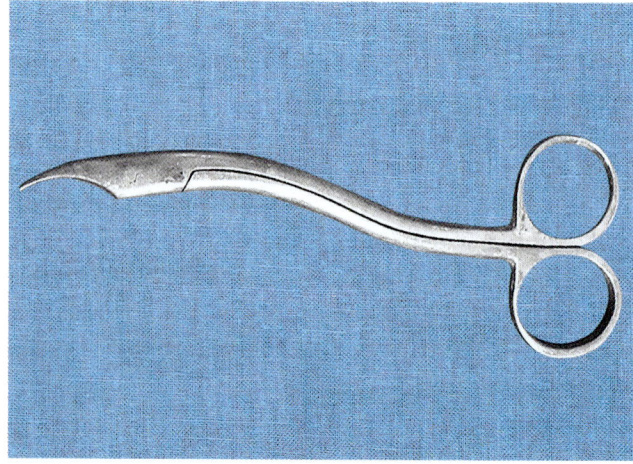

Fig. 52: Stitch removal scissors.

CHAPTER 24: Identify the Instruments—Know Your Instruments

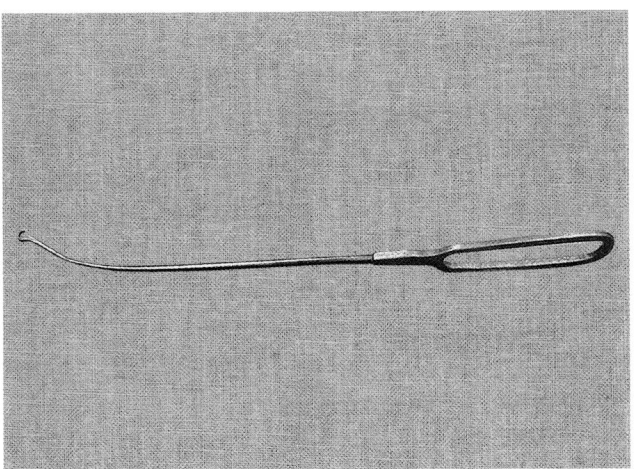

Fig. 53: Loop removal hook—used for removal of intrauterine contraceptive device in missing thread.

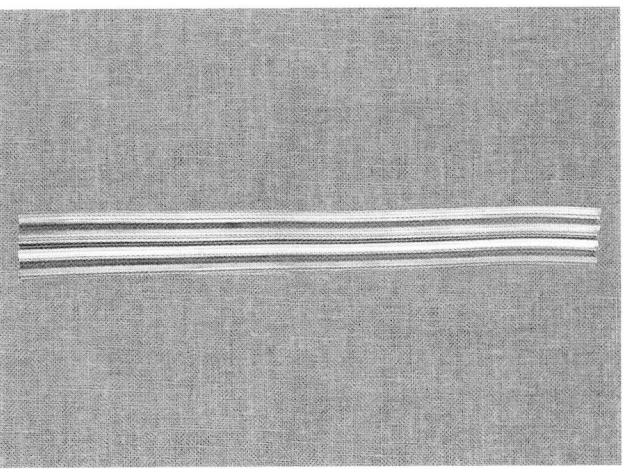

Fig. 56: Corrugated rubber drain.

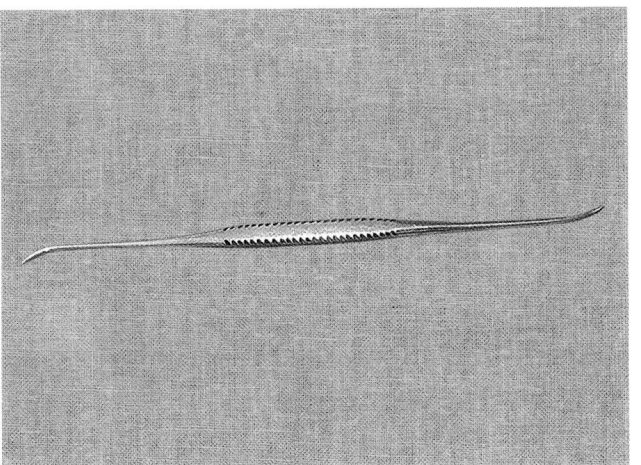

Fig. 54: Lymph node dissector.

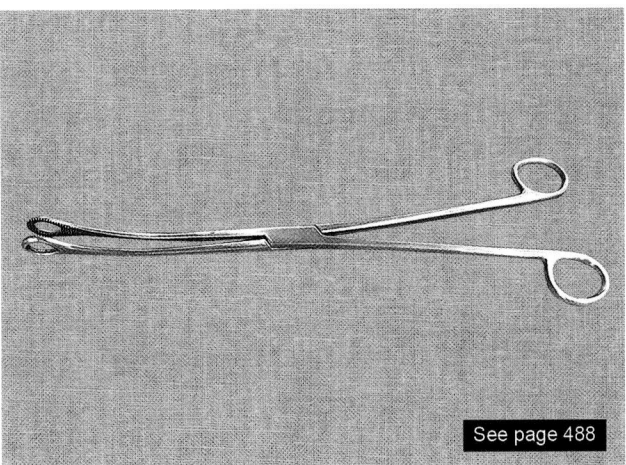

Fig. 57: Kelly placenta forceps for postpartum intrauterine contraceptive device (PPIUCD) insertion.

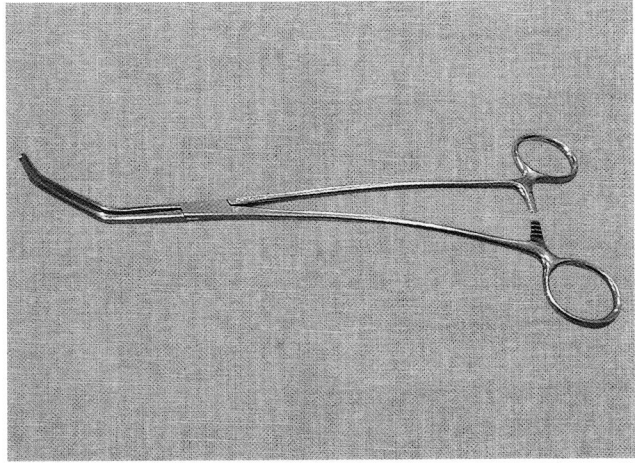

Fig. 55: Wertheim's clamp.

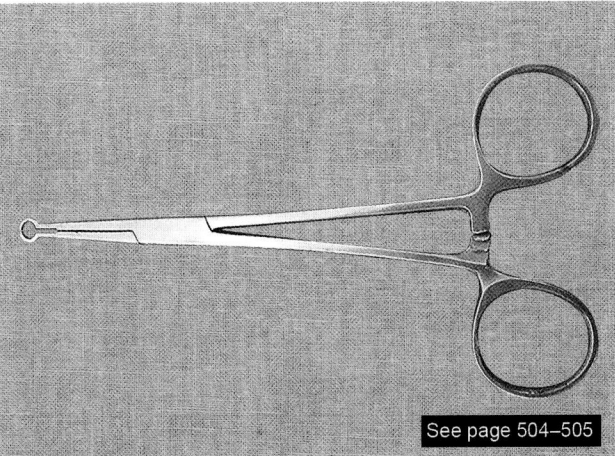

Fig. 58: Ringed clamp for nonscalpel vasectomy (NSV).

SECTION 5: Instruments and Operation

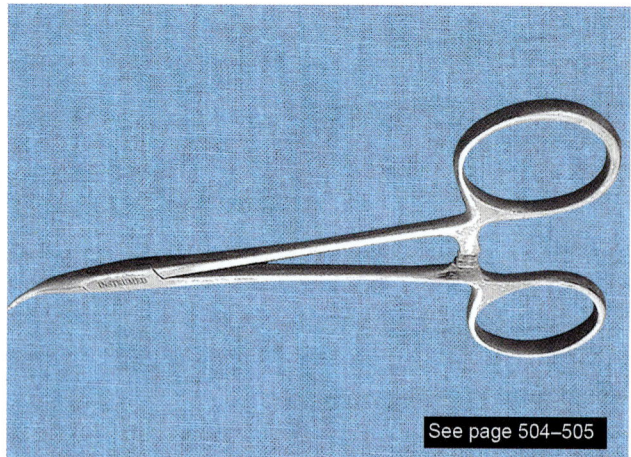

Fig. 59: Dissecting forceps for nonscalpel vasectomy (NSV).

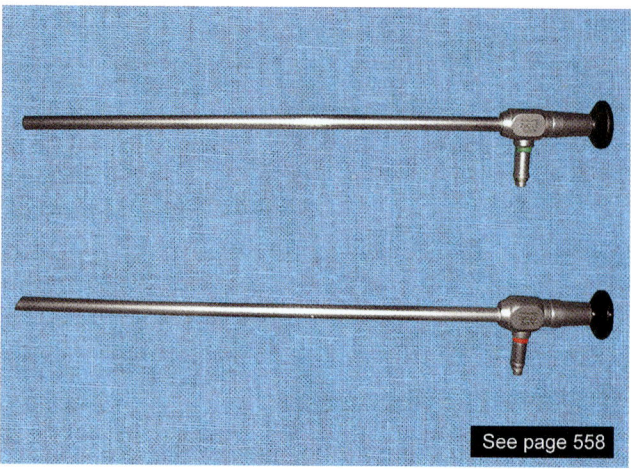

Fig. 62: Telescope of laparoscope.

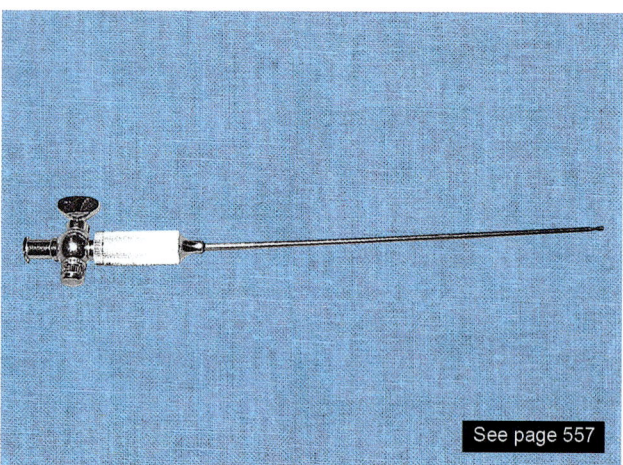

Fig. 60: Veress needle—used for pneumoperitoneum in laparoscopy.

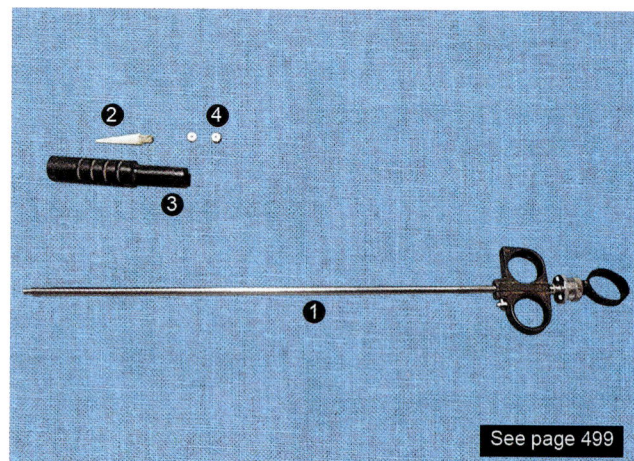

Fig. 63: Laparoscopic ligation set: (1) Tong, (2) loader, (3) pusher and (4) Falope ring.

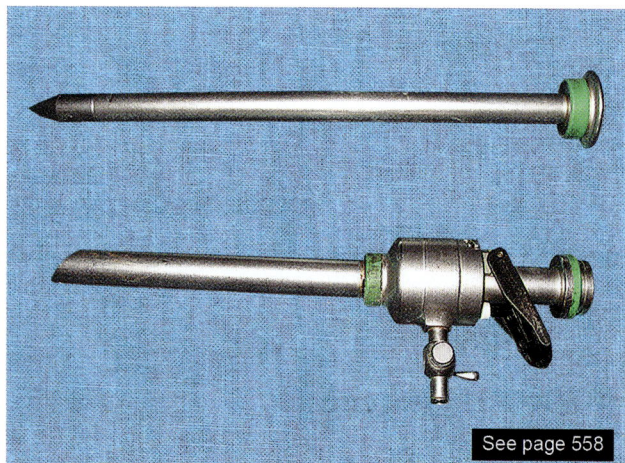

Fig. 61: Trocar and cannula for laparoscope.

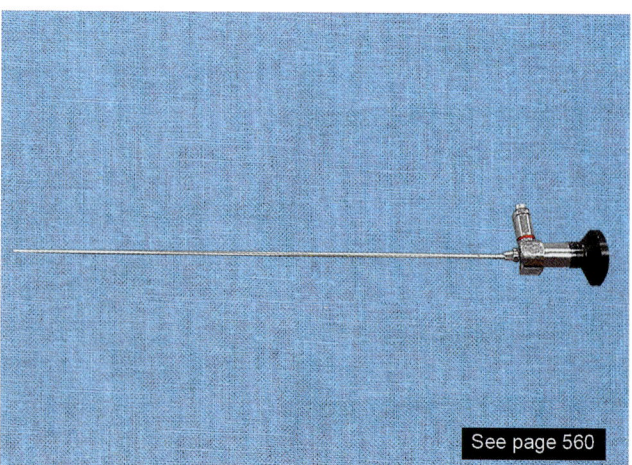

Fig. 64: Hysteroscopic telescope.

CHAPTER 24: Identify the Instruments—Know Your Instruments

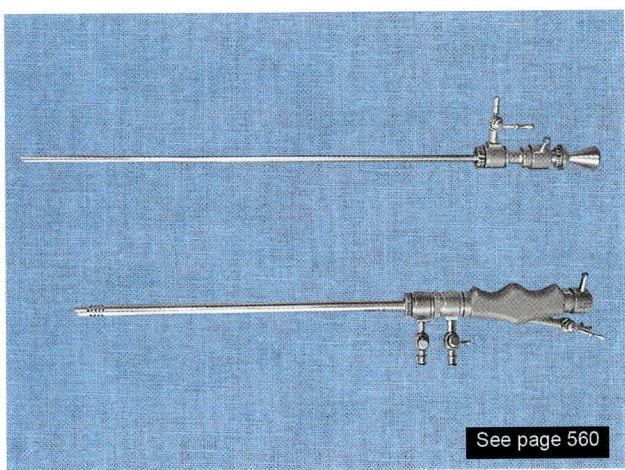

Fig. 65: Operative hysteroscope.

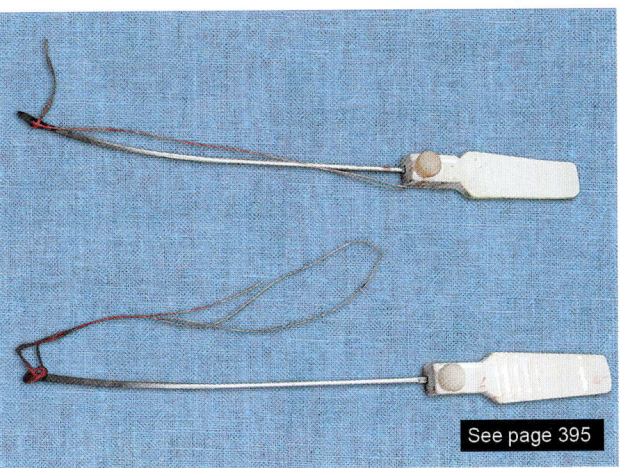

Fig. 66: Tension-free vaginal tape (TVT) needle.

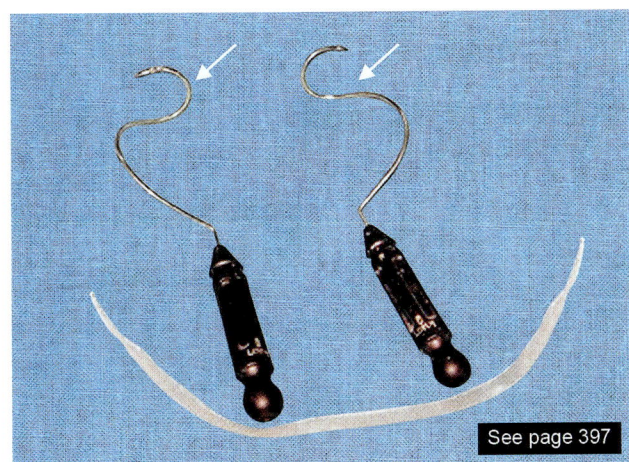

Fig. 67: Transobturator tape (TOT) needle and tape (outside in).

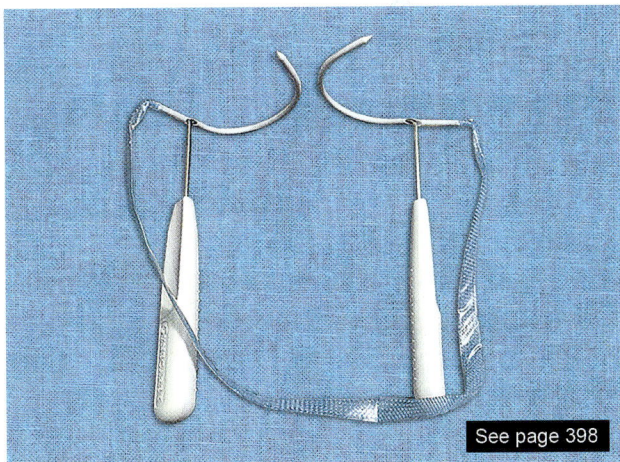

Fig. 68: Composite set of obturator device, helical passars and atraumatic-winged guide for TOT (for inside out).

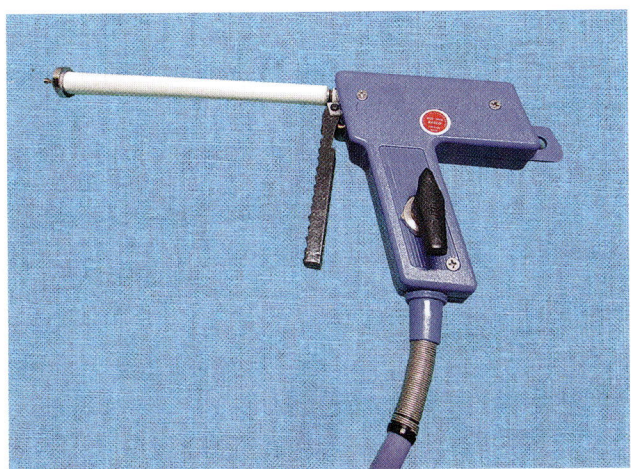

Fig. 69: Cryoprobe with cryogun for cyocautery of cervix.

SECTION 5: Instruments and Operation

SPONGE HOLDING FORCEPS (ALSO CALLED SWAB HOLDING OR RING FORCEPS) (FIG. 1)

It is a long forceps with rings at the anterior end and with a catch near handle which differentiates it from ovum forceps which has no catch.

Uses of Sponge Holding Forceps in Gynecology

- Antiseptic dressing in abdominal and vaginal operations
- Polypectomy
- Packing of roller gauze in secondary hemorrhage following vaginal or abdominal hysterectomy
- To hold the lip of cervix in pregnant uterus, e.g., cerclage operation
- Can be used instead of ovum forceps
- Can be used to anterior vaginal wall retractor
- To occlude the ovarian vessels during myomectomy.

Sterilization

Autoclaving or boiling.

OVUM FORCEPS (FIG. 2)

Uses

- To remove the product of conception in dilatation and evacuation (D and E) operation
- To remove the retained bits of placenta and membranes.

Q. How to differentiate from sponge holding forceps?

- In sponge holding there is catch, in ovum forceps there is no catch.
- In ovum holding forceps the tip is spoon-shaped, in sponge holding forceps the tip is ring-shaped with grooves.

Sterilization

Autoclaving or boiling.

FEMALE METALLIC CATHETER (FIGS. 3A AND B)

Uses

- Evacuation of bladder routinely before vaginal operation
- Retention of urine
- To diagnose vesicovaginal fistula (VVF)
- To differentiate VVF and ureterovaginal fistula (UVF)
- To note the limit of bladder in anterior colporrhaphy operation.

Q. What are the causes of retention of urine in gynecology?

- Cervical fibroid
- Cryptomenorrhea
- Retroverted gravid uterus
- Ovarian tumor impacted in pouch of Douglas (POD)

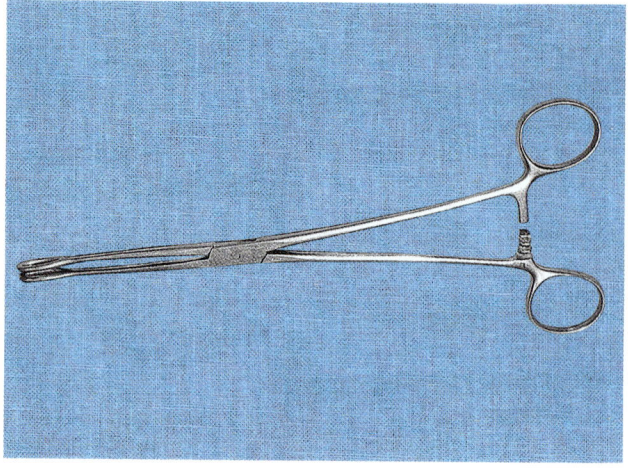

Fig. 1: Sponge holding forceps.

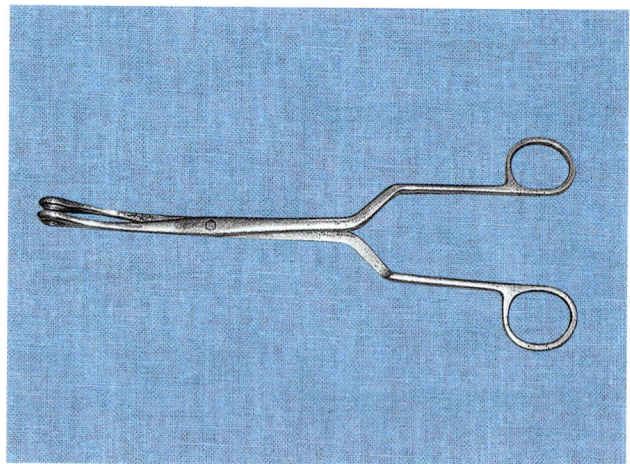

Fig. 2: Ovum forceps.

- Pelvic hematocele due to chronic ectopic
- Postoperative retention following any vaginal surgery
- Pelvic organ prolapse (POP)
- Urethra stricture
- Urethral caruncle.

Q. How to hold the female catheter during evacuation (Fig. 3B)?

- Patient in dorsal position with thigh abducted or lithotomy position.
- With glove hands—left thumb and index finger—labia are retracted. Swabing of external urethral meatus is by using cotton soaked in antiseptic solution from anterior to posterior. For collection of urine for culture and sensitivity purpose, normal saline or distilled water is used instead of antiseptic solution.
- Urethral meatus is a longitudinal slit situated 2.5 cm below and behind the clitoris and identified by pink mucosa.
- Catheter is held on no touch technique holding the flat disk with thumb and index finger keeping convexity upwards.

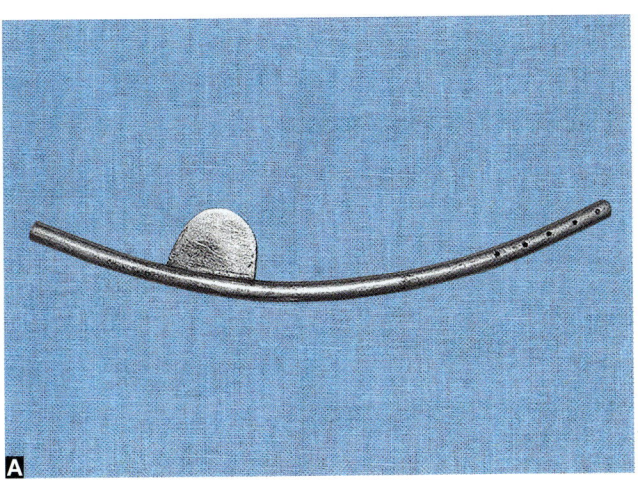 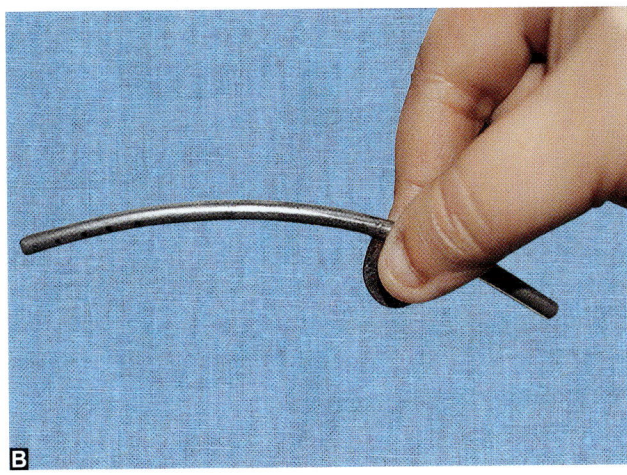

Figs. 3A and B: (A) Female metallic catheter; (B) Procedure of holding metal catheter during evacuation.

Q. How the metal catheter is sterilized?
By autoclave or by boiling for half an hour.

Q. Why does retention of urine occur in retroverted gravid uterus? When does it occur?
In retroverted gravid uterus, uterus is impacted in POD, hence the anterior vaginal wall becomes stretched causing stretching of urethra and the lumen of the urethra becomes narrowed.
Commonly occurs at 12th week of gestation.

Q. How will you manage urinary retention in retroverted gravid uterus?
Patient is admitted and continuous catheterization done with Foley catheter. Patient is asked to lie in prawn position or exaggerated left lateral position. After 14 weeks when the uterus becomes abdominally palpable, spontaneous correction occurs and patient can pass urine herself.

Complications of Catheterization

- Urinary tract infection
- Trauma by metal catheter.

FOLEY CATHETER (FIG. 5)

It is used for continuous drainage of urine available of different sizes made of rubber silicone. Commonly 14, 16 and 18 sizes are used. 8 size is used for sonohysterosalpingography. It is a two-channel tube, one for drainage of urine and other for inflation of bulb with distilled water, 5–10 mL water is given. The size of catheter and capacity of bulb are written on pack.

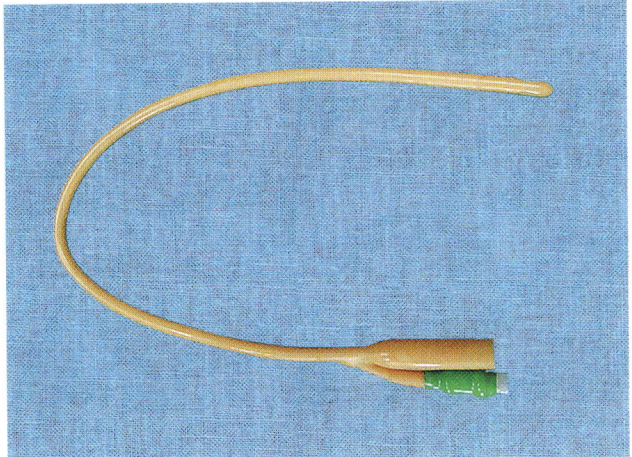

Fig. 5: Foley catheter.

Uses

- For evacuation of bladder in retention of urine.
- For continuous drainage of urine following gynecological surgery like pelvic floor repair, vaginal hysterectomy, Wertheim's operation, repair of VVF and vaginoplasty.
- To monitor output in ill patients where it is required.
- Sonosalpingohysterography (with 8-0 size)
- As tamponade—in abnormal uterine bleeding
- In obstetrics—to control postpartum hemorrhage (PPH) with multiple Foley, induction of labor, in obstructed labor, amnioinfusion.

Sterilization

It is available in sterilized pack—gamma-sterilized or by ethylene tetraoxide.

SIMS' DOUBLE-BLADED POSTERIOR VAGINAL SPECULUM (FIG. 6)

Uses

Diagnostic and therapeutic.

Diagnostic

- To visualize any lesion over cervix and anterior vaginal wall.
- Investigation—cervical biopsy and PAP smear.

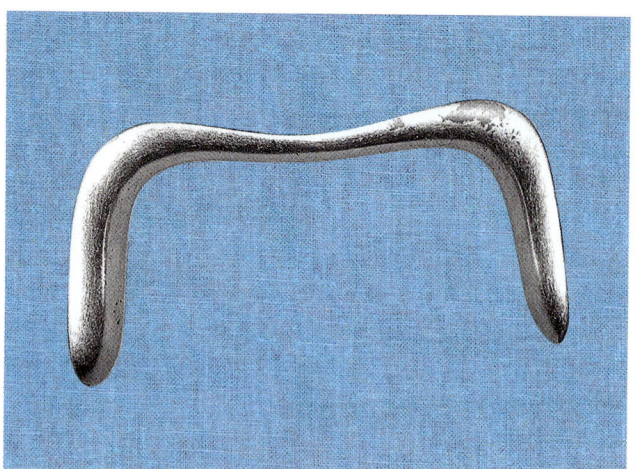

Fig. 6: Sims' posterior vaginal speculum (double-bladed).

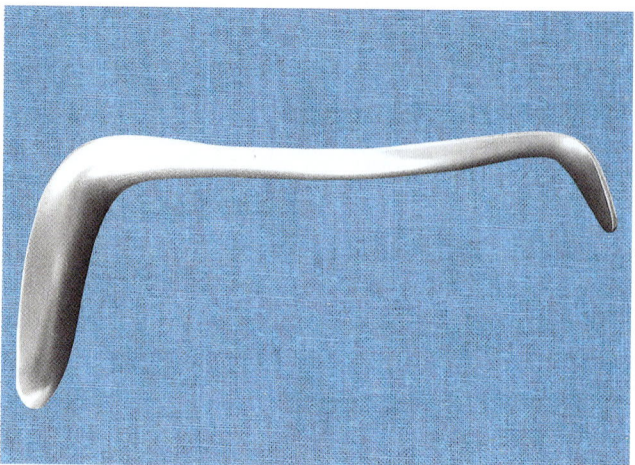

Fig. 7: Single-bladed posterior vaginal speculum.

Q. Tell some lesions on anterior vaginal wall.
Vesicovaginal fistula, cystocele, Gardner duct cyst.

Q. Tell some lesions of cervix.
Cervical erosion, chronic cervicitis, cervical polyp, cervical intraepithelial neoplasia (CIN), cancer cervix, cervical tear, bacterial and fungal cervicitis.

To *see* the cervix anterior vaginal wall may be needed to retract especially in presence of cystocele.

Therapeutic

Any vaginal operation/procedure other than operation on perineum, e.g., D and C, diathermy, cryocautery, intrauterine contraceptive device (IUCD) insertion, anterior colporrhaphy, vaginal hysterectomy, Fothergill's operation, hysteroscopy (diagnostic and operative both).

Q. Why called Sims?
It was after the name of Marion Sims who was the pioneer of VVF repair and used this instrument for VVF repair.

Q. What is Sims' triad?
See details in Chapter 17

Sims' position, Sims' speculum and Sims' silver wire used for VVF repair.

Q. How to introduce Sims' speculum?
Sims' speculum is inserted laterally first and then to be rotated 90° posteriorly to retract the posterior vaginal wall with the blade.

For details of introduction, *see* Chapter 1 (**Figs. 63A and B and 65** of Chapter 1).

Disadvantages of Sims' speculum over Cusco:
- It is not self-retaining, so assistant is needed to retract it in operative procedure.
- In presence of cystocele, an anterior vaginal wall retractor is needed to retract anterior vaginal wall.

Advantage of Sims' speculum over Cusco:
Lesions on anterior vaginal wall (VVF) can be seen whereas by Cusco anterior vaginal wall is not visible.

SINGLE-BLADED (UNIVERSAL) POSTERIOR VAGINAL SPECULUM (FIG. 7)

Same as above, it is single-bladed, universal and in double-bladed two blades are of different sizes. The advantage is that patient may not be needed to come to the edge of the table which is needed in double-bladed.

CUSCO'S BIVALVE SELF-RETAINING SPECULUM (FIG. 8)

Uses
In outpatient department (OPD), the speculum which is mostly used is Cusco's speculum.

Diagnostic
- Mostly diagnostic.
- To see the lesions over cervix as described in Sims' speculum—cervical erosion, chronic cervicitis, cervical polyp, CIN, cancer cervix, cervical tear, bacterial and fungal cervicitis.
- Lesions over lateral vaginal walls.

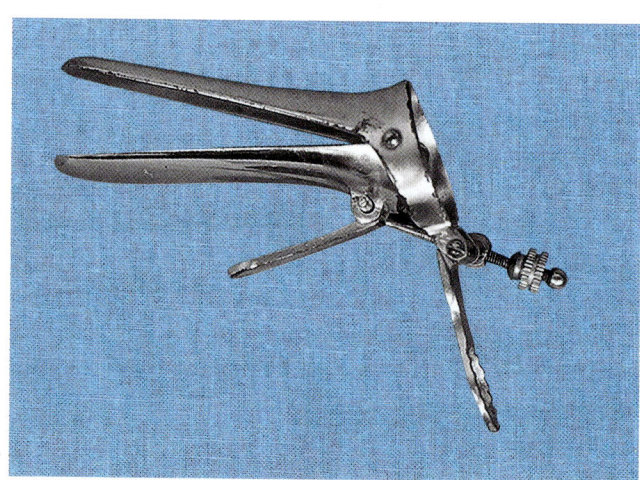

Fig. 8: Cusco's speculum.

Diagnostic: Collection of PAP smear, swab, punch biopsy, colposcopy.

Therapeutic: Diathermy cautery.

Advantages: Self-retaining. Less discomfort to the patent.

Disadvantages: Anterior wall of vagina is not visible.

Q. How to introduce?

After separating the labia with left thumb and index finger, transverse blades of Cusco's speculum (lubricated by jelly) is introduced in anteroposterior direction (as vaginal introitus is anteroposterior slit and depressed from side to side) and is rotated 90° to bring the transverse blades transversely (upper part of vagina transversely enlarged). Details in Chapter 1 (**Figs. 57 to 61** of Chapter 1).

AUVARD'S SELF-RETAINING SPECULUM (FIG. 9)

It is like single-bladed posterior vaginal speculum but wide and heavy.

Due to its heaviness and postoperative pain, it is rarely used.

ANTERIOR VAGINAL WALL RETRACTOR (FIG. 10)

In both sides, ring is present and serrated. Shape is like double-ended uterine curette but much larger and heavier.

Use

To retract the anterior vaginal wall along with Sims' speculum used posteriorly to visualize the cervix well.

Sterilization

Boiling or autoclave.

ALLIS TISSUE FORCEPS (FIG. 11)

It has 5–6 teeth with a catch near handle. It has two sizes: (i) smaller and (ii) larger.

Uses

- To hold the lip of cervix in vaginal surgery instead of vulsellum, e.g., D and C, IUCD insertion, vaginal hysterectomy, Fothergill's operation.
- To hold the tough structures like rectus sheath, peritoneum.
- To hold the vaginal cuff during vault transaction and during repair of vaginal cuff.
- To hold the vagina in vaginal incision and to hold the cut margins of vagina in vaginal operation, e.g., Ward-Mayo's, Fothergill and repair of CPT, etc.

Sterilization

Boiling or by autoclave.

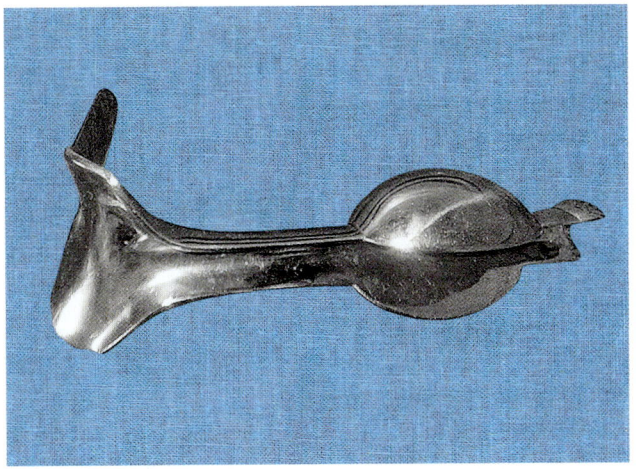

Fig. 9: Auvard's self-retaining speculum.

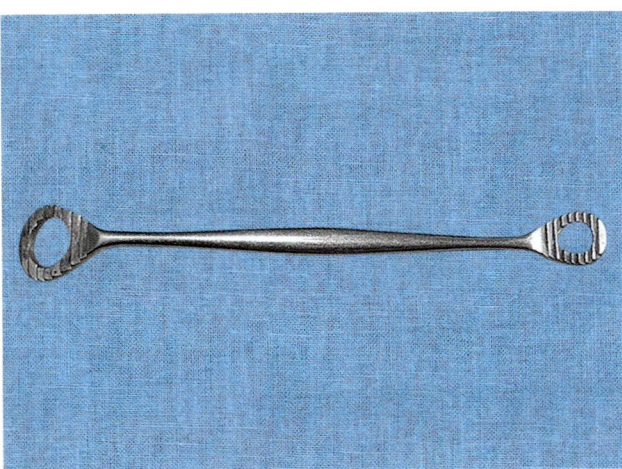

Fig. 10: Anterior vaginal wall retractor.

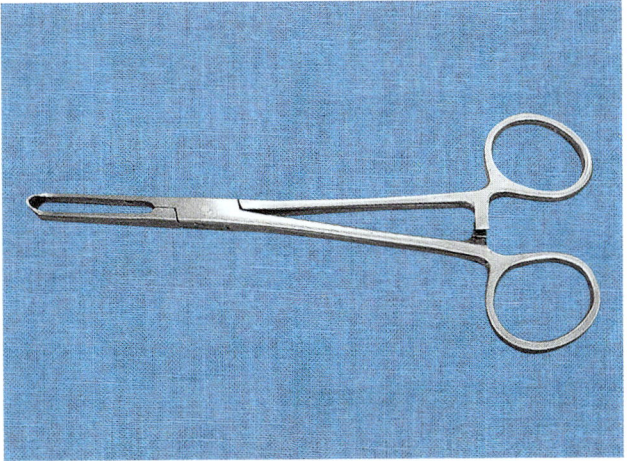

Fig. 11: Allis tissue forceps.

MULTIPLE TEETH VULSELLUM (FIG. 12)

It is tough instrument with 3–4 teeth to grasp any structure and it is provided with catch, much heavier than Allis tissue forceps.

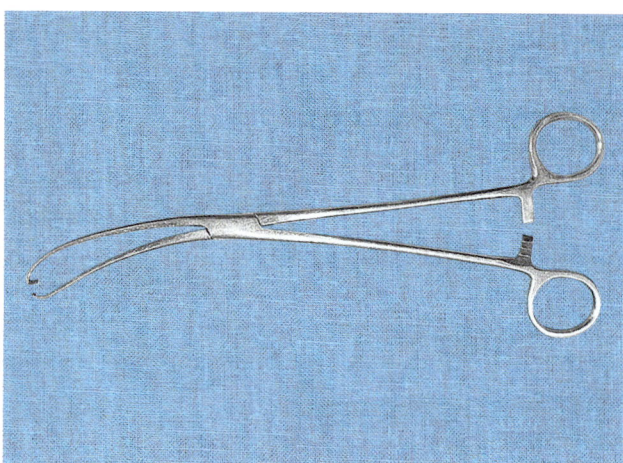

Fig. 12: Multiple teeth vulsellum.

Uses

- To hold the anterior lip of cervix in D and C, vaginal hysterectomy, amputation of cervix and Fothergill's operation.
- To hold the uterus at fundus during abdominal hysterectomy to fix the uterus.
- To hold the myoma during myomectomy.
- To remove large fibroid polyp vaginally.

Q. When you need to hold the posterior lip of cervix?

- Vaginal hysterectomy, Fothergill's operation before incision over posterior fornix
- Posterior colpotomy
- To take biopsy from anterior lip of cervix and anterior lip friable
- Vaginal ligation.

SINGLE TOOTH VULSELLUM (FIG. 13)

It has single tooth and penetrates in tissue much deeper and size is like multiple teeth vulsellum.

Uses

- To catch nulliparous cervix
- To hold cervical stump after amputation of cervix
- To hold the myoma during myomectomy
- During abdominal hysterectomy, after opening the vault of vagina, cervical lip is held to cut the rest of the vault.

UTERINE SOUND (FIG. 14)

It is olive pointed, metallic, graduated, malleable uterine sound.

Q. Why graduated?

To measure the length of the uterus.

Q. Why malleable?

To adjust the position of uterus.

Q. Why olive pointed?

To prevent the perforation of uterus.

Q. Why called sound?

Originally used for sounding of bladder stone.

Uses

- In D and C operation
- Acts as a first dilator
- To detect the position of uterus—anteverted, retroverted or midposition
- To measure the length of uterus.

Q. What is the normal length of uterocervical canal?

- Uterocervical canal is 6.5 cm, cervix—2.5 cm and cavity of uterus—4 cm and fundus—1 cm.
- Total length of uterus including fundus—7 cm, breadth—5 cm and anteroposterior—2.5 cm.
- At childhood cervix:corpus ratio is 2:1 and at puberty and thereafter ratio of cervix: corpus is 1:2.

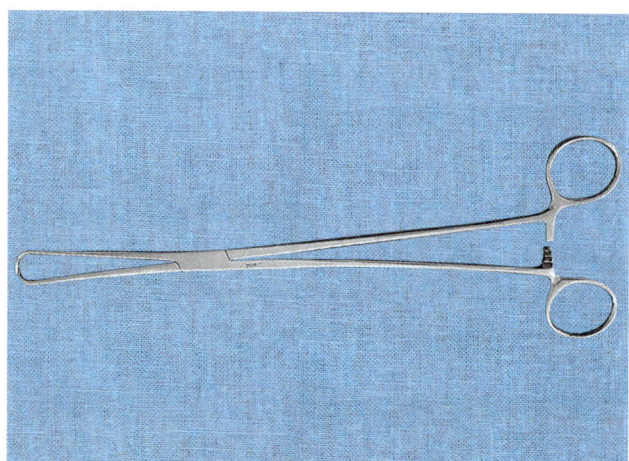

Fig. 13: Single tooth vulsellum.

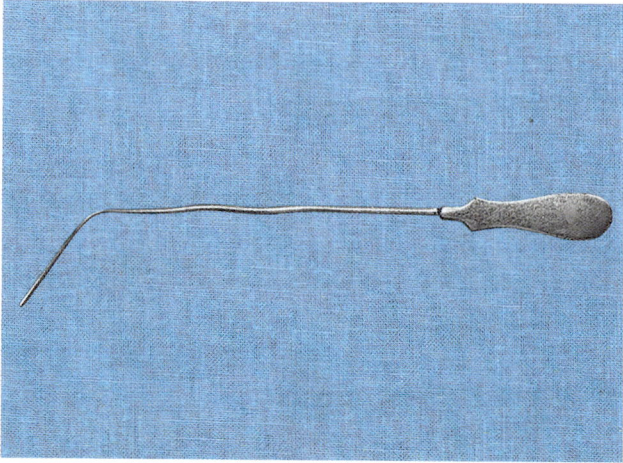

Fig. 14: Olive pointed graduated metallic malleable uterine sound.

Q. Tell the conditions where length of uterus is increased?
- Pregnancy
- Hematometra, pyometra
- Fibroid uterus
- Adenomyosis
- Endometrial cancer
- Uterine prolapse (acquired elongation of cervix)
- Congenital elongation of cervix.

Q. In which conditions the length of uterus is decreased?
- Hypoplastic uterus—Turner syndrome is a condition
- After menopause
- Submucosal polyp
- Uterine inversion.

Q. What is the normal position of uterus?
- It is anteverted and anteflexed.
- Anteversion (V for vagina)—angle between axis of body of uterus and axis of vagina—normal angle is 90°.
- Anteflexion means angle between the axis of body of uterus and cervix—normal angle is 140°.

Sterilization of Uterine Sound
Autoclaving or boiling.

CERVICAL DILATORS (FIGS. 15 AND 16)

Q. What is the use of cervical dilators?
To dilate the cervical canal, external os and internal os gradually.

Q. What are the different types of cervical dilators?
- Das's dilator
- Hegar's dilator **(Fig. 15)**
- Hawkin–Ambler's dilators **(Fig. 16)**

Dilator may be single-ended or double-ended.

Q. What are the measurements of different dilators and what is the total number of dilators in one set?

Das's Dilator or Hegar's Dilator (Fig. 15)
In double-ended dilators the lowest size is 1/2 mm and the largest size is 23/24 mm. So, one set consists of twelve dilators. However, as the larger dilators are not used nowadays, the dilators from 1/2 mm to 15/16 mm sizes (a set of 8 dilators) are sufficient. Single-ended dilators are also available. Das's dilator and Hegar's dilator are similar types. Das's dilator is more gradual (longer) than Hegar's dilator.

The name of Das's dilator is after the name of its inventor, Sir Kedar Nath Das, a famous obstetrician. The length of the uterus is measured by introducing uterine sound before introduction of dilators, otherwise there is a chance of perforation. The purpose of use of dilator is fulfilled when its maximum diameter crosses the internal os.

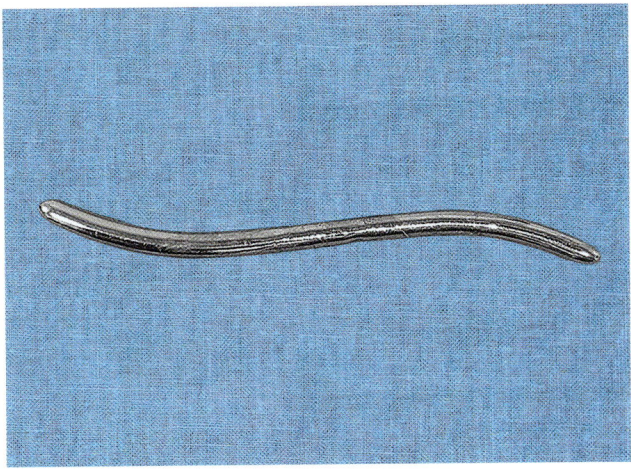

Fig. 15: Hegar's cervical dilator.

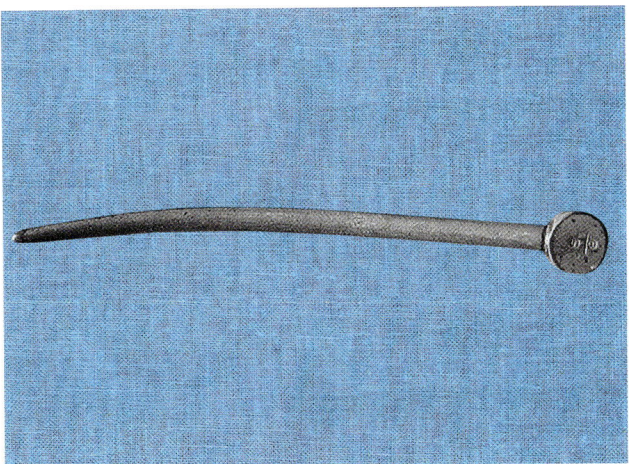

Fig. 16: Hawkin–Ambler's cervical dilator.

Q. How will you understand that maximum diameter has passed through the internal os?
Following resistance at a point, there will be loss of resistance during introduction. There will be gripping of dilator by internal os and it will not fall down if left without any support.

Q. In case of difficult dilatation what will you do?
To start with very small dilator starting with uterine sound and good anesthesia. Once there is false passage there may be a problem. Preoperative administration of misoprostol 200 mg orally or vaginally before 4 hours makes the cervix soft and makes the procedure easy.

Sterilization
Autoclaving or boiling.

Hawkin–Ambler's (H–A) Dilators (Fig. 16)
The lowest size is 3/6 mm and maximum size is 18/21 mm. One set consists of 16 dilators. In 3/6, 3 and 6 denote diameters at the tip and at the widest part behind the tip respectively. H-A dilators are only single-ended.

SECTION 5: Instruments and Operation

UTERINE CURETTE (FIGS. 17 TO 19)

Q. What are the different types of curette?

It may be blunt curette or sharp curette. The curette may be single-ended or double-ended. One curette may be both blunt and sharp types **(Fig. 17)**. Each type in two different ends.

Flushing curette (Fig. 18): It is a special type of blunt curette where there is facility of flushing of uterine cavity with antiseptic solutions.

Sharman's curette (Fig. 19): It is used for taking biopsy from uterine cavity. It is used only for gynecological purpose and can be done as office procedure.

Q. What is the use of sharp curette and blunt curette?

- Sharp curette is commonly used in gynecology for curetting endometrial cavity.
- Blunt curette for D and E.

Q. What is the use of flushing curette?

It is a blunt curette used in dilatation evacuation and especially in old incomplete abortion. Placental polyp can

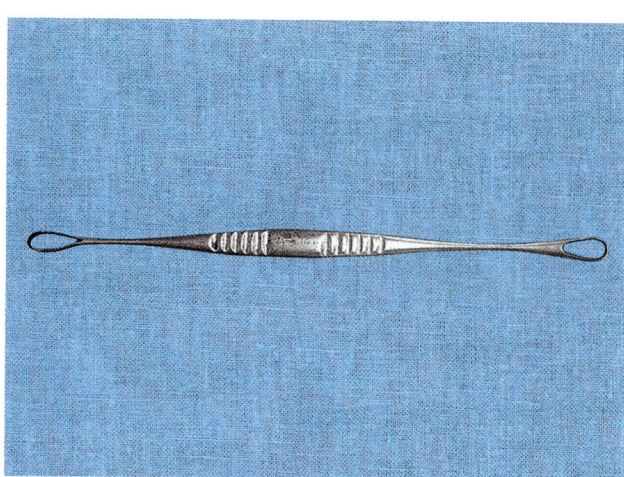

Fig. 17: Uterine curette (blunt and sharp).

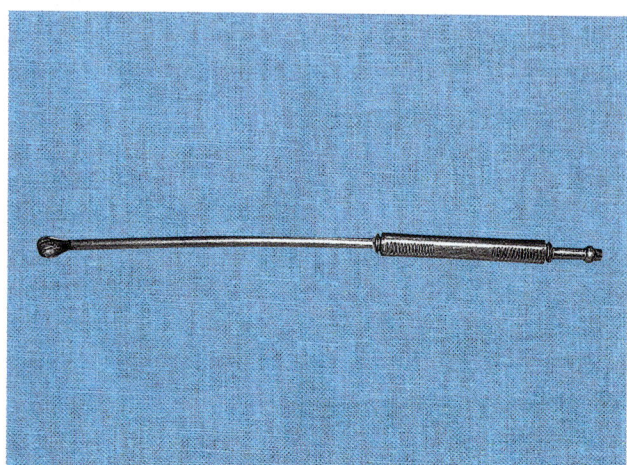

Fig. 18: Flushing curette.

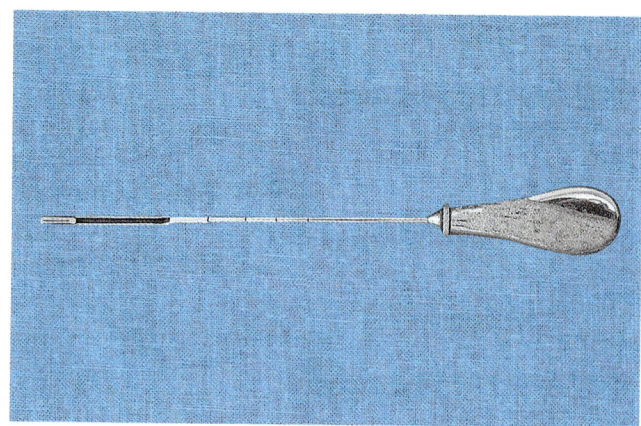

Fig. 19: Sharman's curette.

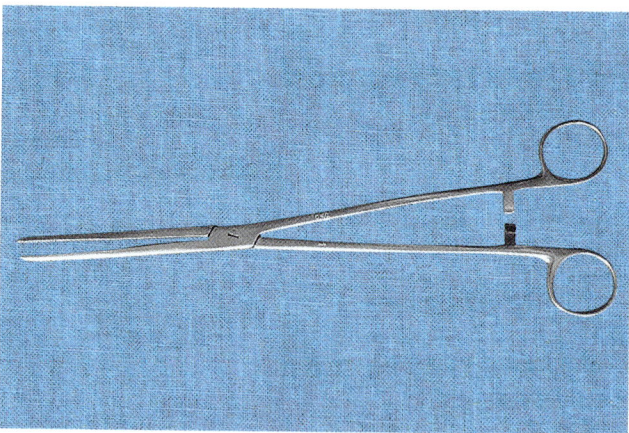

Fig. 20: Uterine dressing forceps.

be curetted with the help of it. Previously, antiseptic solution was used to pass through the channel.

Sterilization

Autoclave or boiling.

UTERINE DRESSING FORCEPS (FIG. 20)

- Its use is less in pure gynecological, mostly in pregnancy-related condition.
- It is used to dress the endometrial cavity following surgical evacuation.
- To dilate the cervix, to drain pyometra or lochiometra in puerperium.
- Pelvic abscess can be drained through posterior colpotomy approach.

LANE'S TISSUE FORCEPS (FIG. 23)

- To retract the upper cut margin of parietal wall during abdominal operation.
- Polypectomy of large cervical fibroid polyp.
- It can also be used in myomectomy to hold the myoma tissue.

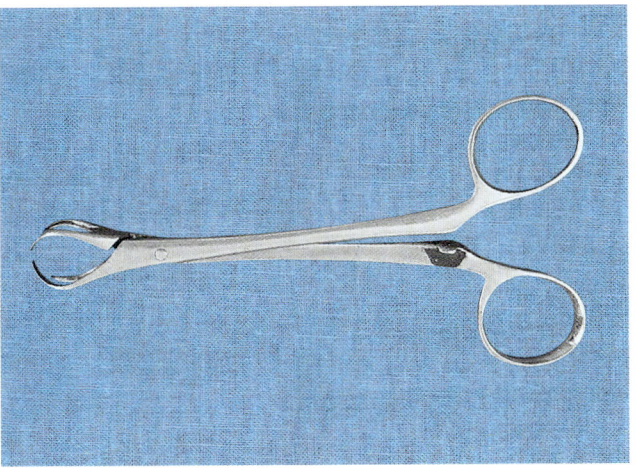

Fig. 23: Lane's tissue forceps.

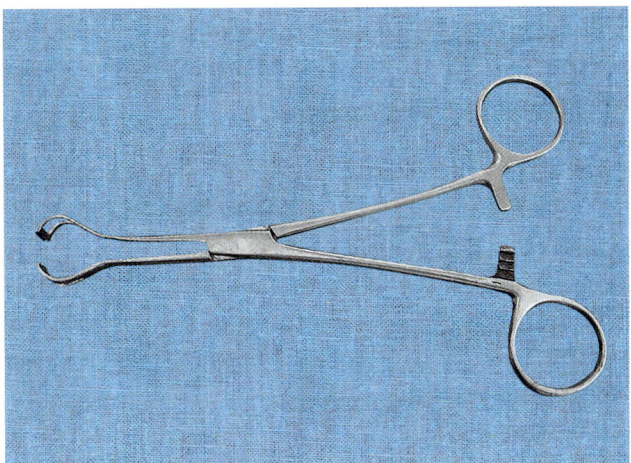

Fig. 27: Babcock's tissue forceps.

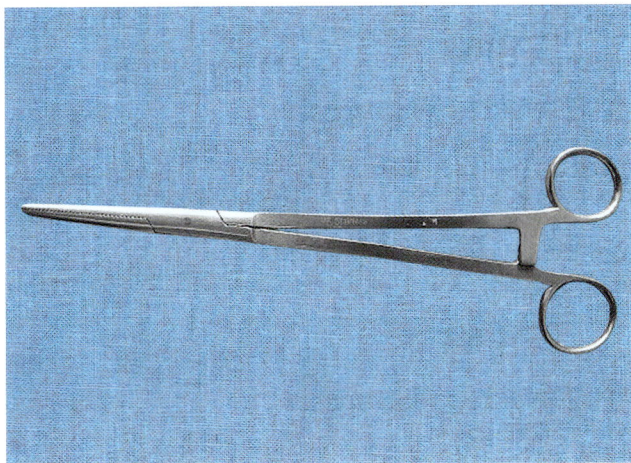

Fig. 26: Hysterectomy clamp (straight).

HYSTERECTOMY CLAMP (STRAIGHT/ CURVE) (FIG. 26)

Uses
- Hysterectomy
- Salpingo-oophorectomy
- Tubal ectopic
- To fix the uterus by holding on two cornua during hysterectomy.
- May be used as hemostatic clamp.

Sterilization
Autoclave or boiling.

BABCOCK'S TISSUE FORCEPS (FIG. 27)

It is used to grasp the structures where gentleness is needed in comparison to Allis tissue forceps as it has no tooth.

Uses
- In surgery of fallopian tube—in tubal ligation and tuboplasty

- To hold the ureter in radical hysterectomy and repair of ureteric injury.
- To hold the bladder margin to repair the VVF.
- To hold lymph nodes in lymphadenectomy.
- To hold the appendix during appendicectomy.
- During internal iliac artery ligation.

Sterilization
Autoclave or boiling.

MYOMA SCREW (FIG. 32)

Uses
- In myomectomy to hold the myoma during enucleation (*see* detail in Chapter 4 Myomectomy) (*see* **Figs. 38 and 39** of Chapter 4).
- In hysterectomy in fibroid uterus to hold and fix the uterus.

Sterilization
Autoclave or boiling.

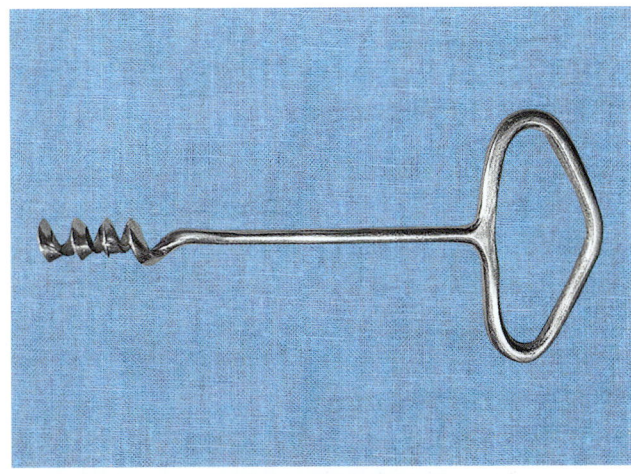

Fig. 32: Myoma screw.

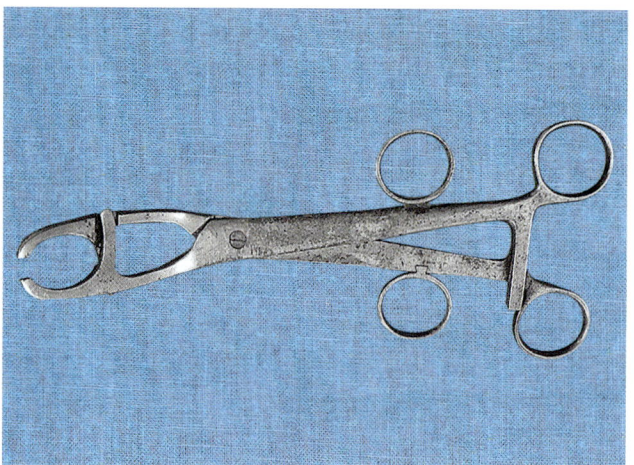

Fig. 33: Bonney's myomectomy clamp.

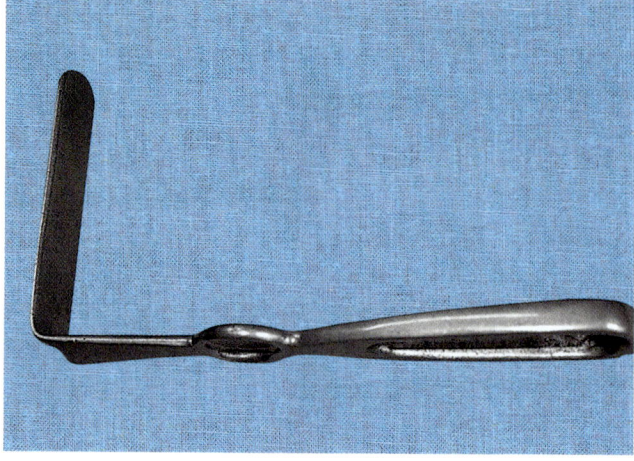

Fig. 34: Landon's bladder retractor.

BONNEY'S MYOMECTOMY CLAMP (FIG. 33)

Uses
- For reduction of blood loss in myomectomy by compressing the uterine arteries temporarily.
- It is applied from the leg ends of the patient keeping the handle in between thighs, the concavity of the instrument fits with the convexity of symphysis pubis. The blades grasp both the round ligaments in the region of isthmus and compress uterine arteries. Inclusion of round ligament prevents slipping. After repair of myoma, blade clamps are released.
- Use of rubber tourniquets (rubber catheter) or local injection of vasopressin almost replaced its use. Before infiltration of vasopressin anesthetist must be informed.

Sterilization
Autoclaving or boiling.

LANDON'S BLADDER RETRACTOR (FIG. 34)

Uses
- To retract the bladder during vaginal hysterectomy after opening of uterovesical fold of peritoneum (*see* Vaginal Hysterectomy in Chapter 10)
- It can also be used to retract lateral vaginal wall in repair of VVF
- Can be used as posterior vaginal wall in narrow vagina.

Sterilization
Boiling or autoclave.

ANEURYSM NEEDLE WITH THREAD (FIG. 39)

Uses
- For internal iliac artery, ligation mostly for obstetric reasons. Sometimes done in radical hysterectomy.
- Venesection.

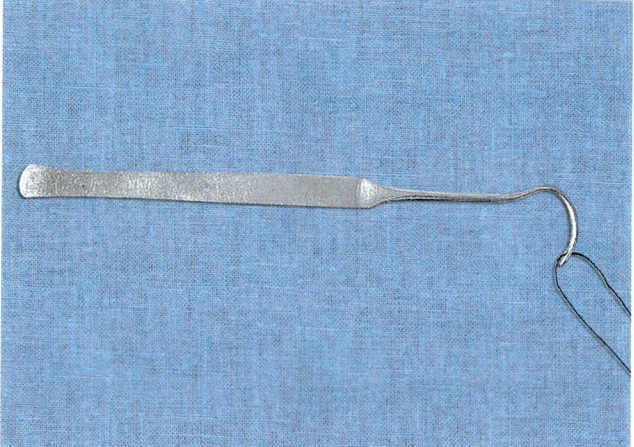

Fig. 39: Aneurysm needle.

Sterilization
Autoclave or boiling.

RING PESSARY (FIGS. 47A AND B)

It is made up of rubber or polyethylene.

Use
In pelvic organ prolapse (POP).

Q. What are the indications of vaginal pessary in POP?

For palliative treatment in POP, it acts by stretching the vaginal wall and elevating the vagina.

The indications are:
- Women who decline surgery
- Medically unfit for surgery
- During pregnancy
- Desires childbearing
- Pending for surgery.

And for pessary test before surgery whether woman will be relieved of symptoms by surgery.

CHAPTER 24: Identify the Instruments—Know Your Instruments

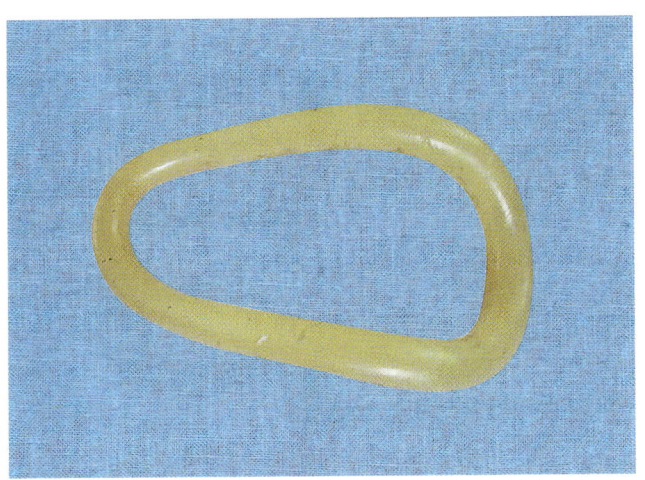

Fig. 48: Hodge–Smith pessary for correction of mobile retroversion.

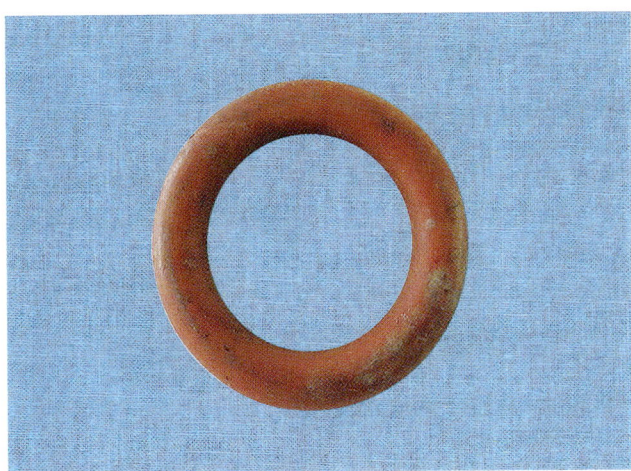

Fig. 47A: Ring pessary used for pelvic organ prolapse (rubber).

Vaginal pessary—types, introduction, follow-up and complications—details are written in Chapter 10, Pelvic Organ Prolapse, Page 223.

Sterilization
By Savlon solution for 12 hours.

HODGE–SMITH PESSARY (FIG. 48)

Uses
- In retroversion (mobile) of uterus
- In retroverted puerperal uterus.

Procedure of Introduction
Measurement: It will be 1.25 cm less between the stretched posterior fornix and symphysis pubis.

Correction of retroversion: Patient is asked to pass urine. Position is lithotomy. By introducing right index and middle finger up to posterior fornix fundus of retroverted uterus is pushed anteriorly and left hand is kept behind the uterus per abdominally to keep it anteverted.

Placing of pessary: Broader end of pessary keeping anteriorly pessary is introduced laterally while the concavity lies medially. Now the pessary is rotated 90° and the broader end is pushed up to posterior fornix and narrow end is pushed behind the symphysis pubis. It stretches the uterosacral ligament and keeps the uterus anteverted.

It is made up of hard rubber or silicone and chemically sterilized.

HYSTEROSALPINGOGRAPHY CANNULA (FIG. 49)

It is a metallic cannula used for hysterosalpingography (HSG) where radiological visualization of uterocervical canal is done.

Q. What are the indications of HSG?
- Tubal patency test as infertility workup—the most common.

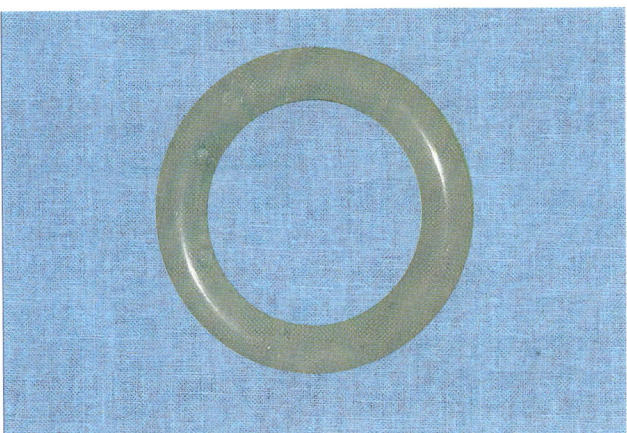

Fig. 47B: Ring pessary made of silicone.

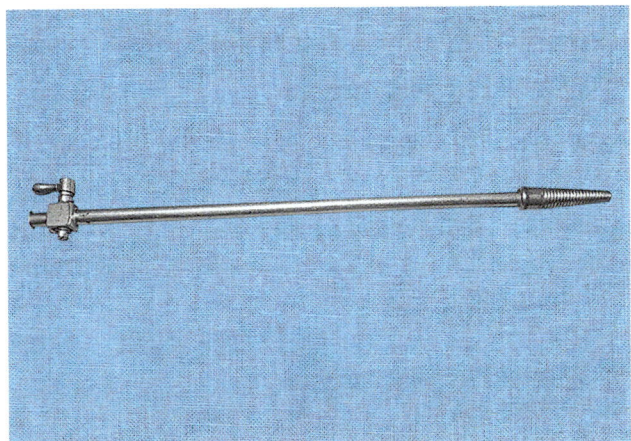

Fig. 49: Hysterosalpingography cannula.

- Recurrent abortion or preterm labor for detection of uterine anomaly—septate, subseptate, bicornuate, unicornuate.

Q. What are the other tubal patency tests?
- Sonohysterosalpingography
- Laparoscopic dye test.

Q. When it is done?

Day 7 to day 10 of menses period.

Q. Which dye is used?

Lipid based or water based. Commonly water-based dye is used as complication is less but delineation is good in lipid based dye. Urografin or conray 420 is used.

Q. Where it is done?

In radiology department.

Q. What are the complications?

- Embolism
- Extravasation
- Pelvic infection.

Q. Describe the procedure.

For details *see* Chapter of Infertility (Chapter 11) and Chapter 29 (HSG)—procedure, advantage, disadvantage and contraindications (*see* Page 258).

AYRE'S SPATULA (FIG. 50)

It is wooden spatula for taking cervical cytology and vaginal cytology. Heart-shaped end is used for cervix and round-shaped side is used for vaginal cytology.

Q. What are the indications of cervical cytology?

- Cytological status of genital cancer.
- Cytohormonal study—mostly lateral wall of vagina.
- Determination of sex chromatin—it is usually done from buccal smear.

Q. Why wooden, not metallic?

As only superficial cells are collected. Plastic spatula is better than wooden spatula as cells enter into micropore of wooden spatula. Three types of plastic devices are used for cervical cytology **spatula**, **cytobrush**, and **broom**. It is available in presterilized pack.

For details and other questions, *see* Chapter of Carcinoma Cervix in Chapter 8—cervical cytology (*see* Page 175).

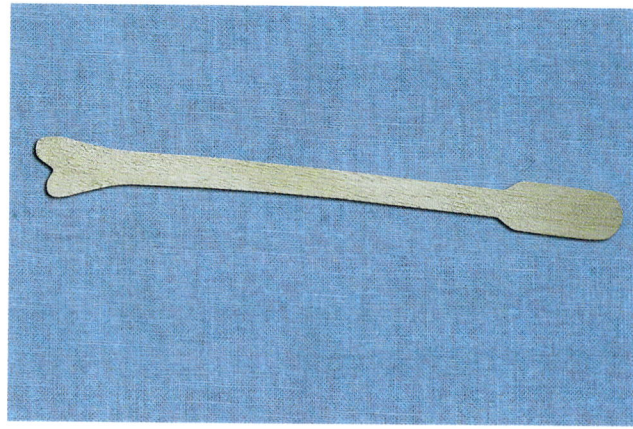

Fig. 50: Ayre's spatula (wooden).

Fig. 51: Cytobrush.

CYTOBRUSH (FIG. 51)

Use

- For taking cytology from the cervical canal.
- It is available in presterilized pack.

For details and other questions, *see* Chapter of Carcinoma Cervix in Chapter 8—cervical cytology (*see* Page 175).

CHAPTER 25

Operative Gynecology

Chapter Outline

- Hysterectomy—Types, Role of Oophorectomy, Salpingectomy, Steps of Abdominal Hysterectomy, Indications and Complications
- Nondescent Vaginal Hysterectomy
- Dilatation and Curettage—Steps, Indications and Complications
- Surgery for Chronic Uterine Inversion—Haultain's Technique, Spinelli's Technique and Kustner's Operation
- Risk of Surgeries with their Location
- Preoperative Assessment of a Patient Undergoing Gynecological Surgery (PAC)

HYSTERECTOMY

Q. What do you mean by hysterectomy?

It is the surgical removal of uterus.

Q. What are the approaches of hysterectomy?

- Abdominal hysterectomy
- Vaginal hysterectomy
- Laparoscopic hysterectomy
- Laparoscopic-assisted vaginal hysterectomy.

Q. What are the different types of hysterectomy?

- *Supracervical hysterectomy (SCH) also called subtotal hysterectomy:* Where only body of the uterus is removed. The term subtotal hysterectomy is not preferred due to its ambiguity.
- *Total hysterectomy (TH):* Uterus and cervix are removed.
- *Total hysterectomy with bilateral salpingo-oophorectomy (TH with BSO):* Uterus, cervix and bilateral adnexae are removed. This was also called panhysterectomy, but the term is not preferred. Rarely, TH with unilateral hysterectomy is done.
- *Extended hysterectomy:* TAH-BSO with upper part of vagina.
- *Radical hysterectomy:* Body, cervix, upper part of vagina, parametrium and draining lymph nodes are removed.

Q. Which type of hysterectomy is done where?

Supracervical (Subtotal) Hysterectomy

- Where TH is technically difficult due to extensive adhesion, such as endometriosis, pelvic inflammatory disease (PID) and ovarian malignancy for fear of adjacent organ damage
- When concurrent sacrocolpopexy is done for prolapse, SCH is done to reduce mesh erosion
- The concept of improving urinary, bowel and sexual function on keeping the cervix is no longer accepted
- Obstetric hysterectomy, e.g., rupture uterus sometimes subtotal hysterectomy done to reduce operative time

Disadvantages: Persistent vaginal bleeding from retained endometrium and difficulty of removal of cervix (trachelectomy) if it is required. Besides there is risk of cancer in the stump (cervical stump cancer).

Radical Hysterectomy

Cancer cervix.

CLASSIFICATION OF HYSTERECTOMY IN RELEVANCE TO SURGERY OF CANCER CERVIX

Q. How hysterectomy is classified in relevance to surgery of cancer cervix?

It is classified into five types depending on the extent of removal of parametrium, paracolpos, vagina, site of cutting of uterosacral ligament and site of uterine artery ligation. Type I is simple hysterectomy (extrafascial hysterectomy) (*see* Chapter 18, "Cancer Cervix").

STEPS OF ABDOMINAL APPROACH OF TOTAL HYSTERECTOMY

Q. Describe the steps of total hysterectomy (Figs. 1 to 18).

- Position of patient—supine position.
- Catheterization (Foley catheter), antiseptic dressing and draping.
- Anesthesia—general anesthesia or regional (usually spinal).

Incision: Transverse (Pfannenstiel incision) or vertical (infraumbilical midline or paramedian). The successive layers are:

Skin, subcutaneous tissue, rectus sheath, retraction of rectus muscles laterally, cutting of extraperitoneal fascia and finally opening of peritoneum to open the abdomen. There is no posterior layer of rectus sheath below the level of umbilicus. Procedure of opening of peritoneum—thin layer of peritoneum is held by two artery forceps at the upper part of incision, excluding by palpation that bowel loop, omentum are not held. A small nick is done by scalpel or scissors and incision is extended by scissors taking care that bladder is not injured.

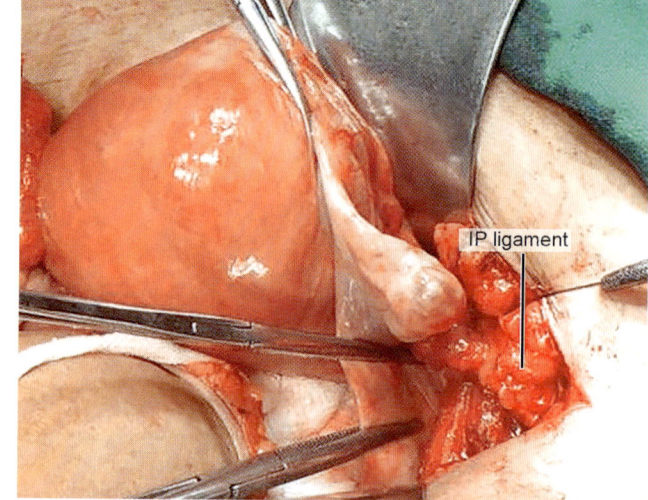

Fig. 2: Clamping, transection and suture of infundibulopelvic ligament.

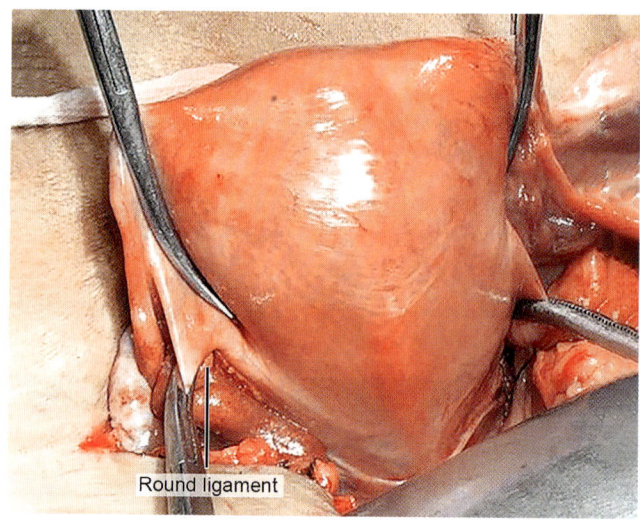

Fig. 3: Clamping, transection and suture of round ligament.

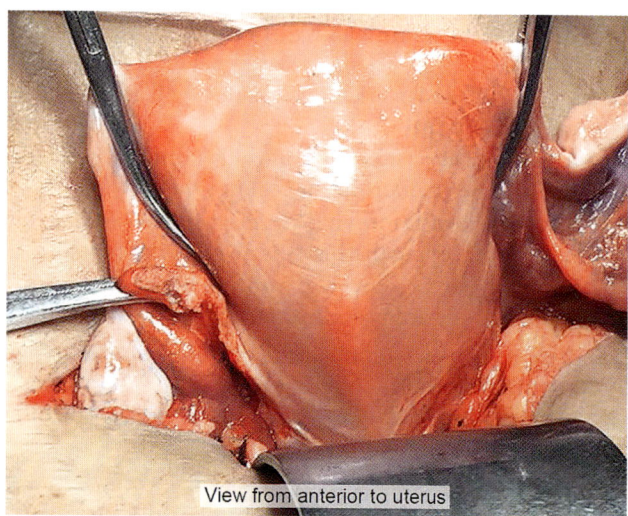

Fig. 1: Uterus is held and fixed by two long clamps on two cornua.

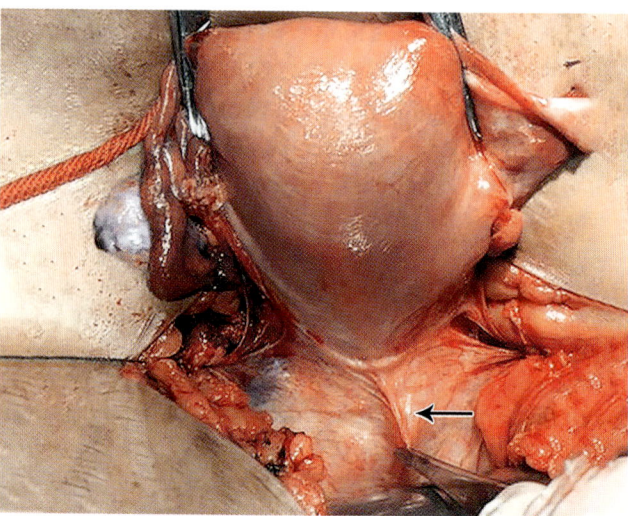

Fig. 4: Loose uterovesical fold of peritoneum.

CHAPTER 25: Operative Gynecology

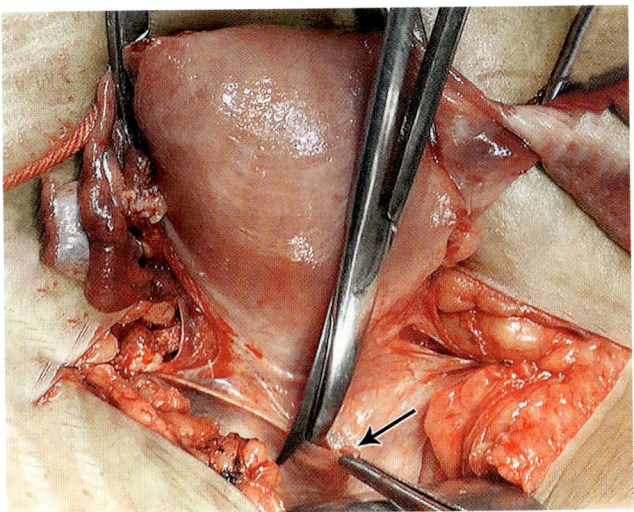

Fig. 5: Cutting of uterovesical fold of peritoneum from one round ligament to other.

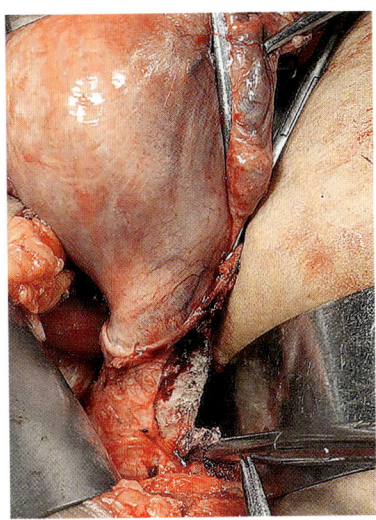

Fig. 8: Clamping and cutting of Mackenrodt's ligament and uterosacral separately or combinedly.

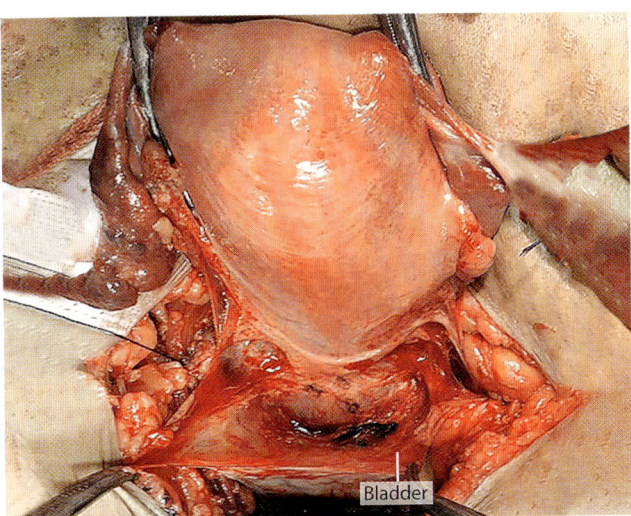

Fig. 6: Bladder is pushed down after cutting uterovesical fold of peritoneum.

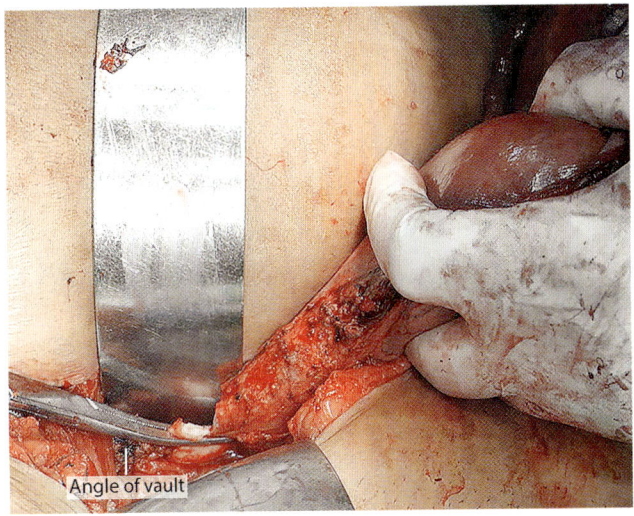

Fig. 9: Cutting the vault of vagina below the level of cervix and vagina is opened (transection of vagina).

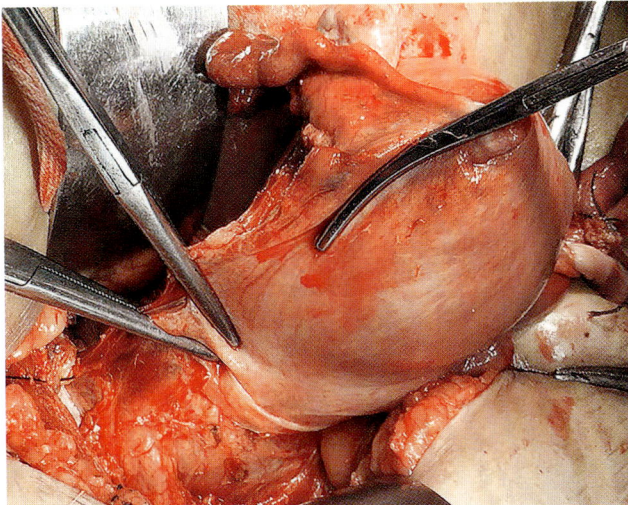

Fig. 7: Clamping of uterine vessels, cut in-between clamps and ligated.

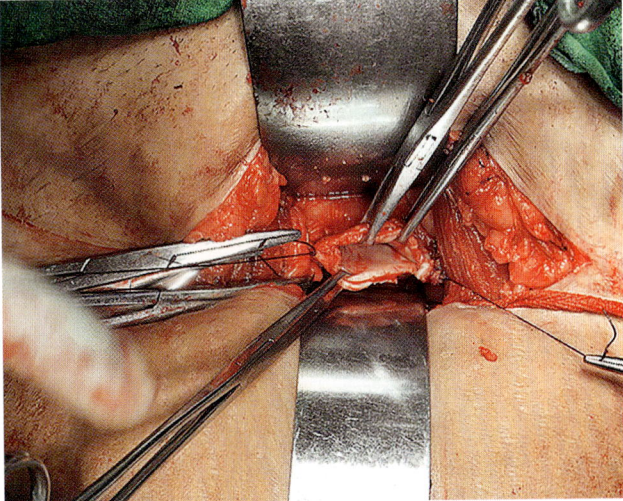

Fig. 10: Vault of vagina after removal of uterus.

Following opening abdomen, a self-retaining retractor (Balfour type) is used or simply Doyen's retractor is used to retract lower margins.

Now the pelvic organs are examined. The fundus is held by two clamps at two cornua or a single multiple teeth vulsellum at fundus to retract it.

The bowel is packed from operative field.

First pair of clamps—if hysterectomy with salpingo-oophorectomy is done, first clamp (two long artery forceps) is placed on *infundibulopelvic ligament (IP) cut and the lateral pedicle is replaced by sutures* **(Figs. 2 and 12)**.

If only hysterectomy is done retaining the tube and ovary *first clamp (two long artery forceps) is placed on broad ligament near the cornu which includes ovarian ligament, fallopian tube and mesosalpinx* **(Fig. 13)**.

Second pair of clamps—placed on *round ligaments and cut in-between clamps and replaced by sutures* **(Figs. 12 and 13)**.

(Alternatively, first pair of clamps is placed on round ligament followed by the IP ligament or at cornu to include ovarian ligament, fallopian tube and mesosalpinx as second pair of clamps).

The same steps are done on opposite side.

Next important step is cutting of uterovesical fold of peritoneum (which is loosely attached) from one round ligament stump to other **(Figs. 4 and 14)**. Attachment of bladder with the cervix is divided with the few snips with the

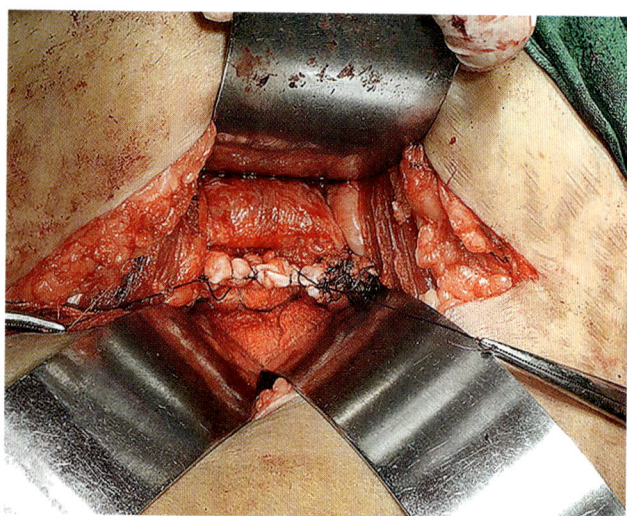

Fig. 11: Vaginal vault after repair—bladder in front and rectum behind.

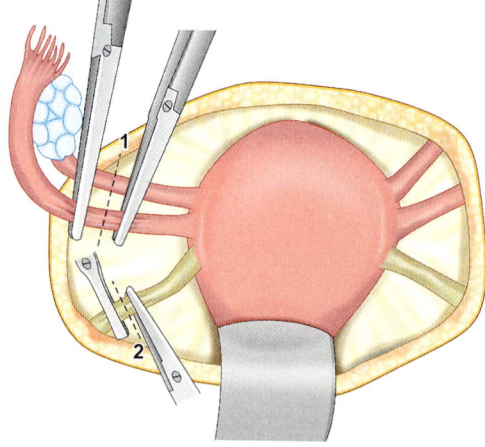

1. Broad ligament structures—fallopian tube and ovarian ligament
2. Round ligament

Fig. 13: (1) Clamping of broad ligament containing ovarian ligament and fallopian tube; (2) Clamping of round ligament—in case of total hysterectomy (TH).

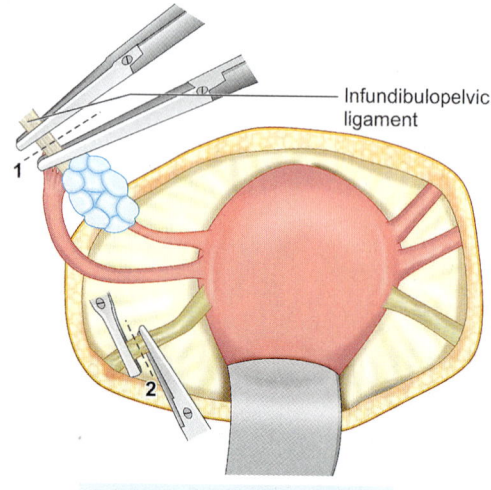

1. Infundibulopelvic ligament
2. Round ligament

Fig. 12: (1) Clamping of infundibulopelvic ligament; (2) Clamping of round ligament—total hysterectomy done—in case of total hysterectomy with bilateral salpingo-oophorectomy (TH with BSO).

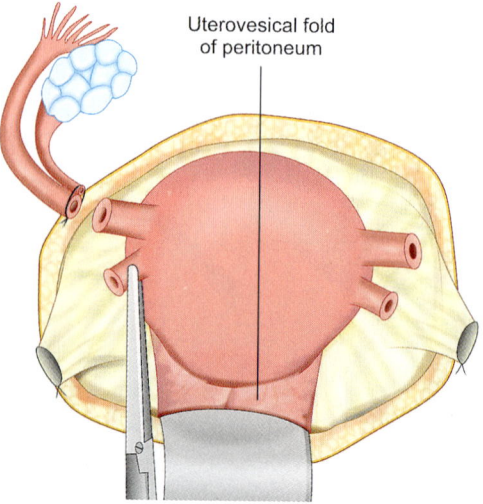

Fig. 14: Uterovesical fold of peritoneum.

help of scissors and bladder is pushed down and ideally be dissected 1 cm below the lower margin of cervix **(Figs. 5, 6 and 15)**. Until and unless this step is done, uterine vessels cannot be clamped as the clamp will injure the ureter and bladder.

Third pair of clamps is given on uterine vessels **(Figs. 7 and 16)** close to the uterus with curved clamps at the isthmus level placing horizontally across the vertical vessels. Skeletonizing the vessel (removing the tissue surrounding the vessel) before clamping has advantages of making smaller vascular pedicle and minimizing the chance of vessel retraction. A clamp is placed above this clamp to prevent retrograde flow. The vessels in-between clamps are cut and the vessels are sutured. Pulling the uterus upward and opposite side will help ligate the uterine vessels well.

Uterine vessels are clamped, cut and stitched on opposite side.

Fourth pair of clamps **(Figs. 8 and 17)** is placed over the Mackenrodt's ligament just below and medial to the uterine pedicle, cut and transfixation suture given. Depending on the length of ligament, multiple clamps may be needed. In last clamp, the uterosacral ligament is included which is identified by upward traction of uterus. Same procedure is repeated opposite side. Both structures can be included in single clamp in small uterus **(Fig. 17)**.

Transection of vagina (Fig. 9): Now curved clamps are placed below the level of cervix on both sides, the tips often near the midline. The bladder must be mobilized sufficiently below before clamping the vaginal vault. The inferior level of cervix is identified by palpating the anterior and posterior vaginal walls. The vaginal tissues above the clamps are transacted and angles are sutured with transfixation suture.

Closure of vaginal cuff (Figs. 10, 11 and 18): Now the vaginal cuff is sutured with running 1-0 delayed absorbable suture. Posteriorly cut margin of peritoneum is included and

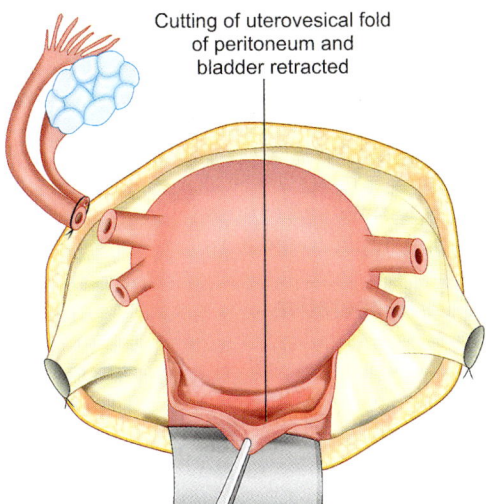

Fig. 15: Cutting of uterovesical fold of peritoneum and pushing down of bladder.

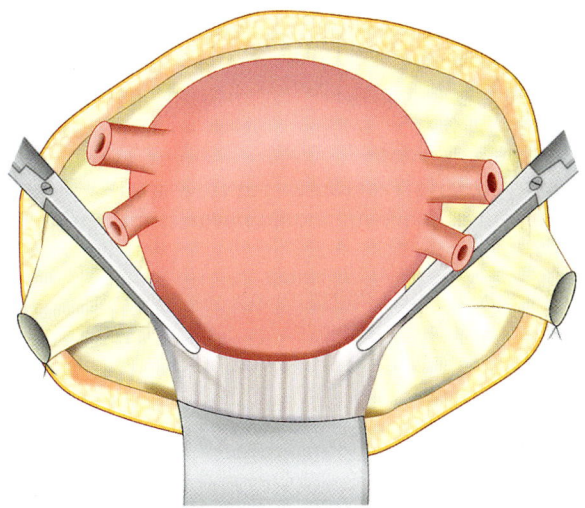

Fig. 17: Clamping of Mackenrodt's and uterosacral ligament (fourth pair of clamps).

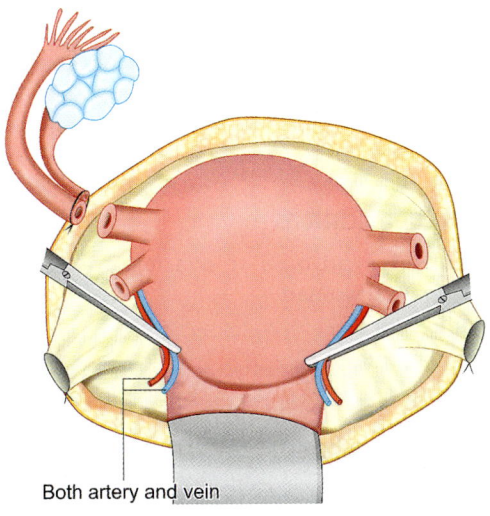

Fig. 16: Clamping of uterine vessels (third pair of clamps).

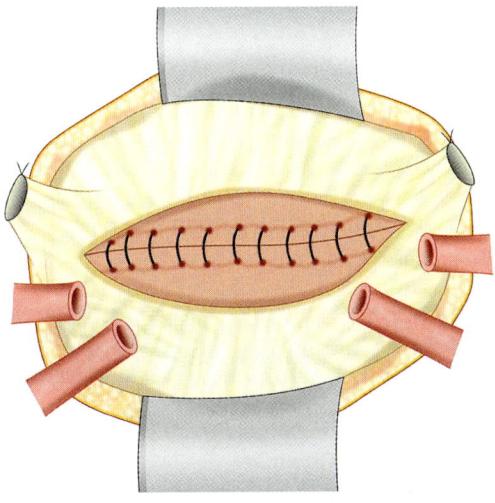

Fig. 18: Repair of vaginal vault after removal of uterus.

anteriorly bladder is kept away from suture. Complete hemostasis is done. Fixing the Mackenrodt's ligament with the lateral angle of vault and fixing the uterosacral ligament with the vaginal walls are suggested to prevent vault prolapse following surgery.

In all the stumps, usually 1-0 delayed absorbable suture is used.

Complete hemostasis is secured. Packs are removed and abdomen is closed in layers.

INDICATIONS OF HYSTERECTOMY

Q. What are the indications of hysterectomy?

The common indications are:
- Dysfunctional uterine bleeding (DUB)
- Uterine leiomyoma
- Adenomyosis
- Pelvic endometriosis
- Ovarian tumor
- Endometrial cancer
- Cervical intraepithelial neoplasia
- Cancer cervix.

Others:
- Uterine perforation
- Obstetric hysterectomy—rupture uterus, morbid adhesion of placenta, atonic postpartum hemorrhage (PPH).

Q. When will you remove ovary during hysterectomy? Advantages and disadvantages.

After 50 years, it should be removed, before 45 years healthy ovary not removed.

Advantages of Keeping Ovary

- Menopausal syndrome (menopausal symptoms, osteoporosis, coronary heart disease) occurs less
- Sexual and mental health not hampered in premenopausal women.

Disadvantages

- Chance of vasomotor symptoms and its severity is more in premenopausal women.
- Sexual function diminished
- Chance of malignancy (0.1–0.75%)
- Benign cyst—chance of relaparotomy
- Residual ovary syndrome.

JUSTIFICATION OF SALPINGECTOMY DURING HYSTERECTOMY

Q. What is the justification of salpingectomy during hysterectomy? Recent thoughts.

As overall evidence suggests that majority of ovarian cancers originate from the fallopian tube, the fallopian tubes should be removed during hysterectomy irrespective of ovarian conservation.

Q. What are the latest views on oophorectomy and salpingectomy at the time of hysterectomy?

- In women with *BRCA1* and *BRCA2* mutations, BSO is clearly beneficial to reduce risk of both ovarian and breast cancers
- Fallopian tubes should be removed during hysterectomy irrespective of oophorectomy as it is widely agreed that majority of ovarian cancers originate from fallopian tube
- Evidence suggests that risk of death, coronary heart disease, and stroke increase in women undergoing BSO and risk increases if it is performed in earlier age
- Women below 45 years who have undergone BSO should be considered for hormone replacement therapy (HRT)
- The benefits and risks regarding removal of healthy ovaries should be discussed before going for hysterectomy for benign condition.

Q. Enumerate the complications of hysterectomy.

Peroperative Complications

- Hemorrhage
- Injury to bladder, ureter (*see* ureteric injury in Chapter 17: Vesicovaginal Fistula)
- Injury of intestines and rectum
- Anesthetic complications.

Immediate Postoperative

- Hemorrhage—reactionary, secondary
- Shock
- Urinary retention, urinary tract infection
- Infection—peritonitis, wound sepsis
- Rectus sheath hematoma
- Wound dehiscence, burst abdomen
- Paralytic ileus, abdominal distension, intestinal obstruction
- Pneumonia
- Thromboembolism—pulmonary embolism
- Secondary hemorrhage from vault on second week onward—granuloma of vault
- Urinary fistula—vesicovaginal fistula (VVF), ureteric fistula.

Long-term Complications

- Menopausal syndrome if ovaries are removed in premenopausal woman
- Band adhesion
- Incisional hernia
- Vault prolapse.

NONDESCENT VAGINAL HYSTERECTOMY (NDVH)

Langenbeck first performed vaginal hysterectomy in 1813. Nondescent vaginal hysterectomy was pioneered by Haene'y in 1934. Vaginal route is preferred as it has less complication, fast recovery with short hospital stay and without any visible scar. Today, NDVH is very popular method of hysterectomy where possible.

Indications of NDVH: NDVH can be done in all patients requiring hysterectomy except few contraindications.

Contraindications: All cases are not suitable for NDVH. The important contraindications are: (1) uterus more than 20 weeks size, (2) adnexal pathology, (3) limited vaginal space, (4) restricted uterine mobility, (5) cervix flushed with wall, (6) previous history of fistula (VVF/RVF) repair.

Advantages: Less hospital stay, less analgesic requirement, early recovery, surgery through natural orifice causing no visible scar and cost effectiveness in comparison to laparoscopic hysterectomy are the main advantages. It is also convenient for obese patients.

Disadvantages: It requires expertise, not preferred in some cases like endometriosis, pelvic adhesions, bigger uterine size (>20 weeks size).

Preoperative evaluation for suitability of NDVH: Uterine mobility, size, descent of cervix, mobility of vaginal mucosa mainly in posterior vaginal wall should be evaluated. In case of scarred abdomen, if there is dimpling over abdomen following traction to cervix, NDVH should be abandoned. This evaluation is done on operative table before proceeding to NDVH.

Basic Steps of NDVH

Regional anesthesia is preferred. Patient's position, dressing and draping are done similar to other vaginal surgery.

Incision is given on cervico-vaginal epithelium (approx. 2.5 cm from external OS) in full thickness of epithelium including underlying fascia after injecting 40–50 mL normal saline (NS) or 10 mL NS from adrenaline rinsed syringe for hydro dissection. After cutting vesicocervical ligament, bladder was pushed upwards by blunt dissection.

Then approx. 2.5 cm from external OS in midline in posterior vaginal wall, a sharp bold incision was made by scissors to open POD. Sometimes POD can be opened in single stroke.

After that two single bladed long Sims' speculum was introduced to retract anterior and posterior vaginal walls. First pair of clamps have to be placed to grasp Mackenrodt's-uterosacral ligament complex. Second pair of clamps are placed over uterine artery. Though some may proceed for delivery of uterus through POD following uterine artery clamping, third pair of clamps usually have been applied over ascending branch of uterine artery and part of broad ligament. After third pair of clamps anterior peritoneum is usually opened. If not opened, proceed for its opening. Next step is delivery of uterus through POD.

After delivery of uterus, clamps are placed over cornual structures. Each clamp is cut and tied. Thus, hysterectomy is completed. Then vaginal vault was closed by continuous sutures. During suturing posterior peritoneum should be included along with posterior vaginal wall. Exclusion of anterior peritoneum can be done.

Foley catheterization is done and kept for 12–24 hours. Sometimes another Foley catheter can be placed in vault as drain.

Ideal suture material is No.1 Polygalactin violet (Vicryl). 40 mm ½ circle needle but some surgeons use SRS needle (short straight needle).

Few Modifications in Operative Technique

Clampless procedure: Direct suturing of ligaments done and then cut.

Aqua dissection: 40–50 mL normal saline(NS) is usually used. Some may use up to 150 mL of NS. Principle is that tissue under the mucosa is flooded with fluid, compresses the vascular plane. Advantages are less blood loss and easier dissection.

Vessel sealing system: In place of clamp, LigaSure vessel sealing system can be used.

Volume reductive procedure: Bisection, myomectomy (in presence of myoma) and intramyometrial coring are done. Morcellation can also be done.

Postoperative care: Routine prophylactic antibiotic, IV fluid for 12 hours, oral fluid after 3 hours, catheter is removed after 12 hours. Patient may return home after 24 to 36 hours.

Complications

Intraoperative: Urinary tract injury, bowel injury and hemorrhage.

Postoperative: Vault hematoma, vaginal discharge, wound infection, urinary tract complications like urinary retention, ureteral injury, vesicovaginal fistula.

WERTHEIM'S OPERATION (ABDOMINAL RADICAL HYSTERECTOMY)

Abdominal—*Wertheim's (Ernst Wertheim 1864-1920) operation:* This may be:

- Bonney type (1941)—radical hysterectomy is done first followed by lymphadenectomy
- Meigs (1954) or Okabayashi—lymphadenectomy first followed by hysterectomy.

For details of surgery in cancer cervix please *see* **Chapter 8: A Case of Carcinoma Cervix and Premalignant Lesions of Cervix**

Basic Steps of Radical Hysterectomy

- Cutting of round ligaments and dissecting the paravesical space
- Cutting of uterovesical fold of peritoneum and dissection of uterovesical space
- Clamping and cutting of infundibulopelvic ligament/tuboovarian ligament
- Identification of ureter, identification of uterine artery and ligation of uterine artery

- Dissection of ureter up to ureteric tunnel followed by dissection of ureteric tunnel and displacing the ureter laterally.
- Dissecting the pararectal spaces and rectovaginal space
- Excision of uterosacral—Mackenrodt's ligament complex
- Excision of vaginal cuff
- Removal of pelvic lymph nodes (*see* below).

Steps of Lymph Node Dissection in Radical Hysterectomy—Abdominal Method (Fig. 18A)

- All visible lymph nodes should be removed though extent and techniques differ from surgeon to surgeon.
- Removal starts from bifurcation of common iliac artery and extended downwards. If any enlarged node is detected the dissection is extended cranially for search of common iliac and para-aortic nodes.
- With the help of retractors one above and medially displacing ureter and the other retracted below and laterally the area along the common iliac vessels and external iliac vessels are exposed. Using tooth dissecting forceps fascia over the iliopsoas muscle is incised along the artery up to the inguinal ligament from where lateral external iliac lymph nodes are drawn avoiding the injury of genitofemoral nerve. Individual lymphatic channels are diathermied very cautiously. Any torn small vessels are ligated or diathermied. Dissection of the fascia and nodal tissue were done over the entire length of external artery, the procedure will make the vessel nude. All nodal tissue can be removed en bloc if the tissue is kept under tension with the forceps by left hand and dissection is done by scissor with the right hand.
- Then external iliac artery is retracted laterally to expose the external iliac vein, the fascia and nodal tissue over which is removed in the similar way but very gently.

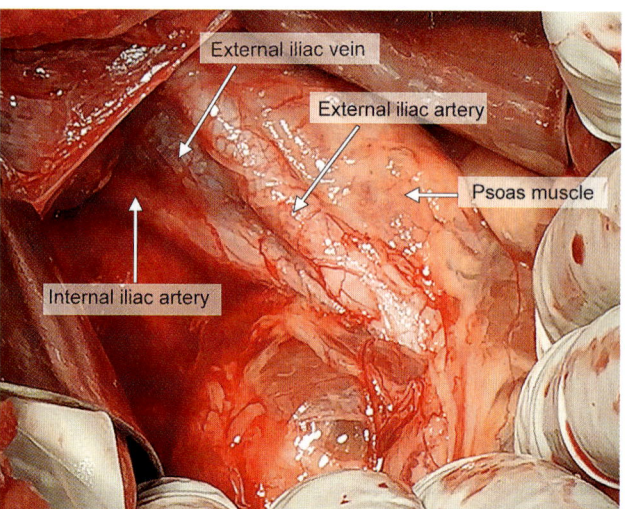

Fig. 18A: Lymphadenectomy in open abdominal approach showing the bifurcation of right common iliac artery along which lymph nodes are situated.

- From the upper end of external iliac vessels the fascial tissue over the internal iliac artery is separated downwards.
- Dissection dipping below the external iliac vein will expose the obturator fossa which can be emptied of all nodal tissue in the final stage. Exposure of obturator fossa becomes easier by retracting the external vein and artery laterally. Following lifting of tissue bulk obturator nerve and vessels are visible. Any bleeding over the area is cauterized or pressed with gauze for hemostasis.

DILATATION AND CURETTAGE

Name the Instruments Used for Dilatation and Curettage (D&C) (Figs. 19 to 21)

1. Sponge holding forceps
2. Catheter
3. Sims' posterior vaginal speculum
4. Multiple teeth vulsellum
5. Uterine sound
6. Cervical dilators
7. Uterine curette.

Steps of Dilatation and Curettage (Figs. 22 to 29)

- *Position:* Patient in lithotomy position (**Fig. 30**)
- *Anesthesia:* Sedation with paracervical block or regional
- Antiseptic dressing and draping (**Fig. 22**)
- Catheterization (**Fig. 23**)
- Bimanual examination—to note the size, position and mobility of uterus (**Fig. 24**). Adnexae are also palpated to detect any other pathology (**Fig. 31**)
- Introduction of Sims' posterior vaginal speculum to retract the posterior vaginal wall and held by an assistant (**Fig. 25**)
- Anterior lip of cervix is held either by multiple teeth vulsellum or Allis tissue forceps (**Fig. 26**)
- Uterine sound is introduced through the cervical canal to note the position and length of uterus (**Fig. 27**)
- Dilatation of cervical os successively with the cervical dilators (**Figs. 28 and 32**)
- First smallest dilator is passed and the size is increased to negotiate the uterine curette
- Curettage of endometrial cavity (sometimes cervical canal) by uterine curette (usually by sharp curette) to curette all the cavity (**Figs. 29 and 33**)
- Sims' speculum and Allis tissue forceps are removed. Cervix is swabbed with antiseptic solution and checked for any unusual bleeding
- An antibiotic is given. After rest of 4 hours, patient may be discharged.

Q. How will you collect and what will you do with the curette material?

Collection of curette material sample is taken on a dry gauze and finally taken in formal saline (10%) and sent

CHAPTER 25: Operative Gynecology

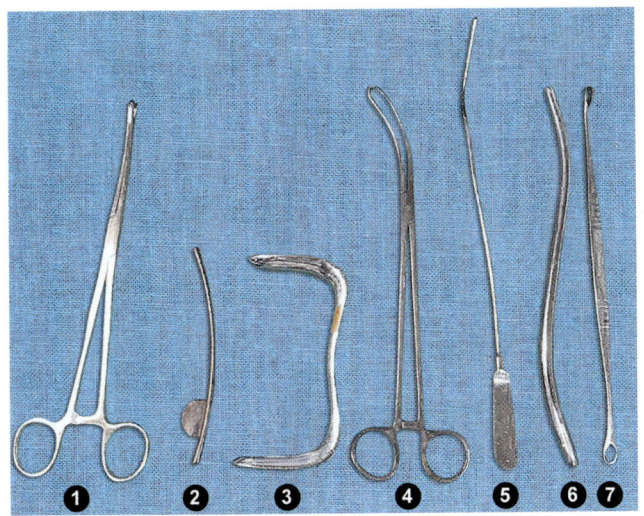

Fig. 19: Instruments. (1) Sponge holding forceps; (2) Female metallic catheter; (3) Sims' speculum; (4) Multiple teeth vulsellum; (5) Uterine sound; (6) Cervical dilator; (7) Uterine curette.

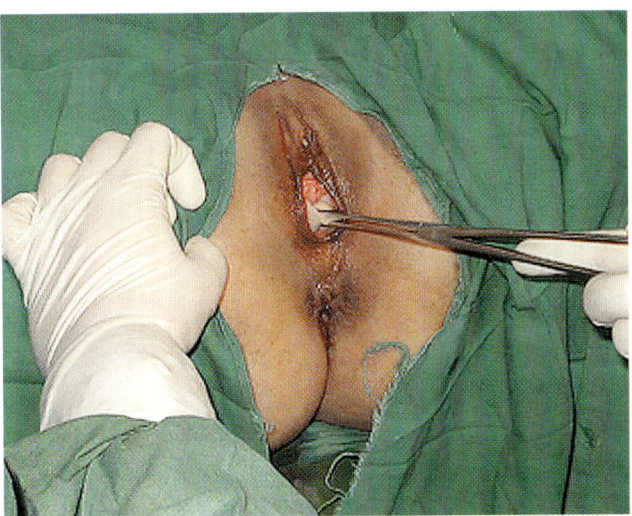

Fig. 22: Swabbing.

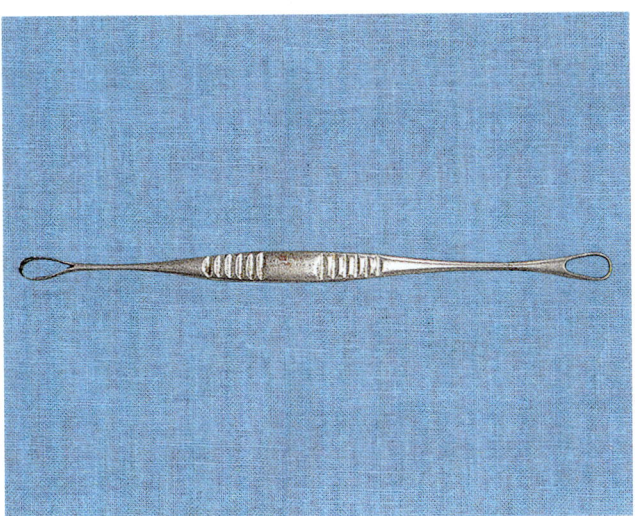

Fig. 20: Uterine curette (blunt and sharp).

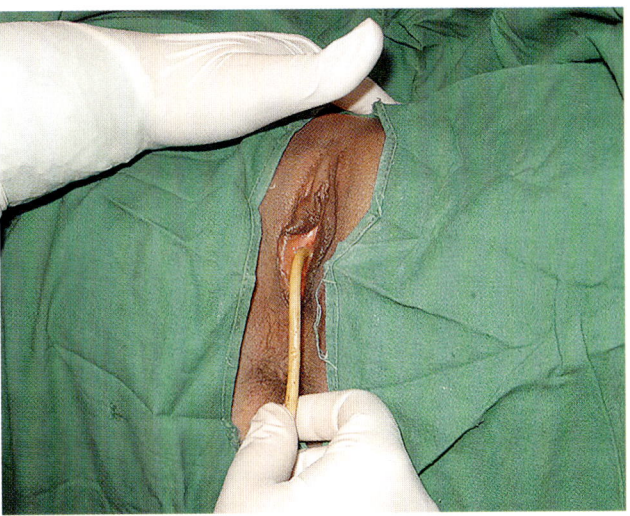

Fig. 23: Catheterization by rubber catheter alternative to metal catheter.

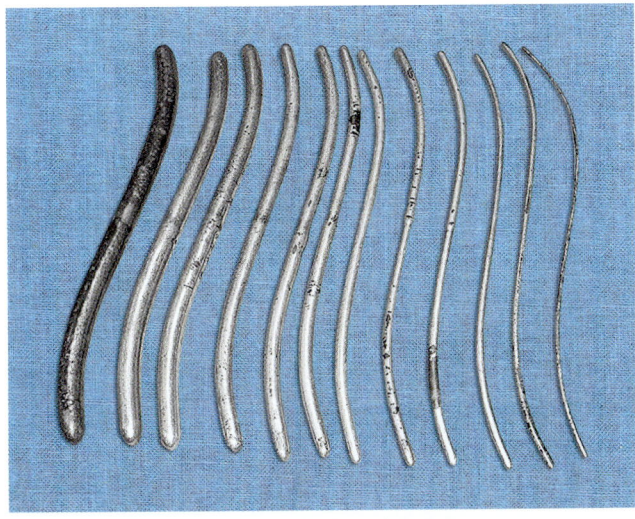

Fig. 21: Set of cervical dilators of different sizes.

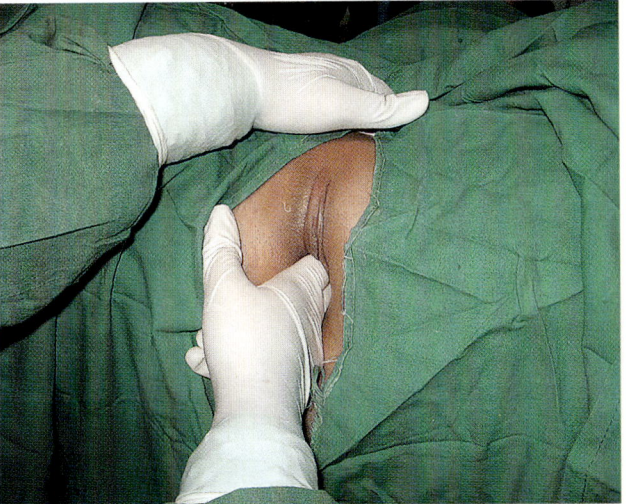

Fig. 24: Bimanual examination to note the size, position of uterus and status of adnexae.

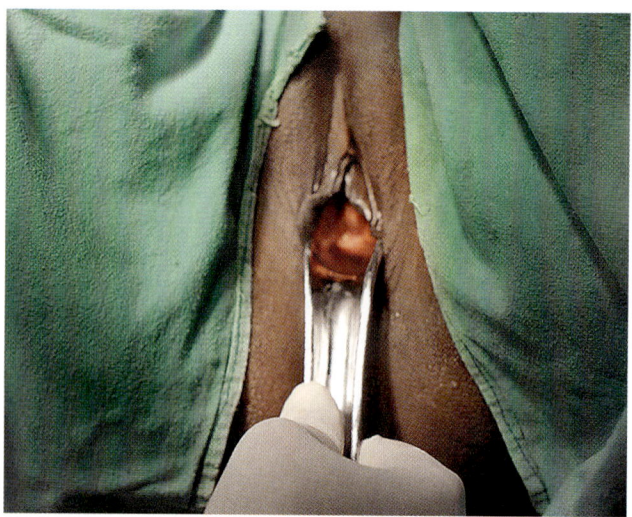
Fig. 25: Application of Sims' posterior vaginal speculum.

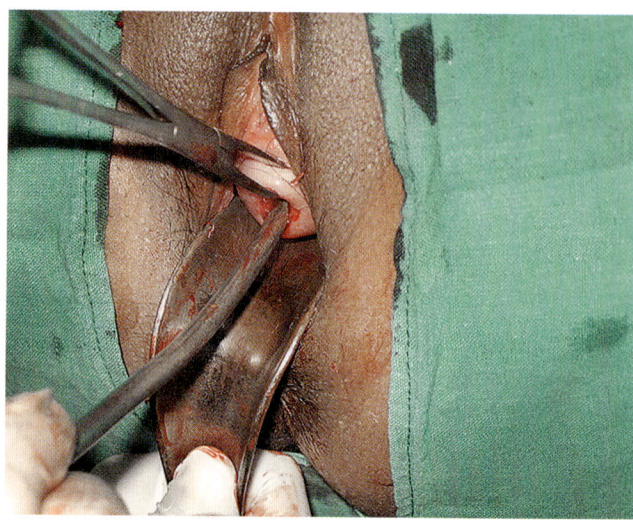
Fig. 28: Gradual dilatation of cervix by one after another to introduce the curette.

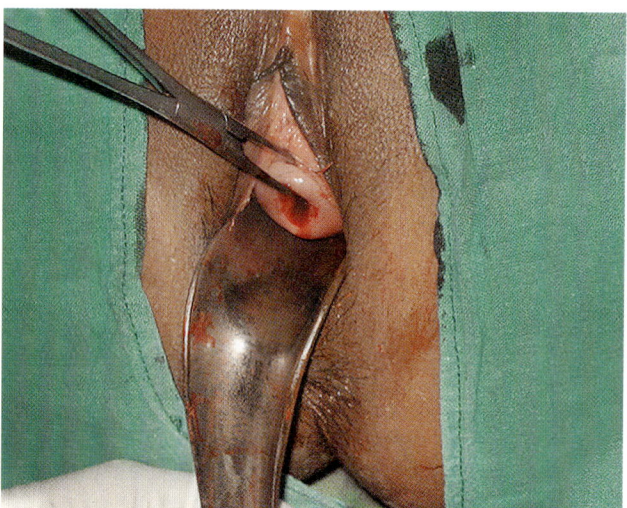
Fig. 26: Anterior lip of cervix is held by Allis tissue forceps instead of multiple teeth vulsellum.

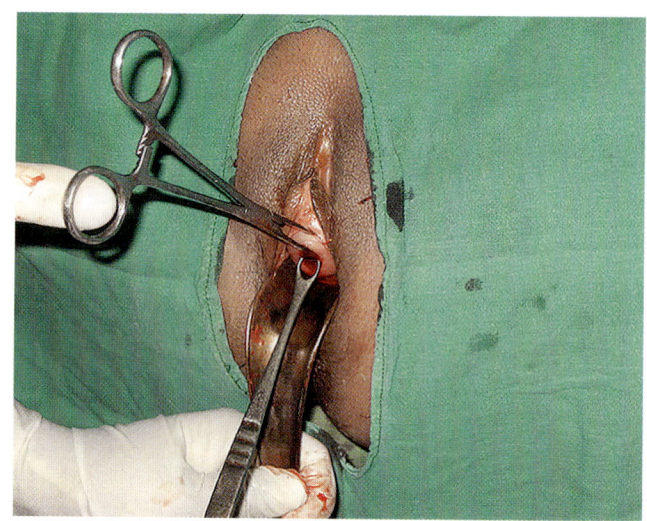
Fig. 29: Curette of uterine cavity.

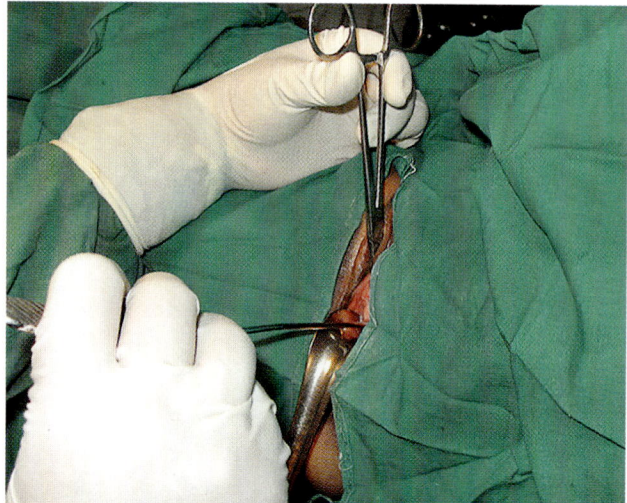
Fig. 27: Introduction of uterine sound to note the length and position of uterus.

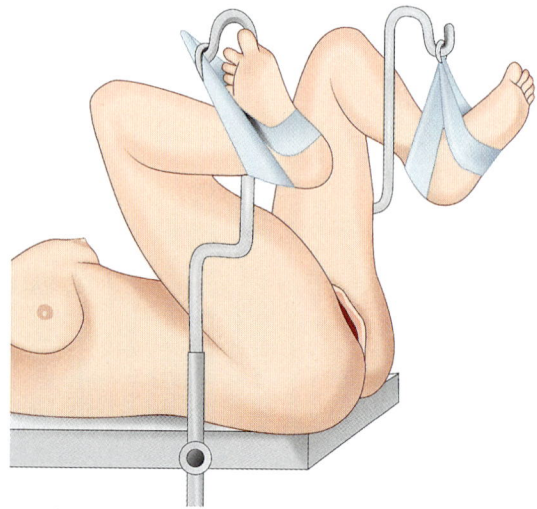
Fig. 30: Lithotomy position.

CHAPTER 25: Operative Gynecology

for histopathological (H/P) examination. In suspected tuberculosis, part of sample is taken in normal saline.

Indications of D and C

Diagnostic
- Infertility
- Abnormal uterine bleeding (dysfunctional uterine bleeding)—to see the cause of bleeding and type of endometrium
- Endometrial carcinoma
- Suspected endometrial tuberculosis.

Therapeutic
- Endometrial polyp
- Dysfunctional uterine bleeding may have therapeutic value.

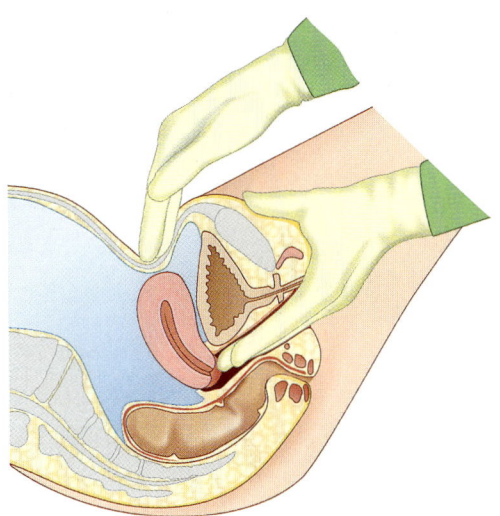

Fig. 31: Bimanual examination.

Adjunct to Other Surgery
- Fothergill's operation
- Amputation of cervix.

Q. When only dilatation is done without curettage?
- Cervical stenosis
- Drainage of pyometra
- Spasmodic dysmenorrhea

Where only curette is done
- For performing endometrial biopsy with Sharman's curette or Pipelle which is outpatient department (OPD) procedure.

Q. When you will do D and C in infertility?

It is done in premenstrual phase to detect the detection of ovulation. In ovulatory woman, the endometrium is expected to be secretory at that time due to the effect of progesterone. If it is proliferative, it indicates nonovulation.

Besides if there is any pathology like tuberculosis that can be detected.

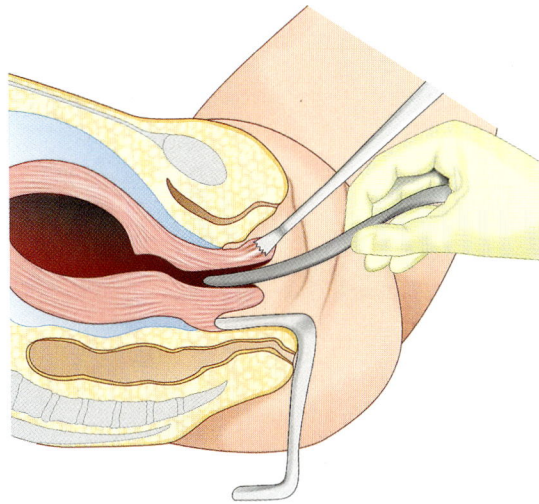

Fig. 32: Dilatation of cervix serially till the size, the curette can be introduced.

Complications of D and C
- Anesthetic complication
- Perforation of uterus
- Intestinal injury
- Cervical injury in forceful dilatation
- Hemorrhage—primary or secondary
- Infection
- Uterine synechia and amenorrhea in excessive curettage
- Morbid adhesion of placenta if vigorous curettage is done.
- Cervical incompetence resulting miscarriage and preterm labor.

Q. Difficulty in dilatation of cervix and how to encounter?

There may be difficulty in dilatation for which nowadays misoprostol 200 µg is given intravaginally or orally at night before operation by which the cervix becomes soft.

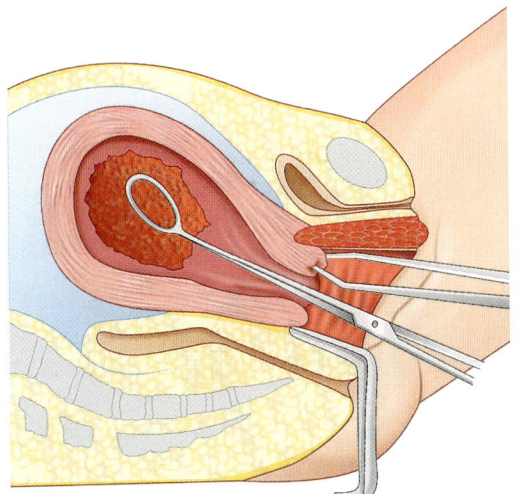

Fig. 33: Curette of uterine cavity.

Q. How would you detect uterine perforation?

Sudden loss of resistance and the instrument goes beyond the length of uterus as measured initially.

Q. What you will do if peroration does occur?

The procedure is stopped. The outcome of perforation depends on the instrument used.

If it is done by uterine sound, usually bleeding stops and monitoring of patient done by observing pulse, BP and pallor, and conservative management is done. If by large dilator or curette or suspected gut injury and chance of bleeding is more. it is better to do laparotomy and repaired in layers followed by exploration of gut to detect any injury. Visualization with the help of laparoscopy is a good strategy before laparotomy.

SURGERY FOR CHRONIC UTERINE INVERSION (FIG. 34)

Uterine inversion occurs due to during delivery of unseparated placenta at liver or dragging down by a mass like large fibroid polyp. Diagnosis is discussed in Chapter 10. The principle of management of chronic uterine inversion is to replace the inverted uterus in normal position which is done by surgery by abdominal method or by vaginal method.

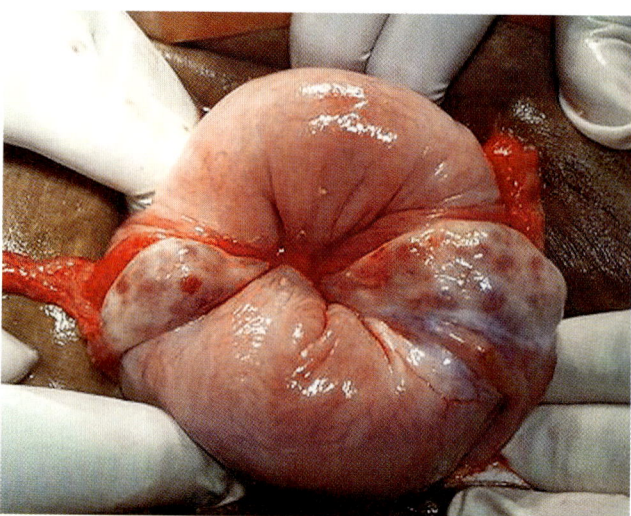

Fig. 34: Uterine inversion—cupping of uterine fundus seen.

Haultain's Technique (Figs. 35A to D)

❖ In this method, following *laparotomy* a vertical incision is given over the middle of posterior margin of the cup-like depression of the inverted uterus **(Figs. 35B and C)**

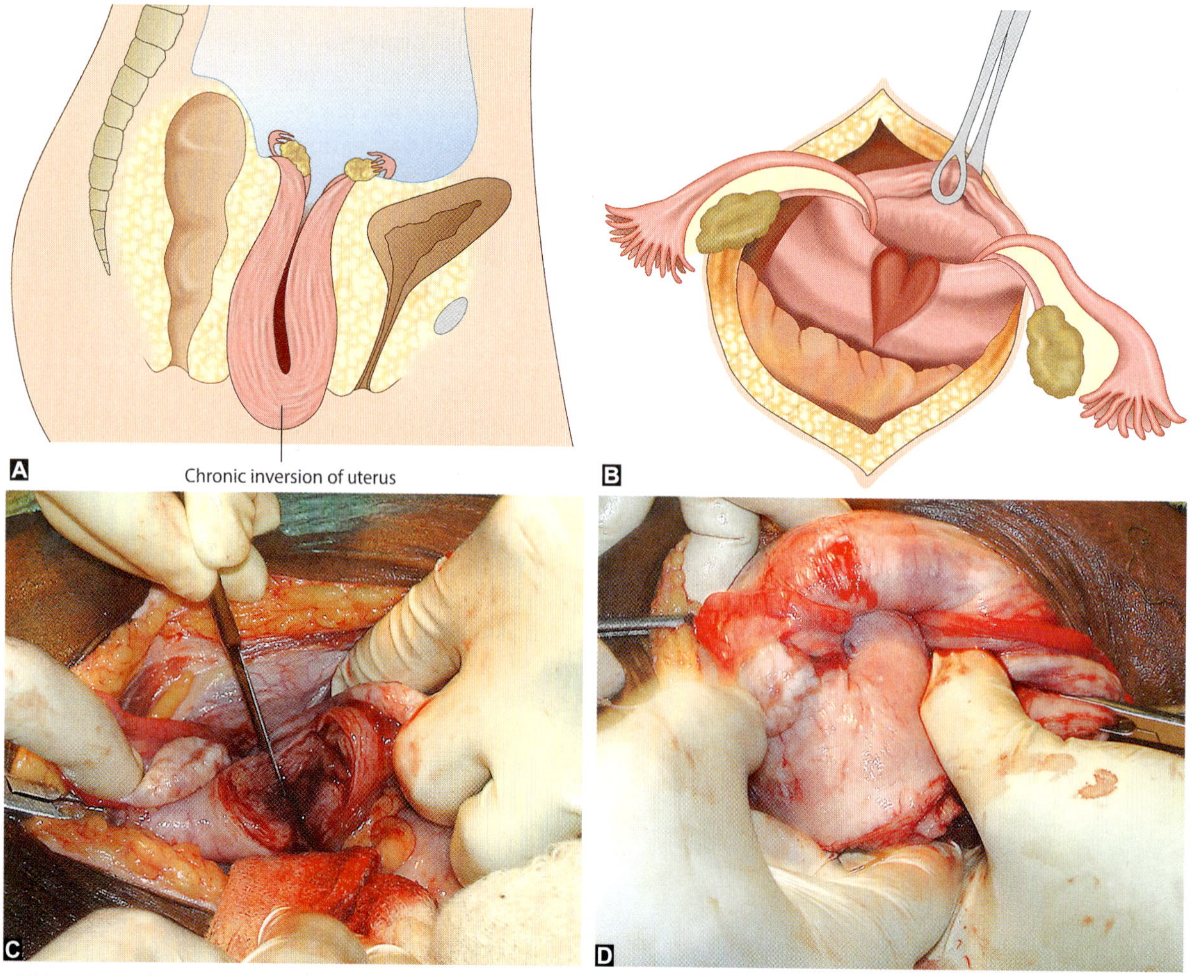

Figs. 35A to D: Haultain's technique: (A) Chronic uterus inversion; (B and C) Surgical method through abdominal route; (D) Reposition of fundus introducing the fingers through the incision wound.

- A finger is introduced to reach the vagina and inverted uterus is pulled up which is a challenging procedure **(Fig. 35D)**
- Now the uterus is repaired in two layers.

Spinelli's Procedure

- This is done in *vaginal approach* and done on anterior aspect. In lithotomy position and under general anesthesia, an inverted T-shaped incision is given like anterior colporrhaphy.
- Vaginal flaps are dissected laterally, uterovesical fold of peritoneum is cut and bladder is pushed upward. Now a longitudinal incision is given on the uterus. Now with the help of both thumbs inverted uterus (fundus) is pushed upward while the index fingers retract the margins of the incision.
- After reposition, uterus is repaired in two layers.
- The uterovesical fold of peritoneum and vaginal margins are repaired.
- The advantages of this method are less chance of infection and repair is on anterior instead of posterior wall with less chance of adhesion.

Kustner's Operation

- This also *vaginal method* but through posterior approach. Through transverse incision pouch of Douglas (POD) is opened and the left index finger is hooked into the inverted uterus inside the POD opening.
- The posterior margin after retracting is cut by a vertical incision and the inverted fundus is turned inside out thus correcting the inversion.
- Uterus is repaired in two layers and POD peritoneum and vagina are repaired.

SURGERY FOR MAKING UTERUS ANTEVERSION

1. Plication of round ligament
2. Gilliam's operation—In Gilliam's operation medial part of round ligament is passed through the broad ligament to bring in front of rectus muscle to fix underneath the anterior layer of rectus sheath with nonabsorbable stitch on each side. It is done in symptomatic mobile retroversion cases, very selected cases of infertility and deep dyspareunia. Now, it is seldom done.

OTHER GYNECOLOGICAL SURGERIES ARE DESCRIBED IN THE RESPECTIVE CHAPTERS AS BELOW

- Anterior colporrhaphy, posterior colpoperineorrhaphy, Ward-Mayo's operation, Fothergill's operation and other surgeries of pelvic organ prolapse—in the Chapter 10 on Pelvic Organ Prolapse (*see* Page 308 and 332)
- Operation on fibroid:
    - Myomectomy—Chapter 4 on Uterine Fibroid (*see* Page 127–132)
    - Polypectomy—Chapter 4 on Uterine Fibroid (*see* Page 141)
- Operations of ovarian tumor—ovarian cystectomy, salpingo-oophorectomy, operation on ovarian malignancy—Chapter 3 on Lump Abdomen (ovarian tumor) (*see* Page 78–81 and 88–90)
- Tubectomy, non-scalpel vasectomy (NSV)—Chapter 22 on Family Planning (*see* Page 699–717)
- Tubal reconstructive surgery including recanalization—Chapter 11 on Infertility (*see* Page 379–382)
- Operations on vulva—vulvectomy—Chapter 9 on Cancer Vulva (*see* Page 259–265)
- Repair of VVF, ureteric injury—Chapter 17 on Vesicovaginal Fistula (For VVF, *see* Page 543–547; for ureteric injury, *see* Page 551–553)
- Operations of stress incontinence—Chapter 17 on Vesicovaginal Fistula (*see* Page 561–569)
- Repair of complete perineal tear (CPT)—Chapter 18 on Complete Perineal Tear (*see* Page 577–582)
- Small procedures on cervix—Chapter 8 on Cancer Cervix (*see* Page 243–245)
- Radical hysterectomy and trachelectomy—Chapter 8 on Cancer Cervix (*see* Page 224–226)
- Ablative procedure on endometrium—Chapter 5 on Abnormal Uterine Bleeding (*see* Page 169–170)
- Ovarian drilling—Chapter 12 on Polycystic Ovarian Syndrome (*see* Page 413)
- Fenton's operation—Chapter 11 on Infertility (*see* Page 401)
- Operation of Bartholin cyst/abscess cyst—Chapter 32 on Vulvar Swelling (*see* Page 822–825)
- Surgery on Müllerian anomaly including vaginoplasty—Chapter 21 on Müllerian Anomaly (*see* Page 640–643).

PREOPERATIVE ASSESSMENT OF A PATIENT UNDERGOING GYNECOLOGICAL SURGERY

Every patient undergoing for surgery should have preassessment in a preassessment clinic (PAC). PAC should be done up to 2 weeks before operation.

Components of Preassessment Clinic (PAC)

1. Full history taking including any risk factors, comorbidities for anesthesia—any medical disorders, such as hypertension, other cardiovascular disease, diabetes, chronic lung disease, coagulation disorder or thyroid disorder and any history of drug intake.
2. General examination of the patient.
3. **Routine investigations:** Complete blood count, blood grouping, cross matching, serum urea, creatinine, postprandial blood sugar, serology including urine examination.
4. X-ray chest, electrocardiography (ECG).
5. If any renal, cardiac and respiratory problems, serum electrolyte and echocardiography are suggested, lung function test may be sought for in severe respiratory problem.

6. Respective interdisciplinary advices are to be taken as and when required.
7. If patient is getting any anticoagulant or suffering from any coagulation disorder, hematologist is consulted.
8. If patient is on oral contraceptive pill (OCP) or HRT, it should be stopped 1 month prior.
9. Patient on thyroxin should be continued till the day of surgery and thereafter.
10. The woman should be assessed for any need of thromboprophylaxis after surgery.
11. In high-risk patients, provision of high dependency or intensive care bed should be kept in immediate postoperative period.
12. Which type of anesthesia will be fit for her is to be reviewed and discussed with the patient.
13. Counseling done and informed consent is taken.

CHAPTER 26: Endoscopic Surgery: Laparoscopic/Hysteroscopic/Robotic Surgery

CHAPTER OUTLINE

- Laparoscopic Surgery—Advantages, Disadvantages, Indications, Contraindications, OT Set-up, Hand Instruments, Laparoscopic Procedure and Complications
- Hysteroscopy—Indications, Instruments and Gadgets, Distension Media, Procedure, Complications and Contraindications
- Robotics in Gynecology—an Overview

INTRODUCTION

Due to several advantages, endoscopic surgery both laparoscopy and hysteroscopy have become popular both for diagnostic and therapeutic purposes. Gynecologic endoscope surgery is a rapidly growing subject and continues to evolve rapidly with technological development and with increase of experience.

LAPAROSCOPIC SURGERY

- Laparoscopic surgery is also called minimally invasive surgery (MIS)
- MIS includes keyhole surgery or no incision surgery.
  The term 'laparoscopy' was introduced by HC Jacobaeus from Stockholm in 1910. The first book in English on laparoscopy in gynecology was written by Patrick Steptoe in 1967.

Advantages of Laparoscopic Surgery

- Minimal scar avoiding large incision more cosmetic
- Hence less parietal blood loss
- Early postoperative recovery
- Less postoperative pain
- Less hospital stay
- Less chance of incisional hernia
- Less postoperative adhesion formation
- Early return to work.

Disadvantages of Laparoscopic Surgery

- Surgeon should have expertise and long learning curve
- Equipment are costly so initial cost is high
- Complications are serious in nature
- No scope of direct palpation of tissue
- Ergonomic
- Instead of natural three-dimensional, one has to depend on two-dimensional view through video monitoring.

Indications

Diagnostic Laparoscopy

- Evaluation of female infertility
- Chronic pelvic pain
- Acute pelvic pain
- Diagnosis of pelvic mass
- Pelvic inflammatory disease
- Evaluation of amenorrhea, Müllerian anomalies
- Follow-up of pelvic surgery.

Surgical Laparoscopy (Minimal Access Surgery)

- Female sterilization
- Adhesiolysis
- Pelvic endometriosis, ovarian endometrioma
- Ectopic (tubal) pregnancy

- Management of benign ovarian cysts, dermoid cyst—ovarian cystectomy, ovariotomy
- Total laparoscopic hysterectomy (TLH), laparoscopic-assisted vaginal hysterectomy (LAVH)
- Laparoscopic myomectomy
- Polycystic ovary syndrome (PCOS)—laparoscopic ovarian drilling (LOD)
- Pelvic organ prolapse—laparoscopic sacrohysteropexy, sacrocolpopexy
- Gynecological malignancy—pelvic lymphadenectomy in early-stage cervical cancer and corpus cancer.

Contraindications

Absolute Contraindications

- Severe heart disease
- Hemoperitoneum with CV instability
- Peritonitis with bowel distention
- A large pelvic mass.

Relative Contraindications

- Extreme obesity
- Extreme thinness
- Peritonitis of any cause
- Inflammatory bowel disease
- Anticoagulant therapy
- Severe chronic illness
- Previous surgery is not a contraindication of laparoscopy; however, one should be cautious and may modify the trocar insertion and approach accordingly, etc.

Set-up an Operation Theater (Figs. 1 to 6)

- Video display monitor
- Camera
- Light source—cable
- Electrosurgical generator
- CO_2 insufflator
- Suction and irrigation system.

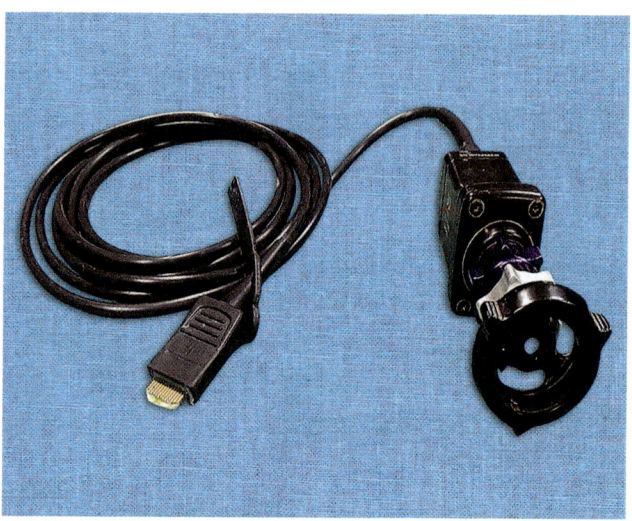

Fig. 1: Camera.

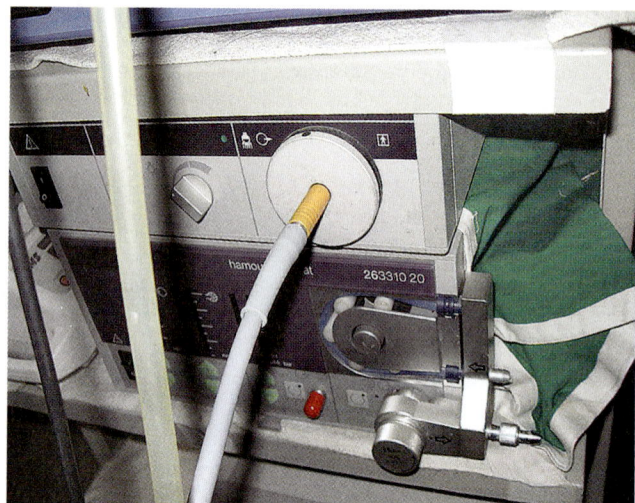

Fig. 3: Light source.

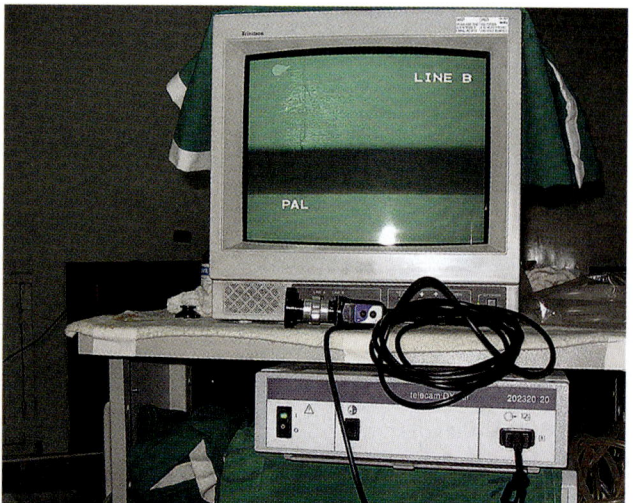

Fig. 2: Video monitor.

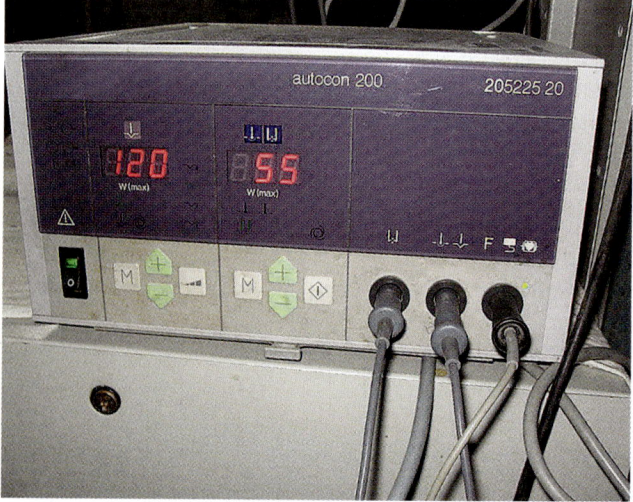

Fig. 4: Electrosurgical generator.

CHAPTER 26: Endoscopic Surgery: Laparoscopic/Hysteroscopic/Robotic Surgery

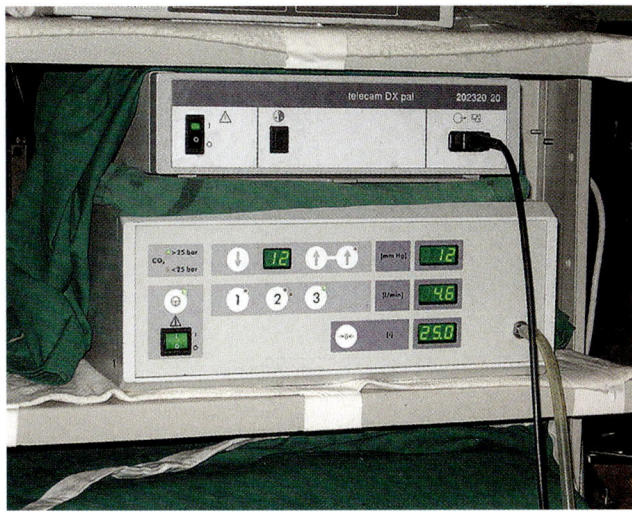

Fig. 5: CO_2 insufflator.

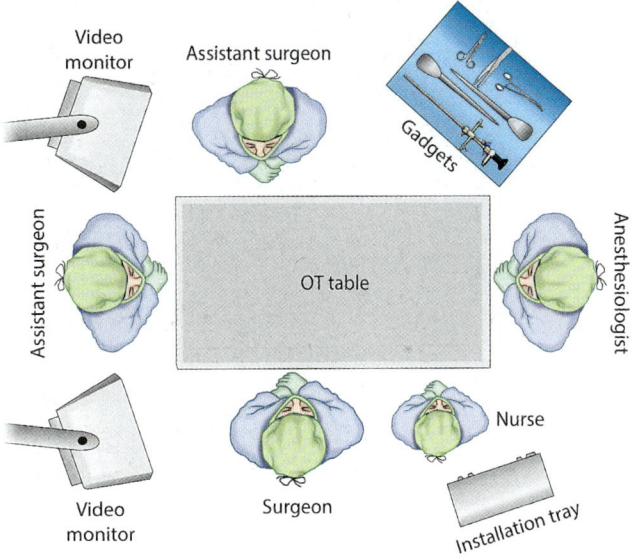

Fig. 7: Arrangement in operation theater.

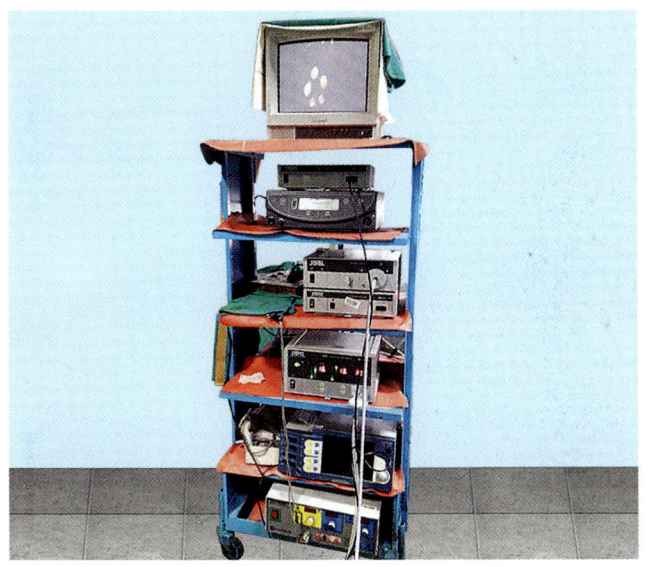

Fig. 6: Gadgets set up in endoscopy cart.

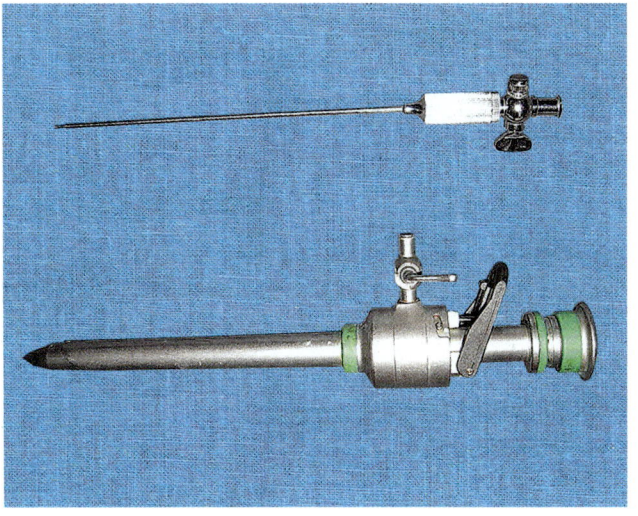

Fig. 8: Veress needle and trocar cannula.

In **Figure 7**, layout shows the arrangement in operation theater.

Hand Instruments (Figs. 8 to 15)

- Veress needle
- Trocars and sleeves—10 mm and 5 mm
- Telescope
- Grasping forceps—atraumatic, traumatic, fenestrated, long and short forceps
- Scissors
- Bipolar cautery—forceps and grasper type with bipolar scissors
- Monopolar—hook, spatula, PCO needle and scissors

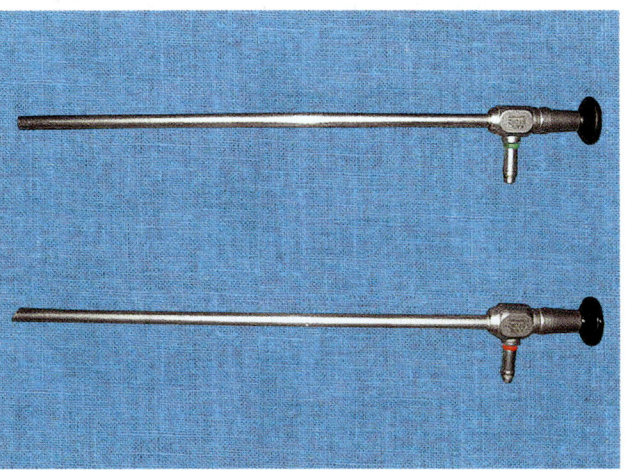

Fig. 9: Telescope.

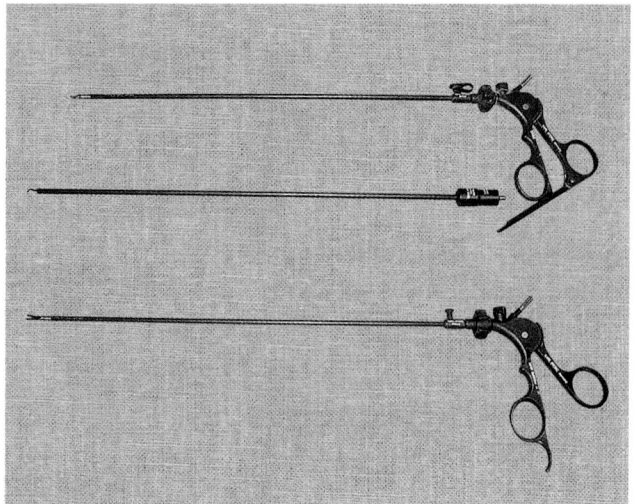

Fig. 10: Hand instruments—grasper, monopolar hook, scissors.

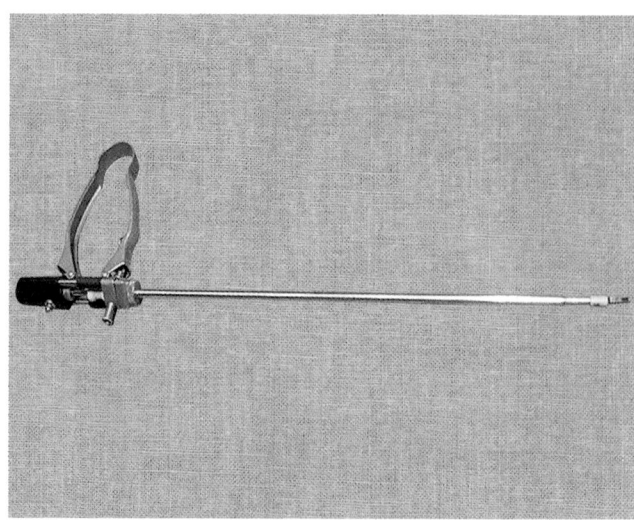

Fig. 13: Bipolar coagulation forceps.

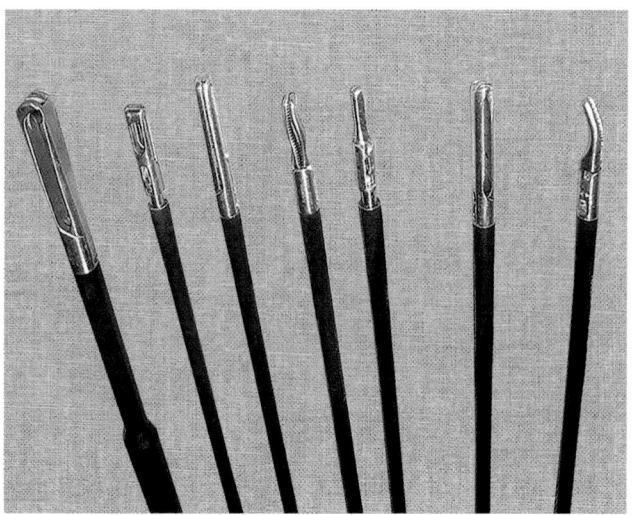

Fig. 11: Hand instruments—varieties of grasping forceps.

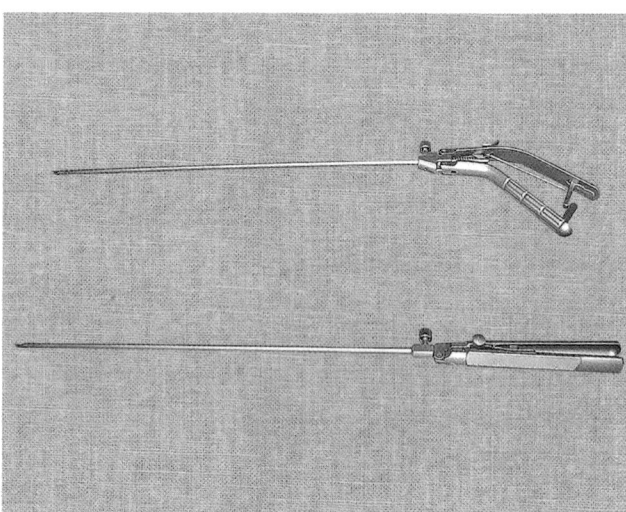

Fig. 14A: Needle holder with ratchet.

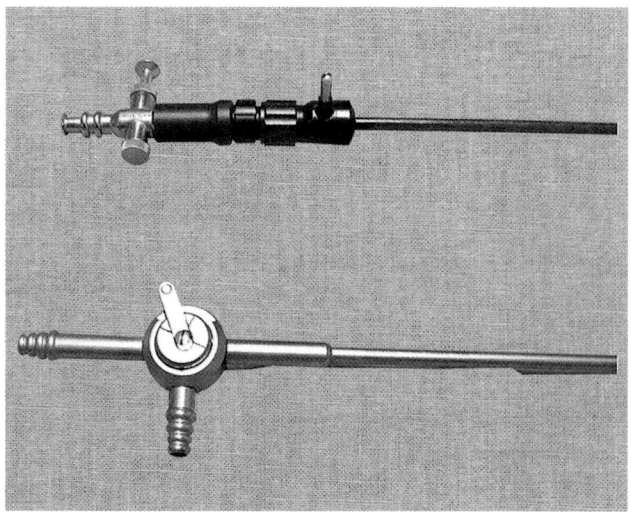

Fig. 12: Suction irrigation cannula.

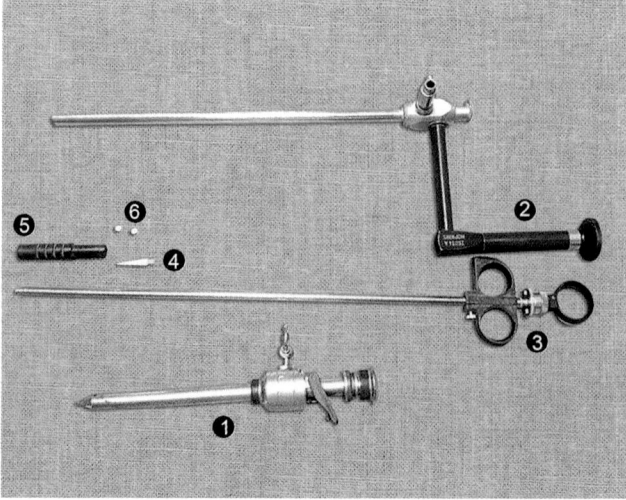

Fig. 14B: Instruments for laparoscopic ligation: (1) Trocar cannula, (2) scope, (3) tong, (4) loader, (5) pusher, and (6) Falope ring.

- Suction, irrigation cannula
- Harmonic scalpel
- Suturing: Szabo-Berci suturing instruments—flamingo assistant's grasper and Parrot needle holder
- Laparoscopic tubal ligation set (tong, loader, pusher and Falope ring).

Informed Consent

- Should be fully informed about the procedure, anticipated outcome, recovery period, possible complications and alternative options.
- If it is for diagnostic purpose and surgeon has intention to do some surgery in the same sitting if needed, that will be clearly explained to patient and party and separate informed consent should be taken other than the routine consent.
- Conversion to laparotomy may be needed in any case of laparoscopy that should be explained and consent taken before operation theater.
- Written consent is signed by the patient, physician and witness.

Laparoscopic Procedure (Figs. 15A and B)

Patient Positioning and Preparation

- Positioning is done after induction of anesthesia.
- Placed in lithotomy position with the legs in padded Allen stirrups to avoid pressure points.
- Buttocks should protrude a few centimeters over the table.
- Legs should be extended, not elevated, to allow the surgeon, room for instrument manipulation.
- Trendelenburg position is not done at this moment, and done only after insertion of primary trocar.
- Per vaginal examination is done before insertion of Veress and trocar to exclude the large mass in the pelvis.
- Bladder evacuation is done and the catheter may be kept in prolonged operative procedure. All the necessary hand instruments are washed, articulated and made ready.
- Trocar is fitted with sleeves.
- Veress needle of proper size is selected and tested for spring action and patency is tested by pushing saline water by syringe.

Insertion of Veress Needle

- It is done in flat position (not in Trendelenburg)
- A small incision, either transverse or vertical is given on inferior aspect of umbilicus as there is little fat or muscle here
- The skin of the lower abdomen is lifted upward and caudad with left hand or with towel clips attached to the umbilical area
- Veress needle is grasped like a pencil with fingers of right hand along the shaft of the needle to act as buffer.
- Verification of Veress needle inside the abdominal cavity: At almost a vertical angle down toward the true pelvis not

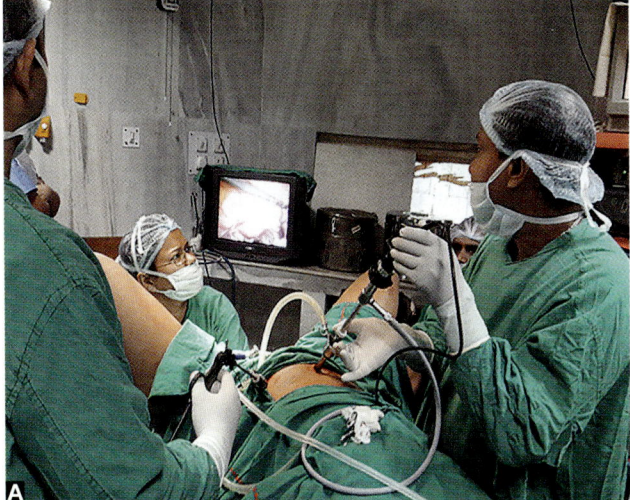

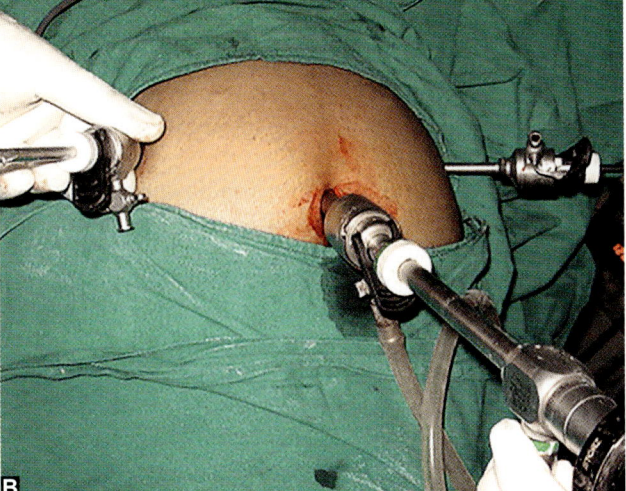

Figs. 15A and B: (A) Laparoscopy on process; (B) Three ports are done.

at a shallow angle to avoid gas being inserted in parietal fats.

- *"Hanging drop" test:* A drop of water is placed on the open end of Veress needle. The abdominal wall is elevated, if the needle is correctly positioned, the water should disappear down the shaft.
- *Water test:* A syringe full of sterile water or saline is attached to Veress needle and 1–2 mL is injected. If it is intra-abdominal, the saline will flow in easily and cannot be withdrawn by aspiration.

Vigorous movement of Veress after its insertion to see its correct position is strongly discouraged.

In case of repeated failure alternative sites are chosen:

- *Palmer's point:* In the line of the left nipple, two fingers below the lower margin of rib cage— least risk of hitting an intra-abdominal structure, left ninth intercostal space in the anterior axillary line or posterior cul-de-sac.
- *Hasson technique:* In this technique, trocar is introduced by open technique (1–2 cm transverse incision at the lower margin of umbilicus) instead of blind way.

Pneumoperitoneum:

It is done by CO_2:

- Initially CO_2 flow is kept at 1 L/minute and intra-abdominal pressure is noted.
- A pressure reading of 12 mm Hg or less and loss of liver dullness to percussion after 1 L of gas insufflations indicates correct needle placement.
- If entry pressure is found very high say 20 mm, needle is withdrawn.
- Gas flow is then be increased.
- During the procedure, abdominal pressure is maintained at 14 mm Hg or below.
- Just before insertion of trocar, pressure is raised little more (18–20 mm) but after which it should be kept 14 or less.

Trocar Placement

- Patient still in horizontal position. The trocar is "palmed" in the dominant hand with the *index finger extended down the shaft* to the point of planned penetration to prevent the tip from being driven too deeply into the pelvis.
- The angle of insertion is always toward the center of true pelvis, aiming toward the uterus.
- Trocar is twisted slightly while firm downward pressure is applied. After the "give" of the fascia is felt, the trocar is advanced slowly to traverse the peritoneum.
- The sleeve is then advanced few centimeters over the trocar, and the trocar is removed.
- A rush of gas through the opened trumpet valve confirms placement.

Number of Ports and Location of Accessory Trocars

- In diagnostic laparoscopy, one accessory trocar is sufficient and placed in the midline 4–5 cm above symphysis pubis.
- In operative procedures, two accessory trocars are commonly placed, each 4–5 cm above the symphysis pubis and lateral to the rectus muscle, thus avoiding deep inferior epigastric artery.
- If 3rd accessory trocar is needed, it is placed in the midline between the symphysis pubis and the umbilicus or at McBurney's point.

Techniques of Making Accessory Port

- Abdominal wall is transilluminated to determine the location of and to avoid the damage of any parietal blood vessel (other lights are switched off).
- Under direct visualization with the laparoscope toward the midline of the true pelvis.
- Pressing a finger on the abdominal wall and viewing its indentation by laparoscopy is very helpful.

Insertion of Laparoscope and Thereafter

- Now the laparoscope is inserted and the gas tube is attached. Camera is fitted with laparoscope. A fiberoptic light is attached to the laparoscope and intra-abdominal structures are observed.
- In case of laparoscope mists, it is gently touched with the nearby bowel.
- If the picture becomes hazy, scope is removed, tip is dipped in warm sterile water or antifogging solution. Correct focusing is done by adjusting the lens and by making white balance. Pelvis/abdomen are evaluated systematically.
- First, the entry areas are inspected to ensure no injury has occurred, then the abdomen is inspected noting liver, gallbladder, diaphragm, intestine, omentum and appendix.
- Then in Trendelenburg position, pelvic organs are inspected.
- In diagnostic laparoscopy, all pelvic structures are visualized and findings are noted in operative note.
- In operative cases, surgical procedures are done accordingly.
- After completion of procedure, all instruments except the scope with camera are taken out under direct vision to be sure of no bleeding from port sites.
- All operative sites are visualized for hemostasis before and during deflation.
- Deflation is completed.
- All port sites are sutured. Any port larger than 5 mm, fascia should be closed separately.

Figures 16 to 19 show few applications of laparoscopy.

Complications of Laparoscopy

Perioperative Complications

- Anesthetic complications—hypercarbia, lung atelectasis.
- Surgical emphysema, omental emphysema.
- Injury to blood vessels, gut, bowel, ureter.
- Thermal injury of any structure
- CO_2 embolism.

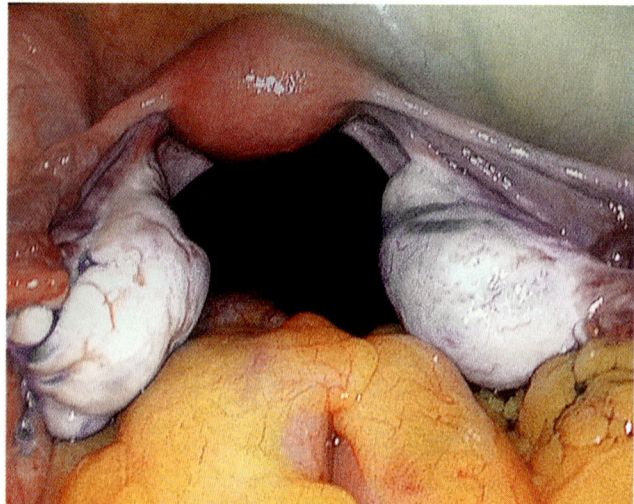

Fig. 16: Laparoscopic dye test—tubal patency test—positive-dye visible.

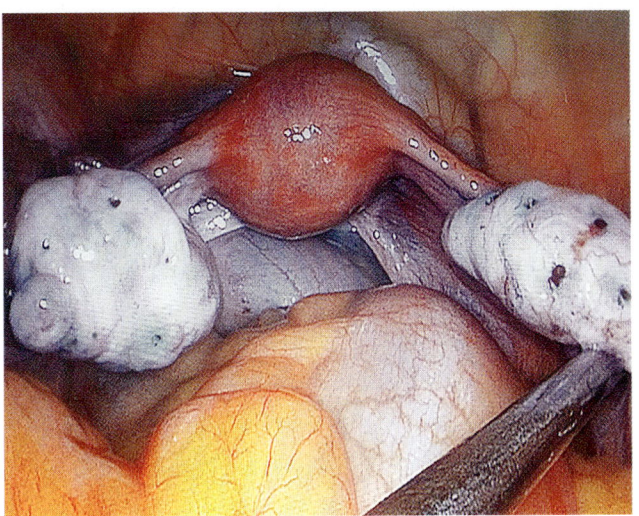

Fig. 17: Laparoscopic ovarian drilling (LOD) in PCOS.
Courtesy: Dr Subhas Halder (Figs. 16 and 17)

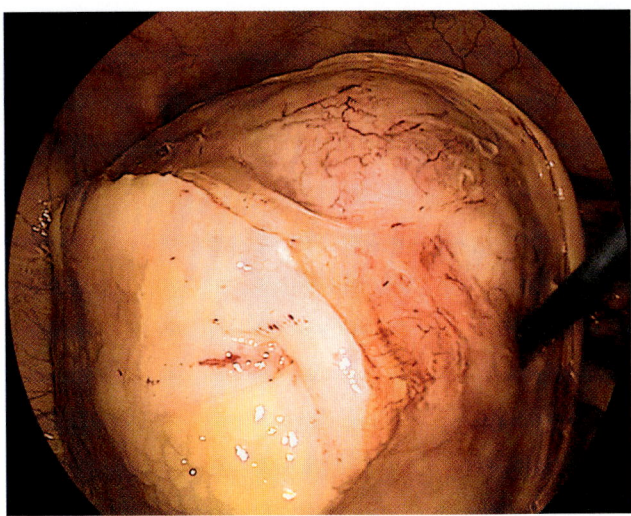

Fig. 19B: Laparoscopic myomectomy.
Courtesy: Dr Abhinibes Chatterjee, Advanced Laparoscopic Surgeon, Kolkata

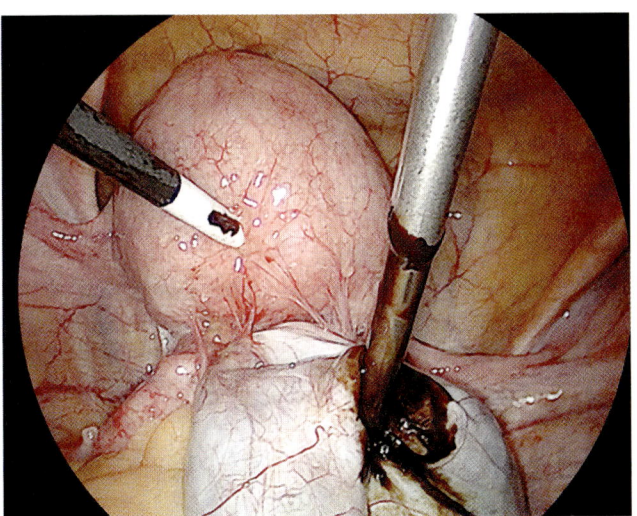

Fig. 18: Endometriosis—ovarian cystectomy and adhesiolysis.

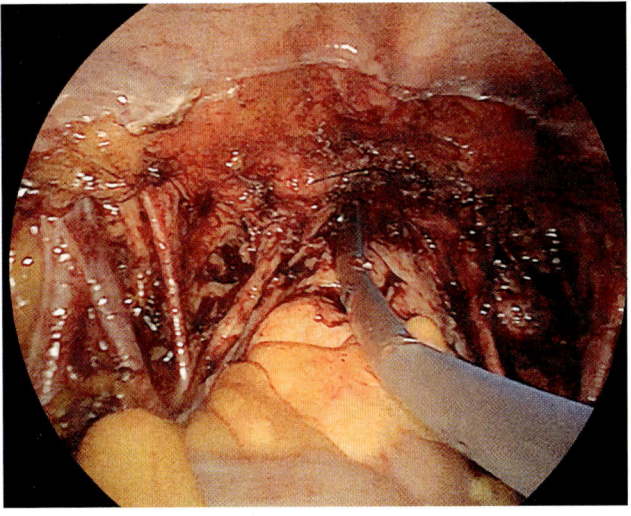

Fig. 19C: Radical hysterectomy.
Courtesy: Dr Abhinibes Chatterji

Late Complications

Infection especially port infection, port hernia.

HYSTEROSCOPE

Visualization of endometrial cavity and endocervical canal with illumination and magnification is called hysteroscopy.

Q. What is ambulatory hysteroscopy, office hysteroscopy or outpatient hysteroscopy?

Ambulatory services, in general are services which are provided in hospital or community settings where the admission of patient is not needed. The terms 'ambulatory' or 'outpatient' are commonly used in UK whereas the term 'office gynecology' is familiar in USA. The terms are synonymous and also used in other procedures like colposcope and surgical management of miscarriages, etc.

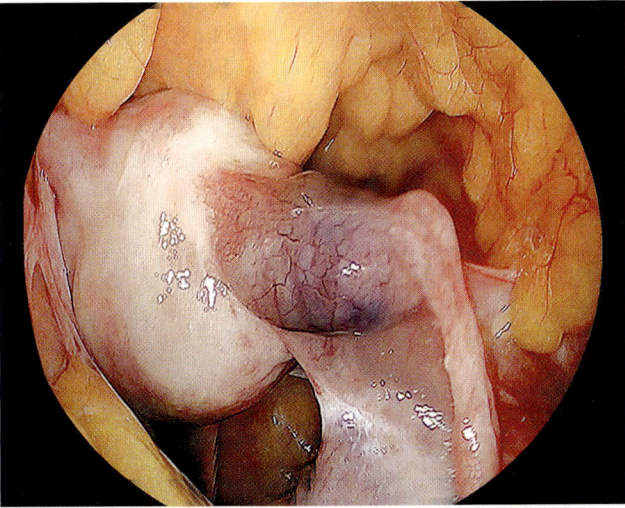

Fig. 19A: Unruptured ectopic.
Courtesy: Dr Abhinibes Chatterji (Figs. 18 and 19A)

In ambulatory, office or outpatient settings hysteroscopy is commonly done for diagnostic purpose, but surgical procedures like endometrial ablation, sterilization (placement of Essure), polypectomy, septal resection, division of adhesions and morcellation are also performed.

Indications

Diagnostic and operative.

Diagnostic

- Endometrial polyp
- Submucous fibroid
- Endometrial growth
- Uterine septum
- Intrauterine contraceptive device (IUCD) in missing thread
- Postmenopausal bleeding
- Abnormal uterine bleeding.

Operative

- Biopsy
- Polypectomy
- Septal resection
- Removal of IUCD
- Endometrial resection transcervical resection of the endometrium (TCRE)
- Hysteroscopic sterilization (Essure)
- Cannulation of tube
- Lysis of uterine synechia.

Instruments and Gadgets (Figs. 20 and 21)

- Diagnostic sheath
- Hysteroscope (Telescope)
- Operative sheath
- Operative accessories—resectoscope, loop, roller ball electrode

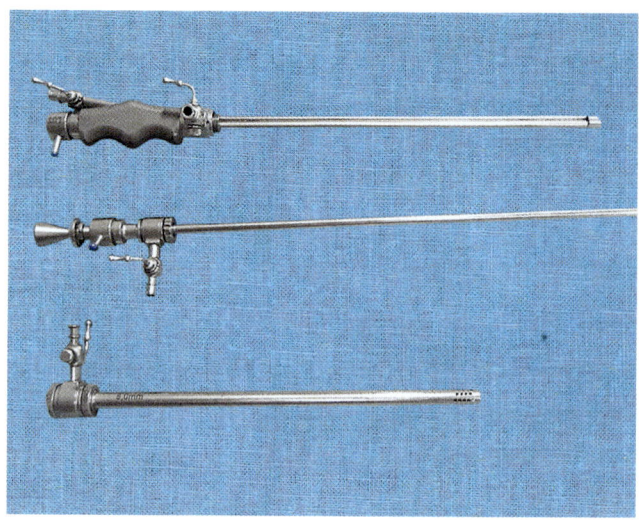

Fig. 21: Operative hysteroscope instruments.

- Light source, fiberoptic cable, camera and monitor like laparoscopy
- Distention media
- Hysteroflator.

Telescope: Telescope may be rigid, flexible or micro-hysteroscope. Commonly used telescope is rigid telescope. Size may be 3 mm or 4 mm. The angle of view is commonly 0° or 30°. Other angle may be 70°/90°.

Sheath: The diameter of diagnostic sheath is 5 mm and that of operative sheath is 8 mm. Operative sheath is provided with two channels one for introduction of distention media and other is for outlet of distention media other than the port for hysteroscope.

Hysteroflator—for controlling flow rate of distention media.

Distension Media

Distension of uterine cavity is needed by any distension media for proper visualization of uterine cavity as the anterior and posterior walls of uterus lie in apposition. The medium is either gaseous, usually CO_2 or liquid which may be electrolyte liquid (0.9% normal saline) or low electrolyte liquid (glycine 1.5%, mannitol 5% or sorbitol 3%), each with advantages and disadvantages. Normal saline and glycine are commonly used. A pressure of 45–80 mm Hg is needed to distend the cavity. At 70 mm of Hg fluid is passed to peritoneal cavity through fallopian tube. To avoid fluid overload (as fluid is absorbed in the process) **fluid deficit** (fluid given-retained fluid) is calculated **(Table 1)**.

Procedure (Fig. 22)

- Patient in dorsal lithotomy position.
- General or regional anesthesia for operative hysteroscope. Office hysteroscope needs only sedation, no anesthesia is needed.
- Vaginal wall is retracted with posterior vaginal speculum, anterior lip is held by Allis tissue forceps, uterine sound

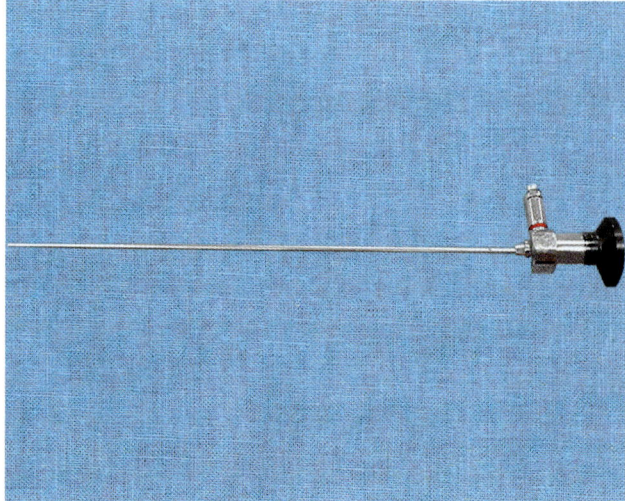

Fig. 20: Hysteroscope (telescope).

Table 1: Description of common media used in hysteroscope.

Media	Characteristics	Use	Complications	Measures taken to avoid danger
Gaseous CO_2	Colourless gas, Poor image quality due to gasbubble formation with blood or mucus	Diagnostic purpose only, no operative use	Embolism, rarely used due to serious gas embolism	To keep pressure <100 mm Hg and flow rate<100 mL/min
Liquid electrolyte 0.9% saline	Low viscosity isotonic, safest of all media Better image quality due to lavage of blood and mucus (in all liquid media)	Mainly diagnostic, operative using mechanical, bipolar, YAG and KTP laser, but **never unipolar**	Fluid overload, pulmonary edema	To complete procedure within 750 mL fluid deficit To stop at 2.5 L deficit
Electrolyte- poor liquid Glycine 1.5%	Low viscosity, hypo-osmolar	Operative with monopolar and resectoscope	Fluid overload, hyponatremia, hypo-osmolarity, hyper ammonia causing neurological damage	To complete procedure within 750 mL fluid deficit To stop at 1.5 L deficit
Mannitol 5%	Low viscocity, Iso-osmolar	Do	Fluid overload, hyponatremia	Do

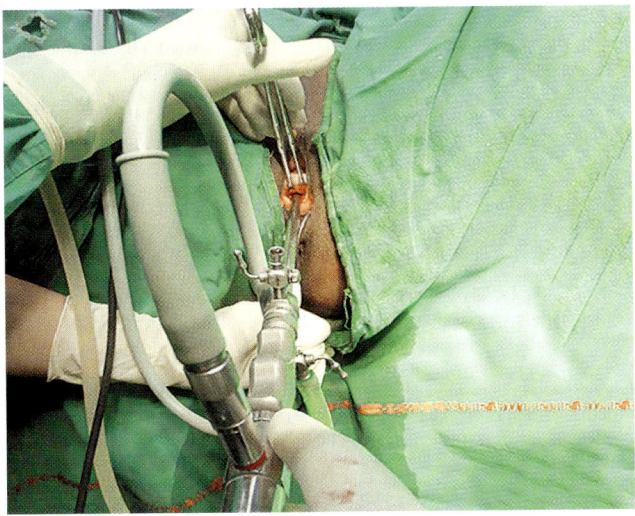

Fig. 22: Procedure of hysteroscopy.
Courtesy: Dr Abhijit Rakshit, Associate Professor

Complications

- Fluid and electrolyte imbalance in prolonged procedure
- Perforation
- Hemorrhage
- Infection
- Anesthetic complication.

Contraindications of Hysteroscope

- During bleeding phase
- Pregnancy
- Infection.

Figures 23 to 25 show few examples of hysteroscopic procedure.

is introduced first followed by dilatation of cervix for operative hysteroscope (which needs 8–10 size Hegar's dilator). For office hysteroscope, no dilatation is needed. Preoperative oral or vaginal administration of 200–400 μg misoprostol at night makes dilatation smooth.

- Diagnostic sheath and telescope are assembled and connected with cable and disension media delivery system and introduced into the uterus.
- Cervical canal is visualized, then uterine cavity, ostium are seen with distension of cavity. In diagnostic procedure, diagnosis is done by proper visualization. For operative procedure, respective procedure is done.
- Input and output of distension media is recorded in operative procedure.

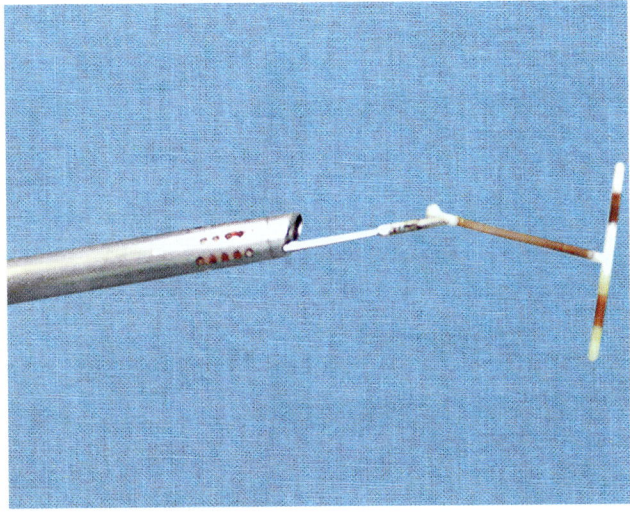

Fig. 23: Hysteroscopic removal of CuT in missing thread due to torn thread.
Courtesy: Dr Sudipto Jana

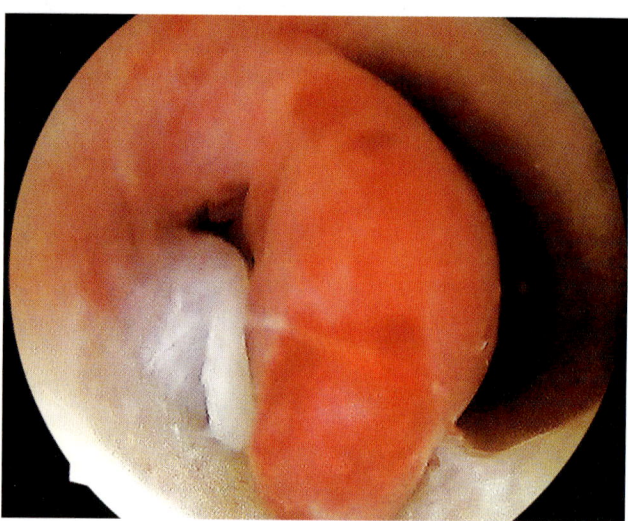

Fig. 24: Endometrial polyp.
Courtesy: Dr Abhinibes Chatterji

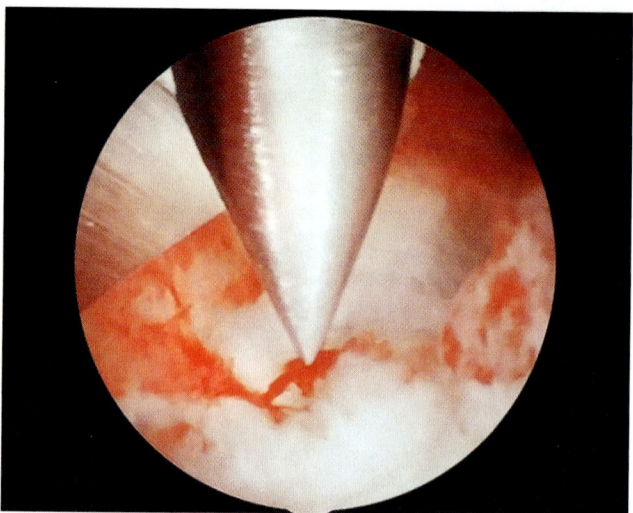

Fig. 25: Hysteroscopic septal resection.
Courtesy: Dr Bani Mitra

ROBOTIC SURGERY

- Robotic surgery is one type of facilitated laparoscopy utilizing the robotic technology.
- The purpose is to increase the quality of the surgery by placing a computerized interface between the surgeon and the patient.
- Robotic surgery consists of:
    - Robotic console where from the surgeon controls the robotic hands
    - Robotic column provided with four robotic arms.
- Surgeon uses both his hands for controlling arms and also his foot to control foot switches. One assistant lies with the patient.
- Basic differences from the conventional laparoscopy are precision of articulation and intuitive movements.
- Robotic surgery was originally approved by the Food and Drug Administration (FDA) (2003) in cardiovascular surgery, later it is done in urology and gynecology and also other branches.
- This surgery in gynecology is particularly useful where high precision and absence of tremor are needed like lymph node dissection, sever endometriosis, tubal anastomosis, urinary and rectal fistula repair. However, the common surgery simple hysterectomy, adnexectomy and myomectomy, etc. are also done with great precision.
- However, high initial cost and lack of facility of training are now important barrier for its widespread availability.
- Quick surgery, increase accuracy, ease of suturing in comparison to laparoscopy, less error and less stress of surgeon may make this surgery popular in future in gynecological practice.

CHAPTER 27: Routine Postoperative Management in a Gynecological Surgery

Chapter Outline

- Anticipated Complications in Postoperative Period
- Parameters to be Observed in Round in a Postoperative Patient, Frequency of Examination, Observation in Second Postoperative Day
- Postoperative Care—Fluid Management, Pain Management, Antibiotic, Thromboprophylaxis
- ERAS Protocol

Q. Which is the most important period after surgery? And why?

It is the first 48–72 hours of which first 24 hours is most important because the patient is at risk of immediate surgical complications.

Q. What complications may occur during this period?

- Hemorrhage
- Sequel of anesthesia—hypoxia
- Thromboembolic complications
- Sepsis.

POSTOPERATIVE ROUND IN FIRST POSTOPERATIVE DAY

Q. Suppose you are in a postoperative round in first postoperative day—what about will you enquire and what are the parameters you will see?

- *Details of surgery:* Time of surgery, type of surgery, duration of surgery, any complication during surgery, whether blood transfusion was given during surgery or immediately after surgery (to review the operative note if necessary).
- Anesthesia—type, any complication.
- Examination parameters:
  - Consciousness of patient (alert and conscious)
  - Patient's complaint—especially regarding pain—site and severity
  - Pallor
  - Pulse
  - Blood pressure (BP)
  - Respiration—oxygen saturation
  - Temperature
  - Dehydration—tongue, eye, amount and color of urine
  - Auscultation of chest/heart sound
  - Abdomen
  - Examination of wound site—whether any wound soakage, if vaginal surgery—any bleeding. In suspected condition, gentle vaginal examination may be needed to detect hematoma.
  - Look for the intravenous (IV) fluid channel and type of fluid she is getting and rate of fluid administration.
  - Urinary bag—urine output
  - Drainage—if any—amount of collection and nature of collection.
  - Input output chart.

Q. In how much frequency a patient is examined routinely in postoperative period?

Regular, usually 4 hourly in first 24 hours—may be more frequent according to the condition of the patient to see the vitals to detect any hypovolemic collapse or signs of infection.

A good strategy is to monitor vital signs (SpO_2, respiratory rate, pulse, BP and temperature) hourly for the first 4 hours, 2 hourly for next 4 hours and 4 hourly thereafter.

After 24 hours, twice daily routine round should be given.

Q. When intravenous fluid is stopped?

Usually after 12–24 hours of surgery when oral feeding can be started, depending upon the individual case. Patient is encouraged to mobilize as early as possible and to start oral intake at earliest it can done.

Q. When the drain is usually removed?

It is after 24 hours when the collection is minimal. Mostly, the drain is removed after 48 hours depending upon the amount of collection in drain.

POSTOPERATIVE ROUND IN SECOND POSTOPERATIVE DAY

Q. What will you look for in the second postoperative day?

- Similar observations like first day.
- Whether feeling hungry or not [listen for the intestinal peristaltic sounds (IPS)].
- Whether passed flatus or not (subjective feeling).
- Whether accepted sips of water of not (which may be started as early as possible).
- Note the wound again and the pressure areas of the body.
- Note the abdominal drain (if any) and whether suitable to remove early.
- Whether ambulation may be started early and catheter may be removed.
- Whether IV fluids may be stopped and oral feeds may be started.

Q. What do you mean by postoperative directions and postoperative care?

- These are instructions and care regarding support of organ systems till gradual re-establishment of normal functions.
- The main objectives should be resuscitation (fluid balance), pain control and prevention of infection, early detection of any complication and resumption to normal condition.
  According to different gynecological surgeries performed, postoperative directions may be customized for individual patients.

Components of Postoperative Care

Done by medical as well as nursing personnel:
1. Physical support
2. Fluid balance
3. *Pain relief*: Balance should be maintained between the degree of pain relief and associated side effects.
4. Antibiotics—prevention of infection
5. *Minimization of complications*: Anticipation of complications is the best way or complications should be caught early to best mange them.
6. Monitoring of patients with the parameters as mentioned above
7. Investigations to be sent as and when necessary— hemoglobin levels (Hb%), blood count, coagulation profile, urea creatinine, electrolytes and blood glucose.

COMPLICATIONS ANTICIPATED IN POSTOPERATIVE PERIOD

Q. What complications you will keep in mind in postoperative period?

- Postoperative hypovolemic shock: Anticipate and prevent.
- Postoperative urinary retention: Anticipate and prevent.
- Postoperative ileus: Anticipate and prevent.
- Postoperative pulmonary complications: Anticipate and prevent.
- *Postoperative nausea and vomiting (PONV)*: One of the most common complications following surgery and should be taken care of primarily. Pantoprazole or ranitidine and metoclopramide or ondansetron 12 hourly will prevent PONV.

ALARMING SIGNS IN POSTOPERATIVE PERIOD

Q. What are the alarming signs in postoperative period?

- Blood pressure <90/60 mm Hg or >160/100 mm Hg.
- Pulse <60/min or more than 120/min.
- Temperature >38°C or 101°F.
- Respiratory rate >20/min.
- Urine output <30 mL/h.

Postoperative Fluid Management

- This is done by an anesthesiologist or a surgeon, or a team formed of both. Management of postoperative fluid therapy should be done considering both patients' status and intraoperative events.
- It should also be kept in mind that stress of surgery causes inappropriate antidiuretic hormone (ADH) release.
- Types of the fluids, amount of the fluid given and timing of the administration are the main topics that determine the fluid management strategy.
- The main goal of fluid resuscitation is to provide adequate tissue perfusion without harming the patient.
- Management is done by either crystalloids or colloids.
- Crystalloids consist of glucose or sodium chloride (saline) solutions. Osmolarity of the solution determines if the solution is hypotonic, isotonic or hypertonic.
- Colloids can be blood products, such as human albumin solution and fresh frozen plasma, or they can also be

synthetic large molecules which are not able to distribute across vascular barrier such as gelatins, dextrans, and hydroxyethyl starches.

Choice of Fluid

- Dextrose saline may produce hyponatremia in a postoperative patient. Alternate bottles of saline and dextrose saline with supplementary potassium give the best balance. Ringer's lactate (RL) is the preferred postoperative fluid usually in all clinical situations.
- Colloids stay in the vascular compartment whereas saline stays in the extracellular compartment. However, dextrose eventually goes in all the compartments.
- Intravenous fluids as RL or normal saline (NS): 5% dextrose (5% D) 2:1 to run 4–6 hourly is a good strategy.
- Administration of blood and blood products as and when required.

Principles of Quantity of Fluids

1. To maintain fluid input required under normal circumstances:
   - Normal adult intake: 1.5 mL/kg/h = 2.5 L/day
   - Normal adult urine output: 1.2 mL/kg/h = 2 L/day
   - Postoperative maintenance fluids in adults: 1.2 mL/kg/h or 1.5 L/24 h.
2. To match any ongoing losses:
   - Quantify output (urine, vomit, drain, diarrhea)
   - Estimate insensible loss (about 600–900 mL; increases in pyrexia).
3. To replace any deficit occurring:

   Laboratory tests for confirming fluid deficits: Hematocrit estimation for the degree of hemoconcentration and urinary Na^+ concentration (<20 mmol/L) and urinary osmolality (>400 mosmol/kg). In cases of fluid deficit, body tries to conserve Na^+ and water thus producing high-colored concentrated urine.

   In such situation, a single dose of fluid (e.g., 500 mL in a previously fit adult over 30–60 minutes) is given as challenge which is as large as possible but not so large to affect patient's heart by causing fluid overload.

Postoperative Infection Prevention—Surgical Site Infection and Sepsis: Use of Antibiotics

- Maintain asepsis and provide antibiotics.
- Single dose antibiotic is given prophylactically in intraoperative period in all gynecological surgery.
- Intravenous antibiotics (e.g., ceftriaxone 1 g 12 hourly after skin test and metronidazole 100 mL 8 hourly ± gentamicin 80 mg 8 hourly for 48 hour followed by oral antibiotic for 3 days. However, routine empirical antibiotic is not recommended.
- In case of suspected infection, a screening (swab, blood culture) for infection is done followed by appropriate antibiotic therapy. Low-grade fever is common in first 12–24 hours due to release of acute phase proteins but resolves spontaneously. Persistent fever or fever above 39°C warrants investigation and antibiotic administration.

Postoperative Pain Management

- Any delivery system like "long-acting local blocks" which reduces peaks and troughs of pain is likely to reduce the overall demand of analgesia and also reduces side effects.
- Best available option is patient-controlled analgesia (PCA).
- Nonopioids like acetaminophen/paracetamol and nonsteroidal anti-inflammatory drugs (NSAIDs) are commonly used and are usually well tolerated but overdosage and the risk of nephrotoxicity should be kept in mind.
- However, in cases of severe pain, the primary choice should be opioids like pethidine, morphine and fentanyl keeping in mind the associated adverse effects like respiratory depression, nausea and vomiting. Opioids should be used when appropriate and no dependency is found when opioids are used specifically in the postoperative period.

Postoperative Venous Thromboembolism

It should be taken care of when indicated like associated risk factors comprising of obesity, prolonged surgery and immobilization and thromboprophylaxis with low-molecular-weight (LMW) heparin is prescribed and is not started within 6 hours.

Postoperative Hypoxia

Postoperative hypoxia is not uncommon and its detection is very important before deterioration of the condition of patient. The causes are residual effect of anesthesia and hypoventilation. Hypoxia occurs more following prolonged surgery particularly following laparoscopic surgery due to the lung complication. Hypoxia is managed with consultation with the anesthesiologist.

Q. Would you administer O_2 routinely following surgery?

Not needed routinely. If the oxygen saturation in room air is more than 92% and other parameters are normal, O_2 administration is not mandatory.

Care of Abdominal Wound

After 48–72 hours of surgery, wound dressing should be removed and fresh dressing is done. In case of Pfannenstiel incision, sutures are removed on day 5 and in longitudinal incision on 7–10 days. Care of vaginal wound is taken daily in vaginal surgery.

Fluid Compartments in Human Body

The approximate "Two-Thirds Rule":
- Total body water in a 70 kg adult is 60% = 42 L
- Two-third is intracellular = 28 L
- One-third is extracellular = 14 L
- Two-third of the extracellular compartment is extravascular = 9 L

❖ One-third of the extracellular compartment is intravascular = 5 L

ERAS

Q. What is ERAS protocol?

ERAS means *enhanced recovery after surgery*. It is a multimodal, multidisciplinary approach to the care of the surgical patient.

ERAS protocol includes: (1) changes from overnight fasting to allow liquid containing carbohydrate 2 hours before surgery; (2) minimally invasive surgical approach instead of large incisions; (3) balanced fluids instead of large volume of IV fluid; (4) early removal of drains and tubes or its avoidance; (5) early mobilization; and (6) early oral fluid and food on the same day of surgery.

It reduces the stress of operation, reduces the period of hospital stay, reduces complication and costs become less. Chance of readmission is also reduced.

Section 6

Specimens

Section Outline

28. Specimens

CHAPTER 28

Specimens

CHAPTER OUTLINE

Common questions asked in a specimen are discussed. Individual sample specimen is shown with probable questions:

- Fibroid—Submucous Variety, Multiple Fibroids, Subserous Variety, Cervical Fibroid, Broad Ligament Fibroid
- Ovarian Tumor:
  - Ovarian Cyst—Following Cystectomy, Following Salpingoophorectomy, or TAH with BSO
- Dermoid Cyst, Serous Cystadenoma, Mucinous Cystadenoma, Benign Variety, Malignant Variety, Bilateral Ovarian Tumor including Krukenberg Tumor
- Hysterectomy Specimen for Benign Condition, Radical Hysterectomy Specimen, Hysterectomy in Endometrial Cancer

INTRODUCTION

While dealing with a specimen in examination every specimen will be analyzed on the following broad points so that the answering will be very easy. The question may vary according to the type of specimen.

1. Description of the specimen.
2. Identification and diagnosis of the specimen.
3. What surgery has been done?
4. Build up the case (clinical)—patients profile, symptoms, signs and examination findings.
5. How to reach a final diagnosis—investigations?
6. What is the alternate management of this case?

SPECIMEN 1: SUBMUCOUS FIBROID (FIG. 1)

Q. Describe the specimen.

It is a specimen of uterus to cut open to show the uterine cavity where a small mass is seen.

Try to see the normal anatomical structures—uterus—body and cervix, tubes and ovaries, myometrium, endometrium and serous coat and to search for whether there is any pathology.

Q. What is your diagnosis?

Submucous fibroid.

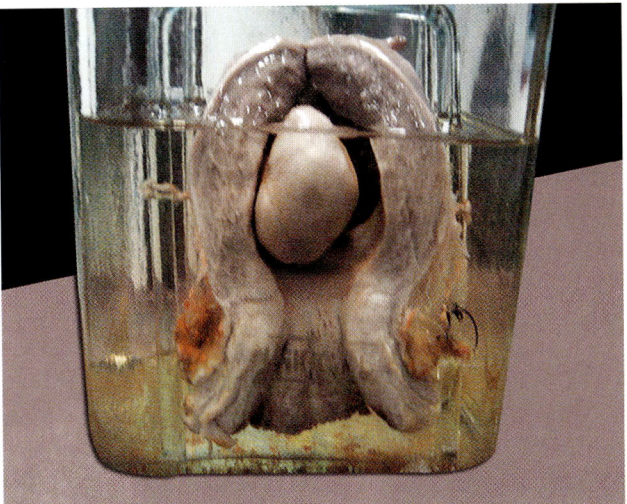

Fig. 1: Submucous fibroid.

Q. What surgery has been done?

Total hysterectomy (TH).

While answering this question see whether along with the body of uterus cervix has been removed or not? If cervix is present in specimen say TH, if not present say "Subtotal hysterectomy" (for classification of types of hysterectomy, *see* the Chapter 25 on Hysterectomy).

Search for whether tubes and ovaries are present on both sides.

If both tubes and ovaries are not present with the specimen, then it is called "Total hysterectomy". When bilateral ovaries and tubes are present (removed) with the specimen, it is called "TH and bilateral salpingo-oophorectomy (TH with BSO)". Sometimes, one-sided tube and ovary are present, then say "TH with unilateral (left or right) salpingo-oophorectomy".

In mounted specimen very often the ovary becomes compressed, so look carefully.

Q. Can you say which one is anterior surface and which one is posterior surface of the uterus? Which side is left and which side is right (adnexa)?

- The relation of round ligament, fallopian tube and ovarian ligament is from anterior to posterior. (Fallopian tube is identified by fimbriae, ovarian ligament identified by attachment with the ovary if oophorectomy done).
- Serous coat is deficient in lower part of anterior surface of uterus due to the bladder attachment while on posterior surface it extends much low down due to pouch of Douglas (POD).
- *Right adnexa or left adnexa?*—the side is determined by the above two points.

Q. How will you identify the cervix in a uterus and what information can you guess on finding of an intact cervix?

- Cervix is identified by the external os.
- Parity can be assessed from the os. In parous woman, cervix looks nearly transverse whereas in nulliparous it is small and circular.

Q. Can you say from this specimen in which age group does the patient lie?

Premenopausal, before 45 years as the tubes and ovaries are not removed here and left with the patient.

Q. Can you guess the parity of the patient?

She is parous, otherwise hysterectomy would not be done in this type of pathology.

Q. If nulliparous which treatment should be offered to her?

Myomectomy, best is hysteroscopic removal in this case.

Q. What was the clinical presentation of this patient, can you guess?

Premenopausal parous woman came with abnormal uterine bleeding (AUB) usually menorrhagia gradually turning into metrorrhagia (due to submucous variety) with dysmenorrhea, weakness and pain lower abdomen and her problem was not responding to conservative treatment.

Menorrhagia is a usual symptom of uterine fibroid. Here there is metrorrhagia as there is submucous fibroid. Pelvic pain and dysmenorrhea is not common symptom of fibroid, submucous variety may cause these symptoms. Pain and fibroid may be due to submucous variety, degeneration and torsion of subserous fibroid.

Lump abdomen and infertility may be presenting features. Here size of the uterus is small, so not the complaint. In infertility, hysterectomy is not done, so never say the patient came with infertility.

Q. On examination what you will get in this patient?

- General examination—pallor.
- *Per abdominal (P/A):* Lump is not palpable here, pelvic lump is palpable above 14 weeks size uterus.
- *Per vaginal (P/V):* uterus—enlarged, adnexae—not palpable.

Q. What investigation is usually done to confirm the diagnosis?

Ultrasonography.

Q. Alternate managements in fibroid uterus other than hysterectomy.

- Conservative—other than hematinic, hormones are tried—progesterone, gonadotropin- releasing hormone (GnRH) and ulipristal, etc., and others—for details *see* Chapter 4 on Fibroid Uterus.
- Myomectomy—if patient is desirous of children. In this type of pathology, hysteroscopic removal of tumor is an option.
- Advanced management—uterine artery embolization (UAE)—it is a uterus preserving surgery, but not for those who want child.

Q. Tell the steps of hysterectomy.

See Chapter 25 on Operative Gynecology.

Q. Tell how myomectomy is done and its preliminaries?

See Chapter 4 on Fibroid Uterus.

Q. Types of fibroid and recent FIGO classification of fibroid.

See Chapter 4 on Fibroid Uterus.

SPECIMEN 2: SUBMUCOUS FIBROID (FIG. 2)

Patient aged 46 years with three children. TH with BSO done. Uterine cavity is opened from posterior surface of uterus—look at the ovarian ligament which lies posteriorly.

SPECIMEN 3: MULTIPLE FIBROID (FIG. 3)

A 47-year parous woman presented with pain abdomen with AUB—total abdominal hysterectomy (TAH) with BSO done. Look here, ovaries were adhered due to endometriosis.

SPECIMEN 4: SUBSEROUS FIBROID (FIG. 4)

Total abdominal hysterectomy with BSO done in multiparous perimenopausal woman shown from in front. Look that lower part of uterus is devoid of serous coat, and ovarian ligament attachment with uterus lies posteriorly and not visible.

There is every possibility of torsion in subserosal pedunculated fibroid.

SPECIMEN 5: LARGE CERVICAL FIBROID (FIG. 5)

This is a specimen of large cervical fibroid. Patient came with something coming down per vagina with occasional retention of urine. TAH-BSO is done. Hysterectomy without myomectomy is a risky procedure with risk of ureteric injury which needs expertization. In this type usually cervical myomectomy is done first followed by hysterectomy.
See the Chapter 4, for details of Cervical Fibroid.

SPECIMEN 6: LARGE CERVICAL FIBROID (FIG. 6)

Large cervical fibroid—myomectomy done first after hemisection of uterus, followed by hysterectomy.

SPECIMEN 7: PSEUDOBROAD LIGAMENT FIBROID (FIG. 7)

Pseudobroad ligament fibroid—small. Note that fibroid originates from the body of uterus and is buried into layers of broad ligament. Posterior surface is shown—ovarian

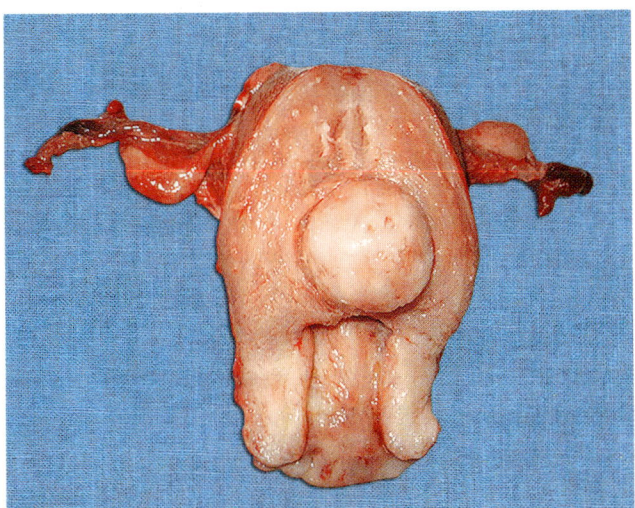

Fig. 2: Submucous fibroid—patient aged 46 years—total hysterectomy (TH) with bilateral salpingo-oophorectomy (BSO) done.

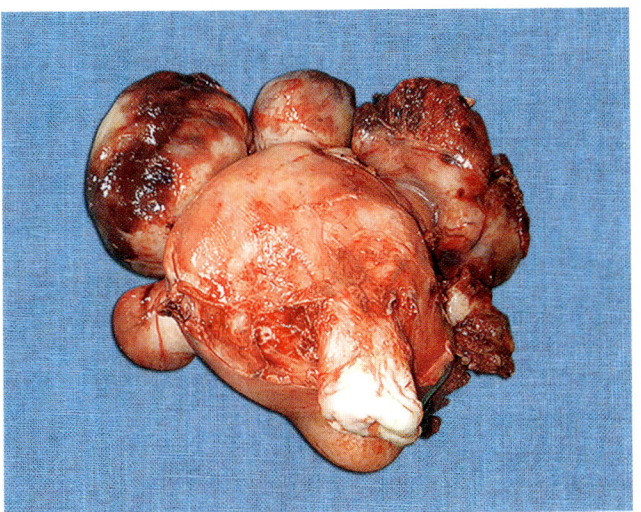

Fig. 3: Multiple fibroid in parous woman—TH-BSO done.

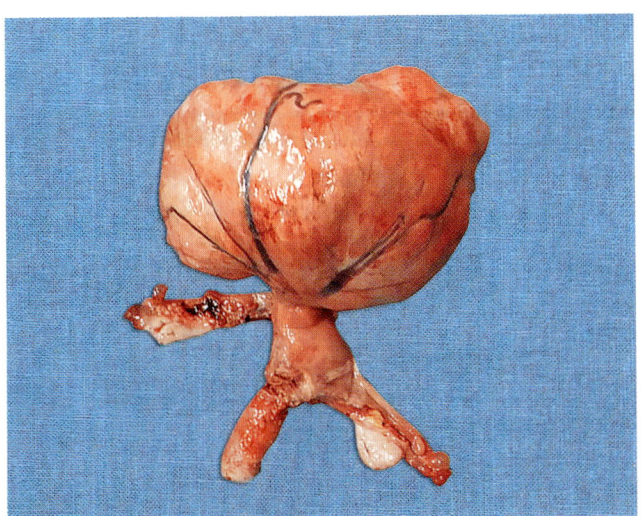

Fig. 4: Subserous fibroid—TAH-BSO done.
Courtesy: Dr Prajit Roy

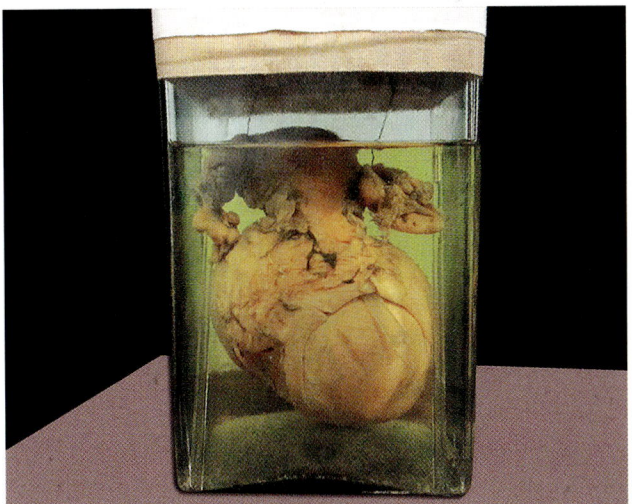

Fig. 5: Large cervical fibroid.

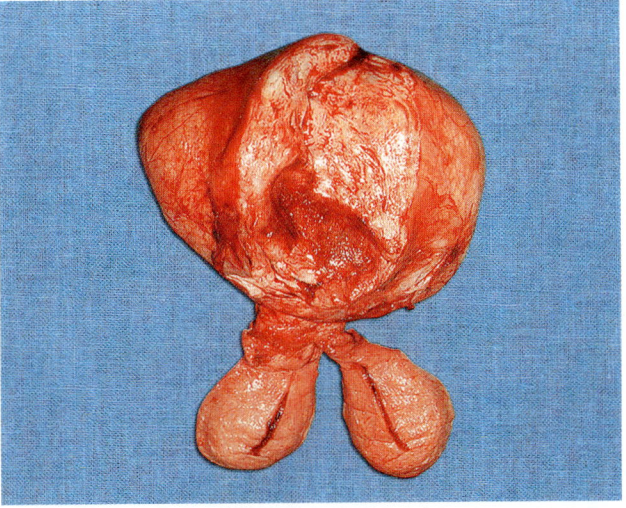

Fig. 6: Cervical fibroid.

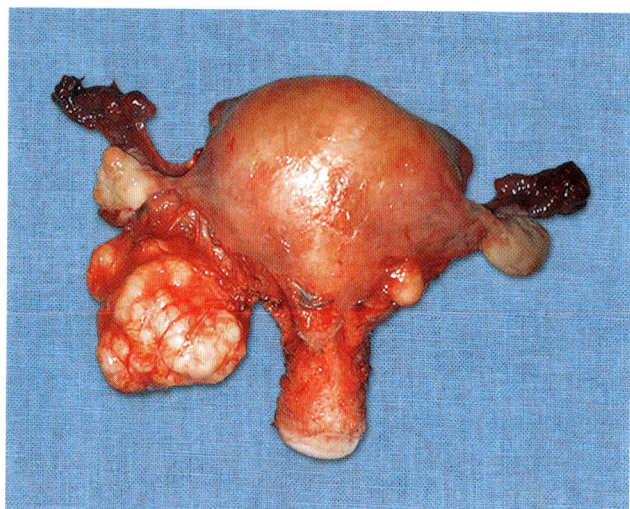

Fig. 7: Pseudobroad ligament fibroid—small. TAH-BSO done.

ligament lies posteriorly and serous coat of uterus extends lower down.

SPECIMEN 8: SIMPLE SEROUS CYST OVARY (FIG. 8)

Q. Describe the specimen.

The specimen is clear cystic mass with smooth surface, no adhesion, uniloculated with fallopian tube attached with it (not well visible but seen behind—inspect all the sides of specimen).

Q. What surgery is done?

Salpingo-oophorectomy.

Q. What is your diagnosis?

Benign ovarian cyst.

Q. What was the presentation?

Patient relatively younger with no or less number of child presented with lump abdomen and heaviness of pelvis. She may have acute pain abdomen due to torsion.

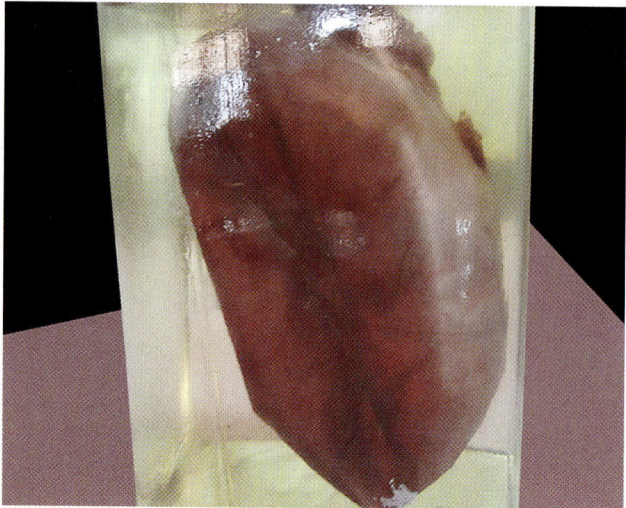

Fig. 8: Salpingo-oophorectomy—in simple serous cyst of ovary.

On examination, general condition is not deteriorated in benign cyst or in early period. Patient complaint of anorexia, looks cachectic in malignant ovarian tumor, but not in this case.

P/A: A lower abdominal cystic, nontender, a smooth-walled mass and mobile from side to side.

P/V: Mass is separated from the uterus—there will be a cleft in between uterus and mass but not in fibroid (*see* Chapter 1 on Bimanual Examination).

Q. Why are you saying benign?

Look of the specimen and also conservative surgery is done.

Q. What more conservative surgery could have been done?

Ovarian cystectomy.

Q. Whether a tumor is benign or malignant—how will you differentiate?

See Chapter 3 on Lump Abdomen.

Q. Name some benign cyst of ovary.

Serous cystadenoma, mucinous cystadenoma and dermoid cyst.

Q. Will you always do surgery in ovarian tumor?

Yes, as there may be complications, most important ones are malignant change, torsion and rupture (*see* Chapter 3 on Lump Abdomen in detail).

Q. What are the different surgeries done in ovarian tumor?

- Ovarian cystectomy—where only cyst is removed retaining the healthy ovarian tissue
- Salpingo-oophorectomy
- Hysterectomy with BSO (TAH-BSO)
- TAH-BSO, infracolic omentectomy and removal of metastasis in malignancy
- In advance malignancy—debulking surgery, removal of metastasis, omentectomy, lymphadenectomy done.

Q. What are the different types of tumor of ovary?

See Chapter 3 on Lump Abdomen.

SPECIMEN 9: BENIGN TUMOR (FIG. 9)

This is a specimen of ovarian tumor—salpingo ophorectomy done in young woman. Questions are like Specimen 8.

SPECIMEN 10: OVARIAN CYST (FIG. 10)

This is a specimen where ovarian cystectomy has been done retaining the healthy ovarian tissue. This is done in young patient who needs further child and the tumor is benign in nature.

SPECIMEN 11: DERMOID CYST OF OVARY (FIG. 11)

- This is a dermoid cyst of ovary.
- Common questions are here.

CHAPTER 28: Specimens

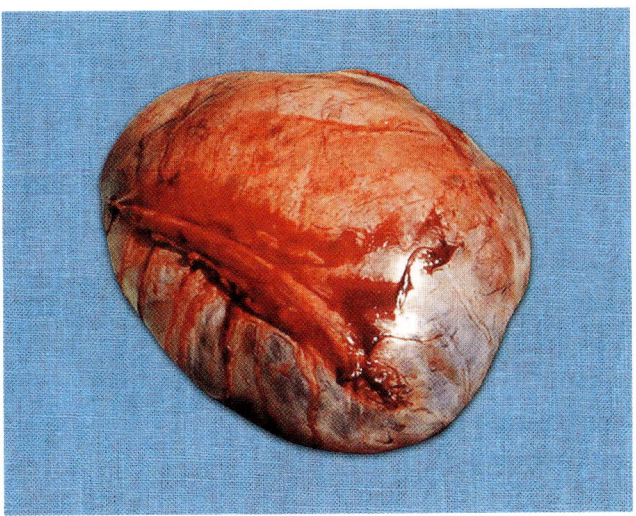

Fig. 9: Salpingo-oophorectomy in benign tumor in young woman.

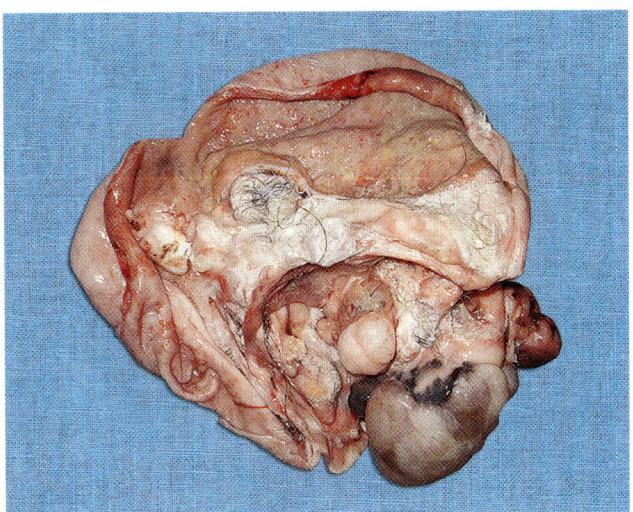

Fig. 11: Dermoid cyst of ovary specimen following ovarian cystectomy.

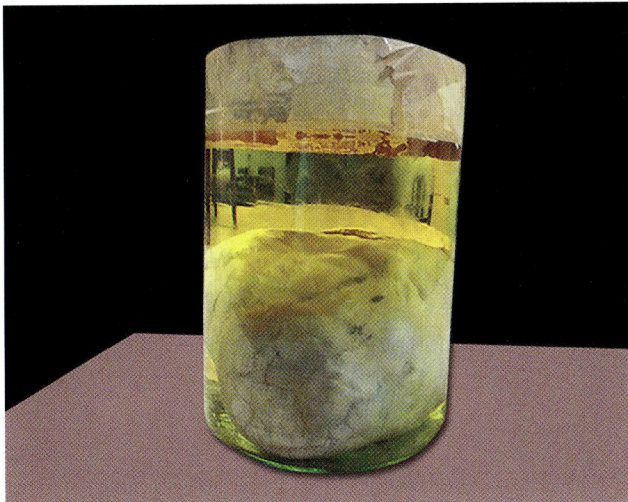

Fig. 9A: Ovarian cyst.

Q. Why are you saying dermoid cyst?

As all three tissue elements are present. Hair, skin, nail, teeth and mandible, etc., are found.

Q. What surgery is usually done?

Cystectomy or salpingo-oophorectomy.

Q. In which group does it lie? What is other name of this tumor?

Germ cell tumor. Benign cystic teratoma.

Q. Tell some uniqueness of this tumor.

- Notorious for torsion—moderate size, heavy tumor and long pedicle.
- Commonly found with pregnancy as it occurs mostly in reproductive age group.
- The most common germ cell tumor (95% of all germ cell tumor).
- Chance of malignancy is less (1–3%), bilaterality less (<10%).

Q. What are the other germ cell tumors?

- *See* Chapter 3 on Lump Abdomen.
- *See* dermoid cyst of ovary in Chapter 3 on Lump Abdomen.

SPECIMEN 12: BENIGN OVARIAN TUMOR (TAH WITH BSO) (FIG. 12)

This is a specimen of TAH with BSO in ovarian tumor. TAH with BSO has been done as the patient is in postmenopausal age even the tumor looks benign.

SPECIMEN 13: MALIGNANT OVARIAN TUMOR (FIG. 13)

This is a specimen following TAH with BSO in a bilateral ovarian tumor. Tumor was in malignant nature (serous cystadenocarcinoma). Infracolic omentectomy is also done in such case.

See Chapter 3 on Malignant Ovarian Tumor—varieties, stages, diagnosis and management.

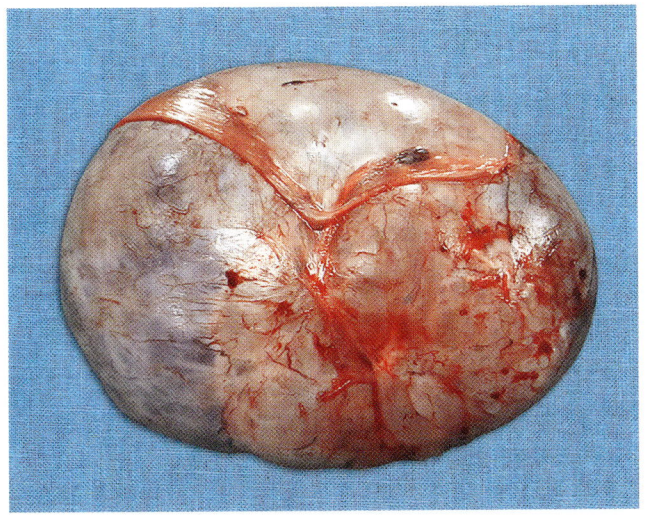

Fig. 10: Ovarian cyst following cystectomy.

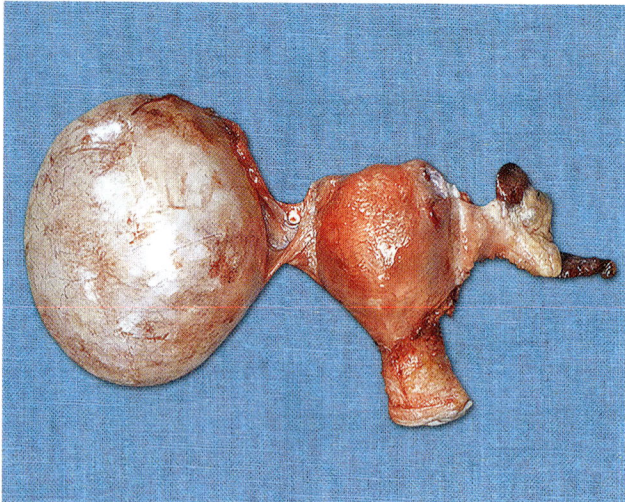

Fig. 12: TAH-BSO in postmenopausal woman in benign ovarian tumor.

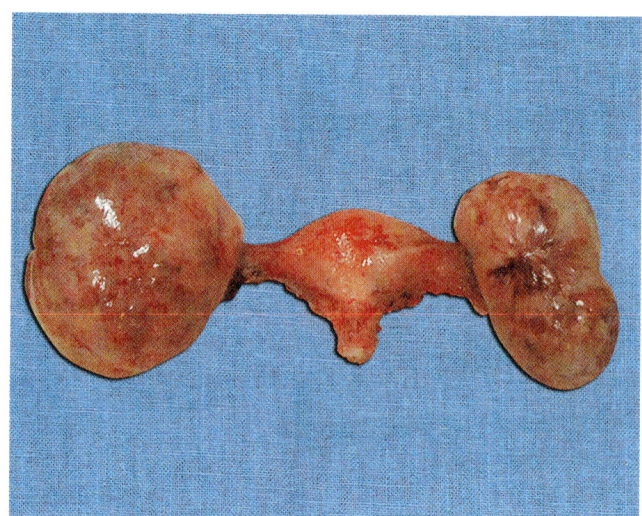

Fig. 14A: TAH-BSO in Krukenberg tumor.

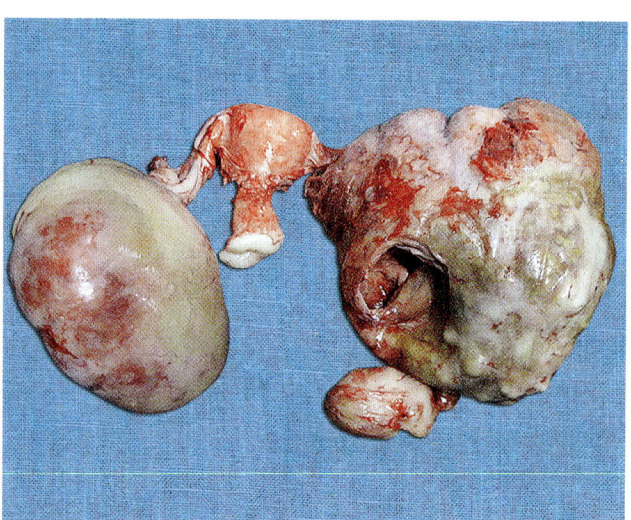

Fig. 13: TAH-BSO in malignant ovarian tumor.

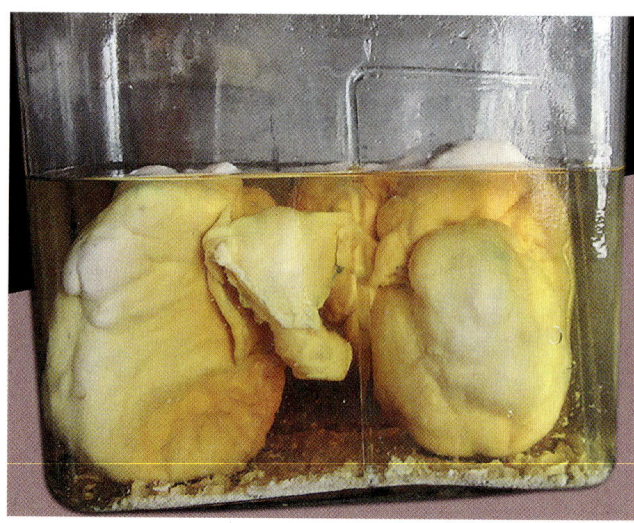

Fig. 14B: Bilateral ovarian tumor (likely to be Krukenberg tumor).

SPECIMEN 14A AND 14B (FIGS. 14A AND B): KRUKENBERG TUMOR

This is a case of bilateral ovarian tumor—TAH with BSO done.

Q. When a bilateral malignant ovarian tumor is diagnosed? What will you keep in your mind?
May be a case of secondary metastatic tumor.

Q. Name one secondary metastatic ovarian tumor.
Krukenberg tumor.

Q. What may be the primaries?
Stomach is the most common, others are intestine, breasts and gallbladder.

Q. In evaluation what will you do?
To search for primary.

Q. What is the histological finding of Krukenberg tumor?
Signet ring appearance. *See* also Krukenberg Tumor in Chapter 3.

SPECIMEN 15 AND 15A (FIGS. 15 AND 15A): CANCER CERVIX

Q. Describe the specimen.
This is a specimen of uterus with bilateral tubes and ovaries, cervix, upper part of vagina and parametrium with a growth on cervix.

Q. What is your diagnosis?
Cancer cervix.

Q. What surgery is done in cancer cervix?
Radical hysterectomy.

CHAPTER 28: Specimens

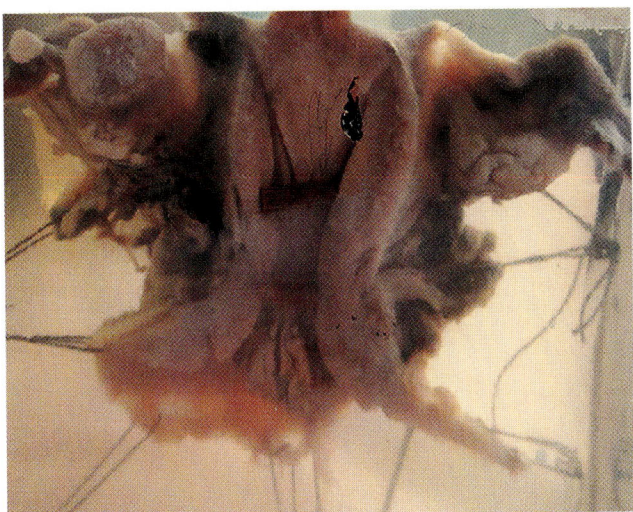

Fig. 15: Radical hysterectomy in cancer cervix (Wertheim's operation—*see* Fig. 16).

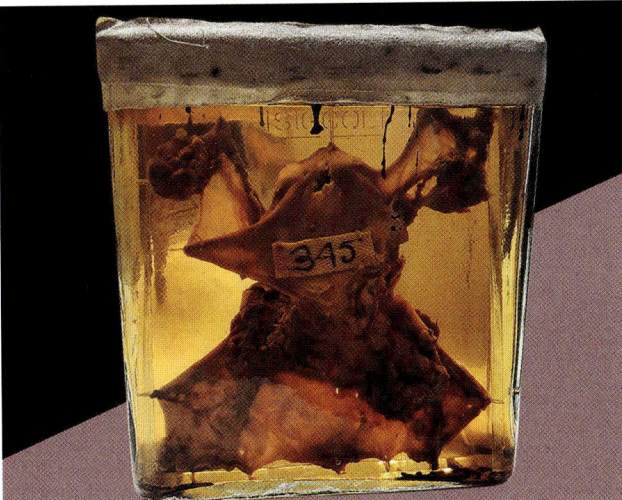

Fig. 15A: Mitra's radical vaginal hysterectomy for cancer cervix. Lymphadenectomy is done by extraperitoneal approach. Parametrium and vaginal cuff can be removed more in vaginal approach.
Courtesy: Professor Ashish Kumar Mukhopadhyaya and Professor Ramprasad Dey, Chittaranjan Sevasadan College of Obstetrics, Gynaecology and Child Health, Kolkata

Q. What are the components of radical hysterectomy? Which structure is deficient in your specimen?

- Removal of uterine body, cervix, upper part of vagina, parametrium, both-sided tubes and ovaries and draining lymph nodes.
- Lymph nodes are deficient here.

Q. In which stage surgery is done?

- Early stage—from stage I to stage IIa. In early stage, surgery or radiotherapy can be done but in late stage surgery could not be possible, radiotherapy is preferred option.
- Other questions (*see* Chapter 8 on Cancer Cervix).

Q. How will you diagnose cancer cervix?

See Chapter 8—Cancer Cervix.

Q. What is the treatment of cancer cervix?

See Chapter 8—Cancer Cervix.

Q. In which route radical hysterectomy is done?

- Abdominal route—Wertheim's operation **(Fig. 15)**.
- Vaginal route: (1) Schauta's operation—the disadvantage is there no provision of lymphadenectomy. (2) Mitra's operation—vaginal radical hysterectomy **(Fig. 15A)** with extraperitoneal lymphadenectomy.

SPECIMEN 16: CANCER CERVIX (FIG. 16)

This is a specimen of radical hysterectomy (Wertheim's operation) in cancer cervix. The patient was of 42 years of age with four children, came with irregular vaginal bleeding and postcoital bleeding.

There was a growth over cervix prominent over anterior lip which bled on touch.

On biopsy, it showed squamous cell carcinoma. Surgery was done by TAH with BSO with removal of upper third of vagina with parametrium.

The draining lymph nodes were removed which is displayed on the sides of the specimen. Lymph nodes became positive on histology.

Postoperative radiotherapy was given. On follow-up of three years, patient is well.

SPECIMEN 17: ENDOMETRIAL CANCER (FIG. 17)

Figure 17 shows specimen of TAH with BSO done in a case of growth of endometrium.

Endometrial cancer—growth looks like a polypoidal mass on left fundal region—a 39-year woman having one issue presented with profuse irregular bleeding per vagina. On

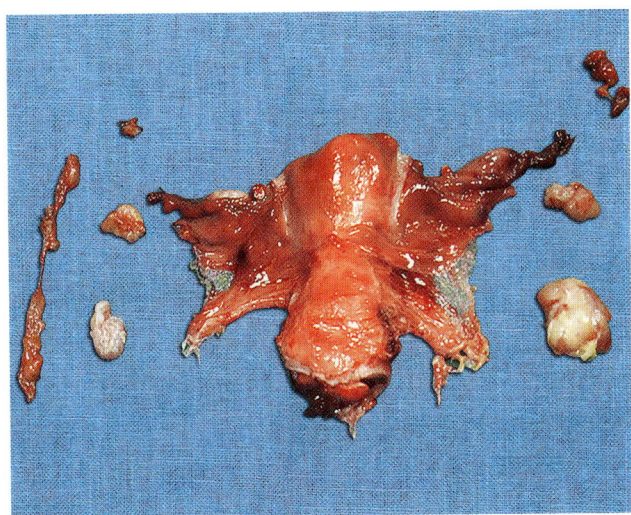

Fig. 16: Specimen following Wertheim's operation including lymph nodes (*see* Fig. 15).

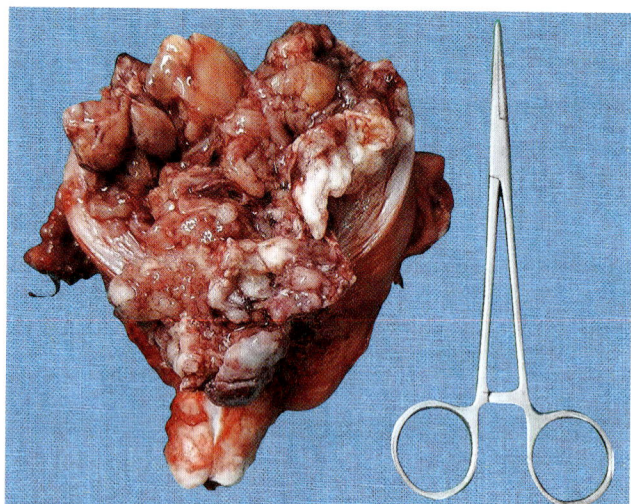

Fig. 17: Endometrial cancer—a 39 years woman having one issue.

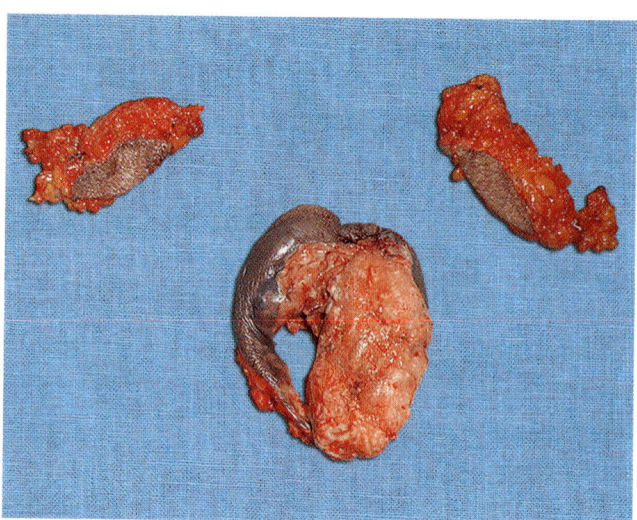

Fig. 18: Radical vulvectomy in cancer vulva showing the radical vulvectomy with growth and removal of bilateral inguinal glands.

endometrial biopsy, histopathology showed endometrioid adenocarcinoma.

The questions related to endometrial cancer:
- Risk factors and etiological factors
- Diagnosis
- Staging
- Role of magnetic resonance imaging (MRI)—for determination of stage preoperatively
- Management including hormone therapy
- Prognosis—overall 5-year survival rate—80%, Stage I near 90%.

See answers and more from the Chapter 6 on Endometrial Cancer.

SPECIMEN 18: CANCER VULVA (FIG. 18)

Specimen of radical vulvectomy in cancer of vulva.

Inguinal lymphadenectomy was done by separate incisions instead of old butterfly incision.

The dissected inguinal lymph nodes with fatty tissue with the skin of inguinal region are displayed by the sides of vulvectomy specimen.

The questions related to cancer vulva:
- Risk factors of cancer vulva—two age group two etiogenesis
- Staging
- Spread and lymphatic drainage
- Types of surgery
- Other therapy.

See answers from the Chapter 9 "Cancer of Vulva".

Section 7

Imaging

Section Outline

29. Hysterosalpingography Plates, X-ray Plates with IUCD and Other Imaging

CHAPTER 29

Hysterosalpingography Plates, X-ray Plates with IUCD and Other Imaging

Chapter Outline

- Hysterosalpingography—All Probable Questions Discussed Including the Procedures
- HSG Plates—Patent Tubes, Block Tube, Unicornuate, Bicornuate, Septate and Arcuate are Displayed with Probable Questions
- X-ray Pelvis with Cu-T—All Probable Questions Discussed
- USG with Cu-T in Normal Position, Misplayed Position and 3D USG with Normal Position IUCD are Displayed
- USG Plate of Chocolate Cyst and MRI of Uterine Fibroid are Displayed. Relevant Questions may be Asked. USG, MRI and CT Scan are Incorporated in Specific Chapters

HYSTEROSALPINGOGRAPHY PLATES

NORMAL SCAN (FIG. 1)

Q. Describe the plate.

It is hysterosalpingogram showing normal uterine cavity with bilateral spillage of dye on both sides indicating that both the tubes are patent.

Q. Why this investigation was done?

It is commonly done as an infertility work-up to check the tubal patency test.

Q. What are the other tubal patency tests?

Laparoscopy and sonohysterosalpingography.

Q. What other factors will you see in infertility?

- Semen analysis
- Ovulatory factor.
  (for other questions on infertility—see Chapter 11)

Q. Where it is done?

It is done in radiology department; dye is usually pushed by gynecologist.

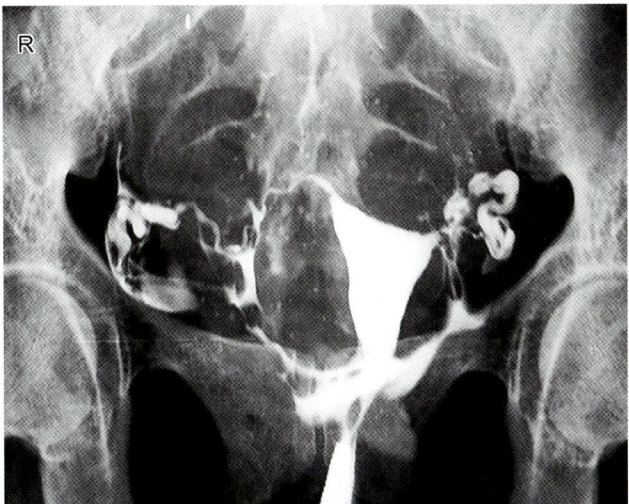

Fig. 1: Hysterosalpingography—bilateral patent tubes.

Q. Is any anesthesia needed?

No anesthesia is needed. Usually, any antispasmodic drug or nonsteroidal anti-inflammatory drug (NSAID) is given half an hour before.

Q. What are the indications of hysterosalpingography (HSG)?

- Infertility for tubal patency test—commonest.

- Recurrent abortion and preterm labor for detection of uterine anomaly, mass in endometrial cavity (filling defect) and cervical incompetence.
- Tubal patency test after recanalization and Essure placement (after 3 months).
- Displaced intrauterine contraceptive device (IUCD)—rarely done nowadays. It is diagnosed by USG.
- Amenorrhea after excluding pregnancy—uterine synechia may be detected.

Contraindication

- Active pelvic infection—in presence of pelvic infection sudden exacerbation of severe type or infection may occur.
- Menstruation
- Suspected pelvic tuberculosis.
- Known allergy to iodine containing compound.
- Suspected pregnancy.
- During abnormal uterine bleeding.

Complications of Hysterosalpingography

- Infection
- Embolism or granuloma formation in oil-based dye.
- Dye allergy.
- Intravasation of dye.
- Perforation of uterus.

Q. Is there any therapeutic benefit of HSG?

Chance of pregnancy is increased in oil-based dye.

Q. When this X-ray is taken and why?

- Within 7–10 days of period.
- At this time, there is no possibility of pregnancy, no chance of interference of pregnancy.
- The endometrium is thin so better delineation of cavity.
- During menstruation, there is chance of retrograde flow of menstrual blood and chance of intravasation is more.
- Chance of infection is also less during this period.

Q. Which types of dye is used?

- Both water soluble and oil-based dye has advantages and disadvantages. Commonly water soluble is used.
- In water soluble dye, the picture quality is not good, and with oil-based dye, better delineation of cavity is found. Complications like embolism and granuloma formation are more in oil-based dye. In water-based media, the procedure is completed within 15 minutes but in oil-based, 3rd film is taken after 24 hours.

Q. What type of cannula is used?

1. Metallic HSG cannula (*see* Page 258, **Fig. 18**).
2. Hysterosalpingography catheter (*see* Page 260, **Fig. 23**).

Q. How many films are taken?

Usually three films:
1. Before dye instillation.
2. Second film immediately after dye instillation to see uterine cavity.
3. Third film to see the spillage of dye after 10 minutes in water-soluble dye.

If in the second film, spillage of dye is seen and tubes are visualized, no need of third film. It is now done in fluoroscopic view which takes less time.

Q. What is your advice immediately after HSG?

No contraindication of sexual intercourse and prophylactic antibiotic (Doxycycline 100 mg BD) is given for 5 days to start 2 days after HSG.

Q. What amount of dye is usually needed?

5–10 mL. Urograffin or Conray 420.

Q. Procedures of HSG.

See Page 258.

BILATERAL TUBAL BLOCK (FIG. 2)

Q. What is your finding?

Hysterosalpingogram showing bilateral tubal block with irregular outline of uterine cavity. This type of finding is suggestive of pelvic tuberculosis.

Q. What are the features of HSG finding in pelvic tuberculosis?

- *Tubes:* Tubes may be blocked at fimbrial end or at corneal end. If tubes are visible, there may be presence of beaded appearance of tube, tobacco pouch appearance due to everted fimbria and/or lead pipe rigidity appearance. There may be hydrosalpinx.
- *Uterus:* Lining of cavity is irregular.
- Intravasation of dye may be present.

Q. What are the causes of tubal block?

- Pelvic tuberculosis
- Pelvic infection
- Surgical adhesions

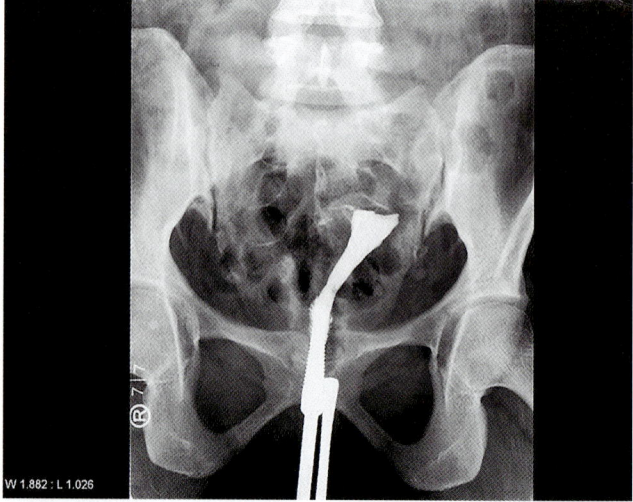

Fig. 2: Hysterosalpingography—bilateral tubal block suggestive of tuberculosis.
Courtesy: Professor Kamal Oswal, Head, VIMS, Kolkata

- In endometriosis tubes are usually patent but there may be distortion of tubes.
- Cornual block may be due to cornual polyp, mucus plug and corneal spasm.

Q. What is the chance of false negative in tubal patency test by HSG?

- There may be false negative due to corneal spasm or plug. Findings of fimbrial block in most of the cases are correct. Diagnosis of distal tubal block by HSG is almost accurate.
- Out of total, 60% of patients of proximal tubal block by HSG shows patency after repeat HSG in subsequent months. On laparoscopy, 50% of patients with proximal tubal block diagnosed by HSG shows tubal patency.

Q. What you will do if you get tubal block in HSG?

Laparoscopic chromopertubation test is done to confirm the tubal block. However, it is not immediately done as HSG has some therapeutic benefit.

Q. If it is really bilateral tubal block by laparoscopy, what is the treatment option?

- Either tubal surgery, preferably microsurgery or in vitro fertilization and embryo transfer (IVF-ET).
- Result of surgery is not satisfactory and there is chance of ectopic pregnancy.
- In presence of hydrosalpinx, the result of IVF-ET is not good. Prior surgical removal or clipping of hydrosalpinx is done as fluid of hydrosalpinx is toxic to gamete and embryo.
- In case of cornual block, hysteroscopic cannulation under guidance of laparoscopy is an option.

LEFT SIDE TUBE BLOCK (FIG. 3)

Hysterosalpingogram showing spillage on right side and left tube is also visible, but without spillage suggestive fimbrial block on left side.

Q. What will you do in this case for treatment of infertility?

- Evaluation of other factor of infertility.
- Intrauterine insemination may be done as one tube is patent.
- If the patient is elderly and married for long period, diagnostic laparoscopy is advised for evaluation of pelvic pathology.

BICORNUATE UTERUS (FIGS. 4 AND 5)

- Hysterosalpingogram showing bicornuate uterus.
- In **Figure 4**, there is no spillage of dye in right tube and in **Figure 5**, spillage of dye is seen in both the tubes.

Q. How can you say it is bicornuate uterus and not septate uterus?

- For confirmation, laparoscopy is needed. In septate uterus, the outer fundal contour is normal but in bicornuate, two separate horns are seen.
- In HSG, the angle between two horns is acute (<75°) in septate uterus but in bicornuate uterus, it is more than 105°.
- Magnetic resonance imaging (MRI) and 3D are helpful to differentiate the two types.
- Fundal invagination bigger than 1 cm by MRI and distinct vascularization in color Doppler testify bicornuate uterus. It is less than 1 cm in septate uterus.

Q. So far as obstetric outcome is concerned, which one is better—bicornuate or septate?

Obstetric outcome is better in bicornuate than septate and surgery is needed more in septate uterus.

Reproductive Outcome in Bicornuate Uterus

- Premature onset of labor may occur around 22–32 weeks as pregnancy grows in half of the uterus.
- Chance of preterm delivery more than 60%. Increased risk of miscarriage, preterm birth and malpresentation.

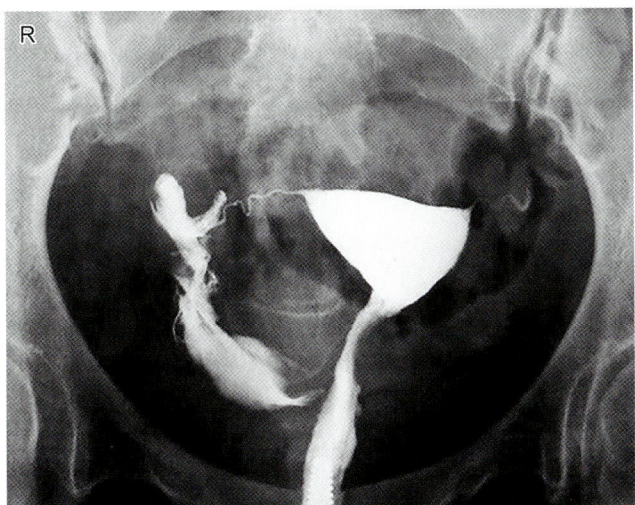

Fig. 3: Hysterosalpingography. Left side—ampullary block; right side—spillage present.

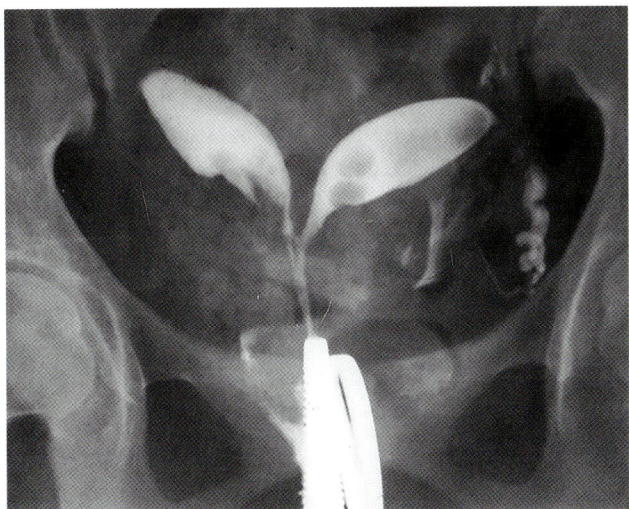

Fig. 4: Hysterosalpingography—bicornuate uterus, no spillage on right tube, spillage on left side.

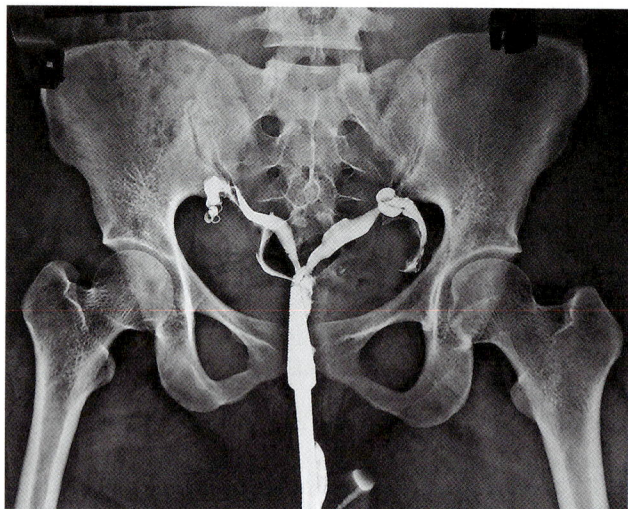

Fig. 5: Hysterosalpingography (HSG)—bicornuate uterus, right side localized spill and left side free spill. [*see* also Fig. 23 in Chapter 11 (Infertility)]

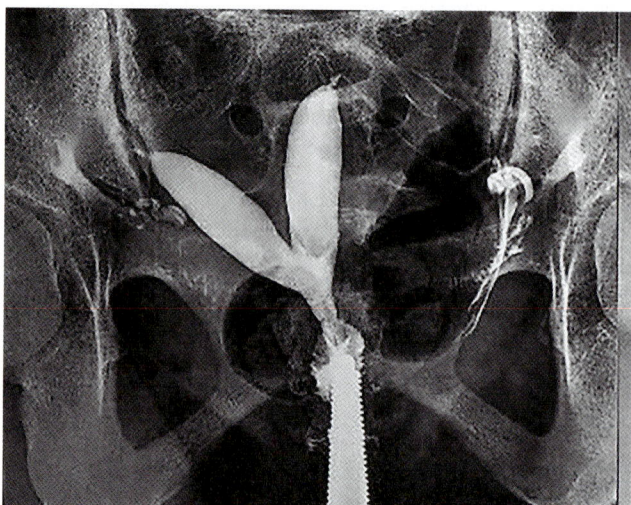

Fig. 6: Hysterosalpingography—septate uterus.

- Other than monitoring of pregnancy, no specific treatment is advocated.
- Success of delivering live baby is 60%.

Indication of Surgery in Bicornuate Uterus

- Unification operation (*Strassman technique*) is indicated with good outcome in women with multiple spontaneous abortions with bicornuate uterus in absence of other cause (*see* Chapter 21, Müllerian Anomaly for details *see* Page 260).
- More than 85% end in live birth following surgery.
- Cesarean section is indicated following metroplasty.

SEPTATE UTERUS (FIG. 6)

Hysterosalpingography showing septate uterus.

Q. How can you say septate, not bicornuate?

It is explained under the heading bicornuate uterus (*see* Page 581).

Q. What is the reproductive outcome in septate uterus?

- Reproductive outcome is poor in comparison to bicornuate uterus.
- Septate uterus is associated with subfertility, more miscarriage, and malpresentation. Preterm delivery is not increased.
- Spontaneous abortion (8–12 weeks) rate is 40%.
- The cause of 1st trimester abortion is diminished blood supply, implantation on avascular septum, distorted uterine cavity and cervical and endometrial abnormalities.

Q. When will you advise surgery? Which type of surgery is preferred?

- Surgical resection via hysteroscopic metroplasty is considered when associated with infertility or recurrent pregnancy loss or infertility in the absence of other factors.
- About 60% pregnancy rate and 45% live births are reported following hysteroscopic resection. (*See* Chapter 21, Müllerian Anomaly for more details).

Q. How to differentiation of bicornuate, septate and arcuate uterus?

- Initial diagnosis is done by 2-D TVS. MRI, 3-D TVS of bicornuate, septate and arcuate uterus in coronal plane can differentiate the three. This differentiation is very important as septate uterus can be managed by hysteroscopic septal resection, not the bicornuate uterus.
- Fundal indent is more than 1 cm, in bicornuate uterus, in ASRM classification. In septate uterus partition depth is more than 1.5 cm and partition angle is less than 90° and in arcuate uterus partition depth is less than 1cm and partition angle is more than 90° (American Society for Reproductive Medicine, 2016). ESHRE/ESGE also made different differentiating features in the same way. *See* Chapter 21, Müllerian Anomaly for more details.

UNICORNUATE UTERUS (FIG. 7)

Hysterosalpingography shows unicornuate uterus with spillage of dye suggesting patency of tube.

Q. What is the cause of adverse pregnancy outcome?

- Impaired uterine blood flow, diminished uterine cavity, less muscle mass of hemiuterus and cervical incompetence are considered to be adverse obstetric outcome.
- These are preterm labor (16%), miscarriage (36%), fetal growth restriction, fetal demise and malpresentation (commonly breech presentation).
- Live birth rate: 54%
- High cesarean rate.

CHAPTER 29: Hysterosalpingography Plates, X-ray Plates with IUCD and Other Imaging

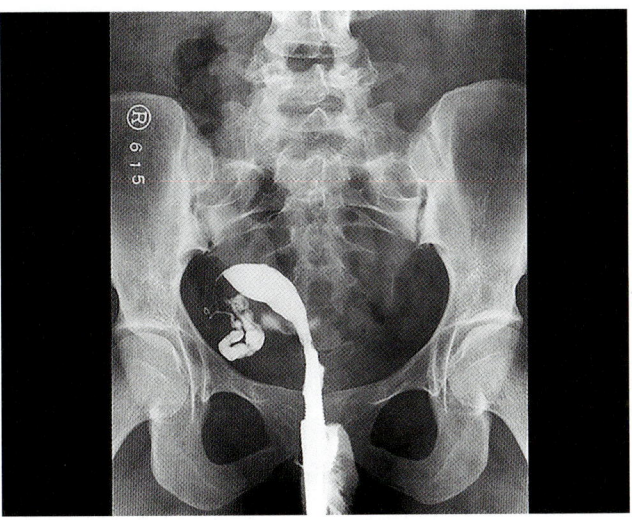

Fig. 7: Hysterosalpingography suggestive of unicornuate uterus with spillage of dye.

Management

- Possibility of rudimentary horn should be kept in mind.
- A noncommunicating horn containing functional endometrium should be resected.
- Pregnancy in rudimentary horn is excised.
- Pregnancy in unicornuate uterus: No specific treatment.

ARCUATE UTERUS (FIG. 8)

- Hysterosalpingography shows arcuate uterus.
- There is slight indentation in the fundus. Ratio of height to fundal indentation to intercornual distance is less than 10%.
- Most women have no adverse reproductive consequences and no treatment needed.
- Surgery is indicated in repeated pregnancy losses when other reasons are not found.

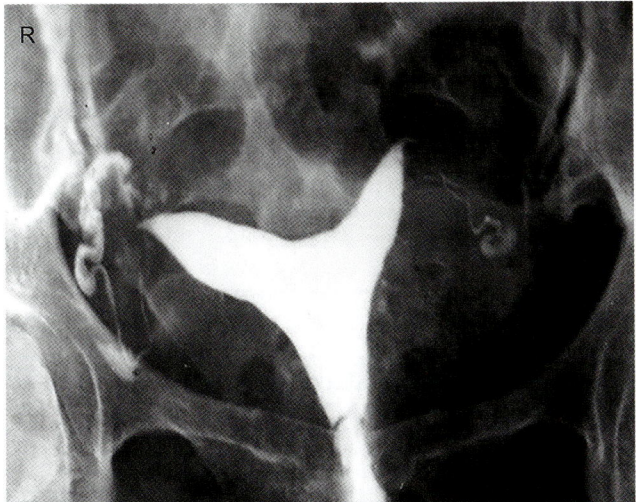

Fig. 8: Hysterosalpingography—arcuate uterus, both tubes are visible, no spillage on left side.

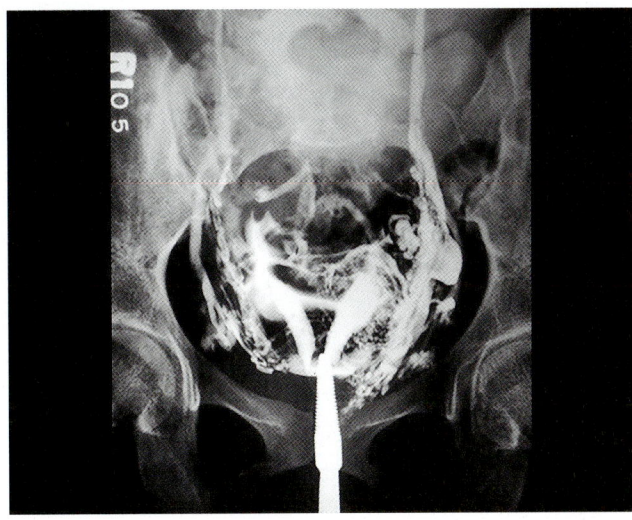

Fig. 9: Hysterosalpingography extravasation of dye in venous and lymphatic route with bicornuate uterus.
Courtesy: Dr Subir Roy, Consultant Gynecologist

BICORNUATE UTERUS (FIG. 9)

Bicornuate uterus with spillage of dye with extravasation of dye in venous and lymphatic channel. Patient was asymptomatic during and after HSG.

For all the Questions of Müllerian Anomaly—*see* Chapter 21.

X-RAY PLATES

CU-T INTRAUTERINE CONTRACEPTIVE DEVICE (FIGS. 10 AND 11)

Q. Describe this X-ray plate.

- Straight X-ray of pelvis showing a Cu-T in pelvis.

Q. Why this X-ray was taken?

- Patient came with missing thread (string) of IUCD.

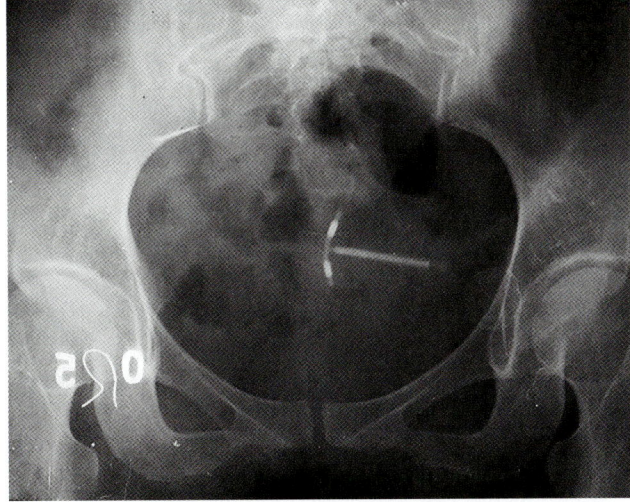

Fig. 10: X-ray pelvis showing intrauterine contraceptive device.

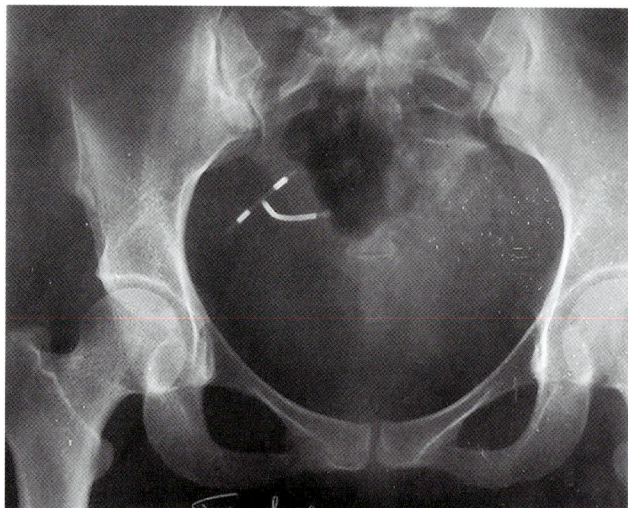

Fig. 11: X-ray showing Cu-T in pelvis. Laparotomy showed Cu-T adhered with right adnexa.

Q. How did she know about missing thread?

After insertion of IUCD, woman is asked to palpate the thread regularly following menstrual period. She failed to palpate it.

Q. What are the causes of missing string (thread)?

The causes of missing thread are:
- Torn of the thread
- Expulsion of device
- Twisting of the thread inside
- Perforation, or
- Pregnancy.

Q. In missing thread, what history will you take?

Whether the Cu-T is expelled, she can remember or she has noticed that a thread is expelled or the patient is amenorrheic or she has any specific complain.

Q. What you will do in order of sequence?

- Do a speculum examination and inspect carefully whether it is visible through external os or not.
- Urinary pregnancy test is done in case of amenorrhea to exclude pregnancy.

Q. Can you say by seeing this plate whether it is the uterus or outside?

No, it cannot be said.

Q. How will you determine it is intrauterine or extrauterine?

By ultrasonography (USG) pelvis (*see* Figs. 13 to 15), hysterogram or hysteroscopy.

Q. Suppose it is intrauterine, what will you do?

- Removal of IUCD is done commonly either by loop removal hook or by hysteroscope (*see* Chapter 22 on Contraception).
- Alternatively, patient is told that it will prevent pregnancy as before if it is kept in situ.
- If she wants it is removed, another IUCD is given or alternate contraceptive is advised if she does not opt for next pregnancy.

Q. Suppose it is outside the uterus, i.e., it is perforated, what will you do?

- It is removed laparoscopically or sometimes laparotomy may be needed.
- Sometimes, the device may penetrate the uterine wall in varying degrees. Hysteroscopically or laparoscopically removal depends on how much it is uterine and how much it has perforated.

Q. What will happen if you do not remove perforated loop?

- Extrauterine copper-bearing device induces local inflammatory reaction and adhesion formation.
- Perforation may occur partial or completely and migrated commonly to omentum, adhered to adnexa or to the parietes. Bowel perforation or fistula is also reported. (*see* Chapter 22 on Contraception).

Q. If there is pregnancy with IUCD in situ what you will do?

- Woman usually comes with amenorrhea.
- On examination, the string is visible up to 14 weeks, thereafter it goes inside.
- As it is contraceptive failure, counseling is needed whether she wants termination or continuation. Medical termination of pregnancy is done if she wants.
- If she wants continuation, woman is counseled that there is increased chances of abortion, infection and preterm birth if the device lies *in situ*.
- If the thread is visible, it is removed with slight increased chance of abortion.
- If continuation is done with device in situ, chance of birth defect is usually not increased.

INERT IUCD (FIG. 12)

Q. Can you identify it?

- X-ray of pelvis showing Lippes loop, an inert IUCD.
- Lippes loop, an oldest intrauterine device made of polythene, made radioopaque by impregnating with barium sulfate, is commonly used in Pakistan, Indonesia and China. Once popular, it is not used in India from 1980s and is gradually being replaced by medicated intrauterine device throughout the world.

For IUCD Related Questions (all types)—*See* Chapter 22 on Contraception

SONOGRAPHY PLATES

IUCD IN UTERINE CAVITY (FIG. 13)

Transvaginal sonography showing normal position of IUCD inside uterine cavity.

DISPLACED CU-T (FIG. 14)

It is USG (transvaginal ultrasound) showing displaced Cu-T.

CHAPTER 29: Hysterosalpingography Plates, X-ray Plates with IUCD and Other Imaging

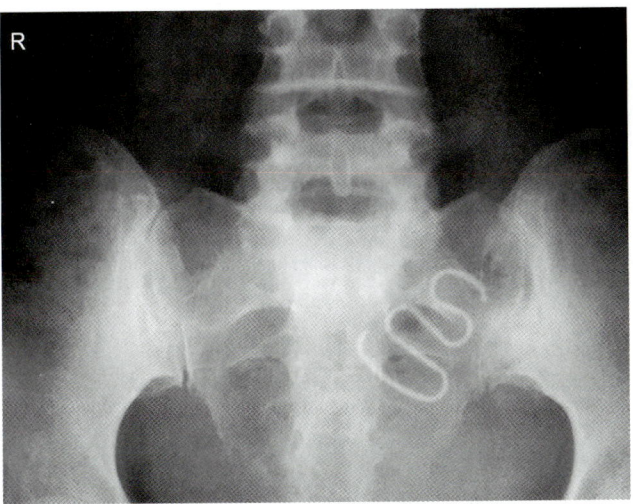

Fig. 12: Lippes loop by straight X-ray pelvis.

3D USG (FIG. 15)

Three-dimensional USG showing normal position of IUCD inside uterine cavity.

CHOCOLATE CYST OVARY (FIG. 16)

Transvaginal ultrasonography showing chocolate cyst of ovary. Questions related to this from endometriosis and adenomyosis (see Chapter 16).

MRI PLATES

FIBROID UTERUS (FIG. 17)

Magnetic resonance imaging showing fibroid uterus—sagittal T2-weighted MRI of pelvis of a 42-year-old lady

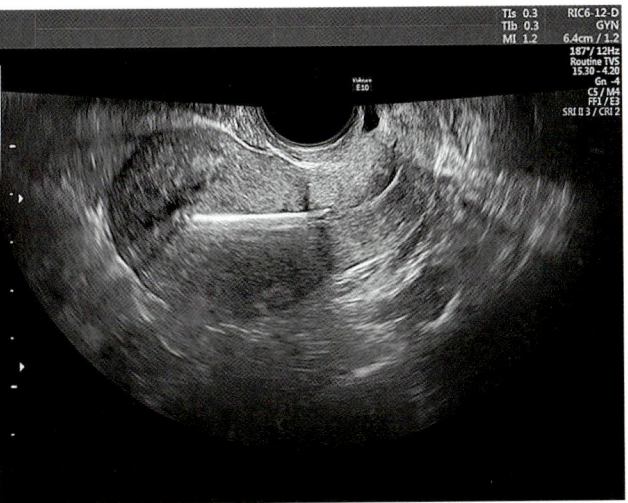

Fig. 13: Transvaginal sonography showing normal position of intrauterine contraceptive device inside uterine cavity. Patient came with missing thread and X-ray pelvis showed IUCD in pelvis.

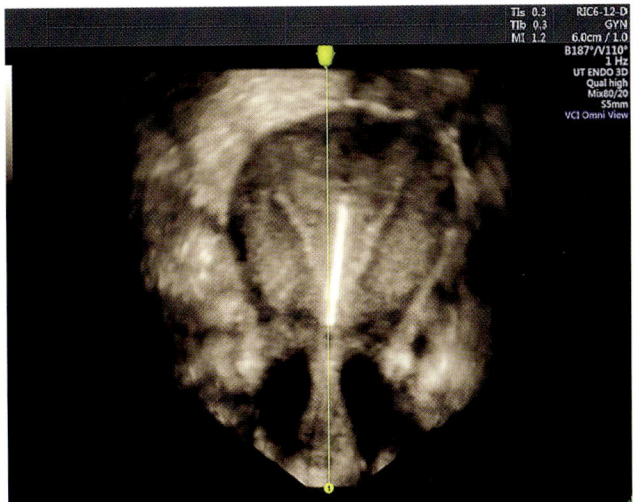

Fig. 15: Three-dimensional ultrasonography showing normal position of intrauterine contraceptive device inside uterine cavity.
Courtesy: Professor Kamal Oswal

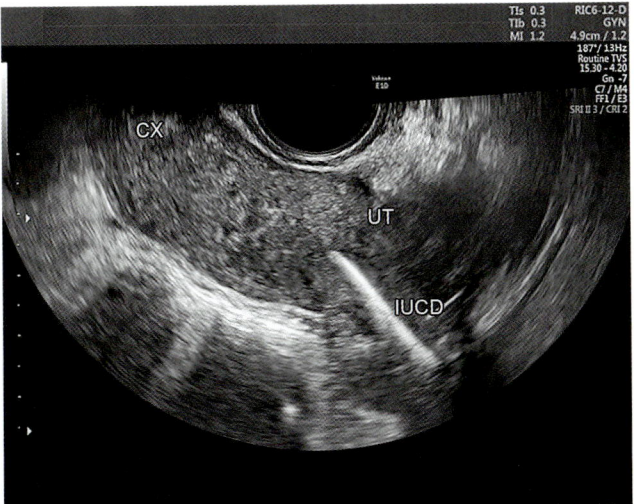

Fig. 14: Transvaginal sonography showing misplaced intrauterine contraceptive device.
Courtesy: Professor Kamal Oswal

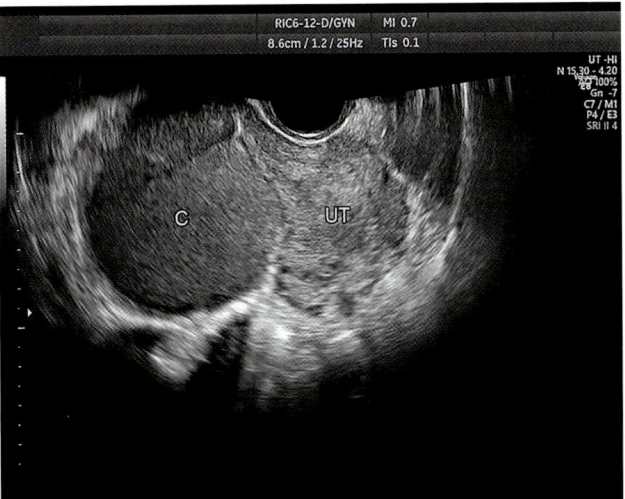

Fig. 16: Transvaginal sonography showing chocolate cyst of ovary.

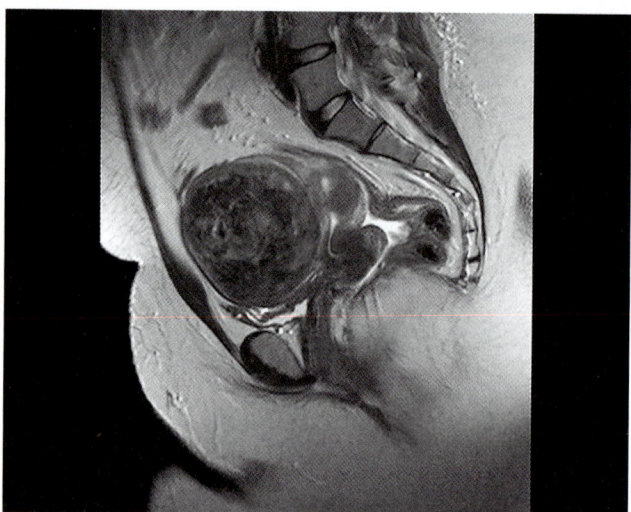

Fig. 17: Magnetic resonance imaging—fibroid uterus.
Courtesy: Dr Shuvro H Roy Choudhury, Consultant Abdominal and Interventional Radiologist

with symptomatic large intramural and subserosal fibroids with a distorted endometrium. This compresses the urinary bladder anteriorly and causes frequency and urgency during periods. Questions relation to this—fibroid and what is the role of MRI in gynecology (*see* Chapter 4 and Chapter 2).

For Sonographic Diagnosis of Ovarian Tumor and Fibroid *see* **chapter 3 and 4.**

Role of Imaging in Gynecology—*See* **Chapter 2**

Section 8

Miscellaneous

Section Outline

30. Research Questions for Students
31. Examination of a Rape Victim: Procedures and Protocols
32. Swellings of Vulva: Bartholin's Cyst and Abscess
33. Pelvic Inflammatory Disease, Sexually Transmitted Infections and Female Genital Tuberculosis

Research Questions for Students

CHAPTER OUTLINE

- Basic Research Questions
- Synopsis, Thesis—How to Start, How to Work and How to Write with their Components with the Concept of IMRaD
- Types of Study, Clinical trials
- CONSORT
- Statistic Related Questions like Specificity, Sensitivity, Positive Predictive Value, Negative Predictive Value, Mean, Median, Mode, p-value, CI, OR and RR are Defined
- Level of Evidence with Classification of Recommendations are Discussed

INTRODUCTION

Research is essential for progress of any science. In biomedical science doing research is an integral part. Every medical student should have basic knowledge on research methodology. In university curriculum, research methodology has been included. In this chapter, very basic questions are discussed in simpler way as far as possible so that it can help the students to write synopsis, to study the work, and to write the thesis and to face the questions on research methodology in examination.

Q. What is research?

The term "Research" refers to using the spirit of scientific enquiry to discover new facts and knowledge as well as to examine and verify old facts and knowledge in order to interpret them in a more modern and practical way.

Q. Why is research needed in medical sciences?

The main purpose of conducting research work is to acquire new knowledge which can be used for the betterment of society in general and patients in particular. The outcomes of such research can influence patient management, administrative policy making, and improve general health.

Study on population → Interpretation → Writing and Publishing → Knowledge → Application of knowledge.

Q. What do you mean by synopsis, thesis or dissertation, and original article?

Synopsis

(Greek word; *syn* means together and *opsis* means seeing) Synopsis refers to a brief summary or gist of the *proposed research project* which has to be approved by the authorities before the actual research work can be started. It is the written document comprising of essential scientific and administrative information submitted by the investigator toward obtaining Institutional Ethical Committee (IEC) approval and funding if applicable.

It should be brief and usually in a prescribed format. The number of words should be 500–1,000 for Master degree and between 1,000 and 2,500 for Doctoral projects.

So, preparation of synopsis has two components—one is writing the research proposal in a prescribed format and the other is to maintain the protocol for its submission and application for approval.

So writing synopsis has two parts: (1) Research proposal in prescribed format which includes introduction, aims and objectives, materials and methods, and few references, etc.; (2) Protocol of submission for approval for performing the study.

Thesis or Dissertation

It is the elaboration of the actual research work done by a student which has to be submitted in support of candidature for awarding an academic degree or professional qualification which he/she is pursuing.

Thesis or dissertation is a document submitted in support of candidature for awarding an academic degree or professional qualification by presenting the author's research findings.

Dissertation is a partial fulfillment for Master's degree whereas thesis is mandatory for awarding Doctoral. MD/MS thesis/dissertation is a test more of scientific rather than clinical ability and normally provides some contribution to medical knowledge. Length of the thesis should be less than 60,000 words.

Original Article

It is the publication of the research work in a journal in a precise manner arranged in a prescribed format.

Sequences of Work

A synopsis is submitted, after acceptance of which study is done. After completion of study the thesis is written and submitted. From the thesis an original paper which is actually the extract of thesis is written for publication in an authentic journal.

Q. What are the components of an original article or thesis? The components of an original article or thesis are as follows:

1. Title
2. Author's name/names (including initials, designations and attachments or positions held along with the names of institutions where the research was undertaken)
3. Abstract (a very brief summary of the study mainly focusing on results)
4. Keywords (helps in easy access to the article while researching similar materials on the internet)
5. Text (the main body written under IMRaD)
6. Acknowledgments
7. Vested interests or conflict of interests (example, if the study was sponsored by a drug company)
8. References (in Vancouver or Harvard style)
9. Pictures, illustrations, graphics, and photographs.

IMRaD

Q. What is IMRaD?

The main body of the thesis is written under four main headings abbreviated as IMRaD. It was first proposed by Bradford Hill in 1950. It stands for:

Introduction (I)—Why this particular research was conducted?
Materials and Methods (M)—How this research was conducted?
Results and analysis (Ra)—What was the outcome of the research?
Discussion (D)—What conclusion was drawn from the research?

Q. How will you choose a topic?

Choosing a topic should be based primarily on one's area of interest and should also depend on the clinical materials and other investigations available in one's institution as well as the area of interest of one's Guide. Ideas may be obtained by consulting seniors, teachers, thesis of previous years from the internet or by attending seminars, conferences, and workshops.

Q. How to write an appropriate title?

The following points must be kept in mind while writing a topic for a thesis/original article.

- It should be short and to the point (without it becoming too short).
- It should be specific and relevant to what is being studied.
- It should be informative and easy to grasp by others.
- Abbreviations should be avoided (except very common ones like HIV).
- Avoid dramatizing the title (Example, Steroids: Boon or bane in inflammatory disorders).
- Name of the institution and number of cases studies should not be mentioned (one may write "Tertiary Care Hospital").
- The hypothesis may be included but it should not be vague.

Q. How to write an introduction to a synopsis/thesis?

It should be short, about 1–2 pages. The main purpose is to bring out the need and importance of the study which is being performed. The following points must be included:

- It should begin by summarizing the current knowledge already present regarding the topic.
- Next, the shortfalls or gaps of the studies must be emphasized and their relevance in the clinical scenario.
- Specific reason for choosing the topic.
- How the study aims to address them should be mentioned.
- Finally, the hypothesis and the study design to test the hypothesis should be presented.
- Only 2–3 references may be used in the introduction part.
- It should be written in the present tense.

Q. What is hypothesis?

Hypothesis is a logic or idea based on which the investigator conducts the study. It is a proposition made as a basis of reasoning. Hypothesis is usually a conjecture, a guess or a supposition which a researcher uses to explain his observations.

Aims and Objectives

The study should have few (about 2–3) objectives. They can be divided into primary and secondary objectives.

The primary objective deals with proving the hypothesis while the secondary objective refers to those assumptions which could be made along the course of the study. Every effort should be made to achieve them.

Review of Literature

Before the beginning of the study, it is expected to review all available literature on the topic and to update it as your study progresses. Review of literature is written with all the existing researches about the topic with plenty of references and cross references. All the cited references are written in the reference according to standard style.

Components of Materials and Methods

This segment contains details of the processes used in completing the study. It should be discussed under the following headings:

1. Type of study (Cohort, case-control, cross-sectional, etc.)
2. Design of study (Experimental or observational)
3. Place of study (Hospital, institution or district, etc.)
4. Inclusion and exclusion criteria of the study subjects
5. Sourcing of the study subjects (from where the study and control populations were obtained).
6. Dropouts from the study and the reasons thereof (including the criteria for compliance).
7. Sample size calculation.
8. Power of the study.
9. Details of interventions carried out (if any).
10. Criteria for assessing the effectiveness of interventions (must include baseline criteria, well-defined endpoints and complications if any).
11. Details during follow up of the patients.
12. Statistical tools employed.
13. Ethics committee approval.
14. Clinical trial registration number.

Sample Size and Calculation of Sample Size

To make the study significant adequate sample size is essential. Hence, calculation of sample size is an integral part of the research work though the need for the sample size estimation in carrying out a study is not beyond debate.

Some important considerations in determination of sample size are the variable and parameter (like mean, proportion, correlation coefficient, sensitivity, specificity, etc.) of interest, minimum degree of precision, minimum clinically important difference, type of research, and power of the study and confidence level. With conventional 95% confidence level, the sample finding-based confidence interval has a probability of 0.95 that it would contain the actual population parameter. The statistical power of the test is an important consideration when the researcher does not want to miss a specified difference.

Sources of different parameter values (like mean, proportion, correlation coefficient, sensitivity, specificity, etc.) can be authentic previous research works or pilot studies.

Depending on those considerations different sample size calculation formulae are used to get the sample size, and softwares are utilized frequently for sample size determination. Softwares commonly used are *SPSS, Medcalc, Strata, and Graphpad priston.*

Results and Analysis

This refers to the findings of the study. It should only contain the facts obtained without going into any discussion or interpretations of the findings.

This can be done by pictorial representation of the data in the form of Tables, Bar diagrams, Pie charts, etc., with the help of softwares as and when required.

Results are given in chronological order. This segment should be written in the past tense. *P* value is calculated to evaluate if study is statistically significant or not. A *P* value of less than 5% or less than 0.05 is considered to be statistically significant. The *P* value reflects the alpha-error.

Discussion

The most important part this segment deals with interpretation of the results and their implications in improving current practice.

It should include a brief recapitulation of the important findings, review of the studies that agree and studies that disagree with the results obtained, and an explanation of the merits and appropriateness of the study design.

The extent to which the objectives of the study are met and how well the research query or hypothesis has been answered should also be discussed here.

Limitation

No study is perfect and this segment should include all the major shortcomings of your study (like inadequate sample size, too short study period, population that could not be included, dropouts, bias, etc.).

Summary and Conclusion

The essence of the entire research paper is a brief, systematic, and clear representations of the findings of the research study along with their significance presented in a point-wise manner. The extent to which the aim of the studies was fulfilled must be emphasized here.

Q. How to write references? What are different styles?

References

There are mainly two types of style for writing the references.

Harvard Style

In the text, references are given in brackets containing author's name and year of publication. In the reference list, they are listed in alphabetical order of the surname of the first author. It is author friendly as the names get prominence.

Flowchart 1: Basic research studies.

```
                    Study design
                   /            \
           Analytical study    Descriptive study
           /        \          (case report and case series)
  Experimental    Observational study
  study              |
  (clinical trials)  ├── Cohort study
                     ├── Case-control study
                     └── Cross-sectional study
```

Vancouver Style

In the text, references are given in brackets containing only a digit in ascending order. In the reference list, they are listed in the order in which they are cited in the text. It is more librarian friendly and easier to catalogue.

References are taken either from the original article, book or many other authentic sources. Specific format should be maintained and they should always be written only in the following format:

Article references: Authors; title of article; name of journal; year of publication; volume number; page number.

Example: Mondal PC, Ghosh D, Santra D, Majhi AK, Mondal A, Dasgupta S. Role of Hayman technique and its modification in recurrent puerperal uterine inversion; Journal of Obstetrics and Gynaecology Research. 2012;38;438-441.

Book references: Authors of the chapter; name of chapter; name of book with edition; place of publication; name of publication with year of printing; page number.

Example: Hay PE, Sharland M, Ugwumadu AHN. Infections in pregnancy; In: Chamberlain G, Steer PJ (Eds). Turnbul's Obstetrics 3rd edn; London; Churchill Livingstone; 2001;356-81.

TYPES OF STUDY

Q. What are the different types of study?

Types of research study may be of different varieties. Strength of the study depends on the type of study chosen. Selecting the type of study depends on the purpose of study and which answers the investigator want to get. However, all types of study may not be applicable to each study.

Basically studies are of two types:
1. Analytical study
2. Descriptive study

Analytical studies are experimental studies (clinical trials) and observational studies (Cohort study, case-control study and cross-sectional study). Descriptive studies include case reports and case series.

In observational study, there is no intervention or exposure, but in experimental study (clinical trials), there will be intervention. Descriptive studies may provide useful information for doing future analytical studies. The **Flowchart 1** shows the basic type of studies.

CLINICAL TRIALS

Q. Clinical trials.

Clinical trials are subtype of clinical research where intervention is done after human participants are assigned prospectively.

Phases of clinical trials

The investigational drugs or therapy are evaluated in phases by clinical trials which start with small trials to assess the safety (phase 1) and tested phase wise the efficacy, and side effects successively in large scale studies. There are four phases of clinical trials given in **Table 1**.

RANDOMIZED CONTROL TRIAL (RCT)

Q. Which type of study is considered the gold standard in clinical trials?

Randomized Control Trial (RCT).

Q. What do you mean by RCT?

RCTs are subset of clinical trials that use a controlled experimental design for the assessment the effectiveness of an intervention of an outcome. The study population is "randomly" allotted into two groups, one of which, known as the "Study group" (treatment/intervention group), is designated to receive a new drug or intervention, and the other group, known as the "Control group", receives either a placebo or the old/established drug or intervention. Then the outcomes of the two groups are compared after an appropriate time period has elapsed. Example: People suffering from rheumatoid arthritis is taken, and divided into two groups, one receiving nonsteroidal anti-inflammatory drugs and the other disease-modifying antirheumatic

Table 1: Phases of clinical trials.

Phase	Aim of the trial	Average number of participants
Phase 1	Evaluation of the safety of treatment to determine the range of safe dose. Data regarding dose, pattern of intake of drug and responds of participants in terms of effects and side effects are collected	20–100 healthy volunteers or people with disease or condition
Phase 2	Evaluation of treatment efficacy and further evaluation of safety and tolerability	Several hundred people with the disease or condition are included
Phase 3	Definite determination of the efficacy of treatment for the intended population, comparison with other available treatments, to note the adverse events and side effects if any	30–3,000 participants are involved mostly with randomized clinical trials
Phase 4	This phase is conducted after the therapy is approved by the FDA. Evaluation is done for uncommon serious adverse effects and side effects, optimal use to identify the subgroups that may benefit from the treatment under trial. This phase is important particularly for rare adverse events when the therapy is given in larger populations	Large trials or observation studies, involving thousands of participants

drugs and their quality of life is assessed after 10 years. The randomized controlled double-blinded clinical trial design minimizes bias and minimizes the influence of confounders. Not all studies are designed with blinding but the procedure used in the trial to minimize bias from nonblinding should be explained.

Q. How to define Cohort study, case–control study, and cross-sectional study?

Cohort study: It is a "prospective" or "forward looking" study in which a definite population is followed from exposure (to a drug/risk factor/protective factor) for a predecided time up to their clinical outcome. Strength of cohort studies include the ability to get attributable and relative risks the outcome is compared in two groups. Truly prospective cohort studies may be expensive and may take longer time for completion.

Example: A group of alcoholic and another non-alcoholic group are taken and after 20 years the development of cirrhosis of liver is compared between the two groups.

Case–control study: It is a "retrospective" or "backward looking" study in which a definite population with the required outcome/effect is first selected and then their history is traced backwards to identify the cause (exposure). Case–control studies are lower in cost and easier to conduct than other analytic studies. The disadvantage is that they may be prone to selection bias and recall bias.

Example: People suffering from acute pancreatitis are taken and risk factors to which they may have been exposed to in last 10 years are studied thoroughly, whether alcohol induced, gallstone induced or due to other causes.

Cross-sectional study: It is a "concurrent" or "snap-shot" study in which both exposure and outcome are determined by studying the population at a specific time, i.e., there is no follow up. Cross-sectional studies are also called prevalence studies as the disease exists at the time of study. Prevalence (PR) is the number of cases present at a specific point of time. During interpretation of a cross-sectional study one must be very careful that causality cannot be established as there is no temporal relationship between the exposure and the outcome.

Example: The percentage of patients suffering from maculopathy after taking chloroquine due to Malaria is studied during the rainy season.

Q. Randomized control trial is a comparative study and Cohort, case–control, and cross-sectional study are also comparative study—what is the basic difference?

All four studies here are comparative studies which mean that in each of these studies, the "study group" with the "control" group is compared to arrive at a conclusion. However, RCT is an "experimental" study, i.e., one where an experiment is conducted by actively introducing a variable (in the form of an intervention or exposure) in the natural course of a disease to see how it modifies or changes it. In other three (Cohort, case–control, and cross-sectional study) are **"observational"** study where investigator acts as an observer only and compares the two groups and no new intervention or exposure is applied and there is no blinding or masking. Observational studies are analytical study that take advantage of "natural experiment" and the exposure is not assigned by the investigator.

Q. What is blinding? What are the different types?

Blinding or masking is the technique of not revealing which is the study group and which one is the control group. It is necessary to prevent Bias, which may arise at different levels. There are three types of blinding.

1. *Single-blind study:* The patient does not know to which group he belongs to.
2. *Double-blind study:* Both the patient and the investigator does not know the identity of the two groups.
3. *Triple-blind study:* The patient, investigator, and statistician all three are unaware of the identities of the two groups.

Q. Case report and case series.

In a case report, an unusual clinical scenario or a procedure undertaken in a single patient is described whereas in case series larger group of patients with similar exposures or outcomes are included. Hypothesis about exposures and disease which is developed from descriptive studies can be explored in analytical study.

SECTION 8: Miscellaneous

Q. Strength of study.

Every study has an inherent strength and weakness. Study's overall quality of evidence is determined by the quality of methods of the individual study and its scientific validity. Scientific validity of a study is assessed by the study question, how the study was designed whether bias, chance and confounding factors were taken into consideration.

Q. Which study has the greatest strength?

Triple-blind study has the greatest strength as it reduces the maximum number of Bias.

Q. Define meta-analysis, systematic review, and multicenter study.

Meta-analysis: It is a statistical analysis in which the results of a number of published studies dealing with the same research hypothesis are plotted together to bring out the ultimate and final result or statistic.

Systematic review: It is a concise form of literature in which all important research evidence pertaining to a single research question are studied and examined thoroughly to arrive at a conclusion. It may/may not include a statistical component unlike meta-analysis which always has a statistical component.

Multicenter study: It basically refers to a research study which is being conducted in many centers simultaneously while following a single protocol. It becomes important in studies involving a rare condition or a large sample size which cannot be obtained from only a single center in the given time period.

Q. Which is the best example of systematic review?

The best example of a systematic review is the Cochrane Collaboration.

Q. What do you mean by Cochrane?

The Cochrane Collaboration is an international organization which compares the results from different RCTs dealing with the same research question and presents it in the form of a systematic review.

The pioneer of this idea was Professor Archibald Lemon Cochrane (1909–1988). Cochrane first (1972) published an article on *Evidence-based medicine* which introduced the concept that healthcare should be evaluated based on scientific evidence rather than clinical opinion.

CONSORT

Q. What do you mean by CONSORT?

CONSORT is an abbreviation of Consolidated Standards of Reporting Trials. CONSORT is an evidenced-based, minimum set of recommendations for reporting on RCT. It was developed by CONSORT group to remove the problems due to inadequate reporting of RCT. There are 25 items in the CONSORT check list under seven broad sections, namely—title and abstract, introduction, methods, results, section/topic, discussions and other information. CONSORT group also developed a flow diagram **(Flowchart 2)** consisting of enrollment, allocation, follow up and analysis. The CONSORT flow diagram and check list provide a standard way to prepare reports of trial findings, with complete and transparent reporting and interpretation.

Q. Define sensitivity, specificity, PPV, and NPV.

Sensitivity: It is a measure of the proportion of people with the disease that are correctly identified by the test as actually having the disease. It reflects the true positives. *Example:* The sensitivity of CB-NAAT (cartridge-based nucleic acid

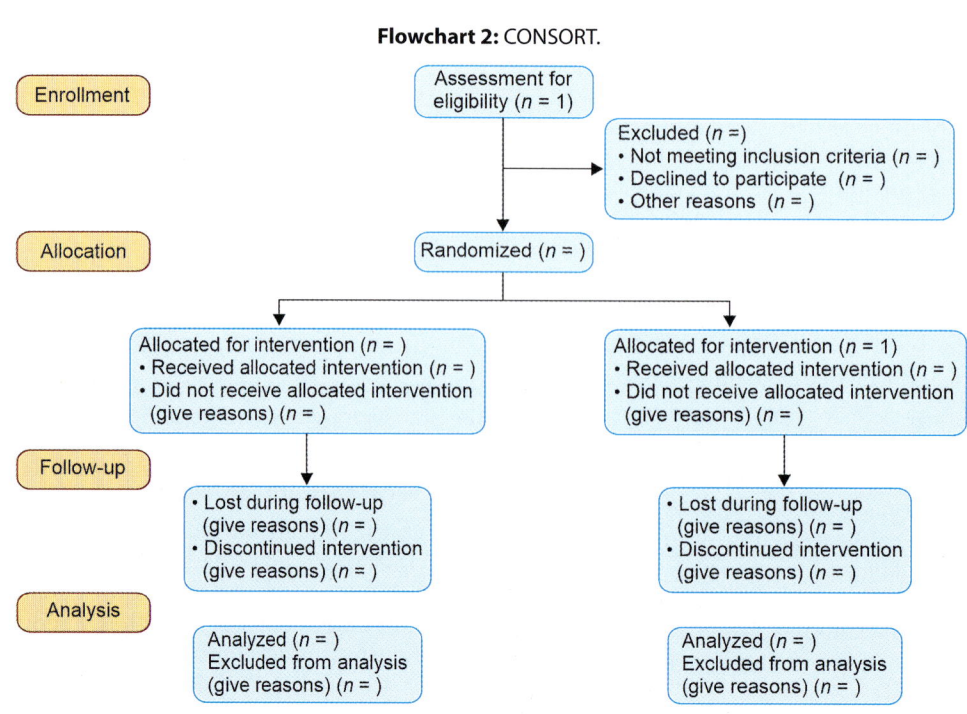

Flowchart 2: CONSORT.

amplification test) for TB is 81% means that this test can identify 81 out of 100 TB patients.

Specificity: It is a measure of the proportion of the healthy people that are correctly identified by the test as NOT having the disease. It reflects the true negatives. *Example:* The specificity of CB-NAAT is 99% means that this test can identify 99 out of 100 people not infected with TB.

PPV: It stands for Positive Predictive Value. It is the probability that the disease is present when the test turns out to be positive. *Example:* The PPV of CB-NAAT is 94 means that if this test turns out to be positive, there is a 94% chance that the subject has TB.

NPV: It stands for Negative Predictive Value. It is the probability that the disease is absent when the test turns out to be negative. *Example:* The NPV of CB-NAAT is 95 means that if this test turns out to be negative, there is a 95% chance that the patient does not have TB.

Q. What do you mean by Mean, Median, and Mode?

Mean: It is the average, calculated by adding up all the observations and dividing by the total number of observations. *Example:* Mean of 5, 7, 2, 8, 3 is 25/5 = 5.

Median: It is the central value which is obtained after arranging all the observations in either ascending or descending order. It reflects the 50th percentile of the distribution. *Example:* Median of 5, 7, 2, 8, 3, 10, 14 is 7 (central value after arranging observations in ascending order—2, 3, 5, 7, 8, 10, 14).

Mode: It is the most commonly occurring value in the list of observations. *Example:* Mode of 2, 4, 5, 6, 4, 4, 6, 4 is 4).

Q. What is *P* value?

Here, the *P* stands for probability. Probability that the result was obtained merely by random accident or chance. Lesser the *P* value, lesser is the chance that the result is obtained by fluke. Larger the *P* value, lesser is the importance or significance of the study. A *P* value of less than 5% or less than 0.05 is considered to be statistically significant. The *P* value reflects the alpha-error.

Q. What is CI, OR, and RR?

CI: It stands for Confidence Interval. It provides an estimated range of values which falls within the confidence limits and can be obtained from the observations of the study. Example: 95% CI with confidence intervals of 40 and 60 means that one can be 95% confident that the mean of the population falls within these values.

OR: It stands for Odds Ratio. It is the ratio of the odds of developing a disease in an exposed group to the odds of developing the disease in the non-exposed group. It is a measure of association between exposure and outcome.
- OR = 1—Exposure does not affect odds of outcome
- OR >1—Exposure associated with higher odds of outcome
- OR <1—Exposure associated with lower odds of outcome.

RR: It stands for Risk Ratio or Relative Risk. It is a measure of the increase in risk of an adverse outcome when exposed to a risk factor compared to when not exposed to the same risk factor.

Example: The RR of smoking with chronic obstructive pulmonary disease (COPD) is 10 means that smokers are 10 times more likely to develop COPD than nonsmokers. It is mainly used in Cohort studies.

LEVELS OF EVIDENCE

Q. How will you categorize different levels of evidence? Based on the levels of evidence, how recommendations are given?

Levels of evidence: Level I, Level II-1, Level II-2, Level II-3, and Level III.

Recommendations: A, B, C, D, and I.

The categories of level of evidence and classification of recommendation are given in **Table 1**.

Table 1: Categories of level of evidence and classification of recommendation.

Quality of evidence assessment	Classification of recommendations
I-1: Evidence obtained from at least one properly randomized controlled trial	A. There is good evidence to recommend the clinical preventive action
II-1: Evidence from well-designed controlled trials without randomization	B. There is fair evidence to recommend the clinical preventive action
II-2: Evidence from well-designed cohort (prospective or retrospective) or case-control studies, preferably from more than one center or research group	C. The existing evidence is conflicting and does not allow to make a recommendation for or against use of the clinical preventive action; however, other factors may influence decision-making
II-3: Evidence obtained from comparisons between times or places with/without the intervention	D. There is fair evidence to recommend against the clinical preventive action E. There is good evidence to recommend against the clinical preventive action
III: Opinions of respected authorities, based on clinical experience, descriptive studies, or reports of expert committees	F. There is insufficient evidence (in quantity or quality or quality) to make a recommendation; however, other factors may influence decision-making

CLINICAL TRIALS REGISTRY–INDIA

Q. What do you mean by CTRI?

CTRI means Clinical Trials Registry-India. Registration of clinical trials in the Clinical Trials Registry-India (CTRI) is now mandatory, as per notification of the Drugs Controller General, India (DCGI) with effect from 15th June 2009.

International Committee of Medical Journal Editors (ICMJE) member journals require submission of the trial registration number prior to consideration of clinical trial data for publication.

CHAPTER 31

Examination of a Rape Victim: Procedures and Protocols

Chapter Outline

This is a burning topic about which everyone should have idea. The topic is written by forensic expert so that reader can gather knowledge about the subject and be able to tackle the situation methodically.

"Doctor is a man of science, he has no victim to avenge, no guilty person to convict and no person to save."

RAPE AND FUNCTION OF A DOCTOR

- Rape is not a medical diagnosis, it is a legal definition only.
- Doctor has no duty to explain or interpret legal Act but he has a duty to help law court in trial of a criminal case by providing scientific medical evidences and opinion bases on medical findings.

Q. Who can do medical examination?

Any registered medical practitioner (RMP) (MBBS), preferably a Government doctor, can examine an adult female victim.

In case the victim is a girl child, the medical examination shall be conducted by a woman doctor. "Child" means any person below the age of eighteen years; the Protection of Children from Sexual Offences (POCSO) Act, 2012.

Q. What are the two important legal guidelines on rape for medical examination of victims or survivor of sexual offense cases?

- Two most important guidelines are: (1) POCSO Act and (2) 164A Code of Criminal Procedure (CrPC).
- One has to work within a framework of legal guidance and medical jurisprudence.

PURPOSE OF MEDICAL EXAMINATION IN FEMALE RAPE VICTIM

Medical examination is done for confirmation of allegation with an objective to:
- Establish the use of force
- Establish the link between victim and the assailant
- Establish a link of the victim with the scene of crime
- Establish the identity of the assailant.

Findings should be recorded and samples collected in such a manner that objectives of medical examination are achieved.

PREREQUISITES FOR EXAMINATION OF VICTIM

- Female attendant
- Valid consent.

Female Attendant

One female attendant is always necessary during examination and she will act as assistant and witness. In case of adult female victim, any disinterested third female can be attendant. In POCSO Act attendant is to be either mother or any female upon which the victim has faith and confidence or any woman deputed by the head of hospital/institution.

Valid Consent

- Valid written informed consent is the single most important preliminary requirement for medical examination of a female victim.
- Mentally sound female of 12 years and above can give valid consent.
- Girl below 12 years or mentally retarded female of any age cannot give valid consent. In this case, consent is given by legal guardian.
- Consent is best if written by the female herself, otherwise written by the legal guardian or a disinterested third party female attendant but never by police personnel.
- In case of an adult female with a suspicion of mental abnormality, doctor should take second signature or finger print of the guardian on the consent paper. Authorize expert trained person/interpreter is required to record consent and history in case of deaf and dumb patient and when victim female does not understand language of any person in medical team or guardian.

Consent must be clear on three components as given in the sample here:

Sample informed consent:

- I, Miss X, 12 years of age. D/O Smt Y, giving my consent for medical examination of my whole body including private parts.
- I also agree to collect necessary samples for medicolegal examination.
- I do give my consent to repot my case to police.
- I have put my signature/finger print after having understood all the above written words which are explained to me in the language I understand.

Female may agree in first part but may refuse in second part and or third part. Whatever may be the situation doctor must take written refusal and do accordingly.

EXAMINATION AND NOTE OF FINDINGS

Only after valid informed consent further examination is done:

- *Identification marks*: Two ID marks must be taken preferably from exposed parts. Marks must be permanent in nature like congenital mark or deformity (mole birth mark), scar mark, permanent tattoo noting their shape, size and external anatomical position in relation to bony landmark or body midline (anterior or posterior). Preferably, two measurements in 'X' and 'Y' axis are taken to fix the point.
- *History by the subject*: It is very important. It decides the planning of examination, collection of samples.

Subject should voluntarily give as far as practicable an exact account of the alleged crime in her own statement mentioning time, place, position, number of assaulter, any struggle, use of force, drugs, condom any discharge and bleeding, etc. Even a girl child of 5 years should be allowed to give her own statement not dictated or assisted even by guardian but doctor can assist her to explain some act or event in her language as per the level of intelligence.

- *Physical examination*: Extragenital body parts and genital examination separately noting any injury, discharge, bleeding, stains, etc., keeping in mind the history.

Injury must be mentioned as required to be mentioned in the injury report, i.e., nature, shape, size, position, vital reaction, etc.

Examples: (1) Linear scratch abrasion 2 cm long almost parallel 1 cm apart vertically placed on the upper surface of left breast, red scabbed; (2) one bruise 2×1 cm on the right lateral vaginal wall from introitus downward, deep red in color; (3) tear of hymen at 6 and 11 o'clock position, red inflamed margin.

Injury pattern on body and/or private parts of female depends upon:
1. Disproportionate size of male genital organs
2. Lack of sexual desire and cooperation in sex act
3. Deflorated/parous
4. Struggle and resistance
5. Use of any kind of vaginal lubricant, cream, gelly etc.

Injury in private parts is common and severe in child virgin girl whereas injury in private parts is nil/minimum in parous woman/deflorate woman. In case of rape, extragenital body injury in adult woman is more extensive unless incapacitated or unconscious.

- *Sample collection*: The samples which are collected are:
1. Wearing apparel which was worn during the crime
2. Swab from suspected blood, semen, salivary stain, etc.
3. Urine or blood in case of intoxication
4. Vulvovaginal swab and smear (mandatory in all cases where crime was likely to have committed within 96 hours from examination). Swab and smear is air dried not heat or sun dried.
5. Any foreign body—hair, thread, button, condom, and tampon, etc.
6. Blood of the victim is not routinely collected but is collected on request of police or direction of court for DNA test following all protocols as laid down by CFSL.

Handover of Samples and Report of Medical Examination

All samples must be sealed, labeled with direction for particular examination and handed over to concerned police personal along with the report of medical examination. No sample or material be handed over to police without seal and label.

Health Advice by Doctor to the Victim

After examination and report preparation, doctor should give necessary advice for:

- Prevention of pregnancy
- If pregnant, advice medical termination of pregnancy (MTP) with preservation of abortus whole in (−20°C)

for forensic DNA profiling. In cases of live birth, chord blood is collected soaked in few layers of sterile cotton gauge pieces and air dried followed by packing in dry uncontaminated clean paper envelope followed by signing, sealing and labeling.
- Prevention of sexually transmitted disease (STD)
- Psychological counseling.

Some Practical Problems

- The victim giving consent for examination and treatment but not for reporting to police.
- Apparently minor female come alone for examination and examination suggestive of injuries due to sexual intercourse but refused to give consent for information to police.
- A 11-year girl complaining of sexual assault but mother refused to give consent for medical examination or to report to police.
- Consent obtained from mother but girl refused and resisting examination or examination of private parts.

Q. What are the duties of a doctor in those problems?

Doctor must not refuse examination if they are legally eligible to do the examination. First examination is very vital and records of injury and sample collection must be done in first examination. Doctor requires to collect swab and smear even after 96 hours of alleged crime to prove STD.

Doctor must not examine a female victim forcefully even after valid consent. Doctor must stop at the point of resistance and record findings up to that point with a note of reason for stopping the examination.

All refusal must be taken in writing and all injuries must be very accurately recorded. If any samples collected in injured victim girl of under 12-year-old girl must be kept confidentially under the hospital authorities custody or in her own custody in case of private practitioner. All those materials must be preserved till it is demanded by Court or police authority, but how long to be preserved is not clearly known.

Q. How opinion/answer to be given to the queries made by police?

- There are evidences of sexual intercourse in the past/recently.
- There are evidences of penetration by things other than penile penetration recently.
- There are injuries on the extragenital body parts and/or private parts as noted.
- No clinical evidences of STD could be detected.
- Final opinion on recent sexual intercourse or STD will be given after receipt of forensic science laboratory reports.

Doctor should never make direct opinion on rape in spite of the fact that police queries directly on frequent occasion. 'Rape is a legal definition, not a medical opinion'.

They should make opinion on violent forceful sexual intercourse/any object penetration.

Doctor should keep this in mind that any pattern or distribution of injury may be found in consensual sexual intercourse also.

ACKNOWLEDGMENTS

This chapter is contributed by:

Professor Sobhan Kumar Das, Head, Department of Forensic Medicine and Toxicology, Santiniketan Medical College, Bolpur, Birbhum, West Bengal, Former Head, Department of Forensic Medicine and Toxicology, RG Kar Medical College, Kolkata, India. (email—*dasdrsobhank@gmail.com*)

CHAPTER 32

Swellings of Vulva: Bartholin's Cyst and Abscess

CHAPTER OUTLINE

- Classification of Swellings of Vulva with Few Illustrations
- Vulvar Lesions have been Illustrated Elaborately in Chapter 1
- Bartholin Cyst and Abscess with Management and Surgical Details

INTRODUCTION

Vulva refers to the female external genitalia which lies on the pubic bones and extends posteriorly. Structures of vulva include mons pubis, labia majora, labia minora, clitoris, urethra, fourchette, vaginal introitus, vestibular bulb, vestibule, Bartholin's gland, anus and gynecological perineum. Due to the presence of various structures of versatile nature tissues, the lesions and pathology are of variable natures.

The lesions of vulva have already been described in Chapter 1 (Gynecological Examinations) with lot of illustrations from Page 21 to 23. In this chapter, the different swellings of vulva are listed with few illustrations.

CLASSIFICATIONS OF SWELLINGS

- **Neoplastic:**
  - *Benign:* Lipoma **(Fig. 1)**, fibroma **(Fig. 2)**, neurofibroma, papilloma, angioma, hemangioma.
  - *Malignant:* Vulvar carcinoma (squamous cell carcinoma, malignant melanoma), sarcoma, metastatic tumor, lymph node metastasis
- **Infective:** Vulvar warts [condyloma acuminata by human papilloma virus (HPV)] **(Fig. 3)**, syphilitic condyloma (by *Treponema pallidum*), furuncle, acute vulvitis, tuberculosis
- **Traumatic:** Vulvar hematoma
- **Developmental:** Clitoromegaly, hypertrophy of labia minora, phimosis, accessory nipple
- **Structural displacement through introitus:** Pelvic organ prolapse, uterine inversion, cervical uterine polyp, elongation and hypertrophy of cervix
- **Endometriosis**
- **Cystic:** Sebaceous cyst, Gartner's duct cyst, epidermoid cyst **(Figs. 4A and B)**, clitoridal cyst, swelling of Bartholin's

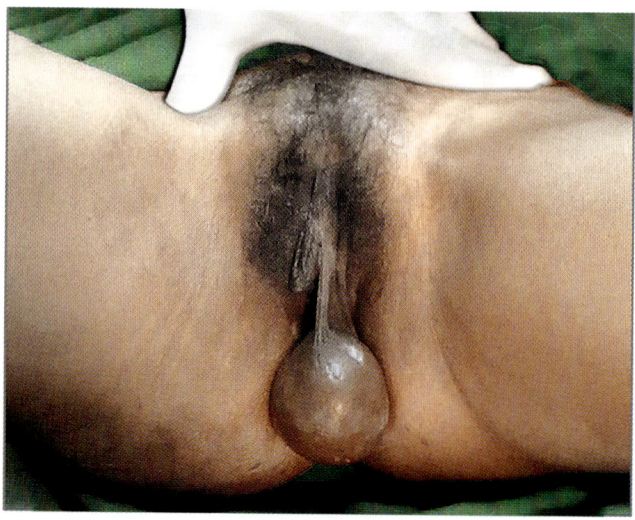

Fig. 1: Lipoma.
Courtesy: Dr Anirban Mandal

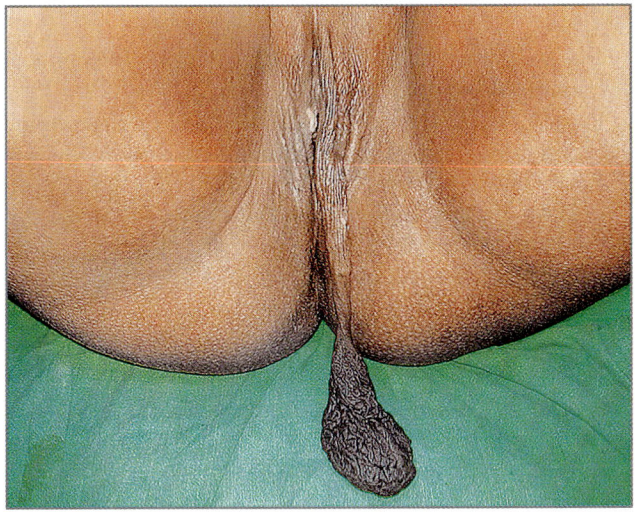

Fig. 2: Fibroma.

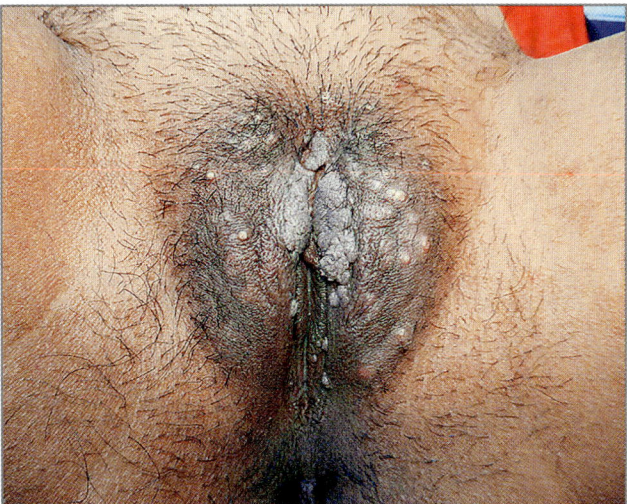

Fig. 3: Vulvar warts in pregnancy.

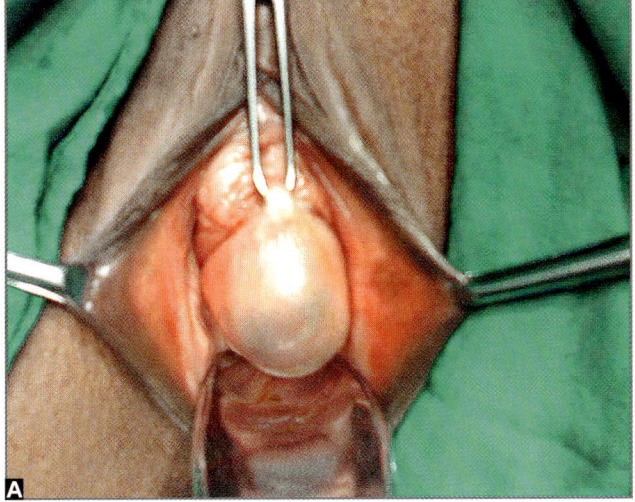
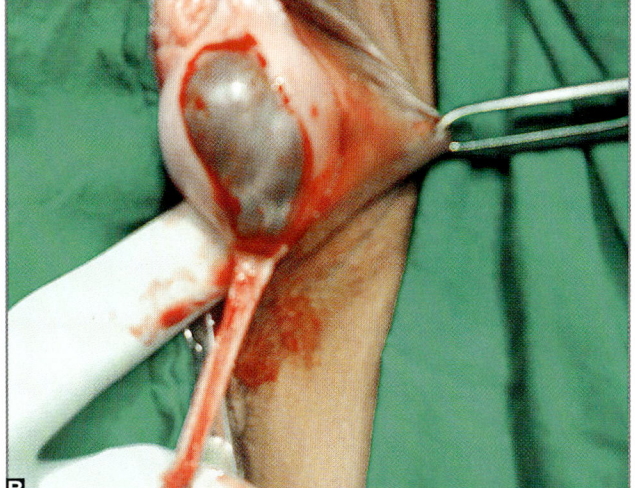

Figs. 4A and B: A 38-year-old woman with vaginal epidermal cyst.

gland—Bartholin's cyst **(Fig. 5)**, Bartholin's abscess **(Fig. 6)**, bartholinitis, Bartholin's adenoma, adenocarcinoma
- Urethra-related swelling: Urethral caruncle, urethral prolapse, diverticulum, carcinoma, swelling of Skene's tubule
- Vascular related: Hamartoma **(Fig. 7)**, vulvar varicosity, elephantiasis, vulvar edema (pregnancy, preeclampsia), postradiotherapy lymphedema
- Inguinal canal and femoral canal related: Inguinal and femoral hernia, hydrocele of canal of Nuck.

BARTHOLIN'S CYST AND ABSCESS

Anatomy of Bartholin's Gland
- Bartholin's glands are bilateral pea-sized oval glands one on each side situated on posterior one-third of labia majus deep to bulbospongiosus muscle and connected to

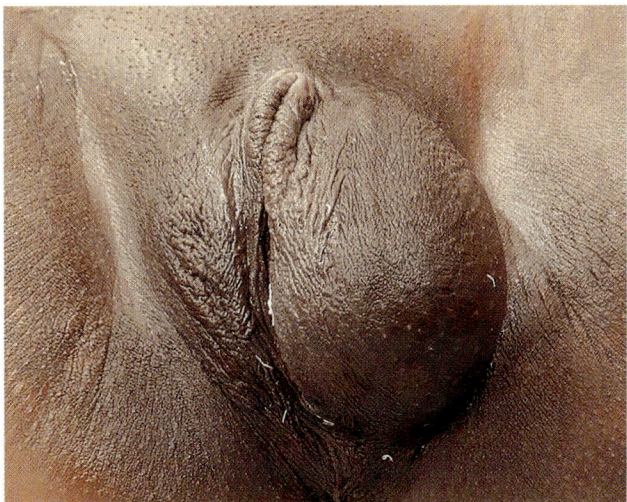

Fig. 5: Bartholin's cyst.

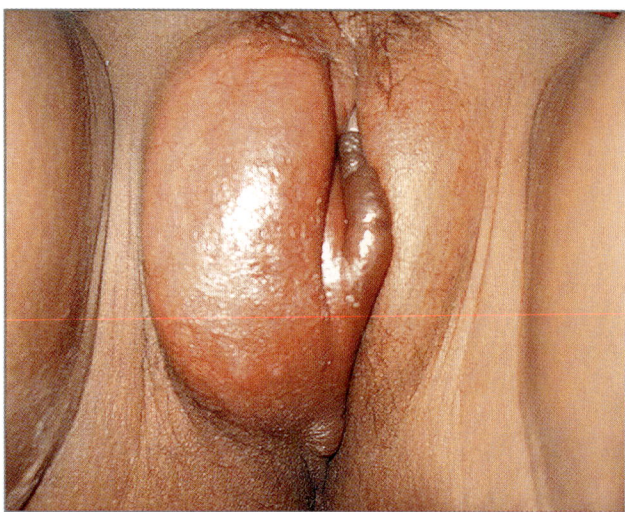

Fig. 6: Bartholin's abscess.

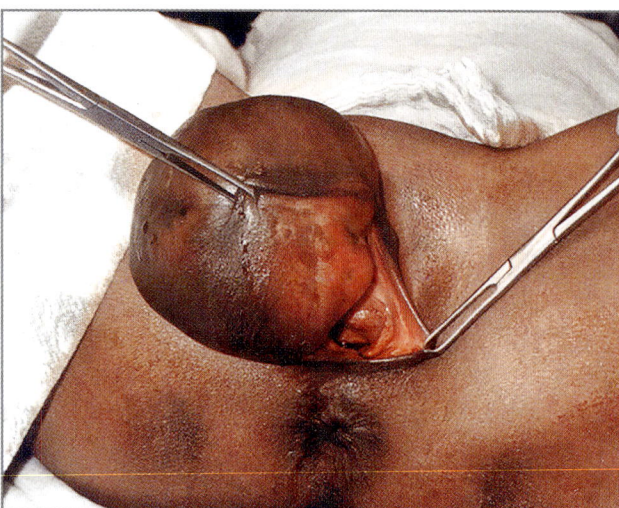

Fig. 7: Hamartoma of vulva (36 years of age)—painless swelling—excision done.
Courtesy: Professor Debashis Bhattacharyya, Director of Medical Education, West Bengal

Etiology

* Due to obstruction of Bartholin's duct by infection or trauma, rarely congenital.
* In many cases, no cause is explored and more common in sexually active woman. Organisms responsible are *Escherichia coli* (most common). Others are Gram-positive and Gram-negative. Previously *gonococcus* was thought to be the most common organism.
* Sudden division or ligation during operation or episiotomy usually is not followed by cyst formation.

Presentation

* *Symptoms:* Mostly asymptomatic. In large woman becomes aware of the swelling, difficulty in walking and sometimes difficulty in coitus.
* *Signs:* A tense swelling situated in posterior part of labia, looks shiny more common on right side. Due to projection inside the swelling looks S-shaped.

Complication

* Infection and Bartholin's abscess formation.

Treatment

* Excision—traditional treatment or
* Marsupialization—the function of the gland is preserved. In abscess formation, incision drainage or marsupialization is done.

Cyst Excision (Cystectomy) (Figs. 8 and 9)

* Done as outpatient procedure under general anesthesia.
* Lithotomy position, antiseptic dressing, draping.
* A sponge holding forceps with a gauze is placed inside the vagina medially and posterior to the cyst so that the cyst becomes prominent.
* A vertical incision is made over cyst wall on medial surface of labia minus and care is taken not to pierce the cyst wall.

vestibule with 2 cm duct to open in between the groove between the labia and hymen at 5 and 7 o'clock positions
* Glands contain columnar cells and secrete clear mucus having lubricating property by contraction of bulbospongiosus particularly at sexual stimulation.

Disorder of Bartholin's glands: Cyst and abscess are common problems. Adenoma and carcinoma are rare.

Bartholin's Cyst

* Bartholin's cyst is the most common cyst of vulva and *mostly cyst of the duct* due to dilatation of duct and cyst of gland is less common.
* Bartholin's duct cyst is usually of 5 cm, sometimes may be large occupying whole labia majus and minus, rarely bigger than hen's egg size.
* Content is mucoid fluid secretion of Bartholin's gland.

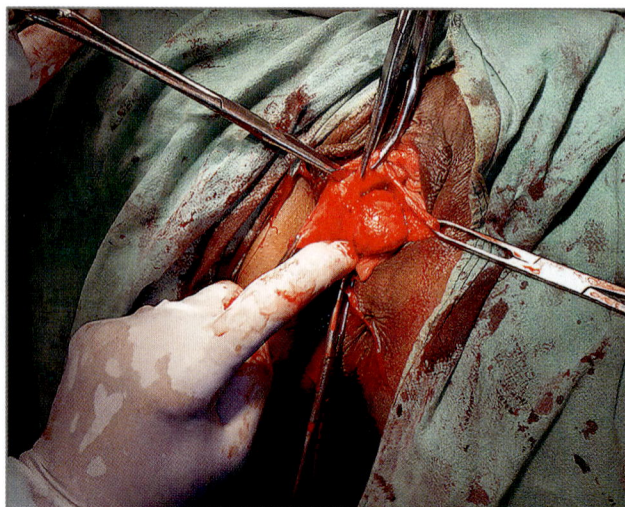

Fig. 8: Excision of Bartholin's cyst

CHAPTER 32: Swellings of Vulva: Bartholin's Cyst and Abscess

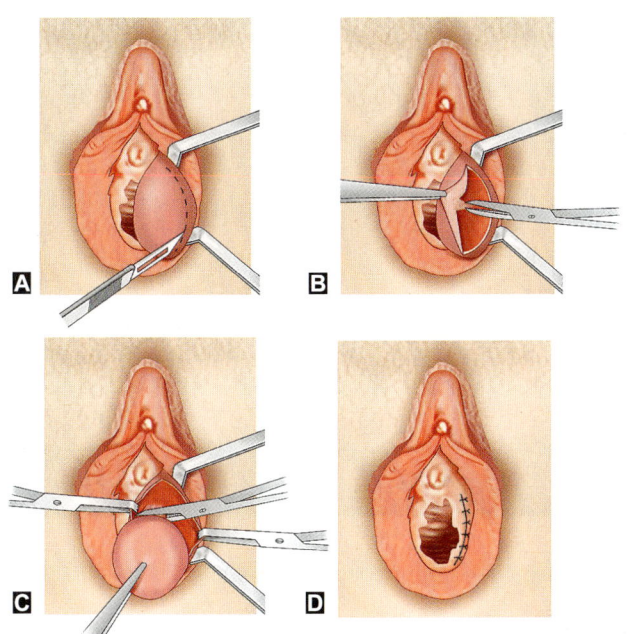

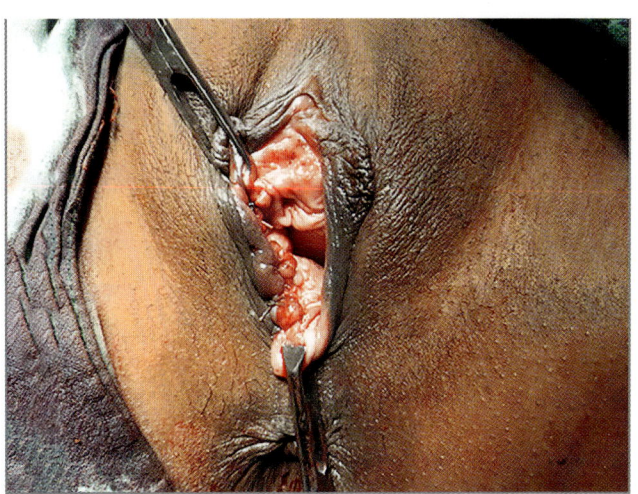

Fig. 10: Skin and mucous membrane repaired with closure of cavity.

Figs. 9A to D: Cyst excision: (A) Incision is given on skin; (B) Dissection done for enucleation; (C) Cyst enucleated; (D) After hemostasis of bed skin is repaired.

- By holding the skin margins with Allis tissue forceps, the cyst is enucleated gradually from the fibrofatty bed. The maximum blood vessels lie on superior aspect, so dissection is done first from below. And the pedicle with blood vessels is clamped, cut and ligated with 3-0 delayed or chromic suture **(Fig. 8)**. All bleeding vessels are secured and the bed is closed with running or interrupted 3-0 delayed absorbable suture, finally the skin is sutured with 3-0 delayed absorbable suture **(Fig. 10)**.
- The cyst wall is sent for histopathology.

Marsupialization (Figs. 11A to C)

- Under general anesthesia, one 2.5 cm vertical or elliptical incision is given across the skin overlying the cystic bulging outside and parallel to the hymen and incision is extended down to the normal opening of Bartholin's duct (5 or 7 o'clock depending on side).
- Another incision is given over cyst wall and its content mucus or pus is drained.
- The margin of the cyst wall is sutured with the skin margin with interrupted 2-0 or 3-0 delayed absorbable suture **(Fig. 12)**. Spontaneous drainage occurs.
- However, closure of the opening may occur and to prevent this, opening of the wound should be adequate. In recurrence, repeat marsupialization or excision is done.

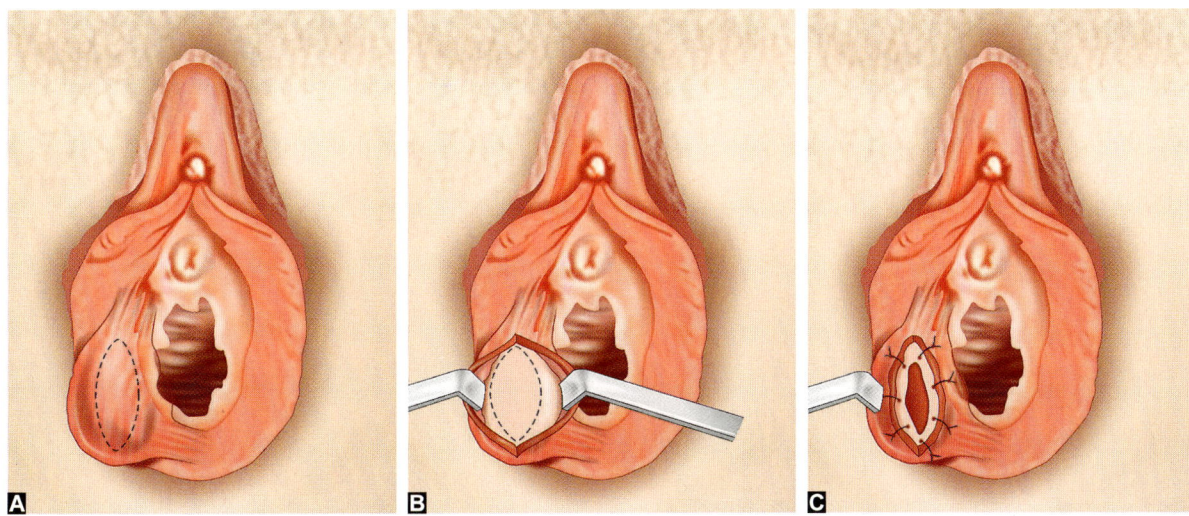

Figs. 11A to C: Marsupialization: (A) Skin incision given; (B) Incision given on the cyst wall; (C) After drainage of cyst content, margins of skin and cyst wall are stitched together with interrupted stitches (marsupialization done) keeping the mouth of the cyst open.

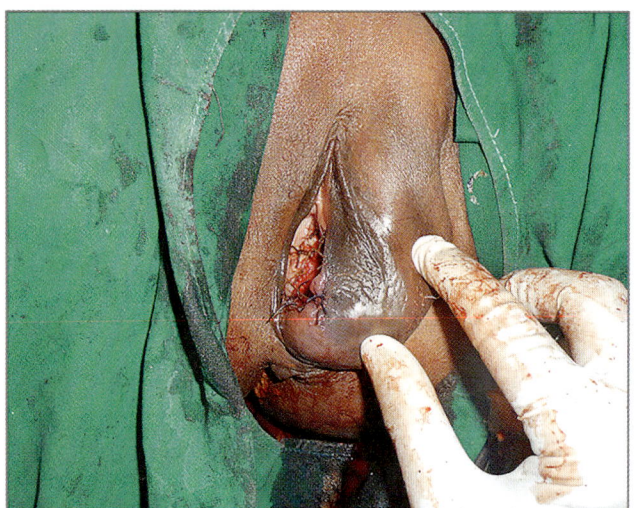

Fig. 12: Marsupialization—margins are repaired keeping the mouth open.

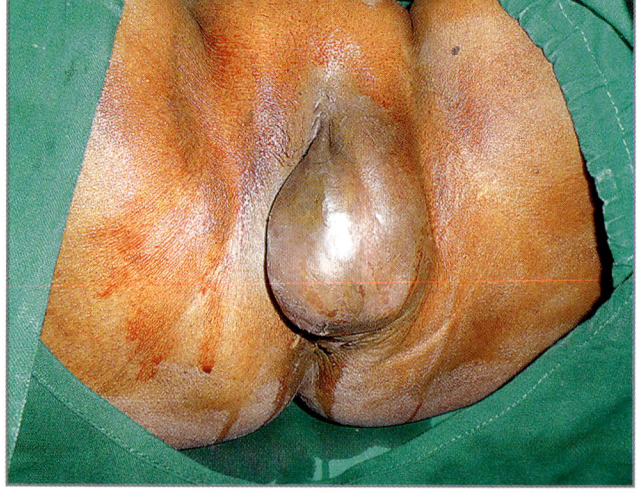

Fig. 13: Bartholin's abscess.

Incision and Drainage for Abscess Drainage

- Incision and drainage (I&D) is done with local lignocaine infiltration with mild systemic analgesia. 1 cm vertical incision is given over abscess up to the 5 or 7 o'clock position and pus is drained
- The cavity is swabbed with a small cotton swab on the tip of small artery forceps to break the loculi. Sometimes "Word catheter" or 14 Foley catheter is placed inside the cavity for few days.

Bartholin's Abscess (Fig. 13)

It is the collection of pus inside the Bartholin's gland resulting a tender and tense mass in labia.

Causative Organism

- The abscess usually occurs in sexual life and polymicrobial in nature, e.g., *E. coli, Staphylococcus, Streptococcus,* anaerobic streptococci and bacteroides. *Previously Gonococcus* was the leading organism.
- Following the blockage of duct by infection accumulation of secretion occurs which becomes infected and pus is formed.

Diagnosis

- Patient complains of swelling over vulva and severe pain, fever and difficulty in walking. The problem appears rapidly.
- The mass becomes tender, hot and fluctuant situated over posterior and medial to labia majus **(Fig. 13)**.

Treatment

Surgery is the treatment. Hot sitz bath may be given for temporary relief. Analgesic and antibiotic are administered.

Surgical options are:

- Incision and drainage as described above.
- *Marsupialization (see Fig. 12):* It is the treatment of choice, but difficult in acute condition, suitable for chronic or recurrent cases. As recurrence is common in I&D, it is preferred as well as gland function is preserved.
- *Excision:* It is done in recurrence or to exclude malignancy in elderly. Whole sac is excised and sent for biopsy. The bed is repaired as described above (*see* **Figs. 9 and 10**).

CHAPTER 33

Pelvic Inflammatory Disease, Sexually Transmitted Infections and Female Genital Tuberculosis

Chapter Outline

- Pelvic Inflammatory Disease—Types, Pathology, Organisms Involved, Clinical Features and Management of Acute PID and Chronic PID, and Syndromic Case Management (SCM)
- STIs—Causative Organisms, Clinical Manifestations and Management—Candidiasis, Trichomoniasis, Bacterial Vaginosis, Gonorrhea, Chlamydia, Lymphogranuloma Inguinale, Chancroid, Granuloma Inguinale, Condyloma Acuminata, Molluscum Contagiosum, Genital Herpes, and Syphilis
- Genital Tuberculosis—Etipathogenesis, Pathology, Sites, Diagnosis and Current Management

PELVIC INFLAMMATORY DISEASE (PID)

Q. How to define pelvic inflammatory disease (PID)?

Pelvic inflammatory disease is defined as infection of the upper genital tract which includes uterus, tubes, ovaries and adjacent pelvic structures not caused by surgery or due to pregnancy.

Q. What are the important features of pelvic inflammatory disease?

- Woman may be critically ill in acute PID—severe form is tubo-ovarian abscess formation and its rupture.
- Women suffer from infertility in long run due to damage of fallopian tube and formation of hydrosalpinx.
- Women become the victim of chronic pelvic pain and other symptoms
- Pelvic mass formation
- Morbidity and even mortality
- Sexual transmission occurs
- Preventable.

Types of Pelvic Inflammatory Disease

Acute PID and Chronic PID.

Natural Barrier of Pelvic Infections

- Acidic pH (4.5) of vaginal discharge is the most important defense due to presence of *Lactobacillus*.
- Cervical mucus and the ciliary movements of endometrium and cervical in opposite direction (descending) inhibit ascending infection.
- Intact hymen in virgin.

Q. How does the natural mechanism break?

- Menstruation: Blood changes the pH.
- Pregnancy related: Abortion, delivery
- Contraception: Intrauterine contraceptive device increases whereas barrier contraceptive and oral contraceptive pill prevents pelvic infection.
- Sexual transmission of disease
- Operative and vaginal procedure: Dilatation and curettage, hysterosalpingography (HSG), major gynecological surgeries.
- Appendicitis may involve pelvic organs
- Tuberculosis: Mostly blood borne from pulmonary tuberculosis.

Q. What are risk factors of PID?

- Women of young age

- Low socioeconomic status
- Multiple sex partners, previous sexually-transmitted infection
- Smoker
- Intrauterine contraceptive device insertion.

Q. What are the organisms responsible for PID?

- Sexually-transmitted disease (STD) organisms are commonest. Three-fourth cases are due to STDs—*Chlamydia* and *Gonococcus* infection are common. Chlamydial infection initially asymptomatic and silently damage the tube after harboring in genital tract especially in cervix.
- Mostly polymicrobial in nature.

The organisms are:
- *Aerobic*
    - STDs—*Neisseria gonorrhoeae, Chlamydia trachomatis, Mycoplasma hominis, Ureaplasma urealyticum, Gardnerella vaginalis*
    - Pyogenic: Staphylococci, streptococci, *Escherichia coli*
    - *Mycobacterium tuberculosis*
- *Anaerobic:* Bacteroides, Peptostreptococcus, Clostridia, Actinomycosis.

Pathology of Acute Pelvic Inflammatory Disease

- Fallopian tube and ovary–acute salpingitis, pyosalpinx looking retort shaped and may form a tubo-ovarian abscess.
- Endometritis
- Pelvic abscess
- General peritonitis.

Q. What is Fitz-Hugh-Curtis syndrome?

It is the inflammation of liver capsule caused by gonococcal and chlamydial infection manifested by pain and tenderness of right upper abdomen simulating cholecystitis.

Stages of Pelvic Inflammatory Disease

Depending upon the severity, PID may be staged from stage 1 to stage 5.

Pathology of Chronic Pelvic Inflammatory Disease

It is the sequel of acute PID after inadequate or no treatment. The changes of organs are:
- Hydrosalpinx
- Chronic interstitial salpingitis
- Formation of tubo-ovarian mass (TO mass)
- Pelvic adhesions.

Clinical Features of Acute Pelvic Inflammatory Disease

There may be silent infection. However, acute manifestations are as follows:

Symptoms
- Pain in lower abdomen on both sides
- Pain in upper right abdomen
- Vaginal discharge
- Pyrexia
- Nausea vomiting
- Abnormal uterine bleeding
- Diarrhea and tenesmus in pelvic abscess.

General Examination

High temperature, toxic look, tachycardia, dehydrated tongue.

Per abdomen: Tenderness in lower abdomen, rigidity, may be tenderness on right upper hypochondrium.

Per vaginal: Foul smelling vaginal discharge, tenderness of movement of cervix, tenderness on palpation of lateral fornices, fullness of posterior fornix is suggestive of pelvic abscess.

Differential Diagnosis

- Ectopic pregnancy
- Acute appendicitis
- Torsion of ovarian cyst
- In both acute PID and disturbed ectopic pregnancy, there is acute lower abdominal pain, tachycardia and tenderness on movement of cervix. But in ectopic pregnancy, there will be amenorrhea, pallor and urinary pregnancy test is usually positive whereas in acute PID patient has temperature, look toxic and pregnancy test is negative and leukocytosis.

Investigation

Blood: Hb%, complete blood count, erythrocyte sedimentation rate (ESR), C-reactive protein, electrolytes, serum urea.

Discharge—from endocervix—for *Chlamydia* and gonorrhea culture. For *Chlamydia,* direct enzyme immunoassay and immunofluorescence examination is possible from the smear.

Gonococcal infection is diagnosed with Gram-staining of discharge collected from cervix, Bartholin gland and urethra by detecting gram-negative intracellular diplococci. It is cultured in agar medium containing antibiotic to reduce growth of other organism which are commonly associated with gonorrhea. It is also diagnosed by nucleic acid amplification tests (NAATs).

Chlamydia cell culture, antigen tests, polymerase chain reaction and ligase chain reaction. High vaginal swab, urethral swab and culture, urine and blood culture.

Vaginal discharge test for bacterial vaginosis (BV): Clue cells and Amsel criteria (*see* Chapter 2, Page 36)

Ultrasonography (transvaginal): Free fluid in pouch of Douglas, TO mass, to exclude ectopic pregnancy and appendicitis. Power Doppler can assess hyperemia in acute PID.

Laparoscopy: Visual findings—inflamed tube, TO mass, pus in the fimbrial end. Pus taken for culture and microscopical examination.

Management of Acute Pelvic Inflammatory Disease

- Treatment of acute conditions
- Medical management: Antibiotics, intravenous fluid if needed and analgesics
- To review for surgical intervention
- Treatment of partner and counseling
- Follow up
- Patient should be offered treatment in early stages as soon as patient comes with clinical manifestations and treated as OPD basis with drugs for chlamydial, gonococcal, aerobic and anaerobic infections and then reviewed after 48–72 hours.

Q. When to admit a patient suffering from acute PID?

- Critically-ill patient
- Surgical condition like appendicitis is suspected
- Not responding to medical management
- Severe nausea and vomiting
- Presence of abscess.

Management in Hospital

- Intravenous fluid
- Antibiotic
- Any of the following regimens of antibiotics can be used for in-patient.

Regimen A

Cefotetan 2 g IV 12 hourly or 2 g IV every 6 hours plus doxycycline 100 mg twice daily orally or IV for 14 days [Centers for Disease Control and Prevention (CDC) recommendation] Alternatively, ceftriaxone 2 g IV daily and doxycycline 100 mg twice daily orally or IV for 14 days.

Regimen B

Clindamycin 900 mg IV every 8 hours plus gentamicin 2 mg/kg intramuscular (IM) or intravenous (IV) (loading dose) followed by 1.5 mg/kg every 8 hourly.

As soon as the recovery occurs, oral clindamycin 450 mg 6 hourly plus doxycycline 100 mg 12 hourly are given and continued for total 14 days.

Q. What is syndromic approach [Syndromic case management (SCM)]?

Syndromic case management is the cornerstone of sexually-transmitted infection (STI) or reproductive tract infection (RTI) management to control STI/RTI in India and in Prevention of Parent to Child Transmission (PPTCT) program endorsed by World Health Organization (WHO).

Pelvic inflammatory disease is very common and its sequel are serious so far as infertility and other morbidity is concerned. Acute PID is difficult to diagnose because of the wide variation in symptoms and signs associated with it.

In developed countries, including India, the initiation of treatment is often delayed if treatment started after complete manifestation of the disease and after full investigations, e.g. laboratory test and other investigations. Hence, an earlier treatment has been suggested by CDC as below.

CRITERIA DEVELOPED AND RECOMMENDED (2015) BY CDC FOR INITIATION OF TREATMENT OF PID

Minimal Clinical Criteria

Minimal clinical criteria for presumptive treatment for PID should be initiated in sexually active young women and other women at risk for STDs if they feel lower abdominal and pelvic pain and if one or more of the following criteria on pelvic examination is fulfilled.

- Cervical motion tenderness, or
- Uterine tenderness, or
- Adnexal tenderness.

Additional Criteria

One or more of the following additional criteria can be used to increase the specificity of the minimal clinical criteria to diagnose PID.

- Temperature (oral) higher than 101°F (>38.3°C)
- Abnormal cervical mucopurulent discharge or cervical friability
- Presence of abundant numbers of white blood cells on saline microscopy of vaginal fluid
- Elevated ESR
- Elevated C-reactive protein
- Laboratory documentation of cervical infection with *C. trachomatis* or *N. gonorrhoeae.*

Definitive Criteria

The most specific criteria for diagnosing PID include:

- Endometrial biopsy with histopathological evidence of endometritis
- Transvaginal sonography or magnetic resonance imaging techniques showing thickened, fluid-filled tubes with or without free pelvic fluid or tubo-ovarian complex, or Doppler studies suggesting pelvic infection (e.g. tubal hyperemia) or
- Laparoscopic findings consistent with PID.

Kits Provided by National AIDS Control Organization

Several kits are provided by National AIDS Control Organization for use in specific indications. In relation to

STIs/RTIs SCM for treatment of PID, the following kits are available:

- **Kit 1 (Gray)** contains Tab azithromycin 1 g and Tab cefixime 400 mg single dose stat for vaginal discharge (vaginitis).
- **Kit 2 (Green)** contains Tab secnidazole 2 g and Cap fluconazole 150 mg single dose for urethral discharge and cervical discharge (cervicitis).
- **Kit 6 (Yellow)** contains tablet cefixime 400 mg—single dose, Tab metronidazole 400 mg twice daily × 14 days and doxycycline 100 mg twice daily × 14 days for lower abdominal pain (PID).

Indications of Surgery in Pelvic Inflammatory Disease

Surgery may be laparotomy, laparoscopy or posterior colpotomy. The indications are:

- Pelvic abscess drainage through posterior colpotomy
- Not responding to all type of medical managements with severe peritonitis
- Rupture tubo-ovarian abscess
- Intestinal obstruction.

Types of Surgery Done

- Drainage of pus
- Laparoscopic aspiration and adhesiolysis and peritoneal toileting
- Salpingo-oophorectomy, usually radical surgery is avoided as patient is mostly young
- Posterior colpotomy.

Clinical Features of Chronic Pelvic Inflammatory Disease

Symptoms

- Chronic lower abdominal pain
- Past history of PID
- Menstrual abnormality
- Dysmenorrhea (congestive)
- Vaginal discharge
- Dyspareunia
- Infertility
- Low back pain.

Signs

- Tenderness lower abdomen and there may be lower abdominal mass
- Per speculum—vaginal discharge.

Bimanual Examination

Pelvic mass on adnexal region, tender and mobility restricted and may be adhered with uterus.

Differential Diagnosis

- Endometriosis
- Old ectopic pregnancy.

Investigations for Chronic Pelvic Inflammatory Disease

Ultrasonography (USG) or laparoscopy or other imaging if indicated.

Management

- Laparoscopic adhesiolysis or salpingo-oophorectomy
- Laparotomy: Removal of TO mass with/without hysterectomy.

Q. BASHH guideline.

This is a guideline by British Association for Sexual Health and HIV (BASHH) where evidenced-based information regarding pelvic inflammatory disease (PID) is obtained. The guideline recommends regarding the diagnostic tests, various therapeutic regimens and health promotion principles required for the effective management of PID, their transmission reduction, to reduce complications and to prevent further infection.

SEXUALLY TRANSMITTED INFECTIONS (STIs)

Q. How will you define STIs?

Sexually transmitted infections are those infections which are transmitted through the sexual contact. However other than the sexual contact, these infections may be transmitted by other route namely, through blood transfusion, needle prick, and vertical transmission.

Q. Recommended STDs for routine screening.

Recommended STDs are *C. trachomatis, N. gonorrhoeae, Treponema pallidum,* HIV, HBV, HCV and HSV (not routinely).

Q. What are the problems with STIs?

- Sexually transmitted diseases (STDs) cause PID, pain, infertility, and ectopic pregnancy.
- Viral STDs like human papilloma virus (HPV) cause cervical and vulvar cancer.
- Obstetric outcome may be poor due to STDs affecting the child.
- AIDS caused by HIV infection results severe immunosuppression, opportunistic infections, and cancer.
- Sexually transmitted infections are one of the most important global health problem.

Candidiasis (Vulvovaginal Candidiasis)

Candidiasis is caused by *Candida albicans*— an yeast, not always transmitted by sexual intercourse and for which *it is not strictly regarded as STIs.*

Symptoms and Signs

In candidiasis, there is creamy white, thick curdy discharge associated with marked vulvar itching, soreness, and dysuria (**Fig. 1**).

CHAPTER 33: Pelvic Inflammatory Disease, Sexually Transmitted Infections and Female Genital Tuberculosis

In the Chapter 2, in evaluation of vaginal discharge the diagnosis of BV, trichomoniasis, moniliasis, and gonorrhea have discussed. Here the STDs are discussed with their management.

Predisposing Factors

Predisposing factors include combined oral contraceptive (COC) pill, diabetes, pregnancy, and antibiotics.

Diagnosis

Typical hyphae and budding spores (yeast-like organism) are seen under microscope on treatment with 10% KOH of the discharge. *Candida* is also diagnosed by Gram staining showing speckled Gram-positive spores. For culture of *Candida albicans*, culture Nickerson-Sabouraud media is used.

Treatment

- Intravaginal pessaries of clotrimazole (100 mg) for 7 days or 500 mg single are given.
- Fluconazole: 150 mg single oral dose.
- For symptomatic relief topical antifungal cream, aqueous cream as emollient, and local steroid cream are applied.
- Treatment of asymptomatic partner is not necessary as in true sense, it is not STIs.

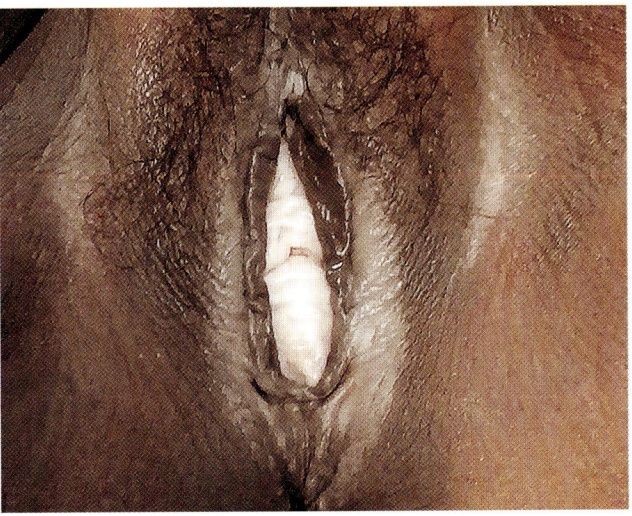

Fig. 1: Vulvovaginal candidiasis.

The common infections are BV, trichomoniasis, and moniliasis. The infections may be bacterial, viral, fungal, and protozoal.

In **Table 1** STIs, causative organisms, and common clinical manifestations are given.

Table 1: Sexually transmitted infection, causative organisms, and clinical manifestations.

Types	Disease	Agent	Clinical effects
Fungus	Moniliasis	Candida albicans	Vulvitis and vaginitis
Protozoal	Trichomoniasis	Trichomonas vaginalis	Vaginitis
Viral	Genital herpes	Herpes simplex virus	Genital ulcers, carcinoma cervix, and neonatal herpes
	Heterotrophic negative infective mononucleosis	Cytomegalovirus	Cervicitis and fetal congenital defect
	Condyloma accuminata	Genital wart virus	Genital warts
	Genital molluscum contagiosum	Molluscum contagiosum virus	Papules with punctum
	AIDS	HIV (type 1 or 2)	Mostly asymptomatic Immunosuppression and opportunistic infections
Bacterial	Bacterial vaginosis	Gardnerella vaginalis	Foul smelling vaginal discharge
	Gonorrhea	Neisseria gonorrhea	Bartholinitis, PID, urethritis, conjunctivitis, ophthalmia neonatorum
	Lymphogranuloma venereum	Chlamydia trachomatis	Genital ulcer, urethritis, proctitis, elephantiasis, and pneumonia of infant
	Syphilis	Treponema pallidum	Manifestation of syphilis— early and late
	Chancroid or soft sore	Haemophilus ducreyi	Congenital syphilis
	Donovanosis or granuloma inguinale	Calymmatobacterium granulomatis	Soft genital ulcers and bubo
	Nongonococcal urethritis	Chlamydia trachomatis, Ureaplasma urealyticum, and Treponema pallidum	Pseudobubo, genital ulcer, and elephantiasis
Infestations	Scabies Pediculosis	Sarcoptes scabiei Crab louse	Discharge from urethra

Trichomoniasis (Fig. 2)

It is caused by flagellate protozoan. *Trichomonas vaginalis* causes vaginal and urethral discharge.

Symptoms and Signs

- There is vaginal discharge of fishy-odor, frothy, clean, sometimes yellowish green and associated with vulvar soreness and itching.
- The vagina looks strawberry appearance due to hemorrhagic punctum.
- Asymptomatic up to 50%.

Diagnosis

For hanging drop preparation, the discharge is collected from the posterior fornix by speculum and one drop is taken on glass slide and mixed with a drop of saline and covered with cover glass and examined under microscope.

Motile protozoal organism with *typical flagella* (cone-shaped flagellated organism in the center, with a terminal spike and four flagella) is detected in hanging drop preparation under microscope **(Fig. 2)**. Feinberg-Whittington or Diamond's media is used for culture of *Trichomonas vaginalis*. Gold standard is NAAT with endocervical, vaginal swab, and urine with sensitivity and specificity up to 95%.

Treatment

- Oral metronidazole (400 mg) thrice daily for 5–7 days, tinidazole 2 g single dose orally or Secnidazole 2 g single dose orally which also acts against BV.
- Partner is also treated.

Bacterial Vaginosis

It is caused by *Gardnerella vaginalis*.

Symptoms and Signs

It is the most *common cause of vaginal discharge (40–50% cases)*. The discharge is clear, homogenous, whitish-gray, and fishy smelling with high pH.

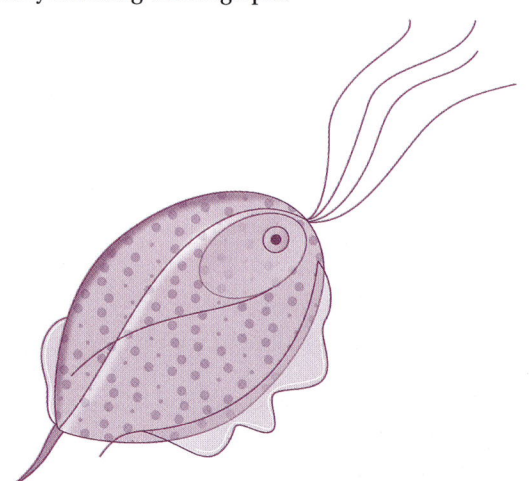

Fig. 2: Trichomonas with four flagella.

Diagnosis

Wet film preparation—*clue cells* are detected in wet film of vaginal discharge under microscope in case of BV. Clue cells are epithelial cells covered with bacteria showing characteristic stippled appearance. A fishy smell after mixing the discharge with KOH indicates BV.

Amsel criteria for diagnosing BV—any three of four:
1. Presence of clue cells on microscopy
2. Creamy grayish-white discharge
3. Vaginal pH above 4.5
4. Characteristic fishy-odor on addition of alkali.

Adverse Effects of Bacterial Vaginosis

- PID and posthysterectomy vaginal cuff cellulitis.
- Pregnancy: Miscarriage, preterm birth, and premature rupture of membranes.
- Increase risk of HIV infection.

Treatment

- Metronidazole (400 mg) twice daily or clindamycin (300 mg) twice daily or tinidazole (500 mg) twice daily for 7 days or tinidazole 2 g single dose orally can also be given. Or, vaginally metronidazole (0.75%) for 5 days or clindamycin (2%) cream for 7 days at bed time can also be used. Excess vaginal wash or douching is avoided.
- Treatment of husband is not required in BV.

Gonorrhea

Gonorrhea is caused by Gram-negative *Diplococcus Neisseria gonorrhoeae*.

Symptoms and Signs

- Asymptomatic up to 50% cases. May present with increase vaginal discharge, pelvic pain, dysuria, endocervical and urethral mucopurulent discharge, low-grade fever, skin rash, and arthralgia. It causes cervicitis and PID. Rarely hematogenous spread occurs resulting purpuric rash and/or arthralgia of monoarticular type.
- There may be perihepatitis due to spread of infection to the liver with formation of adhesion with abdominal wall. The typical "violin string" type adhesion are seen and called "*Fitz- Hugh-Curtis syndrome*".
- Chance of miscarriage, preterm labor, and puerperal sepsis are more. Neonatal ophthalmic infection may occur due to transmission during delivery.

Diagnosis

Gonococcal infection is diagnosed with *Gram staining* of discharge collected from cervix, Bartholin gland, and urethra by detecting *Gram-negative intracellular diplococci*. It is cultured in agar medium containing antibiotic to reduce growth of other organisms which are commonly associated with gonorrhea. It is also diagnosed by *NAATs*.

Screening of other STIs, especially *Chlamydia trachomatis* is essential as coexistence is very common.

Treatment

Third-generation cephalosporin in parenteral route with azithromycin is the treatment. Ceftriaxone 250 mg IM and azithromycin 1 g orally single dose is recommended. Azithromycin is added to prevent early drug resistance.

Chlamydia Infection

Chlamydial infection is one of the most common STDs, caused by *Chlamydia trachomatis*, an obligate intracellular bacterium.

Symptoms and Signs

The most common bacterial STI in women below 25 years and is often asymptomatic. There may be contact bleeding, intermenstrual bleeding, and mucopurulent discharge from cervix or urethra with dysuria. It causes subclinical PID and its complications. There may be monoarticular arthritis in weight-bearing joint. Perihepatitis *(Fitz-Hugh–Curtis syndrome)* occurs more in Chlamydia than gonorrhea.

Diagnosis

It is diagnosed by nucleic acid amplification technique from a vulvar swab or a first-void urine sample. The intracellular organism is seen under microscope. Diagnosis is confirmed by staining by an immunofluorescence technique. It contains both DNA and ribonucleic acid. It multiplies like bacteria, but only inside cell as viruses. Culture is very expensive.

Treatment

- For uncomplicated Chlamydia, azithromycin or doxycycline is recommended. Single dose of azithromycin 1 g orally or doxycycline 100 m twice daily orally given for 7 days.
- Partner is also treated.

Lymphogranuloma Inguinale

It is caused by *Chlamydia trachomatis*—an obligatory intracellular Gram-intermediate organism.

Symptoms and Signs

It starts with papule, ulcer or, pustules. Inguinal lymph nodes are enlarged, matted and there is formation of *bubo* with discharge of pus. "Groove sign" is compression of lymph nodes by inguinal ligament which is found in lymphogranuloma venereum (LGV). In long-standing cases, swelling, ulceration, fistula, and stricture formation occur on vulva, vagina, and rectum due to lymphatic obstruction. Vulvar swelling may result vulvar elephantiasis.

Diagnosis is done by clinical manifestations and compliment fixation test, culture, and isolation of Chlamydia serotypes and detection of LGV antigen.

Chancroid

Also called *soft sore* caused by *Haemophilus ducreyi* which is Gram-negative *Streptobacillus*.

Symptoms and Signs

- Presented with painful small multiple ulcers with foul-smelling purulent or hemorrhagic discharge. Lymphadenopathy occurs which may form pus.
- Culture of *ducreyi* bacillus in specialized media confirms the diagnosis.

Treatment

Single dose of ceftriaxone 250 mg IM or azithromycin 1 g oral single dose is recommended.

Granuloma Inguinale

It is caused by *Calymmatobacterium granulomatis*.

Symptoms and Signs

- Multiple papules over external genitalia followed by formation of red painful ulcer are seen. With fibrosis lymph obstruction occurs with development of lymphedema and elephantiasis.
- Biopsy and detection of Donovan bodies are confirmatory.

Treatment

Treatment includes azithromycin or doxycycline.

Condyloma Acuminata (Genital Warts) (Fig. 3)

It is caused by HPV of type 6 and 11.

Wartic lesions are seen over external genitalia, common during pregnancy, very often cauliflower-like appearance. Most commonly seen on cervix, followed by vulva, vagina, and anus.

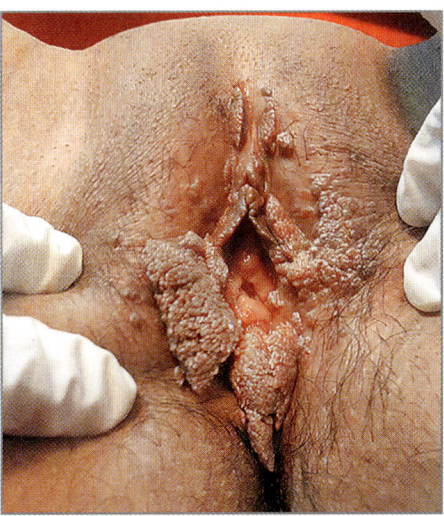

Fig. 3: Vulvar warts (condyloma acuminata).

Treatment

Podophyllin or trichloroacetic acid but are contraindicated in pregnancy. Destructive therapy includes laser, cryotherapy, diathermy or surgical excision. HPV vaccine (type 6 and 11) prevents genital warts.

Molluscum Contagiosum

It is caused by pox virus. The typical feature is centrally umbilicated. It may be transmitted both sexually and asexually and may occur over skin on genital or extragenital area.

Treatment

Treatment includes cauterization with phenol or cryotherapy with liquid nitrogen.

Genital Herpes

It is caused by herpes simplex virus type 1 and 2 (large DNA virus).

Symptoms and Signs

- Pain is severe in nature
- Fever, malaise, dysuria, and discharge
- Over the skin of labia majora, minora, introitus, and other areas of vulva the lesions appear with erythematous plaque which later forms ulcer with yellow base with severe tenderness.
- Acute problems may persist for 3–4 weeks.

Diagnosis

It is done by detection of antigen or by polymerase chain reaction (PCR).

Treatment

- Analgesic—both local and systematic. Saline wash may relieve pain.
- Acyclovir 200–400 mg five times daily for 5 days. Antibiotic is given only where secondarily infected.

Syphilis

- Causative organism of syphilis is *Treponema pallidum*—an anaerobic spirochete.
- Transmission occurs by direct contact or by transplacental transfer of bacteria.
- The infection may be congenital or acquired.

Symptoms and Signs

- *Primary syphilis:* Early lesion is "***chancre***"—a painless well-circumscribed ulcer develops at the site of exposure and gradually develops in other sites. The exudates contain T. pallidum. The inguinal lymph nodes become enlarged and nontender. The lesions heal spontaneously within few weeks. Tubes are not affected with primary syphilis.
- Secondary syphilis: Manifestations of secondary syphilis occur within 6 months of primary lesion. The features are erythematous rash on the palms, soles, and oral and genital mucosa. The raised lesions over the anogenital area are called "**condyloma lata**". Systemic manifestations may be fever, sore throat, myalgia, alopecia, meningitis, uveitis, arthritis, etc. This also spontaneously resolves due to effective host immune response. However, relapse may occur for up to 2 years. In two-thirds of patients, no ill effects occur. Both the stages of primary syphilis and secondary syphilis are infective.
- Latent syphilis: It is the phase after the resolution of secondary phase and may be up to two decades.
- Tertiary syphilis: In one-third of individual's late complications develop in the form of gummatous lesions (deep ulcer with everted margins) of skin and bone, cardiovascular complications which involve aortic valve and ascending aorta and neurological involvements like meningovascular diseases, progressive dementia, tabes dorsalis, and cranial nerve palsies, etc.
- Congenital syphilis: Fetal affection usually occurs after 20 weeks. Fetal affection may be second trimester miscarriage, early congenital syphilis, and late congenital syphilis. As screening in pregnancy is universal at present and so effective treatment is usually advocated.

Diagnosis

- *Detection of organism—T. pallidum* from the serum of lesions of primary or secondary syphilis by dark-field microscopy.
- *By serology:*
  - VDRL (venereal disease research laboratory) and rapid plasma reagin (RPR)
  - More confirmatory tests are *T. pallidum* hemagglutination inhibition test (TPHA) and fluorescent treponemal antibody-absorption test (FTA-ABS)
  - Currently, *enzyme immunoassay tests* to detect IgM and IgG and PCR tests are employed both of which is more sensitive and specific.

Treatment

- Depo preparation of penicillin is the drug of choice
- Benzathine penicillin G 2.4 million units IM in single dose in two divided doses in two buttocks.
- Current sexual partner is also treated.

FEMALE GENITAL TUBERCULOSIS (FGT)

Q. What is the importance of genital tuberculosis in female?

- Tuberculosis of female genital organs is an important cause of infertility and prognosis so far as reproductive outcome is poor.
- Menstrual abnormality
- Long-term health hazard
- Mostly secondary to primary and usually primary is pulmonary tuberculosis.

- Mostly asymptomatic in nature and damage of genital organs occur silently.

Prevalence

Among the infertile women—10%; varies according to population. Less in developed country.

Q. What is the causative organism?

Mostly *Mycobacterium tuberculosis* (95%), a few cases (5%) caused by *Mycobacterium bovis*.

Etiopathogenesis

- Almost secondary to other organs by hematogenous spread. The most common primary focus is the lungs from where it spreads through the hematogenous route. The primary lesion often heals when the feature of genital tuberculosis develops. May occur from abdominal tuberculosis by direct spread.
- Less than 1% cases caused by sexual transmission from male partner. It may occur as a primary disease transmitted by sexual partner with tubercular infection, genitourinary infection or from infected sputum used for sexual lubrication.
- Prevalence of involvement of different genital organs.
    - Fallopian tube—*commonest*—90-100%—in almost all cases of pelvic tuberculosis, fallopian tube is involved.
    - Endometrium—50-60% cases
    - Ovary—25%
    - Cervix—5-10%
    - Vulva and vagina—1-2%.

Pathology

Fallopian Tube (Figs. 4 and 5)

Depending upon the mode of spread, pathological changes occur. The changes in fallopian tube are:
- Endosalpingitis

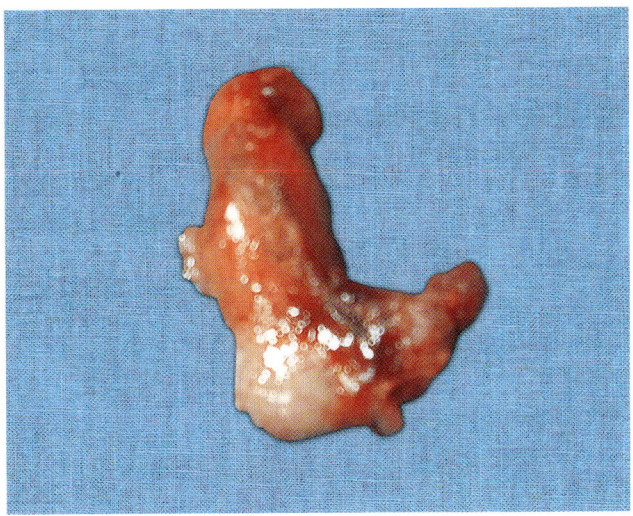

Fig. 5: Excised fallopian tube studded with caseous materials in a parous patient of 41 years.

- Exosalpingitis
- Interstitial salpingitis.

Hematogenous spread causes endosalpingitis and direct spread results exosalpingitis and interstitial salpingitis.

In endosalpingitis, tubercles are not visible on outer surface, but lies deeper. In acute stage, tubes are inflamed and congested followed by formation of pus, pyosalpinx due to caseation. In chronic stage, fibrosis develops with multiple blocks which occur in more than 50% cases and fimbrial block and these blocks result hydrosalpinx.

In exosalpingitis, which occurs by direct contact or by lymphatic spread, there are tubercles on outer wall of tube. Exosalpingitis may occur as a result of intestinal tuberculosis **(Fig. 6)**. There will be peritonitis, ascites, adhesion formation with adjacent structures, ovary and intestines. With progress of disease, tubes become hard and beaded, and adhered with ovary to form TO mass and may result frozen pelvis.

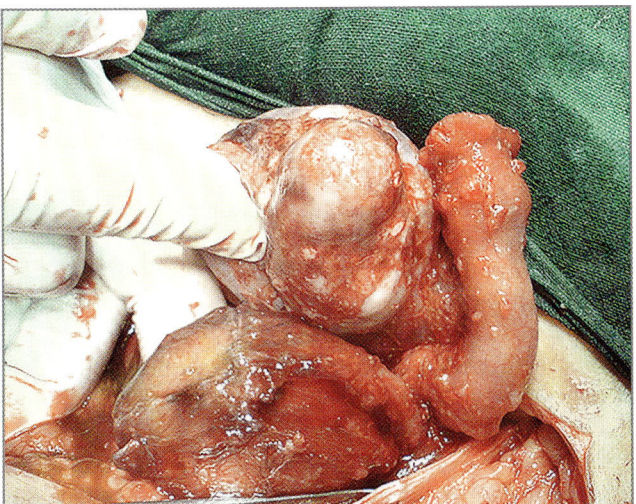

Fig. 4: Tuberculosis of fallopian tube and ovary (pelvic tuberculosis).

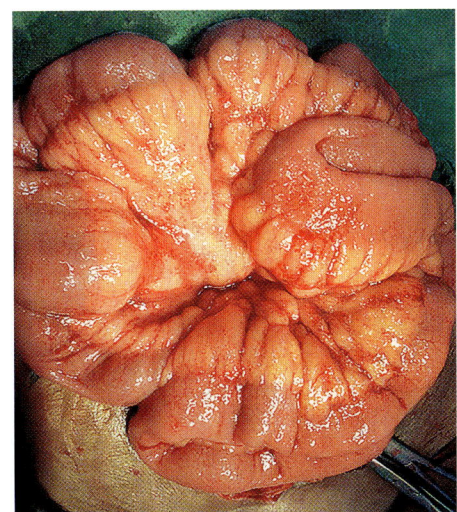

Fig. 6: Tuberculosis of intestines.

Endometrium

Initially, plenty of caseous materials are formed but the spread to myometrium occurs rarely. Later destruction of endometrium results in adhesion formation and synechia. Initially, hypomenorrhea followed by amenorrhea is the typical sequence.

Cervical Tuberculosis (Fig. 7)

In cervical tuberculosis, there may be vegetative, papillary or hypertrophic growth of cervix with/without ulceration mimicking cancer cervix.

Vulva and Vagina

Vulva and vagina are the rare sites of tuberculosis and mostly secondary to extension of the disease from endometrial and cervical tuberculosis. Very rarely, it may be primary, due to direct contact from sexual partner. The lesion may be hypertrophic, ulcerative (nonhealing) and may mimic malignancy. For diagnosis, biopsy is essential. There may be formation of fistula **(Fig. 8)**.

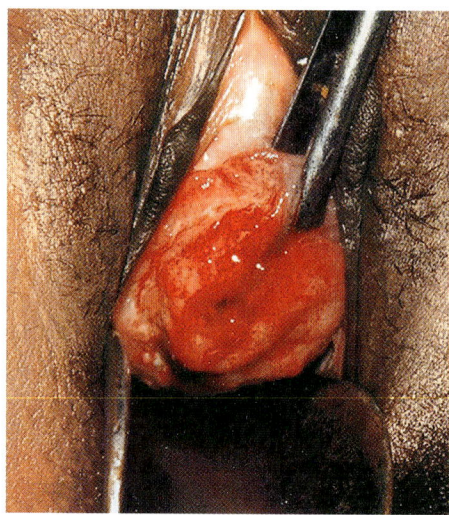

Fig. 7: Cervical tuberculosis.

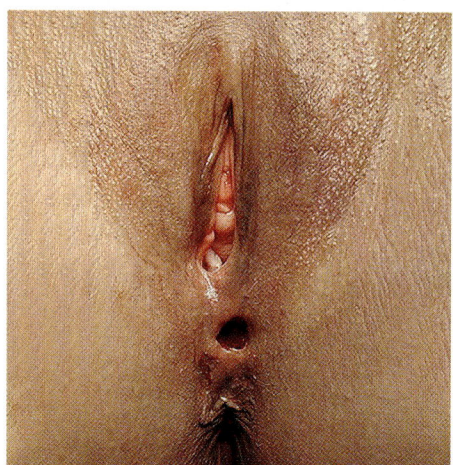

Fig. 8: Tubercular vaginoperineal fistula.

Microscopic Feature

Typical of tuberculosis—granulomatous lesion with caseation, Langhans giant cells and epithelioid cells.

Q. What is the clinical presentation of pelvic tuberculosis?

Symptoms

From the symptoms, it is very difficult to diagnose, typical symptoms are not present and many are asymptomatic.
- May be history of pulmonary tuberculosis
- May present with infertility
- Low-grade fever with malaise
- Menstrual abnormality—amenorrhea, hypomenorrhea, postmenopausal bleeding
- Blood-stained vaginal discharge initially
- Pelvic pain—an inconsistent symptom
- Sometimes, swelling abdomen due to ascites and encysted tubercular peritonitis.

Signs

- Typical features of low genial condition of pulmonary tuberculosis is not found.
- Inguinal lymph nodes may be palpable
- Per abdomen: Doughy feeling is revealed if associated with abdominal tuberculosis. Sometimes, a cystic mass resembling ovarian cyst may be palpable due to encysted tubercular peritonitis.
- Inspection and per speculum examination: A lesion may be seen in case of tuberculosis of cervix, vagina and vulva.

Bimanual Examination

Restricted mobility of uterus, adnexal mass may be palpable. Nodules in the pouch of Douglas may be palpable.

Differential Diagnosis

- Chronic PID
- Endometriosis
- Ovarian cyst
- Old ectopic.

Q. What are the investigations done for diagnosis of pelvic tuberculosis?

- Blood: Complete blood count, lymphocytosis, high ESR
- Chest X-ray: Evidence of old lesion, very rarely active lesion. May be normal.
- Mantoux test: Poor specificity and sensitivity. It is called negative when it is less than 5 mm, positive more than 10 mm, 5–10 mm—inconclusive. Positive indicates infection, may be after bacille Calmette-Guerin vaccination but not necessarily active infection.
- QuantiFERON gamma release assay is a rapid test, does not affected by previous vaccination and is better than Mantoux test due to high specificity.

- Sputum for acid-fast bacilli (AFB) test for consecutive 3 days.
- Deoxyribonucleic acid-polymerase chain reaction (DNA PCR): Endometrial aspirate, menstrual blood or biopsy tissue by laparoscopy are sent for DNA PCR. Less useful for high false-positive result, mostly due to contamination.
- Endometrial biopsy collected in premenstrual phase. Sent in formal saline for histopathology, in normal saline for mycobacterial culture.
- Sonography may show adnexal mass—unilateral or bilateral and hydrosalpinx may be present. Ascites may be present. However, no USG finding is specific for tuberculosis.
- Laparoscopy: TO mass, tubercles over peritoneal surface and over serous coat. Pyosalpinx and caseation may be seen. Biopsy is taken from suspected areas.
- Hysterosalpingography: In case of high suspicion of tuberculosis, HSG is avoided. The features may be found are as follows:
  - Tubes may be blocked at fimbrial end or at corneal end.
  - If tubes are visible, there may be presence of beaded appearance of tube, tobacco appearance due to everted fimbria and/or lead pipe rigidity appearance. There may be hydrosalpinx.
  - Uterus lining of cavity is irregular.
  - Intravasation of dye may be present.
- Human immunodeficiency virus testing: It should be done in patient suffering from tuberculosis after counseling as tuberculosis is more common in immunocompromised patients.

Management

- *Medical management:* Multidrug therapy for 6–9 months is the treatment option.
- Due to noncompliance and fear of multidrug resistance, *directly observed treatment short course therapy* (DOTS) is recommended by WHO.
- According to new guidelines (Guidelines for Extrapulmonary Tuberculosis of India, WHO 2016) in female genital tuberculosis intensive phase HRZE (four drug) for 2 months followed by continuation phase HRE (three drug) for another 4 months are recommended (total 6 months).

Four drug regime [INH (H), rifampicin (R), pyrazinamide (Z), ethambutol (E)] daily for next 2 months in *intensive phase* + **followed by**:

Three drug regime [INH (H) and rifampicin (R) and ethambutol (E)] daily for next 4 months *continuation phase*.
- The dose depends on the weight of the patient as given in Table 2.

Drug Dosage for Adult Tuberculosis (Table 2)

Table 2: Drug dosage for tuberculosis in adults.

Weight category	Number of tablets		Injection streptomycin
	Intensive phase	Continuation phase	
	2HRZE	4HRE	
	75/150/400/275	75/150/275	Gm
25–39	2	2	0.5
40–54	3	3	0.75
55–69	4	4	1
>=70	5	5	1

Q. How will you assess treatment response?

- Improvement of symptoms—patient symptomatically improved
- Size of the mass reduced clinically and by USG
- Blood parameter: White blood cell count and ESR favorable.

Indications of Surgery

- Progression or persistence of the mass size
- Persistence of symptoms in spite of antitubercular drug therapy
- No improvement of laboratory parameters.

Types of Surgery

- Total abdominal hysterectomy with bilateral salpingo-oophorectomy (TAH+BSO) in family completed women
- Removal of adnexal mass in young woman
- Drainage of pyometra and tubo-ovarian abscess.

Contraindications to Surgery

- Dense adhesions may develop fistula due to injury
- Infertility treatment
- Reproductive outcome is not good
- In vitro fertilization (IVF) and embryo transfer result is not good. Clipping or surgical removal of hydrosalpinx is needed to improve success rate in IVF.

Index

Page numbers followed by *b* refer to box, *f* refer to figure, *fc* refer to flowchart, and *t* refer to table

A

Abbe-Wharton-McIndoe operation 454
Abdomen 9, 101, 558
  contour of 14
  examination of 503
  fullness of 14
  inspection of 13*f*
  palpation of 15*f*
  regions of 14
  subdivision of 14*f*
Abdominal lump
  lower 314
  palpation of 14*f*
Abdominal mass 16, 343
Abdominal muscle 14
  laxity of 217
Abdominal open method 97
Ablation 126, 367
Ablative therapy, results of 127
Abnormal bleeding 433
  mechanism of 116
  ovulatory 116
  types of 117
Abnormal glucose tolerance test 289
Abnormal uterine bleeding 10, 38, 39*f*, 84, 110-112, 115-119, 120*f*, 124*t*, 125, 126, 128, 352, 374, 560, 570
  causes of 116
  diagnosis of 117, 120
  etiology of 116
  management of 121, 127, 128, 128*t*
  nonstructural causes of 113
Abortion 113, 338, 477
  medical 495
  recurrent 38
  spontaneous 441, 448
Abscess 20
  cyst, operations of 551
Abstinence 264
Acanthosis nigricans 10, 11*f*, 290, 292, 292*f*, 293*f*, 301
Accessory glands, secretion of 421, 424
Accredited Social Health Activist 511
Acetic acid 178
Acetowhite epithelium 178
Acid-fast bacilli, sputum for 615
Acne 251, 297, 301, 311, 312, 314, 348
  incidence of 297
Acquired immunodeficiency syndrome 189, 328
Acrosomal integrity test 267
Acrosome reaction 267*f*, 422*f*, 424, 425

Actinomycin D 155
Actinomycosis 606
Activin 417
Acute pelvic inflammatory disease
  clinical features of 606
  management of 607
  pathology of 606
Acute pelvic inflammatory disorder 5, 607
Acute pelvic pain 38
  causes of 5
Addison's disease 337
Adenocarcinoma 63, 164, 173
  cervix 165*f*
  endometrial 139*f*
  endometrioid 53, 64*f*, 138, 139
  mucinous 63, 64, 138
  serous 63
Adenoid
  basal carcinoma 164
  cystic carcinoma 164
Adenoma, pituitary 337, 338
Adenomyoma 113
Adenomyosis 30, 37, 40*f*, 84, 87, 114, 115*f*, 262, 369, 371, 371*f*, 372, 372*f*, 373, 544
  features of 84
  focal 371*f*
  types of 370
Adhesiolysis 273, 279, 553
Adhesions 58
  lysis of 367
  separation of 352*f*
Adiana 499
Adjuvant therapy 76, 268
Adnexa 160, 570
  status of 547*f*
Adnexal mass 31, 51, 338
Adnexal pathology 545
Adrenal glands 295
  androgen secreting tumors of 299
Adrenal tumor hypothyroidism 337
Adrenarche, premature 348
Adrenocorticotropic hormone 289, 299, 327, 333
  stimulation test 327
Adrenogenital syndrome 7, 308, 310, 310*f*, 327
Advanced epithelial ovarian carcinoma 69*f*
Advanced ovarian cancer 68
  management of 68, 70
Advisory Committee on Immunization Practices 183

Agenesis 439
Agglutination reaction test, mixed 266, 267
Allis tissue forceps 108, 108*f*, 227, 227*f*, 231, 231*f*, 237, 396, 396*f*, 405, 406*f*, 517, 531, 531*f*, 535
Alopecia 306
Alpha-chlorohydrin 508
Alpha-fetoprotein 51, 76
Alprazolam 430
Ambiguous genitalia 312, 327, 331
  diagnosis of 331
Ambosexual hairs 306
Amenorrhea 34, 38, 78*f*, 110, 117, 149, 158*f*, 290, 313, 321, 338*f*, 339, 341-343, 343*f*, 400, 408
  causes of 6
  exercise-related 261
  functional hypothalamic 343
  hypothalamic 335
  mechanism of 341
  postpill 338, 468
  primary 7, 32, 38, 308, 31-314, 317, 317*fc*, 318, 319, 322, 352, 355
  secondary 7, 291, 335, 337-339, 340*fc*, 342*f*
Aminobutyric acid gabapentin 436
Amplification test 37
Ampulla 426
Amsel criteria 36, 610
Anagen 306
Anal canal 401
  anatomy of 402, 403*f*
Anal incontinence 403
  pathophysiology of 403
Anal sphincter
  anatomy of 402, 403*f*
  internal 402
Anal wink reflex 220
Analgesics 365, 366
Androblastoma 53, 77, 78, 343
Androgen 293, 298, 342, 365, 415
  binding globulin 424
  effects 348
  excess 290
    evaluation of 301
  insensitivity syndrome 7, 8, 308, 309, 309*f*, 310*f*, 314, 315*f*, 316*f*, 317, 315, 322, 323, 323*f*, 324*t*, 325*f*, 326, 326*t*
  producing tumor 343
  progestogen combination 507
  secreting adrenal tumors 300
  sensitivity
    syndrome 323*f*
    types of 324

Index

synthesis 300, 301f
    disorder of 330
Androgenicity 301
Androstenedione 300, 355, 415
Anechoic fluid 55f
Anemia 9, 10f, 93, 160, 217
    causes of 10
Anesthesia 98, 495, 500, 563, 579
    general 242
    regional 545
Aneurysm needle 522, 536, 536f
Angiogenesis 427
Angiogenic agents 366
Angioma 600
Annovera 476
Annular tubules 52, 53, 77
Anorectal mucosa 406f, 407
Anorexia 50, 338
    nervosa 248
Anovular abnormal bleeding 116, 116t
Anovulation 254, 261, 268, 272, 294, 342
    causes of 261
    hypergonadotropic
        hypoestrogenic 261
        hypogonadism 261, 313
Antara 471, 473, 473f, 511
Anterior colporrhaphy 225-227, 230, 234, 234f, 237, 240, 551
    complications of 231
Anterior vaginal wall 205f, 530
    prolapse 215, 219, 225
    retractor 26f, 517, 531, 531f
Antiandrogens 303, 304
Antibiotics
    intravenous 565
    use of 565
Antidepressant drugs 436
Antifertility vaccine 508
Anti-Mullerian hormone 249, 256, 257, 289, 319, 333, 432, 438
Antioxidants 280, 421
Anti-potency pill 286
Antiprogestational agent 365
Antiprogestins 95
Antiseptic dressing 98, 500
Antisperm antibody test 266
Antral follicle 414, 416
    count 257
Anus 20
Aorta 69f
    coarctation of 314, 320
Aortic dissection 320
Apoplexy, ovarian 54, 418
Appendicectomy 8
Appendicitis, acute 606
Appetite 8, 150, 158
Aqua dissection 545
Arcus tendineus fascia pelvis 230
Aromatase excess syndrome 347
Aromatase inhibitor 85, 268, 269, 294, 365, 367

Arrhenoblastoma 78, 291, 297f, 299f, 300, 300f, 337, 343, 343f, 344f
Arteriovenous malformation 38, 113, 130, 154f
Artery
    arcuate 418
    forceps 398f
    ovarian 418
Artificial insemination 280, 283, 286
    types of 283
Artificial urinary sphincters 393, 395
Ascites 16, 17f, 40, 47, 48, 66, 81, 84, 217
    dragging of 38
Ascitic fluid 61
Asherman syndrome 313, 321, 337, 342, 481
Aspermia 266
Assisted reproductive technology 267, 274, 275, 279, 280, 285
Asthenospermia 266
Asthma, bronchial 8
Atherosclerosis 296
Atresia, vaginal 316f
Atretic cervix 451
Atrophic cervix, postmenopausal 181f
Atrophy 198, 210
Atypia 131
Atypical squamous cells 171
Autoimmune disorders 199
Autoimmune functional ovarian cysts 347
Autosomal recessive genetic disorder 263
Auvard's self-retaining speculum 517f, 531, 531f
Auvard's weighted speculum 237
Axillary hair 309, 310, 315
Axillary tail 12
Ayer's spatula 35f, 175f, 176f, 220, 220f, 251, 524, 538, 538f
Azithromycin 611
Azoospermia 265-267, 280, 286, 287
    nonobstructive 286
    obstructive 286

B

Babcock's tissue forceps 520, 535, 535f
Bacterial vaginosis 20, 27, 35-37, 606, 610
    adverse effects of 610
    diagnosis of 36
Bacterium, intracellular 36
Bacteroides 606
Baden-Walker halfway system 213
Bagshwe regime 155
Baldness 306
Barrier methods, types of 491
Bartholin's abscess 21f, 600, 601, 602f, 604, 604f
Bartholin's adenoma 601
Bartholin's cyst 20, 600, 601, 601f, 602
    excision of 602f
    operations of 551
    palpation of 24f

Bartholin's gland 20, 23, 600, 601
    anatomy of 601
    carcinoma 188
    disorder of 602
    swelling of 600
Basal artery 418
Basal body temperature 250, 251, 252f
    method 494
Basal cell carcinoma 188
Basophilic cells 253f
Bazedoxifene 367, 436
Benign ovarian cyst 54, 59
    malignant transformation of 59
    management of 59
Benign ovarian tumor 48, 52f, 54, 59, 574f
    diagnosis of 48
Beta-human chorionic gonadotropin 149
Bethesda system 170, 171, 177
Bilateral patent tubes 41f, 258f, 579f
Bilateral tubal
    block 580, 581
    obstruction 280
Billing's method 494
Biopsy 34, 64, 66, 136, 161, 179, 188, 197, 200, 365, 372, 520f, 611
    excisional 188
    frozen section 66
    gonadal 324, 332
    incisional 188
    out of phase 255
Bipolar coagulation forceps 556f
Birth control methods 457, 461, 462t
    classification of 462
Bisphosphonates 436
Bivalent vaccine 183
Bladder 8, 150, 158, 239f, 502
    filling and emptying 389
    flap 389, 389f
    function evaluations 223
    injury 395f
    mucosa 384f
    pillars 237f
    retraining 392
    sulcus 218
    wall 384f
Blastocyst 278f, 427f, 428
    development of 426
    formation 425, 426
Bleeding 30, 113
    abnormalities 467
    acute 129
    amount of 7, 82, 110, 157
    disorders 128
        prevalence of 128
    infrequent 112, 113
    irregular 112, 157, 473
    ovulatory 117t
    per vagina 7, 133
    postcoital 117
    postmenopausal 145
    rectal 158
Bleomycin 75, 155

Blind vagina, causes of 315, 316f
Blood 606, 614
   dyscrasia 8
   loss
      quantity of 7
      reduction of 536
   pressure 11, 312, 346, 563
      high 93
      measurement of 11
   sugar 189
   transfusion 8
   vessels 418
Blunt curette, use of 534
Boari's flap method 389, 389f
Boari's technique 388
Body mass index 9, 83, 111, 134, 248, 289, 312, 346, 433
Bone
   age determination 349f
   loss, postmenopausal 434
   marrow density 434, 367, 434
   mass, markers of 435
Bonney's hood operation 99, 99f, 100f
Bonney's myomectomy clamp 99, 100f, 521, 536, 536f
Bonney's stitch 235, 235f
Bonney's test 391, 393
Borderline ovarian tumor 72
Bowel 8, 150, 158
   distention 554
   fistula 502
   function, evaluation of 223
   preparation 405
   problems 217
   small 358
Bowen's diseases 198
Brain, magnetic resonance imaging of 315
Braxton Hicks contraction 33
Breastfeeding 63, 495
Breasts 8, 12, 251, 309, 310, 322, 351, 467
   atrophy 310f
   development 317, 320
      absent of 314319
      normal 314
      sequence of 318f
   examination 12, 12f, 46, 111, 134, 136, 150, 158, 186, 204, 248, 312, 315, 357, 378, 401
      clinical 12
      self 12
   growth of 351f
   regression of 343f
   sizes, reduced 297f
Brenner tumor 56
   left-sided 56f
   malignant 63, 64
British Hypertension Society 11
British Society of Clinical Cytology 170
Broad ligament
   clamping of 542f
   cysts 105
   fibroid 32, 47, 84, 90, 105, 106f, 107f
   tumor 32, 105
Bromocriptine 270, 303, 341
Broom devices 176
Budding spores 36
Buffalo hump 312, 314
Bulbocavernosus reflex 220
Bull's eye target 58
Burch colposuspension 393, 394, 394f
Butterfly incision 193f

C

Cabergoline 270, 341, 367
Cachexia 160
   ovarian 9f, 65f
Café-au-lait spots 347, 348, 365
Caffeine 93
Calcium 436
Calendar rhythm method 493, 494
Camels, uteri of 461
Cancer 143, 474
   cervix 28f, 32, 134, 135, 144, 144f, 159, 161, 163f, 170, 177, 189, 207f, 544, 574, 575, 575f
      complications of 161
      early 6
      lymphatic drainage of 165
      management of 166
      prognosis of 170
      stages of 161, 161t, 162f, 163
      surgery of 540
      treatment of 575
   characteristics of 138, 139
   death, incidence of 170
   endometrium 144f
   ovary 141f
   peritoneal 67
   risk 268
   vulva 576, 576f
   vulvar 20, 22f, 187-190, 195t, 196
Candida 609
   albicans 6, 34-36, 608
Candidiasis 20, 27, 35-37, 608
   diagnosis of 36
   vulvar 22f
Cannon balls appearance 153
Cannula 500, 526f
   types of 580
Carboplatin 72
Carcinoma 53, 64, 138
   adenosquamous 164
   cervix 32, 40, 157, 182
      microinvasive lesions of 171f
      preinvasive lesions of 171f
      stage of 165, 165t
   embryonal 52, 53, 74, 76
   endometrial 143
   endometrium 140
   in situ 170, 172, 198
   mixed 138
   serous 139, 164

Carcinosarcoma 63, 138, 139, 146, 147
Cardiac disease 8
Cardinal ligament 208, 209
Cardiovascular anomaly 321
Cardiovascular disease 434, 435
   prevalence of 437
Cardiovascular system 12, 83, 134, 150, 158, 186, 203, 248, 312, 314, 357
Carnett test 375
Catagen 306
Catgut, pack of 523f
Catheterization 227f, 500
   complications of 529
Cavitational ultrasonic surgical aspiration 197, 198
Cavity
   endometrial 87f
   peritoneal 240
Ceftriaxone 565
Cell
   adhesion molecule 255, 429
   carcinoma, small 63, 64, 164
Cellular pleomorphism 72
Centchroman 472
Central nervous system 83, 134, 150, 158, 186, 203, 248, 311, 313, 314, 335, 357, 467
   tumor 338, 346
Central precocious puberty 348
   causes of 375t
   diagnosis of 347
   etiology of 346
   problems of 347
Cerclage, role of 449
Cerebral metastasis 40
Cerebrovascular accident 125
Cervical agenesis 352, 441, 451, 451f
Cervical atresia 280, 321
Cervical biopsy 146
Cervical cancer 146, 170, 173
   causes of 172
   epidemiology of 170
   etiology of 170
   pathology of 164
   risk factors of 170
   screening 174
      advantages of 174
   spread of 164
   stages of 163
Cervical cap 493, 493f
Cervical carcinogenesis 173
Cervical condyloma 179f
Cervical cytology 35f, 172t, 175, 175f, 176f, 189
   cytobrush 35
   indications of 538
   methods of 175
Cervical dilators 533, 547f
   set of 547f
   types of 533
   use of 533
Cervical ectopy 179f

Cervical erosion 159, 159f
Cervical factor 261
    infertility 262, 268
        treatment of 279
Cervical fibroid 20, 22f, 37, 102, 102f, 103, 103f, 104f, 105, 206f, 210f, 213f, 571, 571f
    anterior 103f
    central 102f-104f
    diagnostic clinical criteria of 104
    incidence of 102l
    management of 104
    polyp 206f
    posterior 103f
    varieties of 102
Cervical intraepithelial lesion
    diagnosis of 179
    management of 179
    system 177, 178
Cervical intraepithelial neoplasia 170, 171f, 172, 174, 189, 196, 544
    development of 172
    high-grade 180f
    low-grade 180f
    risk factors of 173
Cervical mucus 253f, 254f, 339, 466
    amount of 253
    estrogenic 254
    method 494
    study 251
Cervical neoplasia 172
Cervical polyp 20, 107f, 108f, 146, 159, 159f
Cervical smear 27
    normal 175f
Cervical squamous cell carcinoma 154
Cervical stump cancer 539
Cervical syphilitic ulcer 159
Cervical vertebra malformation 452
Cervicitis 280
Cervicography 174
Cervicovaginal junction 237f, 238f
Cervix 23, 27, 28, 34, 141f, 145, 165f, 178f, 187, 189, 217, 230f, 237f, 321, 338, 353, 360, 425, 439, 451, 520f, 613
    abnormalities of 312
    amputation of 234, 234f, 235f
    anterior lip of 29f, 548f
    carcinogenesis of 170
    carcinoma of 162t
    cauliflower growth of 164f
    cyocautery of 527f
    development of 438
    dilatation of 549f
    double 445f
    elongation of 20, 206, 207, 207f
    gradual dilatation of 548f
    hypertrophic 207f
        elongation of 205
    large malignant growth of 205-207
    lesions of 530
    level of 541f
    lips of 30f

    looks 160
    lymphatic drainage of 166f
    normal 28f, 178f
    old tear of 27
    palpation of 30
    Pap smear of 145
    posterior lip of 30f, 532
    preinvasive lesions of 170, 182, 183fc
    premalignant lesions of 157, 170
    small procedures on 551
    strawberry appearance of 27
    vaginal part of 102f
Cesarean
    ligation 495
    section 97, 361
Chancre 612
Chancroid 611
Chemoradiation 169
Chemotherapeutic agents 71, 74
Chemotherapy 8, 62, 69, 70, 74, 142, 154, 155, 166, 169, 311
    intravenous 71
    neoadjuvant 69, 70
    response score 71
    standard adjuvant 71
Chest
    auscultation of 83, 134, 150, 158, 186, 203, 248, 357
    broad-shield 320
    X-ray 138, 151, 614
Chhaya 471, 472, 472f, 511
Chimerism 331
Chlamydia 37, 172, 353, 606, 611
    infection 36, 611
    trachomatis 36, 272, 611
Chloro-6-deoxy sugars 508
Chocolate cyst 32, 47, 48, 84, 359f, 364f, 368f, 585, 585f
    bilateral 359f, 368f
    calcified 360f
    causes of 365
    dragging of 368f
Cholecystectomy 8
Choriocarcinoma 40, 52, 53, 74, 76, 149, 151, 152, 152f, 153
    diagnosis of 153
    gestational 152, 152f
    treatment of 153
Chorionic frondosum 429
Chorionic laevae 429
Chronic pelvic inflammatory disease 358, 608
    clinical features of 608
    pathology of 606
Chronic pelvic pain 38, 358, 363, 375
    causes of 5, 375t
Chronic respiratory disease 263, 263f
Chronic uterine inversion 20
    surgery for 550
Cilia, loss of 272
Cimetidine 304
Cisplatin 75, 155

Clamps
    first pair of 542
    fourth pair of 543
    pairs of 239
    pedicle 61
    second pair of 542
Clear cell
    adenocarcinoma 63, 64, 138
    carcinoma 139, 164
    tumors 53
Cleft 31
Clindamycin 610
Clitoridal cyst 600
Clitoris 20, 439, 600
    enlarged 20, 23f, 299f, 311f, 312, 315, 326f
    lymphatic drainage of 190
    skin of 190
Cloacal extrophy 331
Clomiphene 261
    citrate 250, 268, 294
        challenge test 257
    risk of 269
    side effects of 269
Clostridia 606
Clot 7, 110
Clubbing 10
Clue cells 36, 610
Coagulation disorder 113, 352
Coagulopathy 114
Cohort study 593
Coital function 319, 321, 363
Coitus 452
    interruptus 494
Cold coagulation 181
Colles' fascia 404
Colles' Rogen deficiency 434
Color Doppler 151
Colpocleisis 241
Colpoperineorrhaphy, posterior 225, 231, 232f, 233, 234, 237, 241, 551
Colporrhaphy, posterior 225, 231, 241f
Colposcopy 34, 177, 177f, 178t, 179, 188, 189, 197
    advantages of 177
Colposuspension, laparoscopic 393
Combined oral contraceptives 85, 94, 118, 125, 128, 135, 294, 355, 365, 369, 459f, 464
    benefits of 467
    noncontraceptive uses of 467
    pill 462, 464, 469
        absolute contraindications of 468
        types of 465, 466t
    role of 54
    use of 467
Complete androgen insensitivity syndrome 334
Complete blood cell count 266
Complete perineal tear 20, 32, 378, 402, 403, 404f
    causes of 404

repair of 405, 551
risk factors of 404
treatment of 405
Computed tomography scan 37, 40, 189
Computer-assisted semen analysis 264, 267
Condom 460, 491
benefits of 492
development of 491
female 463, 492, 492*f*
male 460*f*, 463, 491, 491*f*
Condyloma 187
acuminata 20, 21*f*, 196, 353, 600, 611, 611*f*
lata 612
Cone biopsy 182, 182*f*
Congenital adrenal hyperplasia 7, 23*f*, 289, 298, 298*f*, 299*f*, 308, 310, 310*f*, 315*f*, 327, 329, 347
adult-onset 338
clinical presentation of 327
late-onset 343
management of 327
treatment of 327
Conjunctiva, upper bulbar 10
Conservative cryotherapy, role of 180
Conservative surgery 367, 451
Constipation 158, 200, 203
Contraception 459, 461
broad categories of 462
hormonal method of 464
long-acting reversible 123, 490
methods of 462
permanent 495
postcoital 476, 477
Contraceptive 459, 468*t*, 492, 511
barrier methods of 491
hormonal 111, 465
ideal 462
injectable 338, 472
male 507
prevalence rate 510
sponge 493
Controlled ovarian hyperstimulation 275
protocols of 276
Conventional glass slides method 175
Cooper ligament 394
Copper-containing intrauterine device 478, 481
mechanism of action of 480
Core biopsy 66
Cornified cells 252*f*
Corona radiata 416
Coronary heart disease 544
Corpora cavernosa 190
Corpus albicans 418
Corpus cancer syndrome 9, 136
Corpus luteum 358
cyst 53, 54
formation of 417
Corticosteroid 294, 304
Cotte's operation 374

Cramps 352
Creamy discharge 160
Crohn's disease 358
Crude birth rate 509
Cryogun 181*f*
Cryoprobe 181*f*, 527*f*
Cryotherapy 181*f*
Cryptomenorrhea 311, 315*f*, 316*f*, 323, 352, 355
dragging of 450*f*
Cryptorchidism 262
Cubitus valgus 309, 309*f*, 319
Cumulus
cells 417*f*
oophorus 416
Curette, types of 534
Cusco's speculum 23, 24*f*, 25, 25*f*, 160, 254, 517*f*, 530, 530*f*
Cushing's syndrome 291, 298, 302, 312, 314, 337, 347
signs of 301
Cu-T 380a 479*f*, 480, 511
insertion of 482
Cu-T
intrauterine contraceptive device 583
plunger of 220*f*
Cyanosis 10
Cyclic adenosine monophosphate 416
Cyclic progesterone 123
Cyclofem 474
Cyclophosphamide 155
Cyclosporine 300
Cyproterone acetate 304, 348, 465
Cyst 20
blue-domed 363*f*
endometriotic 38
excision 602, 603*f*
follicular 53, 54
hemorrhagic 358
mesenteric 47, 48, 84
neoplastic 38
paraovarian 32
parasitic 59
parovarian 105
sebaceous 20, 21*f*, 205*f*, 600
simple 55*f*
Cystadenoma
benign
mucinous 55, 56*f*
serous 49*f*, 55, 55*f*
multiloculated mucinous 56*f*
serous 52*f*, 55*f*
Cystectomy 55*f*, 59, 368*f*, 602
ovarian 59, 60, 60*f*, 349*f*, 551, 559*f*, 573*f*
Cystic degeneration 93, 93*f*
Cystic endometrial changes 39, 132
Cystic fibrosis 250, 263
transmembrane conductance regulator gene 267
Cystic teratoma, benign 56, 57*f*
Cystocele 27, 204, 210, 211*f*, 212, 218, 218*f*, 219, 219*f*, 228, 229*f*, 237

displacement 211, 212*f*
distension 211
midline 212, 212*f*
repair of 230*f*
Cystometry 391
Cystoscopy 146, 200, 395
Cystourethroscopy 380
Cytobrush 175, 176, 524, 538, 538*f*
Cytokines 429
Cytology 64, 66
classification 176
systems of 177*t*
liquid-based 175, 176
Cytoplasmic syngamy 425
Cytoreductive surgery, secondary 72
Cytotrophoblast 428

D

Danazol 122, 123, 128, 300, 365, 366
Darifenacin 393
Das's dilator 533
Daytime urinary frequency 217
Death, causes of 161
Deaver's retractor 522*f*
Decidua basalis 418
Decidua functionalis 418
Decubitus ulcer 216, 216*f*, 219, 219*f*, 223
management of 223
site of 223
Deep dyspareunia 362
causes of 8
Deep inguinal nodes 189
Dehydration 563
Dehydroepiandrosterone sulfate 293, 300, 312, 339
Delivery, preterm 448
Dementia 434
Denonvilliers fascia 228
Density gradient centrifugation technique 280, 281
layers method of 282
Denys-Drash syndrome 330
Deoxyribonucleic acid 36, 189, 196, 615
double-stranded 172
Depilation, temporary 303
Depo-provera 473
Depot medroxyprogesterone acetate 94, 123, 126, 510
benefits of 474
mechanism of action of 473
Depression, treatment of 436
Dermal papilla
destruction of 305
enzyme of 305
Dermoid cyst 56, 57*f*, 74, 214*f*, 573, 573*f*
diagnosis of 40
Desmopressin 122
Desogestrel 471
Detrusor overactivity 243, 389
diagnosis of 392
surgery for 395

Dexamethasone 268, 271, 303, 304
   test 303
Diabetes mellitus 8, 93, 135, 248, 250, 262, 263, 289, 293, 296, 311
Diaphragm 463
Diazoxide 300
Didelphic uterus 446f
Dienogest 366, 465
Diethylstilbestrol 439
Digital vaginal examination 338
Dihydroepiandrosterone 346
Dihydrotestosterone 300, 301, 355
Dilatation, Frank method of 453
Diploid cells-46 422
Disorder of sexual differentiation, management of 332, 355
Dissecting forceps 505f, 523f, 526f
Disseminated peritoneal adenomucinosis 64
Distension media 560, 561
Diverticulitis 358
DNA fragmentation index 267
Dominant follicle 416, 420
Donor oocyte 326
Donovan bodies, detection of 611
Dopamine agonist 268, 270
   pregnancy rate of 270
Dorsal supine position 14, 18f, 217, 378
Double-blind study 593
Double-layer method 282
Douglas pouch 32, 46, 102, 158, 225, 238f, 256f, 357, 359
Doxycycline 611
Doyen's retractor 521f
Drospirenone 465, 470
Drugs
   interaction 468
   side effects of 393
Dryness, vaginal 434
Ducreyi bacillus, culture of 611
Duhrssen's incision 246
Dydrogesterone 366
Dye
   test 251, 258, 380
   types of 580
Dynein bands 422
Dysfunctional uterine bleeding 5, 84, 117, 304, 544, 549
   status of 117
Dysgenesis, gonadal 319, 329
Dysgerminoma 52, 53, 74, 7575f
Dyskaryosis 170, 171
Dyslipidemia 8, 296
Dysmenorrhea 7, 82, 86, 123, 352, 362, 371, 373
   congestive 374
   membranous 374
   primary 7, 373, 374
   secondary 7, 373, 374
   severe 359f, 373f
   spasmodic 374
Dyspareunia 8, 118, 362, 371

   causes of 6
   superficial 8
Dysplasia 170, 177
Dysuria 158, 200, 434

E

Ectocervix 164
Ectopic pregnancy 32, 38, 113, 444, 487, 502, 553, 606
   relation of 487
Ectovaginal septum 32
Edema 9, 160
   demonstration 9f
   vulva 9f
Edge-pairing technique 385
Eflornithine 304
   hydrochloride 303, 305
Egg, transport of 425
Ejaculated semen 421f
Ejaculation 424
   treatment of premature 286
Ejaculatory duct obstruction 265
Ejaculatory dysfunction 286
   treatment of 285, 286
Ejaculatory failure 285
Elagolix 367
Electrocoagulation 181
Electrolysis 305
Electrosurgical loop 182
Elephantiasis, vulvar 187
Embryo 285, 429
   donation 285
   third day cleaved 278f, 427f
   transfer 250, 275, 279, 279f
      catheter 279f
Embryoendometrial synchronization 428
Emergency contraceptive 464, 476, 477t, 482
   effects of 478
   methods 478
   pill 461, 461f, 470, 471, 477, 477f
Empirical therapy 280, 294
Encephalitis 311
Endocervical adenocarcinoma 28f
   in situ 171
Endocervical canal 35f, 175
Endocervix 164, 172
Endocrinal disorder 113
Endocrine disorder 263
Endocrine profile 293
Endodermal sinus tumor 52, 53, 74, 76
Endometrial ablation 97, 102, 126
Endometrial biopsy 118, 120, 120f, 136, 138f, 145, 146, 251, 254, 255, 615
   future of 255
   indications of 146
   methods of 120
Endometrial cancer 8, 9, 38, 40f, 134, 135, 136, 138f, 141f, 143, 144, 146, 433, 544, 575, 576f
   incidence of 135

   lymphatic spread of 140f
   prevalence of 143
   prognosis of 143
   spread of 139
   types of 138
Endometrial carcinoma 30, 40, 84, 115f, 133, 135, 139, 143, 144
   curettage of 136
   management of 140
   stages of 140
Endometrial cycle 252f, 413, 415f, 420
Endometrial dysfunction, primary 127
Endometrial hyperplasia 110, 113, 130, 130f, 131, 131f, 132, 134, 135, 144, 146, 480
   varieties of 131
Endometrial intraepithelial neoplasia 131
Endometrial pathology 38
Endometrial polyp 30, 37f, 38, 39f, 41, 86f, 87f, 113, 117, 119f, 120f, 121f, 134, 135, 144, 146, 560, 562f
   small 118f
Endometrial sampling 35, 118, 132
Endometrial stromal sarcoma 147
Endometrial thickness 145, 257f, 339
Endometrioma 359f
   aspiration of 368f
Endometriosis 32, 47, 48, 62, 84, 88, 113, 262, 272, 352, 354, 358, 360, 362-366, 368, 369, 369fc, 372, 374, 559f, 600, 614
   adenomyosis 356
   causes of 362
   classification of 362, 370f
   clinical features of 362
   diagnosis of 363, 364
   etiology of 361
   fertility index score 362
   incidence of 358
   management of 368
   prevalence of 365
   risk factors of 358
   signs of 363
   site of 358, 359f
   surgical management of 367
   symptoms of 362
   treatment modalities of 365
   umbilical 361f
   varieties of 372
Endometritis 280
Endometrium 39, 363, 418, 428, 429, 433, 613, 614
   ablative procedure on 551
   absence of 321
   atrophic 41, 144
   curettage of 137f
   defective 294
   homogeneous thickened 39, 132
   preparation of 426
   proliferative 254f, 419f
   thickness of 130f, 137f, 418
   transcervical resection of 126

Endomyometrial junction 371*f*, 372*f*
Endtz test 266
Enterocele 210, 211, 211*f*, 219*f*, 220, 222, 222*f*
 formation 454
 management of 245
 repair of 225, 234, 237
Enucleation 100, 101*f*
ENZIAN staging system 362
Eosin nigration test 265
Eosinophilic cells 252*f*
Epicanthal folds 319
Epididymal obstruction 263
Epididymal sperm aspiration 283
Epididymis 263, 421
Epididymitis 250
Epigastrium 14
Epilation 305
 temporary 303
Epilepsy 8
Epimenorrhea 7, 113
Episiotomy scar 361
Epithelial cells 54
 proliferation of 151*f*
Epithelial ovarian cancer 51, 62, 71
 early 70
 prognosis of 72
 spread of 66
 treatment assessment of 71
Epithelial stromal tumors 53
Epithelial tumors, mixed 53
Epithelial vulvar diseases, classification of 198, 199*t*
Epithelioid trophoblastic tumor 151, 154, 155, 155*f*
Epithelium
 normal 170
 stratification of 72
Equine estrogen 125
Erectile dysfunction 285
 treatment of 285, 286
Erectile failure 285
Erosion 20
Erythrocyte sedimentation rate 85
Escherichia coli 602
Essure 498
Estradiol 255, 256, 257, 342, 346
 early 257
 serum 339
 transdermal 436
Estrogen 94, 144, 298, 301, 342, 415, 416, 420, 432, 433, 436, 437, 464, 470, 472
 cream 352
 deficiency 338
 dose of 122
 effects of 253*f*, 254*f*
 extraovarian production of 362
 high-dose 122
 injectable 122
 lowering dose of 465
 progesterone 366, 369
  contraceptives, use of 122

 pill, combined 122, 466*f*
 therapy 435
 treatment 343
 protection 434
 receptor modulator, selective 95, 135, 268, 367
 status 339
  assessment of 339
 therapy 135, 435, 436
  contraindications of 437
Ethinyl estradiol 304, 355, 476
Ethiodol 258
Etonogestrel 476
Etoposide 75, 155
Eugonadotropic eugonadal anovulation 261
Excision 197, 198, 604
Exercise 268
Exfoliation 66
Exophytic growth 164*f*
Exosalpingitis 613
External anal sphincters 402
External beam radiotherapy 142
External genitalia 23*f*, 187*f*, 290, 311*f*, 320, 439
 examination 315, 332
 inspection of 19, 20, 158, 249, 401
 observations of 20
 palpation of 19, 20, 158, 249, 401, 403
Ezy-pill 471, 511

F

Facies, examination of 10
Fallopian tube 61, 61*f*, 67, 68*t*, 320, 359, 438, 499*f*, 542*f*, 544, 570, 613, 613*f*
 cancer 73, 73*f*
 carcinoma 38
 fimbriae 61
 sperm perfusion 283
 tuberculosis of 613*f*
Falloposcopy 261
Family planning 459, 461, 510
 methods, use of 510
 programs 509
  milestones of 510
Fascia
 endopelvic 208
 laxity of 209*f*
 paravaginal 394
 prerectal 231, 232*f*, 233*f*, 406*f*, 407
Fatty degeneration 92, 92*f*
Female condom 463, 492, 492*f*
Female infertility 257, 275, 279
 management of 268
Female metallic catheter 516*f*, 528, 529*f*, 547*f*
Female sterilization 463, 495, 502, 503, 553
 effects of 502
 failure of 502
 health benefits of 502
Femilon 467

Femoral vessels 193
Fenton's operation 279, 287, 551
Fern test 252-254
Ferning pattern 254
Ferriman-Gallwey scoring system 302, 302*f*, 336
Fertility
 awareness 493
  methods 494
 control 461
 highest time of 417
 indicators 509
 outcome following tubal surgery 275
 potential for 332
 rate, total 509
 sparing conservative management 144
Fertilization 267*f*, 413, 422*f*, 424, 426*f*
 impaired 294
Fesoterodine 393
Fetal growth restriction 292, 444
Fetal heart sound 46
Fibroid 30, 37, 50, 98, 262
 cystic degeneration of 93*f*
 degenerations of 93*f*
 fatty degeneration of 92*f*
 infected 102
 multiple 91*f*, 101*f*, 102, 571*f*
 parasitic 90
 polyp 28*f*, 107, 108, 205-207
 solitary 86*f*
 subserous 90*f*, 570, 571*f*
 types of 115*f*
 uterus 30, 32, 47, 84, 85, 86, 113, 570, 585, 586*f*
  diagnosis of 84
  management of 94
 varieties of 88*f*
Fibroma 80*f*, 81, 600, 601*f*
 ovarian 80*f*
 vaginal 22*f*, 205*f*
 vulvar 20
Fibrous histiocytoma, malignant 189
Filshie clip 500*f*
Fimbrial cyst 32, 105
 bilateral 105*f*
Fimbrioplasty 273, 275
Finasteride 304
Fine-needle aspiration cytology 38, 189
Fistula 378, 379*f*
 margin scar tissue 383
 perineal 20
 urethrovaginal 381*f*
 varieties of 381*f*
Fitz-Hugh-Curtis syndrome 606, 611
Flap splitting method 383
Flat condyloma 179*f*
Fluid
 balance 392
 choice of 565
 compartments 565
 deficits 565
 intravenous 564

management, postoperative 564
  principles of quantity of 565
  thrill 16
  thrill, demonstration of 18f
Fluorodeoxyglucose positron emission tomography 200
Flushing curette 518, 534f
Flutamide 304
Foley catheter 98, 384f, 516, 529, 529f, 540
  guidewire for 395f
  tourniquets of 98
Follicle
  cohort of 415
  depletion of 433
  maturing multiple 270f
  multiple 38f, 291f
  ovulatory 415
  preovulatory 414
  secondary 413
  stimulating hormone 122, 249, 252, 261, 266, 289, 295, 311, 313, 314, 317, 333, 424, 336, 340, 416, 417, 432
    recombinant 269
    serum 346
  tertiary 413, 416
Follicular development 416
Fornix
  anterior 32
  lateral 31, 32
  posterior 32
Fothergill's operation 8, 225, 231, 233, 234f, 236, 236f, 245, 551
  complications of 236
  components of 234
  indications of 234
  steps of 234
Fothergill's stitch 235, 235f, 236f
Frasier syndrome 330
Fructose 266
Functional cyst 38, 53, 54
  characteristics of 53
  different varieties of 53
Fundus 238f, 438, 551
Fusion, cranial ends of 438

G

Gait, examination of 217
Galactorrhea 12, 248, 251, 263, 301, 338, 340
  amenorrhea syndrome 340
  causes of 340
Gamete intrafallopian transfer 279, 285
Ganirelix 367
Gardnerella vaginalis 6, 35, 36, 610
Gartner duct cyst 20, 22f, 27, 205, 205f, 207, 600
Gastrointestinal lump 47, 84
Gastrointestinal system 83, 12, 134, 150, 158, 186, 203, 248, 357, 467
Gastrointestinal tract 359
Gellhorn pessary 224

Gem cell tumor 76
Genetic disorder 8, 250, 285
Genetic sex 328
Genital fistula 380
  milestones of 381
Genital hiatus 215, 221f
Genital malignancy 170
Genital organs, development of 438
Genital prolapse 32, 202, 216, 223, 445f
  examination of 204f
Genital system 467
  female 438
  male 438
Genital tract
  anomalies 439
  female 424, 507
  male 504f
Genital tuberculosis 37, 605, 612
Genitalia
  external 20f, 600
  internal 332
  prepubertal external 319, 319f
Genitourinary fistula 378, 380, 454
  classification of 380, 381
  diagnosis of 379, 380
Germ cell 52, 53f, 414f
  layers 76f
  mixed 53, 74
  primary 422
  sex cord 53
  tumor 53, 54, 56, 74, 573
    diagnosis of 74
    malignant 62, 75
    mixed 52, 76, 354f
    treatment of 74
Gestation, multiple 268
Gestational trophoblastic disease 37, 53, 54, 151, 481
  classification of 151
Gestational trophoblastic neoplasia 7, 149, 151, 153f, 154
  treatment of 154
Gestodene 469
Gestrinone 365, 366
Gilliam's operation 279, 551
Glands 419
  bulbourethral 421
  endometrial 418
Glandular cell 171
  atypical 171
Glandular growth 418
Glandular lumen 419
Glassy cell 164
Glucose 564
  tolerance test 293
Gluteal pain 243
Glycine 560
Glycophilic squamous epithelium 180f
Gonadal dysgenesis
  mixed 331
  pure 319, 325
Gonadal function 332

Gonadal sex 328
Gonadectomy 323f, 334t
  timing of 334
Gonadoblastoma 53
Gonadotropin 34, 268, 269, 294, 317, 337, 420
  dependent precocious puberty 349
  dose of 269
  independent precocious puberty 347, 349
    problems of 347
  indications of 269
  levels of 317
  preparation of 269
  regulators of 417, 417f
  releasing hormone 125, 126, 268, 276, 277, 295, 304, 319, 333, 339, 346, 351, 366, 369, 417, 424, 432
    agonists 94, 122, 123, 272, 303, 365, 366
    analogs 268
    antagonist 95, 276, 365, 367
    etiology of 347
    stimulation test 332, 349
  results of 270
  risk of 270
  stimulation 270f
  use of 424
Gonads 331
Gonorrhea 36, 37, 610
  diagnosis of 36
Gossypol 508
G-protein alpha subunit, genetic mutation of 347
Graafian follicle 413, 416
Graft rejection 454
Gram stain 36, 37
Gram-negative intracellular diplococci 36, 37, 610
Granuloma inguinale 611
Granulosa cell 415
  tumor 52, 53, 77, 77f, 348f-350f,
Grave's disease 199
Groin dissection 193f
Growth
  endometrial 560
  factors 429
  hormone 321
  hypertrophic 164f
  malignant 27
  over vulva 186f
  tuberculous 27
Grumbach syndrome 351f
Gum 10
Gunshot lesion 364
Gynandroblastoma 53, 77, 80
Gynecological disease 8
Gynecological emergencies 93
Gynecomastia 263
Gynefix intrauterine device 490

H

Hair
- balding loss of 315f
- distribution 251
- duration of survival of 306
- excessive growth of 338
- follicle, structure of 306f
- length of survival of 306
- loss, permanent 305
- pattern, male 298f
- phases of 306, 306f
- physiology of 305
- removal
  - permanent 303
  - physical methods of 305
- structure of 305
- terminal 305, 306
- types of 305

HAIR-AN syndrome 292, 293f, 301, 338f
Hamartoma 601, 602f
- hypothalamic 347f

Hand instruments 556f
Hanging drop test 557
Hard stool 32
Hart line 188
Hasson technique 557
Haultain's technique 550, 550f
Hawkin-Ambler's cervical dilator 518f, 533, 533f
Headache 338
Healthy skin, margin of 195f
Heart
- auscultation of 83, 134, 150, 158, 186, 203, 248, 357
- disease
  - ischemic 8, 125
  - severe 554

Heavy menstrual bleeding 7, 82, 89f, 110, 112, 115, 117, 125, 126, 128, 342f, 369, 371, 373f
- causes of 7, 128

Hegar's cervical dilator 518, 533, 533f
Hemangioma 600
Hematocrit estimation 112
Hematoma 563
- hypothalamic 349
- vulvar 600

Hematometra 30, 37, 315f, 316f, 451
Hematuria 158, 200
Hemoglobin 84
Hemogram, complete 189
Hemoperitoneum 358
Hemorrhage 52f, 88, 93, 161, 236, 243
- intracystic 58
- intraperitoneal 502
- postpartum 4, 373, 443
- secondary 195
- severe 98
- torrential 152f

Hemorrhoids 402
Hemostasis 98

Hepatoblastoma 347
Hereditary nonpolyposis colorectal cancer syndrome 8, 62, 135, 145
Hermaphrodite 330
Hernia 263
- incisional 502
- indirect inguinal 20

Herpes simplex virus 172, 189
High-arch palate 319, 320f
HIPEC therapy 71
Hirsutism 10f, 34, 38, 78f, 251, 297, 298f, 299f, 300, 302, 303, 311, 312, 314, 315f, 338, 348
- causes of 297, 298
- evaluation of 301, 303
- idiopathic 300
- therapy for 303, 303t

Hodge-Smith pessary 524f, 537, 537f
Hook effect 340
Hormone 34, 85, 122, 249, 346, 365, 373, 435
- antidiuretic 564
- assays 266
- changes, sequence of 433
- estimation 251, 255, 256, 266
- levels 290
- profile 266
- replacement therapy 135, 186, 435
- synthesis 299f
- therapy 435-437
  - goals of 334
  - indications of 143, 334
  - risks of 437

Horse-shoe kidney 320
Hulka-Clemens spring clip 500f
Human chorionic gonadotropin 119, 155, 155f, 276, 277, 332, 333, 346
Human epididymis protein 51
Human immunodeficiency virus 172
- testing 615

Human leukocyte antigen 327
Human papilloma virus 174, 178, 179f, 183, 189, 196, 197, 467, 600
- infection 170, 172, 189
- role of 172
- testing 176
- transmission of 173
- types of 173
- vaccination 355
- vaccine 183, 197

Hyaline degeneration 92
Hydatidiform mole 113, 151, 151f, 152
Hydrocele 263
Hydrocortisone 300, 343
Hydrodissection 228
Hydronephrosis 161, 217
Hydrosalpinx, diagnosis of 38
Hydroureter 217
Hydroxyprogesterone 289, 299, 346
Hymen 279, 439
Hyperandrogenemia 295fc, 296, 298, 301

Hyperandrogenism 292, 294, 342
- features of 251, 290

Hyperinsulinemia 295, 295fc, 298f
- testing of 293

Hyperplasia 38, 39, 131, 433
- complex 131
- endometrial 110, 113, 130, 130f, 131, 131f, 132, 134, 135, 144, 146, 480
- simple 131

Hyperprolactinemia 7, 40, 250, 261-263, 294, 300, 335, 337-341
- causes of 340
- effects of 341
- treatment of 341

Hypertension 8, 135, 136, 250, 289, 296, 311, 312, 314
Hyperthecosis, ovarian 292
Hyperthyroidism 291, 337
Hypertrichosis 297, 300, 300t
Hypertrophy 27, 333
- myometrial 130

Hyphae, typical 36, 609
Hypochondrium 14
Hypoestrogenism 352
Hypogastrium 14
Hypoglycemia 310f
Hypogonadism
- eugonadotropic 313
- hypogonadotropic 250, 261, 308, 310, 311f, 313, 327
- idiopathic hypogonadotropic 328

Hypogonadotropic hypogonadism 250, 261, 308, 310, 311f, 313, 327
- causes of 328t

Hypomenorrhea 7, 112, 113
Hyponatremia 310f
Hypo-osmotic swelling test 265, 267
Hypoplasia 322
Hypospadias 263, 326f
Hyposperm 266
Hypothalamic-pituitary-ovarian 117, 128
Hypothalamus 313, 337
- arcuate nucleus of 420

Hypothesis 590
Hypothyroidism 113, 250, 261, 263, 291, 294, 311, 335, 341, 342f
- severe primary 347

Hypoxia 565
- postoperative 565

Hysterectomy 62, 85, 97, 104, 105, 107f, 126, 132, 142f, 144, 154, 155, 180, 182, 361, 373, 374, 539, 544, 570
- abdominal 69f, 140, 362, 368f, 369, 445f
- approaches of 539
- clamp 520f, 535, 535f
- classification of 540
- complications of 544
- extrafascial 142
- indications of 544
- obstetric 544
- steps of 570
- subtotal 539, 569

Index

supracervical 539
total abdominal 369
types of 166, 167*t*, 539, 569
vaginal 8, 102*f*, 107*f*, 203, 227, 236, 237, 240*f*, 245
Hystero-laparoscope 261
Hysterosalpingo-contrast-sonography 260
Hysterosalpingography 34, 37, 41, 41*f*, 249-251, 258, 258*f*, 260, 579*f*-583*f*, 615
cannula 258*f*, 537, 537*f*
catheter 260*f*
complications of 580
indications of 537, 579
plates 579
Hysteroscope 87, 372, 499, 559, 560*f*
contraindications of 561
Hysteroscopic septal resection 449*f*, 562*f*
Hysteroscopy 34, 85, 121, 136, 559
ambulatory 559
procedure of 561*f*
role of 87
Hysterosonography 120
Hysterosonosalpingography catheter 447*f*
Hysterotomy 361

I

Iceberg sign, tip of 57
Iliac artery 95*f*
internal 522*f*
Iliac fossa 14
Iliac lymph nodes 165
external 546
Iliococcygeus colpopexy 225
Iliopectineal ligament 394
Imipramine hydrochloride 393
Immature teratoma 52, 54, 74, 75, 76*f*
Immotile cilia syndrome 250, 263, 422
Immune tolerance 429
Immunobead test 266
Immunological test 266, 267
Immunomodulation 429
Immunosuppression 189
Impaired glucose tolerance 296
Imperforate hymen 20, 23*f*, 313-315, 315*f*, 316*f*, 321, 323, 323*f*, 352
Implantation 426
bleeding 113
failure 294
luteolysis, absence of 420
morphological steps of 428
window 427
In vitro fertilization 38, 250, 255, 275, 278, 279, 369
steps of 277*f*
In vitro maturation 285
Incision, vertical 99, 237, 396
Incontinence 390, 393, 434
Infections 58, 88, 92, 161, 216, 262, 487
gonococcal 36, 606
prevention 482
postoperative 565
vaginal 34

Infertility 38, 82, 247, 249, 250, 261, 262, 272, 292, 362, 368, 369, 369*fc*, 372, 373, 579
causes of 86, 262, 294
female 249, 257, 275, 279
incidence of 249
male 262
reasons of 363
treatment of 581
types of 249
unexplained 269, 287
Inflammatory bowel syndrome 358
Infracoccygeus vaginal sling, posterior 226, 243, 244*f*
Infundibulopelvic ligament 61, 61*f*, 540*f*, 542
clamping of 542*f*
Inguinal gland enlargement 160
Inguinal incision, repair of 194*f*
Inhibin 432
A 417
B 257, 417
Injectable contraceptives 338, 472
contraindications of 474
types of 472
Injury
ureteric 387
vulvar 353*f*
Inner cell mass 426
Insemination 280, 282
intraperitoneal 283
Insler score 253
Insomnia 378
Insulin 298
like growth factor-1 351
resistance 292, 296
sensitizing agents 268, 294, 303, 304
Intact cervix 570
Intermenstrual bleeding 7, 89*f*, 110, 113, 115, 157
causes of 85
Intersex 38
Intestinal peristaltic sounds 564
Intestines, tuberculosis of 613*f*
Intracytoplasmic sperm injection 280, 283, 284*f*
advantages of 284
indications of 283
procedure of 283
results of 284
Intrafollicular insemination 283
Intramural fibroid 86*f*, 90*f*, 93*f*
Intraperitoneal chemotherapy 71
dose of 71
Intraperitoneal collection, detection of 40
Intrauterine contraceptive device 8, 35, 111, 119, 461, 464, 477, 478, 481, 487*f*, 489*f*, 491, 525*f*, 560, 583*f*, 584, 585*f*
advantages of 481
complications of 485
disadvantages of 481

frameless 490*f*
in situ 487
insertion 482
procedure of 488
misplaced 585*f*
noncontraceptive uses of 481
postpartum 488, 489*f*, 525*f*
remove 477, 488
types of 478
Intrauterine insemination 248, 275, 279, 280, 283, 283*f*, 286, 368, 369
basic steps of 280*fc*
cannula 283*f*
indications of 280
set-up 281*f*
Intrauterine progestogen-releasing systems 123
Intrauterine system, hormone containing 122
Intrinsic sphincteric defect 390
Introitus 279
Invasion, depth of 196
Invasive cancer 178
cervix
management of primary 166*t*
treatment modalities of 166
Invasive carcinoma, development of 174*fc*
Invasive mole 151, 152
Involution, stage of 418
Iron therapy 122
Irving technique 498, 498*f*
Isthmocele 130

J

Jadelle and Sino-implant 474
Jaundice 10
Jones metroplasty, modified 453

K

Kallmann syndrome 261, 311, 328
Kartagener's syndrome 263, 263*f*, 265, 422
Karyotype 287, 315, 332, 343
Kelly's forceps 488, 489*f*, 525
Kelly's operation 394
Kelly's plasty 226
Kelly's suture 230
Ketoconazole 303, 304
Keyes punch biopsy 188, 197
Khanna's abdominal sling operation 241
Kidney 12, 204, 456
enlarged 79
function 189
palpation of 15, 16*f*
Kiss ulcer 188, 188*f*
Klinefelter syndrome 250, 263, 264, 264*f*, 267, 287, 330
Knee
chest position 378
elbow position 16

Koch's peritonitis 47, 48, 84
Kocher's artery forceps 519f
Koilocytosis 172
Korotkoff phase 11
Kraurosis vulvae 198
Kroener's fimbriectomy technique 498, 499f
Krukenberg tumor 53, 79, 79f, 574f
    primary of 79
Kustner's operation 551

L

Labia
    fusion of 352f
    majora 20, 190, 439, 600
        anterior part of 190
        shrinkage of 435
    minora 20, 190, 231, 352, 405, 435, 439, 600
        anterior part of 190
    separation of 24f
Labial adhesion 352, 352f
Labiaplasty 334
Labioscrotal fusion 326f
Labor, preterm 38, 444
Lactate dehydrogenase 51
Lactation 337, 338, 400
    failure 338
Lactational amenorrhea method 494
Lactobacillus 605
Landon's retractor 221, 237, 239f, 521f, 536, 536f
Lane's tissue forceps 519, 534, 535f
Lanugo hair 305
Laparoscope 309, 526f
    insertion of 558
    telescope of 526f
    trocar for 526f
Laparoscopic chromopertubation test 260
Laparoscopic dye test 261f, 558f
Laparoscopic ligation 500f
    instruments for 499f, 556f
    set 526f
Laparoscopic ovarian drilling 272, 294, 294f, 559f
Laparoscopic procedure 557
Laparoscopic sterilization 499
    advantages of 501
    disadvantages of 501
Laparoscopic surgery 553
    advantages of 553
    disadvantages of 553
Laparoscopic uterine
    artery occlusion 85, 102
    nerve ablation 374, 376
Laparoscopy 34, 59, 85, 251, 256, 257, 261, 290, 312, 332, 364, 367, 372, 501f, 607, 615
    adjunctive 449
    chromopertubation test 251, 258
    complications of 558
    role of 88, 364
    surgical 553
Laparotomy 56f, 65f, 80f, 97, 349f, 367, 550
    steps of 60
Large bowel disorder 358
Laser 182
    ablation 181, 197, 198
    hair removal 303, 305
Last menstrual period 6, 82, 110, 133, 149, 157, 247, 288
Latent syphilis 612
Latzko vaginal repair 385
Lawson Wilkins Pediatric Endocrine Society 328
Lax perineum 210, 231f
Le Fort's operation 225, 226, 241
Lead pipe 390
Leg
    raising test 15
    veins 11
Leiomyomas 38, 86, 91f, 92, 92f, 98, 114, 115f, 455
    uterus 41
    submucosal 38
Leiomyomatosis 86
Leiomyosarcoma 147, 147f, 148t, 189
Lesions 187, 360, 530
    endometrial 34
    types of 364
Letrozole 261, 268, 269
Leukemias 53
Leukocytes 266
Leukocytospermia 266
Leukoplakia 20, 178, 198, 207f
    vulva 21f
Leukorrhea 35
    causes of 35
Leuprolide acetate 124
Levator ani 231, 404
    muscle 208
Levonorgestrel-intrauterine system 122, 123, 125, 126, 128, 129, 143, 366, 480f
    contraindications of 481
    emily 480
    mirena 367, 480, 480f
    noncontraceptive uses of 480
Leydig cell 423
    tumor 53
Lichen sclerosus 189, 196, 199, 352, 353
    et atrophicus 20, 198
Life table method 463
Ligaments
    laxity of 209f
    ovarian 61, 61f, 90, 542f
Lip, posterior 30f, 235f, 532
Lipid profile 189
Lipoma 20, 600, 600f
Lippes loop 478, 478f, 585f
Lithotomy position 218, 396, 548f
Live birth rate 444
Liver 15, 134, 158, 186, 203, 248, 347, 357, 456
    function test 189
    metastasis 340
    palpation of 15f
Local vaginal estrogen, low-dose 437
Local vasopressin injection 99
Loop electrosurgical excision procedure 163, 181, 182f, 183
L-ornithine decarboxylase 305
Lower uterine fibroid, posterior 32
Lugol's iodine, application of 180f
Lumbar vertebra 452
Lump
    abdomen 45, 75f, 78f, 82, 147f, 343f, 344f, 570
        differential diagnosis of 47, 84
    growth of 88
    lower abdomen, causes of 6, 47
Lung metastasis, detection of 41
Luteal phase
    defect 255, 262
    progesterone 123
Luteal support 279, 283
Luteinizing hormone 249, 252, 261, 266, 269, 289, 295, 313, 317, 333, 340, 346, 416, 417, 424
Luteolysis 418
Lymph node 69f, 165, 165f, 167f
    dissection, steps of 168, 546
    dissector 525f
    inguinal 187, 189
    involvement 163, 196, 340
    paracervical 165
    parametrial 165
    rectal 165
    superficial 194f
Lymphadenectomy 142, 168f, 169, 169f, 546f
    bilateral inguinofemoral 193f
    inguinal 576
    inguinofemoral 191
    para-aortic 140
Lymphatic
    spread 66, 139, 140f, 165
    vulvar 190
Lymphogranuloma
    inguinale 611
    venereum 187
Lymphography 189
Lymphoma
    malignant 53
    retroperitoneal 47, 84
Lynch syndrome 62, 135, 143

M

MacKenrodt's ligament 208f, 209, 231, 234, 234f, 235, 236, 240f, 245
    clamping of 541f, 543f
    cutting of 541f
    tightening of 234
Macroadenoma 337, 341
Macroprolactin 340, 341

Madlener technique 498
Magic pill 461
Magnetic resonance imaging 37, 40, 85, 97, 189, 200, 315, 317, 341, 392
Maine coast 347, 348
Mala N 466f, 467, 471, 511
Male condom 460f, 463, 491, 491f
Male contraceptive
    hormonal method of 507
    summary of 508
Male fertility regulation 507
Male infertility 262, 267
    assessment of 266
    causes of 250, 262, 262t, 285
    etiology of 250
    management of 280
Male sterilization 503
    eligibility of 506
    medical eligibility criteria for 506
Male subfertility 266, 266t, 267
    treatment of 280
Male-balding pattern 312, 314
Malignancy 87, 88, 92, 93, 102, 114
    chance of 56
    gynecological 135
    index, risk of 51, 51t
Malignant melanoma 188, 600
    vagina 200f, 201f
Malignant ovarian tumor 40f, 50, 52f, 64, 65f, 66f, 574, 574f
    extent of 40
Malnutrition 161, 217
Manchester operation 233
Mantoux test 614
Marshall's test 391, 393
Marshall-Marchetti colposuspension 393
Marsupialization 327, 603, 603f, 604, 604f
Masigna 474
Mass 16, 31, 32
    causes of 32
Matrix metalloproteinases 429
Maturation index 435
Maturity, stage of 418
Mayer-Rokitansky-Küster-Hauser syndrome 308, 309, 309f, 315, 321, 321f, 322t, 329, 451
    incidence of 452
Mayo's scissor 521f
McCall's culdoplasty 225, 226, 244
McCune-Albright syndrome 347, 348
McIndoe vaginoplasty 454f
McIndoe-Reed operation 452
Medroxyprogesterone acetate 125, 126, 334, 366
Meigs syndrome 81
Meigs-Navratil forceps 522f
Meiosis 413
Melanoma, malignant 188, 600
Membrana granulosa 416
Menarche 250
    age of 7, 82, 110, 149, 157, 289
    early 93
    late 62

Meningitis, childhood 311
Menometrorrhagia 112, 113
Menopausal hormone therapy 435
Menopausal syndrome 544
Menopausal transition 431, 436, 437
Menopause 7, 160f, 210, 337, 431, 433, 434, 437
    consequences of 433
    early 62
    effects of 433t
    late 62, 432
    management of 435
    physiology of 432
    premature 8
    transition 433
Menorrhagia 7, 82, 84, 112, 128, 352, 362, 485
    causes of 85, 113
Menstrual abnormality 342
    types of 290
Menstrual bleeding, normal 116
Menstrual calendar 112
Menstrual cycles, normal 471
Menstrual disorders 352
Menstrual function 318, 321
Menstrual irregularity 50, 292
Menstruation 117, 337, 413, 420
    control of 313fc
    duration of 7, 82, 110, 149, 157, 288
    normal 112
    physiology of 418
    resumption of 452
Mesh
    traction of 244f
    use of 245
Mesovarium 61, 61f
Metabolic syndrome 292, 296
    diagnostic clinical criteria of 296
    management of 296
    monitoring for 296
Metal catheter 529, 547f
Metallic malleable uterine sound 518, 532f
Metastasis over peritoneum 69f
Metformin 271, 294, 304
Methotrexate 155
Methyldopa 300
Metoclopramide 300
Metronidazole 610
Metropathia hemorrhagica 129
Metroplasty 279
    hysteroscopic 449
Metrorrhagia 7, 85, 112, 113
Metzenbaum scissor 227, 237, 521f
Microadenoma 337, 341
Microinvasive disease, staging of 163
Microsurgery 274
    epididymal sperm aspiration 280, 283
    principle of 274
Microwave ablation 126, 127
Micturition
    cystourethrography 392
    mechanism of 389

Midurethral sling 394, 394f
Mifepristone 95, 365, 367
Minerals 430
Minimal access surgery 553
Minimal invasive surgery, role of 70
Minoxidil 300
Mirabegron 393
Mirena insertion 483, 485f, 485f
Miscarriage 250, 280, 444, 448
    management of 559
Missing pill 468
    management of 469t
Mitosis 413
Mitra's operation 167, 169
Mitra's radical vaginal hysterectomy 575f
Miya hook 243
Mobile retroversion, correction of 524f
Molluscum contagiosum 20, 612
Monophasic combined oral contraceptive pills 129, 465, 466
Mons pubis 600
Mood disturbance 352, 433
Morning after pill 476, 477
Morphology, ovarian 291f
Morula, formation of 426
Mosaic pattern 178
Moschcowitz operation 225
Mosquito forceps 409f, 520f
Motile protozoal organism 36, 610
Mucinous cystadenoma ovary 56f
Mucinous epithelial ovarian carcinoma 51
Mucosa, nonneoplastic epithelial disorders of 198
Müllerian agenesis 313, 314
    complete 321
Müllerian anomaly 37, 38, 40, 322, 352, 438, 441, 453
    classification of 439, 440f, 441f
    diagnosis of 443
    effects of 441
    management of 322, 355
    prevalence of 441
    surgery on 551
Müllerian duct 438, 439
Müllerian hypoplasia, segmental 439
Müllerian tissue 90
Müllerian tumor, malignant mixed 147
Müllerian, renal, cervicothoracic somite syndrome 322
Multichannel cystometrics, procedure of 392
Multiload copper 375 460f, 471, 478, 479f, 511
    insertion of 483
Multiphasic pill 465
Multiple cystic bone lesions 347
Multiple pregnancy 269, 295
    rate 279
Multiple small hypoechoic cysts 38f, 290f
Mumps 262
Muscle, perineal 231, 233f
Mycobacterium tuberculosis 613

Mycoplasma hominis 272
Myohyperplasia 130*f*
Myoid cells 423
Myolysis 85, 97, 102
Myoma 87
    bed, closure of 99*f*
    enucleation of 101*f*
    screw 521, 535, 535*f*
        traction of 101*f*
    staging system of 99*f*
Myomatous erythrocytosis syndrome 86
Myomectomy 85, 97, 98*f*, 100*f*, 101, 101*f*, 104, 105, 126, 279, 551, 570
    abdominal 98
    disadvantages of 101
    hysteroscopic 97
    laparoscopic 97, 98*f*, 559*f*
    open 98
    robotic 97, 98
    route of 97
    vaginal 97, 98
Myometrium 39, 141*f*
Myxoid degeneration 93

N

Nabothian cyst 172
Nabothian follicle 172
Neck 421
    gland 10, 160
    veins 10
    webbing of 309*f*, 319, 320*f*
Necrosis 92
Necrozoospermia 265, 266
Needle
    aspiration 161
    holder 522*f*, 556*f*
    suspension 393, 395
Neisseria gonorrhoeae 36, 272, 353
Neocervix 236*f*
    formation of 234, 236*f*
Neoplastic disease 467
Neovagina
    construction 334
    creation of 322
Nestorone 465
Neurectomy, presacral 367, 374, 376
Neurofibroma 600
Neurofibromatosis 347
Neurological disorder 203
Neurological systems 12
Nevi 319
Nexplanon 475, 475*f*
    insertion of 475
Nickerson-Sabouraud media 36
Nipple
    examination of 111, 134, 150, 158, 186, 204, 248, 357, 401
    hypoplastic 320
Nirodh 460, 471, 511
Nocturnal penile tumescence study 263
Nodules 27
Nomegestrol 465
Noncommunicating rudimentary horn 443*f*
Noncyclic hormone pattern, development of 295
Nondescent vaginal hysterectomy 544
    basic steps of 545
    indications of 545
    suitability of 545
Nonhormonal agent 125, 125*t*, 508
Nonhormonal drug 436
Nonopioids 565
Nonoxynol-9 493
Nonscalpel vasectomy 504, 505*f*, 506*f*, 525*f*, 551
    dissecting forceps for 505*f*, 526*f*
Nonsexual hairs 306
Nonsteroidal anti-inflammatory drugs 41, 85, 111, 122, 125, 126, 366, 369
Nontouch technique 489*f*
Norethindrone 300
    acetate 127, 366
Norethynodrel 465
Norgestrel 300
Normozoospermia 266
Norplant
    rods 474*f*
    system 474, 491
Novelon 467
Nuclear
    abnormality 170
    atypia 72
    syngamy 425
Nucleic acid amplification technique 36, 611
Nulliparous 5, 55*f*, 373*f*, 570
    cervix 179*f*
    prolapse 210*f*
Nutrition 9
Nuvaring combined hormonal ring 476*f*

O

OASIS 402, 405
OASIS occult 405
Obesity 93, 135, 136, 289, 290, 292, 296, 342
    central 296, 312, 314
Obstructed hemivagina and ipsilateral renal anomaly syndrome 446*f*
Obstruction 358
    intestinal 502
Obturator
    device 527*f*
        composite set of 398*f*
    foramen 394
    fossa 169*f*
    nodes 165
Office aspiration biopsy 136
Office hysteroscopy 559
Old complete perineal tear 6*f*, 400, 401*f*
    diagnosis of 403
Oligoasthenoteratozoospermia 266
Oligomenorrhea 7, 112, 113, 247, 290, 291, 338*f*
Oligoovulation 268, 272, 294
Oligospermia 265
Oligozoospermia 266
Omentum, part of 486*f*
Oocyte 277*f*, 285, 415
    depletion 433
    donation 285
    maturation inhibitor 414
    mature 416, 417*f*
    ovulated 414*f*
    pick-up 425
    primary 413, 416
    retrieval 38, 276
    secondary 413, 414*f*, 416, 417
Oogenesis 414*f*
    process of 413
Oophorectomy 59-61, 570
    unilateral 78
Oophoropexy 59
Operative hysteroscope 527*f*
    instruments 560*f*
Oral contraceptive 63, 122, 126, 174, 300, 303
    contraindications of 468
    pill 8, 127, 363, 368
    types of 470, 470*t*
Oral progesterone, regimen of 122
Oral progestins 122
Orchidectomy estrogen therapy 324
Orchitis 250
Organism, detection of 612
Ortho cervical cap 493
Osteoporosis 434, 437, 544
    prevalence of 436
    treatment of 436
Ostitis 195
Otoxynol-9 493
Ovarian cancer 8, 62-64, 73
    diagnosis of 64
    early 68
    metastatic nodule of 32
    pathology of 63
    prognostic factors of 73
    recurrent 71
    risk of 51
    screening of 62
    stages of 67, 67*f*
    types of 53, 63
Ovarian carcinoma, epithelial 72
Ovarian cycle 252*f*, 413, 415*f*, 420
Ovarian cyst 17*f*, 32, 46, 47*f*, 56*f*, 60*f*, 62, 358, 573*f*, 614
    adhesion of 59
    infections of 59
    rupture of 59, 59*f*
    torsion of 38, 58, 58*f*, 606
Ovarian development, disorder of 330
Ovarian drilling 551
Ovarian endometrioma
    criteria for 365
    management of 368

Index

Ovarian endometriosis
　surgery for 272
　types of 359
Ovarian failure
　premature 250, 261, 294, 314, 334, 335, 337, 342
　primary 261, 294
Ovarian follicles 414
　depletion of 433
Ovarian function 363
Ovarian hormone 415f, 416
　cyclical changes of 252f
Ovarian hyperstimulation syndrome 38, 255, 268, 271, 271f, , 295
　diagnosis of 271
　pathophysiology of 271
　prediction of 272
　treatment of 271
Ovarian insufficiency, primary 335
Ovarian malignancy 32, 38, 38f, 51, 66, 71, 353, 551
　grading of 68
　risk of 51
Ovarian mass 58f
　causes of 52
　unilocular 55f
Ovarian neoplasms 52, 353
　types of 354
Ovarian pedicle, clamping of 61f
Ovarian remnant syndrome 376
Ovarian reserve 257
　markers of 257
Ovarian response, monitoring of 270
Ovarian retention syndrome 376
Ovarian tumor 32, 45, 47, 49-52, 54, 57, 58, 60, 65f, 66f, 84, 135, 299f, 353, 544, 572
　benign features of 51t
　bilateral 574f
　classification of 52, 54
　complications of 58
　diagnosis of 48
　malignant 70f
　　features of 51t
　management of 81, 354
　metastatic 79, 574
　operations of 551
　pedicle of 61f
　pure solid 54
　surgery in 354, 572
Ovarian volume 38, 257, 258
Ovariotomy 60
Ovary 32, 67, 295, 359, 613
　androgen secreting tumors of 299
　benign cyst of 572
　chocolate cyst of 32, 373f, 585, 585f
　connective tissue of 52
　dermoid cyst of 56, 57f, 573f
　dysgerminoma of 75f
　enlarged 79
　malignant tumor of 76
　simple serous cyst of 572f
　staging of 68t
　thecoma-fibroma of 80
　tumors of 53f
Overactive bladder 389, 390
Ovral-L 467
Ovulation
　detection of 251
　diagnosis of 250, 251
　folliculometry 38
　induction 268, 294
　　indications of 268
　infrequent 294
　medical induction of 268
　phase 417
　physiology of 413
　prediction kit 255
Ovulatory dysfunction 268
　management of 268
Ovum forceps 515, 528, 528f
Oxidoreductase deficiency 329
Oxybutynin 393

P

Paclitaxel 72, 75
Pad test 391
Paget's disease 189, 196, 198, 199
Pain 352, 362, 363
　causes of 85, 363, 374
　during period 7, 110, 157
　management, postoperative 565
　relief 365, 564
Pallor 9
PALM COEIN classifications 113, 114f
Palmer's point 557
Palpation, superficial 14
Pap smear 27, 34, 35f, 145, 175
　screening 118
Pap stain, role of 138
Papanicolaou classification 176
　grades of 176t
Papanicolaou grades 176
Papanicolaou slide method 175
Papanicolaou system 177
Papanicolaou test 33, 35
Papillary serous adenocarcinoma 138
Papilloma 600
Papules 20, 27
Para-aortic lymph node dissection 69f, 165
Paracentesis 66
Paramesonephric ducts 438
Parametrium 167
Pararectal space 244f
Paravaginal defect 221
　repair of 227, 228, 393
Parkland technique 498, 498f
Partial androgen insensitivity syndrome 323, 324, 325, 326f, 334
Pediatric gynecology 352
Pegylated liposomal doxorubicin 72
Pelvi-abdominal cavity 49
Pelvic adhesions 374
Pelvic cellular tissue 404

Pelvic congestion syndrome 376
Pelvic endometriosis 32, 359, 368f, 544, 553
　surgery for 272
Pelvic examination 33, 62, 375, 391
　examination of 503
Pelvic floor
　exercise 223, 286
　repair 225, 236
　strengthening 392
Pelvic infection 502, 580
　natural barrier of 605
Pelvic inflammation 358
Pelvic inflammatory disease 62, 88, 113, 125, 249, 250, 272, 374, 605, 608
　features of 605
　risk factors of 605
　stages of 606
　types of 605
Pelvic lymph nodes 167
Pelvic lymphadenectomy, indications of 140
Pelvic mass 352, 554
Pelvic organ 542
　prolapse 20, 27, 188f, 202, 203f, 207f, 211, 212, 214f, 215, 215b, 216, 217, 226, 245, 434, 524f, 537f, 551
　　anatomical classification of 210
　　compartment 210
　　diagnosis of 217
　　etiology of 209
　　grading systems of 212
　　management of 223
　　prevalence of 245
　　quantification 214, 214f, 215, 215b, 220
　　stages of 215, 215b
　　surgery in 225
　　symptoms of 217
Pelvic pain 5, 5t, 118, 200, 250, 352, 444
　characteristics of 5
Pelvic pressure 202
Pelvic surgery 381
Pelvic tuberculosis 272, 580, 613f
　clinical presentation of 614
　diagnosis of 614
Pelvis 31, 40f, 66f, 208f, 434, 558
　heaviness of 103
　transvaginal sonography of 111
　ultrasonography of 249, 289, 312, 315
Penicillamine 300
Penile urethra 311f
Percutaneous epididymal sperm aspiration 280, 283, 284f
Perineal body 215, 221f
　repair of 407
　tone of 204, 220
Perineal pouch 455
Perineal skin 233f
Perineal talc, regular use of 62
Perineal tear 404
　prevalence of 404
　types of 402

Perineorrhaphy 231
  layer method of 405
Perineum 190, 219
  deficient 20
  gynecological 20, 32
  uterovesical fold of 238f
Perirectal fascia, site specific-repair of 225
Peritoneal carcinoma, primary 64, 67, 68t
Peritoneal surfaces 66
Peritoneum, uterovesical fold of 238f, 542, 542f
Peritonitis 502, 554
Periurethral injection 394
Persona 495
Pessary
  placing of 537
  test 223, 393, 536
Pfannenstiel incision 242, 540
Pharmacologic therapy 303
  role of 303
Phenazopyridine hydrochloride 380
Phenothiazines 300
Phenotype 332
  sex 328
    determination 329
Phenytoin 300
Phimosis 263
Phytoestrogens 436
Phytoprogestogens 436
Pills, selection of 469
Pinopodes 427
Pipelle
  advantages of 41
  biopsy 34, 41, 41f, 121f
  device, disadvantages of 41, 121
Pituitary disease 313
Pituitary hormone 415f, 416
  cyclical changes of 252f
Placenta
  adhesion of 130
  polyp 107, 108f
  site trophoblastic tumor 151, 153, 153f, 155, 155f
Plasmacytomas 53
Plastic vaginal mold 455f
Platelet aggregation 420
Platinum refractory 71
Pneumoperitoneum 558
Polycystic ovarian syndrome 7, 93, 113, 116, 117, 128, 135, 261, 288, 290, 291f-294f, 295, 296f, 298f, 311, 314, 317, 335, 337, 338f, 339f, 342, 342f, 348, 352, 355
  clinical presentation of 292
  complications of 292
  diagnosis of 290
  diagnostic clinical criteria of 290, 290t
  differential diagnosis of 307
  etiology of 292
  incidence of 292
  management of 295, 355

  pathophysiology of 295
  phenotypes of 292t
Polycystic ovary 38f, 261f, 291
  bilateral 291f
Polyembryoma 52, 53, 74
Polyhedral cells 75f
Polymenorrhagia 7
Polymenorrhea 7, 112, 113
Polymerase chain reaction 615
Polyostotic fibrous dysplasia 347
Polyp 27, 38, 114, 262
  malignant 107
  mucous 107
  submucous 374
  types of 107
Polypectomy 146, 551
  steps of 108
Polyspermia 425
Pomeroy technique 496, 496f
Portio vaginalis 22f
Postabortal ligation 495
Postcoital test 250, 261, 262
Postgonadectomy 334
  vault prolapse, prevalence of 245
Postmenopausal bleeding 7, 133, 134, 144, 145, 146, 560
  causes of 7, 135, 144
  therapy 62
Postmenopausal period 27
Postradiation fistula temporary colostomy 410
Post-tubal sterilization syndrome 502
Postvasectomy syndrome 506
Postvoid residual urine 223, 391
Potassium hydroxide 37
  solution 36
Powder burn 364
Prader staging 332
Preantral follicle 415
  stages of 414
Precocious puberty 38, 77, 345, 346, 348, 351, 353
  evaluation of 348
Precordium, palpation of 12
Prednisolone 304
Pregnancy 4, 30, 37, 47, 84, 109, 210, 245, 321, 337, 444
  antecedent 155
  cervical 37
  cornual 37
  ectopic 32, 38, 113, 444, 487, 502, 553, 606
  failure 472
    early 363
  medical termination of 250, 336, 461, 495
  molar 151
  multifetal 54
  multiple 269, 295
  outcome 169
  rate 270, 275, 279
  termination of 461

  test 312, 315
  tubal 553
Preinvasive lesion 171f, 185, 196
Premenstrual dysphoric disorder 429
Premenstrual syndrome 429
  diagnosis of 429, 430
  etiology of 429
Pressure
  abdominal 210
  diastolic 11
  systolic 11
Primary amenorrhea 7, 32, 38, 308, 31-314, 317, 317fc, 318, 319, 322, 352, 355
  causes of 313
  clinical classification of 314t
  diagnosis of 314
  etiology of 313
  management of 318
Primary dysmenorrhea 7, 373, 374
  treatment of 374
Primordial follicle 413, 414
  development of 413
Primordial germ cells 75f
Probe test 410
Procidentia 210f, 212, 220f
Proctoscopy 146
Progesterone 94, 122, 132, 143, 255, 256, 415, 420, 432, 433, 436, 437, 464, 472, 473
  antagonist 365
  challenge test 339
  effects of 254f
  influence of 427
  injectable 123
  level 418
  only contraceptives 473, 474
  only pill 135, 461f, 470, 471, 471t
    missing 472
  receptor modulator 367
    selective 122, 366
  secretion, maximum 420
  therapy 130
  vaginal ring 476, 476f
Progestins 300, 365, 464
  fourth generation 465
  second generation 465
  third generation 465
Progestogen 300, 470
  discovery of 461
  only pill 461
Prolactin 34, 249, 256, 289, 298, 312
  measurement of 341
  source of 341
  structure of 341
  types of 341
Prolactinemia 340
Prolapse
  different degrees of 213f
  recurrence of 243
  surgery, use of 245
Prophylactic surgery, role of 63
Propionibacterium acnes 297

Prostaglandins 429
Prostatic secretion 421
Prostatitis 250
Proteolytic digestion 428
Protozoa 36
Proximal femur 434
Pruritus 187
Psammoma bodies 63
Pseudobroad ligament
   cyst 105, 105*f*
   fibroid 105, 106, 571, 572*f*
      small 106*f*
Pseudocapsule 91
Pseudocervical fibroid 103
Pseudodecidua 419
Pseudohermaphrodite
   female 330
   male 330
Pseudo-Meigs syndrome 86
Pseudomyxoma peritonei 58, 59, 64
Psoraleas 300
Psychosexual therapy 286
Pubertal development tanner staging, sequence of 351
Puberty 346, 350, 351
   delayed 7, 308, 313, 319
   development of 317
   idiopathic precocious 347*f*
   incomplete precocious 348, 350
   menorrhagia 128
   onset of 350
   precocious 38, 77, 345, 346, 348, 351, 353
Pubic hair 299*f*, 309, 310, 315, 351
   development, sequence of 318*f*
   growth of 317
   Tanner staging of 315
Pubocervical fascia 208, 228, 229*f*
   repair of 229*f*
Pubocervical ligament 207*f*, 208*f*, 228
Pubovaginal sling 393, 394
Pulse 11, 346
Punch biopsy forceps 161*f*, 520*f*
Purandare's abdominal sling operation 241
Purandare's sling 225
Pyelogram, intravenous 37, 322, 380
Pyelonephritis 217
Pyknotic nuclei 252*f*
Pyometra 30, 37, 144, 144*f*, 161
   causes of 144
   dragging of 144*f*

Q

Q-tip test 221, 391
Quadriphasic pill 465
Quadrivalent vaccine 183
Quantiferon gamma release assay 614
Queyrat erythroplasia 198
Quinacrine pellets 499

R

Radial arteries 418
Radial pulse 11
Radiation 8, 166
Radical hysterectomy 146, 164*f*, 165, 167, 168, 539, 540, 546, 551, 559*f*, 575, 575*f*
   abdominal 545
   basic steps of 545
   components of 575
   laparoscopic 169
   modified 142
   steps of 168
   vaginal 169, 575
Radical vulvectomy 191, 193, 196*f*, 576*f*
   complications of 195
   steps of 193
Radiofrequency-induced thermal ablation 126, 127
Radiotherapy 311
   role of 155
Raloxifene 436
Randomized controlled trial 449, 592
Rape victim, medical examination of 597
Reactive oxygen species 267, 421
Rectal buttonhole tear 402
Rectocele 27, 210, 211*f*, 219*f*, 220, 222, 231*f*
   repair of 233*f*
Rectovaginal examination 32, 33*f*, 46, 50, 65, 380
Rectovaginal fascia 208
Rectovaginal fistula 381*f*, 389, 402, 408, 408*f*, 409*f*
   causes of 408
   prevalence of 410
   signs of 410
   symptoms of 409
Rectovaginal septum, examination of 249
Rectovaginal space, dissection of 406*f*
Rectovaginal wall, mass of 32
Rectum 232*f*, 406*f*
Red lesion 20, 365
Reflexes 204, 220
Regular normal ovulatory menstrual cycle, mechanism of 432
Reifenstein syndrome 325, 330
Renal angle tenderness 12, 204
Renal disease 8
Renal lump 47, 84
Renin-angiotensin-aldosterone system 429
Reproductive function 319
Reproductive tract
   bleeding, causes of 113
   female 438*fc*
   infection 607
   male 425*f*
Reserpine 300
Respiration 11, 346
Respiratory system 12, 134, 150, 158, 186, 203, 248, 357
Rete ovarii, tumors of 53

Retrograde ejaculation 286
   treatment of 286
Retroversion, correction of 537
Rhabdoid tumor, malignant 189
Rhabdomyosarcoma 353
Rheumatic fever 8
Ribonucleic acid 36
Ring forceps 528
Ring pessary 224*f*, 409*f*, 524*f*, 536, 537*f*
Ringer's lactate 565
Ritumala 494, 494*f*
Rizzoli's operation 410
Rodent ulcer 188
Rokitansky-Küster-Hauser syndrome 7, 262, 316*f*, 321*f*, 452*f*
Round cells 266
Round ligament
   clamping of 542*f*
   fibroid 90
   suture of 540*f*
Rubber catheter 547*f*
   simple 98, 516*f*
Rubin's cannula 251, 258
Rubin's test 251, 258
Rudimentary horn 444, 444*f*

S

Sacral vertebra, lumbarization of 452
Sacrocolpohysteropexy 241, 242*f*, 243
Sacrocolpopexy 241, 242*f*, 445*f*
   abdominal 225, 226, 241, 242, 242*f*
   infracoccygeus 225
Sacrospinous colpopexy 225, 226
Sacrospinous ligament 244
   fixation 243, 243*f*
   right 243
Sacrum 9
Saheli 472
Saline
   infusion sonography 39, 39*f*, 119, 120, 260
      role of 120
      transverse section 119*f*
   normal 545
Salpingectomy
   justification of 544
   opportunistic 61, 63
Salpingitis, interstitial 613
Salpingo-oophorectomy 59-61, 542*f*, 551, 572*f*, 573*f*
   bilateral 59, 60, 60*f*, 140, 142, 167, 368*f*, 369, 539, 570
   left-sided 344*f*
   right-sided 299*f*
   unilateral 76, 79
Salpingo-ovariolysis 275
Salpingoscopy 261
Salpingostomy 273, 273*f*
Salvage chemotherapy 72
Saphenous vein 193, 194*f*
Sarcoma

epithelial 147, 189
vulvar 189
Scalp hair, asynchronization of 306
Scar endometriosis 360, 361, 361*f*
Schauta's operation 167, 575
Schiller test 176, 178
Schroeder's disease 129
Sclerotic dermatoses 198
Scrotal ultrasound 266
Scrotum 263
Scybella 32
Secondary amenorrhea 7, 291, 335, 337-339, 340*fc*, 342*f*
    causes of 291, 337, 337*f*
    diagnosis of 338
    physiological causes of 337
Secondary dysmenorrhea 7, 373, 374
    causes of 373
    treatment of 374
Secretory endometrium 255*f*, 419*f*
Segesterone acetate 476
Seizure disorder 8
Semen 266, 281*f*, 421
    absence of 266
    analysis 250, 264, 287
    collection 264, 281
    composition of 421
    cryopreservation of 285
    culture 266
    low volume 266
    normal composition of 421
    preparation 282*f*
    sample 264
    volume 265
Seminal plasma, functions of 421
Seminal vesicle
    congenital absence of 265
    secretion of 265
Seminiferous tubule, cross section of 423*f*
Seminopathy, severe 280
Sepsis, puerperal 8
Septate 581
    uterus 279, 439, 441, 444, 448, 448*f*, 581, 582, 582*f*
    vagina 446*f*
Septum
    transcervical resection of 453
    transvaginal 321
Serkal syndrome 330
Serotonin-reuptake inhibitors, selective 430
Serous cancer, low-grade 68
Serous cyst adenocarcinomas, high-grade 61, 63
Serous cystadenoma 60*f*
    high-grade 61
    simple clear 55*f*
Serous ovarian cancer, high grade 68
Serous tubal intraepithelial carcinoma 63
Sertoli cells 332, 423
Sertoli-Leydig cell tumor 52, 53, 77, 78, 78*f*, 79, 343, 343*f*

Serum progesterone, midluteal 255
Serum testosterone 339, 355
    level 300
        total 301
Sex
    chromosome 329
    cord 53*f*
        stromal tumors 52, 53, 77
        tumor 52, 53, 77
    hormone binding globulin 295, 433
    steroids 34, 347
Sexual assault 476
Sexual behavior 183
Sexual character 263
    secondary 10, 12, 315, 321
Sexual development
    disorder of 308, 328, 329, 329*t*, 331*t*, 351
Sexual differentiation 328
    disorder of 328, 329, 333*fc*, 333*t*, 354
Sexual dysfunction 217, 434
    male 280
    treatment of 436
Sexual hair 306
    quantification of 301
Sexual orientation 332
Sexual precocity 347
Sexuality, potential for 332
Sexually transmitted
    disease 8, 33, 35, 174, 189, 196, 197, 262, 606
    infection 37, 125, 605, 607, 608, 609*t*
Shallow placentation 429
Sharman's curette 120*f*, 518, 534, 534*f*
Sheath 560, 561
Sheehan's syndrome 261, 291, 337, 338
Shirodkar's abdominal sling operation 241
Shirodkar's sling 225
Short stature 309*f*, 319
Sigmoidoscopy 200
Signet-ring appearance 79
Silastic ring 501
Sildenafil 286
    citrate 286
Silicone 224*f*
Simple vulvectomy 192*f*, 198*f*
    incision 192*f*
    repair of 192*f*
Sims' double-bladed posterior vaginal speculum 529
Sims' position 25, 218, 218*f*, 378, 379*f*, 382, 382*f*
Sims' posterior vaginal speculum 237, 516, 530*f*, 546
    application of 548*f*
Sims' saucerization 385
Sims' semi-prone position 16, 19
Sims' speculum 23, 25, 26*f*, 227*f*, 379*f*, 382, 382*f*, 530, 545, 547*f*
    double-bladed 24*f*
    insertion of 25
    over Cusco
        advantages of 530
        disadvantages of 530
Sims' triad 382, 530

Sims-Huhner test 261
Single puncture technique 500
Single tooth
    tenaculum 100*f*
    vulsellum 235*f*, 517, 532, 532*f*
Sinusitis 263*f*
Skeletal system, examination of 204
Skin 195*f*, 404, 603
    biopsy, gonadal 332
    changes 434
    condition of 14
    examination of 10
    excision of 192*f*
    incision 98
    labial 379
    nonneoplastic epithelial disorders of 198
    pigmentation of 10
Sleep 8, 150, 158
Sling operation 225
Smooth muscle tumor 147
Snow storm appearance 153
Sodium chloride 564
Soft palate 10
Soft tissue tumors 53
Solid epithelial tumor 56*f*
Solid ovarian
    mass, triad of 81
    tumor 80*f*
Solid silicone plugs 507
Solifenacin 393
Solitary myoma, removal of 98*f*
Sonography 57, 58, 74, 86, 372, 439, 615
    plates 584
    transabdominal 37
Sonohysterography 85, 120, 137
Sonohysterosalpingogram 260
Sonohysterosalpingography 34, 251, 258, 260*f*, 272
Sonosalpingography 249
Sore, painful 185, 187
Sound 532
Spatula 175
Sperm 263, 265*f*, 425
    centriole 421
    cervical mucus contact test 262, 267
    chromatin structural assay 267
    concentration 265
    deoxyribonucleic acid
        damage, tests of 267
        integrity test 267
    deposition of 507
    fertilization 424
    function 363
        tests 266, 267
    granuloma 506
    head, structure of 422*f*
    immotile 261, 263*f*, 267
    insertion, subzonal 285
    maturation 508
    morphology 265
    motility 265

oocyte fusion 267f, 422f, 424, 425
penetration assay 267
preparation techniques 281
reversible inhibition of 508
transport 424
viability test 267
vitality test 267
zona pellucida binding tests 267
Spermatids 423
Spermatocyte
    primary 422, 423, 423f
    secondary 422, 423f
Spermatogenesis 413, 423f, 424, 507
    hormonal control of 424, 424fc
    physiology of 422
Spermatogonia 422, 423f
Spermatozoa 421, 423
    mature 266f, 421f, 423f
    structure of 421
Spermiation 424
Spermicides 493
    vaginal 492
Spermiogenesis 422
Sphincter, external 407
Sphincteroplasty, layer method of 405
Spine 434
    examination of 217
Spinelli's procedure 551
Spinnbarkeit test 252, 253, 253f
Spiral artery 418, 419
    spasm of 420
Spironolactone 304
    cyproterone acetate flutamide finasteride 303
Spleen 15, 134, 158, 186, 204, 248, 357
    palpation of 15f
Splenic enlargement 47, 84
Sponge holding forceps 108f, 220, 515, 528, 528f, 547f
    use of 528
Squamocolumnar junction 172, 172f, 173f, 174, 175
Squamous cell 171
    carcinoma 20, 63, 138, 160f, 165f, 171, 173, 188, 189, 600
        in situ 198
        primary 64
    hyperplasia 20, 196
    tumors 53
Squamous epithelial lesion, high grade 197
Squamous intraepithelial lesion
    high-grade 171, 172, 178, 179, 197, 198
    low-grade 171, 172, 178, 197, 198
Squamous metaplasia, normal 180f
Squatting position 16, 218, 218f
Squeeze techniques 286
Standard days method 494
Stein-Leventhal syndrome 292
Stenosis 321
Sterilization 495, 528, 529
    certificate of 503
    female 463, 495, 502, 503, 553

    male 503
    microsurgical reversal of 274
    permanent 502, 511
    procedure 272
    transcervical 498
Steroid
    adrenal 433
    anabolic 300
    cell tumors 53
    contraceptives 470
    hormones 417
        production of 433
    ovarian 420
Steroidal contraceptives 464fc, 470t
    classification of 464
Stimulation, ovarian 280, 281
Stool, incontinence of 6, 404
Strassman metroplasty 453, 453f
Strassman technique 448, 582
Streak ovaries 320
Streptomycin 300
Stress 261
    incontinence 204, 219, 222, 226, 230, 243, 389, 391-393, 434
        diagnosis of 391
        operations of 551
        pathophysiology of 390
        risk factors of 390
    management 430
    psychosocial 347
    urinary incontinence 217
    treatment of 393
Stroma 419
    cells 53f
    growth 418
    luteoma 53
    ovarii 54
Stumps, cut ends of 241f
Subdermal implants 474
Subfertility 448
    male 266, 266t, 267
Submeatal sulcus 218
Submucosal myoma, hysteroscopic resection of 97
Submucous fibroid 87f-89f, 560, 569, 569f, 571f
Suction irrigation cannula 556f
Supine position 98
Surgery 97, 223, 225, 305, 393, 563
    aim of 225, 393
    endoscopic 553
    extent of 61
    feminizing 334
    gynecological 8, 381, 551, 563
    hysteroscopic 553
    indications of 97, 225, 341, 448, 582, 608, 615
    placing of 226
    primary 70
    principles of 405
    Robotic 553, 562
    role of 154, 155

    route of 143
    types of 97, 191, 192t, 367, 582, 608, 615
Surgical resection 142, 449, 450
Surrogacy 279
    gestational 279, 456
    issues of 280
Swede score 178
Swelling 20
    abdomen 354f
    adnexal 32
    classification of 600
    vulvar 197
Swim-up technique 280, 281, 282f
Swyer syndrome 319, 325, 326t, 330
Symphysis pubis 394
Symptothermal method 494
Syncytiotrophoblast 428
Synechiae 262, 337, 338
Synopsis 589, 590
Syphilis 172, 612
    congenital 612
    primary 612
    secondary 612
    tertiary 612
Syphilitic condyloma 600
Systemic lupus
    disease 113
    erythematosus 125, 199

T

Tadalafil 286
Tamoxifen 135, 143, 268, 269
    therapy 135
Tampon test 380
Tanner staging 315, 317, 318f, 348
Teeth 10
    vulsellum, multiple 109f, 517, 531, 532f, 547f, 548f
Telescope 526f, 555f, 560
Telogen 306
    effluvium 306
Tension, premenstrual 429
Tension-free vaginal tape 390, 394, 394f-396f, 527f
    advantages of 398
    surgical procedure of 395
Teratomas 53, 74
    ovarian 54
Teratozoospermia 266
Testes 263
    cut section of 325f
    removal of 325f
Testicular biopsy 266
    role of 267
Testicular development, disorder of 330
Testicular feminization syndrome 308, 309, 312, 322t, 323
Testicular secretion 421
Testicular sperm
    aspiration 283
    extraction 267, 280, 283

Testicular volume 263
Testosterone 293, 300, 312, 346, 438, 507
    deficient 319
    high injectable-dose of 424
    low-oral dose of 424
    use of 424
Tetrachlorodibenzodioxin 361
Theca
    cells 415
    externa 415, 416
    interna 415, 416
    lutein cyst 53, 54
Thecoma 80
    fibroma 53, 77, 80, 81
Thelarche, premature 347, 348f
Therapeutic donor insemination 287
Thermal balloon therapy 126
Thread test 253
Threadability test 253f
Three swab test 380
Thrombi control blood loss 420
Thrombocytopenia 113
Thromboembolism 125
Thyroid 313
    disorder 8, 248, 289, 341
    gland 251, 263
        examination 314
    hormones 298, 301
    profile 346
    stimulating hormone 85, 249, 250, 289, 312, 317, 336, 340
    serum 256
Thyroxin 268, 351f
    therapy 351f
Tibolone 436
Tinidazole 610
Tissue
    abdominal 148
    ovarian 285
    subcutaneous 194f, 407, 540
Tolterodine 393
Tompkins procedure 453
Tongue 10
    under surface of 10
Tonsils 10
Torsion 58, 59, 93
    ovarian 38, 58f
Total hysterectomy 59, 60, 167, 539, 540, 542f, 570
    specimen of 60f, 61f
    steps of 540
Touch technique 482
Trabecular bone 434
Trachea, position of 12
Trachelectomy 166, 169, 551
    procedure of 169
    selection criteria of 169
Tranexamic acid 85, 122, 125, 128
Transcutaneous nerve stimulation 374
Transdermal combined hormonal patch 476f
Transdermal patch 366, 464

Transformation zone 172, 174
    large loop excision of 181, 183
    needle excision of 183
Transgender 330
Transitional cell
    carcinoma 63, 64
    epithelial tumors 53
Transobturator
    needle 397f
    procedure 394
    tape 396f-398f, 527f
        advantages of 398
        surgical procedure of 396
Transureteric ureteroureteric anastomosis 388f
Transvaginal sonography 37, 62, 87f, 111, 119, 119f, 132, 134, 136, 256f, 290f, 364f, 372, 419f, 487f, 585f
    role of 120
Transverse incision 227f, 237
Transverse sulcus 218
Transverse vaginal septum 312, 313, 315, 323, 352, 352f, 441, 449, 450f
    management of 450t
Trauma 353
Treponema pallidum 600
Trichomonas 20, 36f, 610f
    vaginalis 6, 34-36, 353, 610
Trichomoniasis 27, 35-37, 610
    diagnosis of 36
Triple-blind study 593
Trocar 500
    cannula 475f, 499f, 555f, 556f
    placement 558
Troglitazone 304
Trophectoderm 426
Trospium 393
Tru-cut biopsy 66
True broad ligament
    cyst 105f
    fibroid 105, 106
Tubal block 274f, 581
    causes of 262, 272, 580
Tubal defect, congenital 262, 272
Tubal disease 38
    classification of 272
Tubal embryo transfer 285
Tubal factor infertility 262, 268, 272, 274
    surgery for 273
    treatment of 273
Tubal function 363
    assessment of 272
    diagnosis of 272
Tubal insufflation test 251, 258
Tubal ligation 62, 495, 496f, 502
    approaches of 495
    failure rate of 498
    laparoscopic 500
Tubal patency test 34, 250, 258, 272, 537, 558f, 579, 581
    methods of 251
Tubal reconstructive surgery 551

Tubal sterilization
    complications of 501
    techniques of 498
Tubectomy 262, 503, 551
Tubercular vaginoperineal fistula 614f
Tuberculosis 8, 32, 250, 258f, 262, 311, 337
    cervical 159, 160f, 614, 614f
    drug dosage for 615, 615t
    genital 612
    vulvar 187
Tubocornual anastomosis 274, 275
Tubo-ovarian mass 32
    large 47, 48, 84
Tubotubal anastomosis 273, 273f, 275
Tumor 53, 105, 160, 573
    benign 573f
    endometrioid 53
    genital 353
    low malignant potential 72
    malignant 68, 76
        nature of 52
    management of 59
    marker 34, 51
        measurement of 50
    mesothelial 53
    metastatic 188
    mucinous 53
    pituitary 261
    secondary 53
    serous 53
    size of 196
    trophoblastic 151
Turner's syndrome 7, 8, 11, 261, 308, 309f, 319, 314, 314f, 319, 319f, 320, 320f, 321, 330, 334, 533
    classic stigma of 319
    clinical presentation of 319
    management of 321
Two-gonadotropin theory 415, 416f

U

Uchida technique 498
Ulceration 187
Ulcerative colitis 358
Ulcers 20
Ulipristal 367
    acetate 95
Ultrasonography 37, 84, 85, 118, 136, 276, 277, 309, 317, 358, 374, 392
    folliculometry 251, 256
    guided cyst aspiration 38
    hematometra 316f
    role of 37
    transvaginal 37f, 38, 38f
Ultrasound 37, 51
    guided biopsy 38
    scan 145
    transperineal 223
    transrectal 266, 268
Umbilicus 360
    condition of 14

Unicornuate uterus 439, 441, 443, 443f, 444, 444f, 582, 583f
   adverse impacts of 444
Unification operation 448
Upper legs, paresthesia of 195
Uremia 161
Ureter 92, 385
   course of 386f
   injury of 386f, 387
   pelvic part of 385
   types of 387
   vasculature of 386f
Ureteric catheter 388f
Ureteric fistula 381
   management of 388
Ureteroureteric anastomosis 388f
Ureterovaginal fistula 6, 385, 387, 389
   causes of 387
   incidence of 385
Ureterovesical anastomosis 388, 388f, 389, 389f
   procedure of 388
Urethra 20, 23, 222, 379, 600
   fistula 381
   glands 421
   mucosa 390
   prolapse 353
Urethrocele 204, 210, 218, 219
Urethrocystometry 391, 392
Urge incontinence 389
   causes of 390
Urinary beta-human chorionic gonadotropin 118
Urinary bladder 32, 88f
Urinary follicle-stimulating hormone 269
Urinary frequency 434
Urinary human
   chorionic gonadotropin 269
   human menopausal gonadotropin 269
Urinary incontinence 377, 389, 393
   management of 392
Urinary luteinizing hormone monitoring 255
Urinary pregnancy test 339
Urinary system 12, 83, 217
Urinary tract infection 433
   lower 434
Urine
   analysis 266
   examination 391
   incontinence of 6
   retention of 93, 528, 529
Uroflowmetry 391, 392
Urogenital sinus 439
Uterine 337, 418
   abnormality 37
   anomaly 449
   artery 545
      crossing ureter 168f
      embolization 41, 85, 95, 95f, 96, 126
      ligation 166, 167
   cavity 425, 426f, 484f, 485f, 584
      curette of 548f, 549f
   cervix 438
   classification of 440t
   corpus 438
   curette 137f, 518, 534, 534f, 547f
   descent 211f, 219f
   didelphys 439, 445, 445f, 446, 446f
   dressing forceps 519, 534f, 534
   factor 262
   fibroid 31, 48f, 50, 82, 85, 92, 93, 97, 109, 279
      classification of 90
      common associations of 92
      complications of 93
      degenerations of 92
      diagnosis of 87
      etiology of 93
      nomenclatures of 84
      risk factors of 93
      types of 91t
   fundus 154f
      cupping of 206f
   inversion 93, 550f
   leiomyoma 82, 544
      incidence of 93
      location of 88
      macroscopic features of 91
      management of 85, 94
      types of 89
   mass 31
   origin 118
   papillary serous carcinoma 139
   perforation 544, 550
   polyp 107, 112
      management of 108
   procedures 126
   prolapse 6f, 211, 219f
      exact degree of 220
      three degree of 213f
   rupture 444
   sarcoma 133, 147f
      staging of 147
   septum 453, 560
   size 338
   sound 532, 547f
      sterilization of 533
   synechia 279, 321, 335, 342, 481
   tamponade 126
   transplantation 452, 455, 456
      indications of 455
   unification, surgical techniques of 448
   vessels 543
      clamping of 541f, 543f
Uterocervical canal, length of 532
Uterosacral ligament 32, 90, 208, 209, 226, 237, 239f, 359, 364f, 543f
   posteriorly 207f, 208f
Uterosacral nerves, ablation of 367
Uterosacral suspension, abdominal 226
Uterotubal junction 425
Uterovaginal prolapse 210, 211
Uterovaginal surgery 279
Uterus 30, 31f, 92, 98, 136, 160, 208f, 217, 225, 320, 321, 418, 425, 437, 451, 540f, 570, 580, 584
   abnormalities of 315
   anteverted 28, 29f
   arcuate 444, 449, 449f, 582, 583, 583f
   bicornuate 439, 441, 444, 446, 447, 447f, 448, 581, 581f, 582, 582f, 583
   bimanual examination 30f
   bulky 155f
   chronic inversion of 205-207
   complete septate 39f, 448f
   cut section of 90f, 131f
   delivery of 545
   descent of 219
   development of 438
   didelphys 441, 446f
   different positions of 30f
   double 445f
   dragging of 210
   enlarged 131f
   fundus of 238f, 438
   globular enlarged 371
   hemisection of 104f
   holding forceps 522f
   incision over 99
   inversion of 206f
   length of 533
   lower part of body of 163f
   mobility of 30
   normal 30
      position of 207, 533
   outside 584
   palpation of 30
   position of 548f
   posterior surface of 32, 365f
   prolapse of 210
   removal of 541f, 543f
   retroverted 28, 30f, 32
   rupture 539
   sarcoma of 146
   septate 279, 439, 441, 444, 448, 448f, 581, 582, 582f
   serosal coat of 99f
   specimen of 240f, 569
   straighten 489f, 490f
   subseptate 279, 448f, 449f
   supports of 207, 208, 209f
   thumbs inverted 551
   unicornuate 439, 441, 443, 443f, 444, 444f, 582, 583f

V

Vacuum pump 286
Vagina 27, 34, 90, 187, 189, 310, 321, 322, 338, 360, 401, 439, 613, 614
   anterior wall of 242f
   cutting vault of 541f
   development of 438
   double 445f
   eversion of 216f

Index

examination of 145
level of 541*f*
longitudinal septum of 441, 450, 451*f*
lower third of 410
palpation of 19, 20
pathology of upper 353
posterior wall of 242*f*
stenosis of 338
supports of 207, 209*f*
transection of 541*f*, 543
upper part of 312, 315, 451
vault of 242*f*, 541*f*
Vaginal agenesis 20, 23*f*, 32, 312, 316*f*, 451, 451*f*
Vaginal anomaly 440, 440*t*
Vaginal approach 225, 383, 551
  advantages of 382
Vaginal atresia, isolated 321
Vaginal bleeding 160, 200, 351*f*, 352, 353
  causes of 353
Vaginal blunt manipulator 243
Vaginal cancer 28*f*, 185, 199, 200*f*
  diagnosis of 200
Vaginal cuff, closure of 543
Vaginal cytology 251, 252*f*, 253*f*
Vaginal diaphragm 492, 493*f*
Vaginal discharge 6, 200, 203, 217
  causative organisms of 36, 36*t*
  causes of 610
  evaluation 35
  examination 34
  study of 35
  test 606
Vaginal disinfection 405
Vaginal epidermal cyst 601*f*
Vaginal examination 16, 46, 83-85, 108, 111, 134, 150, 158, 160, 186, 204, 249, 357, 378, 401
  sequence of 19
Vaginal flaps 229*f*, 235*f*, 551
  cut 230*f*
Vaginal intraepithelial neoplasia 197, 200
Vaginal introitus 20, 205, 310*f*, 600
Vaginal length, total 215, 221*f*
Vaginal ligation, contraindications of 501
Vaginal longitudinal septum 446*f*
Vaginal margins, repair of posterior 407
Vaginal mucosa 204, 228*f*, 231, 232*f*, 233*f*, 236*f*, 407*f*
  cut, redundant part of 230*f*
  cutting redundant portion of 230*f*
  exfoliated cells 435
  redundant portion of 228
  repair of 229*f*
  separation of 228*f*, 232*f*
Vaginal mucous membrane 216
Vaginal opening, absence of 312, 315
Vaginal pessary 223, 537
  indications of 223, 536
  types of 223
Vaginal prolapse 210
Vaginal ring 366, 464, 470
  combined 463

Vaginal route 167, 234
Vaginal rugosity 218
Vaginal septum 20, 23*f*, 314, 446*f*
  low transverse 450*f*
  removal of 279
Vaginal space, creation of 454*f*
Vaginal speculum
  posterior 482
  single bladed posterior 25*f*, 516, 530, 530*f*
Vaginal sulcus, lateral 219
Vaginal surgery, types of 383
Vaginal swab, high 34
Vaginal tubal ligation 501
Vaginal vault 210, 226, 542*f*
  carcinoma 200*f*
  repair of 543*f*
Vaginal wall
  bulging of posterior 219
  flaps of 383
  posterior 25, 26*f*, 227*f*, 379*f*, 382*f*
  prolapse 32
    posterior 32, 215, 216*f*, 225
Vaginismus 8, 287
Vaginitis, atrophic 134, 135, 146
Vagino-perineal fistula 22*f*
Vaginoplasty 322, 452, 455*f*, 551
  laparoscopic 453
  methods of 322, 452, 453
Vaginouterine prolapse 210
Van Wyk and Grumbach syndrome 347, 350
Vanishing testes syndrome 330
Vardenafil 286
Varicocele 250, 262, 263
Vas deferens, congenital bilateral absence of 286
Vas ligation 504*f*
Vascular endothelial growth factor 116, 367
Vascular pattern, atypical 178
Vascularization, stage of 418
Vasectomy 250, 463, 503, 504*f*, 506, 507
Vasography 266, 268
Vasomotor symptoms, treatment of 436
Vault prolapse 211, 226*f*
  management of 225
  repair of 225
Vecchietti's technique 453
Vellus hair 305, 306
Vena cava, inferior 69*f*
Venous thromboembolism, postoperative 565
Verbal descriptor scales 5
Veress needle 500, 526*f*, 555*f*
  insertion of 557
Verrucous carcinoma 188
Vescicovaginal fistula 7
  repair 384*f*
Vesicocervical fascia 228, 237
Vesicocervical fistula 161

Vesicocervical ligament 228*f*
Vesicouterine fistula 6, 26*f*, 161, 377, 381, 381*f*, 382, 383*f*, 389
Vesicovaginal fistula
  repair 384*f*
    methods of 384*f*
  types of 381
Vessel
  ovarian 61
  sealing system 545
Vestibular anus 410
Vestibular bulb 600
Viagra 286
Videocystourethrography 392
Vincristine 155
Virchow's gland 10
Virgin, rectal examination for 338
Virilization
  degree of 332
  signs of 301
Visual analog scale 5
Visual defect 338
Visual detection 179
Visual field defect 263
Vitamin 430
  A 352
  B_6 430
  D 352, 430, 436
  E 436
Voice, hoarseness of 78*f*, 297*f*
Volume reductive procedure 545
von Willebrand's disease 113, 116, 352
Vulva 9, 34, 90, 189, 338, 360, 379, 614
  carcinoma of 185, 191*t*
  disfigurement of 195
  examination of 145, 186
  hamartoma of 602*f*
  lymphatics of 189
  palpation of 24*f*
  preinvasive lesion of 185, 196
  sebaceous cyst of 21*f*
  swellings of 20, 185, 187, 600
Vulvar cancer 20, 22*f*, 187-190, 195*t*, 196
  develops 188
  incidence of 189
  lesion 188
  management of 191
  prognosis of 195
  risk factors of 189
  spread 189
  staging of 190
  treatment of 191, 193*t*
Vulvar carcinoma 600
  diagnosis of 187
  premalignant lesions of 196
  prognostic factors of 196
Vulvar dystrophy, chronic 198
Vulvar growth 187*f*, 188*f*
  recurrence of 196*f*
Vulvar hematoma, traumatic 353*f*
Vulvar intraepithelial disease 198

Vulvar intraepithelial neoplasia 187, 189, 196-198
    classification of 197
    diagnosis of 197
Vulvar lesion 188
Vulvar tissue, removal of 195f
Vulvectomy 193, 551
    radical
        complete 193f
        partial 192f
Vulvitis
    atrophic 198
    hyperplastic 198
Vulvodynia 199
Vulvoscopy 188, 197
Vulvovaginal candidiasis 608, 609f
Vulvovaginitis 35, 352
    bacterial 353
    treatment of 353

W

Walthard bodies 56
Ward Mayo's operation 102f, 225, 231, 236, 238f, 239f, 551
    complications of 241
Warts
    genital 611
    vulvar 20, 21f, 600, 601f, 611f

Water test 557
Weight
    gain 338
    loss 268, 294, 338, 392
    reduction of 294
Wertheim's clamp 525f
Wertheim's operation 166, 167, 167f, 168, 168f, 545, 575, 575f
White discharge 160
White lesion 20, 365
Whorl appearance 91f
Williams' vaginoplasty 455f
Williams' vulvovaginoplasty 452, 455
Withdrawal technique 482
Wolffian structure 329
Wound
    abdominal 565
    dehiscence 195, 502
    hematoma 502
    infection 195
    repair of 453f

X

X-ray 583
    abdomen 486f
    chest 37, 80f, 161, 189
    pelvis 583f
        straight 585f

    plate 579, 583
    straight 486f
XX gonad ovarian structures 438
XXY karyotype 287f

Y

Y chromosome
    deletion 250
    short arm of 438
Yeast-like organism 609
Yolk sac tumor 52, 74, 76
Young's syndrome 263

Z

Zona
    binding 267f, 422f
    dissection, partial 285
    hatching 428
    pellucida 267, 415, 425
        loss of 428
    penetration 422f, 424, 425
    reaction 425
    recognition 424
Zygote intrafallopian tube transfer 279, 285, 451